NURSING
BASIC DEGREE

NURSING

MATERNITY CARE
THE NURSE AND THE FAMILY

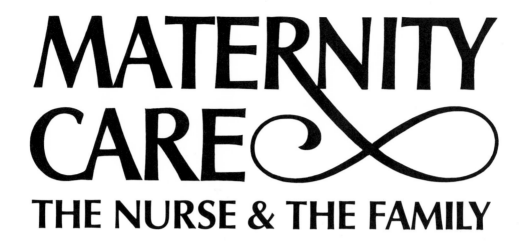

THE NURSE & THE FAMILY

MARGARET DUNCAN JENSEN, R.N., M.S.

Associate Professor, California State University at San Jose,
San Jose, California

RALPH C. BENSON, M.D.

Formerly Professor and Chairman, Department of Obstetrics and Gynecology,
University of Oregon Medical School,
Portland, Oregon

IRENE M. BOBAK, R.N., M.S.

Associate Professor, California State University at San Francisco,
San Francisco, California

with 684 illustrations

THE C. V. MOSBY COMPANY

SAINT LOUIS   1977

Printed in the United States of America

Distributed in Great Britain by Henry Kimpton, London

The C. V. Mosby Company
11830 Westline Industrial Drive, St. Louis, Missouri 63141

Library of Congress Cataloging in Publication Data

Jensen, Margaret, 1921-
    Maternity care.

    Bibliography: p.
    Includes index.
    1. Obstetrical nursing. I. Benson, Ralph Criswell,
1911-   joint author. II. Bobak, Irene M., 1933-
joint author. III. Title. [DNLM: 1. Infant, Newborn—
Nursing texts. 2. Pregnancy—Nursing texts. 3. Ob-
stetrical nursing. 4. Family—Nursing texts. WY157
J54m]
RG951.J57   610.73'678   76-48641
ISBN 0-8016-2489-4

GW/VH/VH 9 8 7 6 5 4 3 2

Contributors

CHERYL HALL HARRIS, R.N., B.S.

Formerly Infant Care Coordinator,
The Children's Mercy Hospital,
Kansas City, Missouri

HELEN READEY, R.N., M.S.

Coordinator of Fundamentals of Nursing
and Medical and Surgical Nursing I,
St. Vincent's Hospital School of Nursing,
Bridgeport, Connecticut

To **Emma Erin (Peppiatt) Duncan,**
pioneer in maternity nursing, who graduated from
St. Mary's Hospital, Praed St., London W2,
in 1914 and was certified in 1915 by the Central Midwives Board.
In 1917 she was named to the College of Nursing Limited, Cavendish Sq., London W1,
and served in the British nursing corps,
Queen Alexandra's Imperial Military Nursing Service,
during World War I, 1914-1918.

M. D. J.

To my mother, **Margaret Rinner Benson,**
a grand old lady of 100 years to whom I owe so much

R. C. B.

To **Susan** and **Joseph Bobak,**
who provided a good beginning

I. M. B.

Preface

Caring for and about the childbearing family demands a constant awareness that the greatest common denominator of patient, family, and nurse is their humanness. *Maternity Care: the Nurse and the Family* emphasizes the human qualities implicit in birth. It was written to help the nurse function competently and sensitively, recognizing the individuality of mother, father, infant, and all significant others.

Birth is intensely personal as well as universal. It holds a uniqueness and a sameness for all participants. Each baby thrusts myriad alterations into an already changing world; each replicates and perpetuates humanity's countless generations. The child born today enters a family that may bear little resemblance to any traditional pattern. The communities rippling from that family change are changed by it and by each other, creating a dynamic cultural setting. Nursing moves within that setting to render specific health care services to individuals and to families.

Today's maternity nurse can participate in the birth experience more actively and creatively than ever before. Increased knowledge—physiologic and psychosocial—offers an opportunity for the nurse to gain increased competence, accountability, and personal and professional satisfaction. This current, pertinent knowledge and its application in actual patient care situations form the framework of this book. Plans for nursing intervention based on diagnostic, therapeutic, and educational objectives are included throughout. The entire presentation points up the importance of (1) knowing the goal of care before planning that care or trying to assess its results and (2) knowing what others on the maternity care team are doing to correlate, integrate, and initiate nursing action.

Accessibility of information has been a primary objective in developing this book. It follows the chronological sequence of pregnancy, beginning with the bio-psychosocial components of human sexuality and family planning, through pregnancy, birth, and the postnatal period. Normal phenomena are explained prior to complications. Capable illustrator J. P. Tandy has created many drawings expressly for this book. These outstanding illustrations, together with photographs, charts, tables, diagrams, and care plans, clarify and enrich the text. Careful cross-referencing to eliminate duplication, an extensive glossary, and a detailed index add to the book's usefulness.

The dimension of human sexuality affects many facets of maternity nursing and therefore has been integrated throughout the text. This significant contribution is the effort of Marianne K. Zalar, R.N., M.S.

Continued change in the health care delivery system affects every aspect of maternity nursing. That is why the concluding unit contains a chapter on "Problem-oriented System" by Helen Readey and a chapter on "Legal and Ethical Aspects of Maternity Nursing" by Cheryl Hall Harris. Neither attempts exhaustive treatment of the subject; each presents a succinct survey of the nursing implications in these areas.

We are fully cognizant of the increasingly important contribution men are making to the nursing profession and have tried to eliminate all sexism from text and illustrations. However, for clarity and simplicity, the feminine pronoun has been used to refer to the nurse. For the same reason, the terms *husband* and *father* have been used even though it is recognized that the existence of a family relationship does not depend on a legally sanctioned union. The term *patient* was preferred to *client* because the patient-nurse relationship seems to suggest greater human concern.

Every birth holds pain as well as joy, and the emergence of this book is no exception. We believe that the emphasis on the human dimension will make the scientific, clinical content more meaningful and its assimilation and application more enjoyable for both student and practitioner. We believe that this book is uniquely significant in the literature of maternity nursing and that comments from instructors who use it will increase its usefulness in future editions.

Margaret Duncan Jensen
Ralph C. Benson
Irene M. Bobak

Acknowledgments

This book represents the concern, support, and assistance of many valued friends, colleagues, and family members. It also reflects what we have learned from our students and patients. Without these contributions, the project could not have been successfully completed.

We are especially grateful to those who reviewed our efforts while the manuscript was in progress and offered detailed, thoughtful criticism. Particular thanks go to Elsie Lang, A.B., M.S.N., who patiently and thoroughly reviewed the first draft of the manuscript, and to Kathy Rose-Pendleton, R.N., M.S., who reviewed much of the psychosocial material and provided valuable input.

We are deeply indebted to June Brady, M.D., and Patricia Ryan, R.N., of Children's Hospital, San Francisco, and to Roberta Ballard, M.D., of Mount Zion Hospital and Medical Center, San Francisco, for their assistance in obtaining original photographs. We also wish to thank photographers Kathleen Whaley and Donna Duell for their dedicated efforts. To the staffs of Kaiser-Permanente Hospital and Santa Clara Valley Medical Center, Santa Clara, California, we offer thanks for their shared expertise.

Three families outside of our own have made unique contributions to the original photographic illustrations in this text. We wish to thank Gregory and Allyn Westermeier and their daughter Shannon Michelle (photographer: Martha Thompson); Mr. and Mrs. Floore-Bennett and sons Zaalen and Ezekiel (photographer: Alan Tolhurst); and Theresa and Timothy Kilduff and their son Cass and daughter Kristin.

We are grateful to Lucille Whaley who graciously granted permission for us to use many illustrations from her text on genetics, *Understanding Inherited Disorders*. To Gail Marlow, who typed the manuscript, and Carol Monlux, who contributed to the glossary, belong our lasting gratitude. Particular thanks are also due Jane Adams for her continued support and encouragement in the development of the manuscript. For their enduring love and support and for patience beyond all understanding, we thank Emil Jensen and Jean Benson, feeling truly blessed by their presence in our lives.

Margaret Duncan Jensen
Ralph C. Benson
Irene M. Bobak

Contents

UNIT ONE

Maternity nursing today— emergence, dynamics, challenges

CHAPTER 1

A time to be born

Slowly the head emerged, first the top—I could see wisps of hair, next the forehead, nose, mouth, and then the whole head was born. Such a puckered little face, so blue. The doctor cleared the nose and mouth, and with the next few pushes I could see a shoulder, then an arm came free, and suddenly SHE WAS HERE, OUR CHILD! I was overcome with awe, I wanted to laugh and cry and shout out our joy.

Since recorded time, birth has occasioned such emotions. It is one of the dramatic episodes in life—a moment in time when the past merges with the present and the present holds all the potential for a future. Wonder and excitement, awe and reverence are stirred by evidence of creation of another human, a creation that began with conception, moved through an orderly process of biologic development, and culminated in birth. Each culture, concerned as it must be with the care and rearing of future generations, develops patterns of behavior associated with the birth process and describes the social roles of the participants—mother, father, and infant—and the persons designated to offer assistance.

These patterns vary widely throughout the world. Some cultures develop rituals of birth that include separation of the mother and infant; others view the process as one to be shared by immediate family and friends. Some exclude the father; in other cultures the father's role is proclaimed by his ceremonious cutting of the umbilical cord. In societies such as those of North America, the cosmopolitan makeup of peoples and changing life-styles result in wide divergence in role expectations and procedures even within a small community. Even so, being born, being cared for by parents, and in turn caring for others in a like manner are events shared by all of us. They form part of life's continuum and are universal experiences.

These life events are therefore as much a part of the nurse's personal experience as they are the patient's. This means that when we describe the childbearing family and its health needs, we are describing ourselves and our own health needs. When one elects to nurse maternity patients, one is in a sense nursing oneself.

MATERNITY PATIENT

Potentially all sexually mature adults are candidates for reproductive care. Many of these, both men and women, will seek assistance for alternative methods of contraception. In the United States approximately 15% of couples will seek help for infertility problems, and 3.5 million women will give birth each year. These women range in age from 12 to 52 years. They come from all racial, economic, and social groups. Approximately 70% are white and 30% nonwhite. They or their forebears came to this continent mainly from Europe, Africa, or Asia or were native-born Indians or Eskimos. Although a majority of women experience normal pregnancy and give birth to normal newborns, at least 500,000 will be designated as *high-risk* for either maternal, fetal, or familial reasons.

Maternity health services are initiated in response to individuals seeking care for biologic or psychologic events that have a bearing on their reproductive processes. These events appear to cluster about the tasks of decision making, adaptation, and/or participation in a critical life episode.

All individuals have to make certain major decisions that will affect themselves and others for the remainder of their lives. A crisis may develop for the sexually mature adult who must make such decisions as whether to have intercourse, whether to become pregnant, whether to sustain a pregnancy or abort the fetus, whether to become a parent or give up a child for adoption, or whether to utilize health facilities and the health supervision of professionals.

Such decisions are not made in a vacuum; all the values, beliefs, and attitudes of the culture that have shaped and made these individuals aware enter the process. For some, decisions are made with much thought for the consequences and are based on carefully gathered information. For others, decisions are made without thought for the future and are based on ignorance, prejudice, or myth.

3

The response of an individual and family to the biologic reality of gestation may be both physiologic and psychologic, adaptive or maladaptive. The physiologic processes involved are the adaptation of the mother to the pregnancy, and the adaptation of the newborn to extrauterine existence, and the adaptation of both organisms to preexisting or presently existing physical or genetic insult. Psychologically the assumption of parental roles may overtax the coping mechanisms that each parent believed he or she may have developed, and anxiety about the ability to master new tasks, behaviors, attitudes, and sentiments inherent in the role may precipitate a crisis.

Generally, everyone regardless of the level of income or social esteem wishes to function in the best possible manner when confronted with a life event that has great personal implications. The ability to participate wholeheartedly in situations that result in growth, joy, and pleasure to the self and others and, conversely, to face pain, separation, disability, or death adequately and well comes in part from the feelings one has about one's ability to maintain control, in part from the sharing of these critical periods with those who care, and in part from the nurturing provided by others in the environment.

Statistics

The birthrate, the number of live births per 1000 population, varies from year to year depending on a variety of factors. The rate was low during the severe financial depression of the 1930s. This period predated the availability of modern contraceptive methods and seems to represent a determined mass decision not to have children during a time of great economic stress. The advent of World War II and the subsequent martial involvement of total populations resulted in initial downward trends and then an upsurge after the cessation of hostilities and reestablishment of regular family patterns.

The more recent and dramatic fall in birthrate would appear to stem directly from the accessibility of contraceptive techniques and abortion to young and poor persons, as well as the more affluent members of society. Surveys conducted by the United States Census Bureau in 1967 and 1972 demonstrate this change. In 1967 the average number of births expected by wives 18 to 39 years old was 3.1. In 1972 the group expected to have only 2.7 children.

Families apparently are limiting the number of offspring to one to three children. Contraceptive techniques are preventing unwanted pregnancies, and it is hoped that eventually every child born will be a wanted child.

In light of this, parents are looking increasingly to the health professions for protection of the infant from trauma before, during, and after birth.

A maternal death is the death of a woman from any cause during pregnancy or within 42 days of the termination of the pregnancy, irrespective of the duration or site of the pregnancy. The maternal mortality rate measures the number of maternal deaths per 100,000 live births. The rate remained relatively static between 1916 and 1929. By the end of the 1920s a downward trend became apparent, and by approximately 1936 the rate of decline in maternal mortality became rapid. Within 9 years (1936 to 1945) the rate was cut by almost two thirds. A combination of factors stimulated this decline: availability of sulfa drugs for the control of infections, availability of blood and blood substitutes for treatment of hemorrhage, and formation of hospital and community committees to investigate causes and circumstances of each maternal death and assign responsibility.

The rate of decline further accelerated after World War II as antibiotics became available and hospitalization for deliveries increased. By 1949 the rate was 90.3 maternal deaths per 100,000 live births (Fig. 1-1). Between 1957 and 1964 the rate of decline slowed. After 1964 the downward trend again became evident until 1972 when the maternal mortality rate stood at 18.8 per 100,000. This rate reflects the decrease in maternal deaths from abortion as the states legalized the abortion procedure and safer techniques were employed.

There continue to be differences between white and nonwhite maternal mortality rates. In 1972 the mortality rate for nonwhite women was 170% higher than for white women. Currently the mortality rates for nonwhite women approximate the rates for white women in 1954. The young and poor members of any racial group also represent a population vulnerable to maternity complications and maternal death. Many women still do not receive adequate antenatal care, and many women categorized as "high risk" are still without specialized treatment. More equal distribution and utilization of health resources to all citizens will be necessary to effect a beneficial change within these categories.

The infant mortality rate is usually expressed as the number of deaths per 1000 live births and is the ratio between the number of deaths of infants before their first birthday during any given year and the number of live births occurring in the same year. In 1973 it was 17.6 infant deaths per 1000 live births in the United States (Fig. 1-2 and Table 1-1). The United States is experiencing a slow but continuing downward trend in infant mortality dating from 1964. That year new public health programs which affected the health of mothers and chil-

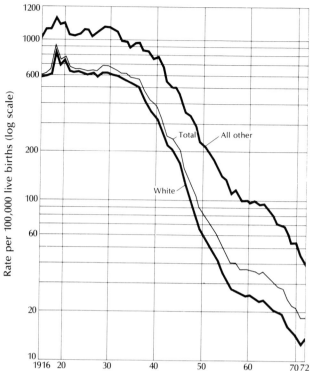

Fig. 1-1. Maternal mortality rates per 100,000 live births by race: United States, 1916-1972. (From Garfinkel, J., Chabot, M. J., and Pratt, M. W. 1975. Infant, maternal, and childhood mortality in the United States, 1969-1973. Rockville, Md., U.S. Department of Health, Education, and Welfare, Public Health Service, Health Services Administration, Bureau of Community Health Services.)

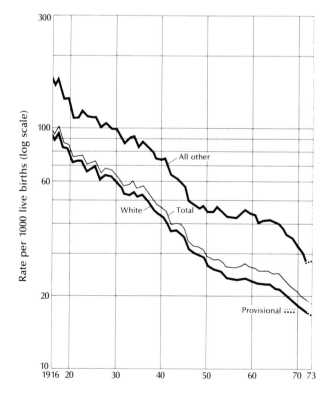

Fig. 1-2. Infant mortality rates per 1000 live births by race: United States, 1916-1973. (From Garfinkel, J., Chabot, M. J., and Pratt, M. W. 1975. Infant, maternal, and childhood mortality in the United States, 1968-1973. Rockville, Md., U.S. Department of Health, Education, and Welfare, Public Health Service, Health Services Administration, Bureau of Community Health Services.)

Table 1-1. Infant, neonatal, and postneonatal mortality rates per 1000 live births and maternal mortality rate per 100,000 live births, by color: United States, 1949-1973*

Year	Infant			Neonatal			Postneonatal			Maternal		
	Total	White	All other	Total	White	All other	Total	White	All other	Total	White	All other
1973	17.6†	15.2†	28.8†	12.9	11.5†	19.8†	4.7	3.7†	9.0			
1972	18.5	16.4	27.7	13.6	12.4	19.2	4.9	4.0	8.5	18.8	14.3	38.5
1971	19.1	17.1	28.5	14.2	13.0	19.6	4.9	4.0	8.9	18.8	13.0	45.3
1970	20.0	17.8	30.9	15.1	13.8	21.4	4.9	4.0	9.5	21.5	14.4	55.9
1969	20.9	18.4	32.9	15.6	14.2	22.5	5.3	4.2	10.4	22.2	15.5	55.7
1968	21.8	19.2	34.5	16.1	14.7	23.0	5.7	4.5	11.5	24.5	16.6	63.6
1967	22.4	19.7	35.9	16.5	15.0	23.8	5.9	4.7	12.1	28.0	19.5	69.5
1966	23.7	20.6	38.8	17.2	15.6	24.8	6.5	5.0	14.0	29.1	20.2	72.4
1965	24.7	21.5	40.3	17.7	16.1	25.4	7.0	5.4	14.9	31.6	21.0	83.7
1964	24.8	21.6	41.1	17.9	16.2	26.5	6.9	5.4	14.6	33.3	22.3	89.9
1963	25.2	22.2	41.5	18.2	16.7	26.1	7.0	5.5	15.4	35.8	24.0	96.9
1962	25.3	22.3	41.4	18.3	16.9	26.1	7.0	5.4	15.3	35.2	23.8	95.9
1961	25.3	22.4	40.7	18.4	16.9	26.2	6.9	5.5	14.5	36.9	24.9	101.3
1960	26.0	22.9	43.2	18.7	17.2	26.9	7.3	5.7	16.3	37.1	26.0	97.9
1959	26.4	23.2	44.0	19.0	17.5	27.7	7.4	5.7	16.3	37.4	25.8	102.1
1958	27.1	23.8	45.7	19.5	17.8	29.0	7.6	6.0	16.7	37.6	26.3	101.8
1957	26.3	23.3	43.7	19.1	17.5	27.8	7.2	5.8	15.9	41.0	27.5	118.3
1956	26.0	23.2	42.1	18.9	17.5	27.0	7.1	5.7	15.1	40.9	28.7	110.7
1955	26.4	23.6	42.8	19.1	17.7	27.2	7.3	5.9	15.6	47.0	32.8	130.3
1954	26.6	23.9	42.9	19.1	17.8	27.0	7.5	6.1	15.9	52.4	37.2	143.8
1953	27.8	25.0	44.7	19.6	18.3	27.4	8.2	6.7	17.3	61.1	44.1	166.1
1952	28.4	25.5	47.0	19.8	18.5	28.0	8.6	7.0	19.0	67.8	48.9	188.1
1951	28.4	25.8	44.8	20.0	18.9	27.3	8.4	6.9	17.5	75.0	54.9	201.3
1950	29.2	26.8	44.5	20.5	19.4	27.5	8.7	7.4	17.0	83.3	61.1	221.6
1949	31.3	28.9	47.3	21.4	20.3	28.6	9.9	8.6	18.7	90.3	68.1	234.8

*From Garfinkel, J., Chabot, M. J., and Pratt, M. W. 1975. Infant, maternal, and childhood mortality in the United States, 1968-1973. Rockville, Md., U.S. Department of Health, Education, and Welfare, Public Health Service, Health Services Administration, Bureau of Community Health Services; based on data from "Vital Statistics of the United States, 1940-60" (annual volumes) and "Vital Statistics of the United States" (monthly vital statistics reports).
†Provisional data.

dren received support from federal, state, and local funds. Maternal and infant care projects provided antenatal care and infant care for high-risk mothers and infants through the first year of life. The children and youth project extended pediatric care from birth to 21 years of age. Family planning services increased with support from the Maternal and Child Health Service, Office of Economic Opportunity, and the Family Planning Service and Population Research Act of 1970. The development of intensive care units for the newborn and of regional perinatal centers increased.

Despite these efforts, mortality rates for different segments of the population and differing socioeconomic groups still show gross inequities (Fig. 1-3). The United States and Canada seem to share similar problems in the utilization and distribution of health services as reflected in the ranking of rates for infant mortality for selected countries and years (Table 1-2).

MATERNITY NURSE

Nursing care of the maternity patient forms an integral part of the federal and community health systems. Maternity nursing has been defined as a "direct service to individuals, their families, and the community during childbearing and the childbearing phases of the life cycle" (American Nurses' Association, 1973). During the

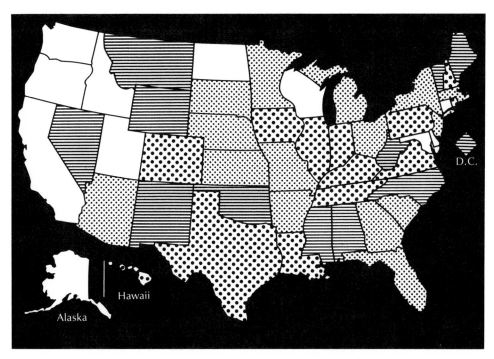

Fig. 1-3. White neonatal mortality rates per 1000 live births: each state, 1968-1970. (From Garfinkel, J., Chabot, M. J., and Pratt, M. W. 1975. Infant, maternal, and childhood mortality in the United States, 1968-1973. Rockville, Md., U.S. Department of Health, Education, and Welfare, Public Health Service, Health Services Administration, Bureau of Community Health Services.)

Table 1-2. Infant mortality rates for selected countries and years: 1950, 1960, 1969*

	Rates per 1000 live births			Rank		
	1950	**1960**	**1969**	**1950**	**1960**	**1969**
Sweden	21.0	16.6	11.7	1	1	1
Australia	24.5	20.2	17.9	2	4	9
Netherlands	25.2	17.9	13.2	3	2	2
New Zealand	27.6	22.6	16.9	4	9	8
Norway	28.2	18.9	13.8	5	3	3
United States	29.2	26.0	20.9	6	10	15
Denmark	30.7	21.5	14.8	7	7	6
Switzerland	31.2	21.1	15.4	8	6	7
United Kingdom	31.4	22.5	18.6	9	8	10
Canada	41.5	27.3	19.3	10	11	11
Finland	43.5	21.0	14.0	11	5	4
Ireland	46.2	29.3	20.6	12	13	14
France	52.0	27.4	19.6	13	12	12
Japan	60.1	30.7	14.2	14	14	5
Eastern Germany†	72.1	38.8	20.3	15	15	13

*From Garfinkel, J., Chabot, M. J., and Pratt, M. W. 1975. Infant, maternal, and childhood mortality in the United States, 1968-1973. Rockville, Md., U.S. Department of Health, Education, and Welfare, Public Health Service, Health Services Administration, Bureau of Community Health Services; based on data from Chase, H. C. 1972. Am. J. Public Health **62:**581.
†Includes East Berlin.

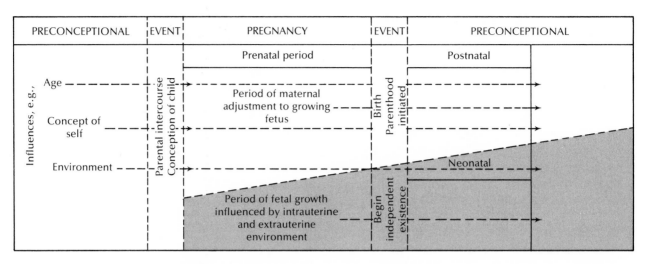

Fig. 1-4. Maternity nursing scope: continuum of life.

past few decades maternity nursing has evolved from an occupational role limited to skilled technical care offered during the antenatal, natal, and postnatal periods of the maternity cycle in clinics and hospitals to one which is concerned with the psychosocial as well as the physiologic needs of patients. Nursing care of the maternity patient is offered through a multiplicity of national and local agencies and spans a time period beginning with the preconceptional planning for children through the early adjustment period of the family to the newborn child (Fig. 1-4).

Roles

The maternity nurse practices a unique type of nursing service. Patients include those of varying age groups from the fetus and neonate, to the adolescent, to the young adult, to individuals approaching middle age. Their significant others include young children, peers, parents, or grandparents. Their health needs range from health maintenance to detection of physical or emotional disability and institution of corrective measures. In meeting these needs, the maternity nurse utilizes the skills of technician, teacher, counselor, supervisor, and advocate as an integral part of nursing care. Technical skills include assessment of health status, setting up environments that afford safety and comfort to patients and others, initiating therapeutically effective nursing measures, and being aware of the implications of efficient use of time, energy, and materials both for patient and nurse. The technical competence of a nurse generates a feeling of confidence and security within the patient and is an important part of the emotionally supportive care patients require. The skills of

teaching, counseling, and supervising have much in common, since they are focused on the behaviors of others and whether such behaviors are to be initiated, sustained, or modified. In her capacity as teacher, counselor, and supervisor, the nurse functions as a change agent, and interventions are directed toward assisting patients in their acquisition of knowledge, providing an environment conducive to decision making, or establishing evaluative processes to ensure the completion of assigned or assumed tasks.

The expanded role of the nurse in maternity care is not a new concept. Until the nineteenth century, few people, including physicians, were concerned with providing women in childbirth with other than untrained women attendants. By the middle of the nineteenth century, the medical profession was taking an increasing interest in obstetrics, and educational programs for nurse-midwives were started in Britain. Standards were not high, and in 1891 concerned persons united to form the Midwives Institute. In 1902 the Midwives Act was passed to secure the better training of midwives and to regulate their practice. In 1925 Mary Breckinridge, who had completed a midwifery course in Britain, was instrumental in organizing the Frontier Nursing Service in Kentucky. In 1939 the Frontier Graduate School of Midwifery opened, and recently it has added "and Family Nursing" to its title to better reflect the scope of the preparation nurses receive. Numerous educational programs throughout North America are undertaking the preparation of nurses for several expanded roles in maternity nursing (see Appendix M for list of nurse-midwife programs).

Although there are no official definitive statements that serve to categorize the various personnel engaged in maternity nursing, the following three definitions illustrate the scope of maternity nursing and the need for nurses prepared at different levels.

Women's health care specialist. The women's health care specialist may be a registered nurse. The length of specialist training for a registered nurse is approximately 3 months and for a licensed practical nurse or medically experienced woman, 6 months. Women health care specialists can screen for physical abnormalities and refer any suspected abnormality to the physician. They perform routine gynecologic examinations, provide birth control counseling, and can insert and remove intrauterine devices. Under a physician's standing orders or contingency orders, these health care specialists also treat certain simple abnormalities such as uncomplicated vaginal infections.

Obstetric-gynecologic nurse practitioner. These persons are registered nurses who have completed a formal education program that meets the professional criteria of an obstetric-gynecologic nurse practitioner. They may have a master's degree. These persons are licensed and certified by the state of residence but function in collaboration with physicians. They are able to take a complete health history and perform and complete physical examination with special focus on the reproductive system. They can provide antenatal care, including counseling and teaching of patients. Evaluation of and supportive care during labor is included along with postnatal care, which includes family planning. Obstetric-gynecologic nurse practitioners provide immediate and continuing assessment of the newborn in collaboration with the health team and assist the family in assuming its new responsibility. They can also provide primary health care to normal, nonpregnant women for health maintenance.

Nurse-midwife. Certified nurse-midwives are registered nurses who have additional knowledge and skill gained through an organized program of study and clinical experience recognized by the American College of Nurse Midwives. They must pass a certification process before beginning practice. They are able to perform the tasks and care for the patient in the same way as obstetric-gynecologic nurse practitioners, but their primary focus is in the area of management and care of mothers and babies throughout the maternity cycle (including delivery), so long as maternal progress meets criteria accepted as normal. The nurse-midwife is prepared to teach, interpret, and provide support as an integral part of her services.

In 1970 the American College of Obstetricians and Gynecologists (ACOG), the Nurses' Association of the American College of Obstetricians and Gynecologists (NAACOG), and the American College of Nurse Midwives (ACNM) issued a joint statement to the effect that in "medically-directed teams, qualified nurse-midwives may assume responsibility for the complete care and management of uncomplicated maternity patients." This position has opened the door to the increased use of nurse-midwives in North America, and in a number of states in the United States, which have not permitted the full functioning of these nurses, legislative bills are pending that will provide the necessary license to practice.

The professional role of the midwife as defined by the World Health Organization and amended by the Working Party on Midwifery Training in European Countries is as follows:

A midwife is a person who is qualified to practice midwifery. She is trained to give the necessary care and advice to women during pregnancy, labor and the postnatal period, to conduct normal deliveries on her own responsibility and to care for the newly born infant. At all times she must be able to recognize the warning signs of abnormal or potentially abnormal conditions which necessitate referral to a doctor and to carry out emergency measures in the absence of a doctor. She may practice in hospitals, health units or domiciliary services. In any one of these situations she has an important task in health education within the family and the community.

Nurse-patient identification

The universal nature of birth and parenting experiences creates an inevitable identification of nurse with patient. This identification process can function either to augment or detract from the care afforded the childbearing family. Being able to picture oneself in the roles of others makes some of their needs more obvious and more reasonable. Nurses are able to enter more completely into their patients' experiences and share in the joy and sorrow. They are ready to give their patients the kinds of correct, pertinent information nurses would expect themselves and provide the supportive care and interest they would consider their due. However, the fact that the patient and the nurse share similar health needs and are confronted with similar health problems can highlight the nurse's anxieties and needs for reassurance, and the disparate expectations of each other's behavior can cause conflict. Those who would hope to provide maternity care that is both therapeutic and supportive need to accomplish certain tasks. First, they must come to terms with their own sexuality. Reproduction is a function of sexuality, and nursing related to reproduction necessarily concerns itself with this aspect of an individual's life. For many students the experience in maternity nursing represents an introduction to this nursing responsibility, and the overt intimacy of woman-man relationships and the intrusive nature of some nursing interventions can be disquieting. For others who are sexually active, the contrast between their experienced sexuality and that of their clients may call forth feelings of envy or rejection. Students will need freedom to discuss these reactions so that they can become aware of and accept their own biases and gain insight into how to function from their own perspectives.

The second task relates to the concept of pain. Pain and the thought of pain are frightening to all, and every society devises ways for individuals to behave when confronted with a painful experience. These range from stoic acceptance to the "warding off of evil by loud cries." Control of one's responses to painful stimuli is part of the process of maintaining control of one's destiny. In Western culture, physical pain has long been associated with childbirth, and this association has persisted in spite of modern advances in the control of pain. It remains a central issue in accepting or rejecting the birth process, and control of pain is a component in all childbirth education programs. Pain can, of course, be psychologic, as well as physical. Death or deformity comes as a shock in maternity practice; neither is expected. It comes to the young and vital, a group to which society affords much worth. Discussions concerning the meaning of pain in childbirth to both patient and nurse should be included in the educational plan for students. Instructors must be aware of the potential or realized childbearing activities of the nursing student and that the learning experience in this nursing area acts as childbirth preparation for many women and men. Students need time to examine their responses in coping with another's pain to become aware of their own modes of self-protection, acceptance, rejection, and denial and to become aware of helpful approaches to pain control.

The third task is the acceptance of variations in parent-child-family relationships. To witness parental rejection of a child can be a shattering experience. Not only are we made conscious of a possible deprived future for a vulnerable newborn, but also we are shaken by memories that come unbidden, of what we meant to our parents or of what we may mean to our own children. These thoughts are unsettling, and students may anticipate that they will arise. Society permits open discussion of the desirability of having children, and the existence of conflicts between childbearing and consequent changes in desired life-styles are openly recognized and discussed. This can give rise to haunting thoughts about being wanted by one's own parents and what this has meant to oneself.

REFERENCES

American Nurses' Association. 1973. Standards of maternal and child health nursing practice. Kansas City, Mo., The Association.

Chase, H. C. 1972. The position of the United States in international comparisons of health status. Am. J. Public Health **62:**581.

Committee to Study Extended Roles for Nurses. 1972. Extending the scope of nursing practice: report to the Secretary of Health, Education, and Welfare. Nurs. Outlook **20:**46.

Garfinkel, J., and Pratt, M. 1975. Infant, maternal, and childhood mortality in the United States, 1968-1973. Washington, D.C., U.S. Department of Health, Education, and Welfare, Public Health Service, Health Services Administration, Bureau of Community Health Services.

Hilliard, M. E. 1967. New horizons in maternity care. Nurs. Outlook **15:**33.

Hunt, E. P. 1967. Infant mortality and poverty areas. Wel. Rev. **5:**1, Aug.-Sept.

The maternity and infant care projects. 1975. Washington, D.C., U.S. Department of Health, Education, and Welfare, Public Health Service, Health Services Administration.

Nurse practitioner—preparation and practice. 1974. Nurs. Outlook **22.**

Nurse practitioner—preparation and practice. 1975. Nurs. Outlook **23.**

Nursing at the crossroads. 1972. Nurs. Outlook **20.**

Slatin, M. 1971. Why mothers bypass prenatal care. Am. J. Nurs. **71:**1388.

World Health Organization. Technical report series No. 331. Geneva, Switzerland.

CHAPTER 2

Maternity nursing

The enlarged scope and nature of the care offered the maternity patient and her family has made mandatory a collaborative approach to the delivery of the service. Nurses, physicians, nutritionists, and other health professionals work with the patient for mutual assessment of maternal and infant needs, formulation of goals for their health maintenance or attainment, effective use of therapies based on clinical assessment of their needs, and rehabilitative treatment to prevent maternal and infant disability and to assist them in realizing their potentials. No one group of health practitioners possesses either the competence or the time to act as the sole dispenser of health care—full utilization of all groups is needed.

ASSUMPTIONS

The conceptual framework for maternity nursing reflects the expansion of care. It is now predicated on assumptions such as the following:

1. Childbearing is in essence a normal physiologic function, and for most women and their offspring, pregnancy and birth represent a physically and emotionally safe process.

2. The childbearing process has a cultural significance, which introduces elements capable of producing crisis situations for women and their families.

3. The rapid physiologic development of the fetus and the newborn and the profound physiologic adjustments the infant is required to make in the transfer from intrauterine to extrauterine existence make him particularly vulnerable to hazardous environmental conditions rarely noxious to older individuals.

4. The total response of the maternal organism to the presence of the developing fetus means that a significant deviation from normal in any of the physiologic systems is reflected in the whole.

5. Modes of fertility control now available to an increasingly large number of persons within our society means parenthood is becoming increasingly a voluntary state.

6. Care and socialization of children is recognized and accepted as a functional prerequisite of any society.

CONCEPTUAL FRAMEWORK

Because of the complexity of the real world, one can conceptualize only small parts of it at any one time. The various theories that are part of the conceptual framework of maternity nursing cannot in and of themselves provide all knowledge and thereby all answers to nursing problems. What they can do is provide perspectives from which to view the totality of maternity care. The choice of content is therefore an eclectic one, and the necessity to maintain a pure approach is secondary to selecting content on the basis of its practical applicability.

The natural and physical sciences provide information that acts as the rationale for care of a biologic nature and as such forms a critical basis for the selection and practice of much of maternity care. The behavioral sciences provide knowledge basic to understanding the holistic and dynamic nature of maternity nursing, the cultural and social context of patient-nurse interactions, and the psychologic responses of both to the reproductive process. Selected theories from the behavioral sciences that have proved particularly helpful appear as recurring themes within this text and are reviewed briefly.

Role theory and self-concept

Growth in social role. Social roles may be defined as prescriptions for interpersonal behavior. Persons who share common attitudes and beliefs and assume responsibilities for certain tasks are performing a social role. These roles are learned in the process of social interaction, which begins at birth and continues throughout life. An individual's concept of a role (role expectations) governs how he expects others to act and how he expects to act. Every society sets up cultural norms for essential roles that serve as models for individuals to emulate in developing their personalized versions. The exact process entailed in accomplishing this has yet to be unraveled, but certain elements of the process are known.

Awareness of the idea of a role comes from myriad sources. Individuals use all their senses in doing this—hearing, seeing, touching, and smelling—as well as their cognitive powers—assessing, planning, and evaluating. The process is accomplished over time and may be described as having three phases: a preparatory phase, an assumption phase, and a reality phase.

The *preparatory phase* is a time for playacting, taking stepping-stone roles, fantasizing, daydreaming about the role, and seeing oneself in the mind's eye acting the role. During this time an individual compares his version of the role against the patterns exhibited by others. Options as to acceptance or rejection of certain tasks and behaviors are taken, with some aspects of the role deleted, some added, and some delegated to others. Doubts as to one's ability to master the role adequately come and go, and ambivalence toward eventual participation is therefore a common finding. In this phase, a person's need to assume a role, for whatever reason, can make that individual seemingly deaf and blind. Because of this narrowed perceptual field, the implications such a role holds for these persons or others involved are explored only in part.

Once committed to the idea of a role, it is incorporated into the self, and values are assigned to particular aspects of it. Certain aspects are viewed as basic and become defensible, and their loss is accompanied by much stress. Other aspects are seen as expendable, and the individual remains open and flexible about them. Still others are ignored completely either consciously or unconsciously. Validation of one's ability and the correctness of one's decisions is sought from many sources, including individuals or groups seen as knowledgeable and interested.

The antenatal period of pregnancy acts as a preparatory phase for the new role of parenthood. The idea of the role of parent arises much earlier, but when individuals are faced with eventual reality, the actual preparatory process is speeded up. Nursing interventions directed toward helping women and men with these activities are not only sought after by potential parents but expected as part of their health care.

The *assumption phase* can be either psychologic or physiologic in nature or a combination of both, for example, the marriage ceremony or the birth process. It is usually characterized by a period of high excitement and great personal involvement.

The *reality phase* of adaptation to a role begins immediately after role assumption and takes place in three stages. In the first stage, dependency needs predominate, and one relies on others for nurturative support and acceptance, input of various kinds, and release from coping with everyday problems. This period of suspended involvement enables an individual to concentrate energy on assuming the new role.

In the second stage, a more active involvement in role adaptation necessitates fluctuating between satisfying dependent and independent needs. Much learning takes place as the activities associated with the role are attempted; a feeling of trust in the ability to perform adequately begins and as a result, self-esteem rises. This stage requires from others those attitudes and actions which permit and support independence and give feedback to enhance a feeling of accomplishment.

In the third stage, interdependency reasserts itself. The feeling of success grows as essential tasks and behaviors are mastered, and this permits relaxation in attitudes toward oneself and significant others. Relationships begun in the first stage are expanded, and these are realigned with past relationships. Flexibility in assuming responsibilities is more apparent and stems from the needs the self and others exhibit. Loss of some past relationships may evoke feelings of grief, anxiety, or anger. Gain of new relationships may bring great pleasure, as well as new commitments to others and involvement of the self. Life patterns are reorganized with the new role as part.

During the second and third stages, unresolved conflicts regarding the role begin to reappear. It is necessary to confront and deal with the implications of the new role. These conflicts may be resolved with little difficulty if an individual comes to terms with reality and, as indicated, redefines the role and his playing of it. For others who are unable to cope with these conflicts, crises may develop, and the resolution or nonresolution of these crises affects the outcome for all involved. The reality phase of role assumption is evident during the postnatal period as the mother adjusts to the new tasks and responsibilities of the new role of parent. Her family adjusts also; father and children have to assume and function in changed roles.

The concept of a life role, with the various responsibilities and relationships it entails, is not a static one. Change is inevitable as new life situations occur. If the initial adaptation results in a satisfactory outcome, subsequent alteration in role structure comes with less stress. The individual can trust his ability to adjust, modify, or enlarge his role commitments; the foundation for growth in the role has been established.

Role conflict. Since growth in a social role and the concomitant development of role expectations are a normative process, nurses must become aware of their expectations and the expectations of their patients. These may not be congruent, since each has developed a personalized version of the role in question and acts in accordance with that premise. When there is reasonable congruence, expectations are similar, and the nurse-patient interaction can flow smoothly. When there is lack of congruence, stress arises, and results of the ensuing conflict might include a mutual inability to achieve goals, forfeiture of self-respect, or a feeling of failure.

Certain social roles become stereotyped to such a degree that modification of the role by a player is construed as betrayal, and the deviant individual can be viewed with much disfavor. The roles of mother and father fall into this category. Changes in life-styles can cause conflict in role expectations, for example, if the mother contributes to the family income and the father shares in the caretaking activities in the home. The mother can be labeled inadequate because she does not act in a "true motherly fashion." Both actor and audience are involved. Our self-esteem is linked to what others think of us, and we respond to their evaluations with pleasure or pain.

The patient, or *sick role,* has been well defined in our society. Patients are assigned specific roles, and sets of expectations about their behavior have arisen. They are expected to take a dependent role, accede to hospital regulations and rules, and be relieved of normal role responsibilities because of illness. The care and treatment afforded is not to be based on external power and prestige but given without consideration for color, race, or creed. Suffering and pain are to be expected and accepted stoically. Finally, patients should want to recover their health as quickly as possible.

The average pregnant woman has difficulty fitting into that particular definition. She is well, not sick. She is ambulatory, attends offices or clinics for most of her care, is hospitalized for only a few days and participates in her own care and in the care of her child within 24 hours after delivery. Yet her needs and those of her family require nursing and medical management that can be described as intensive, critical, long-term, and rehabilitative. One of the challenges of maternity nursing is this paradox.

Expectations of the patient with regard to medical and nursing roles may be at as great a variance as those of the nurse with regard to the patient. The health values, norms, attitudes, and behaviors of the indigenous group within a community affect the utilization of health resources.

For example, "The primary source of medical care in most Mexican villages as well as in the poorer sections of the cities is folk medical practitioners whose knowledge is based upon an elaborate and well developed system of beliefs acquired outside of any regular educational institutions" (Bullough and Bullough, 1972). The medical practitioner is the *curandero* (female: *curandera*) who is expected to evince a warm human interest in the sick person and his family as much as he is expected to dispense cure. In contrast the scientific approach of North American medicine with its batteries of laboratory tests and impersonal responses of its technicians tends to alienate the newcomer.

The self. Man's quest for identity, a sense of who he is, is a lifelong process. The idea of a self arises as individuals act out others' roles. This acting is noted and commented on by *significant others,* who have been described as (1) persons controlling rewards and punishments, (2) persons possessing power or competence, (3) persons loved, and (4) persons with whom one is currently interacting. The significance of these persons rises and falls on the basis of the issues involved and the importance of these issues to the individual. The nature of the verbal or nonverbal interaction is also relevant, since its intensity, frequency, and clarity have a bearing on its effect on the development of the self-concept. The self may be construed as having two dimensions: an *evaluative self,* consisting of feelings one has about oneself ("I am great," "I am a failure," "I am a good mother"), and a *cognitive self* ("I am a woman," "I am American," "I am a lawyer") (Heiss, 1968). The evaluative dimension gives rise to feelings of self-worth or self-esteem. Satir (1967) maintains that the adult needs to have esteem for himself in two areas: as a masterful person and as a sexual person. The masterful person is one who has become adept in such areas as working, thinking, reading, problem solving, and experimenting. The sexual person is one who can accept and esteem his own and other's sexuality and give and receive expressions of love and nurturance. Numerous studies have indicated that negative feelings of self-esteem may be determining factors in an individual's use of health facilities, particularly those relative to preventive care (Morris, 1966; Milo, 1967; Watkins, 1968). This has a telling impact on maternity nursing, since much effort is directed to the early detection of abnormalities, as well as to health maintenance. Regardless of the source of events calculated to lower feelings of self-worth, such as ethnic identity, poverty, or experiencing an unsanctioned or unwanted pregnancy, nursing management must attempt to counteract such feelings to be successful in the delivery of health services.

The cognitive identities that make up the second dimension of the self are arranged in a hierarchy based on their relative importance to the individual involved. Two persons may share the same set of identities but, by arranging them in different orders, vary considerably in how they would react to the same situation. Two nurses, for example, may share identities of nurse and mother. However, by ordering them as *nurse, mother* versus *mother, nurse,* one may react in a different way to happenings such as illness in the family and work attendance. Cognitive identities are intimately connected with the concept of life-style. This concept is now recognized as an important component in acceptance or rejection of health services.

Communication

Communication occurs during interactions between persons or between components of a person's self. It is central to all one does in life. The way individuals dress, their behavior and speech patterns, where they were born, their church affiliations, their choice of magazines, in short, every aspect of their lives conveys information about them to others. Every culture sets up an entire repertoire of communication patterns, most of which are acquired by members of that culture as a result of mingling with various social groups and informally learning these patterns. The failure on the part of a stranger to the culture to recognize these and operate within their context can lead to misunderstandings and the inability to carry on meaningful exchanges.

The communication process consists of verbal, non-verbal, and written messages conveyed by one individual to another and received and interpreted by the other in light of his own perceptions. Response is made to those parts of the message that one deems important to oneself. This feedback triggers another response on the part of the sender and so the process repeats. Satir (1967) comments, "Communication is a complex business. The receiver must assess all the different ways in which the sender is sending messages as well as being aware of his own receiving systems, that is, his own interpretation system."

Such a process is too complex and extensive to consider in detail in this text; however, certain components of the process considered particularly important to the maternity nurse will be briefly discussed.

Language. The social or lay language of any culture contains elements that are known and recognized by all who speak it. Each subgroup, however, develops a language of its own. These subgroups may be determined by ethnic origin, age, or profession. The nurse speaks a number of languages. A professional language is learned as part of being initiated into the nursing group. For transactions between colleagues, it provides for a pre-cise, meaningful exchange of information. Between nurse and patient it can serve the same purpose if the patient has the requisite background. If the patient has not been schooled in medical terminology, use of the professional language can be effective as a screen to guard the real thoughts of the nurse or as a "put-down" to remind the patient of his place. It may also mean that the nurse is unable to translate the ideas into the social language familiar to another individual.

Working with teenagers in a family planning clinic is illustrative of this. Their "in" language has differences that need to be recognized, commented on, and used if at all possible. Many slang terms are used for sexual intercourse, and some young people do not know and do not use the medical terms for genital organs. Unless the information given is couched in their language and feedback for mutual understanding is sought, much of what is said is either unclear or lost.

North American culture also supports ethnic groups that use foreign languages in the greater part of their daily living, and their knowledge of English may be limited. After being in North America for a few years, a hybrid language develops that is part original and part English; frequently, the terms relating to medical care become part of the graft. In a prenatal clinic in a predominantly Mexican-American community, the pamphlets relating to care were written in Castillian Spanish. Unfortunately the people spoke a mixture of Spanish and English ("Spanglish" as one nurse described it), and the information was therefore still not available to them.

Language may also be used defensively. Nurses who maintain a joking relationship with patients regardless of the patient's condition and thereby call forth a similar response on the part of patients may be acting to defend themselves against the hurt and weight of involvement in the pain of others. This is often an unconscious act. According to Luft (1970), "The individual, like the group of which he is a part, has limited awareness of the sources of his own behavior and the effects of his behavior on others."

Space. Hall's study (1966) of man's use of space, *proxemics,* showed that middle-class North Americans utilize the space between communicators in defined ways. There are definite distances used to connote varying interpersonal relationships, and the voice range and tone, the topic discussed, and the body language employed are specific for each range. Hall described four distances as follows: *intimate,* 3 to 18 inches; *personal,* 1½ to 4 feet; *social,* 4 to 12 feet; and *public,* beyond 12 feet. Voice tones progress from a murmur to a loud voice; topics discussed range from top secret to information considered in the public domain; and the body language changes from caresses, stroking, and eye contact to exaggerated gestures and change in body stance.

Such findings have many implications for nursing. Nursing activities, particularly those of the intrusive type, are carried out within the intimate distance, indicating personal involvement. At times, the nurse uses this cultural connotation to an advantage. This was apparent to one of us (M. J.) when watching a skillful nurse in the delivery area coach a patient on how to bear down with a contraction. The nurse placed her face close to that of the patient, spoke softly and gently, and had the full attention and cooperation of the woman, who appeared trusting of this comforting and protective person. At other times, one uses metacommunication channels to bring these intimate activities into an impersonal range. One method is to give the purpose of the procedure before beginning. Another is by the use of a definite body set; the face becomes impassive and preoccupied, the touch firm but gentle and precise, and the eyes directed away from the patient's eyes.

Frequently, the nurse consciously or unconsciously violates the norms of distance to prevent true communication with patients. The nurse pauses in the doorway and calls, "How goes it?" The reply is usually noncommittal. An individual is unable to discuss personal matters in a public distance range and may feel frustrated at being placed in this unsuitable position.

Another example of the use of space is the procedure adopted in a physician's office. Once an examination is completed, the patient is given time to dress and is then seated in a chair by the physician's desk. This breaks the pattern of intimate distance and establishes the one of personal distance, wherein personal matters may be discussed in a soft voice while maintaining eye contact. This engenders a feeling that the physician has a warm and friendly interest in the patient, as well as a professional one.

Another aspect of space is the idea of territoriality. Sommers (1959) alludes to this as "personal space"; it moves with the individual, with the body as its center. Violations of this personal space arouse defensive responses, either covert or overt. The allocation of space in a delivery room is illustrative of this. The patient, nurse, and physician have their appointed spots, and if others move into these areas, they are subtly or openly asked to move. The nurse's territory consists of the head of the delivery table, the worktable, and the cupboards. The physician's territory is the area at the foot of the delivery table bounded by the instrument table and sterile solution basin. The receiving crib for the infant is the nurse's territory unless medical intervention is necessary, in which case it is shared by physician and nurse. If another

physician enters the area and occupies the nurse's territory, much frowning and obvious reaching around occurs until the physician moves into a neutral zone. When the father was introduced into the delivery room, decisions had to be made as to just what territory he was to occupy. It could not be on the periphery (the traditional neutral area into which most observers are placed), since the goal was to promote a closeness between father and mother-to-be. In most units, the father is seated near the head of the table and is expected to remain there. Freedom to move about is not often permitted. All these space assignments may have a rational basis, but once assigned they become territories to be defended.

A third aspect of space is how it is utilized. In North America, the outer areas of a room are traditionally used for sitting, leaving the center clear for activity. This pattern is found in clinic waiting rooms. From a psychologic point of view, grouping of chairs or even single chairs would better answer the patient's need to cluster or to be alone, but the normative pattern persists. If patients change the chair arrangement of their own accord, the personnel often become uneasy and make comments regarding the liberties some will take—the message of nonconformity has been communicated.

Time. Another element in communication is time—its meaning and use. Many aspects of North American culture are related to time. Appointments are made at definite times, and although a little leeway is allowed, the person is expected to be on time and, conversely, does not expect to be kept waiting. To be kept waiting is interpreted as a slight, as an indication that one is of an inferior status. This can be particularly enraging if individuals suspect that there may be reasons to assume others are downgrading their status. Frequently, one sees such reactions in government-sponsored health clinics, where patients suspect that the personnel are "looking down on them as charity cases."

Patients who do not keep appointments are assumed to be shiftless and unconcerned. One of us (M. J.) visited an Indian village on the west coast of British Columbia to carry out a previously planned immunization program. Only a few older residents were found there; the others had left because the salmon were running. No offenses were intended—one project could wait; the other could not. Being guided by the timing of natural events rather than by hours, days, weeks, months, or any other division of time seems incomprehensible to many North Americans. Communication can break down on such provocation.

Perceptions. The perceptions individuals hold in relation to concepts such as health, illness, time, and role behaviors of health professionals profoundly affect the

GUIDELINES FOR CROSS-CULTURAL HEALTH PROGRAMS*

A common problem in improving the delivery of health services to culturally diverse groups is that frequently the programs are planned and implemented by professionals of a culture different from that of those they are trying to help. It is important, therefore, for the "outside" professionals to realize that they cannot *make* changes but can only supply new approaches or create a desire in others for change.

For a number of years Project HOPE nurses have been planning and implementing health teaching programs overseas and—in more recent years—in this country, as they have attempted to help solve some of the health problems of certain minority groups within our society. It is on the basis of both these experiences that these guidelines have been developed.

1. Beware the temptation to arrive at a project with a specific proposal in hand (immediately giving the impression to the local people that "mother knows best"). Instead, come prepared with ideas to be discussed and subsequently molded into a program, with clearly defined mutual objectives that are related to the perceived needs of the particular community.

2. Develop an awareness of your own culture and values. In working in a cross-cultural setting you will first be accepted as a person and only later as a professional. The converse is also true; that is, before attempting to judge the professional capabilities of those with whom you will be working, you must first accept them as people.

3. Familiarize yourself with the actual work situation. Observe and become actively involved in daily routine. Attempt to gain an understanding not only of how care is delivered but also why a certain method or procedure is used. Is it because of lack of equipment, knowledge, money? Do you question it only because it is different from what you are used to?

4. Identify your own strengths and limitations. Try not to make commitments that you or your team will be unable to fulfill. Obvious limiting factors to what one may accomplish are time and money; less obvious but equally important restraints are the limits of one's personal expertise.

5. Identify the areas of excellence of local professional personnel with whom you are working. Learn from them and do not duplicate their efforts. In some areas, for example, midwives will undoubtedly be skilled in deliveries due to years of practice; accordingly, the obstetric nurse will be wiser to concentrate her efforts on planning for continuity of care, patient teaching, resuscitation of the new-born, or other areas in which the local midwife is probably less proficient.

6. Attempt to identify specifically what you as an individual have to offer those of another culture and the ways in which you will share your knowledge. You may do this as a professional role model or by more formal methods. Utilize the knowledge gained from your own experience in previous, similar situations, at the same time recognizing the uniqueness of each new situation and individual.

7. Be flexible and compromise, but only to the point where you feel personally comfortable. To compromise is not to surrender, but to blend or modify one's objectives or set ideas. An operating room nurse once asked me how I could expect her to be "flexible" in teaching sterile technique, which appeared to be the biggest problem in the hospital where she was working. "Either something is sterile or not sterile" was a statement very difficult to deny. But, as the same nurse became more aware of the local problems and needs, she was able to establish her own priorities, neither becoming "just like" those whom she was attempting to teach, nor removing herself from a situation that would never be identical to the corresponding situation in her own country.

8. Take into account that trying to change people's attitudes is usually less productive than changing the circumstances around them. A public health nurse in Peru found that despite a concentrated health education campaign, mothers from poor barrios were not bringing their children back for their second and third doses of DPT vaccine although they brought the children to the clinic time and time again when they were acutely ill. The nurse and the physician with whom she worked decided to study the effect of immunizing a number of these ill children. When no unfavorable reactions occurred, immunization procedures were changed accordingly.

9. Timing is important: learn when to push and when to wait. In one instance, monthly reports from a health team eager to help set up an ICU in an area where this was an entirely new concept indicated that even though the plan was accepted and preparation begun early in the year, little mention was made of this project for a number of months thereafter. As time drew near for the entire team to leave, the local personnel themselves began to push for help in completing the project; the unit was opened several weeks before the team left. I am firmly convinced that had the team done all the pushing, the results would have been different, with progress being made only to "please" the outsiders.

10. Finally, and perhaps most important, set short-term goals within the framework of long-range objectives. You, as well as the people with whom you will be working, need to see concrete results. Those who recognize that only rarely is a long-range objective reached by a narrow, straight path will be able to construct a broader, winding one, which still has guard rails in the form of clearly defined objectives. Also important are reflectors, in the form of frequent evaluation, to keep one from falling over the edge and leading one eventually to a predetermined end.

These guidelines, it is hoped, will be useful to those involved in the planning and implementation of cross-cultural health programs. They are guidelines only, however, for it is our belief that the success of such programs depends, to a large extent, upon the individual initiative; attitudes, and skills that are developed with time and experience.

*From Aeschliman, D. 1973. Guidelines for cross-cultural health programs, Nurs. Outlook **21:**660.

use made of available health resources. Communication processes set up to encourage their use must take differing perceptions into account. A study of Spanish-speaking villagers of New Mexico and Colorado showed they did not seek medical care unless the illness was pronounced and their health severely debilitated. Another group whose idea of time was present oriented rather than future oriented were not committed to the concept of preventive health care.

Communication across the cultural gap is one problem health professionals face in establishing quality care for all citizens. Some guidelines for cross-cultural health programs are given on p. 16.

Crisis

Successful resolution of a crisis increases a person's ability to resolve future ones successfully. Three factors act as determinants in crisis resolution (Aguilera and Messick, 1974): (1) perception of an event, (2) availability of situational support, and (3) presence of adequate coping mechanisms (Fig. 2-1). Nursing interventions directed toward augmenting these three factors are necessary components in nursing care plans. Since crisis resolution proceeds in phases, which include the crisis event, a period of disorganization, a period of recovery, and a period of reorganization, intervening in any phase may prove therapeutic. In terms of mental health, Cap-

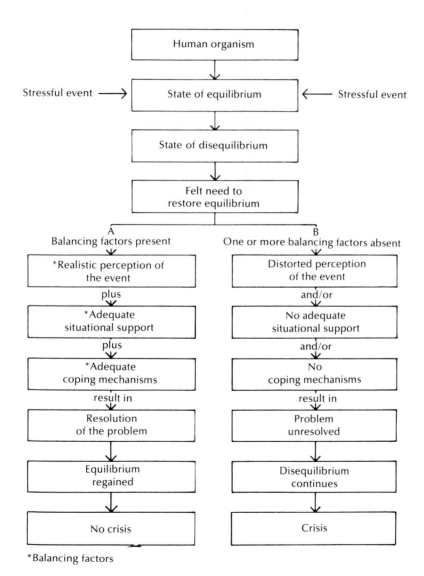

Fig. 2-1. Paradigm of effect of balancing factors in stressful event. (From Aguilera, D., and Messick, J. 1974. Crisis intervention: theory and methodology [ed. 2]. St. Louis, The C. V. Mosby Co.)

lan (1959) maintains that the outcome is governed to a critical degree by interactions between the individual or family and significant others in the environment, and frequently only minimal intervention is necessary to effect recovery in a positive sense.

Perception of event. What one person considers a crisis may not be perceived as such by another. Such factors as health, age, previous experience, educational or social background, and emotional states such as anxiety or hostility alter individuals' perceptual fields. In some instances, intervention by health workers will be instituted regardless of whether an individual perceives an event as threatening. For example, women who daily experience hunger and who have little understanding of nutrition accept as normal the fact that their antenatal diet is lacking in essential nutrients that safeguard their health and that of the developing child. The nurse instituting health care under these circumstances would need to include efforts to teach the fundamentals of nutrition, as well as to utilize community resources to provide the necessary nutrients.

Other individuals will differ in their perception of a crisis event because of coping mechanisms previously developed. An illustration of this is in the contrasting responses of two women to the pain experienced in labor.

A 28-year-old primigravida's behavior became progressively disorganized with each contraction. She changed from a calm, pleasantly excited woman to one bordering on a panic state. She screamed that she could "not stand the pain," thrashed about in bed, and cried uncontrollably. The pain experience was a crisis situation for her. Any of the coping mechanisms she had used previously to maintain composure during a pain episode were not adequate. Interventions aimed at controlling pain and reinstituting self-mastery were indicated.

In another case a 35-year-old multiparous patient was offered medication for pain. She refused it, saying, "Oh, not yet, I can feel the pains, but I just ride them out. I keep thinking each one brings the baby closer." Pain was not a crisis experience for her and to treat it as such would have represented an error in patient care.

Other persons' perceptions of precipitating factors in the crisis may be distorted. Such distortion minimizes the individual's ability to mobilize the necessary situational support or the correct coping mechanisms. In these instances the first step in intervention is to clarify the antecedents to the crisis situation so that those involved attempt to solve the real problems.

Situational support. This refers to the support persons may expect others in their environment to provide during a time of crisis. These others include members of the immediate family, friends, and/or neighbors. In times of stress, those persons closest to an individual become necessary to the patient's well-being. An example of this occurred after the delivery of an apparently normal infant. The father and mother were very excited and happy and were waiting to hear the baby's first cry. When this did not occur, tension became noticeable. The health team initiated resuscitation measures for the baby, and their attention, interest, and concern were focused on the infant. The parents seemed to huddle together in their response to this threat. The husband clasped his wife's hand and shoulder as they murmured to each other. Then the mother was observed to reach out and take a fold of the nurse's uniform in her fingers, thus establishing a link from the father and mother through the nurse to the baby. When queried about this later, she remarked, "We needed to be in touch with him; it was all we could do to help."

Other individuals who function as situational supports are health personnel, or "community caretakers," as Caplan (1959) refers to them. These persons are located in various agencies and represent the organized health resources of a community. Because of their knowledge and experience, they may be able to assist those unable to handle crises on their own or with the help of family and friends. This assistance may take the form of being supportive in themselves or by knowing the procedures for enlisting the help of community agencies.

Coping mechanisms. These may be characterized as patterns of behavior that individuals or families have devised for dealing with threats to their sense of well-being. Some of these mechanisms are intrinsic, developed on a trial-and-error basis and gradually incorporated into the unconscious; they become habitual. It may require considerable effort to bring such responses into conscious focus to enable individuals to change or to adapt them. Behaviors that serve to restore equilibrium in one situation may be inadequate in another.

The grieving process

How often one hears that the "maternity ward is the happiest place in the whole hospital." This type of comment is most often expressed by those with no experience on a maternity service. However, experienced maternity nurses recognize the need to be prepared to meet the grief and grieving needs of mothers and their families.

Pregnancy and birth comprise an identity crisis situation when everything is expected to proceed normally. During this natural transition in the woman's life cycle, she examines and actively relates to her femininity, sexuality, and capacity for motherhood, motherliness, and mothering. An unnatural or unexpected interruption in the process poses a potential threat to a woman's self-esteem and femininity. Possible threats to maternal mental health include abortion (spontaneous, therapeutic, or both), unsanctioned pregnancy, premature or postmature delivery, birth trauma, placing the baby for adoption, stillbirth, neonatal death, or the birth of a child with a defect.

When expectations of birth and joy are replaced by loss, the nurse's role is critical. The nurse must be able to cope constructively with her own response to loss and grief to meet the mother's needs. As in any crisis situation, the nurse's problems may be reactivated by those the patient presents; the nurse too becomes more vulnerable as these internal conflicts emerge in the face of the patient's problems. An understanding of the normal grieving process is fundamental to the nursing process. Suggestions are presented throughout the text for nursing management of loss and grief on a maternity unit to assist the nurse in developing, implementing, and evaluating therapeutic care plans.

In the face of a loss or the threat of a loss, the individual's reactions follow a predictable pattern. Phases of mourning have been described by Lindemann (1944) and Kübler-Ross (1969) and may be compared as follows:

Lindemann (three phases)	Kübler-Ross (five stages)
1. Shock and disbelief	1. Denial and isolation: ''No, not me!''
2. Developing awareness and acute mourning	2. Anger: ''Why me?'' 3. Bargaining: ''If I . . .'' 4. Depression and acute grief: ''How can I . . .''
3. Resolution or acceptance	5. Acceptance: ''I can, I must.''

The phases of mourning according to Lindemann are explained further.

Shock and disbelief. During the period immediately after the loss the individual struggles with the reality of the event and may even deny its existence. Mental symptoms may include restlessness, confusion, and apathy. The following somatic manifestations are common: dizziness, light-headedness or syncope, pallor, perspiration, tachycardia, palpitations, nausea, and other gastrointestinal tract symptoms.

Developing awareness and acute mourning. Reality of the loss begins to penetrate awareness; interest in daily affairs and activity diminishes. Feelings of sadness, self-depreciation, depression, guilt, helplessness, and hopelessness surface. Intense feelings of loneliness or emptiness, a strong urge to cry, and preoccupation with

the loss are common. Blame may be internalized or projected onto significant others. Anger is a common characteristic in this phase. Exhaustion and shortness of breath may occur occasionally.

Resolution or acceptance. Recovering from grief may take a year or longer, although the acute period lasts approximately 6 weeks. With resolution of the mourning process, the individual gradually resumes daily activities, reestablishes all precrisis relationships in light of the crisis event, forms new relationships, and becomes less preoccupied with the loss.

Systems theory

The systems theory, which originated in the physical sciences, was applied to the industrial complex during World War II and permitted the necessary production and distribution of essential goods. It provided a model which assumed that any particular operation was goal oriented, the components of the operation could be analyzed as tasks or activities, and the energy to initiate and maintain the process arose from a need that required satisfaction, whether it arose intrinsic or extrinsic to a system.

Systems are *open* or *closed* in that they are open to the external environment and can develop system linkage or are self-sufficient and closed. Components of the system are related in a causal network so that each component ''is related to at least some others in a more or less stable way within a particular period of time'' (Buckley, 1968).

From this perspective, health care and the services so contained can be viewed as a system within itself or a subsystem within the larger cultural matrix. The system may be viewed as a whole or its components—patients, health personnel, agencies, or facilities—may be examined as individual elements or processes, regardless of position at the national, community, or interpersonal level. The external or internal forces that affect change can be predominantly political, social, or economic in nature, but change in any one of the components eventually affects the whole.

This approach permits a more patient-responsive type of nursing care. Both patient and nurse can view themselves as variables within an open system. Their actions have an impact, one on the other and on the system as a whole, and conversely, changes on the national level necessitate planning for changes on the personal level. This theory is basic to a holistic concept of health care and emphasizes goal-directed activities, as well as promoting continuous analysis and evaluation of the effects of health care strategies.

MATERNITY NURSING PROCESS

Once confronted with a patient's problem, whether it is generated by the patient or noted by another individual, the task of devising a *plan of care* begins. An example of the plan of care form that will be used throughout this text is shown below. The task of developing a plan of care for the maternity patient involves a number of steps.

Development of a data base

The collecting of sufficient data to serve as a basis for nursing assessment is an essential first step. The sources of data are the maternity patient, her family, friends, records, reports, and other documents. Areas to be assessed include the patient's biologic status, the patient's perception of her condition, the expectations of the patient and her family of what constitutes health care, situational factors (e.g., family socioeconomic status, availability of health resources) that may prove supportive or nonsupportive, and her patterns of coping and interacting that can act as assets or liabilities for her care.

Systematic recording of this information in the patient's record as the medical history, reproductive history, and patient profile forms the *data base* for subsequent planning of care. The process of data collection and assessment is a continuous one, and input of new data can alter the original plan at any time (Fig. 2-2).

Nursing assessment *

After sufficient data has been collected, they can be analyzed and a nursing assessment made. This may represent any one or combination of the following:

---

* Various terms are currently being used for nursing assessment (e.g., client-centered problem, nursing diagnosis, nursing impression).

- A normal biologic process (e.g., pregnancy, antenatal period)
- A pathophysiologic process or disease entity (e.g., preeclampsia)
- A symptom perceived as a problem by the patient or health personnel (e.g., sore nipples)

Patient care objectives

Once the assessment is made and the goals or outcomes made explicit, the steps required to meet the goals (patient care objectives) are stated as objectively and specifically as possible to permit their use as criteria for evaluating the effectiveness of selected nursing interventions. For example, patient care objectives for successful transition of the neonate from intrauterine to extrauterine existence with regard to respirations would be written on the plan of care as follows:

Airway is open and respirations stabilized at 40 to 60 breaths/min. Breathing is quiet (no grunting or wheezing). Chest and abdomen rise and fall in synchronized motion with no sternal retraction.

Nursing interventions

Nursing interventions include activities that are diagnostic, therapeutic, or educational in nature. They are *selected* on the basis of anticipated therapeutic effectiveness, the amount of risk involved for the safety of the patient, and the availability of health resources, facilities, and personnel. They are *instituted* on the basis of priority of need. For example, the following nursing intervention is appropriate in a situation in which a newly born infant given to his mother to hold turns dusky in color, and his respirations are grunting:

Immediately return infant to receiving crib; resuscitation process initiated involving all available personnel.

PLAN OF CARE: _____

PATIENT CARE OBJECTIVES

_____

NURSING INTERVENTIONS

Diagnostic	Therapeutic	Educational*

*In some cases, there will be no educational interventions. This is true particularly in the section on the high-risk neonate, since interventions are performed only in the hospital setting and require no follow-up by parents.

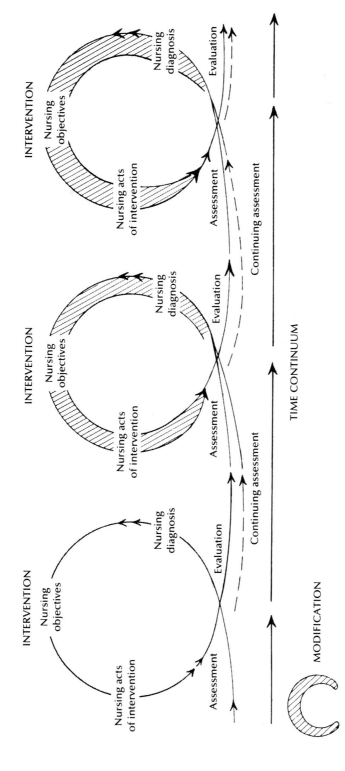

Fig. 2-2. Model: nursing process. (From Turner, M. 1974. In Hall, J., and Weaver, I. [eds.]. Nursing of families in crisis. Philadelphia, J. B. Lippincott Co.)

The rationale for this intervention is that the need to initiate and maintain respirations is more vital to the infant's health than his need for emotional closeness to the mother.

Evaluation

Assessing the effectiveness of the interventions used by utilizing the patient care objectives as criteria is a constant process. Failure to satisfy these criteria results in an immediate change of plan.

REFERENCES

Aeschliman, D. 1973. Guidelines for cross-cultural health programs. Nurs. Outlook **21:**666.

Aguilera, D., and Messick, J. 1974. Crisis intervention: theory and methodology (ed. 2). St. Louis, The C. V. Mosby Co.

Anderson, R., and Carter, J. 1974. Human behavior in the social environment. Chicago, Aldine Publishing Co.

Arieti, S. 1958. The process of planning nursing care. St. Louis, The C. V. Mosby Co.

Bradford, L. P., Gibb, J. R., and Benne, K. D. 1964. T-group theory and laboratory method. New York, John Wiley & Sons, Inc.

Brink, P. (ed.). 1976. Transcultural nursing. Englewood Cliffs, N.J., Prentice-Hall, Inc.

Buckley, W. (ed.). 1968. Modern systems research for the behavioral scientist. Chicago, Aldine Publishing Co.

Bullough, B., and Bullough, V. 1972. Poverty, ethnic identity and health care. New York, Appleton-Century-Crofts.

Bureau of Community Health Services. 1974. Infant, maternal, and childhood mortality in the United States, 1968-1973 (Publication No. [HSA] 75-5013). Rockville, Md., U.S. Department of Health, Education, and Welfare.

Caplan, G. 1959. Concepts of mental health and consultation. Washington, D.C., U.S. Department of Health, Education, and Welfare, Childrens Bureau.

Chase, H. C. 1972. The position of the United States in international comparisons of health status. Am. J. Public Health **62:**581.

Duhl, F. R. 1964. Grief. Paper presented to the Ohio League for Nursing Convention, Columbus, Ohio.

Duval, E. V. 1967. Family development. Philadelphia, J. B. Lippincott Co.

Erikson, E. H. 1959. Identity and the life cycle; selected papers. In Psychological issues. New York, International Universities Press.

Hall, E. 1966. Hidden dimensions. Garden City, N.Y., Doubleday & Co., Inc.

Hall, J., and Weaver, B. 1974. Nursing of families in crisis. Philadelphia, J. B. Lippincott Co.

Hearn, G. (ed.). 1969. The general systems approach: contributions toward a holistic conception of social work. New York, Council of Social Work Education.

Heiss, J. 1968. Family roles and interaction. Chicago, Rand McNally & Co.

Hill, R., and Hansen, D. 1960. The identification of conceptual framework utilized in family study. Marr. Fam. Liv. **22:**299, Nov.

Jourard, S. 1964. The transparent self. New York, Van Nostrand Reinhold Co.

Kübler-Ross, E. 1969. On death and dying. New York, Macmillan, Inc.

Leininger, M. 1971. About interdisciplinary health education for the future. Nurs. Outlook **19:**791.

Lindemann, E. 1944. Symptomatology and management of acute grief. Am. J. Psychol. **101:**141.

Luft, J. 1970. Group processes: an introduction to group dynamics (ed. 2). Palo Alto, Calif., National Press Books.

Lysought, J. 1971. An abstract for action, National Commission for the Study of Nursing and Nursing Education. New York, McGraw-Hill Book Co.

Mayer, M. 1973. Home visit—ritual or therapy. Nurs. Outlook **21:**328.

Mead, M. 1956. Understanding cultural patterns. Nurs. Outlook **4:**260.

Mead, M. 1961. Determinants of health beliefs and behavior. Am. J. Public Health **51:**1552.

Meglen, M., and Burst, H. 1974. Nurse-midwives make a difference. Nurs. Outlook **22:**386.

Milo, N. 1967. Values, social class and community health services. Nurs. Res. **16:**26, Winter.

Morris, N., Hatch, M., and Chapman, S. 1966. Alienation, a deterrent to well-child supervision. Am. J. Public Health **56:**874.

Paynich, M. L. 1964. Cultural barriers to nurse communication. Am. J. Nurs. **64:**87.

Perkins, M. R. 1974. Does availability of health services ensure their use. Nurs. Outlook **22:**496.

Polacca, K. 1962. Ways of working with Navajos who have not learned the white man's ways. In Reinhardt, A., and Quinn, M. (eds.). 1973. Family-centered community nursing. St. Louis, The C. V. Mosby Co.

Rapapart, L. 1957. Motivation in the struggle for health. Am. J. Nurs. **57:**1455.

Committee to Study Extended Roles for Nurses. 1972. Extending the scope of nursing: report to the Secretary of Health, Education, and Welfare. Nurs. Outlook **20:**46.

Satir, V. 1967. Conjoint family therapy, Palo Alto, Calif., Science and Behavior Books, Inc.

Schulman, S., and Smith, A. 1963. The concept of health among Spanish-speaking villagers of New Mexico and Colorado. J. Health Hum. Behav. **4:**226, Winter.

Sevcovic, L. 1973. Health care for mothers and children in an Indian culture. In Reinhardt, A., and Quinn, M. (eds.). Family-centered community nursing. St. Louis, The C. V. Mosby Co.

Smoyak, S. 1968. Cultural incongruence: the effect on nurses' perception. Nurs. Forum **7:**234.

Sommer, R. 1959. Studies in personal space. Sociometry **20:**247.

Walker, F. 1974. Bridging a cultural gap for better patient care. Milit. Med. **139:**26.

Watkins, E. 1968. Low-income Negro mothers—their decision to seek prenatal care. Am. J. Public Health **58:**655.

Whiting, B. E. 1973. Six cultures and studies of childbearing. New York, John Wiley & Sons, Inc.

Williams, F. 1974. Intervention in maturational crisis. In Hall, J., and Weaver, J. B. (eds.). Nursing of families in crisis. Philadelphia, J. B. Lippincott Co.

UNIT TWO

Biopsychosocial components of human sexuality

CHAPTER 3

Biologic components

The maternity nurse shares in an experience as old as humanity—the emergence of new life. She enters that experience with a rich heritage of knowledge, skills, and technology, as well as greater freedom to apply that heritage than ever before. Maternity nursing holds unparalleled opportunity to care for and care about the childbearing family. However, to do and be all that she can, the maternity nurse must begin with a sound knowledge of the basic components of life and its continuity—the anatomic structures and their functions in conception, pregnancy, and birth.

Although the male and female reproductive systems differ markedly in appearance, their structures are analogous (Fig. 3-1). Each performs a vital role in the propagation of the human species and the generation and maintenance of secondary sexual characteristics. Each system consists of the following four principal components:

1. External genitals
2. A pair of primary sex glands (gonads)
3. Ducts leading from the gonads to the body's exterior
4. Secondary (accessory) sex glands

In the normal course of events, life begins and is sustained for 9 months within the protective environment of the female. Therefore those organs will be considered first, beginning with the external genital structures.

FEMALE REPRODUCTIVE SYSTEM

Following are the external female genitals (vulva) (Fig. 3-2):

1. Mons veneris or mons pubis
2. Labia majora and minora
3. Clitoris
4. Vestibule
5. Hymen
6. Fourchette
7. Vulvovaginal or Bartholin's glands
8. Fossa navicularis
9. External urethral meatus
10. Paraurethral or Skene's glands
11. Perineum or perineal body

All these structures can be seen easily without special instruments.

The internal female genitals include the following:

1. Vagina
2. Cervix
3. Uterus
4. Oviducts or fallopian tubes
5. Ovaries

A speculum must be used to inspect grossly the vagina and cervix. A potent light source, speculum, and culdoscope (a magnifying viewing instrument) are required to appraise the vulva, vagina, or cervix for abnormal surface changes such as precancer or early cancer. The intrapelvic organs of a supine patient (Fig. 3-3) can be visualized by means of a culdoscope or laparoscope, an instrument with a narrow, tubular body, electric light, and compound lens system, introduced through an incision 1 to 2 cm long in the lower anterior abdominal wall. The culdoscope, a similar shorter instrument, can be used to inspect the pelvic viscera when it is introduced through a small incision in the posterior vaginal fornix and the peritoneum with the woman in the knee-chest position. In complicated cases or those in which extensive surgery may be required, larger vaginal or abdominal incisions are necessary.

External structures

The *mons veneris* or *pubis* is the rounded, soft fullness over the symphysis pubis. It develops coarse dark hair at pubarche 1 to 2 years prior to the onset of the menses at menarche (average 13 years). Moderately heavy hair during the functional years thins considerably after the menopause (average 50 years) and ovarian hormone production declines. Concomitantly there is flattening of the mons veneris due to the loss of adipose tissue.

Sudoriferous or sweat glands and sebaceous glands are present in the skin over the mons veneris. Disorders typical of other hairy areas affect the mons veneris such

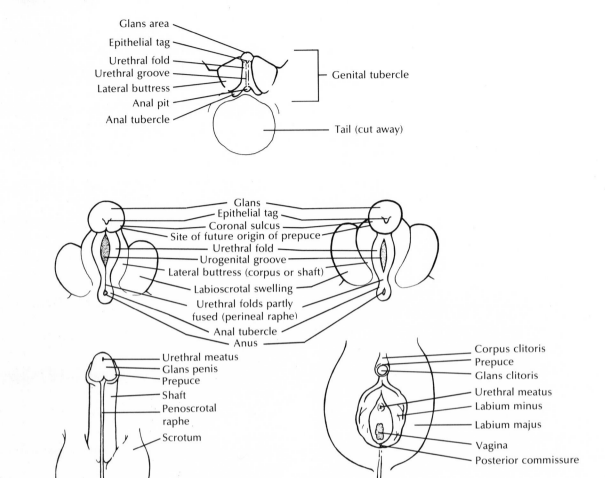

Glans area
Epithelial tag
Urethral fold
Urethral groove
Lateral buttress
Anal pit
Anal tubercle
Genital tubercle
Tail (cut away)

Glans
Epithelial tag
Coronal sulcus
Site of future origin of prepuce
Urethral fold
Urogenital groove
Lateral buttress (corpus or shaft)
Labioscrotal swelling
Urethral folds partly
fused (perineal raphe)
Anal tubercle
Anus

Urethral meatus
Glans penis
Prepuce
Shaft
Penoscrotal
raphe
Scrotum

Corpus clitoris
Prepuce
Glans clitoris
Urethral meatus
Labium minus
Labium majus
Vagina
Posterior commissure

Perineal raphe
Perineal tissues including
external sphincter

Fig. 3-1. Homologues of external genitals.

as furunculosis and pediculosis. Edema of the mons veneris accompanies severe eclamptogenic toxemia of pregnancy.

The *labia majora* are sparsely hairy, often pigmented, crescentic, fatty tissue–containing folds of skin that extend downward from the mons veneris around the external vaginal opening or introitus, terminating in the perineum in the midline. The labia majora are homologous to the scrotum in the male. The labia majora approximate and obscure the introitus in the nulliparous woman. Some labial separation and even gaping of the introitus follow childbirth and perineal or vaginal injury.

Like the mons veneris, the labia majora lose their fullness and much of their hair during old age. Dermatitis and cysts such as a sebaceous cyst or cyst of the canal of Nuck (of the terminal inguinal canal) may develop on the labia majora. Obstetric trauma such as hematomas may involve the labia majora.

The *labia minora* are narrow folds of skin and fibroareolar tissue extending from the clitoris to the fourchette between the labia majora and the vaginal introitus. Fusion or maldevelopment of the labia suggests anomalous sexual differentiation.

Increased estrogen causes development of the labia

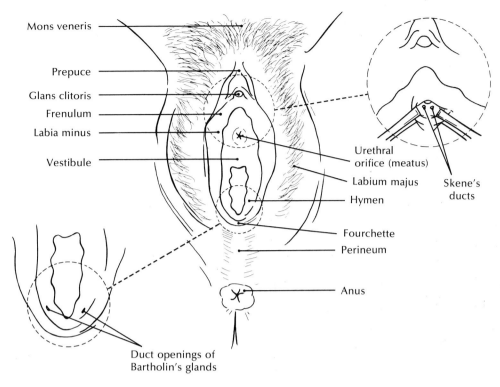

Fig. 3-2. External reproductive organs.

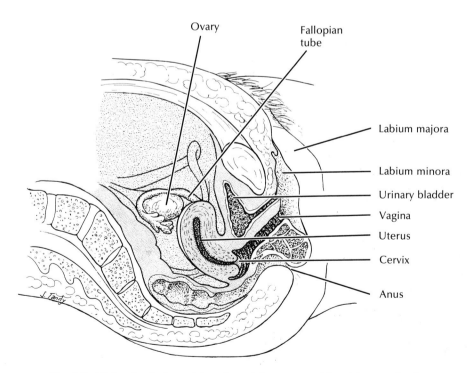

Fig. 3-3. Midsagittal view of female pelvic organs with subject on back.

minora at menarche; after the menopause, they diminish in size, even with the usual hormonal supplement.

A transition from skin on the lateral aspect to mucosa on the inner surface of the labia minora is gradual. Suffusion of the labia occurs with irritation, sexual arousal, or pregnancy. Vulvovaginitis always involves the labia minora, which contain many tactile nerve endings. Hence irritation in this region generally is most uncomfortable.

The *clitoris*, homologous to the penis, is a short (approximately 1 to 2 cm) erectile organ fixed just beneath the arch of the pubis, slightly above the urethral meatus. It is highly sensitive to temperature, touch, and pressure sensation that may stimulate sexual arousal. Lower genital tract inflammation or cancer may involve the clitoris.

The *vestibule* is an ovoid area formed between the labia minora, clitoris, and fourchette. The thin, almost mucosal, surface of the vestibule is easily irritated. The *urethral meatus*, a pink or reddened slitlike opening, often with slightly puckered margins, marks the terminal or distal urethra. Urinary, vulval, or vaginal infections may cause inflammation of the urethral meatus. Caruncles, reddened everted urethral mucosal tags, occur frequently in postmenopausal women. Caruncles often are tender and may bleed. These irregularities must be differentiated from cancer.

The *paraurethral (Skene's) glands* are two very short tubular structures, vestiges of prostatic glands, situated posterolaterally just inside the urethral meatus. Acute gonorrhea or, less commonly, other vulvovaginal pathogens may cause infection of these glands. Dysuria generally will be reported, and a few drops of pustular fluid may be expressed for culture and sensitivity.

The *hymen* is a partial, rarely complete, elastic but tough mucosa-covered septum in virginal patients. The hymen may mark the junction between the lower primitive urogenital hiatus and the descending müllerian duct system in embryologic development. In virginal females, the hymen may be an impediment to vaginal examination, insertion of internal menstrual tampons, or coitus. When complete, vaginal obstruction (gynatresia) by an imperforate hymen may be associated with menstrual pain, amenorrhea, and lower abdominal fullness. Incision of the hymenal membrane or ring will relieve obstruction. Such minor surgery may be necessary premaritally. After instrumentation, coitus, or vaginal delivery, residual tags of the hymen (carunculae myrtiformes) may be identified.

The muscles of the *perineum* (transverse, bulbocavernous, sphincter ani externus, two levator ani, and perineal) and subdermal and dermal tissues comprise the perineal body. These muscle layers are interwoven and superimposed on each other. Their movement makes it possible for full dilatation of the birth canal during emergence of the fetus and closure following delivery.

The *fourchette* is the ridge or line of convergence of the labia majora and minora in the midline. A small depression, the *fossa navicularis,* lies between the fourchette and the hymen. These structures are subject to laceration or are purposely incised (episiotomy) during vaginal delivery. Considerable blood loss can occur unless meticulous hemostasis is accomplished. Proper repair after delivery is important. If the defects are overly corrected, dyspareunia may result; inadequate surgical reapproximation often is followed by perineovaginal relaxation, including rectocele.

Internal structures

Vagina. The vagina is a thin-walled, partially compressed, musculofascial tube lined by aglandular mucous membrane characterized by transverse rugae. The vagina extends from the introitus to the cervix and measures about 10 cm in length and 4 cm in width in the nullipara. The width is increased in multiparas. The vagina curves backward and upward. Prior to childbearing, the vagina is compressed by the levator ani musculature laterally and anteroposteriorly by the puborectal muscle, so that it resembles the letter "H." Because the cervix protrudes at least 2 cm into the vagina, fornices or recesses are present all around the cervix, the right, left, anterior, and posterior fornices. The posterior fornix is the deepest, the others being about the same depth.

The vagina is situated between the bladder and rectum and is supported mainly by its attachments to the pelvic floor musculature and the associated endopelvic fascia. It has three principal functions: it acts as a passageway for the sperm's entrance to the uterus, for menstrual discharge from the uterus, and for the fetus emerging from the uterus. During coitus, the erect penis is inserted into the vagina, and with ejaculation, the sperm are deposited at the external cervical os. They swim through the cervical canal and enter the uterus.

The peritoneum of the posterior cul-de-sac (the pouch of Douglas) closely approximates the posterior vaginal fornix, a site of entry into the peritoneal cavity for culdoscopy, culdotomy, or surgical drainage of the peritoneal cavity.

The vaginal mucosa responds promptly to estrogen and progesterone stimulation. Moderate exfoliation of the vaginal mucosa occurs, particularly during the menstrual cycle and pregnancy, so that vaginal cytology or, even better, a fixed, stained scraping from the lateral vaginal wall generally provides a satisfactory estimate of the steroid sex hormone level. Vaginal fluid may also contain bacteria, parasites, or neoplastic cells derived from the lower or upper genital tract. A spread of vaginal mucus from the posterior vaginal fornix and a scraping from the mucosquamous (squamocolumnar) junction of the cervix, fixed in ethyl ether and alcohol and then treated with trichrome nuclear-cytoplasmic stain, constitute the Papanicolaou (Pap) smear used throughout the world for gynecologic cancer detection.

The sensory nerves to the vagina are derived from the pudendal nerve and middle hemorrhoidal nerve.

The copious blood supply to the vagina is derived from the descending branches of the uterine artery, the middle hemorrhoidal artery, and the internal pudendal arteries. The venous return of vaginal blood is through the pudendal, external hemorrhoidal, and uterine veins.

The lymphatics of the upper vagina drain to the presacral, external iliac, and hypogastric nodes. The lower vaginal lymphatics are directed to the superficial inguinal nodes. The spread of vaginal sepsis and malignant disease follows these routes.

Leukorrhea, literally a "whitish vaginal discharge," usually is a symptom of local disease such as vaginal moniliasis, although a systemic problem such as varicella (chicken pox) may infrequently be responsible. In other instances, cervical or uterine abnormality may be responsible. In the postnatal or postmenopausal woman, estrogen deficiency may be a cause of leukorrhea.

Primary vaginal malignancy is rare, but secondary cancer spread to the vagina from the uterus, ovary, or rectum, for example, is not uncommon.

Cervix. The cervix of the nulliparous woman (one who has never borne children) is a rounded, almost conical, rather firm body of approximately 2 to 2.5 cm external diameter. The cervix is of about the same length as its width, and it protrudes into the vault of the vagina. The cervix, or "neck of the womb," is the inferior extension of the uterus and feels much like the end of one's nose with a dimple in the center—the narrow cervical canal. This canal joins the uterine cavity and the vagina.

Lacerations of the cervix almost always occur during the birth process. With or without lacerations, the cervix has an anterior and a posterior lip and resembles a slit (Fig. 14-2).

Cervical supports are the thin pubocervical ligaments anteriorly, the sturdy wide transverse cervical ligaments (Mackenrodt's ligaments) laterally, and the moderately developed uterosacral ligaments posteriorly.

Squamous epithelium covers the cervical canal usually to the external ostial area; the endocervical canal with its many infoldings has a surface layer of tall, columnar, mucus-producing cells. This mucus changes at ovula-

tion, becoming thin and copious, thereby permitting the passage of sperm. The peripheral circular musculature of the cervix actually is an extension of the myometrium of the uterine body.

The sensory nerves of the cervix are derived from S2-4 and the pelvic sympathetic nerves. The cervical circulation is through the right and left cervical arteries and veins, branches of the uterine vessels.

Chronic cervicitis is a principal cause of infertility. Leukorrhea is a prominent sign of cervicitis, as well as vaginitis. Poor cervical dilatation (cervical dystocia), frequently due to fibrosis or scarring, may impede labor and delivery. Cervical lacerations are a major cause of postnatal hemorrhage and puerperal sepsis. Cancer of the cervix is the second most common malignancy of women, exceeded only by cancer of the breast, and is a major cause of death from malignant diseases in women.

Uterus. The uterus (corpus and fundus) and cervix have the shape of an inverted pear (Fig. 3-4). The uterus is a thick-walled, muscular, pelvic organ with a cavity flattened anteroposteriorly. It is situated between the bladder and rectum. The uterus of the adult, nonpregnant woman is about 4×8 cm in maximal dimensions. The two fallopian tubes, or oviducts, merge with the uterus, one on each side, at the cornua at a level 1 to 2 cm from the top of the uterus. That portion of the uterus superior to the level of tubal insertion is termed the *fundus,* whereas that below is called the *corpus,* or body. The juncture of the corpus and the cervix, the *isthmus,* forms the internal os of the cervix.

The uterus is angulated forward on the cervix in most women so that the fundus rests on the dome of the collapsed bladder. The peritoneum covers the uterus, except for a small part of the corpus anteriorly where the bladder is attached. The uterus is supported by the levator musculature and fascia of these muscles. The uterus is a part of the obturator in the pelvic aperture, or hiatus, together with the urethra and rectum. Slight elevation, direction, or support may be ascribed to the uterine ligaments, which include the broad ligaments, the transverse cervical ligaments (Mackenrodt's or cardinal ligaments), the uterosacral ligaments, and the pubocervical ligaments (Fig. 3-5).

Smooth muscle (the myometrium), which interdigitates throughout the uterine wall, together with fibrous tissue and blood vessels, make up the bulk of the uterus, which is particularly thick in the fundal region but thin in the isthmic portion. The uterine cavity is lined by a specialized mucous surface, the *endometrium,* which responds to estrogen and progesterone during the menstrual cycle. The endometrium is the primary site of

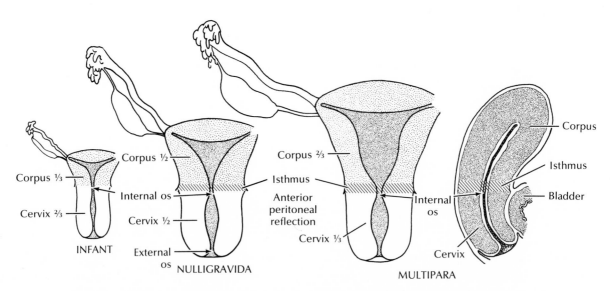

Fig. 3-4. Frontal and sagittal sections of normal uterus and adnexa showing comparative size of infant's, adult nulligravida, and adult multiparous uteri.

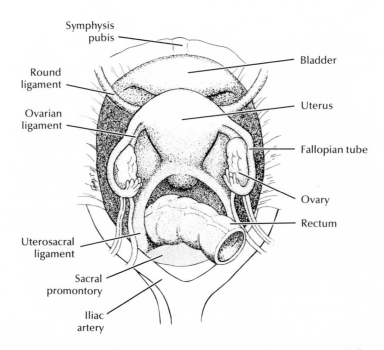

Fig. 3-5. Position of pairs of ligaments and their relationship to uterus, fallopian tubes, and ovaries.

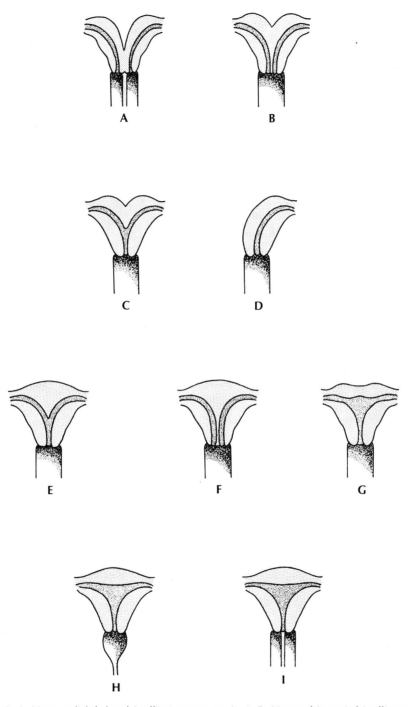

Fig. 3-6. A, Uterus didelphys bicollis (septate vagina). **B,** Uterus bicornis bicollis (vagina simplex). **C,** Uterus bicornis unicollis (vagina simplex). **D,** Uterus unicornis. **E,** Uterus subseptus. **F,** Uterus septus. **G,** Uterus arcuatus. **H,** Congenital stricture of vagina. **I,** Septate vagina. (Modified from Willson, J. R., Beecham, C. T., and Carrington, E. R. 1975. Obstetrics and gynecology [ed. 5]. St. Louis, The C. V. Mosby Co.)

implantation for the fertilized ovum. Afferent nerve impulses to the uterus travel through T5-12 and S2-4. The sacral nerves carry efferent stimuli from the uterus.

The uterus and ovarian arteries and veins are responsible for the copious uterine circulation, especially remarkable during pregnancy. Contraction of interlacing myometrial strands that surround the blood vessels controls blood loss after abortion and childbirth.

Lymph drainage from the uterus is directed to the sacral, iliac, periaortic, and inguinal lymph nodes.

Uterine anomalies. Minor developmental anomalies of the uterus such as arcuate or subseptate uterus are fairly common; major anomalies such as bicornuate and unicornuate uterus occur rarely. The cause of uterine anomalies is unknown, but errors of embryonic maturation are blamed. Uterine anomalies are important because the incidence of infertility, spontaneous abortion, or premature labor and delivery is higher in patients with such problems in direct proportion to the degree of maldevelopment. Many variations are possible (Fig. 3-6).

Plastic surgery, for example, the unification operation for bicornuate uterus, often improves a woman's ability to conceive and carry the fetus to term.

Fallopian tubes. The fallopian (uterine) tubes or oviducts are two small tubular intraperitoneal structures that measure about 10 cm in length and extend laterally from their juncture with the uterus at the cornua almost to the ovaries. The distal tubal extremities are fimbriated and bell-shaped. At ovulation, the fimbriated portion of the tubes is turgescent, almost erectile. The tubular diameter within the uterine wall (interstitial or proximal portion) measures less than 1 mm, whereas at the distal or fimbriated extremity, there is an almost cornucopial widening approximately 1 cm in diameter. The fallopian tubes are attached to the broad ligaments by a peritoneal extension, the mesosalpinx.

The delicate tubes are made up of external transverse and internal circular smooth muscle coats. The lumen is lined by low cuboidal and midcuboidal cells, a few of which are ciliated. These, together with a sparse stroma, make up the endosalpinx, which slightly resembles endometrium. Many delicate longitudinal plicae, or folds, are found in the distal portion of the oviducts.

The fallopian tubes are innervated by the same nerves that serve the uterus. The circulation of the tubes involves the uterine arteries and veins for the proximal portions and the ovarian arteries and veins for the distal segments. The lymphatics of the tubes are directed to the hypogastric, iliac, sacral, and inguinal nodes.

Ascending spermatozoa meet the descending ovum in the middle third of the fallopian tube where fertilization takes place.

Over a 3- to 4-day period, peristaltic and ciliary action carries the zygote or fertilized ovum down the tube for implantation in the endometrium of the fundus. Enzymes produced by the endosalpinx make fertilization possible (capacitation of the sperm).

Salpingitis often destroys or alters cells of the endosalpinx so that pregnancy may not occur despite normal sperm and ova. More often, however, salpingitis (usually gonorrheal or postabortal sepsis) may occlude one or both tubes partially or completely. Partial closure of the tubes is associated with infertility, but fertilization may occur. If tubal transit of the zygote is impossible, however, an ectopic (tubal) pregnancy may be the ultimate disastrous sequel. With complete tubal occlusion, sterility will result.

Ovaries. The ovaries, which contain ova or female germ cells, are a pair of whitish, rounded but flattened, intraperitoneal pelvic organs that measure approximately $2 \times 3 \times 3.5$ cm. Each ovary is suspended from the lateral pelvic sidewall by the meso-ovarium, a portion of the uterine broad ligament. The ovary is not covered by the peritoneum but by the so-called ovarian germinal epithelium, a derivative of the primitive celomic epithelium. Another thin peritoneal strand, the ovarian ligament, attaches each ovary to the uterus.

Beneath the single cuboidal cell layer of the ovarian germinal epithelium is the outer or cortical zone of the ovary. The cortex comprises slightly more than one third of the thickness of the ovary. The stroma of the cortex is made up largely of spindle-shaped cells. Larger, darker cells surround numerous randomly situated peripheral vesicular spaces (graafian follicles), each of which contains an ovum. Depending on the phase of the menstrual cycle, certain follicles appear to be more mature, with several far advanced about the time of ovulation.

The medullary portion of the ovary contains connective tissue, blood vessels, and ovarian stroma. Occasional clusters of epitheloid cells may be seen in the medulla—a possible source of androgenic hormone.

The genetic endowment of the normal female neonate is at least 40,000 primordial ova.

Estrogens, progestogens, and even small amounts of androgens normally are produced by the ovaries beginning a few years prior to puberty. The primordial follicles become graafian follicles after puberty in response to the increased amounts of the pituitary gonadotropic hormones, follicle-stimulating hormone (FSH) and luteinizing hormone (LH). If ovulation occurs following an LH surge, one or rarely more than one mature follicle releases its ovum. This follicle now develops into a corpus luteum ("yellowish body") in response to pituitary LH. Certain cells lining the corpus luteum develop into large granulosa lutein cells, which produce progesterone. Other smaller elements, theca lutein cells, secrete estrogen in greater amounts than did their follicular cell antecedents. This buildup would seem to be in anticipation of a pregnancy.

Once a zygote implants, the corpus luteum becomes much larger (the corpus luteum of pregnancy). This ductless gland is even more productive of the estrogen and progesterone needed to support early pregnancy.

If pregnancy is not achieved, degeneration of the corpus luteum begins about the twenty-fourth day of the cycle, and menstruation usually follows by the twenty-eighth day. Months afterward, the corpus luteum will have passed through a stage called the corpus albicans, and finally, only a small scar, a corpus fibrosum, can be identified. Incompletely mature follicles with their unreleased ova degenerate concomitantly.

The nerve supply to the ovary is through T10-L1, together with fibers of the pelvic sympathetic nervous system. The ovarian arteries are derived from the aorta and carry a rich blood supply to the ovaries. The ovarian veins, like the arteries, traverse the ovarian suspensory ligaments; the left ovarian vein empties into the left renal vein, but the right drains into the inferior vena cava.

The ovarian lymphatics extend to the iliac and periaortic nodes. Although normal women may skip an occasional ovulation despite menstruation each month, nonetheless, many infertile women will be found to ovulate rarely, if at all, for long periods because of physical or emotional disorders. Congenital absence of ova is the rule in the ''streak ovaries'' of the female with ovarian dysgenesis, also called *ovarian agenesis of Turner* (XO chromosomal designation).

Ovarian failure may be primary, caused by a disorder in the pituitary, or secondary, resulting from anomalous development, injury, disease, or neoplasia of the ovary. If this occurs in infancy or in early childhood, dwarfism, lack of secondary sex characteristics, amenorrhea, sterility, and symptomatology such as osteoporosis, usually associated with the postmenopausal period, can be expected. After adolescence and the achievement of full growth, ovarian failure will result in all these changes except reduced stature.

The pelvis

Maternity care emphasizes not a detailed consideration of the pelvic bones but those bony relationships that are of special importance in the birth process.

The pelvis is an articulated bony ring that is supported by the lower extremities and that in turn bears the weight of the trunk and upper body. In the female, normal delivery of the offspring requires an adequate size and shape of the pelvic aperture.

There are two parts to the pelvic basin: the shallow upper or false pelvis that supports the enlarged uterus and the lower, smaller, but deeper true pelvis that must be adequate for the delivery process. The true pelvis lies below the linea terminalis and is the bony birth canal (Fig. 3-7).

The pelvis is composed of the following bones: the right and left innominate bones, each of which is made up of the right or left pubic bone, the ilium, and the ischium; the sacrum; and the coccyx.

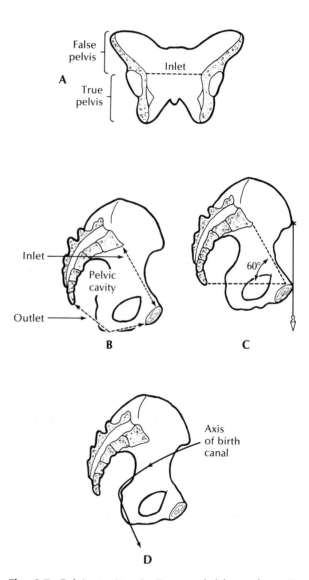

Fig. 3-7. Pelvic cavity. **A,** True and false pelves. **B,** Cavity of true pelvis. Note curve of sacrum and tilt of pelvis posteriorly. **C,** Pelvic inclination with patient standing. **D,** Axis of birth canal.

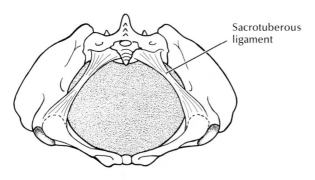

Fig. 3-8. Female pelvic outlet (from below).

The pelvic inlet, or brim of the pelvis, is bounded by the pubic crest and spine, the iliopectineal line along the innominate bone, and the anterior border of the body and promontory of the sacrum.

The pelvic cavity is a curved passage having a short anterior wall and a much deeper concave posterior wall. It is bounded by the pubis, the ischium, a portion of the ilium, and the sacrum and coccyx.

The obturator foramen in the female is a large, almost triangular opening in the wall of the cavity anterolaterally. Nevertheless, the opening is covered by the tough obturator membrane and is lined by the internal obturator muscle and its fascial covering.

The great and small sciatic foramens form a large notch posterolaterally, and these accommodate structures

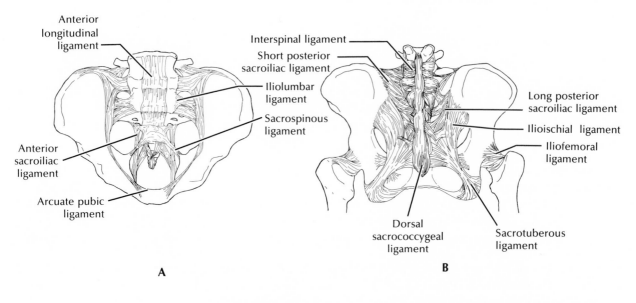

A

B

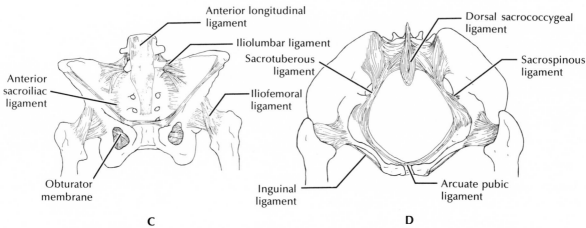

C

D

Fig. 3-9. Bony pelvis with ligaments. **A,** Superior view. **B,** Posterior view. **C,** Anterior view. **D,** Inferior view.

that leave the pelvis: the sciatic nerves, the piriform muscles, and tendons of the internal obturator muscles.

The pelvic outlet when viewed from below is ovoid, bounded by the pubic arch anteriorly, the arcuate pelvic ligament, the ischial tuberosities and sacrotuberous ligaments laterally, and the tip of the coccyx posteriorly (Fig. 3-8).

The four pelvic joints and similarly named ligaments of the pelvic bones, excluding the femoral articulations, are the symphysis pubis, the right and left sacroiliac joints, and the sacrococcygeal joint (Fig. 3-9).

The intrinsic pelvic joints of the pelvic bones are synchrondroses and allow little movement in the nonpregnant state. Nonetheless, the hormones of pregnancy cause considerable mobility to develop. Widening of the symphyseal joint often can be demonstrated by x-ray films, and instability may cause pain in any or all the joints in extreme cases. No appreciable increase in any of the internal diameters of the pelvis can be expected as a result of relaxation of the pelvic joints or position of the patient.

The pelvic canal varies in size and shape at various levels. The diameters at the plane of the pelvic inlet, midpelvis, and outlet (Fig. 3-10) determine whether vaginal delivery is possible and the manner by which the fetus may traverse the birth canal (mechanism of labor).

The pelvic axis is a line projected through the center of each of the planes of the pelvis. It is J-shaped and influenced especially by the curve of the sacrum. The pelvic axis is not the exact course taken by the fetal head

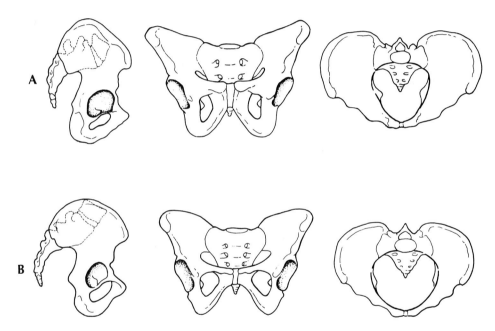

Fig. 3-10. Contrast of male **(A)** and female **(B)** pelves, especially shape of pubic arch and inlets.

Table 3-1. Female and male pelves

	Female	Male
Sacral promontory	Flattened	Prominent
Ischial spines	Widely spaced	Narrowly placed
Shape of inlet	Rounded, ovoid, or bean shaped	Wedge or heart shaped
Pelvic cavity	Commodious	Constricted
Sacrum	Wide, deep	Narrow, curved
Sacrosciatic notch	Wide	Narrow

through the pelvis; hence it has little more than anatomic and historical interest.

In contrast, the axis of the birth canal charts the course normally followed by the fetal head or breech during delivery. Moreover, it is the all-important directional guide for traction in forceps delivery.

Pelvic variations. Race, sex, and age are responsible for the greatest variations in pelvic shape and size. Diminutive people have smaller, lighter bones than larger people. Moreover, the male pelvis in all population groups is heavier, deeper, and more angular and the pelvic cavity is less commodious than in the female (Fig. 3-10). Some loss of strength was traded for an adequate birth canal in the female. As a consequence, the internal contours of the woman's pelvis are rounder and the diameters of the pelvic canal are significantly greater than those of the man. The male and female pelves are compared in Table 3-1.

The pelvis changes greatly during growth and development. Pelvic ossification is not complete until 20 years of age or older. Pelvic architecture is largely dependent on weight bearing in the erect posture. The pelvis must carry much of the weight of the body. Thus an upward force and a downward thrust are operative; this is reflected ultimately in the architecture of the pelvis. In patients with rickets, osteomalacia, or paralysis of one or both extremities, the pelvis may be grossly deformed and the pelvic canal so distorted as to preclude vaginal delivery of a full-term fetus.

External measurement yields little worthwhile information regarding the size and shape of the true or internal pelvis, except in gross deformity. Consequently, except for pelvic outlet dimensions, external obstetric pelvimetry has been abandoned. In contrast, great importance now centers on radiographic or ultrasonographic internal pelvimetry, cephalometry, and the internal configuration of the birth canal.

Obstetric measurements

Plane of inlet (superior strait). The principal pelvic diameters of the plane of the inlet are as follows:

1. The *diagonal conjugate* (12.5 to 13 cm) is the distance from the inferior border of the symphysis pubis to the promontory of the sacrum (Fig. 3-11). The diagonal conjugate is the only dimension of the superior strait that can be obtained clinically. It is 1.5 to 2 cm greater than the obstetric conjugate.

2. The *obstetric conjugate* is the shortest distance between the posterior surface of the symphysis and the sacral promontory. The obstetric conjugate determines whether the presenting part can engage or enter the superior strait. Hence this diameter is the most important measurement of the inlet. Unfortunately it can only be obtained by x-ray examination or ultrasonography.

3. The *true conjugate* or conjugata vera is the distance from the upper margin of the symphysis to the sacral promontory (11 cm or more). This dimension, like the obstetric conjugate, usually is a radiographic measurement.

The transverse diameter of the inlet (13.5 cm or more), an important determinant in assessing the shape of the inlet, may not be truly available to the presenting part, which usually is thrust forward by the sacral promontory. For this reason, the head (vertex), for example, often enters the superior strait in the oblique diameter because the colon occupies the left pelvis.

The oblique diameter (12.75 cm or larger) is directed from the sacroiliac joint on one side to the opposite iliopectineal prominence. The designation *right or left*

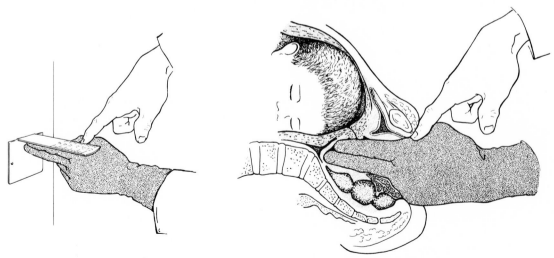

Fig. 3-11. Metal wall scale to determine length of diagonal conjugate.

oblique diameter refers to the sacroiliac articulation from which this dimension extends.

Inclination of pelvic inlet (brim). The plane of the pelvic inlet (brim) normally describes an angle of approximately 60 degrees with the horizontal when the patient is standing (Fig. 3-12). The pelvic inclination or *tilt* of the pelvis, measured by x-ray examination, is altered with exaggerated posture. Straightening of the lumbar curve reduces the inclination; increasing the curve increases pelvic inclination. This inclination may greatly influence the progress of labor.

Midplane of pelvis. The midplane of the pelvis normally is its largest plane and the one of greatest diameters. Anteroposteriorly the greatest dimension is from midsymphysis to the sacrum (at the fused second and third sacral vertebrae). This measurement should be 12.75 cm or more. The transverse diameter is drawn across the midpelvis from the top of one acetabulum to the other and should be 12.5 cm or more. The ischial spines are bony attachments of the pelvic floor muscles and are at the same level as the vaginal vault.

The ischial interspinous diameter averages 10.5 cm, making this the narrowest transverse diameter of the normal pelvis.

The posterior sagittal diameter of the midpelvis normally is approximately 4.5 cm and represents that segment of the anteroposterior diameter dorsal to a line between the ischial spines. Although the midplane is comparatively large, critical shortening of the interspinous or posterior sagittal diameter of the midplane may cause pelvic dystocia.

Plane of pelvic outlet. The outlet presents the smallest plane of the pelvic canal. It encompasses an area including the lower portion of the symphysis, the ischial tuberosities, and the tip of the sacrum. The significant diameters are as follows:

1. The *anteroposterior diameter* of the outlet is measured from the lower border of the symphysis to the tip of the sacrum (11.9 cm or more). The coccyx may be displaced posteriorly during labor and is not considered to be a fixed bone. Therefore it is not a proper reference point.

2. The *transverse diameter* of the outlet is measured from the inner border of one ischial tuberosity to the other (greater than 8 cm) (Fig. 3-13).

3. The *posterior sagittal diameter* of the outlet is projected from the tip of the sacrum to a point in space where the intertuberous diameter transects the anteroposterior projection.

The subpubic angle, which indicates the type of pubic arch, together with the length of the pubic rami and the intertuberous diameter, is of great practical importance.

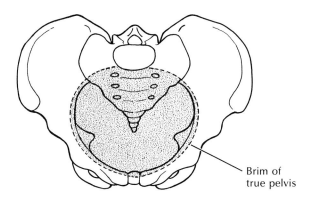

Brim of true pelvis

Fig. 3-12. Female pelvis from above pelvic brim (inlet or linea terminalis).

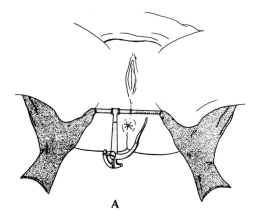

A

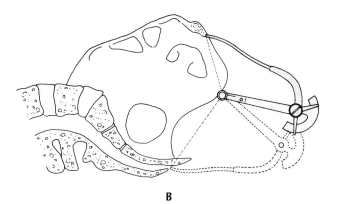

B

Fig. 3-13. A, Thoms pelvimeter. Measurement of transverse diameter of outlet (i.e., distance between ischial tuberosities). **B,** Side view of Thoms pelvimeter. Measurement of anterior and posterior sagittal diameters with free-swinging arm of instrument.

Table 3-2. Comparison of pelvic types

	Gynecoid	Anthropoid	Platypelloid	Android
Brim	Slightly ovoid or transversely rounded	Oval, wider antero-posteriorly	Flattened antero-posteriorly, wide transversely	Heart-shaped, angulated
Depth	Moderate	Deep	Shallow	Deep
Side walls	Straight	Straight	Straight	Convergent
Ischial spines	Blunt, somewhat widely sepa-rated	Prominent, often, with narrow inter-spinous diameter	Blunted, widely separated	Prominent, nar-row interspi-nous diameter
Sacrum	Deep, curved	Slightly curved	Slightly curved	Slightly curved, terminal por-tion often beaked
Subpubic arch	Wide	Narrow	Wide	Narrow

Because the presenting part must pass beneath the pubic arch, a narrow subpubic angle suggesting a gothic arch will be less favorable than a rounded, wide, Roman arch. If the subpubic angle is narrow, the head, for example, is forced backward toward the coccyx, and the extension of the head may be difficult. This is known as *outlet dystocia* (difficult labor). Forceps delivery frequently is required, and fetal injury or deep maternal lacerations may ensue.

Descent of the fetus through the birth canal follows an orderly process. Generally, the descent of the head (usually presenting first) occurs at right angles to the plane of the pelvic brim. Descent continues in a slightly backward and downward direction to the ischial spines, which mark the midpelvis or midplane.

An almost right-angled anterior turn occurs in the birth canal at the ischial spines. When the head turns to pass between the ischial spines, it contacts the forward-sloping pelvic floor musculature and is generally directed forward and downward. The fetal head thus is guided into the vagina, which is in the axis of the pelvic outlet.

Classification of pelves. X-ray studies of many pelves by Caldwell and Malloy (1933) disclosed four basic types (Table 3-2):

1. Gynecoid (the classic female type)
2. Anthropoid (resembling the pelvis of anthropoid apes)
3. Platypelloid (the flat pelvis)
4. Android (resembling the male pelvis)

Classic types occur in only about one third of all women. Therefore the majority of patients will have variations or mixed types (Fig. 3-14). For example, a patient may have a gynecoid posterior pelvis and an android anterior pelvis. These types and their significance in labor will be discussed in Chapter 24.

Pelvic floor. The pelvic viscera are retained but only slightly supported by the muscular pelvic floor, coccyx, bony pelvis, and an obturator mass (the urethra, cervix, uterus, and rectum in the pelvic aperture).

Pelvic floor muscles include the right and left levator ani group that arise from the anterolateral pelvic walls, from the fascia over the internal obturator muscle (e.g., the iliopectineal line), and from the ischial spines. These muscles are inserted into the anococcygeal ligament and into the terminal portion of the sacrum. The anococcygeal ligament, or median raphe, extends from the distal sacrum to the posterior limit of the pelvic floor aperture, the "weak spot" in the anterior pelvis.

The right and left pubococcygeal muscles together are V-shaped, and the puborectal muscle is U-shaped. These muscles tend to compress and close the pelvic aperture both anteroposteriorly and laterally and prevent sacropubic hernias (e.g., prolapse of the uterus).

The pelvic fascia is not a single layer of fibrocollagenous tissue nor does it line the pelvic cavity. Fascial condensations are found at the origins and insertions of muscles and attachments to bones. The fascia is extremely thin in certain areas. Numerous partitions are formed about muscles and blood vessels, but there are no firm connections with the viscera.

The pelvic floor, like the abdominal wall and diaphragm, is controlled by the nervous system for harmonious function. By concerted action, a pressure equilibrium is maintained, even during breathing, coughing, and straining, so that uterine prolapse will not occur

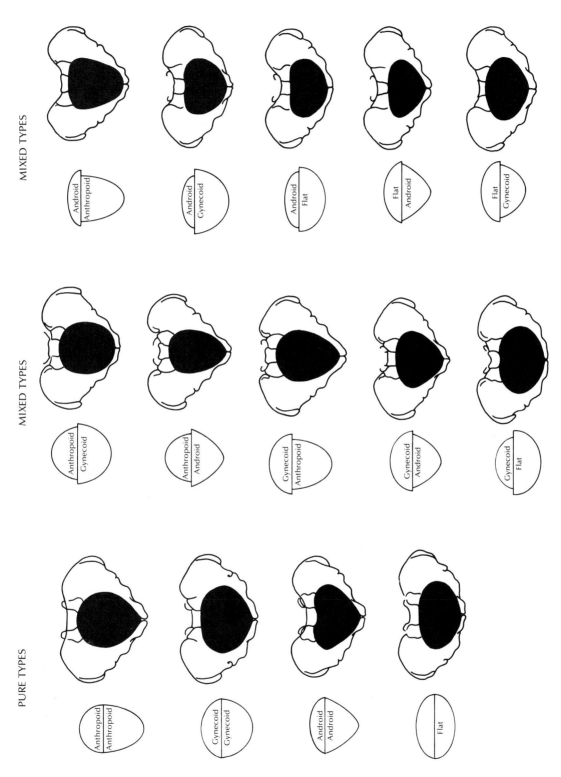

Fig. 3-14. Female pelves: pure and mixed types. Note differences in shape of inlets.

unless some injury or distention of the pelvic aperture has occurred.

The pelvic floor components are contrived so that they glide upon one another like a trapdoor arrangement. During labor certain parts may even be drawn out of the way. The planes are changed and the pelvic floor aperture becomes enormously dilated, allowing conversion of the aperture into a large urogenital hiatus for delivery of the fetus. The soft tissue birth canal begins to dilate at the top (cervix); closure is in the reverse order. Damage to the pelvic floor may alter this sequence, however.

Menarche

Although young girls secrete small, rather constant amounts of estrogen, a marked increase occurs between 8 and 11 years of age. Moreover, increasing amounts and variations in gonadotropin and estrogen secretion develop into a cyclic pattern at least a year prior to menarche or the first menstrual period. This occurs in most girls in North America at about 13 years of age.

Initially periods are irregular, unpredictable, painless, and anovulatory in the majority of young patients. After one or more years, a hypothalamic-pituitary rhythm develops, and adequate cyclic estrogen is produced by the ovary to mature a number of graafian follicles. Approximately 14 days before the beginning of the next menstrual period, pituitary FSH rises, a surge of LH is released by the anterior hypophysis, and ovulation (extrusion of the ovum) occurs.

Ovulatory periods tend to be regular, monitored by progesterone. Although not universal, ovulatory periods may be associated with slight uterine cramping (dysmenorrhea), which may be an effect of progesterone and/or prostaglandins. This discomfort is rarely serious, readily relieved by simple analgesics, and, when viewed in its proper perspective, may be reassuring to the girl and her parents as an indication of normal ovulatory function.

Although pregnancy may occur in exceptional cases of true (constitutional) precocious puberty, most pregnancies in very young patients occur well after the normally timed menarche. Nevertheless, all girls should be educated to the fact that pregnancy can occur any time after the onset of the menses.

Menstrual cycle

Menstruation is periodic uterine bleeding associated with the shedding of secretory endometrium beginning approximately 14 days after ovulation. The first day of menstrual bleeding is the first day of the cycle, which averages 28 days for the mature female but the range is 24 to 32 days. The average duration of menstrual flow is 5 days, and the average blood loss is approximately 70 ml, but this varies greatly. It is generally assumed that the purpose of the menstrual cycle is to prepare the uterus for pregnancy. When this fails to occur, menstruation ensues. The individual's age, physical and emotional status, as well as her environment influence the regularity of the periods.

The three phases of the menstrual cycle are (1) the menstrual phase, (2) the proliferative phase, and (3) the secretory phase. During the *menstrual phase,* shedding of the superficial two thirds of the endometrium (the compact and spongy layers) is initiated by periodic vasoconstriction of the spiral arterioles most marked in the upper layers of the endometrium. The basal layer is always retained, and regeneration begins near the end of the cycle from cells derived from the remaining glandular remnants or stromal cells in the basalis.

The *proliferative phase* is a period of rapid growth and extends from about the fifth day to the time of ovulation; for example, day 10 of a 24-day cycle, day 14 of a 28-day cycle, or day 18 of a 32-day cycle. The endometrial surface is completely restored in approximately 4 days or slightly before bleeding ceases. From this point on, an eightfold to tenfold thickening occurs, with a leveling off of growth at ovulation. During the proliferative phase, the glands are tubular, and the columnar cells lining the glands have oval nuclei centrally placed. The stroma is moderately dense and only slightly vascular. Active mitosis increases rapidly until ovulation. Three or 4 days prior to ovulation, moderate tortuosity of the glands has developed, and although the stroma maintains its cellularity, vascularity is increased also. The proliferative phase is dependent on estrogen stimulation derived from ovarian follicles.

The *secretory phase* extends from the day of ovulation to about 3 days before the next menstrual period. After ovulation, larger amounts of progesterone are produced. This hormone causes the glands to become tortuous, serrated, and widened. An edematous vascular stroma is now apparent. The cells lining the glands, which have basally placed nuclei, secrete a thin, glycogen-containing fluid. Finally, in the fully matured secretory endometrium, three strata are noted: the superficial or compact layer, an intermediate or spongy layer, and the basal or inner inactive layer.

At the end of the secretory phase, the uterine lining is prepared to receive and nourish the fertilized ovum, should one be available. Implantation of the fertilized ovum generally occurs about 7 to 10 days after ovulation. If fertilization is not accomplished, the corpus luteum and endometrium regress. Just before menstruation begins, ischemia develops in the endometrium, and this is followed by necrosis of the two superficial layers. Sep-

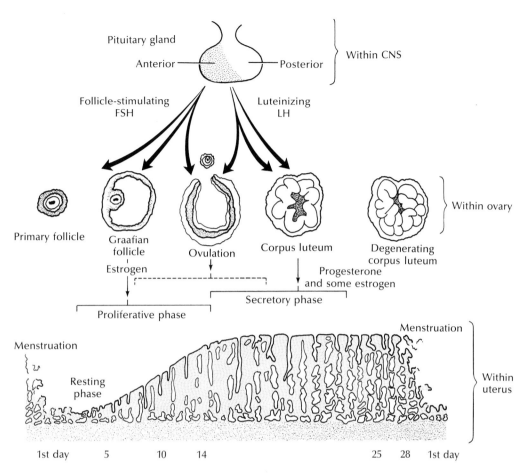

Fig. 3-15. Hormonal control of menstrual cycle.

aration of tissue soon occurs, and menstrual bleeding begins once again.

The function of ovulation is regulated by a complete interplay of hormonal secretion and action (Fig. 3-15). Releasing (RH) or inhibitory (IH) hormones are produced in various areas of the hypophysis and are transmitted to the anterior pituitary through a minute vascular portal system. A single RH has been identified as triggering the production of the gonadotropins FSH and LH.

With the proper coordination of releasing and inhibiting substances, the anterior lobe of the pituitary secretes still other tropic hormones: thyrotropin (TSH), corticotropin (ACTH), growth hormone (HGH), melanocyte-stimulating hormone (MSH), all of which are important to reproductive physiology. Another hormone produced by the anterior pituitary is prolactin, which is responsible for lactation. Its production is inhibited until after birth and thus plays no part in the normal menstrual cycle.

The posterior pituitary lobe is linked with the hypothalamus by nerves in contrast with the anterior. The posterior pituitary hormones, vasopressin and oxytocin, are secreted in the hypothalamus and stored in the posterior pituitary. Vasopressin, or antidiuretic hormone, controls plasma osmolarity and is released by impulses from the supraoptic nuclei. Oxytocin, stimulatory for labor and lactation, is released by discharges from the supraventricular nuclei.

Normal menstrual cycles are carefully regulated by gonadotropin secretion. FSH, at low levels during menstruation, rises slightly in the proliferative phase of the cycle until just before ovulation when both FSH and LH become variable and, finally, rise rapidly. The most marked is the dramatic LH surge on about the fourteenth day of the 28-day cycle, which triggers rupture of the follicle and ovulation. Slight bleeding occurs, and the empty follicle soon becomes filled with clotted blood and is termed an *hemorrhagic follicle*. LH and FSH stimulate luteinization of the granulosa cells, and a corpus luteum is thus formed. The granulosa lutein cells produce progesterone, which peaks about the twenty-third or twenty-fourth day of a 28-day cycle. If fertilization and nidation of the ovum (pregnancy) has not occurred by this time, regression of the corpus luteum follows. Therefore the levels of progesterone and estrogen decline to reach a critical level at approximately the twenty-eighth day when endometrial bleeding (menstruation) occurs.

If pregnancy occurs, however, active secretion and even greater tortuosity of the endometrial glands develop. Edema of the stroma is apparent, and much greater vascularity is notable. The stromal cells become large and polygonal in shape and are known as *predecidual cells*.

The exact biochemical or endocrine mechanism that results in uterine bleeding is still speculative. It may be that steroid sex hormones may alter the production or metabolism of specific enzymes or other substances necessary for cell function. When catabolic products accumulate, release of prostaglandins (PG), largely $F_{2\alpha}$, causes spasm of the arterioles, which may be responsible, at least in part, for hypoxia, necrosis, and, finally, separation and dissolution of the superficial endometrium (see pp. 47 and 48 for further discussion of prostaglandins).

Physiologic response to sexual stimulation

Anatomic and reproductive differences notwithstanding, men and women are more alike than different in their physiologic response to sexual excitement and orgasm (Tables 3-1 and 3-2). Not only is there little difference between male and female sexual responses, it is now accepted that the physical response is essentially the same whether the source of stimulation is coitus, fantasy, or mechanical or manual masturbation. Physiologically all sexual response can be analyzed in terms of two processes: vasocongestion and myotonia.

1. *Vasocongestion.* Sexual stimulation results in reflex dilatation of penile (erection) and circumvaginal (lubrication) blood vessels, causing engorgement and distension of the genitals. Venous congestion is localized primarily in the genitals, but it also occurs to a lesser degree in the breasts and other parts of the body.

2. *Myotonia.* Arousal is characterized by increased muscular tension resulting in voluntary and involuntary rhythmic contractions. Examples of sexually stimulated myotonia are pelvic thrusting, face grimacing, and spasms of the hands and feet (carpopedal spasms).

Table 3-3. Four phases of male human sexual response*

Organs and body functions	Excitement phase	Plateau phase	Orgasmic phase	Resolution phase
Penis	Erects	Diameter of coronal ridge increases		Loss of erection
Nipples	May erect			Slow return to normal
Muscles	Tense		Contractions and spasms	Relaxation
Pulse rate	Increases		Reaches peak	Gradual return to normal
Blood pressure	Increases		Reaches peak	Gradual return to normal
Skin of scrotum	Tenses and thickens			Returns to normal state
Scrotal sac	Elevates			Returns to normal state
Testes	Draw up	50% increase in size		Return to normal state
Sex flush	May appear		Is most pronounced	Disappears rapidly
Breathing rate		Increases	Reaches peak	Gradual return to normal
Other			Contractions of seminal vesicles and ampullae	
			Filling of bulb in urethra near base of penis	Returns to normal state
			Contractions of bulb, urethra, and penis	
			Ejaculation	Refractory period is experienced before another cycle may be resumed

*Courtesy Victor J. Des Marais, Jr., National Sex Forum, San Francisco, Calif.; based on data from Masters, W. H., and Johnson, V. E. 1966. Human sexual response. Boston, Little, Brown & Co.

Four successive phases of the sexual response cycle have been identified through observational research (Tables 3-3 and 3-4). It is important to note that although there are four describable phases, the response cycle is a continual process.

Excitement phase. The most obvious changes resulting from sexual stimulation are the following:

1. Tumescence of the clitoral glans marked by elongation and increased diameter of the clitoral shaft
2. Vaginal lubrication, a process similar to sweating, caused by vasocongestion
3. Expansion and lengthening of the inner two thirds of the vaginal barrel and elevation of the uterus and cervix
4. Elevation and flattening of the labia majora and extension of the labia minora
5. Erection of the nipples and increase in breast size
6. Appearance of the sex flush, a measles-type rash attributable to generalized vasocongestion, on the face and upper torso of some women
7. Development of some intracostal and abdominal muscle tension
8. Increase in heart rate and blood pressure

Plateau phase. With continued stimulation the following changes occur:

1. Elevation of the clitoral body and retraction under the clitoral hood
2. Engorgement of the labia minora with blood, causing them to become darker in color (nulliparous women, bright red; multiparous women, dark red)
3. Development of the orgasmic platform (a characteristic enlargement of the vaginal wall) at the outer one third of the vagina
4. Further engorgement of the nipples and areolas
5. Possible spreading of the sex flush to the abdomen, thighs, and back

Table 3-4. Four phases of female human sexual response*

Organs and body functions	Excitement phase	Plateau phase	Orgasmic phase	Resolution phase
Wall of vagina	Moistens (sweats)			Returns to normal state
Glans clitoris	Swells	Elevates		Returns to normal state
Clitoral shaft	Diameter increases			Returns to normal state
Areolas around nipples	Enlarge			Return to normal state
Nipples	Erect and increase in size			Slowly return to normal
Breasts	Increase in size			Slowly return to normal
Labia majora (outer lips)	Open	May swell		Return to normal state
Labia minora (inner lips)	Swell	Color darkens		Return to normal state
Cervix	Pulled up and back			Returns to normal
Uterus	Pulled up and back	More elevation, size increases	Contracts rhythmically	Begins to shrink
Inner two thirds of vagina	Balloons (vaginal barrel)	Balloons further		Returns to normal
Outer one third of vagina	Contracts (vaginal platform)	50% decrease in diameter	Spasm, then contraction	Relaxes after clitoris
Breathing rate		Increases	Reaches peak	Returns to normal
Pulse rate	Increases		Reaches peak	Returns to normal state
Blood pressure	Increases		Reaches peak	Returns to normal
Muscles	Tense		Contractions and spasms	Relax
Sex flush	May appear		Is most pronounced	Rapidly disappears
				No refractory period is necessary before another orgasm

*Courtesy Victor J. Des Marais, Jr., National Sex Forum, San Francisco, Calif.; based on data from Masters, W. H., and Johnson, V. E. 1966. Human sexual response. Boston, Little, Brown & Co.

6. Increased myotonia of facial, abdominal, and intracostal muscles with occasional voluntary contractions of the rectal sphincter
7. Some hyperventilation as well as further increase in heart rate and blood pressure
8. Rising of cervix, producing a tenting effect on the inner part of the vagina

Orgasmic phase. Orgasms have been divided into three subjective stages: (1) sensation of "suspension" followed immediately by a feeling of "intense sensual awareness, clitorally oriented but radiating upward in the pelvis," (2) "suffusion of warmth" primarily in the pelvis and moving to the rest of the body, and (3) pelvic throbbing in the vagina or lower pelvis (Masters and Johnson, 1966). Physiologically there are from three to fifteen rhythmic contractions of about 0.8-second duration in the orgasmic platform and the uterus; minor or no change in the breasts, labia majora, labia minora, or clitoris; generalized voluntary and involuntary myotonia; and hyperventilation and peaking of heart rate and blood pressure. Some women may be multiorgasmic (two or more orgasms without appreciable loss of plateau phase excitement levels).

Resolution phase. After orgasm the woman begins to return to the unexcited state. The loss of congestion and myotonia result in the following:

1. Loss of the orgasmic platform
2. Return of the labia majora and labia minora to their normal size and color
3. Disappearance of the sex flush
4. Reemergence of the clitoris from under the clitoral hood
5. Return of nipples and breasts to normal size
6. Lowering of respiration, heart rate, and blood pressure levels

Subjectively the response cycle may vary considerably depending on such factors as a woman's energy level, sexual interest, surrounding circumstances, and her level of health (Table 3-5). Although there are many possible response patterns, the three most common patterns are (1) mild or minor orgasms, (2) intense orgasms and (3) multiple orgasms.

Table 3-5. Female sexual response during and after pregnancy*

First trimester	Second trimester	Third trimester	After childbirth
Severe breast tenderness in some women if first pregnancy Intercourse and masturbation to orgasm may be harmful to "habitual aborters" (three or more abortions in first trimester)	During orgasm, rhythmic contractions of orgasmic platform felt but not observable Orgasmic platform more noticeable and grips penis tightly During orgasm, uterus only contracts once (for approximately 1 min) Resolution takes longer and is less complete Some have cramping in lower abdomen related to orgasm and some have backache after cramping Fetal heartbeat sometimes slows a little during orgasm Level of sexual interest and responsiveness increases Orgasmic contractions do not relieve sexual tension for long	Intercourse harmful if baby's head engages in cervix and cervix descends into axis of vagina late in final month Orgasm will not cause premature birth	Breast-feeding can stimulate mother to orgasm and cause release of oxytocin (a hormone that causes uterus to return to original position for renewed sexual intercourse) Most women may resume sexual intercourse 3 weeks after giving birth Mother's sexual responses during breast-feeding may cause guilt feelings Prohibition of intercourse can frustrate—should be resumed when agreeable to both partners

*Courtesy Victor J. Des Marais, Jr., National Sex Forum, San Francisco, Calif.; based on data from Masters, W. H., and Johnson, V. E. 1966. Human sexual response. Boston, Little, Brown & Co.

MALE REPRODUCTIVE SYSTEM

The *penis,* or external male reproductive organ, which enters the vagina during coitus, is composed of three cylindrical layers of erectile tissue, two lateral *corpora cavernosa* and a *corpus spongiosum,* which contains the urethra. These corpora terminate distally in the smooth, sensitive *glans penis,* which is the counterpart of the female clitoris. Skin and fascia loosely envelop the penis. The *prepuce* (foreskin), an extended fold of skin, covers the glans in uncircumcised males. With sexual arousal, neurocirculatory factors cause considerable increase in blood flow to the erectile tissue of the corpora, and enlargement and erection of the penis occur.

The urethra, which transverses the glans penis and extends the length of the male organ, is the *penile urethra.* The *membranous urethra,* a segment of urethra within the perineum, joins the prostatic or *posterior urethra* just below the vesicourethral junction (Figs. 3-16 and 3-17).

The *scrotum,* a wrinkled, pouchlike fullness of skin, muscles, and fascia, is divided internally by a septum, and each portion normally contains one *testis,* one *epididymis* and one *vas deferens* (seminal duct). The testes' two principal functions are spermatogenesis and hormone production. The epididymes are storage sites for maturing spermatozoa and produce a small part of the seminal fluid (semen). The vas deferens are the sperm conduits, contained within the fibrous spermatic cords, extending from the epididymes up through the inguinal canal to the ejaculatory ducts. These two short tubes pass through the prostate and terminate in the urethra. The sperm move from the epididymis through the vas deferens and ejaculatory duct and exit through the urethra. Thus in the male a single terminal system serves both the urinary and the genital tracts.

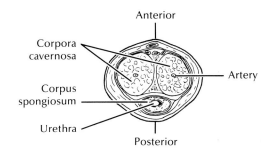

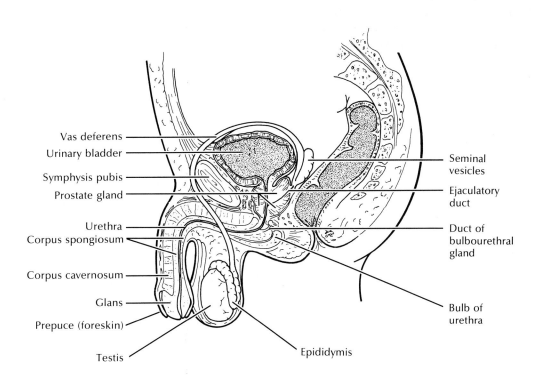

Fig. 3-16. Fascial planes of male lower genitourinary tract. *Top,* Transverse section of penis. *Bottom,* Relationship of bladder, prostate, seminal vesicles, penis, urethra, and scrotal contents. (Modified from Smith, D. R. 1975. General urology. Los Altos, Calif., Lange Medical Publications.)

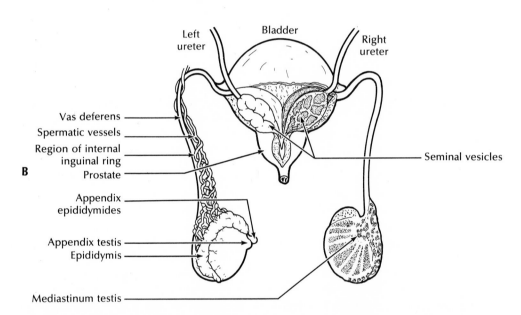

Lower tract

Vas deferens

Seminal vesicles
Prostate

Verumontanum
Urethra

A

Corpus
cavernosum

Testicle

Midtract
bladder

Vas deferens

Trigone

Left
ureter

Bladder

Right
ureter

Vas deferens

Spermatic vessels

Region of internal
inguinal ring
Prostate

B

Appendix
epididymides

Appendix testis
Epididymis

Mediastinum testis

Seminal vesicles

Fig. 3-17. A, Frontal section of lower male genitourinary tract. **B,** Enlarged frontal section
of lower male genitourinary tract. (Modified from Smith, D. R. 1975. General urology.
Los Altos, Calif., Lange Medical Publications.)

The *prostate* is a fibromuscular glandular organ that surrounds the posterior urethra. It occupies a space between the musculofascial urogenital diaphragm and the bladder. The prostate produces an alkaline mucoid vehicle for the spermatozoa released at the time of ejaculation. This alkaline substance comprises more than half the seminal fluid, protecting the sperm from the acid environment of the male urethra and female vagina and enhancing the sperm's motility. Aging often causes enlargement of the prostate, with consequent constriction of the urethra and resultant urinary retention. Sur-

gical removal of the prostate gland may be necessary to relieve this condition.

The *seminal vesicles* are pouchlike structures located along the lower posterior surface of the bladder, anterior to the rectum. These vesicles secrete nearly one third of the volume of the semen, as well as PG.

A pair of *bulbourethral* or *Cowper's glands* are located below the prostate, one at either side of the membranous urethra. They also secrete an alkaline fluid into the semen as a defense against urethral and vaginal acidity.

Testicular function

White fibrous tissue surrounds each testis and divides it into several lobules. Within each lobule are a long, narrow, coiled *seminiferous tubule* and clusters of *interstitial cells* (cells of Leydig). Sperm is produced by the seminiferous tubules and testosterone by the interstitial cells.

Normal male growth and the development of secondary sexual characteristics are largely dependent on androgenic hormones, principally testosterone. The normal adult male produces 4 to 9 mg/day of testosterone. Slight amounts of this and other androgens normally are secreted by the ovaries in women and by the adrenal cortex in men and women. Traces of estrogenic hormones are also produced either by the Leydig or closely associated Sertoli cells.

The anterior pituitary gland in males produces FSH and interstitial cell–stimulating hormone (ICSH) (LH in the female). FSH causes more rapid sperm production by the tubules, and ICSH stimulates the Leydig (interstitial) cells, increasing testosterone secretion. A feedback mechanism from the testes to the anterior pituitary aids in the control of steroid sex hormone secretion.

Spermatogenesis

Primitive sex cells (spermatogonia) are present in the seminiferous tubules of the male newborn. During puberty these cells undergo a maturing process called *spermatogenesis*. This process is a series of meiotic divisions in which one primary spermatocyte divides into two secondary spermatocytes, each of which redivides, ultimately producing four spermatids (sperm cells). Meiosis also reduces the number of chromosomes carried by each spermatid to 23, one of which is either an X or a Y chromosome. Spermatogenesis normally continues throughout a man's lifetime (Chapter 7).

Each mature spermatid has a large head, a smaller neck and midsection, and a long tail that makes it highly motile, particularly in a neutral or alkaline environment. This enables the sperm to move from the tubules into the epididymis where they are stored until ejaculation. At that time, 3 to 5 ml of semen containing secretions from the prostate, seminal vesicles, bulbourethral glands, and at least 125 million spermatozoa per milliliter are released. This fluid soon liquifies as a result of its fructose and enzyme content, and the spermatozoa are no longer clumped.

Many factors influence male fertility, the most important of which are the number of sperm released at ejaculation and their size and shape. Sperm capable of fertilization are uniform in size and shape. Millions of sperm seem to be required for fertilization to occur, even though a single sperm actually fertilizes the ovum. If the sperm count drops to less than 50 million/ml of semen, the male is unable to produce offspring.

PROSTAGLANDINS

Prostaglandins (PG) are oxygenated fatty acids now classified as hormones. They are produced in most organs of the body but most notably by the prostate and the endometrium. Therefore semen and menstrual blood are potent PG sources. PG are metabolized quickly by most tissues and are active in minute amounts in the cardiovascular, gastrointestinal, respiratory, urogenital, and nervous systems. They also exert a marked effect on metabolism, particularly on glycolysis. PG play an important role in many physiologic, pathologic, and pharmacologic reactions; $F_{2\alpha}$, E_1, and E_2 are most frequently used in reproductive medicine.

Role in reproductive functions

PG affect smooth muscle contractility and modulation of hormonal activity. Indirect evidence supports PG effects on the following events:

1. Ovulation
2. Sloughing of the endometrium
3. Cervical changes (e.g., affecting receptivity to sperm)
4. Tubal and uterine motility (and therefore sperm migration)
5. Onset of abortion, spontaneous and induced
6. Onset of labor, term and preterm

PG increase myometrial response to oxytocic stimulation, enhance uterine contractions, and cause cervical dilatation. PG may be one factor in the initiation and/or maintenance of labor. In addition, PG may be involved in the following pathologic states: male infertility (due to diminished amounts of PG), dysmenorrhea, hypertensive states, preeclampsia-eclampsia, and anaphylactic shock.

Uses in obstetrics

PG are utilized in obstetrics in various ways including the following:

1. Transabdominal injection into the amniotic sac to induce abortion during the midtrimester ($PGF_{2\alpha}$)
2. Continuous intravenous administration to induce abortion or delivery of anencephalic or dead fetuses and hydatidiform moles (PGE_2)
3. Intravenous or oral administration to induce or augment true labor

The most frequently encountered side effects of PG administration are nausea (severe) and diarrhea. For an extensive discussion of the place of PG in obstetrics, refer to Brenner (1975).

REFERENCES

Anthony, C. P., and Kolthoff, N. 1975. Textbook of anatomy and physiology (ed. 9). St. Louis, The C. V. Mosby Co.

Benson, R. 1974. Handbook of obstetrics and gynecology (ed. 5). Los Altos, Calif., Lange Medical Publications.

Brenner, W. E. 1975. The place of prostaglandins in modern obstetrics. In Aladjem, S. (ed.). Risks in the practice of modern obstetrics (ed. 2.). St. Louis, The C. V. Mosby Co.

Caldwell, W. E., and Malloy, H. C. 1933. Anatomic variations in the female pelvis and their effect in labor, with a suggested classification. Am. J. Obstet. Gynecol. **26:**479.

Hellman, L. M., and Pritchard, J. A. 1976. Williams obstetrics (ed. 15). New York, Appleton-Century-Crofts.

Masters, W. H., and Johnson, V. E. 1966. Human sexual response, Boston, Little, Brown & Co.

Willson, J. R., Beecham, C. T., and Carrington, E. R. 1975. Obstetrics and gynecology (ed. 5). St. Louis, The C. V. Mosby Co.

CHAPTER 4

Psychosocial components

Preparation for adult sexuality has as its genesis the sexual role development of the child. Although an individual's biologic sexuality is determined at conception by the chance combination of an ovum and a particular sperm, from that moment forward, intrauterine and extrauterine environmental influences play their part in the realization of each human's sexual potential.

This potential pervades the whole of an individual's life; it is more than a sum of isolated physical acts. It functions as a purposeful force in human nature and is observable in everyday life in endless variations. Sharing a sexual relationship with another individual may be viewed on a continuum with the need for intimacy at one end and the need for procreation at the other. It may find expression in the love of parent for child and child for parent, of friend for friend, of woman for man, and man for woman. It can be the source of pleasure or pain, fulfillment or deprivation, and sharing or exploitation. Recognition of the power of such drives has prompted each culture since recorded history to develop social codes, religious dogmas, or legal restraints that delineate the sex-role models and patterns to follow in sex-role identification.

SEX-ROLE IDENTIFICATION

We are born into a sexually oriented world and assume sexual roles. The roles reflect the basic pattern prescribed by society and are learned informally as a result through being part of a social group. The process of sex-role identity begins at an early age and continues as a series of developmental tasks throughout the life span. Newman and Newman (1975) have described four essential components of this process as follows:

Dimension	Sex-role outcome
Learning of the gender label	I am a "boy" I am a "girl"
Acquisition of the sex-role standards	Males are "independent," "achievement oriented," "assertive"

Dimension—cont'd	Sex-role outcome—cont'd
	Females are "interpersonal," "nurturant," and "docile"
Establishment of the sex preference	I like being a boy; I'd rather be a boy than a girl I like being a girl; I'd rather be a girl than a boy
Identification with the same-sex parent	I want to be like "Daddy" I want to be like "Mommy"*

In addition, Newman and Newman state:

The outcome of the process for an individual child depends greatly on the characteristics of his parents, the child's own capacities and preferences, and the cultural and familial values placed on one gender or the other. It should be obvious that a strong, positive identification with the appropriate sex, regardless of the specific standards associated with that sex, is essential for the development of self-esteem and for the elaboration of peer group relationships.*

Gender identity

The efforts to determine the emphasis to be placed on biologic versus environmental contributions to one's gender identity has generated much controversy and research. Although studies indicate there are some different biologic responses in male and female newborns and suggest differences in the infants' responses to the environment and readiness for varying learning experiences, other studies reveal the importance of gender labeling on the eventual acceptance of gender identity. Infants whose sex was indeterminant at birth accepted the sex role assigned by their parents and identified with that role (Maccoby, 1966). From the child's perspective, knowing oneself as either boy or girl begins before full realization of the implications of sexual identity. It is largely accomplished by means of acceptance of parental

*From Newman, B., and Newman, R. 1975. Development through life: a psychosocial approach. Homewood, Ill., The Dorsey Press, p. 111.

labeling, for example, ''be a good boy,'' ''that's my girl,'' and ''this is our big boy.'' By 2 or 3 years of age a child can correctly identify his or her own sex.

Sex role standards

Sex role standards refer to the various behaviors, attitudes, and attributes that differentiate the roles and are accepted as appropriate for the role. Even the 2-year-old is exposed to this conditioning by means of the clothing, kinds of toys, and activities selected by parents which reflect their expectations of sex role standards. It is not until the adolescent stage is reached that the socially and parentally defined sex role is openly questioned. In recent years the changes in the conceptualization of what constitutes male and female roles have had great impact on teenagers as they grope for standards consonant with their peer groups and parental expectations. Because sex role expectations serve as ideals and guides to endeavors, noncompliance with acceptable standards can be a potential source of conflict and crisis. In adolescence, the influence of parents is diluted by a growing acceptance of peer relationships. These begin with intense same-sex relationships and, for most individuals, gradually expand into heterosexual ones. They are accompanied by physical changes that both reinforce and raise doubts about the adequacy of an individual's femininity or masculinity. Even slight variations in body structure or functioning can prompt adolescents to question the adequacy of their sexuality. Their efforts to bolster self-esteem in this area can take many forms ranging from agonizing over hairstyles and racing cars, to drug ingestion, to becoming sexually active. This experimentation is a central process in the developmental task of moving from dependency to independency and eventual assumption of the adult role. Individuals emulate, modify, and adopt adult sex role standards just as they do those related to careers or life-styles. An important outcome of these turbulent adolescent years is the individual's ability to establish intimate relations with another person in terms of mutual empathy and give-and-take in regulating needs. Because of social emphasis on the nurturing nature of their sexual role, women are more ready to assume the emotional demands of intimacy. However, the threat of possible sexual assault makes women less receptive to physical intimacy than men. The challenges of intimacy for the man are in being able to express feelings openly and lovingly; for the woman, in being able to enjoy sex.

As individuals assume the prerogatives and responsibilities of adulthood, most conform overtly to the traditionally defined sexual roles. The adjectives used to describe a feminine individual are predominantly expressive of a mothering capacity, that is, ''gentle, loving, submissive, patient, warm, and concerned.'' These qualities suit an individual whose central reason for being is assumed to be the care and nurturing of the young and, by extension, any who need such care. Those adjectives used to describe the male, ''dominant, aggressive, impatient, objective, and ambitious,'' portray an individual capable of independent decisive actions, having qualities needed in the marketplace and the basis for career orientation.

In reality, individuals of both sexes possess these qualities in common, some personalities leaning more to the socially defined concept of either male or female and others with no clear demarcation of roles, labeled *androgenous personalities*. These individuals utilize those qualities most needed at the moment without feeling guilty over usurping another's role. A male nursing student made the following comment during a discussion of mothering:

It is not a case of one or the other, it is what the time calls forth. The most nurturing behavior of ''mothering,'' if you want to call it that, that I've ever seen was in Vietnam when a man was trying to get a wounded friend out of range of fire. He protected him, covering him with his own body, gave him his food and water. No ''mother'' could have shown more devotion.

Today's young adults are acting out their belief in such ideas. Fathers are involving themselves in the birth process and in parenting activities after the birth of the child, and mothers are planning for continuance of previous work patterns.

Gender preference

Gender preference implies not only a knowledge of one's gender and the appropriate sex role but also a liking for it. The process of developing gender preference involves three main elements: (1) success in the role, (2) liking the same-sex parent, and (3) reinforcement from family, ethnic group, and social institutions as to the value of the role (Newman and Newman, 1975). As with other attitudes, fluctuations in preference can and do occur as individuals are confronted with situations in which one sex role either enhances or hinders personal goals. Deep-seated sex preferences on the part of parents can affect initial parent-child relationships if the child is of the undesired sex. The mothering lag that results can last a day or a lifetime as the parents act to resolve or not resolve the conflicting emotions. Certain ethnic groups have welcoming rituals for one sex and not for the other. These seemingly innocuous societal and personal preferences eventually lead an individual to make value judgments about the worthiness of one's own sex and consequently increase or diminish self-esteem.

Identification with parent of same sex

This identification process results in the child internalizing the values, attitudes, and ideals of the parent of the same sex. The exact method by which the process of identification is accomplished is not yet known. However, the child does perceive actual physical and psychologic similarities and is told about similarities by others. The adoption of the same-sex parent's behaviors may be motivated by fear of loss of the love of the important person or by awareness of that individual's power to control rewards, for example, in a situation in which this parent's expectations of the child's sex role behaviors are not fulfilled. Behaviors of influential persons may also be imitated and eventually taken over and considered one's own. For the girl to forego identification with her father, she must love her mother sufficiently to form a positive identification with her. The boy needs to relinquish his early identification with his mother and form a strong commitment to his father.

HUMAN PURPOSE AND SEXUAL ACTS

Although reproduction, the central issue in this text, is almost entirely a function of human sexuality, the components of the reproductive process—intercourse, pregnancy, birth, and parenthood—may be viewed separately by an individual and endowed with a special meaning. The meaning attached to any one component can profoundly affect the outcome of the total process for woman, man, and child.

Intercourse

Intercourse or related acts may be used by both women and men in a positive sense to convey feelings of tenderness and love, to assuage loneliness by becoming part of another, as well as for the physical relief of sexual tension. In a negative sense, it can also be utilized as a means to belittle or demean a partner by refusal, by giving grudgingly of oneself, or by taking another by force (rape). Intercourse can also be a means of demonstrating to oneself or others one's sexual desirability or prowess. It can be used to conform to the acceptable behavior of one's peer group and thereby enhance social acceptance. It may form part of the experimenting process in movement toward the practice of adult sexuality. The increase in premarital intercourse (Table 4-1) as well as the more unconventional practices of sharing partners

Table 4-1. Adolescent sexual activity*

	Percent having sexual intercourse	
	Before age 16	**By age 19**
Males		
1948	39	72
1973	44	72
Females		
1953	3	20
1973	30	57

*From Newman, B., and Newman, P. 1975. Development through life. Homewood, Ill., The Dorsey Press, p. 195; based on data from Sorenson, R. C. 1973. Adolescent sexuality in contemporary America: personal values and sexual behavior, ages 13-19. New York, World Publishing Co.; Kinsey, A. C., Pomeroy, W. B., and Martin, C. E. 1948. Sexual behavior in the human male. Philadelphia, W. B. Saunders Co.; and Kinsey A. C., Pomeroy, W. B., Martin, C. E., and Gebhard, P. H. 1953. Sexual behavior in the human female. Philadelphia, W. B. Saunders Co.

would appear to testify to the complex meaning attached to a biologic act.

Obviously pregnancy can result from vaginal intercourse regardless of the purpose for either woman or man. Such pregnancies may or may not be wanted and may or may not be accepted. One aspect of functioning as an adult in a sexual sense is the assumption of responsibility for the consequences of the sexual act.

Pregnancy

The need for the physical intimacy that intercourse brings does not cease with pregnancy. Some women, because of the increased vascularity of the pelvic organs, are more sensitive to sexual arousal and experience greater satisfaction. For others, sexual desire is lessened, and anxiety for its loss may be a disquieting element in the adjustment to pregnancy. Both states are normal, and the frequency of intercourse may be increased or decreased without any lasting effect on sexual adjustment as long as the sexual partners can reach mutual understandings. This may be difficult if there has been little or no sharing of the meaning each ascribes to sexual acts.

Birth

The birth of the child is now viewed as a time of unifying the family unit. Partners are insisting on sharing this important event in their life together. For some, the sharing extends beyond the immediate participants and includes friends and community members.

Parenthood

Parenthood, beginning as it does with the excitement of birth, can also serve multiple human purposes. To some individuals, it acts as a life-fulfilling state, an opportunity to nurture and rear other human beings and eventually to let them go as the adults of the future. Children born to such individuals are wanted children, and their dependency needs are recognized and accepted. Although their successes bring much pleasure to their parents, their failures are also accepted, and love and support are forthcoming.

Other children, although wanted, are wanted primarily for the satisfaction of the parents. They will be expected to support the parents' self-concepts and need for love, acceptance, and success. Such expectations are unreal when applied to the young child. Disappointments and frustration ensue, and the child may become a victim of neglect or even assault.

Still other children are born as a result of the sexuality of their parents, but the resultant parenthood is neither planned nor desired. These children may experience both parental and material deprivation. Edwards (1973) contends that one of the greatest needs such children have are parents who have learned the art of "gentle socialization of children," of creating a sustaining environment peopled with interested, concerned, and loving adults.

Unlike other manifestations of human sexuality, parenthood can be both a biologic and psychologic entity or entirely psychologic. Once birth has occurred, the parent by substitution or adoptive parent can function in this socially as well as personally important role. These parents need the same preparation for and support in their role as do biologic parents.

NURSE'S ROLE

The nurse's background and education in the physical, social, and behavioral sciences as well as her training in counseling techniques make her an ideal member of the health team to counsel patients in an area as sensitive and highly charged as human sexuality. Her knowledge of social, emotional, and interactional factors provides the framework for patient-centered intervention.

The following factors influence the nurse's ability to deal with sexual content in clinical practice:

1. Her comfort with her own sexuality and her ability to accept the sexuality of her patients
2. Her awareness of her attitudes and prejudices about the wide range of sexual expression (masturba-

tion, premarital and extramarital sex, oral-genital contacts)
3. Her ability to discuss sexual issues in a language understood by the patient (anatomic language often confuses patients who have not heard these words before)

Sex counseling is a three-part process designed to determine what has gone on in the past, assess what is happening now, and plan an appropriate course of action for the future. Thus the process consists of history taking, problem identification, and problem solving.

History taking

The history provides the baseline data for identifying real or potential problems. In addition, it demonstrates to the patient that the nurse is interested in her sexual concerns.

The following areas are to be covered:

1. *Attitudes.* Attitudes concerning the range of acceptable sexual behavior are defined by such factors as culture, religion, family, and the peer group.

2. *Sexual self-concept.* How one sees oneself sexually influences how one relates to others.

3. *Marital relationships or alternative relationships.*

4. *Physical status.* One's state of health affects both sexual interest and the ability to perform sexually.

Problem identification

Physical, emotional, and interactional factors influence sexual expression. Physical changes or illness, gynecologic problems, and myths about sex have an impact on sexual behavior.

Problem solving

Having gathered data by history taking and identified the problems that have occurred, are occurring, or may occur, the nurse has a framework for counseling the patient or the couple. Counseling includes countering misinformation, providing reassurance of normality, and suggesting alternative behaviors. Chapter 11 offers more specific information relating to sexual counseling during pregnancy.

SEX EDUCATION AND COUNSELING FOR ADOLESCENTS

Special considerations are involved in sexual counseling for adolescents. Many teenagers are confused by the intensity of their sexual urges and find it difficult to describe their concerns. They are also striving for adult autonomy, which frequently makes relating to parents and other adults difficult. Finally, they are striving for and trying on adult sex roles without the maturity to comprehend the broad implications of responsible sexuality.

Children are often uncomfortable talking about sexual matters with their parents. Although parents and children who have an open, loving relationship can deal with factual information easily, they frequently have difficulty dealing with the affective component of sexuality. Adolescents usually discuss feelings about sex with peers—best friends and at pajama parties. Unfortunately much of peer learning is speckled with misinformation.

For these reasons, the nurse can serve as a valuable resource for the teenage girl. The nurse who can function as an accepting, knowledgeable adult can provide an opportunity for the teenager to clarify misinformation, as well as explore feelings about becoming a woman. An opportunity to discover that those feelings are normal and "yes, most women feel like that" can be reassuring.

Nurses must be careful to avoid the pitfall of trying to be a "pal" or "buddy." One nurse described her experience with a group of high school sophomores. She used a few street words thinking that the "hip" approach would make the girls more comfortable. Instead she learned of their embarrassment when "grown-ups" talk that way.

As human sexuality becomes recognized as a component of comprehensive health care, nurses and other health professionals are being asked to provide sex education in schools and churches and for other organized groups. Sex education and counseling is also provided for teenagers in adolescent clinics, pediatrician and other physicians' offices, and family planning clinics.

The nurse working with adolescents must approach sexual counseling from the perspectives of the adolescent's level of knowledge, affective resource, and sexual behaviors as indicated in the following outline:

A. Level of knowledge
 1. How body works—menstruation, ovulation, when one can get pregnant, how the pill works
 2. Sexual anatomy (many girls do not know what female genitals look like and do not know how many openings they have; e.g., the pregnant teenager who thought feces, urine, and babies came out of the same opening)
 3. Myths and misinformation about own body as well as relationships (e.g., the sexually excited boy will become ill if the girl deprives him of relief of sexual tension through intercourse)

B. Affective response
 1. Body image—inability to accept imperfection, anxieties regarding secondary sex characteristics (e.g., breasts too big or too little; too much or not enough pubic hair)
 2. Guilt associated with masturbation (no longer fears acquiring warts but it is still seen as a sign of weakness and undesirable)
 3. Homosexual fears (remembers some earlier event of playing "doctor," single or few same-sex experiences, or even homosexual fantasy and sees oneself as being homosexual)
 4. Normalcy of feelings (wonders if feelings are normal, i.e., how do women feel?)

C. Sexual behavior
 1. Dating—many questions and uncertainties (e.g., How will a boy know I like him? On the first kiss, what do I do with nose, braces, lips, glasses and do I squeeze or let arms rest on shoulder? Do I have to go all the way to be popular?)
 2. Shy and withdrawn (not popular and what that means)
 3. Provocative but "don't touch" (dress and actions are a "come on")
 4. Promiscuity

It is important for the counselor not to assume that because a girl seems sophisticated in one of these areas that she is sophisticated in all of them as illustrated by the pregnant teenager mentioned in the list.

The goal of the counselor is to help the adolescent move toward responsible sexuality. The process includes discussion of ideas, feelings, and desires; openness about sexuality (he made me do it; I'll never do it again; I got carried away this time); and what responsible sexuality entails.

REFERENCES

Adams, M. 1971. The single woman in today's society: a reappraisal. Am. J. Orthopsychiatry **41:**776.

American Association of Sex Educators and Counselors. 1973. The professional training of sex counselors. Washington, D.C., The Association.

Bardwick, J. 1971. The psychology of women. New York, Harper & Row, Publishers.

Bradley, R. A. 1965. Husband coached childbirth. New York, Harper & Row, Publishers.

Brown, F. 1972. Sexual problems of the adolescent girl. Pediatr. Clin. North Am. **19:**759.

Browning, M., and Lewis, E. 1973. Human sexuality: nursing implications. New York, The American Journal of Nursing Co.

Caplan, G. 1964. Psychological aspects of pregnancy. In

Lief, N. (ed.) The psychological basis of medical practice. New York, Harper & Row, Publishers.

Clark, A. L., and Hale, P. W. 1974. Sex during and after pregnancy. Am. J. Nurs. **73:**1430.

Claytor, S. B. 1974. Coitus during pregnancy. Med. Asp. Hum. Sex. **8:**39, July.

Colman, A. D., and Colman, L. 1973. Pregnancy: the psychological experience. New York, The Seabury Press.

Cronenwett, L., and Newmark, L. 1974. Fathers' responses to childbirth. Nurs. Res. **23:**210, May-June.

Derthickh, N. 1974. Sexuality in pregnancy and the puerperium. Birth Fam. J. **4:**5, Fall.

Deutsch, H. 1945. The psychology of women (vol. 2). New York, Bantam Books, Inc.

Edwards, M. 1973. Communications: dimensions in childbirth education. Pacific Grove, Calif., M. Edwards.

Elder, M. S. 1970. Nurse counseling on sexuality—an unmet challenge. Nurs. Outlook **18:**38.

Falicou, C. J. 1973. Sexual adjustment during first pregnancy and post partum. Am. J. Obstet. Gynecol. **117:**991.

Fattich, A., Leach, W., and Wilkinson, C. 1973. Fatal air embolism in pregnancy resulting from orogenital sex play. Forensic Sci. **2:**247, May.

Gadpaille, W. J. 1970. Adolescent sexuality and the struggle over authority. J. School Health **40:**479.

Glenc, F. 1972. Some sex problems in pregnancy. Wiad. Lek. **26:**145.

Goldstein, B. 1976. Human sexuality. New York, McGraw-Hill Book Co.

Goodlin, R. C., Keller, D. W., and Raffin, M. 1971. Orgasm during late pregnancy—possible deleterious effects. Obstet. Gynecol. **38:**916.

Guttmacher, A. F. 1962. Pregnancy and birth. New York, New American Library, Inc.

Hazell, L. D. 1976. Commonsense childbirth. Berkeley, Windhover Press.

Human sexuality feature section. 1976. Am. J. Mat. Child Nurs. **1:**165.

Jessner, L., Weigert, E., and Foy, J. L. 1970. The development of parental attitudes during pregnancy. In Anthony, E. J., and Benedek, T. (ed.). Parenthood: its psychology and psychopathology. Boston, Little, Brown & Co.

Lang, R. 1972. Birth book. Palo Alto, Calif., Genesis Press.

Maccoby, E. E. (ed.). 1966. The development of sex differences. Stanford, Calif., Stanford University Press.

Maccoby, E. E., and Jacklin, C. 1974. The psychology of sex differences. Stanford, Calif., Stanford University Press.

Masters, W. H., and Johnson, V. E. 1966. Human sexual response. Boston, Little, Brown & Co.

Mead, M. 1949. Male and female. New York, William Morrow Co.

Mouey, J., and Ehrhardt, A. A. 1972. Man and woman, boy and girl: the differentiation and demorphism of gender identity from conception to maturity. Baltimore, The Johns Hopkins University Press.

Newman, B., and Newman, R. 1975. Development through life: a psychosocial approach. Homewood, Ill., The Dorsey Press.

Rainwater, L. 1964. And the poor have children. J. Mar. Fam. **26:**457.

The Sex Information and Education Council of the United States. 1967. Sexual relations during pregnancy and the post-delivery period (study guide No. 6). New York, SIECUS Publications.

Solberg, D. A., Butler, J., and Wagner, N. M. 1973. Sexual behavior in pregnancy. N. Engl. J. Med. **288:**1098, 1973.

Vincent, C. E. 1968. Human sexuality in medical education and practice. Springfield, Ill., Charles C Thomas, Publisher.

Witters, W., and Witters, P. 1975. Drugs and sex. New York, Macmillan, Inc.

Wood, N. F. 1975. Human sexuality in health and illness. St. Louis, The C. V. Mosby Co.

Wood, N. F. 1973. Sexual activity during pregnancy. N. Engl. J. Med. **289:**379.

Wood, N. F. 1972. Uterine tension and fetal heart rate during maternal orgasm. Obstet. Gynecol. **39:**125.

UNIT THREE

Family planning

CHAPTER 5

Infertility

The inability to conceive and bear a child comes as a tragedy to a surprising number of otherwise healthy adults. Patients requesting assistance for problems of infertility have already made the decision related to wanting a child. The desire to experience pregnancy and birth, to be a parent, and to express love through the care and nurturing of another represent to them the normal growth of adult sexuality. Also the idea that fertility is a necessary component of mature and adequate sexuality is common throughout the world. Pressures from family or peers by means of overtly or covertly expressed sentiments that it is natural to want babies or that only selfishness is the motivating factor in childlessness can bring much unhappiness to couples. Many patients appear anxious and tense as they relate their problems and are sensitive to real or imagined criticisms of their sexual ability or of their need for a child in this overpopulated world. They look for readily expressed acceptance from the physician and nurse of their need for a child, as well as their infertility problem.

Infertility is the inability to conceive after at least 1 year of adequate exposure to the possibility of pregnancy. Generally, the causes of infertility are multiple, but relatively more female abnormalities than male abnormalities probably are responsible for infertility in the population at large. Approximately 15% of all unions are barren. Treatment is successful in the majority of cases, but when correction is impossible, the individual is sterile.

MALE INFERTILITY

Male reproductive failure may be due to many of the difficulties that also affect women, such as nutritional, endocrine, and psychologic disorders. In addition, male infertility may be due to one or more of the following specific causes:

1. *Coital difficulties.* Chordee or marked obesity may make penile intromission difficult or impossible.

2. *Spermatozoal abnormalities.* These include a small ejaculatory volume (less than 3.4 ml), a low sperm count (less than 50 million/ml), increased viscosity, poor initial or reduced sustained motility of the spermatozoa, and more than 30% abnormal sperm forms.

3. *Testicular abnormalities.* These include agenesis or dysgenesis of the testes, cryptorchidism, poor maturation of the spermatozoa because of endocrine disorder such as hypopituitarism or Klinefelter's syndrome; previous orchitis after mumps or tuberculosis; and physical injury perhaps due to direct trauma, irradiation, or increased temperature for prolonged periods.

4. *Abnormalities of the penis or urethra.* These include hypospadias or urethral stricture.

5. *Prostate and seminal vesicle abnormalities.* Chronic prostatitis or seminal vesiculitis may alter the liquid that contains the spermatozoa. In addition, infection may reduce the number or quality of the sperm.

6. *Abnormalities of the epididymis and vas deferens.* These conduits are reservoirs and transport the sperm specimen. Inflammation or closure may reduce the quantity or viability of the specimen.

7. *Severe nutritional deficiencies.*

A careful history and complete physical examination, with special reference to physical maturation, infection, injuries, and operations on or near the genitourinary tract, should be carried out. A sperm analysis on a specimen obtained by masturbation or a complete catch specimen available during intercourse should be done at least twice to determine whether oligospermia or other abnormalities are likely.

Patients with aspermia or oligospermia should be studied endocrinologically for pituitary, thyroid, adrenal, or testicular aberrations. With maldevelopment or anomalous genitals a buccal smear and perhaps a chromosomal study should be carried out to identify genetic disorders such as Klinefelter's syndrome. Testicular biopsy, prostatic treatment, or other procedures may be necessary.

Medical therapy for male infertility has been disappointing, particularly when pituitary, adrenal, or testicular diseases are discovered. It has been reported that about two thirds of reversal operations after vasectomy should be successful. However, the resultant pregnancies number about 30%, inasmuch as the successful results depend on the skill of the surgeon as well as the availability of the procedures. Voluntary sterilization must be considered a method for terminating reproductive ability. If, after thorough study and completion of logical therapy, pregnancy does not occur after a year, adoption or artificial insemination, perhaps with a donor's specimen, should be considered.

Assuming normal female fertility, artificial insemination at or about the time of ovulation has resulted in pregnancy in as many as 70% of cases. Approximately 1 ml of fresh donor sperm, obtained by masturbation from a healthy man, is introduced into the vagina. In such a program, one to four inseminations over one to four cycles have been required.

If thawed, liquid nitrogen–frozen sperm is used, the pregnancy rate is slightly less. However, even after 10 years' storage using glycerol, the best cryoprotective substance, there have been no proved unfavorable genetic consequences.

In either instance, the spontaneous abortion rate is approximately the same as in a control population, and no increase in maternal or perinatal complications is likely.

It is termed *homologous insemination* if the husband's semen is used and *heterologous insemination* if the semen of a donor other than the husband is used. Insemination with the husband's semen presents no legal problems, but heterologous insemination involves many legal, ethical, and emotional aspects. The decision should only be made after being thoroughly thought out and discussed. The implications for the long-term welfare of the child as well as the parents must be considered (Chapter 39).

FEMALE INFERTILITY

Failure to conceive may be the result of incorrect timing. Ovulation occurs on the fourteenth day (between the twelfth and sixteenth day) in most cycles. Hence unless unprotected intercourse occurs within 12 to 24 hours of extrusion of the ovum, pregnancy may not take place.

The basic factors pertaining to successful pregnancy are as follows: (1) a normal ovum must be released from a mature ovarian follicle; (2) the ovum must enter the fallopian tube promptly after its extrusion; (3) spermatozoa must have migrated into the fallopian tube where fertilization of the ovum normally occurs; (4) a fertilized ovum must find its way down the tube into the endometrial cavity to implant 7 to 10 days after ovulation; and (5) normal segmentation, maturation, and development of the embryo and fetus must occur until viability has been reached and delivery accomplished.

The following causes of infertility are recognized:

1. *Nutritional factors.* A seriously faulty diet may be responsible for infertility.

2. *Endocrine abnormalities.* Pituitary, thyroid, or adrenal disorders of either hyperfunction or hypofunction can cause infertility.

3. *Vaginal disorders.* Abnormalities of development such as absence or stenosis of the vagina or imperforate hymen may prevent vaginal penetration. Vaginitis of any type, if severe, may destroy or inactivate spermatozoa.

4. *Cervical abnormalities.* Cervicitis is extremely noxious to spermatozoa. Cervical tumors such as polyps may obstruct the canal or, because of associated infection and discharge, may block the transit of spermatozoa through the cervix.

5. *Uterine anomalies.* Uterine maldevelopment such as hypoplasia may prevent the implantation or adequate development of the fertilized ovum. Uterine neoplasms, particularly polyps and myomas, may injure the uterus, reduce the blood supply, or compromise the fertilized ovum so that proper development to viability is impossible.

6. *Tubal disorders.* Tubal obstruction, generally the result of infection, may block the tube to the ovum or spermatozoa. External pressure or distortion due to perisalpingial adhesions, as with endometriosis, may obstruct the tube.

7. *Ovarian abnormalities.* Congenital anomalies such as ovarian dysgenesis or agenesis may be associated with few or absent ova. Infections, tumors, or endometriosis may disturb, disrupt, or destroy ovarian function.

8. *Emotional problems.* Severe psychoneurosis or psychosis may be responsible for anovulatory cycles, frequently associated with amenorrhea or oligomenorrhea.

9. *Coital factors.* Lubricants, feminine hygiene preparations, or douches, which increase vaginal acidity, may inactivate or destroy spermatozoa.

10. *Chronic disease states.*

11. *Immunologic reactions to sperm.*

The diagnosis of female infertility requires a careful history with special reference to growth, development, and general health, as well as specific illnesses that might compromise fertility (e.g., gonorrhea, tuberculosis). A careful evaluation of the menstrual history, the occurrence of pregnancy in the past, and the outcome may be helpful. Consideration of the patient's emotional makeup, life-style, and habits, as well as general hygiene, are important. Previous abdominal or vaginal surgery should be recorded, and the reason as well as the outcome of the operations may be of significance. The type of contraception, its duration, and problems in addi-

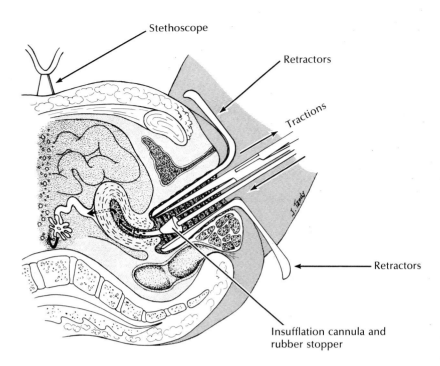

Stethoscope

Retractors

Tractions

Retractors

Insufflation cannula and
rubber stopper

Fig. 5-1. Tubal insufflation: sagittal section. Note that gas flows through intrauterine cannula and escapes through tubes. Cervix is closed by rubber stopper. Resistance to flow is measured by back pressure on mercury gauge (see Fig. 5-6 for results). Attendant listens with stethoscope on abdomen.

tion to the frequency of coitus should be recorded. The family history may be revealing particularly when congenital abnormalities, infertility, and loss of early pregnancies are reported.

A thorough physical examination may disclose medical disorders such as goiter or other endocrine problems causative of infertility. The gynecologic examination must be meticulous for abnormalities.

Laboratory studies should include routine blood and urinalysis, evaluation of the cervical mucus for infection, sperm penetration (Huhner test), and tubal insufflation (Rubin's test) (Fig. 5-1), and laboratory tests for endocrine or other dysfunction may be indicated during the course of study. The patient should be required to take and record her basal body temperature (BBT) each morning to establish whether ovulation occurs and on what day of the cycle (Figs. 5-2 and 5-3).

Treatment of female infertility may be medical or surgical. Medical treatment may relate to nutritional deficiencies, psychologic problems, or medical disorders due to infection or abnormal function.

Surgical treatment of the infertile patient may involve operative correction of developmental anomalies, separation of adhesions, removal of neoplasms, or destruction of endometriosis.

Special therapy may be required for induction of ovulation. Oral clomiphene citrate (Clomid) or intramuscular human menopausal gonadotropin (HMG) (Pergonal) are so-called fertility drugs that often induce ovulation in anovulatory patients.

Special surgical treatment may involve wedge resection of polycystic ovaries in Stein-Leventhal syndrome, excision or fulguration to destroy endometriosis, tubolysis for adhesions, or removal of a pelvic tumor. Reanastomosis of the tubes after tubal sterilization is usually a successful procedure, and pregnancy often ensues (Scheuker and others, 1972; Umezaki and others, 1974). In contrast, tubal surgery to correct obstruction or closure after salpingitis may result in a patent tube, but pregnancy is uncommon because the original inflammatory process often prevents capacitation of spermatozoa, the addition of a substance or substances by the tubal epithelium that makes fertilization of the ovum possible.

The prognosis for the infertile woman is generally good provided serious genital or inflammatory disorders are not identified. Most patients present numerous so-called minor problems that, although compounded, may be relatively easy to correct (e.g., chronic cervicitis, hypothyroidism).

Prolonged treatment of infertility generally is unne-

Text continued on p. 63.

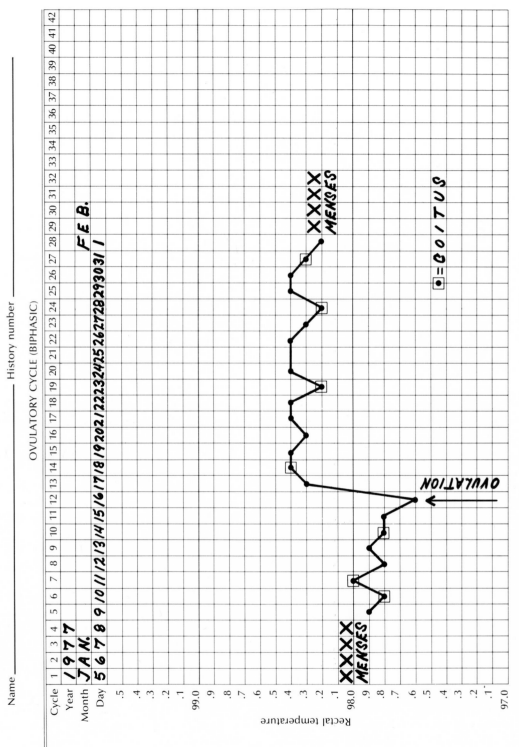

Fig. 5-2. A, Basal temperature record shows drop and sharp rise at time of ovulation. Biphasic curve is indicative of ovulatory cycle.

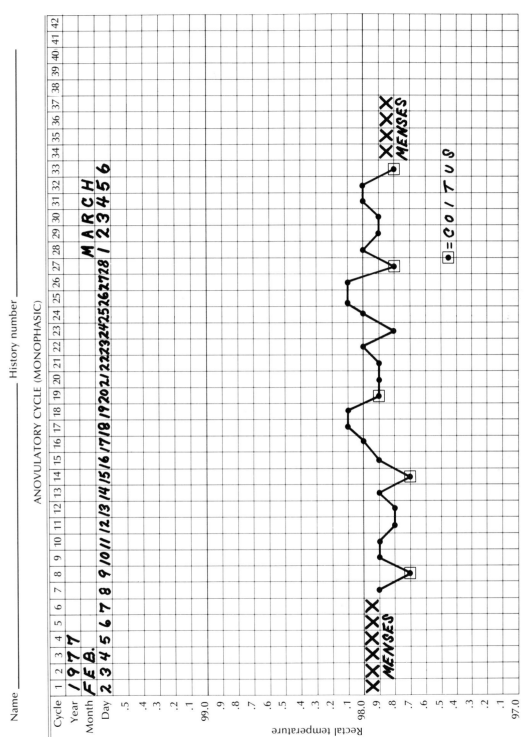

Fig. 5-2, cont'd. **B,** Monophasic (flat) curve is indicative of anovulatory cycle.

B

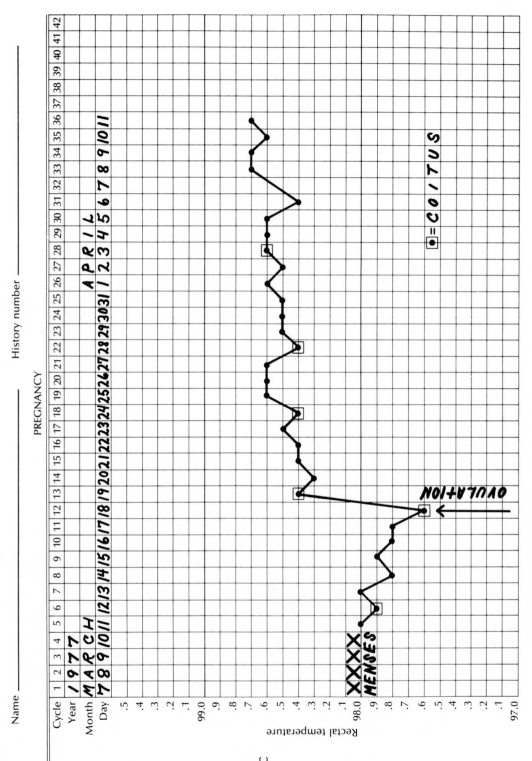

Fig. 5-2, cont'd. **C,** Persistent elevation and amenorrhea are suggestive of pregnancy.

cessary. If successful therapy has not been achieved after a year, for example, adoption should be considered.

PLAN OF CARE

The desired objectives for care are success in conceiving, maintaining a pregnancy, and becoming a parent or, if success in conceiving is not possible, acceptance of alternate routes to parenthood. Nurses are frequently asked questions concerning infertility problems. A description of the basic study for infertility is helpful. The workup requires three to four sessions and includes the following procedures.

FIRST SESSION

1. A complete history is taken with emphasis on menstrual history, sexual history including frequency of coitus and use of vaginal lubricants or douches, illnesses and surgical operations, pelvic infections, and use of drugs.

2. The nurse assists with the general physical and pelvic examination, including cervical and vaginal cytology and microscopic examination of the cervical mucus and vaginal secretions.

3. Instructions are given as to the use of the BBT chart (Figs. 5-2 and 5-3).

4. Written instructions are provided for the man regarding collection of semen samples. The semen specimen should be collected after a 5-day period of abstinence from intercourse by ejaculation into a clean, wide-mouthed glass or porcelain jar after coitus interrputus or masturbation. For Roman Catholic couples a plastic condom with perforations may be used. Rubber condoms should not be used, since the rubber or powder may be spermicidal. The specimen should be kept at room temperature and brought to the laboratory within an hour of emission.

5. The rationale for laboratory procedures (e.g., blood count, urinalysis) is discussed.

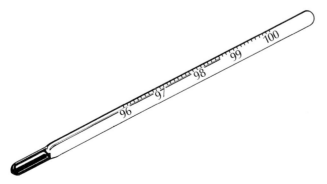

Fig. 5-3. Special thermometer for recording BBT, marked in tenths to enable patient to read more easily.

6. The woman is asked to return near the conclusion of her next menstrual period.

SECOND SESSION

1. If the semen analysis indicates probable male fertility, Rubin's test is performed to ascertain tubal patency (Figs. 5-1, 5-4, and 5-5). After voiding, the woman assumes the lithotomy position as for a pelvic examination. The pelvic area is cleansed and a vaginal speculum inserted. The vaginal lining and cervix are swabbed, and a special cannula is introduced through the cervix into the uterine cavity. A controlled amount of carbon dioxide is administered under pressure. After an initial rise to between 60 to 150 mm Hg, the pressure falls as the gas flows through the fallopian tubes into the abdomen (Figs. 5-5 to 5-7). This can be heard by auscultation. When the woman sits up, the free carbon dioxide rises in the abdominal cavity and, by irritation of the sub-

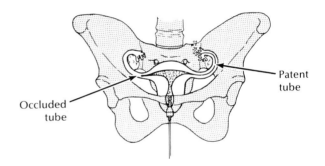

Fig. 5-4. Rubin's test (tubal insufflation).

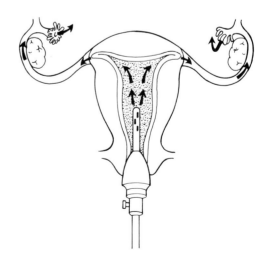

Fig. 5-5. Rubin's test. Enlarged section showing front views and gas escaping through tubes into abdominal cavity.

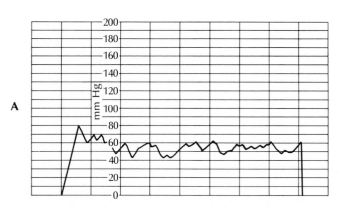

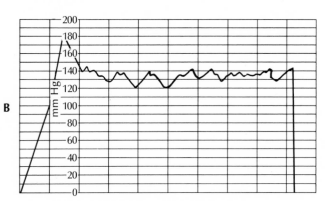

Fig. 5-6. Kymographic record of tubal insufflation (Rubin's test): normal results. **A,** Normal. Gas passes through tube into abdominal cavity demonstrating patency. **B,** High normal. Gas passes through tube into abdominal cavity demonstrating patency.

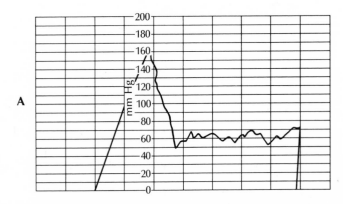

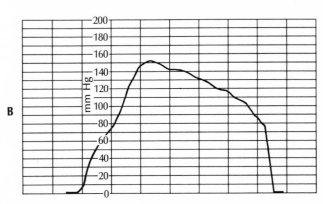

Fig. 5-7. Kymographic record of tubal insufflation (Rubin's test): abnormal results. **A,** Spasm of tube. **B,** Partial tubal stenosis.

diaphragmatic area, results in transient referred pain in the shoulder. This pain should be described prior to the test so as to allay apprehension.

2. The patient is asked to return at her estimated time of ovulation and have coitus 4 to 18 hours prior to the clinical session.

THIRD SESSION

1. The pelvic examination is repeated. At this time the cervical mucus is examined. If ovulation is imminent, the mucus will have the viscosity and clarity of fresh egg white, and a drop allowed to dry on a slide at room temperature forms a fernlike pattern.

2. A microscopic examination of the mucus should reveal mobile spermatozoa.

3. If no definite sterility factors are found to date, she is asked to return 6 to 8 days after ovulation (Fig. 5-2).

FOURTH SESSION

1. The pelvic examination is repeated, and endometrial biopsies are obtained from the uterine fundus by use of a small suction curette and submitted to the gynecologic pathologist for evaluation of the degree of progestational development.

2. Depending on the findings, additional tests or procedures may be necessary. Prompt reporting of the tests is a part of the overall care. The patient and nurse will need to set up times for these contacts.

REFERENCES

Brandl, E., and Mettler, L. 1974. Timing of ovulation in sterility patients. Int. J. Fertil. **19:**13.

Brenner, W. E. 1975. The place of prostaglandins in modern obstetrics. In Aladjem, S. (ed.). Risks in the practice of modern obstetrics (ed. 2). St. Louis, The C. V. Mosby Co.

MacNaughton, M. C. 1973. Treatment of female infertility. Clin. Endocrinol. **2:**545.

Roeoley, M. J., and Heller, C. G. 1972. The testosterone rebound phenomenon in the treatment of male infertility. Fertil. Steril. **23:**498.

Scheuker, J. G., and others. 1972. Fertility after tubal surgery. Surg. Gynecol. Obstet. **135:**74.

Umezaki, C., Katayama, K., and Jones, H. W., Jr. 1974. Pregnancy rates after reconstructive surgery on the fallopian tubes. Obstet. Gynecol. **43:**418.

CHAPTER 6

Contraception

Contraception is the voluntary prevention of pregnancy; it has both individual and social implications. It has been established that more than 90% of couples in the United States have used or intend to use some method of birth control. Family planning is accepted in principle by all religions, but the Roman Catholic Church insists that this be achieved by periodic abstinence alone. The availability of reliable and safe techniques for controlling fertility has meant that parenthood with its tasks and responsibilities, as well as its pleasures, can be willingly assumed by adults who wish to do so. Recent advances in the physiologic safety of prenatal, perinatal, and postnatal existence can now be combined with the psychologic safety of being a wanted child.

Spacing of children is important not only to promote the health of the mother but also that of her progeny. Quality of the offspring rather than quantity is now emphasized. Moreover, to control excessive world population, voluntary limitation of family size has become important.

There is a varied selection of contraceptive techniques in North America. The ideal contraceptive should be safe, easily available, economical, acceptable, simple to use, and promptly reversible. Although no means or method may ever achieve all these objectives, impressive recent progress has been made.

METHODS

Contraception employs one or more of the following methods (Fig. 6-1):

- Biologic periodic abstinence—the "rhythm" method
- Coitus interruptus—withdrawal prior to ejaculation
- Hormonal—estrogen and/or progestogen preparations
- Chemical—spermicidal creams, gels, suppositories
- Mechanical—condoms, sheaths, cervical uterine occlusion by caps or diaphragms, intrauterine contraceptive devices
- Surgical—therapeutic abortion, male and female sterilization

Still under investigation are immunization methods, better procedures to identify ovulation, and hormonal suppression of spermatogenesis for contraception.

Biologic periodic abstinence

Abstinence, although totally effective, is unphysiologic and by and large unacceptable for pregnancy control. Even periodic abstinence, or the "rhythm method," (during the likely period of ovulation), is impractical for the following reasons: it is useless postnatally until regular cycles are established; it depends on the regularity of the woman's menstrual cycles; and it necessitates the cooperation of both the woman and her partner. Nevertheless, the occurrence of ovulation often can be identified by the BBT so that the postovulatory period may in fact be "safe" so far as the onset of pregnancy is concerned. The woman must *accurately* obtain and record her temperature (preferably the rectal reading) immediately on awakening prior to any activity (Figs. 5-2 and 5-3). The BBT during the menses and for approximately 5 to 7 days thereafter usually varies from 97° to 97.8° F. If ovulation fails to occur, this irregular pattern continues throughout the month. However, infection, fatigue, or anxiety may cause temperature fluctuations, altering the expected pattern. About 1 to 1½ days prior to ovulation the temperature may drop 0.2° to 0.3° and then rise 0.7° to 0.8° 1 to 2 days after ovulation, whereupon the temperature plateaus until the day before menstruation when it drops to the low levels recorded during the previous period. The fertile period surrounding ovulation extends from 1 to 2 days before ovulation to 2 days after. Assuming regularity (unlikely for many women), the preovulatory and postovulatory safe periods can be estimated.

Hormonal therapy

Hormonal therapy consists of suppression of ovulation by steroid sex hormones.

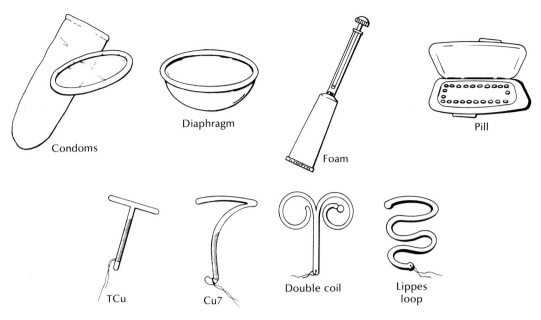

Fig. 6-1. Methods of contraception.

Single hormone therapy. Moderate to large daily doses of estrogen for 3 weeks each month will prevent ovulation by suppressing FSH and LH. Nausea may be a daily problem during treatment, however, and after several months of such therapy, irregular periods and metrorrhagia almost always develop. To eliminate unpleasant side effects and to ensure regular average periods, both an estrogen and a progestogen in sequence or in combination are required. With the availability of synthetic potent progestational agents such as 19-nortestosterone and 17-hydroxyprogesterone, dependable oral contraception is now assured.

Pregnancy protection may be afforded by continuous, small daily doses of progestogen alone, for example, norethindrone (Micronor, Nor-Q-D), without interruption during menstruation. Ovulation continues to occur, but pregnancy is avoided because the cervical mucus becomes thick and impervious to sperm migration. Moreover, the endometrium never achieves normal maturation. Although this medication is not as effective as either the traditional or sequential pill, women who do not tolerate continued estrogen therapy usually can take this preparation. Occasionally breakthrough bleeding, signifying insufficient endogenous estrogen, may necessitate discontinuation of this medication.

Combined hormone therapy. The "pill," originally a combination of a synthetic estrogen, mestranol, and a synthetic progestogen, norethyinodrel (Enovid), is still a popular, successful product. Many subsequent combinations, some of considerably lower dosage (e.g., Loestrin 1/20), now are available. A dosage program common to all these products requires the administration of one tablet daily, beginning on the fifth day, counting from the first day of the period, and continuing for 20 or 21 days. Generally, bleeding begins 1 to 4 days after the last tablet. Resumption of the same treatment program begins again on the fifth day of the cycle. Some pharmaceutical companies have added seven "blanks," lactose or ferrous sulfate tablets, to follow the last combination tablet so that the woman can take one tablet every day, still maintaining the original monthly dosage program to ensure regular average periods.

These drugs prevent conception in several ways. They block the pituitary release of LH, thus preventing ovulation. They maintain the thickness of the cervical secretions, preventing the passage of sperm. In addition, they modify the endometrial maturation, making unlikely implantation of a fertilized ovum. The traditional pill affords the best pregnancy protection of any contraceptive product or method. In addition, oral contraceptives can be used in the treatment of certain clinical problems (Table 6-1).

Contraindications to oral contraceptives include the following:

- Strong family history of stroke
- Severe migraine or convulsive disorder
- Cerebral arterial insufficiency

Table 6-1. When pills can go beyond contraception*

Clinical problem	Type of pill		Comments
	Combined	Sequential	
Acne	+	+ + + +	Avoid androgenic progestogens or use lowest possible dose
Breast pain or cysts	+	+ + +	This condition may improve spontaneously with time; reduce dosage of estrogen and progestogen, aspirate cysts, and order yearly mammography
Chloasma	+ + +	0	The presumptive cause is estrogen excess; use lowest estrogen dose; avoid sun
Dysmenorrhea	0	+ + +	Give maximum estrogen dose
Endometriosis	0	+ + + +	Treat infertility; surgery is best for future pregnancies; inhibition therapy is a good alternative
Lactation	0	0	Avoid pills entirely
Menorrhagia	+ + + +	+	Exclude abnormality; treat for anemia and administer 19-Norsteroids
Migraine	+	+	Estrogen deprivation may be the cause; give added low-dose estrogen during 7-day "rest period" if migraine occurs only at that time each month
Moniliasis	0	+ + +	Poor male hygiene or female diabetes may be a cause; give appropriate antibiotics; order douches and minimal local treatment
Oligomenorrhea	0	+ + +	Make full clinical assessment to rule out pathologic causes
Ovarian pain, cysts, or bleeding	0	+ + +	Inhibit gonadotrophins, and functional cysts should disappear
Polycystic ovary	+ + +	+	Avoid androgenic steroids; adrenal inhibition with dexamethasone may be required
Polymenorrhea	0	+ + +	Limit treatment cycles to 6 months
Premenstrual tension	+ +	+ + +	Recommend low salt, diuretics, and sedation as individually indicated

0 = not preferred; + = fair; + + = moderate; + + + = good; + + + + = excellent.
*From Nursing Update. 1975. **6:**12, May.

- Borderline cardiac decompensation
- Recent hepatitis or hepatic insufficiency
- Severe diabetes mellitus
- Severe renal disease
- Endometrial or breast carcinoma
- Thromboembolic disease or sickle cell disease
- Excessive smoking (more than 2 packs per day)

The patient must be advised concerning possible detrimental effects of the drug, which include blindness and death.

Certain side effects of anovulatory drugs are attributable to estrogen or progestogen (or both) as follows:

1. Estrogen excess—nausea, vomiting, fluid retention, headache, mastodynia, hypermenorrhea
2. Estrogen deficiency—vaginal dryness, vaginitis, dyspareunia, breakthrough bleeding
3. Progestogen excess—tissue weight gain, depression, acne, reduced libido, short or scanty menses
4. Progestogen deficiency—prolonged, heavy menses

Individualization and proper balance of the dosage of the two hormones for each patient is essential (Table 6-2). If intolerance or other problems develop, a different drug content, a different product, or another method of contraception may be required.

Table 6-2. The what, when, and why of currently available oral contraceptives*

Contraceptive	Composition (per pill)	Schedule	Possible advantages
Combinations			
Demulen-21†	Ethynodiol diacetate, 1 mg	1 pill qd for 21 days begin-	Low estrogen
	Ethinyl estradiol, 0.05 mg	ning on day 5 of cycle	
Enovid	Norethynodrel, 5 mg	1 pill qd for 20 days begin-	Anabolic effect
	Mestranol, 0.075 mg	ning on day 5 of cycle	
Enovid-E	Norethynodrel, 2.5 mg	1 pill qd for 20 days	Good cycle control
Enovid-E21	Mestranol, 0.1 mg	(for 21 days)	
Loestrin 1/20	Norethindrone acetate, 1 mg	1 pill qd for 28 days	Minimal estrogen dose
	Ethinyl estradiol, 20 mg; 7 iron tablets		
Loestrin 1.5/30	Norethindrone acetate, 1.5 mg	1 pill qd for 28 days	Low estrogen dose
	Ethinyl estradiol, 30 μg; 7 iron tablets		
Norinyl	Norethindrone, 2 mg	1 pill qd for 20 days	Good cycle control
	Mestranol, 0.1 mg		
Norinyl 1 + 50†	Norethindrone, 1 mg	1 pill qd for 21 days	Low estrogen dose
	Mestranol, 0.05 mg		
Norinyl 1 + 80†	Norethindrone, 1 mg	1 pill qd for 21 days	Balanced low doses
	Mestranol, 0.08 mg		
Norlestrin 21 1 mg†	Norethindrone acetate, 1 mg	1 pill qd for 21 days	Estrogen dominant
	Ethinyl estradiol, 0.05 mg		
Norlestrin 21 2.5 mg†	Norethindrone acetate, 2.5 mg	1 pill qd for 21 days	Progestogen domi-nant
	Ethinyl estradiol, 0.5 mg		
Ortho-Novum 10 mg	Norethindrone, 10 mg	1 pill qd for 20 days	Anabolic effect
	Mestranol, 0.06 mg		
Ortho-Novum 2 mg	Norethindrone, 2 mg	1 pill qd for 20 days	Good cycle control
	Mestranol, 0.1 mg		
Ortho-Novum 1/50†	Norethindrone, 1 mg	1 pill qd for 20 or 21 days	Low estrogen dose
	Mestranol, 0.05 mg		
Ortho-Novum 1/80†	Norethindrone, 1 mg	1 pill qd for 21 days	Balanced low doses
	Mestranol, 0.08 mg		
Ovral†	Norgestrel, 0.5 mg	1 pill qd for 21 days	Minimal progestogen
	Ethinyl estradiol, 0.05 mg		
Ovulen (20 or 21)†	Ethynodiol diacetate, 1 mg	1 pill qd for 20 or 21 days	Good cycle control
	Mestranol, 0.1 mg		
Zorane 1.5/30	Norethindrone acetate, 1.5 mg	1 blue pill qd for 21 days starting on cycle day 5	Low estrogen
	Ethinyl estradiol, 0.03 mg	1 white pill qd for 7 days	
Zorane 1/50	Norethindrone acetate, 1 mg	1 green pill qd for 21 days starting on cycle day 5	Balanced low doses
	Ethinyl estradiol, 0.05 mg	1 white pill qd for 7 days	
Zorane 1/20	Norethindrone acetate, 1 mg	1 pink pill qd for 21 days starting on cycle day 5	Minimal estrogen
	Ethinyl estradiol, 0.02 mg	1 white pill qd for 7 days	
Sequentials			
Norquen	Norethindrone, 2 mg	Mestranol for 20 days, norethin-drone added last 6 days; resume on day 5 of next cycle	
	Mestranol, 0.08 mg		
Oracont	Dimethisterone, 25 mg	Ethinyl estradiol for 21 days, dimethisterone added last 5 days; off 7 days	Improvement in acne
	Ethinyl estradiol, 0.1 mg		
Ortho-Novum SQ	Norethindrone, 2 mg	Mestranol for 14 days, norethin-drone added last 6 days; off 7 days	
	Mestranol, 0.08 mg		
Minipills			
Micronor	Norethindrone, 0.35 mg	Continuously	Minimal constitu-tional effects of progestogens
Nor-QD	Norethindrone, 0.35 mg	Continuously	
Ovrette	Norgestrol, 0.075 mg	Continuously	

*From Nursing Update. 1975. **6:**14, May.
†Also available in 28-day packets containing seven inert or iron tablets.

Chemical contraception

Spermicidal jellies, creams, or suppositories inserted in the vagina 10 to 15 minutes before intercourse cannot be endorsed as good protection against pregnancy. Despite careful application, the medicated cream, for example, may not cover or even collect near the cervical os.

Aerosol contraceptive foam, actually a creamy, water-soluble preparation combining chemical and mechanical methodology, is a moderately effective birth-control method. An applicator is utilized to insert the foam into the vaginal canal precoitally. This method generally has been well received. Vaginal or penile irritation due to the medication may be reported.

Postcoital douches, no matter what the medicinal content, are not methods of contraception. Ejaculation deposits semen in or near the cervical os. By the time a douche can be used, spermatozoa will be within the cervix or uterus—beyond the effect of the irrigation fluid. Spermatozoa have been detected in the cervical mucus within 90 seconds after ejaculation (Sobrero and MacLeod, 1962).

Mechanical contraception

Intrauterine device (IUD) or intrauterine contraceptive device (IUCD). Small plastic rings, coils, shields, or other devices introduced into the uterus are a reliable means of contraception and compare favorably in effectiveness with oral anovulatory drug therapy. The woman continues to ovulate while wearing an IUD, and motile sperm are frequently aspirated from the endometrial cavity. Why these semipermanent IUDs are contraceptive is still under study. It may be that surface contact of the device with the endometrium may cause the release of cytotoxic products that prevent implantation of the zygote or induce an extremely early abortion.

Advantages of the IUD include low cost to produce, no obligation to take or use some preparation, and possible prolonged use. Disadvantages are cramping and metrorrhagia in about 30% of patients for the first few months. Hypermenorrhea and leukorrhea may also occur. There is an increased incidence of salpingitis in IUD patients, probably because of chronic endometritis.

Active cervicitis, salpingitis, and myomata are contraindications to the insertion of an IUD. Complications include perforation of the uterus in about 1% and pregnancy in approximately 3% of women with an IUD in situ (Table 6-3). Others may become pregnant after the undetected loss of the device.

The rate of expulsion is approximately 10% by the end of the first year. Approximately 30% are expelled by women who had an IUD inserted during the puerperium. The woman should be advised to check for presence of

the "tail" of the device before intercourse and after each menstrual cycle. It can be felt in the vagina.

Condom and vaginal diaphragm. If used with a contraceptive cream or gel these devices offer mechanical and chemical protection against pregnancy. Moderate reliability can be expected from this combination. The condom, or "rubber," is used during intercourse and then removed. Failures are due to delayed use of the condom after initial intromission. The condom protects against venereal disease, but because penile sensation is dulled, use is not consistent. The diaphragm can be inserted prior to sexual activity, but once intercourse has taken place it must remain in place for 6 to 8 hours. After removal a postcoital douche may be taken. The woman must be fitted for a diaphragm, since the size varies with the size of the vagina. The diaphragm must be refitted after the birth of each child. It should be checked manually to see if it is correctly positioned covering the cervix. The woman should practice inserting the diaphragm and checking the position before leaving the clinic or physician's office.

Surgical interruption of pregnancy

Therapeutic abortion is the purposeful interruption of a previable pregnancy (before 23 to 24 weeks' gestational age of a fetus weighing less than 500 gm). Indications for therapeutic abortion are as follows:

- Preservation of the life or health of the mother (e.g., Class III or IV heart disease)
- Avoidance of the birth of an offspring with a serious development or hereditary disorder (e.g., Tay-Sachs disease)
- Socioeconomic or voluntary abortion (e.g., inability of the parents to support or care for the child)

Table 6-3. Methods of contraception*

Method	Pregnancy rate per 100 woman years
Coitus interruptus	16
Rhythm	34.5
Vaginal jelly	11 → 39
Vaginal foam	28.3
Diaphragm and spermicide	15
Condom	15
IUD	3
Oral	0.7

*Based on data from Willson, J. R., Beecham, C. T., and Carrington, E. R. 1975. Obstetrics and gynecology (ed. 5). St. Louis, The C. V. Mosby Co.

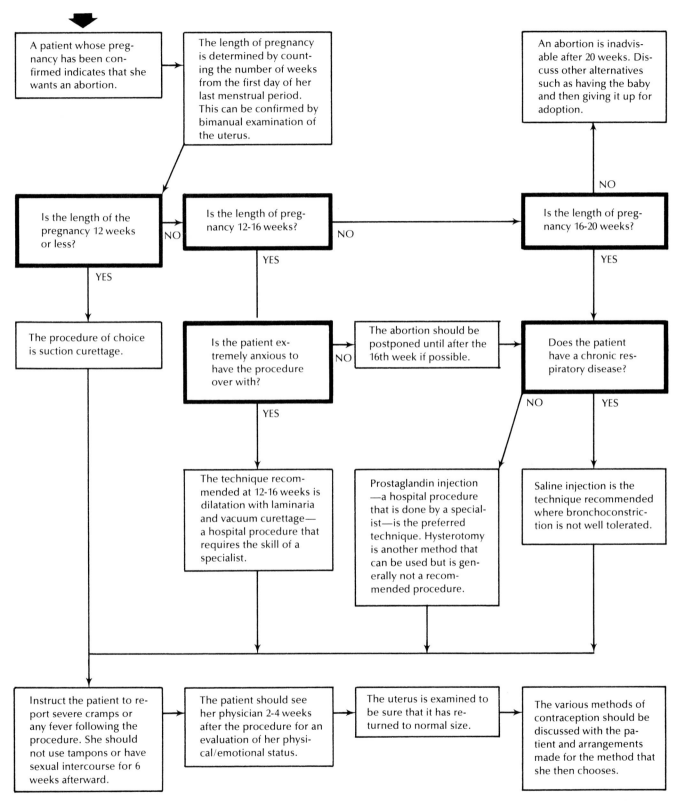

Fig. 6-2. Abortion flow chart to determine what procedures—and when. (Decision points are in heavy outline.) (From Nursing Update. 1975. **6**:5, May.)

Abortion is regulated in most countries presumably to protect the mother from the complications of abortion or because of religious constraints. The U.S. Supreme Court set aside previous antiabortion laws in January 1973, holding that first trimester abortion is permissible in this country inasmuch as the mortality from interruption of early gestation is now less than the mortality after normal term delivery. Midtrimester abortion was left to the discretion of the individual states. Catholic hospitals and some of those maintained by strict fundamentalists forbid abortion (and often sterilization) despite legal challenge. Nonetheless, it is obvious that the final legal ruling on abortion has not yet been written.

In fact, compelling medical, surgical, or psychiatric indications for elective abortion are not numerous but the following probably would qualify: Class III coronary heart disease; fulminating (pelvic) Hodgkin's disease; stage 1B carcinoma of the cervix; and Marfan's syndrome with early aortic aneurysm.

The woman who is diagnosed as Rh negative must receive RhoGAM after an abortion.

The length of pregnancy and the condition of the woman determine the appropriate type of abortion procedure. For a summary of the method of assessment and postabortal instructions, see Fig. 6-2.

Early abortion. Methods for performing early therapeutic abortion include the following:

1. Menstrual extraction—early aspiration of the endometrium in patients who have not yet missed a period
2. Surgical dilatation and curettage (D and C) when newer aspiration equipment is unavailable
3. Uterine aspiration after one or two missed periods

The insertion of a small laminaria tent retained by a vaginal tampon for 6 to 24 hours usually will facilitate the purposeful interruption of a first trimester pregnancy, especially in a young, teenage patient or in an individual whose cervix is unyielding, for example, after cervical conization or extensive coagulation.

On removal of the moist, expanded laminaria, the cervix will have dilated two to three times its original (dry) diameter. Rarely will further mechanical dilatation of the cervix be required because the insertion of an adequate-sized aspiration canula (8.5 to 10.5 mm) almost always is possible. Morbidity probably is not increased; in fact, cervical laceration and bleeding are reduced by the use of laminaria. A disadvantage is the delay necessary and the need for an additional visit to the physician's office or clinic by the patient.

The suction procedure for accomplishing an early therapeutic abortion (ideal time is 8 to 10 weeks since last menstrual period) usually requires less than 5 minutes and can easily be effected under paracervical block anesthesia and single sedation (Fig. 6-3). Bleeding after the operation normally is about the equivalent of a heavy menstrual period, and cramps are rarely severe. Infection such as endometritis or salpingitis occurs in about 8% of patients, and subsequent surgical dilatation and curettage for bleeding or sepsis due to retained placental tissue is necessary in about 2% of patients. With good counseling and proper selection of patients, serious depression or other psychiatric problems are rare.

The patient comes to the clinic or physician's office the day prior to the abortion procedure. The pelvic area is prepared using an antiseptic solution. A vaginal speculum is inserted, and the vaginal canal and cervix are cleansed. Injection of a local anesthetic agent into the cervix follows. Again the area is cleansed, and the laminaria are inserted in the cervix. Prophylactic use of an antibiotic is begun. Some patients experience a mild cramping or have light spotting from the anesthetic injection. Discomfort can be controlled with aspirin. The next day the patient is admitted to the hospital and given preoperative sedation. (Physician and nursing interventions for suction curettage using local anesthetic are given on p. 74.) The vaginal area is cleansed (shaving is not necessary). The anesthetic agent is administered, and the dilatation and suction procedure is completed. The aspirated uterine contents must be carefully inspected to ascertain if all fetal parts and adequate placental tissue have been evacuated. A single dose of oxytocin is usually sufficient to control bleeding. The patient remains in the hospital 3 or 4 hours for detection of excessive bleeding and then is discharged. Instruction is given as to what symptoms to watch for—excessive bleeding, cramps, or fever—and she is warned against using vaginal tampons or having sexual intercourse for 6 weeks to avoid infection. Other contraceptive techniques are reviewed for future use.

Midtrimester abortion. There are four types of techniques used for midtrimester abortion:

1. *Transabdominal intrauterine injection of hypertonic sodium chloride from the fourteenth week until the twenty-third to twenty-fourth week of pregnancy.* The patient is admitted to the hospital for this procedure. Amniocentesis is performed. The physician determines where the needle (an 18-gauge, 3-inch, spinal needle) will be inserted. The area is cleansed, and if desired, a local anesthetic agent is given. Approximately 200 ml of amniotic fluid are withdrawn, and a similar amount of sterile 20% sodium chloride is injected. The patient is instructed to report when uterine contractions begin, which is generally within 8 to 48 hours. In most cases, augmentation with oxytocin is necessary to effect uterine evacuation in a reasonable time. Occasional patients may require reinjection. Labor begins, in theory

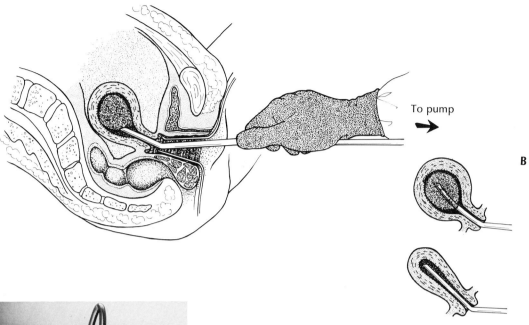

To pump

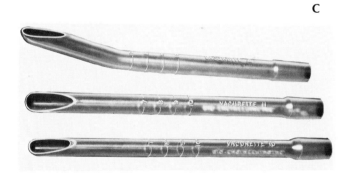

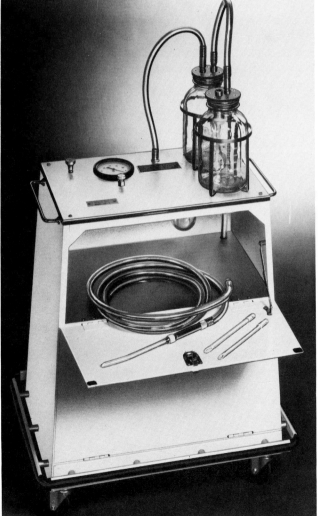

Fig. 6-3. A, Suction (vacuum) curettage machine. **B,** Suction method of therapeutic abortion. **C,** Suction (vacuum) catheters. (**A** and **C** courtesy Berkeley Bio-Engineering, Inc., San Leandro, Calif.)

Suction or vacuum curettage using local anesthetic

Physician interventions	Nursing interventions
	Assist patient to empty bowel and bladder.
	Prepare pelvic area with shave, if ordered. Wash pelvic area with antiseptic solution such as pHysoHex, or povidone-iodine (Betadine).
Prepare patient for what to expect.	Prepare patient for what to expect. Remain at head of table with patient.
Insert sterile speculum and wash vaginal walls and cervix with antiseptic solution (cotton balls and ring forceps).	Explain to patient, "The vagina is being washed. This will probably feel cold."
Inject local anesthetic agent (as for paracervical block) such as lidocaine (Xylocaine), and rewash vaginal vault with antiseptic.	Explain to patient, "You will feel a needle stick as the anesthetic is injected. The vagina is being washed again."
Remove laminaria (if used) and sound size, depth, and position of uterus and configuration of cervix.	Tell patient, "You may feel some cramping."
Dilate cervix until it is 1 mm greater than the number of weeks of gestation (e.g., for a gestation of 8 weeks, dilate to 9 mm).	As largest dilator is inserted, warn patient, "You may feel some heavy pressure for 10 to 15 seconds now."
Insert vacuum tip (of same size in diameter as last dilator or one size smaller) and rotate it around uterine cavity. Suctioning is accomplished within 30 seconds to 3 minutes.	Explain to patient, "The noise you hear is the suction machine. This will last about 2 to 4 minutes. You may feel some menstrual-like cramping."
Examine aspirate to ensure that all products of conception have been removed.	
When indicated, gently scrape with sharp metal curette for any retained deciduate.	

---

at least, because the hypertonic saline releases the placental uterine progesterone blockade that normally prevents the onset of labor. The same careful monitoring of the contractions is as necessary as for a term delivery. Instruction in relaxation and breathing techniques is indicated and analgesia can be administered for discomfort (Chapter 20). The assistance of a supportive person at the time of birth of the dead fetus is essential. If the patient wishes to see the fetus, emotional support before and after should be provided. Many patients are relieved to find the fetus was normal and frequently inquire as to its sex. After the delivery, postnatal observations and care are carried out (Chapter 27). Contraceptive counseling is given before discharge, and the patient is told to return if excessive bleeding should occur.

Complications of hypertonic saline midtrimester abortion with the approximate frequency of their occurrence are as follows:
- Postinjection infection (10%)
- Incomplete separation requiring dilatation and curettage (15%)
- Excessive bleeding necessitating transfusion (2%)
- Consumption coagulopathy (occasional)
- Potentially fatal hypernatremia due to intravascular injection (rare)

- Severe hypotension or cardiac arrest (rare)
- Failure to abort (10%)

2. *Injection of urea solution after amniocentesis.* After the removal of about 200 ml of amniotic fluid, 200 ml of a 30% solution of urea in 5% dextrose in water is given by gravity drip. After 1 hour, 5% oxytocin in 500 ml of 5% dextrose in water is started. Fetal death occurs, and delivery ensues in most cases within 12 hours. Complications are less common and are less serious than with hypertonic saline.

3. *Transabdominal intrauterine injection of $F_{2\alpha}$.* The undesirable side effects of hypertonic saline such as hyponatremia or disseminated intravascular coagulation do not occur with PG; therefore it has become the treatment of choice (Table 6-4). However, nausea and vomiting are common problems. Its use is contraindicated with respiratory problems such as asthma because it has caused marked constriction of the bronchial musculature. The characteristics and actions of PG are as follows:

Characteristics	Actions (partial list)
Soluble in nonpolar solvents	Inhibit secretion of hydrochloric acid
Soluble in water	
Derived in the body from essential unsaturated fatty acids of the diet	Stimulate thyroid gland to produce thyroid hormone
	Cause kidney to lose salt

Table 6-4. Comparison of prostaglandin and saline abortion procedures*

Prostaglandin	Saline
No aspiration is necessary. The obstetrician injects 8 ml of $PGF_{2\alpha}$ into the amniotic sac.	The obstetrician inserts a needle into the introamniotic sac, withdraws 200 cc of amniotic fluid, and injects 200 cc of salt solution.
The procedure takes a minute or two.	Duration of procedure ranges from 15 to 30 minutes.
Contractions usually begin within the first half-hour after injection. Labor usually takes place within 24 hours.	Contractions usually begin approximately 12 hours after salt solution is injected; labor averages 36 hours.
It is not necessary to administer oxytocin IV; therefore patient's movement is not restricted.	To shorten labor, a continuous IV oxytocin drip is often administered. This restricts patient's movement for the reduced period of labor, approximately 24 hours.

*From Nursing Update. 1975. **6**:9, May.

Characteristics—cont'd

Formed by the cells of nearly all mammalian cells thus far examined

Found in menstrual fluids and in amniotic fluid at parturition

Formed in response to physiologic, physical, chemical, inflammatory, and immunologic stimuli

Not stored in tissues, but released in minute amounts by most cells

Metabolized quickly after producing effect*

Actions (partial list)—cont'd

Cause adrenals to secrete cortisone

Cause uterus to contract

Lower blood pressure

Dilate bronchioles

Constrict bronchioles

Increase pulmonary blood flow

Between 40 and 60 mg of PG are required for this procedure. One milliliter is injected slowly over a 5-minute period. The remainder is injected slowly if no side effects have occurred. Should they occur, recovery takes about 30 minutes, since PG has a short half-life and the initial dose is minimal. Abortion usually takes place within 18 to 24 hours. If it does not occur, the procedure is repeated using half the dosage.

The management of the three types of abortion just discussed is the same. All these may require anywhere from 1 to 4 days of hospitalization. Because of this, involvement of the family of the young teenage patient is almost inevitable. Measures taken to foster supportive relationships are part of nursing care.

4. *Abdominal or vaginal hysterotomy.* Hysterotomy may be chosen when pregnancy is more than 14 to 16 weeks, after failure of intrauterine saline or PG injection,

*From Nursing Update. 1975. **6**:10, May.

and when sterilization is desirable. The vaginal approach is employed when transabdominal surgery should be avoided. The patient must remain in the hospital a week to 10 days. The management is comparable to that of cesarean section.

Surgical termination of fertility
FEMALE STERILIZATION

Female sterilization is the prevention of pregnancy by surgical or radiologic means. With regard to surgery, only removal of the ovaries, uterus, or both will result in absolute sterility. All other operations have a small but definite pregnancy failure rate.

Indications for sterilization include virtually all those appropriate for elective abortion, for example, maternal disease, or elective sterilization. Preservation of the life or the health of the mother applies in every state of the United States except Utah, which still requires a threat to the patient's life for sterilization.

Again absolute indications for sterilization are uncommon. Fear of uterine rupture after a third cesarean section (unlikely) has lead to the common recommendation for sterilization. Now many states permit voluntary sterilization of any mature, rational female without reference to her marriage or pregnancy status. Nonetheless, if the woman is married, the husband's permission should be obtained also to avoid marital problems.

Sterilization of minors or mentally incompetent females is restricted by most states, and the operation often requires the approval of a board of eugenics or court-appointed individuals.

The timing of sterilization may be postabortal, postnatal, or interval (interconceptional). The majority of sterilizations are effected after a pregnancy because the patient has made her decision and is in a hospital.

Tubal ligation. Most surgical procedures to accomplish sterilization of the female interrupt tubal continuity. Because more effective operations are radical or are likely to be followed by undesirable loss of function or complications, procedures like oophorectomy or hysterectomy generally are reserved for sterilization in addition to elimination of pelvic pathology such as uterine myomata. Therefore tubal surgery is currently the most common approach to sterilization of women, and the following are popular techniques, in order of probable effectiveness:

1. Uchida operation
2. Kroener fimbriectomy
3. Laparoscopic tubal fulguration
4. Irving sterilization
5. Pomeroy sterilization
6. Madlener sterilization

The Kroener, Pomeroy, and Madlener operations can be accomplished transvaginally also. All these operations have fewer pregnancy failures when accomplished as interval procedures, perhaps because of the absence of tissue edema that may permit the sutures to cut through the tubal wall.

The operation used frequently is the laparoscopic tubal fulguration. The patient is admitted the morning of surgery, and preoperative sedation is given. The procedure often is carried out under local anesthesia. A small vertical incision is made in the abdominal wall below the umbilicus. The patient may experience sensations of tugging but no pain, and the operation is completed within 20 minutes. She may be discharged 4 hours later. Any abdominal discomfort can be controlled with aspirin. Within 10 days the scar is almost invisible.

Major medical complications after elective sterilization are rare. Nonetheless, dysfunctional uterine bleeding or ovarian cyst formation may occur after tubal surgery, presumably because of disturbance of the utero-ovarian circulation. The approximate incidence of pregnancy failure is shown in Table 6-5.

Tubal continuity is not difficult to reestablish, but the incidence of successful pregnancy after reanastomosis is only about 15%, probably because of the loss of a segment of tube necessary for sperm capacitation and fertilization.

Hysterectomy. Hysterectomy, abdominal or vaginal, may be accomplished when other pathology such as in situ carcinoma of the cervix should be eliminated or for sterilization of the patient.

MALE STERILIZATION

Vasectomy. Vasectomy is the easiest and most commonly employed operation for male sterilization. Vasectomy can be carried out under local anesthesia even on an outpatient basis.

In vasectomy, short right and left incisions are made into the anterior aspect of the scrotum above and lateral to each testicle over the spermatic cord. The vas is identified, doubly ligated with fine nonabsorbable sutures, and incised between the ligatures. Many surgeons interpose tissue such as scrotal fascia to lessen the chance of reunion. Then the skin incisions are closed, generally with nonabsorbable sutures, and a dressing is applied. A suspensory or bandage is applied to support the scrotum. Moderate inactivity for about 2 days is advisable because of tenderness. The skin suture can be removed 5 to 7 days postoperatively.

Some spermatozoa will remain in the proximal vas after vasectomy. It requires at least ten ejaculations to

Table 6-5. Success of female sterilization

Sterilization method	Approximate failure rate (literature consensus)	
	At cesarean section	**After vaginal delivery**
Cesarean section hysterectomy	>30 reported abdominal pregnancies	
Cornual resection	?	1 in 20
Madlener	1 in 50	1 in 30
Cooke	?	1 in 250
Pomeroy	1 in 50	1 in 300
Irving	Very rare	Very rare
Uchida	No known failures in about 5000 operations	
Kroener	Exceptional	Exceptional

clear the tract of sperm before unprotected coitus can be permitted.

Vasectomy has no effect on potency, but patients occasionally may develop a hematoma, discharge, or infection. Less common are painful sperm granulomas. Sterilization failures, usually due to recanalization, are rare.

NURSE'S ROLE

The introduction of new members into cultural complexes has always been predominately by birth. The need of a society to protect the welfare of these new members has prompted development of institutions, value systems, and rituals that regulate responsibility and dispense support. These become part of the fabric of a nation, its moral fiber, and changes are faced with reluctance and fear. International consensus for the necessity to limit population levels to those compatible with earth's resources and the subsequent legalizing of techniques for limiting the numbers of children precipitated moral dilemmas for persons such as nurses who have the knowledge and skills that are required for the safe use of these techniques. The values, beliefs, and moral convictions of the nurse are involved to the same extent as those of the patient. Since the conflicts and doubts of the nurse can be readily communicated to patients, who are already anxious and overly sensitive, health professionals need assistance to identify and come to terms with their own feelings.

It is not uncommon for confusion to arise as beliefs are challenged by the reality of care. A student nurse reacted to learning experiences associated with inpatient abortions in the following manner:

I really feel I believe in the rightness of therapeutic abortion but when I watched the physician insert the needle and then inject the dose of prostaglandin I felt an unreasoning rage sweep over me. I could have attacked him. Funny, I felt no anger to the girl at all. I really need to rethink my thoughts.

Responses can also change with life experiences. A nurse who before her marriage had worked as counselor in a municipal clinic established a reputation as a supportive and concerned counselor of young persons with regard to contraception. Four years later she remarked:

I've been trying to get pregnant for the past 3 years. I didn't realize how important it would be to me. You know I can't counsel about abortion any more. I can't be objective, I keep feeling "Have your baby and please give it to me." I am more concerned about myself now, not them, and counseling won't work that way.

Selection of personnel to function in family planning clinics or in hospitals must be carefully done. Studies indicate that attitudes of personnel affect significantly the patient's perception of the quality of care received (World Health Organization, 1971). This is an important consideration in planning for the overall delivery of health services, since seeking help for birth control is frequently the only contact young adults have with the health care system. Positive perceptions of the interest, concern, and technical skill of health workers in this instance may induce wider use of health facilities and care in the future.

Counseling of patients about abortion includes help for the woman in identifying how she perceives the pregnancy; information about the choices available, that is, having an abortion or carrying the pregnancy to term and then either keeping the child or giving it up for adoption; and information about types of abortion procedures. The goal is to assist the woman in coming to a decision that is her own. She will need help to explore the meaning of the various alternatives to herself and her significant others. It is often difficult for the patient to express her true feelings. A calm, matter-of-fact approach on the part of the nurse can be helpful (e.g., "Yes, I know you are pregnant. I am here to help. Let's talk about alternatives."). Listening to what the patient has to say and encouraging her to speak is essential. Neutral responses such as "Oh," "Uh-huh," and "Umm" and nonverbal encouragement such as nodding, maintaining eye contact, and use of touch are helpful in setting an open accepting environment. Clarifying, restating, and reflecting statements, use of open-ended questions, and giving feedback are communication techniques that can be used to maintain a reality focus on the situation and bring the patient's problems into the open. Once a decision has been made, the patient must be assured of continued support. Information as to what is entailed in various procedures, how much discomfort or pain can be expected, and what type of care is needed must be given. If family or friends cannot be involved, time for the necessary support from nursing personnel is an essential component of the care plan.

Individuals desiring sterilization as a means of contraception may be those who have almost come to the end of their childbearing years and have the desired number of children, or they may be young adults who have decided not to bear children. The first group are generally acceptive of the procedure even though there may be some feelings of regret because one of life's phases is over. The second group need the opportunity to explore the consequences of their choice. Many individuals fear sterilization procedures because of the imag-

---

PLAN OF CARE: CONTRACEPTION

PATIENT CARE OBJECTIVES

1. Patient is aware of the biologic and psychologic components of sexuality and possible outcomes of being sexually active.
2. Patient is able to plan for a desired (wanted) pregnancy or prevent an unwanted one.
3. Patient is knowledgeable concerning the advantages and disadvantages of the protective technique selected.
4. Patient is skilled in use of chemical, hormonal, or mechanical techniques or knowledgeable about the technical processes involved in surgical contraception.
5. Patient is aware of community resources for assistance with sexuality problems.
6. Patient is aware of legal rights and responsibilities concerning adult sexuality.
7. Records are established and maintained as a basis for continuity of care.

NURSING INTERVENTIONS

Diagnostic	Therapeutic and educational
1. Assess patient's knowledge of biologic and psychologic components of human sexuality.	1. Refute myths and misconceptions with factual information about the following:
2. Determine need for fertility control in following situations:	a. Biology of sexuality
a. Patient is sexually active or plans to be.	b. Consequences of sexual activity (e.g., women may become pregnant as early as third postnatal week before menstruation resumes; women may become pregnant on first exposure to intercourse; pregnancy can result from deposit of semen on labia minora without vaginal penetration by penis; women may become pregnant after menses have become irregular with approach of menopause)
b. Patient has disease process incompatible with pregnancy (e.g., nephritis).	
c. Patient has recently delivered child.	
3. Assess patient's level of understanding of use of contraceptive techniques.	c. Available contraceptive techniques, their advantages, and disadvantages
4. Determine if method selected meets following criteria:	d. What contraceptive technique selected entails (e.g., consistent use of chemical or mechanical devices) or procedure to be followed for abortion or sterilization
a. Safe for patient's use (e.g., the pill is contraindicated for diabetic patients or for breast-feeding mothers)	2. Provide safe, open, accepting environment to enable patient to come to decision regarding use and choice of method of contraception.
b. Suitable for patient's life-style (e.g., patient wants to become pregnant in future; patient does not want any or more children)	3. Provide safe, physical care for immediate and long-term needs.
c. Compatible with patient's religion or moral convictions	4. Provide supportive nonjudgmental care for patient in clinic or hospital settings, including careful explanation of procedures, relief of discomfort, use of gentle touch, tone of voice, and closeness in space to convey interest, privacy, and presence of family and/or friend, if desired.
	5. Establish with patient a future plan of care (e.g., periodic examinations of individuals using hormonal therapies, counseling sessions for postabortion patients).

---

ined effect on their sexual life. They need reassurance concerning the hormonal and psychologic basis for sexual function and the fact that tubal ligation or vasectomy have no biologic sequelae in terms of sexual inadequacy.

The control of birth, dealing as it does with human sexuality and the question of life and death, is one of the most highly emotionalized components of health care. Abortion as one of the surgical alternatives to contraception has only recently been legalized in North America (1973 in the United States). Prior to the legalization of abortion, many illegal abortions took place, with little-documented sequelae other than death from infection, hemorrhage, or both. Although studies indicate that biologic sequelae do occur after abortion, rates of biologic complications tend to be low, especially if the woman is aborted during the first trimester (Sloane and Harvitz, 1971). Studies related to psychologic sequelae reveal that these are short-lived and related to circumstances surrounding the abortion such as rape and the attitudes reflected by friends, family, and health workers. It must be remembered that the woman facing an abortion is pregnant and will exhibit the emotional responses shared by all pregnant women, even postnatal depressions).

In an attempt to regulate the conflict between professional responsibilities and personal ethics, the Nurse's Association of the American College of Obstetricians and Gynecologists (NAACOG) published a position paper on the nurse's role with the abortion patient in May, 1972, in which the simultaneous rights of each were described (Tyrer, 1973). Patients have the right to expect and receive supportive, nonjudgmental care, and nurses have the right to refuse to assist with abortions or sterilizations in keeping with their own moral or religious beliefs, unless the patient's life is in danger.

REFERENCES

Baudry, F., and Wiener, A. 1974. The pregnant patient in conflict about abortion: a challenge for the obstetrician. Am. J. Obstet. Gynecol. **119:**705.

Corfman, P. A. 1974. Coordinated studies of the effects of oral contraceptives. Contraception **9:**109.

Davis, H. L. 1972. Intrauterine contraceptive devices: present status and future prospects. Am. J. Obstet. Gynecol. **114:**134.

Drill, V. A. 1972. Oral contraceptives and thromboembolic disease. I. Prospective and retrospective studies. J.A.M.A. **219:**583.

Golditch, I. M., and Glasses, M. H. 1974. The use of laminaria tents for cervical dilation prior to vacuum aspiration abortion. Am. J. Obstet. Gynecol. **119:**481.

Gullattee, A. C. 1972. Psychiatric aspects of abortion, J. Natl. Med. Assoc. **64:**308.

Hardeu, G. 1969. Population, evolution, and birth control: a college of controversial ideas (ed. 2). San Francisco, W. H. Freeman & Co.

Harper, M. W., and others. 1972. Abortion—do attitudes of nursing personnel affect the patient's perception of care? Nurs. Res. **21:**327, July-Aug.

Hodgson, J. E., and Portmann, K. C. 1974. Complications of 10,543 consecutive 1st trimester abortions: prospective study. Am. J. Obstet. Gynecol. **120:**820.

Hubbard, C. W. 1973. Family planning education: parenthood and social disease control. St. Louis, The C. V. Mosby Co.

Larsson, C. N. 1975. Oral contraceptives and vitamins. Am. J. Obstet. Gynecol. **121:**84.

McCalister, D. V., Thiessan, V., and McDermott, M. 1973. Readings in family planning. St. Louis, The C. V. Mosby Co.

Mishell, D. R., Jr. 1975. Assessing the intrauterine device. Fam. Plann. Perspect. **7:**103.

Nelson, J. H. 1973. The case of the mini-pill in private practice. J. Reprod. Med. **10:**139.

Nursing Update (entire issue). 1975. **6:**May.

Poulson, A. M., Jr. 1973. Analysis of female sterilization techniques. Obstet. Gynecol. **42:**131.

Rudel, H., and others. 1973. Birth control, contraception and abortion. New York, The Macmillan Co.

Sloane, R. B., and Harvitz, D. F. 1971. The changing practice of abortion. In Sloane, R. B. (ed.). Abortion, changing views and practice. New York, Grune & Stratton, Inc.

Sobrero, G. A., and MacLeod J. 1962. The immediate post coital test. Fertil. Steril. **13:**184.

Stoot, J. E. G. M. and Ubachs, J. M. H. 1973. Sterilization by salpingectomy through posterior colpotomy. Contraception **8:**577.

Tietze, C. 1975. The effect of legalization of abortion on population growth and public health. Fam. Plann. Perspect. **7:**123.

Tyrer, L. 1973. The new morality, ethics, and nursing. J. Obstet. Gynecol. Nurs. **2:**54, Sept.-Oct.

Vancer-Vleit, W. L., and Hafez, E. S. E. 1974. Survival and aging of spermatozoa: a review, Am. J. Obstet. Gynecol. **118:**1006.

Walton, L. A. 1972. Immediate morbidity on a large abortion service. N.Y. State J. Med. **72:**919.

Wheeles, C. R., Jr., and Thompson, B. H. 1973. Laparoscopic sterilization: review of 3,600 cases. Obstet. Gynecol. **42:**751.

Wiggins, P. 1974. Use effectiveness of the diaphragm in selected family planning population in the United Kingdom. Contraception **9:**15.

Willson, J. R., Beecham, C. T., and Carrington, E. R. 1975. Obstetrics and gynecology (ed. 5). St. Louis, The C. V. Mosby Co.

World Health Organization. 1971. Induced abortion as public health program: report on working group. Copenhagen, Regional Office for Europe.

CHAPTER 7

Genetics and genetic counseling

The hoped-for and expected outcome of every wanted pregnancy is a normal functioning infant with a good intelligence potential. Some pregnancies terminate in abnormal, spontaneous abortion; most term pregnancies result in a normal child. In a small, but significant percentage of cases, an abnormal infant is born.

To function therapeutically, the nurse must consider not only the clinical aspects of care but also the psychosocial needs of the patients experiencing the crisis. When a defective child is born, the cause is not always apparent. The parent asks, ''Why me?'' ''What did I do?'' and ''Will it happen again?'' Some abnormalities have a genetic component; others are environmentally induced (p. 112). Frequently, no cause can be identified.

A knowledge of the inheritable and congenital bases for structural or functional disorders must be the foundation for appropriate clinical judgment regarding intervention. The nurse may never choose to become a specialist in genetic counseling, but a fundamental knowledge of genetics, patterns of inheritance, populations at risk, diagnostic methods, and nursing's role in genetic counseling is essential to comprehensive care.

ROLE OF NURSE IN PREVENTIVE INTERVENTION

Nursing's commitment to society is not confined to acute care settings and clinics. Preventive intervention must be an integral part of any health care system. Implementing this concept requires collaborative efforts with many medical specialties and segments of society.

As professionals and as private citizens, nurses can be instrumental in disseminating genetic information to the public. The following avenues are proposed.

First, information concerning the role of genetics in everyday life, the interplay of genetic and environmental factors, and available diagnostic tests should comprise a significant portion of high school biology courses. Second, health education classes, television, films, and articles in popular publications can foster community awareness of and interest in practical genetics.

Genetic counseling is now recognized to be a part of premarital counseling and prenatal clinical service. However, standardization of the counseling provided is still to be accomplished.

Gathering genetic data should become as routine as the taking of the temperature, pulse, and respirations. A complete history and physical examination of the couple often reveal those who are at risk for transmission of a genetic problem. Once the possibility of a problem is disclosed, the prospective parents should be advised of the risk of its appearance in their offspring and the type, extent, and expense (financial and emotional) of study or treatment if a child is born with the defect. The couple must weigh their own feelings, religious persuasion, love for each other, and many other variables against the genetic probabilities. The nurse's interviewing skills and psychologic closeness to patients may assist them in identifying and verbalizing their concerns in a nonthreatening atmosphere. The nurse may clarify misconceptions and provide needed information. The couple should then be equipped to make a value judgment regarding pregnancies, with the option of elective abortion or adoption.

Medical supervision during the prenatal period should routinely include identification of those at risk for having an infant with genetic or acquired congenital defects. Careful history taking in an accepting and unhurried atmosphere results in more complete data on which to evaluate the need for counseling. This method of history taking also affords a natural entry point for anticipatory guidance regarding effects on pregnancy outcome from environmental factors such as nutrition, age, drugs, infections, or smoking.

GENETIC TRANSMISSION IN FAMILIES
Populations at risk

Not everyone will need genetic counseling. Certain populations are known to be at greater risk for having children with genetic defects. Groups who have shown a higher probability include the following:

1. Persons who display structural or functional abnormalities
2. Individuals from high-risk populations—black Americans (sickle cell disease), descendants of northern European or Ashkenazi Jews (Tay-Sachs disease), and those of Mediterranean ancestry (thalassemia)
3. Couples who have already had a child with a defect
4. Individuals whose family history includes a structural abnormality or systemic disease that may be hereditary
5. Prospective parents who are closely blood-related (consanguineous)
6. Older women (over 40 years of age) who are pregnant or who are contemplating pregnancy

Prevalence of genetic disorders

Nurses are frequently confronted with questions about congenital anomalies from women who have a history of repeated spontaneous abortions; who have been exposed to drugs, diseases, or radiation; or who for many reasons fear having an infant with a defect.

The prevalence of malformations is much greater in spontaneously aborted embryos and fetuses than among liveborn infants. Exact figures are difficult to determine, but it is thought that 12% to 15% of all pregnancies abort and that between 25% and 40% of these can be related to chromosomal aberrations. More than 90% of all fetuses with chromosomal abnormalities are aborted. (For a discussion of other causes of spontaneous abortion, see Chapter 16.)

Major malformations of surgical or cosmetic consequence are evident in about 2% to 3% of liveborn infants. Chromosomal abnormalities can be demonstrated in about 10% of all cases of mental retardation. About 15% of all pediatric disorders are genetic; 2% of these are traceable to environmental agents. The etiology of the remainder is unknown.

Appraisal of the liveborn infant with a disorder involves a genetic workup and an evaluation of possible genetic-environmental interaction.

Genetic-environmental interaction

Basic to an understanding of the effects of genetic-environmental interaction on the unborn is a general knowledge of the normal timetable of embryonic development. Each organ or system undergoes a critical period of growth and development when it is most vulnerable to environmental insult (Fig. 7-1). During this critical period, teratogens may interrupt the process of normal tissue growth and differentiation, resulting in fetal malformations or disease syndromes (Fig. 7-2). The teratogenic effects of malnutrition, drugs, disease, and irradiation are in part determined by the time in

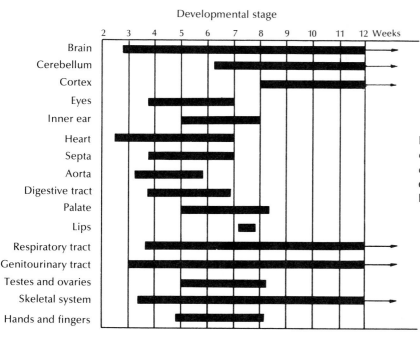

Fig. 7-1. Approximate periods of critical differentiation for some specific organs. (From Whaley, L. 1974. Understanding inherited disorders. St. Louis, The C. V. Mosby Co.)

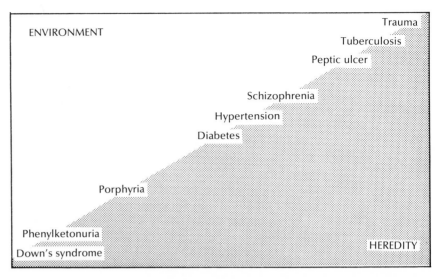

Fig. 7-2. Spectrum of diseases, indicating relative importance of genetic and environmental factors. (From Whaley, L. F. 1974. Understanding inherited disorders. St. Louis, The C. V. Mosby Co.)

ENVIRONMENT

Trauma
Tuberculosis
Peptic ulcer
Schizophrenia
Hypertension
Diabetes
Porphyria
Phenylketonuria
Down's syndrome

HEREDITY

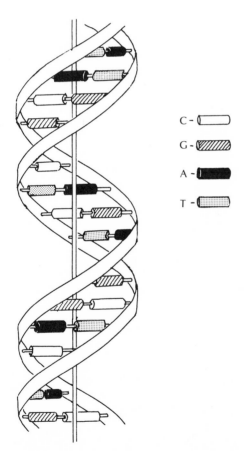

C -
G -
A -
T -

Fig. 7-3. DNA (deoxyribonucleic acid) molecule is composed of chains of smaller molecules called *nucleotides*. Nucleotides have a sugar base (deoxyribose), a phosphate base (phosphoric acid), and a nitrogenous base. *C*, cytosine; *G*, guanine; *A*, adenine; *T*, thymine. (From Whaley, L. F. 1974. Understanding inherited disorders. St. Louis, The C. V. Mosby Co.)

pregnancy at which the mother is exposed, the mother's general health and metabolism, and the dosage and route of entry of the offending agent.

Hereditary transmission

Mendel's laws. Mendel's laws of gene activity during gamete formation and fertilization are the foundation of the science of genetics. Generally, the nurse will not be the one who does in-depth genetic counseling, but a knowledge of Mendel's laws in the transmission of heritable characteristics is an essential tool for health workers.

Genes are the blueprints of life, governing the pattern and timing of the development of all living matter from conception through old age. Thousands of tiny units (genes) carry hereditary material on rod-shaped chromosomes. The double-stranded DNA molecules of gene material contain the genetic code and are capable of self-reproduction (Fig. 7-3).

Human genes are carried on 46 chromosomes in the nuclei of somatic cells. One chromosome from each of the 23 pairs (diploid number) is contributed by the mother, the other by the father. Twenty-two pairs are autosomes. One pair carries the sex trait: the normal female carries two X chromosomes; the normal male, one X and one Y. The presence of the Y chromosome is needed for the early development of male characteristics.

Genetically similar cells are reproduced by a process of cell division called *mitosis*. During mitosis, each chromosome splits into two chromatids connected by a centromere. The chromosomes are then aligned on a central spindle and divide through the center of the centro-

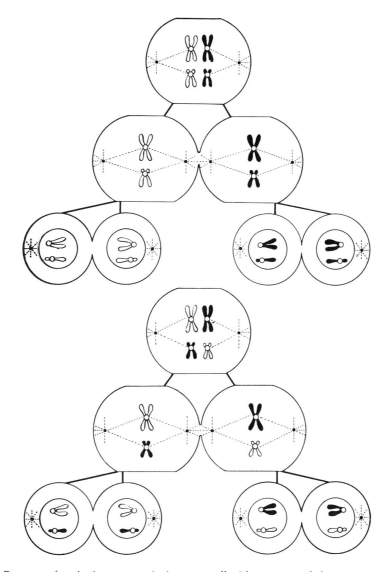

Fig. 7-4. Process of meiosis: a premeiotic germ cell with two sets of chromosomes forms four germ cells, each with single set of chromosomes. Two alternative arrangements of chromosome pairs on first meiotic spindle are diagrammed. (From McLennan, C. E., and Sandberg, E. C. 1974. Synopsis of obstetrics [ed. 7]. St. Louis, The C. V. Mosby Co.)

meres. After the chromatids separate, the cellular material is equally divided by cleavage.

Gametogenesis refers to that process by which germ cells divide and develop into ova and spermatozoa. Each ovum and spermatozoon contains 23 unpaired chromosomes, or the haploid number. *Meiosis* is that process of cell division which reduces the total number of chromosomes from 46 to 23 (Fig. 7-4). Each germ cell contains 23 chromosomes: 22 autosomes plus either one X or one Y sex chromosome. During gametogenesis, meiosis precedes mitosis and ova and spermatozoa formation (Fig. 7-5). Fertilization of an ovum by a spermatozoon

reestablishes a full complement of 46 chromosomes (Fig. 7-6).

Chromosomal abnormalities may occur during either mitotic or meiotic division, resulting in too much genetic material in some cells or too little in others (Fig. 7-7). Abnormalities in chromosomal structure or number occur in both autosomal and sex chromosomes.

Autosomal defects. Down's syndrome (mongolism) is the most frequently occurring autosomal defect (Fig. 7-8). In 95% of cases of mongolism, nondysjunction occurs during meiosis (usually in the female germ cell) of chromosome number 21 (Fig. 7-9). This results in

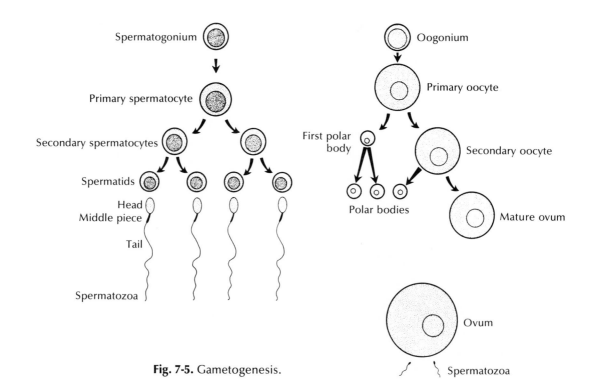

Fig. 7-5. Gametogenesis.

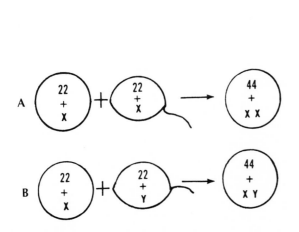

Fig. 7-6. A, Female and, **B,** male zygote. (From Willson, J. R., Beecham, C. T., and Carrington, E. R. 1975. Obstetrics and gynecology [ed. 5]. St. Louis, The C. V. Mosby Co.)

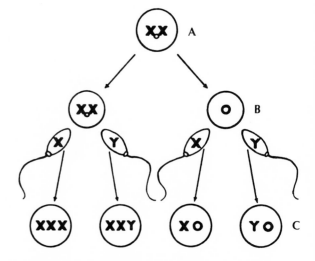

Fig. 7-7. Effects of nondisjunction during gametogenesis. **A,** Haploid daughter cell with two chromatids united by centromere. **B,** Nondisjunction. **C,** Four types of zygotes may be produced during fertilization. (From Willson, J. R., Beecham, C. T., and Carrington, E. R. 1975. Obstetrics and gynecology [ed. 5]. St. Louis, The C. V. Mosby Co.)

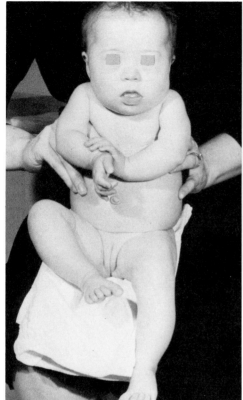

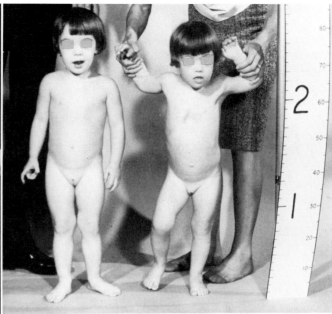

Fig. 7-8. A, Infant with Down's syndrome. **B,** Dizygotic twins: *left,* normal twin; *right,* twin with Down's syndrome. (Courtesy Frederick Hecht, M.D.)

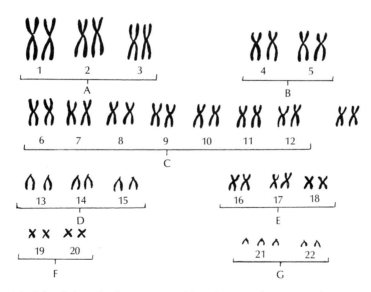

Fig. 7-9. Model of female karyotype with trisomy of 21 (G) chromosome group (47,XX,21+). (From Whaley, L. F. 1974. Understanding inherited disorders. St. Louis, The C. V. Mosby Co.)

germ cells carrying 24 or 22 chromosomes. Cells with 22 chromosomes are nonviable. When the ovum with 24 chromosomes is fertilized, an individual with 47 chromosomes results. Trisomy 21 (three of chromosome number 21) carries the clinical characteristics of Down's syndrome: small, round head with flattened occiput; large fat pads at nape of short neck; protruding tongue; small mouth and high palate; epicanthal folds with slanting palpebral fissures (mongoloid slant of eyes); hypotonic muscles with hypermobility of joints; short, broad hands with inward curved little finger and wide separation between thumb and index finger; transverse simian palmar crease (Fig. 7-10); and mental retardation. Feeding problems arise from poor sucking ability, and

there is a greater risk for upper respiratory tract infections.

The incidence of this type of chromosomal aberration increases with maternal age: in young mothers, 1 per 1000 to 2000 births; in women from 35 to 40 years of age, 1 per 300 births; and in mothers over 45 years of age, 1 per every 30 to 35 births.

In about 5% of cases, Down's syndrome is due to translocation or mosaicism. Translocation Down's syndrome is more common in younger mothers. In this circumstance, there are 46 total chromosomes but part of chromosome number 21 is added to another chromosome, usually number 14. Such a child presents with the same clinical features as in trisomy 21. Mothers of these

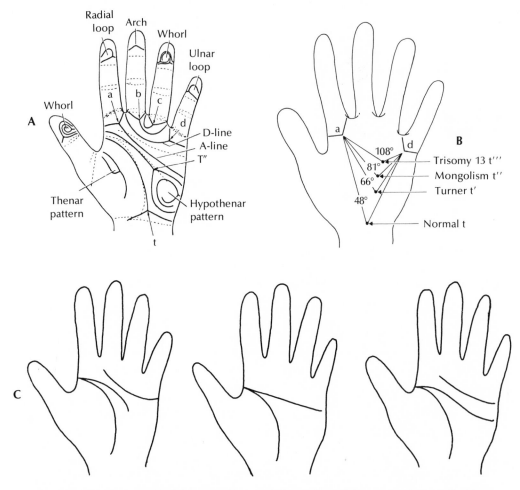

Fig. 7-10. **A,** Dermatoglyphics on palms and fingertips with nomenclature. **B,** Mean position of most triradius *t* in children up to 4 years of age. **C,** Examples of flexion creases on palm. *Left,* normal; *center,* simian line; *right,* Sydney line. (**A** and **B** from Penrose, L. S. 1963. Nature **197:**933; **C** from Whaley, L. F. 1974. Understanding inherited disorders. St. Louis, The C. V. Mosby Co.)

babies are at greater risk for the recurrence of the disorder in subsequent pregnancies.

Mosaicism is a condition in which some somatic cells are normal, whereas others have trisomy 21. The number of abnormal cells determines the degree to which characteristic clinical features of Down's syndrome are expressed.

It should be noted that children with Down's syndrome and their siblings are more prone to develop leukemia. The basis for this fact is unknown.

Cri du chat syndrome is the result of partial deletion of a portion of chromosome number 5. An infant with this disorder can easily be identified by his unique cry. *Cri du chat* is a French phrase meaning ''cry of a cat,'' which aptly describes the child's weak, high-pitched, ''meowlike'' cry. These children have small heads with widely spaced eyes, are profoundly retarded mentally, and fail to thrive.

Sex chromosome defects. Deletion of a sex chromosome may go unnoticed until adolescence or later when the individual seeks counseling for infertility. In Turner's syndrome, the dwarfed female has only 45 chromosomes (44 + X). This defect results in stunted growth, ''streak ovaries,'' and occasionally perceptual problems. A zygote with 45 chromosomes and a single Y chromosome is nonviable.

Males with 47 chromosomes (44 + XXY karyotype) (Klinefelter's syndrome) can appear to be normal, but others are mentally retarded and infertile. They are often taller and more aggressive and may display criminal behavior.

Individuals with 48 chromosomes (karotypes: female, 44 + XXXX; male, 44 + XXXY) generally have severe mental and physical abnormalities.

Individuals with 45 chromosomes, that is, lacking the second X chromosome or the Y chromosome (44 + XO), are hermaphrodites. They may possess genital organs of both sexes, and the diagnosis may be difficult or impossible by examination of external genitals alone.

Dominant trait transmission. For any given trait, an individual has two genes, one from each parent. The dominant or more vigorous of the two genes will be expressed in the identifiable characteristic, or *phenotype,* of the individual. The other, recessive gene will remain hidden but may be passed on to subsequent generations. The dominant gene is manifest whether it is heterozygous or homozygous.

In the example in Fig. 7-11, brown eye color (shaded area) is dominant over blue (white area). The line between the circles is the mating bar. The vertical line from the marriage bar identifies the offspring and the genetic combinations possible.

Recessive trait transmission. The autosomal recessive gene is manifested only in the homozygous state. In Fig. 7-11, blue eye color is recessive and is manifested in the homozygous state. One recessive gene comes from each parent carrier who may not show the trait. Similarly, some diseases that are recessive in nature may be

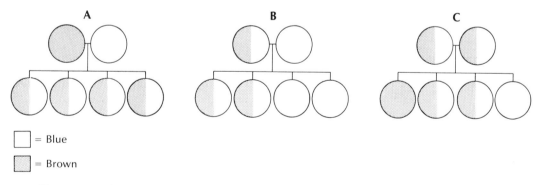

☐ = Blue

▨ = Brown

Fig. 7-11. A, If one parent is homozygous for brown eyes and the other is homozygous for blue eyes, their children's eye color will be as follows: genotype—100% heterozygous for brown and blue; phenotype—all have brown eyes; probability—all have brown eyes. **B,** If one parent is heterozygous for brown eyes and the other is homozygous for blue eyes, their children will present with the following: genotype—50% heterozygous for brown and 50% homozygous for blue; phenotype—two have brown eyes, and two have blue eyes; probability—50/50 for brown, 50/50 for blue. **C,** If both parents are both heterozygous for brown, their children's eye color will be as follows: genotype—25% homozygous for brown, 50% heterozygous for brown, and 25% homozygous for blue; phenotype—three brown-eyed children and one blue-eyed child; probability—75/25 for brown.

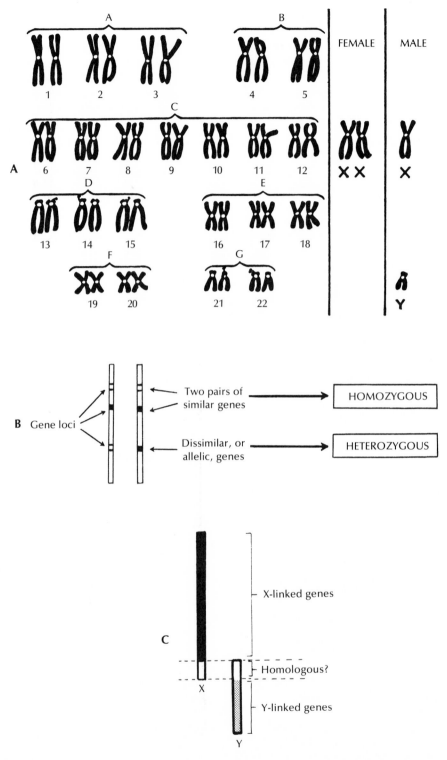

Fig. 7-12. A, Idiogram of human chromosomes—International System of Nomenclature (Denver). **B,** One pair of homologous chromosomes with similar and dissimilar genes at three gene loci. **C,** X and Y chromosomes. (**A** from Eggen, R. R. 1963. Am. J. Clin. Pathol. **39**:10; **B** and **C** from Whaley, L. F. 1974. Understanding inherited disorders. St. Louis, The C. V. Mosby Co.)

carried in the heterozygous state by persons who may seem clinically normal (e.g., cystic fibrosis). In instances of recessive trait transmission, the probability of appearance of the trait in each offspring in only 1:4 or 25%. Despite this favorable risk factor, it is possible for each offspring of a couple to be homozygous for the recessive trait.

Most structural disorders of the infant result from dominant genes, whereas errors of metabolism are primarily the expression of recessive genes (Whaley, 1974).

Some autosomal recessive genes do exert their influence in the heterozygous carrier. The carrier of a recessive gene for cystic fibrosis may be more prone to respiratory problems throughout his life. Persons with sickle cell trait may have less stamina and resilience to physiologic stress such as excessive physical exertion, infection, and high altitude. Women with sickle cell disease may have more pregnancy complications and should never receive general anesthetic agents. Women with the disease or the trait should be cautioned against the use of oral contraceptives because the risk of complications is greatly increased.

Sex-linked transmission. A trait that is carried on a sex chromosome (usually the X chromosome) is known as sex linked (or X linked) and may be dominant or recessive. Mendelian laws prevail in the patterns of transmission. However, unlike autosomes, sex chromosomes are dissimilar in morphology and gene complement. Therefore the pattern of transmission will be affected depending on the sex of the individual. The female sex chromosomes (XX) are homologous, that is, females are heterozygous or homozygous for genes at all loci (or sites) on the X chromosomes. The male sex chromosomes, one X and one Y, are not homologous. Males with only one X chromosome are hemizygous (having only one gene) with no counterpart on the Y chromosome (Fig. 7-12). The single genes on the male's X chromosome are therefore always expressed. One indication for an X-linked (sex-linked) trait is a pedigree that shows no father-to-son transmission of that trait. (For more information, see Whaley, 1974.) An example of X-linked, dominant inheritance is the rarely seen skeletal disease in children, vitamin D-resistant (hypophosphatemic) rickets.

X-linked recessive disorders are more prevalent than the X-linked dominant disorders. Examples of serious conditions with this X-linked inheritance pattern are hemophilia, a disorder resulting in an abnormally prolonged blood-clotting time; Duchenne-type of muscular dystrophy; nephrogenic diabetes insipidus; and one form of hydrocephalus.

An X-linked recessive trait may be identified by its pattern of transmission as follows: (1) the disorder is found primarily in males; (2) the parents of the affected individual, or proband, do not manifest the trait; (3) each daughter will be a carrier, whereas none of the sons will be affected; (4) unaffected brothers of an affected male will not transmit the trait; (5) 50% of all affected males' sisters are carriers; and (6) unaffected sons of a carrier-female do not transmit the trait (Fig. 7-13).

Fig. 7-14 is an example of a pedigree of a family affected by an X-linked disorder.

Inborn errors of metabolism. Disorders of protein, fat, or carbohydrate metabolism reflecting absent or defective enzymes generally follow a recessive pattern of inheritance. Enzymes, the actions of which are genetically determined, are essential for all the physical and chemical processes that sustain body systems. Defective enzyme action interrupts the normal series of chemical reactions from the affected point onward. The result may be an accumulation of a damaging product such as phenylalanine or the absence of a necessary product such as thyroxin or melanin (Fig. 7-15). (See Appendix H for screening tests for inborn errors of metabolism.)

Phenylketonuria (PKU) is an uncommon disorder due to autosomal recessive genes. Heterozygous carriers and affected infants may be identified by genetic screening methods. A deficiency in the liver enzyme phenylalanine hydroxylase results in failure to metabolize the amino acid phenylalanine, allowing its metabolites to accumulate in the blood (Fig. 7-16).

The incidence of this disorder is 1 per every 10,000 to 20,000 births. The highest incidence is found in whites (from northern Europe and the United States). It is rarely seen in Jewish, African, or Japanese populations.

Clinical features of PKU include a normal-appearing newborn, usually with blonde hair, blue eyes, and fair skin. If undetected and untreated, these infants experience vomiting, fail to thrive, and develop eczematous rashes. By about 6 months of age, symptoms of mental retardation and evidence of other central nervous system (CNS) involvement (seizures, abnormal EEG) begin to appear. State laws mandate that screening tests be carried out in newborn nurseries to identify the child with PKU (p. 632 and Appendix H).

Phenylalanine is an essential amino acid found in animal and vegetable protein. Treatment of PKU is dietary. A diet is prepared to limit ingestion of phenylalanine to 10 to 20 mg/kg/24 hr (normal intake is 100 to 200 mg/kg/24 hr) to maintain low blood levels of phenylalanine at 2 to 6 mg/100 ml. A special protein formula such as Lofenalac may be fed to the infant. Lofenalac is a special casein hydrolysate that also provides a balanced

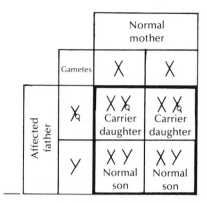

Fig. 7-13. Punnett square illustrating sex differences in offspring ratios in X-linked recessive inheritance. ◯ = Recessive allele on X chromosome. (From Whaley, L. F. 1974. Understanding inherited disorders. St. Louis, The C. V. Mosby Co.)

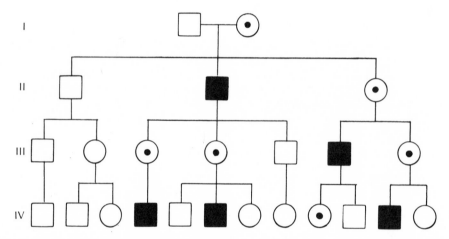

Fig. 7-14. X-linked recessive inheritance pattern. ⊙ = carrier female; ■ = affected male. (From Whaley, L. F. 1974. Understanding inherited disorders. St. Louis, The C. V. Mosby Co.)

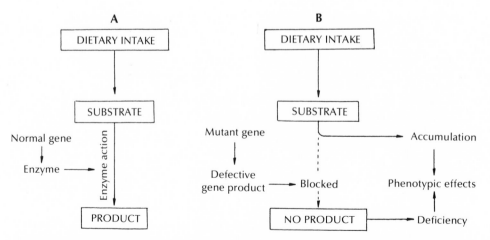

Fig. 7-15. A, Normal metabolic pathway. **B,** Effect of defective gene action. (From Whaley, L. F. 1974. Understanding inherited disorders. St. Louis, The C. V. Mosby Co.)

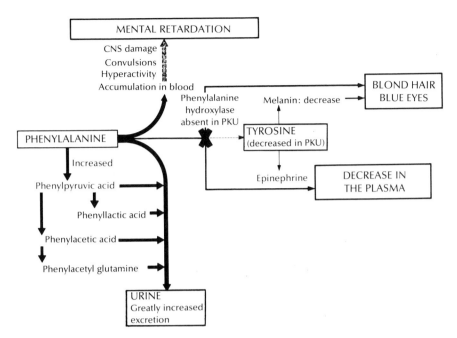

Fig. 7-16. Metabolic error in phenylketonuria. Because of absence of phenylalanine hydroxylase, essential amino acid phenylalanine cannot be converted to tyrosine. (From Williams, S. R. 1973. Nutrition and diet therapy [ed. 2]. St. Louis, The C. V. Mosby Co.)

proportion of fat, carbohydrate, vitamins, and minerals. Food lists are available to assist families with the special diet (Appendix F). If the diet is started before 3 months of age and continued until at least 3 or 4 years of age, damage to the central nervous system can be minimized. This is the period of most rapid myelinization of the central nervous system.

Women with PKU have a higher incidence of spontaneous abortion. If they carry the infant to term and are not on a low phenylalanine diet, infants generally will be small for dates and often display varied abnormalities. Because maternal phenylalanine crosses the placenta during pregnancy, a low-phenylalanine diet should be reinstituted to prevent fetal damage.

Tay-Sachs disease, inherited as an autosomal recessive trait, results from a deficiency of hexosaminidase. It occurs primarily in Jewish families. Until 4 to 6 months of age, infants appear normal; in fact, these infants are considered very beautiful. Then the clinical symptoms begin to appear: apathy and regression in motor and social development and decreased vision. Death occurs between 3 and 4 years of age. There is as yet no known treatment for Tay-Sachs disease. In subsequent pregnancies amniocentesis may be performed on patients who have delivered infants with this condition.

Cystic fibrosis (mucoviscidosis or fibrocystic disease

of the pancreas) is inherited as an autosomal recessive trait characterized by generalized involvement of exocrine glands. It is a serious chronic disease occurring primarily in whites but can appear in those of mixed ancestry. Overall incidence is 1 per every 2000 births. It is thought that the carrier state is 1:20 to 25 (Whaley, 1974). Advances in diagnosis and treatment have improved the prognosis so that now many affected individuals live to adulthood. Some affected women have borne children, but men generally are sterile.

Clinical features are related to the altered viscosity of mucus-secreting glands throughout the body. This thick, inspissated mucoprotein clogs and dilates glands, impairing their function. Digestion and absorption are diminished by the absence of pancreatic enzymes (trypsin, amylase, lipase). Thick mucus threatens ventilatory function. Chronic obstructive pulmonary disease is characteristic. Abnormally large amounts of salt (sodium chloride) are lost through the skin. (This symptom forms the basis for the sweat test, pilocarpine electrophoresis.) Cirrhosis of the liver may result from obstruction of bile ducts. Repeated pulmonary infection and chronic malnutrition affect others.

Although the infant often appears normal initially, deficiency in digestion and absorption is demonstrated eventually. The time of appearance of symptoms varies with the severity of the disease. Occasionally mothers note the first symptom a few months after birth—the infant's skin is salty when she kisses him. A classic symptom is the passage of foul-smelling, bulky, musky, foamy, often clay-colored steatorrheic stools.

Meconium ileus occurs in about 10% of newborns with cystic fibrosis. Although an initial stool may be passed from the rectum with none thereafter, no meconium is usually passed during the first 24 to 48 hours, the abdomen becomes increasingly distended, and eventually the newborn requires a laparotomy for diagnosis and treatment of the condition.

Treatment requires (1) management of pulmonary secretions and respiratory tract infections, (2) dietary replacement of pancreatic enzymes (Cotazyme or Viokase) and salt (sodium chloride), (3) a diet high in calories, protein, and water-soluble vitamins, moderate in carbohydrates, and low in fat.

Polygenic trait transmission. The inheritance pattern for many congenital abnormalities is not clear, but these disorders often cluster in families. The abnormalities may be the result of additive effects of aberrant genes at separate loci on several chromosomes. The recurrence risk varies with the number of members of a family who have the disorder. Some congenital abnormalities in this category are cleft lip, cleft palate, spina bifida and other neural tube defects, and pyloric stenosis.

METHODS OF CLINICAL EVALUATION

Clinical evaluation of heritable or congenital problems can be psychologically threatening. The nurse's critical contribution is in understanding human behavior and responses in this crisis and employing interviewing and explanatory techniques based on this understanding. The nurse should be cognizant of factors that inhibit coping and learning (hate, fear, resentment, anxiety, grief). Anticipatory guidance and teaching are not fact-giving activities. To be effective, teaching must deal first with feelings. The effectiveness of nursing intervention is enhanced by a relaxed, comfortable atmosphere. The nurse should remain sensitive to the individual's or family's attitude toward the disorder and discuss it with them in terms they can understand.

The nurse assists parents in the following ways:
- Helping them identify their concerns and questions
- Sorting out knowledge and facts
- Clarifying misconceptions
- Filling gaps in information
- Repeating information as often as necessary
- Suggesting alternatives
- Referring the family to other resources when appropriate

Since tests used in clinical evaluation are anxiety-producing, the nurse can strengthen the parents' coping strategies by discussing the expected procedures initially. The nurse's technical theory base can be enlarged by an appreciation of the various methods of clinical evaluation.

Effective and appropriate counseling is based on careful clinical evaluation and proper diagnosis. Is the disorder truly genetic? Are there nongenetic etiologies involved? Do other family members need to be examined? A systematic approach is suggested in answering these questions.

Certain of the following procedures and diagnostic tests may be required to identify the genetic or genetic-environmental causes of a disorder. In Table 7-1, congenital heart defects that are apparent in the neonatal period are summarized along with probable diagnostic methods.

Pedigree chart. Constructing a pedigree chart, also known as a *family tree,* aids in discerning patterns of distribution of specific traits in families. The chart is actually a type of shorthand in which data is expressed symbolically (Fig. 7-17). Affected and nonaffected individuals and relationships are indicated by standardized tests.

The *proband,* or *propositus,* is the affected individual. He is the *index case* on whom the chart is developed. His parents are designated by a single line or marriage bar; the male is represented by a square and the female by a circle. A parental consanguineous relationship is shown as a double bar. Siblings are indicated on a horizontal line by Arabic number, with the firstborn on the left. Generations are identified by Roman numeral in a vertical column in the left margin. (For other symbols refer to Fig. 7-17.)

A carefully constructed pedigree may identify mutant genes, as well as recessive genes and carrier states.

The chart should be as extensive as possible, noting normal as well as affected family members. A direct examination of family members may be helpful. If family members are deceased, old records such as family Bibles should be consulted. Photographs may be helpful.

The nurse may not be the one who constructs the chart. Nevertheless, she can be instrumental in encouraging the parents' cooperation and increasing their motivation in supplying data.

Buccal smear. The buccal smear is a simple, convenient, and inexpensive sex chromatin test. Although cells from any tissue are suitable, those on the inside of the cheek are easily accessible. Gentle scraping of the mucosa is sufficient. These cells are spread on a slide, fixed, stained, and evaluated.

Table 7-1. Summary of congenital heart defects (CHD) and clinical diagnostic tools (in addition to physical examination and pedigree)*

Anomaly	Male to female ratio	Definition	Percentage of incidence of CHD in infants†	Disorders associated with increased incidence	Method of clinical evaluation
Ventricular septal defect (VSD)	1:1	Abnormal opening between ventricles	28.3	Down's syndrome (genetic)	Dermatoglyphics Karyotype
Patent ductus arteriosus (PDA)	1:3	Persistence of fetal connection between aorta and pulmonary artery	12.5	Rubella syndrome (environmental)	Viral titer and culture History of exposure
Atrial septal defect (ASD)	1:3	Abnormal opening between the atria	9.7	Holt-Oram syndrome, Down's syndrome (genetic)	Dermatoglyphics Karyotype
Coarctation of aorta	4:1	Stricture in thoracic aorta	8.8	Turner's syndrome (genetic)	Buccal smear Karyotype Dermatoglyphics
Transposition of great vessels (TGV)	3:1	Reversal in origin of great vessels—aorta from right ventricle and pulmonary artery from left ventricle	8.0	Diabetes or prediabetes in the mother (genetic and environmental)	Biochemical studies on mother
Tetralogy of Fallot	1:1	Ventricular septal defect and pulmonic stenosis with right ventricular hypertrophy and aorta overriding ventricular septum	7.0	Thalidomide ingestion (environmental)	History of ingestion
Pulmonic stenosis	1:1	Narrowing of opening into pulmonary artery	6.0		
Aortic stenosis	4:1	Narrowing of opening into aorta	3.5		
Truncus arteriosus	1:1	One large single vessel leaving base of heart	2.7	Thalidomide ingestion (environmental)	History of ingestion
Other			13.5		

*Modified from Whaley, L. F. 1974. Understanding inherited disorders. St. Louis, The C. V. Mosby Co., p. 149; based on data from Perloff, J. K. 1970. The clinical recognition of congenital heart disease. Philadelphia, W. B. Saunders Co.; and Warkany, J. 1971. Congenital malformations. Chicago, Year Book Medical Publishers, Inc.

†Data from Campbell, M. 1968. In Watson, A., (ed.). Paediatric cardiology. London, Lloyd-Luke, Ltd.

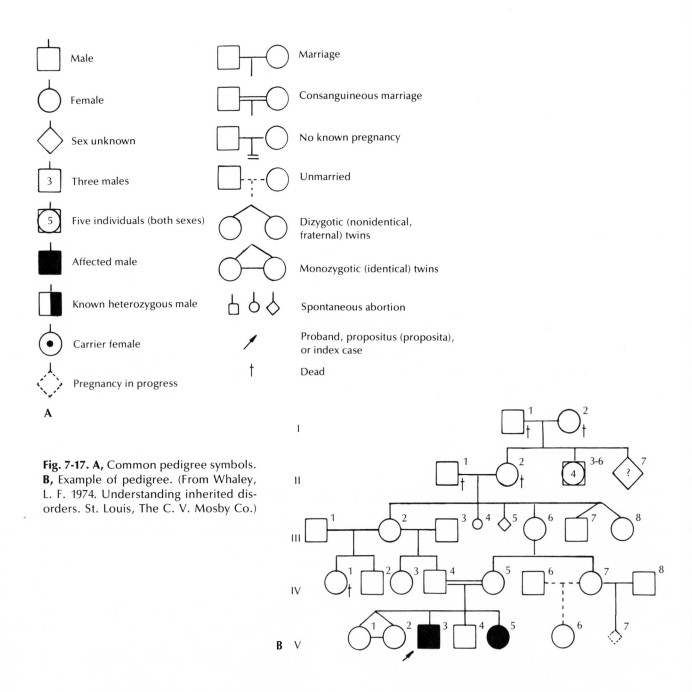

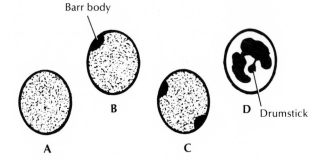

Fig. 7-17. A, Common pedigree symbols. **B,** Example of pedigree. (From Whaley, L. F. 1974. Understanding inherited disorders. St. Louis, The C. V. Mosby Co.)

Fig. 7-18. Sex chromatin, or Barr body. **A,** No sex chromatin is found in normal male somatic cells. **B,** One Barr body is normal in female somatic cells. **C,** Two Barr bodies are found in cells with three X chromosomes (XXX or XXXY). **D,** "Drumstick" is found in many polymorphonuclear leukocytes of normal female. (From Whaley, L. F. 1974. Understanding inherited disorders. St. Louis, The C. V. Mosby Co.)

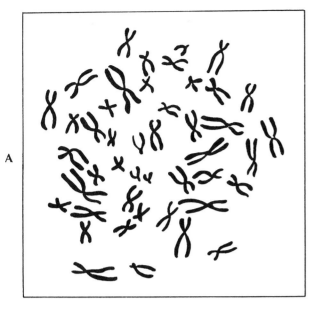

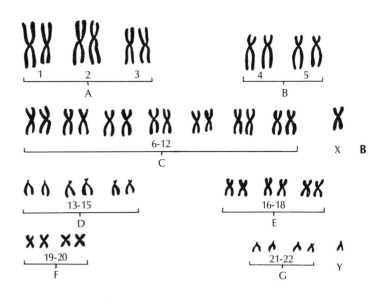

Fig. 7-19. Metaphase spread of male chromosomes. **A,** Example of photomicrograph. **B,** Chromosomes arranged in karyotype. (From Whaley, L. F. 1974. Understanding inherited disorders. St. Louis, The C. V. Mosby Co.)

The sex chromatin lump, or *Barr body,* is found in normal female somatic cells; a single Barr body is observed in the XX female. Females with XO genotype are chromatin-negative (no Barr body is present); males with XXY are chromatin-positive (show one Barr body). The number of Barr bodies is consistently one less than the number of X chromosomes in the genotype (Fig. 7-18).

Many individuals with an excess number of sex chromosomes are mentally deficient, and almost all are sterile. Frequently, this excess is not recognized until adulthood when infertility studies are initiated.

Chromosome analysis. Frequently, chromosomal studies are necessary to prove that a defect has a genetic etiology. Cytogenetic techniques are now available to determine the number, shape, and structural aberrations in the autosomal and sex chromosomes.

Chromosomes can only be identified during the time they are dividing. Cell specimens must be capable of growth and division outside the body. The most suitable cells are taken from skin, fascia, bone marrow, or blood. Leukocytes from peripheral blood supplies are commonly used because they are easily obtained and cultured.

The cells are grown for 3 days in culture tubes at body temperature. Cell division must then be arrested at the metaphase stage when the chromosomes can be most easily identified. Colchicine is the drug most often utilized to arrest cell division.

Placed in a hypotonic solution, the cells swell, causing the chromosomes to spread apart. These cells are placed on a slide, fixed, stained, and photographed under high magnification. The photomicrograph is enlarged, and each chromosome is cut out and arranged in a systematic fashion called a *karyotype* (Fig. 7-19).

Detection of heterozygous states. Tests for determining heterozygous states vary with the condition, only a few of which will be mentioned here.

1. *PKU.* Suspects are given phenylalanine. Carriers demonstrate higher plasma levels of this amino acid.

2. *Tay-Sachs disease.* Carriers demonstrate lower levels of hexosaminidase in blood plasma. Tests are being perfected to detect the affected fetus in utero.

3. *Sickle cell anemia.* The sickle cell trait can be identified in several ways. Two methods are the electrophoretic examination of hemoglobin in the blood and the sickle-turbidity tube test. When an electrophoretic examination is performed, the blood of a person with sickle cell anemia may show two types of hemoglobin: hemoglobin A (normal) and sickle hemoglobins.

The sickle-turbidity tube test (Sickledex) is a quick test that distinguishes sickle hemoglobin from normal hemoglobin. A small amount of blood is placed in a test tube with Sickledex solution and allowed to stand for 5 minutes. The appearance of a cloudy, turbid suspension indicates a positive test; a transparent suspension is a negative test. This test does not distinguish between the

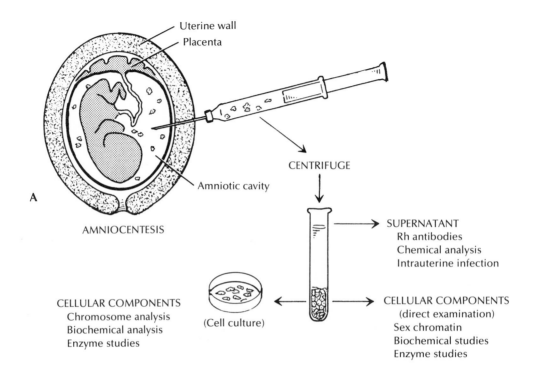

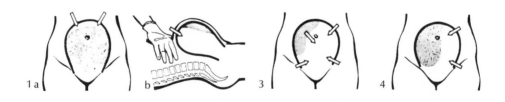

B

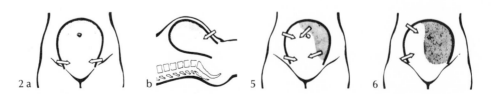

Fig. 7-20. A, Amniocentesis and laboratory utilization of amniotic fluid aspirant. **B,** *1a, 2a, 3, 4, 5,* and *6* are front views with arrows indicating appropriate sites for amniocentesis varying with placental position. *1b* and *2b* are side views. (**A** from Whaley, L. F. 1974. Understanding inherited disorders. St. Louis, The C. V. Mosby Co.; **B** from Hoffbauer, H. 1969. In Huntingford, P. J., Huter, K., and Saling, E. [eds.]. Perinatal medicine. Stuttgart, Georg Thieme Verlag.)

anemia and the trait; in both cases, results are positive. This method is appropriate for mass screening; those whose tests are positive should undergo the electrophoretic test to differentiate between the trait and sickle cell disease.

Amniotic fluid studies. Amniocentesis may be performed between the fourteenth and sixteenth week of gestation. The placenta is located by radiography or sonography to avoid trauma from the needle (Fig. 7-20). Amniocentesis and fluid removal is done under local anesthesia. Amniotic fluid normally contains fetal urine, secretions, cells shed from the respiratory tract, and desquamated skin cells. This material must be centrifuged and cells separated from the fluid component. The cells are then subjected to cytogenetic and enzyme studies and biochemical analysis. Cells may be cultured and prepared to determine karyotypes. The sex of the fetus may be determined by a test for Barr bodies. Fluorescent microscopy of exfoliative fetal cells should reveal the bright Y chromosome in males. The supernatant fluid can also be used for examination for Rh antibodies, presence of degradation products of bilirubin by spectrophotometric analysis, and intrauterine infection.

Amniocentesis is indicated in the following cases:

1. Pregnant women 40 years and older
2. Couples who already have borne one child with a genetic disorder
3. To determine a carrier state of a recessive, single-gene disorder by both parents
4. To determine the presence of an X-linked disorder in a male fetus

5. When one or both parents are affected with a genetic disorder

Amniocentesis is performed to determine the management of the pregnancy. It is often effected on the premise that elective abortion may be performed if an affected fetus is found. If the parents will not consider elective abortion, the procedure may not be warranted.

Dermatoglyphics. The arches, loops, and whorls in finger and toe prints and the palm creases are genetically determined. The numerous genes for dermal ridge patterns occur on many different chromosomes. Abnormalities of chromosomes affect the development of dermal ridge patterns, as well as organs and systems. Dermal ridge patterns that have been analyzed are the palm lines, fingerprints, flexion creases, and soles (Fig. 7-21). This discussion will be limited to characteristic alterations in dermal patterns in a small number of clinical syndromes (Fig. 7-22).

A person with Down's syndrome, or trisomy 21, characteristically presents with a single palmar crease, or simian line (Fig. 7-10, *C*) and an excess of ulnar loops.

Characteristic palm creases have been noted in a significant number of children with rubella syndrome and leukemia. The Sydney line (Fig. 7-10, *C*) has been observed more frequently in children with rubella syndrome than in controls and in 16% of children with leukemia (Whaley, 1974). Certain fingerprint patterns may be found in individuals who suffer cardiac valvular problems later in life.

Microbial detection. Some fetal dysfunctions or malformations result from maternal infection that is trans-

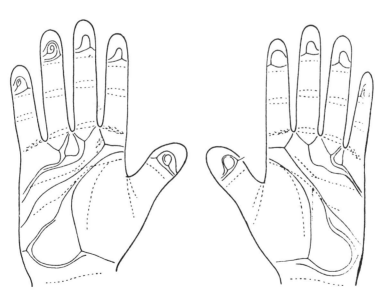

Fig. 7-21. Examples of dermatoglyphics in male with XXXXY sex chromosomes. (From Levine, L. 1971. Papers on genetics—a book of readings. St. Louis, The C. V. Mosby Co.)

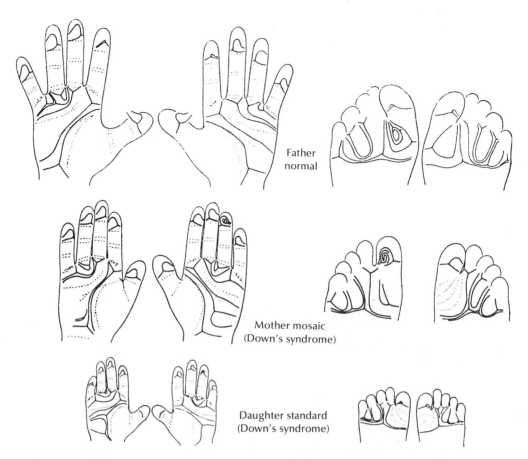

Fig. 7-22. Palms and soles in family with mosaic Down's mother and standard Down's daughters. (From Levine, L. 1971. Papers on genetics—a book of readings. St. Louis, The C. V. Mosby Co.)

mitted to the fetus through the placenta or acquired by the fetus from infected amniotic fluid and the birth canal. Infections with teratogenic potential should be ruled out prior to extensive genetic testing. Table 7-2 contains laboratory tests useful in detecting infection.

GOALS OF GENETIC COUNSELING

One goal of genetic counseling is to identify genetically transmissible malformations and disease syndromes and determine probability risks for their recurrence. A second goal is antenatal identification to anticipate potential fetal and/or neonatal problems and assure early diagnosis and management of the fetus or newborn. A third goal of genetic counseling is the ultimate reduction in the number of births of children with inheritable disorders.

Meanwhile, researchers continue to develop therapies for heritable diseases. Some possible methods of future management include replacement or stabilization by pills, injections, or other methods, altering intracellular

DNA, and other projected feats of genetic engineering (Whaley, 1974). Cloning, or gene grafting, a new frontier in the science of gene manipulation, has been furthered by the development and production of a molecular glue from thymus glands. Now it is possible not only to separate but also to recombine the DNA molecule. Given this ability to recode the instructions within body cells, techniques may be developed to correct faulty DNA causing various genetic diseases such as sickle cell anemia and acquired diseases such as cancer.

These goals pose many medical, legal, and ethical issues. Societies will have to grapple with basic questions regarding man and his destiny and his rights as an individual versus the rights of society. These issues become paramount as the world's ecologic problems grow in scope and magnitude.

The third goal of genetic counseling can be accomplished by means of restricted reproduction, appropriate mating, intrauterine diagnosis, and elective abortion. It

Table 7-2. Detection of maternal infection

Infection and causative microbe	Specimen		Laboratory tests
	Mother	**Fetus/newborn**	
Coxsackievirus (B) disease		Throat washings Stools	Culture of the virus
Cytomegalic inclusion (CID) disease Salivary gland virus	Sera Saliva Urine Vaginal Breast milk		Complement-fixation antibodies Fluorescent antibody test
		Cells from CNS and viscera	Intracellular inclusion bodies seen within cells
Infectious hepatitis (virus A)	Blood	Blood	Complement-fixation antibodies Culture of the virus
Rubella (virus)	Blood		Hemagglutinin inhibition (HI) IgM fluorescent antibody test
		Pharyngeal washings Urine	Viral culture (difficult)
Syphilis (spirochete *Treponema pallidum*)	Blood Lesions	Blood Lesions	STS (serum test for syphilis) Dark field
Toxoplasmosis (parasite)	Blood	Blood	IgM fluorescent antibody test Sabin-Feldman dye test

is the responsibility of health professionals to correct misconceptions or false assumptions and to provide information and support; the final choice remains with the individual or couple.

ROLE OF NURSE IN INTERVENTION WITH PARENTS AFTER BIRTH OF CHILD WITH DISORDER

The birth of a child with an obvious defect is a shattering experience for parents and a disturbing experience for those who attend the birth. Parents feel devastated and inadequate; anticipated joy ends in despair and confusion. A flurry of activity often follows such a birth. The child may then be examined by specialists, often at a facility far from the mother's hospital. Physicians and others (e.g., clergy) may talk with the parents. The natural order of postnatal psychologic tasks is disrupted. The new parents are in crisis. The nurse is in a unique and critical position. Of all the members of the health team, the nurse alone can be available to the patient 24 hours a day. A nurse can help plan for discharge and postdischarge care. Although the nurse's clinical inter-

vention will vary with each situation, in every case she must establish herself as a caring, knowledgeable, resourceful person.

Whether the child is premature, ill, or has a defect, the parental responses and needs are similar in many respects. In general, the couple's needs can be summarized to include (1) mourning the loss of the fantasized perfect baby, (2) immediate diagnosis and management of the neonate, (3) clinical evaluation and diagnosis of the causes of the infant's disorder, (4) when appropriate, preparation and planning for the continued care of the affected newborn, (5) redefinition of their parental role in their social network (i.e., reentrance into their society), and (6) family planning and genetic counseling. Nursing management is planned to help parents meet these needs.

Mourning loss of the perfect child

Grieving is the first difficult task of the new parents of a child with a malformation or disorder. Psychologic shock frequently coupled with the necessity of physical separation from the infant make this a trying and vulnerable period. Resolution of grief for the lost, assumed-perfect child precedes the development of acceptance or attachment to the real imperfect child or any decisions regarding his placement. The period of acute grief is usually about 6 weeks; however, in the continued presence of a child with a defect, grief may become chronic and persist for a lifetime.

The parents are profoundly affected by the manner and attitudes of those around them, especially the medical and nursing personnel. Parents are sensitive to and respond quickly to nonverbal cues from others that may connote nonacceptance, revulsion, or blame. Voice inflections, facial expressions, or the posture of the nurse who witnesses parental grief reactions or views the infant is quickly noted and internalized. Nurses also are representatives of society and may reflect society's reactions to them as parents of a child who is less than perfect.

Early mother-child relationship. Interaction between parent and child in the immediate postnatal period is important in the development of potential maternal feelings. If a parent does not have the opportunity to see, hold, and fondle the child early and often after birth, parental feelings and the development of parenting skills are adversely affected. The very small premature infant, the sick infant, or a child with a serious congenital disorder may have to be taken to another institution immediately after birth, an event that can cause the mother to feel psychologically estranged from her infant.

Continuing parent-child relationship. The skilled medical and nursing care required by the infant in this period, which the parents cannot provide, may be overwhelming. In fact, they may focus on the gadgetry—the machines, tubes, and bottles—associated with the infant's care rather than on the infant.

Parents need to ''keep in touch'' with the infant somehow. This may be accomplished by viewing the infant frequently and at close range and hearing frequent progress reports and answers to their questions. At other times, parents may be permitted to touch, fondle, and stroke the infant when it is still not practical to involve them in actual feeding and bathing. During these initial contacts, and until parents gain in self-confidence, the nurse should remain nearby, offering support as needed.

If the infant's hospitalization is prolonged, the nursing staff should keep the parents informed of the infant's progress with telephone calls and notes ''from the baby.''

Parents and nurse may feel frustrated, uncomfortable,

and even helpless when faced with the birth of a child with a defect. However, parents and nurse can grow from this mutually shared experience. Touching and sharing another's experience of loss can be threatening but also rewarding.

Families' grief reactions. Grandparents may take this opportunity to blame the other parent's family, with remarks such as ''We've never had this happen in *our* family before—ever.'' Other comments that are frequently heard include, ''The women in *our* family have never had problems having babies'' and ''I told him (her) that nothing good would come of this marriage (relationship).''

Comments such as these from members of the parents' families may mask hidden feelings of inadequacy about themselves, a deep concern for the young mother or couple, feelings of helplessness in the situation, concern by the grandparents that there may be no grandchild and therefore no immortality for them, and many other emotional reactions.

The nurse must avoid the pitfall of ''taking sides.'' Patience, tact, and warm sympathy coupled with efforts to help family members identify and explore feelings, clarify misconceptions, and provide simple cogent explanations may contribute to the comfort, strength, and unity of the entire family.

Immediate diagnosis and management of child

Diagnosing the disorder and initiating appropriate therapy is the physician's responsibility; however, the nurse must be conversant with diagnostic techniques and rationales for therapy to reinforce and clarify the physician's explanations. If possible, the nurse should sit in with the parents and physician during their sessions to know what is being said. Open lines of communication between physician and nurse, always essential, are vital now. One nursing function is to assist parents to identify and verbalize their questions, as well as their misgivings and fears. The nurse must deal with those questions and concerns within her realm of expertise and channel others to appropriate team members.

Clinical evaluation and diagnosis of causes

The history taking and diagnostic procedures necessary to uncover the etiology are exacting. One is asked to look for disorders in ancestors, to explore acts of omission and commission prenatally (e.g., nutrition, drugs), and to seek out other environmental factors.

Parents may express feelings of shame and embarrassment lest they be carrying a "bad" gene or be responsible for exposure to a devastating environmental agent. Others are anxious to fix the blame somewhere. Many women remember transient (or persistent) negative feelings about the pregnancy or baby and interpret this as punishment for their real or imagined transgressions.

The nurse's role must be supportive: preparing parents for what to expect and allowing for anticipatory worry, listening actively, and assisting with the formulation of questions and the ventilation of feelings.

Long-term management of child

Long-term management of a child with a disorder necessitates multidisciplinary planning and cooperation and a coordinated program of continual guidance and counseling of the parents. The emotional, physical, and financial status of the parents, available community resources, and the child's condition must be evaluated.

The nurse's role varies with the situation: Is the defect obvious? Is it curable? Is it treatable? How do parents perceive the disorder? Skillfully executed, the nurse's supportive function aids parents in decision making and in self-acceptance regarding their decisions (e.g., surgeries, institutionalization).

If the child requires medications, diet, or physical manipulation, the nurse should assist in the teaching of how, when, and why. Parents will benefit from supervised practice prior to discharge and frequent positive reinforcement of their ability to perform necessary tasks.

Community resources should be tapped to assist with the financial burden, equipment, drugs, and psychologic support (Appendix N). For example, in the San Francisco Bay Area, there is a group of parents of children with cleft lip and palate who meet to share feelings, problems, techniques, and new developments. A social worker may have the prime responsibility in this area of management, but the nurse should be cognizant of re-

---

PLAN OF CARE: GENETICS AND GENETIC COUNSELING

PATIENT CARE OBJECTIVES
1. Parents use the decision-making process to come to an acceptance of their problem to enable them to live with the decision.
2. There are no physical sequelae that would harm either the mother or father if abortion is not contemplated.
3. If abortion is the method of solution selected by parents, the necessary physical and emotional support is given for the process.

NURSING INTERVENTIONS

Diagnostic	Therapeutic and educational

1. Birth of infant with disorder
2. Pedigree chart
3. Chromosome analysis
4. Detection of heterozygous state
  a. Tay-Sachs disease
  b. Sickle cell anemia
  c. Rh factor
5. Amniocentesis with examination of supernatant fluid and cells
6. Buccal smear
7. Viral titers and cultures
8. Dermatoglyphics
9. Urinary clearance tests (PKU)
	1. Identification of populations at risk and developing and encouraging mass screening
	2. Public education
	  a. Hereditary transmission
	  b. Genetic-environmental interaction
	  c. Spontaneous mutations
	3. Prepregnancy counseling
	  a. Populations at risk
	  b. Risk probabilities based on individual's family history
	  c. Amniocentesis with option of selective abortion
	4. Care of families after birth of child with defect: supportive care*
	  a. Mourning
	  b. Immediate diagnosis and management of child
	  c. Clinical evaluation and diagnosis of causes
	  d. Long-term management of child (whether home or institutional)
	  e. Redefinition of parental role and social network and reentry into network with child with defect
	  f. Family planning and genetic counseling

*Supportive care includes assisting family to mourn effectively and to identify, formulate, and verbalize concerns; providing information, filling in gaps, and clarifying misconceptions; facilitating parental (and familial) problem-solving; identifying community resources for family to use as needed; and keeping an open channel of communication between family and medical-nursing–social service personnel.

sources also, and visiting nurse associations may be involved in the follow-up care in the home.

Continued guidance and counseling are essential in helping the family and its members to live in harmony with each other, increasing their comfort, and strengthening their unity. The child with a defect needs love, affection, and social and physical stimulation as much as or more than any other child. At the same time, his special needs and reactions must be considered. Other family members also need love, a sense of fulfillment, and recognition as worthwhile persons. All this requires much energy from each family member. The nurse can help family members understand the special dynamics of their situation and cope with the inevitable tensions and resentments.

Redefinition of parental role and social network

A society expects adults to produce healthy children to perpetuate that society. A social stigma is attached to bearing a defective child, a reality with which the parents must learn to cope.

After parents grieve and come to terms with their failure to produce a healthy offspring, they still face several hurdles. One is to make a decision regarding the disposition of the child—institution or home. If the child comes home, they must learn to meet his special needs and introduce him to society.

Another hurdle is facing others—the other children, family, friends, and strangers. Even during the hospital stay, parents experience society's adverse reaction. Subtle or blatant expressions of social isolation are evident. The cards, flowers, and other gifts of congratulation are sparse. Frequently, the cheery forms of congratulations come only from those unaware of the "situation." Telephone conversations are guarded. Even medical personnel, unhappily, may shun these parents. Families may be insinuating blame on each other. At home, callers do not ask to see the baby. If they do, verbal response may be stilted, although nonverbal response is poignant.

The entire health team and community resources such as clergy must accept the task of helping parents reenter the outside world. Several of the techniques already discussed are helpful, but others may prove helpful also.

One simple technique is role playing. The anticipated meetings with the other children, family, and friends are acted out. Another approach is to discuss how parents will handle the curiosity of friends, acquaintances, and strangers. These techniques help in several ways. First, by anticipating the words and reactions of others, they verbalize their own. Second, the practice augments their store of coping strategies. Both techniques may uncover

feelings that can be dealt with here and now, although resolution of these feelings may not come until much later. Each encounter may serve to strengthen coping mechanisms and bring the resolution of feelings a step closer.

Family planning and genetic counseling

Clinical evaluation and diagnosis of causes form the basis of counseling. The genetic counselor is best qualified to discuss risks of recurrence. Should the disease be genetic, the couple ultimately must make their own decision regarding future pregnancies and their medical management. Other couples may be reassured that a recurrence is not likely.

Individual needs and desires govern the type and

Table 7-3. Characteristic onset of some genetic diseases*

Age of onset	Condition
Lethal during prenatal life	Some chromosome aberrations Some gross malformations
Present at birth	Congenital malformations Chromosomal aberrations Some forms of adrenogenital syndrome Some forms of deafness
Soon after birth	Phenylketonuria Galactosemia Sometimes cystic fibrosis
Infancy	Tay-Sachs disease Werdnig-Hoffman disease Maple syrup urine disease
Early childhood	Cystic fibrosis Duchenne muscular dystrophy
Near puberty	Limb-girdle muscular dystrophy Some forms of adrenogenital syndrome
Young adulthood	Acute intermittent porphyria Hereditary juvenile glaucoma

Variable onset age	Diabetes mellitus (0 to 80 years)
	Facioscapulohumeral muscular
	   dystrophy (2 to 45 years)
	Huntington's chorea (15 to 65
	   years)

*From Whaley, L. F. 1974. Understanding inherited disorders. St. Louis, The C. V. Mosby Co., p. 183; based on data from Porter, I. H. 1968. Heredity and disease. The Blakiston Division, McGraw-Hill Book Co., Inc.; and Thompson, J. S., and Thompson, M. W. 1966. Genetics in medicine. Philadelphia, W. B. Saunders Co.

amount of counseling. For some, knowledge about contraceptive techniques is pertinent. Others may seek sterilization.

DISORDERS NOT APPARENT AT BIRTH

Some disorders do not appear until some time after birth (Table 7-3). The severity of the psychologic impact varies with the disorder and the time when it appears. Parents and the affected child, if old enough, experience the mourning, restructuring of self-image, and the reaction to stigmatization by society together. Parents who had other children prior to the appearance of a disorder in an older child fear for the younger children. The middle-aged individual who develops Huntington's chorea, perhaps even after he has become a grandfather, fears for two generations of descendants. In many cases, affected individuals may experience anger and resentment toward the offending parents, just as parents of a child with a disorder feel resentment toward the child that "did this to us."

EXTENDED ROLE OF NURSE

The parameters of nursing practice are expanding. Interested nurses can develop expertise in history taking, pedigree charting, printing and evaluating dermatoglyphics, as well as in-depth counseling of individuals coping with genetic and congenital disorders. Genetic clinics, family planning clinics, and national organizations for heritable disorders are but a few of the possible choices in which the professional nurse can develop an expanded role.

REFERENCES

Babson, S. G., Benson, R. C., Pernoll, M. L., and Benda, G. I. 1975. Management of high-risk pregnancy and intensive care of the neonate (ed. 3). St. Louis, The C. V. Mosby Co.

Barton, B. K., Gerbie, A. B., and Nadler, H. L. 1974. Present states of uterine diagnosis of genetic defects. Am. J. Obstet. Gynecol. **118:**708.

Clausen, J. P., and others. 1973. Maternity nursing today. New York, McGraw-Hill Book Co., Inc.

Doran, T. A., Rudd, N. L., Gardner, H. A., and others. 1974. The antenatal diagnosis of genetic disease. Am. J. Obstet. Gynecol. **118:**314.

Dumars, K. W. 1975. Genetics and apathy concern U. C. professor. U. C. Clip Sheet **50,** Jan. 28.

Foster, S. 1971. Sickle cell anemia: closing the gap between theory and therapy. Am. J. Nurs. **71:**1952.

Holtzman, N. A., Meck, A. G., and Mellits, E. D. 1974. Neonatal screening for phenylketonuria. I. Effectiveness. J.A.M.A. **229:**667.

Kaback, M. M. 1972. Perspectives in the control of human genetic disease from genetics and the perinatal patient. In Mead Johnson Symposium on Perinatal and Developmental Medicine, Vail, Colo., June 9-13.

Korones, S. B. 1976. High-risk newborn infants: the basis for intensive nursing care (ed. 2). St. Louis, The C. V. Mosby Co.

Levine, L. 1971. Papers on genetics: a book of readings. St. Louis, The C. V. Mosby Co.

Lin-Fu, J. S. 1972. Sickle cell anemia: a medical review (HEW Pub. No. [HSM]72-5111). Washington, D.C., U.S. Department of Health, Education, and Welfare.

McKusick, V. A. 1969. Human genetics (ed. 2). Englewood Cliffs, N.J., Prentice-Hall, Inc.

Naiman, H. 1975. Screening for Tay-Sachs disease. Am. J. Nurs. **75:**436.

Pediatric currents: perspectives in genetic counseling (vol. 20). 1971. Columbus, Ohio, Ross Laboratories.

Perinatal pharmacology. 1974. In Mead Johnson Symposium on Perinatal and Developmental Medicine (No. 5). Vail, Colo., June 9-13.

Pierog, S. M., and Ferrara, A. 1976. Medical care of the sick newborn (ed. 2). St. Louis, The C. V. Mosby Co.

Pochedly, C. 1971. Sickle cell anemia: recognition and management. Am. J. Nurs. **71:**1948.

Ratliff, R. 1975. Gene grafting: great benefits; great risks. U. C. Clip Sheet **51,** Dec. 2.

Waechter, E. H. 1970. The birth of an exceptional child. Nurs. Forum **9:**202.

Whaley, L. F. 1974. Understanding inherited disorders. St. Louis, The C. V. Mosby Co.

Williams, S. R. 1973. Nutrition and diet therapy (ed. 2). St. Louis, The C. V. Mosby Co.

UNIT FOUR

Pregnancy

CHAPTER 8

Conception and fetal and neonatal maturation

Each human life begins with the union of two single cells. Once united, these cells divide, differentiate, and grow into a person, a replica of humanity's continuing generations yet a unique individual. The growth that takes place from conception to birth is more rapid than at any other time in an individual's life; the microscopic union of sperm and ovum increases in size more than 200 billion times during this period.

Before conception can occur, a process called *gametogenesis* occurs. Gametogenesis is the production of specialized sex cells or *gametes*. As these cells mature, the number of chromosomes that they contain is reduced by half (meiosis) to the haploid number of 23, as discussed in Chapter 7. Continuous spermatogenesis in the male testis produces small, highly motile spermatozoons. Cyclic oogenesis in the female ovary produces large, nonmotile ova.

FERTILIZATION

During sexual intercourse, 3 to 5 ml of semen usually containing more than 300 million spermatozoa are ejaculated into the female vagina. By flagellar movement, the sperm make their way through the fluids of the cervical mucus, across the endometrium, and into the fallopian tube to the ovum. A few thousand sperm may survive in the tube for several days. The method by which a single spermatozoon reaches and penetrates the ovum is called *fertilization* and generally occurs in the middle third of the fallopian tube. During the "wait" for the ovum, conditioning (capacitation) of the sperm, presumably by enzyme factors, makes fertilization possible. Only one spermatozoon is required for actual fertilization, but the presence of many increases the probability.

Each normal spermatozoon carries either 22 autosomes and an X chromosome or 22 autosomes and a Y chromosome. Each normal ovum contains 22 autosomes and an X chromosome. When the sperm and the ovum meet and fuse to form a *zygote* (fertilized ovum), the diploid number of chromosomes (44 autosomal and 2 sex chromosomes) is restored, and the sex of the new human is determined. An ovum fertilized by a sperm bearing a Y chromosome normally results in a male zygote, whereas an ovum fertilized by an X-bearing sperm normally results in a female zygote. Fertilization initiates the first of the following three stages of human prenatal development:

1. *Ovum*—the period from fertilization until primary villi appear, approximately 12 to 14 days of gestation
2. *Embryo*—the period from ovum until the embryo measures approximately 3 cm from crown to rump, normally 54 to 56 days of gestation
3. *Fetus*—the period from embryo stage until the pregnancy is terminated

IMPLANTATION

After fertilization, the zygote starts to move through the fallopian tube into the uterine cavity propelled by ciliary action and irregular peristaltic contractions. As it migrates, the zygote begins a process of rapid cell division called *mitosis* or *cleavage*. The initial division of the zygote results in two *blastomeres*, which subsequently divide into progressively smaller blastomeres. At the end of 3 or 4 days, the developing individual comprises about sixteen blastomeres arranged in a ball-like structure called a *morula*. After the morula enters the uterus, a cavity forms within the dividing cells, changing the morula into a *blastocyst*. The blastocyst remains free in the uterus for 1 to 2 days, and then the exposed cells of the *trophoblast* (cellular wall of the blastocyst) implant, generally in the endometrium between the mouths of two uterine glands in the anterior or posterior fundal region. About 7 to 10 days elapse between fertilization and the completion of implantation.

The attaching portion of the trophoblast differentiates into two primitive layers: the *cytotrophoblast,* an inner germinative layer of cells, and the *syncytiotrophoblast,* an outer synctial layer. This outer layer invades the maternal epithelia, stroma, and blood vessels, creating an irregular cavity into which the blastocyst sinks. These invasive trophoblastic cells are the beginning of the primitive placenta, the vital embryo-maternal interface. Implantation is aided by the *chorionic villi* (fingerlike projections) that cover the trophoblast. The chorionic villi produce human chorionic gonadotropin (HCG), the hormone that causes continued secretion of progesterone and estrogen by the corpus luteum, thus preventing additional ovulation and menstruation.

The endometrium has been prepared for implantation by the corpus luteum's secretion of copious amounts of progesterone. After implantation, the endometrium is referred to as the *decidua.* It comprises three parts: that which overlies the embryo is called the *decidua capsularis,* or *reflexa;* that beneath the embryo is the *decidua basalis;* and that which lines the rest of the uterine cavity is the *decidua parietalis,* or *vera.*

The period of rapid cell division (from conception through 8 weeks' gestation) is the most critical time in the development of an individual. All the principal organ systems are being established and are highly vulnerable to environmental agents (viruses, drugs, radiation, infection) (Fig. 7-1). Developmental interferences during this time can result in major congenital abnormalities (Table 8-1). At the end of 8 weeks' gestation, the normal embryo has developed recognizable human characteristics and is referred to as a *fetus,* a Latin word meaning "offspring" (Fig. 8-1).

PLACENTATION

The placenta functions as a transport mechanism between embryo and mother through which nutrients pass to the embryo and waste materials move from the embryo. This process may be referred to as *hematotrophic anabolism* and *catabolism.* The placenta also produces hormones and enzymes (pp. 134 and 135).

During implantation, enzyme action occasionally opens a maternal vein and artery so that lacunas (small blood lakes) are formed in the decidua basalis. This rich blood supply causes the adjacent villi to multiply rapidly. These villi become the *chorion frondosum* or fetal portion of the future placenta. Those villi adjacent to the decidua capsularis become the atrophic *chorion laeve.*

As the *chorion* (outer layer of fetal membranes) develops, the *amnion* (inner layer of fetal membranes) is also forming rapidly around the growing embryo (Fig. 8-2).

Table 8-1. Potential malformations related to time of insult*

Week since ovulation	Potential malformation	Week since ovulation	Potential malformation
Third	Ectopia cordis Omphalocele Ectromelia Sympodia	Sixth	Microphthalmia Carpal or pedal ablation Hairlip, agnathia Lenticular cataract Congenital heart disease Gross septal and aortic anomalies
Fourth	Omphalocele Ectromelia Tracheoesophageal fistula Hemivertebra	Seventh	Congenital heart disease Interventricular septal defects Pulmonary stenosis Digital ablation Cleft palate, micrognathia Epicanthus, brachycephaly
Fifth	Tracheoesophageal fistula Hemivertebra Nuclear cataract Microphthalmia Facial clefts Carpal or pedal ablation	Eighth	Congenital heart disease Epicanthus, brachycephaly Persistent ostium primum Nasal bone ablation Digital stunting

*From Babson, S. G., Benson, R. C., Pernoll, M. L., and Benda, G. I. 1975; Management of high-risk pregnancy and intensive care of the neonate (ed. 3). St. Louis, The C. V. Mosby Co., p. 134; modified from Kaiser, I. H. 1971. In Danforth, D. N. (ed.) Textbook of obstetrics and gynecology (ed. 2). New York, Harper & Row, Publishers.

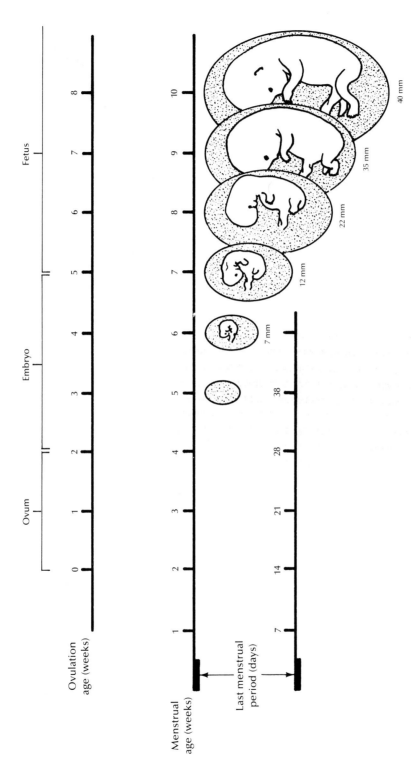

Fig. 8-1. Growth during early weeks of pregnancy.

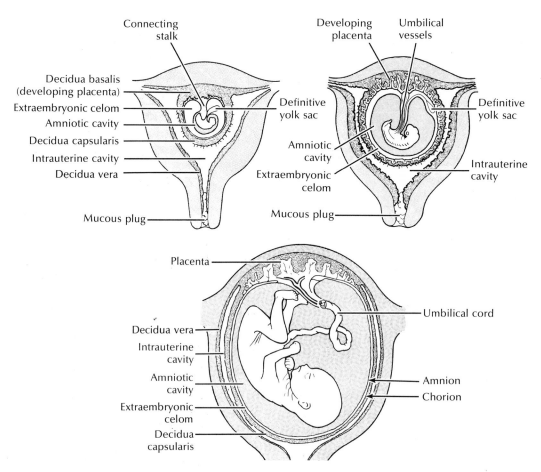

Fig. 8-2. Development of fetal membranes. Note gradual obliteration of uterine cavity as decidua capsularis and decidua vera meet. Also note thinning of uterine wall. Chorionic and amniotic membranes are in appositon to each other but may be peeled apart.

The amnion's rapid expansion forces the body stalk, rudimentary blind allantois, vessels, and vitelline duct into a single pedicle, which eventually becomes the *umbilical cord,* or *funis.* This cord links the embryo and the placenta. At term this light gray, smooth, vascular attachment is 50 to 55 cm long and approximately 2 cm in diameter.

The surface of the cord is a thin, squamous, epithelial extension of the skin of the fetus; however, it contains no pain receptors. The cord normally contains two umbilical arteries and one umbilical vein (Fig. 8-3). The vein carries oxygenated blood to the fetus and the arteries return deoxygenated blood to the placenta. Frequently, these vessels are longer than the cord and consequently become coiled on themselves, giving the cord a coiled appearance. They are supported by a loose connective tissue containing a cushioning mucoid ma-

terial called *Wharton's jelly.* The high water content of Wharton's jelly causes the cord to shrink quickly after birth. It is always important for the physician or nurse to count the vessels in the cord because in at least 1% of neonates, a two-vesseled cord (one vein and one artery) will be noted. Various anomalies are present in at least 10% of these neonates and are more common in multiple births.

The maturing placenta develops into fifteen to twenty subdivisions called *cotyledons.* Each of these is partially separated from other cotyledons by fenestrated septa, so in essence each cotyledon is a functioning unit.

Growth of the thickness of the placenta continues until 16 to 20 weeks' gestation; then the syncytiotrophoblast begins to thin and only the cytotrophoblast remains. However, the placental circumference continues growing until late pregnancy.

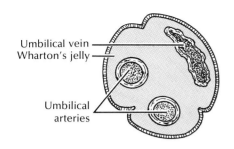

Umbilical vein
Wharton's jelly

Umbilical
arteries

Fig. 8-3. Cross section of umbilical cord. Note collapsed appearance of uterine vein and contour of arteries.

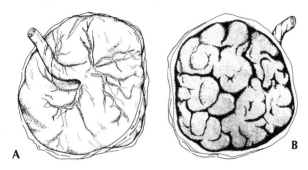

A   B

Fig. 8-4. A, Fetal surface of placenta. **B,** Maternal surface of placenta. (From Taylor, E. S. 1966. Beck's obstetrical practice [ed. 8]. Baltimore, The Williams & Wilkins Co.)

The fully developed placenta (afterbirth) is a reddish, discoid organ 15 to 20 cm × 2.5 to 3 cm. The weight of a term placenta is 400 to 600 gm (approximately one-sixth that of the newborn). About four fifths of the placenta by weight is of fetal origin; the remainder is maternal. The umbilical cord extends from the fetal surface of the placenta to the umbilicus of the fetus. The fetal membranes cover the fetal surface of the placenta and extend from the placental margins to envelope the fetus and its amniotic fluid (p. 116).

The fetal surface of the placenta is shiny and slightly grayish (Fig. 8-4, *A*). The umbilical vessels that enter the cord can be seen as a branching system just beneath the membranes. The insertion of the cord is eccentric. A peripheral insertion, the so-called battledore placenta, is not unusual.

The maternal surface of the placenta is rough and beefy red, the area originally adherent to the uterus (Fig. 8-4, *B*). The cotyledons stand out as segments with shallow clefts between.

In multiple pregnancy, one or more placentas will be present. The number depends on the number of fertilized ova and the manner of ovum segmentation. Several placentas may be fused and appear as one, but inspection should reveal their individuality.

Placental physiology

In addition to its anabolic and catabolic functions, the placenta serves as an effective lung, kidney, stomach, and intestine, as well as an endocrine gland for the fetus. It also serves as a protective barrier against the harmful effects of certain drugs and microorganisms.

Placental function depends almost entirely on maternal circulation. The placenta's life span is measured by its oxygen consumption, which reflects intense metabolic activity until term is approached, whereupon function progressively decreases until delivery.

Contrary to popular assumption, the placental lakes fill during uterine contraction (Braxton Hicks), not during relaxation. This is accomplished by closure of the maternal venous aperture beneath the placenta. In contrast, the heavier arteries to the placental site remain open during uterine contractions. Hence blood flows in. With uterine relaxation, blood drains out of the placental sinusoids into the maternal circulation.

This suggests a sluggish circulation. However, the placental capacity is large, and a considerable volume of maternal blood (approximately 500 ml/min) at term clears the placenta. In contrast, only about 400 ml/min of fetal blood pass through the placenta, obviously advantageous to the fetus.

Optimum circulation to the placenta and fetus is possible when the patient is lying on her left side. When supine, the third-trimester uterus compresses the vena cava, and the venous return from the uterus and lower extremities is significantly impeded.

Placental transfer

Only two layers of cells, the outer syncytiotrophoblast and the inner cytotrophoblast, separate maternal and fetal circulation for the first 12 weeks of gestation. After this time, the cytotrophoblastic cells become fewer and widely separated so that during the second and third trimester, only one cell layer separates the two bloodstreams. Thus the term *placental barrier* must be qualified. There is a barrier of sorts, and some protection of the fetus by the placenta results from enzyme deamination of substances such as epinephrine and histamine.

Passage of materials to and from the fetus is effected by four principal mechanisms:

1. *Diffusion,* such as across a membrane, allows passage of oxygen, carbon dioxide, anesthetic gases, water,

electrolytes, and other substances of low molecular weight.

2. *Selective transfer,* often by enzyme action, results in the passage of glucose, amino acids, calcium, iron, and other substances of higher molecular weight.

3. *Pinocytosis* is a mechanism by which minute particles may be engulfed and carried across the cell, including fats and complex proteins.

4. *Leakage* as a result of small defects in the trophoblastic surface allows slight mixing of maternal or fetal blood cells and plasma.

The transfer of vitamins to the fetus is only partially understood, but vitamins A, B complex, C, E, and K are transmitted to the fetus. It is not known whether vitamin D is produced by the fetus or supplied by the mother.

Many drugs cross the placenta readily (e.g., antibiotics, narcotics, analgesics, anesthetics). Viruses traverse the placenta with ease; bacteria rarely involve the fetus except when placentitis develops. Placentitis is generally the result of an intranatal infection associated with ruptured membranes and prolonged labor. Vaginal pyogenic bacteria cause amniochorionitis and fetal pneumonia, which may result in fatal fetal and even maternal septicemia. Isolated incidences have been reported of placentitis resulting from a systemic maternal infection of nongestational cause such as tuberculosis.

Drugs during pregnancy. Most drugs promptly cross the placenta, and many are deleterious to the human fetus. Harmful drugs may be grouped into categories as follows:

- Established teratogenic drugs
- Possible teratogenic drugs
- Fetotoxic drugs

Examples of these drugs, to which may be added vaccines and excessive amounts of certain vitamins, are given in Table 8-2.

Other medications may contain elements noxious to the fetus. All factors considered, the physician should exercise a special caution in prescribing new, unfamiliar, or multiple drugs. Hence all but the most essential medications should be avoided, particularly during the first trimester of pregnancy.

Table 8-2. Human fetotoxic chemical agents*

Maternal medication	Reported effect on fetus or neonate
Analgesics	
Indomethacin	Prolongs gestation (monkey)
Narcotics	70% of maternal level; death, apnea, depression, bradycardia, hypothermia
Salicylates	Death in utero; hemorrhage, methemoglobinemia, ↓ albumin-binding capacity, salicylate intoxication, difficult delivery, ? prolonged gestation
Anesthesia	
Conduction	Indirect effect of maternal hypotension; direct effect—convulsions, death, acidosis, bradycardia, myocardial depression, fetal hypotension, methemoglobinemia
General	Apnea, depression (prolonged inhalation by gravid female), ? congenital malformations, chromosome abnormality†; ether has direct narcotic effect on infant
Ether	
Halothane (Fluothane)	
Trichloroethylene (Trilene)	
Hypnosis	Indirect effect of maternal hyperventilation and excessive bearing down
Local	
Paracervical	Methemoglobinemia, fetal acidosis, bradycardia, neurologic depression, myocardial depression
Anticoagulants	
Coumarins	Fetal death; hemorrhage; calcifications

*Modified from Babson, S. G., Benson, R. C., Pernoll, M. L., and Benda, G. I. 1975. Management of high-risk pregnancy and intensive care of the neonate (ed. 3). St. Louis, The C. V. Mosby Co., p. 133; and Perinatal pharmacology. 1974. In Mead Johnson Symposium on Perinatal and Developmental Medicine (No. 5). Vail, Colo., June 9-13.

†Pregnant nurses working in operating rooms have shown a higher incidence of abortion, stillbirths, and congenital anomalies for unknown reasons.

Table 8-2. Human fetotoxic chemical agents—cont'd

Maternal medication	Reported effect on fetus or neonate
Anticonvulsant agents	
Barbiturates	Irritability and tremulousness 4 to 5 months postdelivery; hemorrhage; enzyme inducer
Diphenylhydantoin and barbiturate	Congenital malformations; cleft lip and palate; congenital heart disease (CHD); CNS and skeletal anomalies; failure to thrive; enzyme inducer, hemorrhage
Paradione	CHD, microophthalmia, mental retardation, abortion
Tridione	
Antidiabetics	(See hypoglycemic agents)
Antimalarial	
Quinine	? Congenital anomalies of CNS and extremities, thrombocytopenia, hypoplastic optic nerve, congenital deafness
Antimicrobials	All antimicrobials cross placenta
Ampicillin	↓ Maternal urinary and plasma estriol levels
Cephaloridine	Blood levels maintained for hours after delivery; ? false positive direct Coombs' test
Chloramphenicol	Crosses placenta with no reported effect; interferes with biotransformation of tolbutamide, diphenylhydantoin, biohydroxycoumarin (i.e., hypoglycemia may occur if used in combination)
Chloroquine	Death; deafness; retinal hemorrhage
Erythromycin	Possible hepatic injury
Nitrofurantoin	Megaloblastic anemia; G6PD deficiency
Novobiocin	Hyperbilirubinemia
Quinine, quinidine	Possible ototoxicity; thrombocytopenia
Streptomycin	Therapeutic levels reached; nerve deafness
Sulfonamides	
Long and short acting	Icterus, hemolytic anemia, kernicterus, ? growth retardation, thrombocytopenia
Tetracycline	Placental transfer after 4 months' gestation; enamel hypoplasia, delay in bone growth, ? congenital cataract
Antituberculous	
Isoniazid	Toxic blood level in fetus; no reported effect; mother should be on pyridoxine supplement
Pyridoxine	See vitamins
Belladonna derivatives	
Atropine	Intrauterine tachycardia; dilated nonreacting pupils
Scopolamine	? Delays labor, ? delays respiration, deleterious to premature infant
Cancer chemotherapeutic agents	
Aminopterin	Abortion, congenital anomalies (1st trimester); combination of drugs detrimental to fetus; skeletal and cranial malformations, hydrocephalus; questionable long-term effects = slow somatic growth; ovarian agenesis; ↓ immune mechanisms
Busulfan	
Cyclophosphamide	
6-Mercaptoparine	
Methotrexate	
Cardiovascular agents	
Digitoxin	Placental transfer; no reported effect
Propranolol	Indirect effect of delay in cervical dilatation
Cholinesterase inhibitors	Myasthenia-like symptoms for 1 week; muscle weakness in 10% to 20% of infants
Cigarette smoking	Effect equal to number of cigarettes smoked; ↑ incidence of stillbirth; low birth weight; ? effect on later somatic growth and mental development; reduction in O_2 transport to fetus

Continued.

Table 8-2. Human fetotoxic chemical agents—cont'd

Maternal medication	Reported effect on fetus or neonate
Diuretics	
Ammonium chloride	Maternal and fetal acidosis; thrombocytopenia, hemorrhage, hypoelectro-
Benzothiazides	lytemia, convulsions, respiratory distress, death, hemolysis
Chlorothiazide	
Thiazide	
Diazoxide	Hypertrichosis lanuginosa, alopecia, ? hypoglycemia
Drugs of abuse (usually multiple drugs consumed)	
Alcohol	Blood level equal to mother's; convulsions, withdrawal syndrome, hyperactivity, crying, irritability, poor sucking reflex, low birth weight; cleft palate, ophthalmic malformation; malformation of extremities and heart; poor mental performance; microencephaly, small-for-dates, growth deficiency
Barbiturates	Withdrawal symptoms, convulsions, onset immediately after birth or at 2 weeks of age
Glutethimide	Small-for-dates; irritability
LSD (lysergic acid)	Chromosome breakage, limb and skeletal anomalies
Narcotics	Small-for-dates, 4% to 10% mortality, habituation, withdrawal symptoms, con-
Heroin	vulsions, sudden death, indirect effect of maternal complications (i.e., infec-
Methadone	tion, hepatitis, venereal disease), ? permanent effect on somatic growth
Fluorine	Placental transfer—utilized for growth and development of bones and teeth of fetus
Hormones	
Androgens	Labioscrotal fusion prior to 12th week, after 12 weeks' phallic enlargement;
Estrogens	? anomalies; ? ↑ bilirubin, vaginal cancer; cleft lip and palate, CHD, TE fistula,
Progestins	anal atresia, cancer of prostate, testes, and bladder
Corticosteroids	Adrenal insufficiency, cleft palate, small-for-dates infant
Ovulatory agents	? Anencephaly; ? chromosome abnormalities in abortus, multiple pregnancy
Hypoglycemic agents	
Chlorpropamide	Higher fetal mortality, prolonged hypoglycemia, competes for albumin-binding sites
Insulin	Insulin coma; ? increased fetal damage
Tolbutamide	? Potentiates hypoglycemia in newborn, thrombocytopenia
Hypotensive agents	
Hexamethonium	Paralytic ileus, perforation, death
Reserpine	1% to 15% of infants have symptoms; nasal stuffiness, bradycardia, respiratory distress, hypothermia, abnormal muscle tone (in mice, hyperactivity and increased emotionalism)
Insecticide and pesticides	
Organochlorine	Present in fetus, ? enzyme induction, ? premature labor
Intravenous alcohol	Hypoglycemia; abnormal bone marrow morphology in premature infant
Intravenous fluids	Excessive fluids—hyponatremia, seizures
Muscle relaxants	
Curare	Paralysis in utero (prolonged use), position deformities
Narcotic antagonist	
Nalorphine (Nalline)	Not effective unless large doses of narcotics administered to mother; act as re-
Levallorphan (Lorfan)	spiratory depressant if cause of depression is other than narcotic

Table 8-2. Human fetotoxic chemical agents—cont'd

Maternal medication	Reported effect on fetus or neonate
Oxytocin	Thrombocytopenia, fetal bradycardia, water intoxication, ? ↑ bilirubin level; abortions (ergot)
Psychotropic drugs Antidepressants Aventyl Chloropyramine Imipramine Nortriptyline	Withdrawal; coliclike syndrome, cyanosis, irritability, weight loss, hyperhydrosis, respiratory distress, craniofacial anomalies, CNS and skeletal anomalies; urinary retention
Diazepam (Valium)	High fetal levels; hypotonia, poor sucking reflex, hypothermia; ↑ low Apgar score infants; ↑ resuscitation, ↑ assisted deliveries; dose related
Lithium	Neonatal serum levels reach adult toxic range; lethargy, cyanosis for 10 days; teratogenic—dose related
Phenothiazine	? Effect on eyes; withdrawal; extrapyramidal dysfunction; delay in onset of respiration; maternal hypotension, ? prolongs labor, effective uterine contraction; ? chromosomal breakage; hypotonia, hyperactivity
Radiation	Microencephaly, mental retardation, many unknown effects; nondisjunction of chromosomes
Radiopaque media	Elevated PHI, depressed ^{131}I uptake
Sedatives Barbiturate	Apnea, depression, depressed EEG, poor sucking reflex, slow weight gain; concentration of drug in brain; enzyme inducer = lower bilirubin level
Bromides	Growth failure, lethargy, dilated pupils, dermatitis, hypotonia, ? effect on mental development
Magnesium sulfate	Neonatal blood level does not correlate with clinical condition; respiratory depression, hypotonia, convulsions, death; exchange transfusion may be required
Paraldehyde	Apnea, depression
Thalidomide	Administered between 34th and 50th day of gestation causes phocomelia, malformation of cord, angiomas of face, CHD, intestinal stenosis, eye defects, absence of appendix
Thyroid medications Iodine Thioureas	Normal or goitrous infants; euthyroid, hyperthyroid or hypothyroid; respiratory distress due to tracheal compression; thrombocytopenia
^{131}I	Uptake by fetal thyroid after 12 weeks' gestation; exophthalmus, arrest of brain development
Toxins Carbon monoxide	Stillbirth, brain damage equal to anoxia
Heavy metals Arsenic	Concentrated in brain
Lead	Abortions, growth retardation, congenital anomalies, sterility
Mercury	Cerebral palsy, mental retardation, convulsions, involuntary movements, defective vision; mother asymptomatic
Naphthalene	Hemolysis
Vitamins A and D	Congenital anomalies
K (water-soluble analogues)	Icterus, anemia, kernicterus
Pyridoxine	Withdrawal seizures

Fetal-neonatal immunology. Immunity is an organism's ability to resist and overcome infection or disease and may be described as *natural* or *acquired.* When the infective agents causing a particular disease fail to grow in an individual's tissues or when the toxins of those agents are harmless to him, that individual is said to have *natural immunity* to that particular disease.

If natural immunity is not effective, the body produces substances to destroy the invading organism. These substances are called *antibodies,* and the ability to produce them is known as *acquired immunity.*

Two types of acquired immunity are recognized: *active,* which is produced by an individual as the result of an infectious disease such as typhoid fever, and *passive,* which is achieved by transferring to an individual the blood serum of an immunized animal or immune person.

Passive immunity of the fetus to maternal infections results from placental transfer of maternal immunoglobulin IgG. This transfer is an active process unrelated to molecular size and occurs largely during the third trimester. Infants born prior to 34 weeks' gestation may be deficient in IgG. The cord serum of term infants generally contains higher concentrations of IgG than does the maternal blood, and the infant receives the specific antibodies occurring in the IgG class.

Thus the infant's passive immunity depends on the quantity of IgG antibody in the maternal system and the sensitivity of the particular agent to antibody. Most infants receive diphtheria and tetanus antitoxins and antibodies to various bacterial and viral agents. Immunity to certain bacterial diseases such as pertussis may last only a month or two; however, protection against measles and other viral infections may continue for 4 to 8 months.

Unlike IgG, other immunoglobulins such as IgA and IgM are blocked by the placenta, and the embryo-fetus cannot produce these substances in amounts sufficient to combat numerous intrauterine infections such as rubella during the first trimester. These protective mechanisms are still inadequate in the neonate, making it highly vulnerable to certain septic processes.

At one time, the neonate was regarded as incapable of producing antibodies in response to specific antigens. Recent research has demonstrated that this is not accurate. The normal infant is capable of producing an antibody response to immunizing agents or naturally occurring infections; however, the response is generally less vigorous than that of the older child or adult.

Much remains to be learned concerning the role of nonspecific immunity in the infant. It is apparent that the skin serves as an important barrier. Increasingly frequent generalized infections due to enteric organisms, usually not invasive, suggest that the gastrointestinal mucosa may be a portal of entry. Local or generalized circulatory changes may change this intestinal lining, which is normally impermeable to bacteria. Contrary to earlier theory, there is only slight absorption of immunoglobulins from colostrum and breast milk.

Placental variations

Major placental variations include the double but separate bipartite placenta and the succenturiate placenta, which has a smaller accessory lobe or lobes. In the succenturiate placenta the vessels from the major to the minor lobe(s) are supported only by the membranes. During delivery of the placenta, an accessory lobe may remain attached, causing subsequent bleeding or infection.

A velamentous insertion of the cord is a rare placental anomaly in which the cord vessels begin to branch at the membranes and then course on the placenta. Rupture of the membranes or traction on the cord may tear one or more of the fetal vessels. As a result the fetus may quickly exsanguinate (bleed to death). On rare occasions, when slight antenatal bleeding occurs and fetal red blood cells or hemoglobin are identified, prompt rescue of the offspring, usually by cesarean section, may be feasible.

Occasionally a fibrous, grayish brown ring is noted around the periphery of the fetal surface of the placenta. This is called a *circumvallate,* or *circummarginate placenta,* an extrachorionic variation in development sometimes associated with abortion, bleeding in late pregnancy, or low birth weight infants.

Fetal membranes

Two closely applied but separate membranes surround the developing embryo-fetus (Fig. 8-5). The amnion (inner membrane) and chorion (outer membrane) are also attached to the fetal surface of the placenta. These strong, translucent membranes contain not only the fetus but the amniotic fluid.

The point of rupture of the membranes generally is approximately over the internal cervical os. By referring to this point, the general area of placental implantation can be determined. The membranes may be abnormally adherent, especially in the fundus. All the membranes should be recovered after delivery to avoid puerperal infection.

Amniotic fluid

The term fetus is immersed in about 1000 ml of clear liquid. The amniotic fluid approximates water in specific

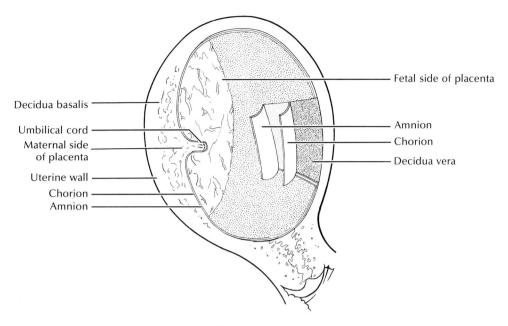

Decidua basalis

Umbilical cord

Maternal side
of placenta

Uterine wall

Chorion

Amnion

Fetal side of placenta

Amnion

Chorion

Decidua vera

Fig. 8-5. Fetal membranes.

gravity (1.007 to 1.025) and is neutral to slightly alkaline (pH 7.0 to 7.25). It contains albumin, urea, uric acid, creatinine, lecithin, sphingomyelin, bilirubin, fat, fructose, inorganic salts, epithelial cells, a few leukocytes, various enzymes, and lanugo hairs. Amniotic fluid is thought to have multiple origins and a composition that changes during pregnancy. It accomplishes numerous functions for the fetus including the following:
1. Protects from direct trauma by distributing and equalizing any impact the mother may receive
2. Separates the fetus from the fetal membranes
3. Allows freedom of fetal movement and aids in musculoskeletal development
4. Facilitates symmetrical growth and development of the fetus
5. Protects from loss of heat and maintains a relatively constant fetal body temperature
6. Is a source of oral fluid
7. Acts as an excretion collection system

There is still much to be learned about amniotic fluid. However, its study has provided a great deal of knowledge concerning the sex, state of health, and maturity of the fetus. Amniocentesis (p. 97) has made it possible to detect diseases and abnormalities that may suggest the options of therapeutic abortion or intrauterine treatment.

During pregnancy the amniotic fluid volume increases at an average rate of 25 ml/wk from 11 to 15 weeks' gestation and 50 ml/wk from 15 to 28 weeks' gestation.

There is great variation within the normal volume; however, more than 1.5 ℓ (polyhydramnios) or less than 500 ml (oligohydramnios) is usually associated with fetal disease or abnormality (Behrman, 1973) (p. 513).

FETAL-NEONATAL MATURATION
Circulation

The first system to function in the developing human is the cardiovascular system (Fig. 8-6). At the end of 3 weeks' gestation, circulation of blood has begun the fetomaternal exchange of oxygen, nutrients, and waste products. This exchange is necessary because the fetal lungs and digestive system are not functional until after birth.

The single umbilical vein carries oxygen-enriched blood from the placenta. This vein divides at the edge of the fetal liver, allowing about half the oxygenated blood to bypass the liver through the ductus venosus into the inferior vena cava. There it mixes with deoxygenated blood from the fetal lower extremities, abdomen, and pelvis. Most of this blood then enters the right atrium and is pumped through the foramen ovale into the left atrium where it mixes with a small amount of deoxygenated blood returning from the lungs through the pulmonary veins. The blood then flows into the left ventricle and exits through the ascending aorta. As a result, the vessels leading to the fetal heart, head, neck, and upper limbs receive well-oxygenated blood. This circulatory pattern is the reason for the embryo's cephalocaudal

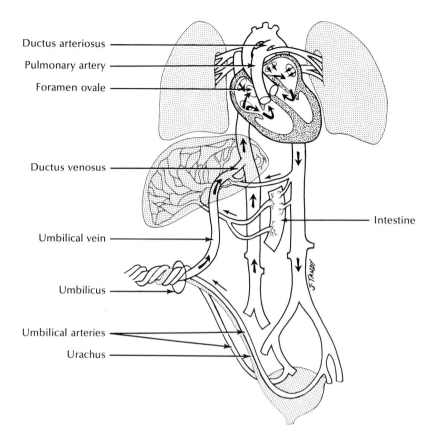

Ductus arteriosus

Pulmonary artery

Foramen ovale

Ductus venosus

Intestine

Umbilical vein

Umbilicus

Umbilical arteries

Urachus

Fig. 8-6. Fetal circulation.

(head-to-tail) development, which persists in subsequent motor development, making it possible for the infant to manipulate his hands long before he can walk.

A small quantity of oxygenated blood from the inferior vena cava remains in the right atrium and mixes with deoxygenated blood from the superior vena cava and coronary sinus. It then flows into the right ventricle and pulmonary artery, passing through the ductus arteriosus into the aorta; a small amount is diverted to the nonfunctional lungs.

The paired umbilical arteries return most of the mixed blood from the descending aorta to the placenta through the chorionic villi. There the fetal blood simultaneously gives up carbon dioxide and waste materials and takes up oxygen and nutrients. The remaining blood circulates through the lower part of the fetal body and ultimately enters the inferior vena cava.

The proportionate amount of blood in the placenta changes with the developing pregnancy. During early gestation, more than half the circulating blood in the placenta is maternal. However, at term, more than half of placental blood is fetal.

Profound physiologic changes occur at birth which make possible the infant's transition from intrauterine to extrauterine life. The most important and dramatic of these changes involve the baby's heart and lungs.

The infant's first breath inflates the lungs, markedly reducing pulmonary vascular resistance, increasing pulmonary blood flow, and initiating a progressive thinning of the walls of the pulmonary arteries. As a result, the ductus arteriosus closes because of increased oxygen (elevated Po_2) pressure changes. The increased pulmonary blood flow elevates the pressure in the left atrium above that in the right atrium, thus closing the foramen ovale.

At birth the circulation of fetal blood through the placenta ceases, eliminating the need for the ductus arteriosus, ductus venosus, and the umbilical vessels. These vessels constrict and are modified to become ligaments (Table 8-3).

Following are a number of compensatory circulatory factors that benefit the fetus:

1. The fetal heart rate is 120 to 140 beats/min, and the fetal cardiac output approximately 20 ml/kg/min or about three times that of the adult at rest.

Table 8-3. Changes in cardiovascular system at birth	
Fetal structure	**Neonatal structure**
Umbilical vein	Ligamentum teres
Umbilical arteries	
Intra-abdominal portions	Hypogastric or lateral umbilical ligaments
Proximal portions	Superior vesical arteries
Ductus venosus	Venous ligament
Ductus arteriosus	Ligamentum arteriosum

2. Oxygen saturation of fetal blood is only about two-thirds that of the neonate. This suggests that the fetus is able to develop in a slightly hypoxic state. Actually, during moderate hypoxia, the fetus can shift to anaerobic metabolism briefly without jeopardy.

3. Fetal hemoglobin concentration is 18 gm/100 ml and the red blood cell count (RBC) is about 5.7 million/mm^3, both higher than in infancy. The dissociation of fetal hemoglobin is greater than that of the adult type, which increases transport and release of oxygen.

4. Carbon dioxide transfer from fetal to maternal blood is augmented because maternal blood has the greater affinity for carbon dioxide.

Respiration

As previously mentioned, the fetal lungs do not function until after delivery. Simple diffusion (passing from higher to lower concentration across a semipermeable membrane) explains the exchange of oxygen and carbon dioxide across the placenta.

Development of human lungs occurs in four overlapping phases:

1. *Pseudoglandular period* (5 to 17 weeks' gestation) —formation of bronchi and terminal bronchi

2. *Canalicular period* (13 to 25 weeks' gestation)— enlargement of lumina of bronchi and terminal bronchioles, development of respiratory bronchioles and alveolar ducts, increased vascularity of lung tissue

3. *Terminal sac period* (24 weeks' gestation to birth) —growth of primitive alveoli (terminal air sacs) from alveolar ducts

4. *Alveolar period* (late fetal period to approximately 8 years of age)—formation of characteristic pulmonary alveoli as the lining of the terminal air sacs thins, with the number of alveoli increasing six to eight times between birth and age 8 years

During the terminal sac period, pulmonary surfactants are produced by alveolar cells. These phospholipid substances cover the internal surface of the alveoli before birth. They reduce the alveolar surface tension during extrauterine respiratory expiration, facilitating expansion of the lungs at birth. If insufficient surfactants are present, the lungs cannot be properly inflated, and respiratory distress syndrome (RDS) may develop.

Lecithin, a major component of surfactant, builds up in the amniotic fluid from about the twenty-fourth week, and sphingomyelin, another pulmonary phospholipid, remains the same. Hence by determining the amount of lecithin present, or the lecithin-sphingomyelin (L/S) ratio, an appraisal of fetal lung maturity is possible. RDS is unlikely when the L/S ratio is greater than 2:1.

Periodic fetal hiccough can be seen and palpated, and rhythmic fetal respiratory movements can be demonstrated by ultrasonography in advanced pregnancy. Fetal squamae and lanugo fragments are commonly found in the fetal respiratory passages. Hence respirations at birth appear to be an extension of intrauterine respiratory activity.

At birth, air must be substituted for fluid that has filled the respiratory tract to the alveoli. During the course of normal vaginal delivery, between 7 and 42 ml of amniotic fluid are squeezed or drained from the neonate's lungs (Aladjem and Brown, 1974). After delivery, most of the remaining fluid may be absorbed into the circulation due to reduced pulmonary vascular resistance that accompanies the onset of respiration. Thus delayed or abnormal respiration may retard normal pulmonary function.

Initial breathing probably is the result of a reflex triggered in part by pressure changes, chilling, noise and light, and other sensations related to the birth process. In addition, the chemoreceptors in the aorta and carotid bodies initiate neurologic reflexes when the P_{CO_2} is increased and the pH is reduced. (When these changes are extreme, however, depression ensues.) In most cases, an exaggerated respiratory reaction follows within 1 minute of birth, and the infant takes his first gasping breath and cries.

With the first breath, the infant develops a considerable negative intrathoracic pressure. Air is drawn in and about half of this remains as residual pulmonary volume. Normally it requires only a few breaths to expand the lungs well; subsequently the pressures will be lower than at the onset of respiration.

A reduction in the rate and depth of maternal respiration may be reflected in fetal oxygenation. Excessive amounts of barbiturate, narcotic analgesia, or maternal hypoxia during anesthesia may reduce the fetal P_{O_2}. Moreover, heavy maternal sedation by those drugs that readily cross the placenta may depress the fetal CNS respiratory center to further jeopardize the baby. Breathing of pure oxygen by the mother prior to delivery and cessation of pulsation in the cord may aid the infant.

If ventilation is reduced, hypoxia and hypercapnia ensue. Combined respiratory and metabolic acidosis, augmented by anaerobic metabolism, soon result. Acidosis and hypoxia combine to cause marked vasoconstriction in the neonate. Pulmonary vasoconstriction results in increased vascular resistance, which may even exceed the systemic pressures. If this develops, a right-to-left shunt through a patent ductus arteriosus or patent foramen ovale or both may develop to further complicate the infant's early life. Cyanosis may then be evident. Once respirations are established, they are shallow and irregular, ranging from 40 to 60/min, with short periods of apnea.

Hematology

Groups of blood cells can be identified by the sixth week of life in the yolk sac, but definite hematopoiesis begins in the liver and spleen about the eighth week when vascular channels become canalized.

Initially, all red blood cells are nucleated. The fetal erythrocytes are larger than those of the adult, but as maturity approaches, newly produced red blood cells are smaller, and at term about 5% remain nucleated.

The placental or fetal blood volume must be determined indirectly because of safety factors. At term birth the placenta contains almost 150 ml of blood— less than half the blood volume of the neonate. The newborn has approximately 10% greater blood volume, nearly 20% greater red blood cell mass, but about 20% less plasma volume when compared by kilogram of body weight with the adult. In further contrast, the infant born about the thirty-fifth or thirty-sixth week will have a greater blood volume than the term neonate. This is because of the baby's greater plasma volume, not to a greater red blood cell mass.

Laboratory values for the mature newborn include the following: RBC, 5 million/mm³; hemoglobin (Hgb) concentration in the red blood cells is 50%; and Hgb, 24 gm/ml. The last two values especially are much higher than those of the adult.

Leukocytosis, with the white blood cell count (WBC) approximately 18,000/mm³, is usual at birth. The number, largely polymorphs, increases to about 23,000 to 24,000/mm³ during the first day after birth. A resting level of 10,000 to 11,000/mm³ normally is maintained during the neonatal period. Serious infection is not well tolerated by the newborn, and a marked increase in the WBC is unlikely even in critical sepsis.

In the first 4 months after birth, the RBC normally falls to approximately 4.5 million/mm³. The hematocrit (Hct) and hemoglobin concentrations are slightly reduced also. The infant simply does not need all the blood it had during fetal life, and obvious adjustments take place, initiated by early blood destruction as evidenced by icterus neonatorum. Fortunately iron stores generally are sufficient to sustain normal red blood cell production for 6 months, so that the slight brief anemia is not serious.

The blood coagulation of the newborn baby may be slightly prolonged over that of the adult. Although the number of blood platelets and amount of plasma fibrinogen compare well with older subjects, the newborn's prothrombin may be slightly lower and the prothrombin time somewhat prolonged until the end of the first week, especially if vitamin K was not given to the mother before delivery or to the infant shortly after delivery. Studies indicate that vitamin K stores are virtually absent in the neonate as are the intestinal microflora that produce this vitamin. During the first few days of life, there is limited intake of foods containing vitamin K. Breast milk is a poor source of this vitamin, and hemorrhagic disorders are more common in breast-fed infants than those receiving cow's milk on the first day of life (Behrman, 1973). Hemorrhage is rarely a problem, but ideally the infant's bleeding and clotting time should be checked before surgery, even for circumcision.

Renal function

The placenta is the major fetal excretory organ and effectively eliminates waste products from fetal blood. The placenta in collaboration with maternal lungs and kidneys maintains fetal water, electrolyte, and acid-base balance. Kidneys are unnecessary for fetal growth and development. In fact, a rare infant may be born without kidneys. Renal excretory and regulatory functions must begin immediately after delivery to maintain life and health.

Thus in preparation for extrauterine existence, the fetal kidney develops rapidly and by the thirty-sixth week, the individual units, or *nephrons,* are of the adult type. The tubules, particularly the loop of Henle, is not completely differentiated until after the fortieth week. Moreover, the length of the proximal tubules and the diameter of the glomeruli continue to grow until adult life.

Because of the relative physiologic immaturity of the kidney at term, glomerular filtration in the newborn is about 50% that of the adult, and other kidney functions such as urine concentration and tubular reabsorption of sodium and phosphate also are deficient. Maturation of renal function comparable with the adult is well advanced only after the first year of life. Despite renal immaturity at birth, however, great fluid and electrolyte variability can be managed successfully by the infant if intake of fluids is adequate, food is nutritionally balanced, and no serious infection is present.

Neurologic function

During the third week of gestation, the *neural plate* (a thickened area of embryonic ectoderm) appears, from which the infant's nervous system develops. The *neural tube* and *neural crest* evolve from this structure, the first differentiating into the CNS (brain and spinal cord) and the second into the peripheral nervous system.

The brain is formed at the cranial end of the neural tube, and it consists of the forebrain, midbrain, and hindbrain. The cerebrum develops from the forebrain; the adult midbrain develops from the midbrain; and the pons, cerebellum, and medulla oblongata evolve from the hindbrain. The longest part of the neural tube ultimately becomes the spinal cord.

The human brain is only partially developed and functional at birth. It doubles its weight during the first year and triples its weight by the sixth year. After this the growth rate slows, and the adult level is reached about puberty.

Actually the fetus is a spinal animal with basic reflexes. In fact, the normal term infant behaves in many ways like an anencephalic newborn (having only a brain stem and basal ganglia). Postnatally developed voluntary control of movement and posture soon replaces the primitive neonatal reflexes. The late pregnancy and early neonatal phases of maturation are especially critical to later achievement. Disease, trauma, or unfavorable environmental factors may irreparably alter the development of the CNS. Developmental defects of the CNS may involve not only the nervous system but also bone, muscle, and connective tissue. Most of these malformations probably result from an interaction of genetic and environmental factors. Some gross abnormalities such as anencephaly preclude survival of the infant. Severe malformations such as myelomeningocele cause functional disability (paralysis and mental retardation).

Hypoxia attributable to maternal causes (e.g., premature separation of the placenta), fetal causes (e.g., cord entanglement), or iatrogenic problems (e.g., hypotension after spinal anesthesia) may be critical to the infant. Many of the survivors of severe asphyxia develop cerebral palsy, mental retardation, or other neurologic deficits. This is especially true of newborns of 36 weeks or less gestational age, who are even more sensitive to hypoxia or trauma than mature newborns. Fortunately, however, the infant has remarkable powers of recuperation, and many depressed babies appear to recover satisfactorily. See Chapter 30 for more information on newborn neurologic function.

Gastrointestinal function

Intrauterine nutrition and elimination occur through the placenta, making it unnecessary for the slowly developing gastrointestinal system to function prior to birth. This system is still physiologically immature at birth; however, during the second trimester, the fetus begins to swallow and subsequently excrete amniotic fluid by way of the kidneys. As term is approached, increasing amounts of *meconium* are found in the fetal intestinal tract. Normal meconium is a sterile, dark greenish brown, semisolid residue of bile and embryonic secretions plus squamous epithelial cells and hair swallowed in utero. The presence of meconium in amniotic fluid prior to delivery indicates fetal hypoxia or maternal narcotic intoxication.

Although limited in function, the intestinal tract of the normal infant is proportionately longer than that of an adult. Its elasticity, musculature, and control mechanisms continue to develop until the child is 2 to 3 years of age when adult levels of gastrointestinal function are achieved.

Normally bacteria are not present in the newborn's gastrointestinal tract. Soon after birth, oral and anal orifices permit entrance of bacteria and air. Bowel sounds can be heard within 4 to 6 hours. Generally, the highest bacterial concentration is found in the lower portion of the intestine, particularly in the large intestine. The normal intestinal flora help synthesize vitamin K, folic acid, and biotin.

A special mechanism present in normal newborns weighing more than 1500 gm coordinates the breathing, sucking, and swallowing necessary for oral feeding. The infant is unable to move food from his lips to pharynx; therefore it is necessary to place the nipple (breast or bottle) well inside the baby's mouth. Peristaltic activity in the esophagus is uncoordinated in the first few days of life but quickly becomes coordinated in normal infants. Persistent uncoordinated motility patterns and swallowing difficulties may indicate brain damage.

The capacity and emptying time for the stomach of the normal newborn is highly variable. Several factors such as time and volume of feedings, type and temperature of food, and psychic stress may affect the emptying time (between 1 and 24 hours).

Two principal types of cells comprise the stomach: *chief cells,* which synthesize and secrete pepsinogen, aiding in protein digestion; and *parietal cells,* which secrete hydrochloric acid. The infant's gastric acidity at birth normally equals the adult level but is reduced within a week and may remain reduced for 2 to 3 months. Gastric acidity and the enzyme pepsin are necessary for preliminary digestion of milk prior to its entrance into the small intestine.

Further digestion and absorption of nutrients from the stomach occur in the small intestine. This complex process is made possible by pancreatic secretions, secretions from the liver through the common bile duct, and secretions from the duodenal portion of the small intestine.

The infant's ability to digest carbohydrates, fats, and proteins is regulated by the presence of certain enzymes. Most of these are functional at birth. One exception is *amylase,* produced by the salivary glands after about 3 months and by the pancreas at about 6 months of age. This enzyme is necessary to digest starch into maltose. The other exception is *lipase,* also secreted by the pancreas; it is necessary for the digestion of fat. Thus the normal newborn is capable of digesting simple carbohydrates and proteins, but it has a limited ability to digest fats.

Liver function

Liver function begins at about the fourth week of gestation as a prelude to erythropoesis, which starts at about the eighth week of intrauterine life.

The fetal liver at term is proportionately much larger than that of the 1-year-old infant. It is a metabolic and glycogen storage organ, that also acts as a depot for iron. Full liver function is not achieved until well after delivery, however. For example, coagulation factors contributed to or produced by the liver and fibrinogen are low at the time of delivery but adjust in early infancy.

The production of fetal liver enzymes is limited, especially in the fetus that is less than 36 weeks gestational age. Hence the conjugation and excretion of bilirubin is impaired in the premature infant. (See Chapter 36.) Poor metabolism of drugs such as sulfonamides by the immature fetal liver also may pose problems for the infant. The congenital absence of certain liver enzymes causes inborn errors of metabolism.

Adrenal function

The fetal adrenal gland is larger than the kidney during much of its development, attesting to the relatively greater importance of the adrenals at that time. The adrenal *medulla* or central portion of the gland produces small amounts of catecholamines, which have important vascular functions. Control of fetal catecholamine production is still under investigation.

The fetal adrenal *cortex,* or outer part of the gland, is composed of a rather thin external layer, which will become the adult cortex, and an inner zone that is four times as thick, which normally disappears after the first year of life.

Maternal ACTH does not cross the placenta to regulate the adrenal cortex as one might suppose, but HCG and LH do enter the fetal circulation. Cortisol is produced by the outer or adult zone, and increasing amounts of this substance may be important in the initiation of labor. The major hormone from the inner or fetal zone is dehydroisoandrosterone (DHA). Fetal ACTH, absent in anencephalic fetuses, stimulates the adult zone but not the fetal zone. HCG and prolactin also help to regulate the fetal zone, although this as yet is poorly understood.

Genitals

Female genital development and function. The fetal ovary with many primordial follicles produces small but increasing amounts of estrogen, and the development of the external genitals and female characteristics are complete at term. The hyperestrogenism of pregnancy followed by estrogen withdrawal after delivery account for the brief mucoid vaginal discharge and even slight bloody spotting that may be noted in female neonates.

During childhood, small but continuing secretion of estrogen occurs. Prior to puberty a much greater production of estrogen accounts for the development of female secondary sex characteristics.

Male genital development and function. Early in embryologic development, the gonads of the genetically male fetus play a critical role in the formation of the genital tract. As the gonads evolve in the testicular pattern, presumably under the influence of maternal HCG, LH, and fetal adrenal hormones, the testes produce androgenic hormones that result in growth and differentiation of the wolffian ducts into a right and left epididymis, vas deferens, and seminal vesicles. Concurrently the embryonic testes also begin to secrete independently a polypeptide material, *müllerian-inhibiting substance* (MIS), which suppresses the müllerian ducts. Eventually these are almost completely resorbed.

During the latter part of fetal life, the testes produce small amounts of androgenic hormone. Normal external male genitals develop under the influence of androgens. After delivery, a slow increase in the production of androgen and traces of estrogen continue until just before puberty when much larger amounts of testosterone particularly are secreted. This causes development of the male secondary sex characteristics.

Table 8-4. Embryonic and fetal growth and development*

Fertilization age (weeks)	Crown-rump length (approx.)	Crown-heel length (approx.)	Weight (approx.)	Gross appearance	Internal development
Embryonic stage					
1	0.5 mm	0.5 mm	?	Minute clone free in uterus	Early morula; no organ differentiation
2	2 mm	2 mm	?	Ovoid vesicle superficially buried in endometrium	External trophoblast; flat embryonic disk forming 2 inner vesicles (amnio-ecto-mesodermal and entodermal)
3	3 mm	3 mm	?	Early dorsal concavity changes to convexity; head, tail folds form; neural grooves close partially	Optic vesicles appear; double heart recognized; fourteen mesodermal somites present
4	4 mm	4 mm	0.4 gm	Head is at right angle to body; limb rudiments obvious, tail prominent	Vitelline duct only communication between umbilical vesicle and intestines; initial stage of most organs has begun
8	3 cm	3.5 cm	2 gm	Eyes, ears, nose, mouth recognizable; digits formed, tail almost gone	Sensory organ development well along; ossification beginning in occiput, mandible, and humerus (diaphysis); small intestines coil within umbilical cord; pleural, pericardial cavities forming; gonadal development advanced without differentiation
Fetal stage					
12	8 cm	11.5 cm	19 gm	Skin pink, delicate; resembles a human being, but head is disproportionately large	Brain configuration roughly complete; internal sex organs now specific; uterus no longer bicornuate; blood forming in marrow; upper cervical to lower sacral arches and bodies ossify
16	13.5 cm	19 cm	100 gm	Scalp hair appears; fetus active; arm-leg ratio now proportionate; sex determination possible	Sex organs grossly formed; myelinization; heart muscle well developed; lobulated kidneys in final situation; meconium in bowel; vagina and anus open; ischium ossified
20	18.5 cm	22 cm	300 gm	Legs lengthen appreciably; distance from umbilicus to pubis increases	Sternum ossifies

*From Benson, R. C. 1974. Handbook of obstetrics and gynecology (ed. 5). Los Altos, Calif., Lange Medical Publications.

Continued.

Table 8-4. Embryonic and fetal growth and development—cont'd

Fertilization age (weeks)	Crown-rump length (approx.)	Crown-heel length (approx.)	Weight (approx.)	Gross appearance	Internal development
24	23 cm	32 cm	600 gm	Skin reddish and wrinkled; slight subcuticular fat; vernix; primitive respiratory-like movements	Os pubis (horizontal ramus) ossifies; viability is reached, but only few survive, even with expert care
28	27 cm	36 cm	1100 gm	Skin less wrinkled, more fat; nails appear; if delivered, may survive with optimal care	Testes at internal inguinal ring or below; astragalus ossifies; less than 10% survive
32	31 cm	41 cm	1800 gm	Fetal weight increased proportionately more than length	Middle 4th phalanges ossify; about 60% survive with specialty care
36	35 cm	46 cm	2200 gm	Skin pale, body rounded; lanugo disappearing; hair fuzzy or woolly; ear lobes soft with little cartilage; umbilicus in center of body; testes in inguinal canals, scrotum small with few rugae; few sole creases	Distal femoral ossification centers present; about 70-80% survive with individual care
40	40 cm	52 cm	3200 + gm	Skin smooth and pink; copious vernix, moderate to profuse silky hair; lanugo hair on shoulders and upper back; ear lobes stiffened by thick cartilage; nasal and alar cartilages; nails extend over tips of digits; testes in full, pendulous, rugous scrotum (or labia majora) well developed; creases cover sole	Proximal tibial ossification centers present; cuboid, tibia (proximal epiphysis) ossify; over 95% survival with good care

VIABILITY

The chronology of pregnancy may be referred to in several ways, for example, 10 lunar months (of 4 weeks each), 40 weeks of gestation, or 9 calendar months (three trimesters of 3 months each). Table 8-4 summarizes the development of the embryo and fetus during the 40 weeks of gestation, and Fig. 8-7 illustrates the stages of growth.

The earliest gestational age at which a fetus can survive outside the uterus is termed *viability*. Until recently, it was believed that viability was reached when the fetus weighed more than 1000 gm and was at least 28 weeks' gestational age. Improvement in maternal and neonatal care now suggests that a new standard of viability must be established. On the basis of current published literature and personal experience, viability is now determined to be a weight of 601 gm or more and at least 24 weeks' gestational age.

Most infants at term weigh about 3200 gm (7 pounds 1 ounce). Wide variation is observed in mature neonates, with weights ranging from 2500 to 4500 gm (5 pounds 8 ounces to 9 pounds 15 ounces). The weight depends on numerous factors, including race, height, and weight of parents; the infant's place in the birth sequence; and maternal weight before and during pregnancy. Boys usually are about 100 gm (3 ounces) heavier than girls.

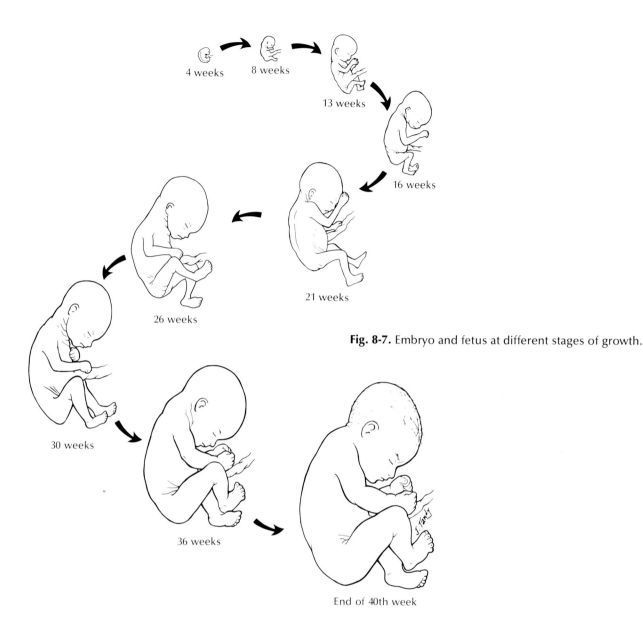

4 weeks　　8 weeks

13 weeks

16 weeks

21 weeks

26 weeks

30 weeks

36 weeks

End of 40th week

Fig. 8-7. Embryo and fetus at different stages of growth.

REFERENCES

Aladjem, S., and Brown, A. K. (eds.). 1974. Clinical perinatology. St. Louis, The C. V. Mosby Co.

Behrman, R. 1973. Neonatology. St. Louis, The C. V. Mosby Co.

Bolognese, R. J., and others. 1973. Evaluation of possible transplacental infection with vaccination during pregnancy. Am. J. Obstet. Gynecol. **117:**939.

Cibils, L. A. 1974. The placenta and newborn infant in hypertensive conditions. Am. J. Obstet. Gynecol. **118:**256.

Dawes, G. 1973. The distribution and action of drugs on foetus in utero. Br. J. Anaesth. **45:**766.

Diczfalusy, E. 1974. Endocrine functions of the human fetus and placenta. Am. J. Obstet. Gynecol. **119:**419.

Edwards, R. G. 1973. Studies on human conception. Am. J. Obstet. Gynecol. **117:**587.

Fleet, W. F., Jr., Benz, E. W., Jr., Karzon, D. T., and others. 1974. Fetal consequences of maternal rubella immunization. J.A.M.A. **227:**621.

McLennan, C. E., and Sandberg, E. C. 1974. Synopsis of obstetrics (ed. 9). St. Louis, The C. V. Mosby Co.

Moore, K. 1974. Before we are born. Philadelphia, W. B. Saunders Co.

Prenatal care: which drugs for the pregnant patient (editorial). 1974. Patient Care **8:**54, March.

Rugh, R., and Shettles, L. 1971. From conception to birth. New York, Harper & Row, Publishers.

Williams, P., and Wendell-Smith, C. 1966. Basic human embryology. Philadelphia, J. B. Lippincott Co.

CHAPTER 9

Maternal physiology

Pregnancy affects every organ system. The genital tract reflects the earliest and most obvious changes; other system variations develop later and frequently are more subtle.

CHANGES IN THE GENITAL TRACT
Vasculature

A prompt, excessive increase in the vasculature of the internal female genitals begins in early gestation. The uterine arteries and veins particularly become more enlarged, elongated, and tortuous after establishment of pregnancy. Hence the blood supply to the pregnant uterus increases progressively throughout pregnancy. The other pelvic organs are similarly, although not as markedly, affected. Considerable dilatation of the pelvic veins and the development of a wide collateral circulation provide a venous reservoir and a protective mechanism against a sharp increase or sharp decrease in uterine blood flow. As a result, the blood flow to the uterus and contained products of conception is maintained at about 10 ml/100 gm of unit weight per minute.

Uterine contractions provide another regulatory circulatory mechanism. The frequency, duration, and intensity of the contraction pattern alter the blood flow to the uterus, placenta, and fetus.

Other internal organs that increase their circulation considerably during pregnancy are the kidneys and adrenal glands. The skin, breasts, and lower extremities also participate in marked circulatory expansion during pregnancy.

Cervix

Increased vascularity and softening of the cervix begins soon after the first missed period (Ladin or Hegar's sign). The endocervix, which is composed of a vast number of crevices, clefts, and tunnels (but no tubular or branching glands), is covered by columnar mucus-producing cells that are supported by a light, musculofibrous, supporting structure. During pregnancy, under the influence of estrogen and progesterone, hyper-

trophy and hyperplasia of all elements occur and edema of the connective tissue becomes notable (Fig. 9-1). The tissues soon lose their rigidity; the folds thin and become more delicate. Considerable mucus is produced, and because of the progesterone effect, ferning does not occur in the dried cervical smear. On the other hand, estrogen causes some eversion of the endocervical cells of the cervical canal normally during pregnancy. The changing consistency of the cervix may be likened to the feel of the following: prepregnant—the tip of the nose, pregnant (early and midterm)—the ear lobe, and pregnant (term)—the lips.

At term, the now spongelike cervix thins (effaces), and the os widens (dilates) to allow the insertion of a fingertip in primigravidas and even several fingertips in multigravidas.

Ovaries and fallopian tubes

Ovulation is suspended during pregnancy, but the corpus luteum associated with gestation remains 3 to 4 cm in diameter until almost midpregnancy when it gradually diminishes in size and function. The corpus luteum of pregnancy remains recognizable until termination of gestation. The fallopian tubes elongate during pregnancy and, together with the ovaries, appear suspended from the sides of the greatly enlarged uterus. Many widely dilated veins develop within the parametrial and broad ligament areas.

Uterus

Uterine enlargement to accommodate the growing fetus is the most distinctive characteristic of pregnancy. Its growth is remarkable, and it causes significant changes in the physiology of adjacent structures (Figs. 9-2 to 9-5). During the course of pregnancy, the uterus increases from approximately 6.5 to 32 cm long, from 4 to 24 cm wide, and from 2.5 cm to 22 cm deep. Its weight increases twentyfold from 50 to 1000 gm. It develops from a small, almost solid organ with a capacity of perhaps 4 ml into a thin-walled muscular sac that can

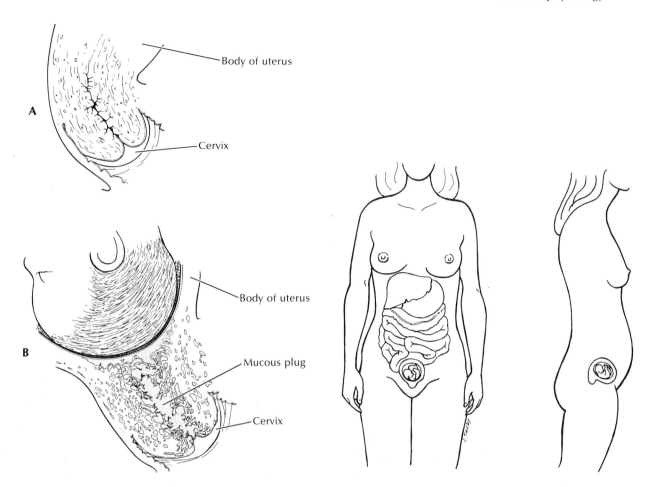

Fig. 9-1. A, Cervix in nonpregnant woman. **B,** Changes in cervix during pregnancy.

Fig. 9-2. Relative size of growing uterus at 16 weeks.

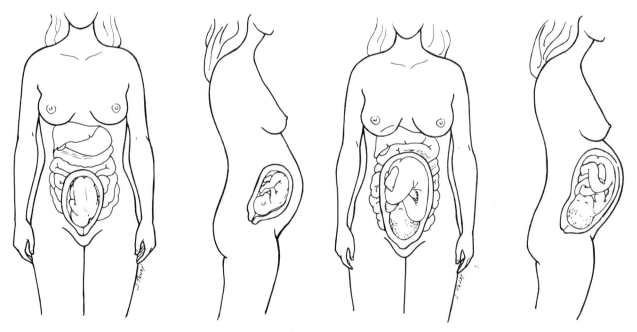

Fig. 9-3. Relative size of growing uterus at 6½ months.

Fig. 9-4. Relative size of growing uterus at 9 months.

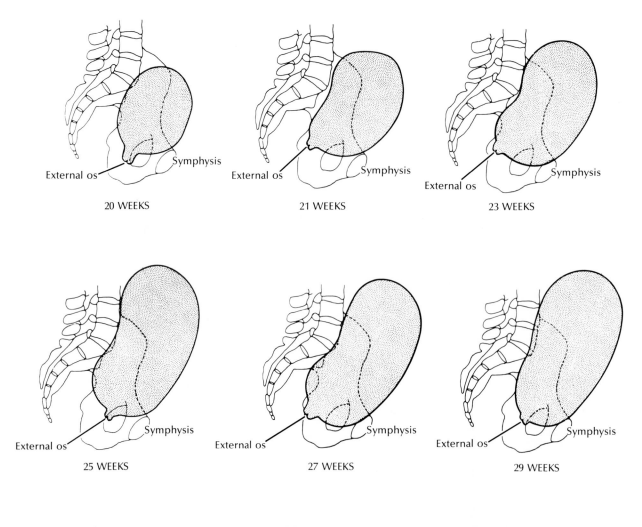

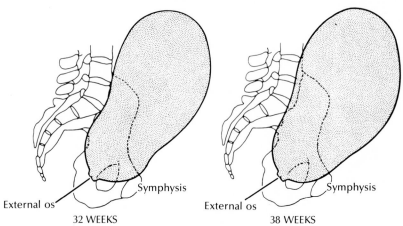

Fig. 9-5. Changes in shape of uterus during pregnancy.

contain fetus, placenta, and more than 1000 ml of amniotic fluid.

New muscle fibers formed in early pregnancy are partially responsible for this phenomenal growth. However, the most significant single factor is the enlargement of preexistent muscle fibers—from seven to eleven times longer and two to seven times wider than those in the nonpregnant uterus. As these bands of muscles enlarge, new fibroelastic tissue develops to form a network between them, strengthening the uterine walls (Fig. 9-6). Uterine hypertrophy in early pregnancy may be attributed to estrogen stimulation of muscle fibers. From a thickness of 1 cm at conception to almost 2 cm at the end of the first few months of pregnancy, the uterine wall then thins to 0.5 cm or less. At term it is thin and soft, permitting effective palpation of the fetus by the examiner.

The musculature of the uterus is unique, since not only does it provide for support and delivery of its contents but also a natural physiologic defense against postnatal hemorrhage. There are three layers of muscle fibers: a thin outer layer curving over the fundus, a thin internal layer around the openings of the fallopian tubes and the internal os, and a thick middle layer of obliquely interlacing fibers. It is through this interlacing network that blood vessels pass to the endometrium from the external

vascular zone. When the uterus contracts and retracts after expulsion of the fetus and placenta, muscles in this middle layer constrict the vessels, shutting off the blood supply to and from the placental lake. (This characteristic is the reason why the uterine musculature is often referred to as the *living ligature*.) Each time contraction and retraction occur, the muscles remain shortened, gradually decreasing the size of the uterine cavity and maintaining muscle tone.

As the uterus grows, it is elevated out of the pelvic area, and may be palpated above the symphysis pubis sometime between the twelfth and sixteenth week of pregnancy (Figs. 9-7 to 9-9). It rises gradually to reach the umbilicus at the end of 20 to 22 weeks and nearly impinges on the xiphoid process at term.

Generally, the uterus is rotated to the right as it elevates, probably due to the presence of the rectosigmoid colon on the left side. Eventually the growing uterus touches the anterior abdominal wall and displaces the intestines to either side of the abdomen. Approximately 2 weeks prior to delivery, the fetus descends into the pelvic cavity, referred to as *lightening*, causing the uterus to sink slightly and fall forward (Fig. 9-10). This shift in positioning relieves the pressure formerly exerted on the diaphragm, making it possible for the patient to breathe and to eat more. This phenomenon does

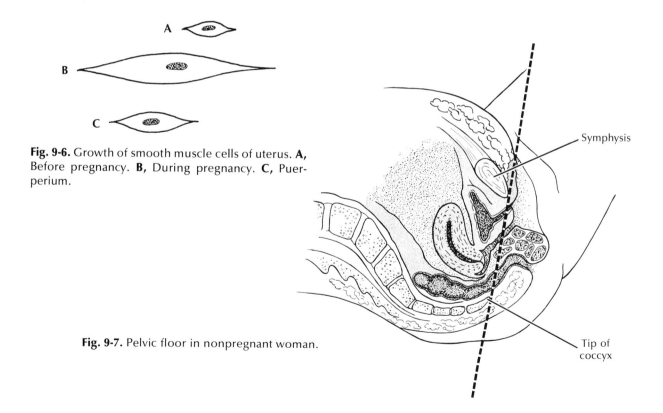

Fig. 9-6. Growth of smooth muscle cells of uterus. **A,** Before pregnancy. **B,** During pregnancy. **C,** Puerperium.

Symphysis

Tip of coccyx

Fig. 9-7. Pelvic floor in nonpregnant woman.

Fig. 9-8. Pelvic floor at end of pregnancy. Note marked projection (growth of tissue) below line joining tip of coccyx and inferior margin of symphysis.

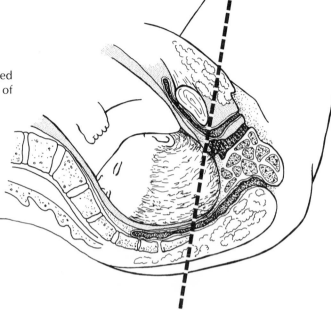

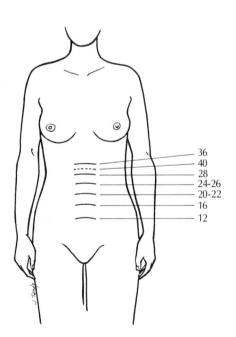

Fig. 9-9. Height of fundus by weeks of gestation.

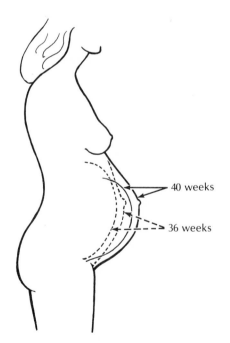

Fig. 9-10. Lightening: descent of presenting part into true pelvis. Pressure on diaphragm is relieved, and breathing is easier; pressure on bladder increases as does urinary frequency.

not usually occur in multigravidas until the onset of labor.

The weight of the gravid uterus and its contents causes an instinctive backward tilt of the patient's torso. This posture places increased strain on muscles and ligaments of the thighs and back and thus contributes to the musculoskeletal aches and cramps so characteristic of late pregnancy.

The most significant observation during sexual arousal in the third trimester is the occurrence of tonic spasms of the uterus during orgasm. This spasm may last for as long as 1 minute. Contractions often continue for some time after orgasm and may be accompanied by backache.

Vagina

In established pregnancy, the vascularity of the vagina imparts the purplish hue of Chadwick's sign. The mucoid vaginal fluid is whitish because it contains many exfoliated epithelial cells. Vaginal cytosmears during pregnancy characteristically reveal folded, clumped, navicular (boat-shaped), precornified cells. Rarely are cornified parabasal or basal cells noted. Leukocytes are numerous; red blood cells are absent, and a mixed bacterial flora, perhaps with lactobacilli predominating, is typical. Therefore pregnancy frequently can be confirmed by vaginal cytology.

This increased vascularity of the vagina and other pelvic viscera results in a marked increase in sensitivity and may lead to a high degree of sexual interest and arousal during the second trimester of pregnancy. As pregnancy progresses, there is more venous engorgement of the entire vaginal canal so that the orgasmic platform becomes almost completely obtruded. During orgasm the rhythmic contractions of the orgasmic platform are felt but not observable. Because of the increased congestion and resolution period that is less complete, some women become multiorgasmic for the first time.

Breasts

Fullness, heightened sensitivity, tingling, and heaviness of the breasts are progressive after the second missed menstrual period. About the same time, a secondary pinkish areola may be apparent. Nipples and areolas become more pigmented, nipples more erectile. Hypertrophic sebaceous glands in the primary areola, called the *tubercles of Montgomery,* may be seen around the nipples. Venous congestion in the breasts is more obvious, especially for nulliparous women. When sexually stimulated vasocongestion is superimposed on increased breast size resulting from pregnancy, the breasts may become extremely tender. The tenderness is frequently localized in turgid nipples and engorged areolas. Colostrum, a premilk fluid, may be expressed from the nipples during the third trimester. Near term, protection may be needed because colostrum often leaks from the breast, soiling the clothing.

CARDIOVASCULAR CHANGES

The heart rate slowly increases by approximately 10 beats/min from about the fourteenth through the thirtieth week of pregnancy. Subsequently, the rate is maintained at this level until after delivery when the normal prepregnancy rate may be expected. The blood pressure shows typical changes. There is a fall in blood pressure during the second trimester and then a rise not exceeding 15 mm Hg in either diastolic or systolic pressure. The study by MacGilivray and others (1969) of 226 primigravidas on the first obstetric visit early in pregnancy showed blood pressures of 113 ± 10 mm Hg (systolic) and 57 ± 10 mm Hg (diastolic) when supine and 103 ± 11 mm Hg (systolic) and 56 ± 10 mm Hg (diastolic) when sitting. By the twenty-eighth week, all showed increases that continued to term, reaching 116 ± 10 mm Hg (systolic) and 71 ± 12 mm Hg (diastolic) when supine. Because of these apparently low readings, the nurse must be alert to minimal rises in blood pressures because they may be indicative of pathophysiology.

The "roll-over test," although not completely valid, can act as a simple screening test for hypertension. When an individual rolls from the prone to the supine position, there is a normal drop in measured blood pressure. However, in an expectant patient with preeclampsia, the reverse happens; the blood pressure goes up.

The venous blood pressure does not change in the arms, but a gradual, rather marked, increase occurs in the legs after the eighth week.

The cardiac output increases by one third to one half by the thirty second week but declines to a 20% increase by term (Fig. 9-11).

The total body water is increased after the tenth week, and plasma and blood volume both rise about 25% to 40% between the twelfth and thirty-second week with a slight decline thereafter. The increase in total body water acts as a safeguard against loss of blood during delivery. The volume of circulating blood and cardiac output can be maintained by drawing on fluid reserves in the tissues.

The hemoglobin may decline slightly during pregnancy as a result of hemodilution, but the red blood cell mass is augmented 10% to 15% after the eighth week of pregnancy. The decline in hemoglobin results in the "pseudoanemia" of pregnancy.

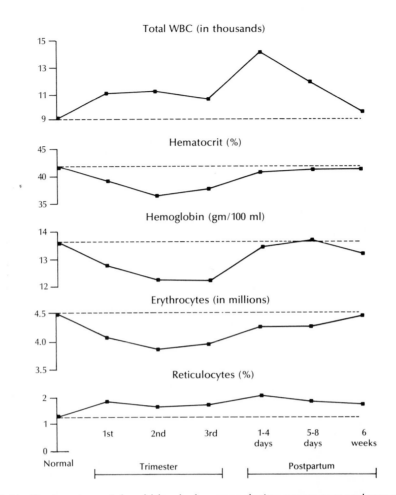

Fig. 9-11. Changes in peripheral blood of woman during pregnancy and puerperium.

The circulation time decreases slightly by the thirty-second week and then returns to normal near term.

Cardiac displacement and cardiac murmurs are normal findings in pregnancy, and return to the prepregnant state occurs after delivery.

RESPIRATORY SYSTEM CHANGES

The nasal mucosa, also responsive to estrogens, become slightly hyperemic and edematous in well-established pregnancy. As a consequence, nasal "stuffiness" and epistaxis (nosebleeds) are common.

Despite the progressive elevation of the diaphragm during late pregnancy, flaring of the ribs increases the anteroposterior and transverse diameters of the chest to accommodate the lungs. Although there may be a slight increase in *vital capacity* during pregnancy, oxygen consumption is increased by about 15% between the sixteenth and fortieth weeks. The respiratory rate, minute volume, and tidal air are increased slightly during pregnancy.

After the twenty-fourth week, thoracic breathing replaces abdominal breathing. Most women exhibit slight dyspnea during late pregnancy. Hyperventilation may be indicative of a greater need for oxygen rather than a reaction to excessive PCO_2, however.

URINARY TRACT CHANGES

The pelvic congestion of pregnancy is reflected in hyperemia of the urethra and bladder. Frequency of urination is due to increased bladder sensitivity and later to compression of the bladder by the enlarging uterus. The bladder is pulled up out of the true pelvis into the abdomen and elongates from 1½ to 3 inches. The vascularity of the bladder mucosa increases, and trauma during delivery may cause hemorrhage. As a response to hormonal influences on the smooth muscle of the bladder, there is a decrease in bladder tone. The capacity increases gradually to 1500 ml, and overdistention is not an uncommon problem in the postnatal period.

Dilatation and slight elongation of the ureters, together with slight pyelectasia of the kidneys are characteristic of second and third trimester pregnancy. The hydroureter, most notable on the right, is due to a slight compression of the ureters by the pregnant uterus, which normally is displaced slightly to the right by the descending colon, and to the suppressive effect of the steroid sex hormones on smooth muscle of the urinary tract. Hypotonia, hypoperistalsis, and even vesicoureteral reflux occur during pregnancy. Thus pyelonephritis is more common and more difficult to treat during pregnancy.

Augmented renal function is progressive during pregnancy. The renal blood flow is increased by approximately 25% during the first and second trimesters, returning to prepregnant levels during the last trimester. The glomerular filtration rate increases by almost 50%, declining somewhat during the last month of pregnancy but returning to normal during the early puerperium. Plasma renin and angiotensin increase slightly during pregnancy. An increased excretion of creatinine and urea is accomplished, but reduced tubular absorption of sodium particularly is necessary to maintain homeostasis.

GASTROINTESTINAL CHANGES

Excessive salivation (ptyalism) may develop during early pregnancy—particularly among women who have nausea and vomiting. This so-called morning sickness actually may occur at any time of day and is often associated with a disagreeable or cooking odor. If vomiting persists beyond the first trimester or is excessive anytime, it is termed *hyperemesis gravidarum* (Chapter 18).

Strange aversions to food or curious food cravings, may develop during gestation. *Pica* is defined as a bizarre appetite. The most common examples of pica in the United States are the eating of red clay or starch (Argo laundry starch is most commonly used) by pregnant women. The type of food seems to be based in local tradition and availability. The danger of this practice lies in substituting nutritionally empty foods for the needed, well-balanced diet.

Esophageal regurgitation or pyrosis (acid indigestion, heartburn) is common during pregnancy, but hypochlorhydria rather than excessive gastric acidity is the rule. Decreased emptying time of the stomach and gallbladder is typical. This feature, together with slight hypercholesterolemia from progesterone levels, may account for the frequent development of gallstones during pregnancy. Constipation is secondary to hypoperistalsis, unusual food choice, lack of fluids, abdominal distention by the pregnant uterus, displacement of intestines with some compression, and effects of progesterone on smooth muscles.

Hepatic function is difficult to appraise during gestation. However, only minor changes in liver function develop during pregnancy. Occasionally a woman may develop cholestasis and pruritus gravidarum during late pregnancy. High levels of estrogen and progesterone may affect liver cells to produce these symptoms, which clear promptly after delivery.

TEETH, BONE, AND JOINT CHANGES

Hypertrophy of gingival papillae (epulis) may be an estrogen effect. Gingivitis or calculus may be responsible for periodontic problems.

Demineralization of teeth does not occur during pregnancy. Hence the old adage "for every child a tooth" is untrue. Poor dental hygiene during pregnancy may contribute to dental caries.

The pregnant woman requires about 1.2 gm of calcium and approximately the same amount of phosphorous every day during pregnancy. This is an increase of about 0.4 gm of each of these elements over the nonpregnancy needs. With a well-balanced diet, these requirements are satisfied. Serious dietary deficiency, however, may deplete the mother's osseous stores of these elements. Except in extreme cases (e.g., osteomalacia), maternal disability or deformity is most unlikely.

Hypermobility of pelvic joints due to slight relaxation of the periarticular structures, possibly an effect of the hormone relaxin, may develop during advanced pregnancy. Rarely, considerable separation of the symphysial synchondrosis may cause a painful, waddling gait. Slight widening of the joint space at the symphysis pubis frequently can be disclosed by x-ray film.

Accentuation of the dorsal and lumbar spinal curvatures because of the altered posture of pregnancy may cause backache.

ENDOCRINE CHANGES
Fetoplacental hormone production

After fertilization, the woman's hormonal pattern differs greatly from that observed during the menstrual cycle. Estrogens continue to rise after nidation. Placental production of estrogens is evidenced by ovarian inactivity during pregnancy. In contrast, progesterone rises rapidly at ovulation. The steroid sex hormone effects are clearly reflected in the endometrium after implantation, as shown in Fig. 9-12.

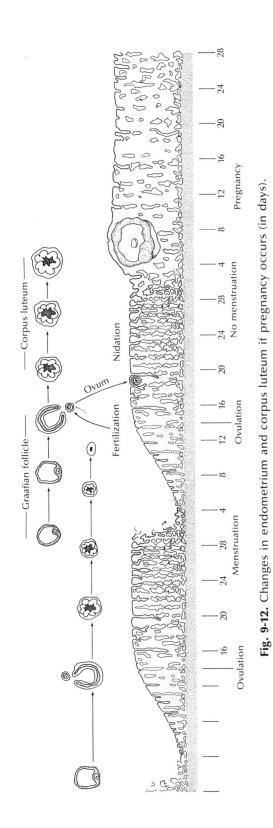

Fig. 9-12. Changes in endometrium and corpus luteum if pregnancy occurs (in days).

However, instead of a maintained elevation for about 10 days followed by a fall to negligible levels as at the onset of menstruation, progesterone production continues to rise until the third or fourth week of pregnancy. Then the level decreases until the sixth to eighth week of pregnancy, perhaps evidence of transfer of progesterone production from the corpus luteum to the placenta. Thereafter the titer rises rapidly again as pregnancy continues.

Although the level plateaus during the last month, it may fall just prior to the onset of labor. Pregnanediol, the major metabolic progesterone, is excreted in the urine, and its pattern follows that of plasma progesterone during gestation.

The placenta synthesizes steroid hormones, but to accomplish this, it must receive some essential steroid precursors from other sources. Certain of these essential materials are fetal such as estriol; others are maternal derivatives such as cholesterol. This interdependency is implicit in the commonly used term *fetoplacental unit.*

Estrogens initially produced by the ovarian theca cells are produced in far greater quantity by the fetal trophoblast. Estradiol is conjugated from maternal and fetal DHA. Estrone is also a placental product, but estriol probably is a much more important substance during pregnancy because it constitutes a major portion of plasma estrogen.

Fetal estriol, derived from 16α-hydroxydehydroisoandrosterone, is significant in fetoplacental metabolism. The maternal organism also produces some estriol, and urinary estriol values continue to rise from conception to term. Nonetheless, because the fetal contribution is so considerable, the measurement of the excreted urinary estriol has become an important index of fetal well-being (p. 196).

HCG as measured in the peripheral plasma rises sharply about 10 days after ovulation to an initial peak at about the sixteenth or seventeenth day of pregnancy, indicative that even at nidation, the blastocyst is producing this new luteinizing hormone. The titer then sinks to a slightly lower level by the twelfth week where it remains for the duration of pregnancy. Although HCG appears to support the corpus luteum early in pregnancy, the function of this hormone later in gestation is unknown. HCG consists of an α and a β subunit, the second probably being similar to the luteinizing prepregnancy ovarian hormone LH. HCG is of large molecular size. Hence excretion of this hormone is slow, and measureable amounts remain in the circulation until about 2 weeks after parturition.

Technically, inadequate estrogen or progesterone may

be a cause of spontaneous abortion. Hormone levels are rarely available before and during the course of a failing pregnancy, however. Therefore endocrine therapy for threatened abortion, on the assumption of hormone deficiency, is purely empirical and almost never beneficial. On the other hand, bleeding during an early pregnancy in which high levels of HCG are reported may indicate hydatidiform mole or choriocarcinoma.

In addition to HCG, chorionic somatomammotropin (HCS), or placental lactogen (HPL), is the other hormone of strictly placental origin. A protein hormone immunologically akin to HCG, HCS has an anabolic effect similar to growth hormone and is measured in gradually increasing amounts during pregnancy. Like HCG, HCS is slowly dissipated after delivery.

Chorionic thyrotropin (HCT), a glycoprotein similar to thyroid-produced TSH, is also produced in small amounts by the trophoblast. The thyroid-stimulatory activity of the serum of pregnant women may be due in part to HCT.

Pituitary

Slight enlargement of the anterior lobe of the pituitary occurs during pregnancy. On rare occasions, compression of the optic chiasm may cause bilateral hemianopsia (blindness in half the visual field). Numerous acidophilic granulocytes appear in the anterior pituitary gland soon after the last menstrual period. The function of these so-called pregnancy cells is unknown.

During pregnancy, the anterior pituitary continues to produce all the tropic hormones exhibited in the nonpregnant state, but these may be noted in slightly different amounts. This relative inactivity of the anterior pituitary is seemingly due to suppression, principally by HCG. Further support for this opinion is the observation that the levels of FSH fall to clinically undetectable levels by the tenth day after ovulation to remain there during the entire pregnancy. Gonadotropins are inhibited but thyrotropic and adrenocorticotropic hormones may be increased slightly. Melanotropic hormone is increased, causing the added pigmentation of pregnancy. Pituitary somatomammotropin (growth hormone) production is suppressed. Concomitantly with pregnancy, pituitary prolactin production begins a marked increase that continues to term and is maintained throughout lactation. Oxytocin is produced in increasing amounts as the fetus matures, but vasopressin production is essentially unchanged during pregnancy.

Thyroid

Pregnancy induces slight hyperplasia of the acinar cells of the thyroid, which results in an increase in iodine metabolism. This is apparent in increased radioactive iodine uptake by the thyroid in experimental animals. Slight but recognizable thyroid gland enlargement occurs by the third month, usually without progression. Return to normal size and function can be expected by the sixth postnatal week.

The pregnant patient's basal metabolic rate (BMR) increases almost 20% by term. The BMR actually indicates greater oxygen utilization by the mother and fetus than the degree of increase of thyroid function.

Laboratory determinations during pregnancy indicate reduced plasma inorganic iodine as a consequence of increased iodine uptake by the thyroid. The protein-bound iodine (PBI) and butanol-extractable iodine (BEI) in the plasma are increased largely because of doubling of the thyroid-binding α globulin. Total thyroxin is increased slightly and the red blood cells' triiodothyronine (T_3) uptake is reduced. However, the level of free thyroxin, the true index of general metabolism, is unaltered. Hence the pregnant patient normally remains euthyroid.

Radioactive iodine must never be administered to a pregnant woman for testing or therapy because this substance is incorporated into the fetal thyroid as early as the twelfth week, and congenital hypothyreosis of the fetus may result.

Parathyroid glands

Pregnancy induces a slight secondary hyperparathyroidism, a reflection of increased requirements for calcium and vitamin D. When the fetal needs are greatest (during the last half of pregnancy), plasma parahormone levels are elevated. Tetany due to calcium deficiency or phosphorus excess is indicative of hypoparathyroidism. Hypercalciuria and nephrolithiasis may be due to hyperparathyroidism.

Adrenal glands

The adrenal cortex thickens slightly, and a "pregnancy zone" has been described. Little change in adrenal function occurs during pregnancy, however. Circulating cortisol is increased during gestation; most of it is bound, with only a small excess of free cortisol demonstrable. The adrenal medulla shows no change during pregnancy, and its function continues without significant alteration.

Pancreas

A gradual increase in the production of insulin by the hyperplastic islets of Langerhans begins in early pregnancy likely due in part to the anti-insulin effect of HPL. A reduced tissue sensitivity to insulin is normal during gestation, but the glucose tolerance is raised only slightly.

The lowered renal threshold for glucose is an expression of the increased production of glucocorticoids by the adrenal cortex and placenta. An augmented glomerular filtration rate and a reduced tubular absorption alter glycogen metabolism during pregnancy.

Glycogen storage during gestation is limited, and patients whose pancreatic reserve is also marginal may develop gestational or even true diabetes.

Because of the tendency for the normal pregnant woman to spill small amounts of glucose (and lactose) in the urine, definite reducing substances in the urine (greater than 1+, Dextrostix) require a fasting blood sugar and a 2-hour postprandial blood sugar determination. If fasting blood sugar is greater than 90 mg/100 ml or the postprandial blood sugar is greater than 140 mg/ 100 ml, a tentative diagnosis of diabetes mellitus must be considered, and a complete 2-hour glucose tolerance test (GTT) will be required to support or reject this possibility.

METABOLIC CHANGES DURING PREGNANCY

Normal pregnancy is an hypermetabolic state as evidenced by weight gain and increased function. Hence nutritional demands are increased. Because pregnancy is a physiologic function and not a disease, most pregnant women maintain good health despite brief annoying problems such as early nausea and vomiting.

Weight gain

It is impossible to recommend average weight gain for all expectant women. Some patients are overweight; others are underweight. Hence individualization is necessary.

Normal pregnancy is responsible for a considerable weight gain. This has been identified by Hellman and Pritchard as follows:

	Kilograms	Pounds
Uterine growth	1.1	2.5
Breast increase	1.4	3.0
Protein retention	1.8	4.0
Increased blood volume	1.5	3.5
Conception products	5.1	11.2
Interstitial water	2.0	4.5
Total	12.9	28.7

Women who are grossly underweight or those who are carrying a multiple pregnancy should gain more than this amount. Obese women may gain less, but they must avoid ketosis, associated with sudden drastic weight reduction, because this complication may jeopardize the fetus.

The patient's prepregnant weight is directly related to weight gain and is inversely related to the percentage of low birth weight infants of women delivered at term. These infants have a higher neonatal mortality than the control group. Gain in weight during pregnancy is also related to increased size of the newborn, with a decline in the percentage of low birth weight infants concomitant with increasing weight gain.

Generally speaking, uncomplicated patients should gain about 3 to 4 pounds during the first trimester, approximately 12 to 14 pounds in the second, and 8 to 10 pounds during the third trimester.

By and large, a more liberal diet for the average woman during pregnancy is good policy. However, one should emphasize the food constituents rather than calories.

Protein metabolism

A positive nitrogen balance, as evidence of protein anabolism, is evident after the third month of pregnancy. Nitrogen losses in the urine (e.g., urea, ammonia) are less during well-established pregnancy than in the nonpregnant state. The growing fetus and enlarging uterus and breasts, together with increased blood elements, account for the mother's increasing nitrogen stores.

Carbohydrate metabolism

Carbohydrate needs during pregnancy are considerably increased, and fetal utilization is obvious, especially during the last two trimesters. Because of factors including glycosuria, reduction in alkali reserve, and maternal lipemia, however, ketosis can be a serious problem. Ketosis also complicates the treatment of pregnant women with diabetes mellitus or those who develop hyperemesis gravidarum. Lactose normally is excreted in the urine during late pregnancy concomitant with breast development preparatory to possible lactation. Therefore lactose must be distinguished from glucose in the urine. (Dextrostix identifies glucose but not lactose.)

Fat metabolism

Increased plasma-neutral fats, phospholipids, and free cholesterol are the basis for a relative lipemia during pregnancy. Why the blood lipids are enhanced is unclear, but there is good reason to conclude that fetal needs and possibly lactation are served.

Mineral metabolism

Approximately 1.2 gm of calcium and 1.2 gm of phosphorus are required every day during pregnancy. This quota is easily met, assuming proper food choice and good digestion. Most of the calcium and phosphorus required by the fetus is utilized during the last 1 to 2 months of gestation.

About 1000 mg of elemental iron are needed during gestation for a greater maternal red blood cell mass, as well as for hemoglobin synthesis by the woman and her fetus. About 18 mg of iron each day is required. This usually must be supplemented by an iron preparation such as ferrous sulfate or ferrous gluconate during the second and third trimesters.

Water metabolism

The pregnant patient has a greater need for water than a nonpregnant individual. An increase in extracellular water of up to 3ℓ in late pregnancy is usual. Fluid retention is explained in part by increases in the adrenocorticosteroids during pregnancy, increased tubular resorption, retention of sodium, and circulatory stasis (in the lower extremities).

Although edema of the legs may be uncomfortable, in the absence of hypertension or proteinuria, treatment other than forced fluids and elevation of the legs may be harmful. Diuretics during gestation should be discouraged. These drugs may lead to dehydration, hyponatremia or thromboembolization.

• • •

Pregnancy is not a parasitic state because a depletion of maternal stores does not develop under normal circumstances. Even so, most pregnancy requirements are obligatory. Hence if a maternal organ is damaged or is unable to adequately increase its function during gestation, it will decompensate and threaten the health or life of the mother or her offspring.

Normal and abnormal physiology will be considered further in subsequent chapters under specific disease entities.

REFERENCES

Atlay, R. D., Gillison, E. W., and Horton, A. L. 1973. A fresh look at pregnancy heartburn. J. Obstet. Gynaecol. Br. Commonw. **80**:63.

Carr, M. C. 1974. The diagnosis of iron deficiency in pregnancy. Obstet. Gynecol. **43**:15.

Cochrane, W. J. 1972. Early obstetric diagnosis by diagnostic ultrasound. Med. Ann. D.C. **41**:148.

Danforth, D. N. 1971. Textbook of obstetrics and gynecology (ed. 2). New York, Harper & Row Publishers.

Desforges, J. 1973. Anemia complicating pregnancy. J. Reprod. Med. **10**:111.

Donald, I. 1968. Sonar in obstetrics and gynecology. In Greenhill, J. B. (ed.). The year book of obstetrics and gynecology, 1967-1968. Chicago, Year Book Medical Publishers, Inc.

Edelman, D. A., Brenner, W. E., Davis, G. L. and others. 1974. An evaluation of the Pregnosticon Dri-Dot test in early pregnancy. Am. J. Obstet. Gynecol. **119**:521.

Fanfera, F. J., and Palmer, L. H. 1968. Pregnancy and varicose veins. Arch. Surg. **96**:33.

Gal, I. 1972. Risks and benefits of the use of hormonal pregnancy test tablets. Nature **240**:241.

Hellman, L. M., and Pritchard, J. 1975. Williams obstetrics (ed. 15). New York, Appleton-Century-Crofts.

MacGilivray, I., Rose, G. A., and Rowe, B. 1969. Blood pressure survey in pregnancy. Clin. Sci. **37**:395.

Marias, V. 1969. Female sexual response during and after pregnancy. San Francisco, National Sex Forum.

Mingeat, R., and Herbant, M. 1973. The functional status of the newborn infant. A study of 5,370 consecutive infants. Am. J. Obstet. Gynecol. **115**:1138.

Moore, K. L. 1973. The developing human. Philadelphia, W. B. Saunders Co.

Sabbagha, R. E., Turner, J. H., and Rockette, H., and others. 1974. Sonar biparietal diameter and fetal age: definition and relationship. Obstet. Gynecol. **43**:7.

Smith, C. A. 1975. The physiology of the newborn infant (ed. 4). Springfield, Ill., Charles C Thomas Publishers.

Stave, H. (ed.). 1970. Physiology of the perinatal period (vols. 1 and 2). New York, Appleton-Century-Crofts.

CHAPTER 10

Psychosocial components of pregnancy

Pregnancy involves not only the mother-to-be but also the father-to-be, prior offspring, parents, and other family members. As Colman and Colman (1971) explained, "Pregnancy is more than simply a biologic event; it is a time of crisis for those involved, a time when identities are changing and new roles are being explored." All the persons involved react to the event from their own perspective and interpret its meaning in light of their own needs, as well as the needs of the others affected.

PERCEPTION OF THE EVENT

Each woman brings to a pregnancy a personalized version of the role of the pregnant woman and the eventual mother. This unique perception has evolved from past experience and will continue to evolve throughout her lifetime. Certain events such as her own pregnancy accelerate, intensify, and bring this lifelong process into conscious awareness. Her perception of the roles may be congruent with the models acceptable to her cultural subgroup or at variance with it. This perception will color her expectations of persons deemed supportive and important to her. Those who are expected to provide support and care have their own versions also, and the congruence between these and the expectant mother's will help determine the effectiveness of the support offered and accepted.

One model that is subscribed to by certain women and professional workers can be described as follows:

1. *Beliefs and attitudes*. Motherhood and pregnancy are states wanted and needed by women to fulfill a natural life cycle. Therefore acceptance of a pregnancy, wanted or not, comes eventually, along with a desire to provide loving and competent care to the child to be born.

2. *Tasks and responsibilities*. The woman will seek, accept, and act on medical advice and care and take participant action in preparing for childbirth and parenthood, that is, obtain antenatal care, arrange for birth in a hospital setting, and attend parent-craft classes.

3. *Relationships and behaviors*. The pregnancy is a shared event in a family, strengthening it as a unit and permitting the acceptance of atypical maternal behaviors such as increased dependency needs, bizarre desires for food, and rapid mood changes.

Such a model is, of course, adapted by each individual. Certain life experiences seem crucial in the adaptative process including the following:

- Memories of mothering experienced as a child and the subsequent nature, supportive or nonsupportive, of the mother-daughter relationship
- The emphasis placed on the primary expression of the feminine role (e.g., dependency vs independency; motherhood vs career)
- The experiences needed to bolster her self-esteem or that act to lower her feelings of self-worth
- Stepping-stone roles that have been played (e.g., caretaker of siblings, baby-sitter, playing with dolls)
- Individuals from the peer group or an older group who acted as negative or positive models and their behaviors that were noted and either emulated or discarded
- Options open for planning to have children and the here-and-now implications of this pregnancy
- The use of sexual activity and consequent pregnancy as mechanisms to satisfy needs not necessarily related to the creation of a child and parenthood
- Economic and/or social conditions so adverse that the care of another person represents a great burden
- Social isolation with no family or friends to act as supports

For the woman, a positive diagnosis of a suspected pregnancy may be the time when the first overt reactions to its biologic reality are manifested. The emotional response to the confirmation of her suspicions may range from expressions of great delight to those of shock, disbelief, and despair as seen in the following statements:

I was just delighted when I heard I was really pregnant. I was so excited I could hardly wait to tell Ron—we talked and talked. I'm still way up there.

I thought, it can't be—it just can't be; I'm too old! What will he say—we have just finished with the other kids—now to start all over. I can't face it—those 2 AM feedings, diapers, and those terrible 2-year-olds into everything. I feel guilty, but I hate the whole idea.

I have a terrible time when I'm pregnant; my legs are so swollen and painful and I feel so lumpy and unattractive, but when I am most down I think of the baby and how much she will mean to us, and I get through another day.

Rubin (1970) describes the reaction of many women when their pregnancy is confirmed as the ''someday but not now'' response:

There is a real pleasure in finding oneself functionally capable of becoming pregnant. There is pleasure in learning that others are pleased with the promise of having, and being given, a child. But these feelings exist independently of the question of time. Personally and privately she is not ready, not now.*

Caplan (1959) also reported that the majority of his patients were initially dismayed at finding themselves pregnant. This dismay gave way to an eventual acceptance of the pregnancy that paralleled the growing acceptance of the reality of the child. He cautioned, however, against assuming that the nonacceptance of the pregnancy state can be equated with the rejection of the child, since he believed that women can separate the state of being pregnant from the idea of being a parent. A woman may dislike being pregnant but be full of love for the child to be born. Other research indicated that a woman with an unwanted pregnancy who is unable to resolve her deep feeling of anger and despair may carry over these attitudes to the postbirth period, with deleterious effects on the child and other family members.

Whether the pregnancy is accepted, pregnant women exhibit certain behaviors in common, and these can be said to be characteristic of pregnancy. One such behavior, as disconcerting to the mother-to-be as to those around her, is the increased sensitivity to actions, verbal or otherwise, of those significant to her. Increased irritability, explosions of tears and anger, or feelings of great joy and cheerfulness alternate apparently with little or no provocation. According to one father-to-be:

I sometimes think she is crazy—we're going somewhere she wants to go—out to dinner or a concert. She goes upstairs happy as a lark and in 2 minutes is down again in a regular temper, won't go, and shouts at me. I really feel bewildered by it all.

Many reasons have been postulated to explain this seemingly erratic behavior. The profound hormonal changes that are part of the maternal response to pregnancy may trigger mood changes much as they do prior to menstruation or during the menopausal period. For some women, recognition of increasing dependency needs when independency has just been attained may give rise to conflicts.

Colman and Colman (1974) state:

Pregnancy involves us in a confrontation with our uncontrollable biologic states and with irreversible change. Furthermore, it shatters the illusion of our separateness and reminds us of our interconnectedness with others. We tend to define growth through separation and individuation. We use terms like ''cutting the apron strings'' in the assumption that the goal of living is individual autonomy. ''Grown up'' is synonymous with being ''on your own.'' Being mature means to ''know who you are.'' The process of emerging from the womb into the arms, from the arms to lap, from lap to yard to school and finally to leaving home is indeed a continuous progression of increasing individuation. The illusion, however, is that this pinnacle reached in adolescence is a stable condition that we achieve on our own. Pregnancy may then seem like a throwback to infancy, for a pregnant woman is never alone. From the inside, the mother has the baby with her always as part of her body consciousness. From the outside, she needs the emotional and economic support of her husband to help her through the child bearing and rearing. Suddenly she is not independent, not on her own. She may become confused about who she is and what is happening.*

Pregnancy offers an opportunity to obtain nurturing care from others and proofs of love, or it can be a desperate attempt at opening up communication channels with significant persons, partner, or parent. Pregnancy may offer acceptable opportunities to withdraw from some of the stress of living. One nursing supervisor remarked, ''As soon as I'm pregnant I'll stop working.'' When she was asked, ''How will you feel about that— not working?'' she replied, ''What a relief.'' A minister's wife reported, ''The only times I could get out of being chairman of this or that or attending all meetings was when I was pregnant.''

The state of being pregnant may represent a period of great creativeness for the woman. She possesses feelings and sensations she never possessed before and may expe-

---

*From Rubin, R. 1970. Cognitive style in pregnancy. Am. J. Nurs. **70:**502.

*From Colman, A. D., and Colman, L. L. 1974. Pregnancy as an altered state of consciousness. Birth Fam. J. **1**(1): 8.

rience a state of fulfillment, a process that goes toward making her a complete woman. To some, the close relationship of mother and child is felt deeply, even by those deliberately terminating an unwanted pregnancy, as illustrated by one woman who said, "my baby would no longer be there to assure me that I was not alone."

Body sensations may come into conscious awareness for the first time. These women's concept of pregnancy becomes a set of symptoms—tingling breasts, increased vaginal discharge, frequency and urgency of urination, nausea, vomiting, bizarre food desires, and shortness of breath—all of which under other circumstances would be interpreted as abnormal and in need of treatment. To those who have little knowledge of physiologic responses of the maternal organism to the growing fetus, such symptoms can be alarming as well as uncomfortable and give rise to concern about personal safety.

Other responses that can be disturbing to those women who are pleased with and accepting of their pregnancies are the feelings that come and go of hostility toward and a wishing away of the unborn child. If birth of a healthy child ensues, memories of these ambivalent feelings are dismissed, but if a defective child is born, some women look back at the times of not wanting the child and feel intensely guilty. Even the most enlightened individuals tend to give credence in times of stress to the "magical powers of thought," and what is a perfectly normal and natural response experienced by all persons preparing for a new role is seen as instrumental in causing the defect in this child.

Other areas that undergo many changes are related to the self-image of the individual. Some women see pregnancy as ultimate proof of their femininity and sexual desirability; others have serious doubts about their sexual attractiveness. Some question their capability to withstand pain, to behave appropriately during the birth process, and to function in a new role as parent, with these thoughts leading to feelings of inadequacy. These feelings can result in a sensation of being "trapped into the pregnant state" (Bobak, 1969).

Pregnancy represents a maturational crisis, since the woman must acknowledge the event of her first pregnancy as an end of girlhood and the advent of womanhood. More than any other happening, it functions as a rite of passage indicative of reaching maturity in a society that has no other obvious rituals. In many states the pregnant woman is legally an adult regardless of age. She may give personal consent for any type of care of her newborn. She is entitled to financial and other aid from a government source if needed and, if unwed, is considered the sole legal guardian of her child. As such she retains the right to care for the child herself, place the child in a foster home, or give the child up for adoption. Pregnancy may serve as a means to establish an independent life, escape from a distasteful environment, or displace a no longer desired love object. Realization of the implications of adult status, its tasks, and responsibilities can come as a surprise to some individuals and can be a stress to many young women.

As the woman progresses through the months of pregnancy, certain overall psychic trends can be observed. Early in pregnancy, concern centers around the mother's "self." There is little real appreciation of the child. The pregnancy is experienced as "something happening to *me*." By the fifth month, most women have accomplished the task of identifying the fetus as a separate being, although very much a part of themselves. With this acceptance of the reality of the child (hearing the heartbeat and feeling the child move) and with a subsidence of early symptoms, the woman enters a quiet or latent period. At this time, she becomes more introspective, and the fantasy child takes shape. She seems to withdraw from relationships and to concentrate her interest on the unborn child. Husbands and children seem to sense this withdrawal, and sometimes husbands comment on feelings of being "left out" and children become more demanding in their efforts to redirect the mother's attention to themselves.

Toward the last part of pregnancy, this quiet period is superseded by another, more active one that is characteristically oriented to reality for both mother and child. A recurrence of symptoms brings the physical nature of pregnancy back into the woman's focus. Breathing is difficult, and movements of the child become vigorous enough to disturb her sleep. Backaches, frequency and urgency of urination, constipation, and problems with varicose veins can prove troublesome. The bulkiness and consequent awkwardness of her body can make more difficult the care of other children, routine housekeeping duties, and finding a comfortable position in which to sleep and rest. Sexual desire and satisfaction are often heightened during pregnancy; some women may experience orgasm for the first time, but intercourse in the face-to-face position is hampered by the woman's greatly enlarged abdomen. Fears of harming the infant or causing premature labor may also act to block the sexual response of either partner. The need to explore other methods of sexual action may be unacceptable to either the mother or father, and this interruption in their sexual bond can cause stress to both.

Anxiety about her personal safety during the birth process can be present if expressed only in the preparation most women make for the care of the new baby and/or other children in case "anything should happen." These feelings persist in spite of the known statistical evidence of the safe outcome of pregnancy for the mother. Many women talk about the pain of labor, concern over what behaviors will be appropriate during the birth process, and how those who will be caring for them will accept them and their actions. Anxiety about reaching the hospital in time for the birth, practical concerns for the care of children at home, and the uncertainty of being able to plan specific dates for outside help or the husband's vacation combine to make these last few months a time of tension compounded by a lack of real rest.

As the time for delivery approaches, the mother must reconcile the fantasy child and real child in terms of sex, appearance, weight, and health. Parental concern about the child's health is directed toward defects in either the mental or physical abilities of the child. Parents are open about these anxieties and press for confirmation that "the child will be all right." Less identifiable is the fear about the death of the child; this possibility is evidently a remote one to parents. Death of the infant comes as a great shock; little or no anticipatory grief work has been done.

As pregnancy progresses, another trait becomes noticeable. This is the mother-to-be's openness about her feelings toward herself and others (Caplan, 1959). The layer of reserve society has hitherto imposed is lifted, and she exhibits a willingness to talk about matters previously not discussed or discussed only within the family confines. She seems to believe that expression of her thoughts and ideas or description of her symptoms will be of interest to and welcomed by the listener. She appears ready to enter into a trusting relationship to the outsider she deems protective. This openness, coupled with a learning readiness, makes working with pregnant

women a delight and increases the likelihood of supportive care being therapeutically effective.

Whether birth is anticipated with joy, dread, or a mixture of both, the majority of women are impatient for labor to begin about the ninth lunar month. There is a strong desire to have the state of pregnancy end, "to be over and done with it." They are ready to move on to the next phase: childbirth and assuming their new role as mother.

SITUATIONAL SUPPORTS

Each society sets up organized patterns or institutions to ensure the introduction and socialization of new individuals and support for those responsible for this vital function. The family represents one of these institutions and, in spite of the stresses and strains to which it now is being subjected, remains one of the most potent sources of support.

A family group is incomplete without the presence of an adult (Fig. 10-1). From an adult's perspective, the family can be comprised of persons of any age or sex bound by a blood and/or love relationship. From the child's perspective, the family is a set of relationships between his dependent self and one or more protective adults (Aries, 1962; Erikson, 1968; Goode, 1964).

Varying approaches can be utilized to analyze the function of the family group (Hill and Hansen, 1970). One such approach, which provides a method of assessing the modes of support the family unit can offer to the pregnant woman, is that of regarding the family as a social system with emphasis on the effects of the interactions of family members (Anderson and Carter, 1974).

Just as does any other social system, a family must perform some crucial tasks if it is to survive and pro-

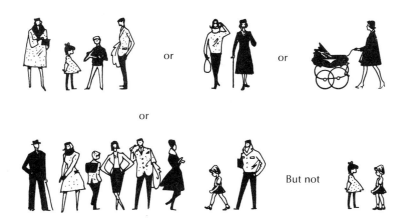

Fig. 10-1. Family configurations: presence of adult is basic to family group.

gress. It must (1) provide for the introduction and socialization of new members; (2) develop a protocol for problem solving, including assessment, decision making, and evaluation; (3) develop communication patterns and channels; and (4) concern itself with key activities related to such matters as defining its boundaries and areas of openness and privacy, seeking compliance from external social systems, local or national, to defend its interests, providing for the health and welfare of its members, and supporting an environment that permits at least a modicum of personal growth.

The family possesses goals, overt or covert, to which members are expected to subscribe and patterned ways of attaining these goals, known as *norms*. Members of the system are positioned into certain *statuses* either by acquisition or ascription and play out these statuses by assuming various *roles*. As a supporting structure for these functional prerequisites, each family develops certain *beliefs, values,* and *sentiments* in common, which are used as criteria in the choice of alternative actions. Those individuals who accept and follow the family's blueprint are esteemed; those who rebel are labeled *deviant* and, depending on the power they possess, are either ignored or have sanctions directed against them. Throughout these everyday interactions, the family uses its own patterns of verbal and nonverbal communication, and these patterns give insight into the feeling exchange within a family and act as "reliable indicators of interpersonal functioning" (Satir, 1967).

In terms of the structure that the family assumes, Boulding (1972) places all family forms on a continuum, from a single person maintaining a household to groups of persons associated by birth or by choice. She maintains there is no discernible difference between the "expanded family" and the "intentional community." Classification of families according to their form provides insight into stresses that families may experience as they differ from the normative structure dictated by the society.

Nuclear family

The nuclear family is the one that is considered "normal" in contemporary Western society, since it represents the largest number of actual families and the goal for the largest number of adults. This family group lives apart from either the husband's or wife's family of orientation. As defined by Parsons and Bales (1955):

The members of the nuclear family, consisting of parents and their still dependent children, ordinarily occupy a separate dwelling not shared with members of the family of orientation of either spouse, and . . . this household is in the typical case economically independent, subsisting in the first instance from the occupational earnings of the husband-father.*

The parents in this family are expected to play complementary roles of husband-wife and father-mother in giving emotional and physical support to each other and the offspring to accomplish family goals. Ideally this family institution provides for the care and socialization of children and social control for its members and is flexible enough to survive in an industrial world. Such a family can be perceived as "existing to fulfill the cultural dictates of its society as that society seeks to perpetuate itself" and in times of crisis may become "a workshop in social change" (Anderson and Carter, 1974). The family is being held together not so much by structure as by strong social bonds (Boulding, 1972).

The nuclear family has been described as "isolated," but there is increasing evidence that kinship ties to previous family structure are not broken. Frequently, sons and daughters, although established in their own nuclear family, remain in the same community as their families of orientation, and visiting relatives is part of their social life. The increased mobility of all segments of the population means grandparents, sisters, uncles, cousins, and other relatives can be more readily available to the isolated family. One often hears new mothers say, "My mother is going to fly in to help me for a week or so."

Reinhardt and Quinn (1973) portray the nuclear family as "characterized by the following descriptive terms: high mobility; changing values and attitudes; communication gaps between grandparents, parents, and children; high divorce rates; increasing rates of illegitimacy; and role reversal and role blurring between the sexes as more women enter the labor force and join the women's liberation cause."

Extended family

By definition, the extended family includes three generations, is family centered rather than individual centered, and through its kinship network provides supportive functions to all members. This family structure acts to proscribe the responsibilities and actions of family members. Some individuals regard the extended family as impeding the free mobility necessary in an industrialized society with its economic demands.

Persons who have experienced such a family grouping may chafe at the bonds it creates but, when they leave, regret the absence of a wider sense of acceptance and recognition such a family provides. In changing to a more socially functionable group, individuals from such

---

*From Parsons, T., and Bales, R. 1955. Family socialization and interaction. New York, The Free Press, p. 16.

''old-fashioned'' families may need help in viewing the social structure as an alternative family to which they can legitimately turn for help and sustenance in times of stress. As pointed out by Anderson and Carter (1974), ''Other institutions such as social welfare services that provide income maintenance, health care, emotional support, and day care, have grown up to specialize in functions previously fulfilled by the extended family.''

Single parent family

The single parent family is becoming an increasingly recognized form in our society. It may result from loss of a spouse by means of death, divorce, separation, or desertion; from the out-of-wedlock birth of a child; or from the adoption of a child. Whatever its source, the single parent family tends to be a vulnerable grouping economically and socially and, unless buttressed by a concerned society, may provide an unstable and deprived environment for the growth potential of children. It represents for many of the persons involved a lonely existence in which decision making and other family tasks depend on a single adult. As with individuals from extended families, these adults may need help in learning how to use community resources in developing or maintaining satisfactory family life.

For other adults, it is a chosen life-style that provides a free and open system for development of parents and children. In these families, decision making and communication are seen as joint commitments between parent and child, and the parent-child relationship is considered a major source for life fulfillment.

Commune family

Communal family groupings may be as varied as any within the societal context, and they vary from the highly formalized structure of the Amish community in Lancaster County, Pennsylvania, to loosely knit groups such as are found in the Santa Cruz Mountains near Boulder Creek, California. These communities of persons are formed for specific ideologic or societal purposes and frequently are considered an alternative life-style for individuals feeling alienated from a predominantly economically oriented society. Some communes consist of nuclear groups living in an extended or expanded family community and are envisioned as persisting over time. Others may provide temporary shelter for single parent families or may be a mixture of dual parent and single parent families. In some communes, all parents participate in caretaking activities for all the children. In many of these groups, the combination is a fluid one; individuals and families are free to come and go as their needs dictate. Just what the outcome of such communities will be with regard to the children is yet to be determined. For the groups that lack some permanence, the difficulties associated with the highly mobile nuclear family in seeking stability and continuity in social contacts may be perpetuated. Those communes composed solely of young adults and their children may be reproducing the ghettolike aspects of suburbia, with its limited contacts with diversified age, cultural, and economic groups.

Expanded family

The expanded family resembles the extended family and the commune family. It consists of varying age groups, kinship groups, or unrelated family members that have become a part of the household. Boulding (1972) uses the term *expanded* to stress the similarities ''between the biologically related extended family and the household as a voluntary association.''

Because the family acts as a primary force in generating support for the pregnant woman, knowledge of this unit forms an essential part of the data basic to the nursing care plan. Not only must the family be identified, but also an awareness of the functioning of the family is indicated. According to Dyer (1973), this functioning is similar to that of any group in that it takes place on two levels, the first being ''what the family is doing, and who is doing what, to whom and how,'' and the second being ''the area of feeling, or how people feel about what is being done.''

REFERENCES

Anderson, R., and Carter, J. 1974. Human behavior in the social environment. Chicago, Aldine Publishing Co.

Aries, P. 1962. Centuries of childhood. London, Jonathan Cape, Ltd.

Bobak, I. 1969. Self-image: a universal concern of women becoming mothers. CNA Bull. **9:**7, April.

Boulding, E. 1972. The family as an agent of social change. The Futurist **6:**186, Oct.

Caplan, G. 1959. Concepts of mental health and consultation. Washington, D.C., U.S. Department of Health, Education, and Welfare.

Colman, A. D., and Colman, L. L. 1971. Pregnancy the psychological experience. New York, Herder & Herder, Inc.

Colman, A. D., and Colman, L. L. 1974. Pregnancy as an altered state of consciousness. Birth Fam. J. **1**(1):7.

Duvall, E. V. 1967. Family development. Philadelphia, J. B. Lippincott Co.

Dyer, W. 1973. Working with groups. In Reinhardt, A., and Quinn, M. (eds.). Family-centered community nursing. St. Louis, The C. V. Mosby Co.

Erikson, E. 1967. Childhood and society (ed. 2). New York, W. W. Norton & Co., Inc., Publishers.

Erikson, E. 1968. Identity: youth and crisis. New York, W. W. Norton & Co., Inc., Publishers.

Goode, W. J. 1964. The family. Englewood Cliffs, N.J., Prentice-Hall, Inc.

Hill, R., and Hansen, D. 1970. The identification of conceptual frameworks utilized in family study. Marr. Fam. Liv. **22:**311, Nov.

Jackson, D. 1970. The study of the family. In Ackerman, N.W. (ed.). Family process. New York, Basic Books, Inc., Publishers.

Kanter, R. M. 1970. Communes. Psychology Today **4:**2, July.

Otto, H. 1973. A framework for assessing family strengths. In Reinhardt, M., and Quinn, A. (eds.). Family-centered community nursing. St. Louis, The C. V. Mosby Co.

Parsons, T., and Bales, R. 1955. Family socialization and interaction. New York, The Free Press.

Reinhardt, M., and Quinn, A. (eds.). 1973. Family-centered community nursing. St. Louis, The C. V. Mosby Co.

Rainwater, L. 1965. Family design: marital sexuality, family size, and contraception. Chicago, Aldine Press.

Reissman, F. 1964. Acceptance or difference. Panel for National Conference on Social Welfare, Urban Studies Center, Rutgers University, New Brunswick, N.J.

Rubin, R. 1970. Cognitive style in pregnancy. Am. J. Nurs. **70:**502.

Satir, V. 1967. Conjoint family therapy. Palo Alto, Calif., Science and Behavior Book, Inc.

Sumner, P. 1976. Six years experience of prepared childbirth in a homelike labor delivery room. Birth Fam. J. **3:**79, Summer.

CHAPTER 11

Psychosocial nursing intervention

The nurse functions in a collaborative manner with other members of the health team in providing emotional support for the pregnant woman and her family. In the process of providing such support, she assumes many roles: consultant, counselor, teacher, and advocate.

The extent of the nurse's involvement with the mother-to-be, the family, or both varies with the needs of the individuals concerned. With some, her actions may consist of noting the presence of adequate situational supports developed by the family and the use of successful methods of coping with stress, commending the individuals for their foresight and planning, and serving as a resource person for information about services available either locally or nationally or in the public or private sector that may be useful for the mother-to-be and her family. With others, stressful periods may necessitate either intermittent or sustained nursing interventions. For those patients who have symptoms indicating a deep and traumatic rejection of the pregnancy or of parenthood, the nurse may be instrumental in securing the intervention of other health workers—psychiatrist, psychologist, psychiatric nurse specialist, or psychiatric social worker. Decisions about the extent of therapy required are of necessity constantly recurring stratagems in the nursing process.

ASSESSMENT

The following information is useful in assessing the family:

A. Family identification
1. Who are the family members? Ages? Kinship?
2. Where do they live?
3. What family boundaries have been established? What family-community interchange exists? Who is permitted to be a family member?
4. What relatives and/or friends are available?

B. Family activity
1. What are the family goals? Plan for the future?
2. Who assumes responsibility for resources such as food, clothing, and housing?
3. How are decisions made? What criteria are used?
4. Who does what family work? Is there men's work, women's work, child's work, or anybody's work?
5. How will the new baby be cared for?

C. Family feeling
1. What communication patterns are used?
2. What are the attitudes toward health care and particularly care during pregnancy?
3. What relationships exist between mother, father, siblings, and in-laws? Is the pregnancy "hers" or "theirs"? Who acts as the mother's primary supporter?
4. What does the "new baby" mean to the family?

The *process* of such an assessment is often more difficult and complicated than that involved in assessing the physical health of the mother and fetus (Fig. 11-1). It requires skill in communication and the ability to establish a trust relationship. In every family group, areas of openness and privacy exist, and any group resents interrogation by an outsider. The reasons for obtaining the following information should be made explicit: Who can be supportive to this woman and her unborn baby at this time? What kinds of support are available? What changes might be attempted to produce the needed support now or in the future? What preparation is being made for the care of the infant once born?

Although some data, for example, address, marital status, and family members' ages can be readily obtained, since it is usually freely given, other information comes from *observing* and noting relationships, at-

145

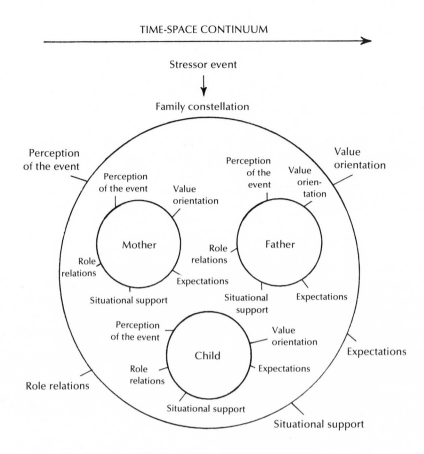

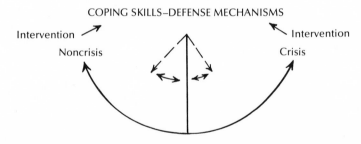

Fig. 11-1. Family assessment model. (From Oehrtman, S. 1974. In Hall, J., and Weaver, B. [eds.]. Nursing of families in crisis. Philadelphia, J. B. Lippincott Co.)

titudes, and stress responses (who is doing what); (2) *listening*, to conversations about community and family involvements or hopes and aspirations, for example; and (3) *being aware* of matters such as who have missed appointments or refused to utilize existing health care facilities.

In providing adequate prebirth support to individuals, a major problem is the difficulty in determining those whose emotional status will prove vulnerable to the stress of pregnancy and parenthood. Larsen and associ-

ates (1967) found that those women holding negative attitudes stemming from the areas of interpersonal relationships (the husband, the mother-in-law, the mother) and self-esteem (my body) were more prone to develop severe personality problems.

Gordon and Gordon (1960) theorized that adverse reactions to childbearing stem from the cumulative effect of social stresses. They categorized these stresses as belonging to three groups:

1. *Sensitizers*—stresses happening early in life that

act to reduce and render inadequate an individual's defense mechanisms (e.g., loss of one's mother before age 21)

2. *Pressurizers*—stresses arising from an individual's everyday environment whether in the home or marketplace (e.g., inadequate income for basic needs)

3. *Precipitators*—unexpected stresses that overwhelm the individual's emotional defenses (e.g., moving to a new community with no relatives or friends to help)

Gordon and Gordon's subsequent research indicated that women who experience ten or more of the fifty identified social stresses are in need of support to prevent emotional breakdown in the postnatal period. Those particularly prone to stress were identified as presenting two key patterns, one centering around the amount of personal insecurity and the other around the amount of maternal role conflict present.

Steele and Pollock (1968) used a questionnaire to assist in detection of parents-to-be possessing traits in common with those parents known to have distorted parent-child relationships. Undue anxiety about the crying of infants, the necessity to assume sole responsibility for a child, negative reactions to supervision of child care, and rigid expectations of a child's behavior can be used as indicators for providing additional emotional support.

Although research is going forward to develop more precise methods of assessing individuals' capabilities in relation to successful coping with the tasks of pregnancy and parenthood, much still must be done. Unfortunately for many nulliparous patients, fantasy about pregnancy and parenthood precludes a real understanding of future commitments. Assessment will therefore need to continue throughout the antenatal, natal, and postnatal periods if those for whom we have sufficient knowledge to help are actually to receive that help.

EXPECTED OUTCOMES

The goals of supportive care relate to developing, augmenting, or changing the mechanisms used by women in coping with stress. An effort is made to promote active participation by the individuals in the process of solving their own problems by gathering pertinent information, exploring alternative actions, making decisions as to choice of action, and assuming responsibility for the outcomes. These outcomes may be any or all of the following:

- Living with a problem as it is
- Mitigating the effects of a problem so it can be accepted more readily
- Eliminating the problem through effecting change

Expectations of success in the area of emotional supportive care must of necessity be flexible. It is not within the province of any outsider to assure another of a rewarding, satisfying experience. The mother and those significant to her are crucial elements in that process, and many of their problems are beyond the scope or capabilities of any professional worker. In describing her work with young and poor persons, Edwards (1973) noted, "They did not usually change their living situation and I was not instrumental in modifying home or drug problems." However, this did not deter her from encouraging them to use the decision-making process as a means of coping with problems rather than merely complaining about injustice.

At other times, a successful outcome can be readily documented. A patient who early in her pregnancy had predicted a severe depressive state in the postnatal period, was elated when such a state did not materialize. She remarked to the nurse who had provided support during the pregnancy and birth, "You are the best nerve medicine I have ever had!"

In counseling it must be remembered that both individuals are contributing to the relationship. The nurse has to accept her own responses as a factor in trying to be of help. An example of one nurse-patient relationship follows:

Mrs. _____ had been very forthright in saying that this pregnancy was unplanned but countered this statement with comments such as "all things happen for the best," "we always wanted the boys to have a family to turn to," "children bring their own love." Over a period of time as our relationship developed to one of *mutual* trust, she complained increasingly of her fear of pain, her hating having to wear maternity clothes, and her having to give up helping the family. Finally I *ventured* to say, "Sometimes when a pregnancy is unplanned, women resent it very much and are angry about it." Her relief was evident. She said, "Oh, you don't know how angry I've been." As a result, the whole tenor of support being offered changed and the plan was adjusted to meet her real needs.

The nurse must also accept the fact that the patient must be a willing partner in a relationship that is a purely voluntary one. As such, it can be refused or terminated at any time by the pregnant woman or her family.

NURSING INTERVENTIONS

The interventions the nurse chooses to use in providing emotional support will depend in part on her orientation to the process and in part on her ability to convey interest and a desire to be of help. These may include such strategies as patient support, development of behavior acquisition or modification, promotion of patient decision making as crucial in solving problems, and providing pertinent information or teaching caretaking activities (Osipow and Walsh, 1970).

The initiation of the nurse-patient relationship is crucial in setting the tone for further interactions. The techniques of listening with an attentive expression, touching, and use of eye contact have their place, as does recognition of the patient's feelings and her right to express them. The intervention may occur in varied settings, formal or informal. For certain individuals, involvement in goal-directed health groups is not feasible or acceptable. Encounters in hallways or clinic examining rooms, home visits, or telephone conversations may provide the only opportunities for contact and can be used effectively. One nurse described her intervention with a maternity patient as follows:

I tried to teach her about relaxation and breathing techniques during childbirth but she was not interested. When she phoned to tell me she was at the hospital in labor she said, "What was all that stuff you were saying about breathing." In between the next few contractions I repeated the salient points.

At other times, patients may seek information about a particular problem repeatedly, not so much for the advice given but to direct the nurse's attention to themselves. Edwards (1973) discourages such mechanisms by making it a rule to give advice three times and then if it is not acted on, to ask for a patient-generated solution and a reporting of its effectiveness. The need for additional attention is recognized and provided in other ways.

Formalized classes in childbirth and parenthood education have proved successful for some patients.* The various methods (e.g., Lamaze, Bradley), have certain premises in common:

1. The partners wish to share the birth of their child as part of their concept of family unity.

---

*Information concerning specific teaching content and strategies can be obtained by writing to the following organizations or individuals: International Childbirth Education Association, P.O. Box 5852, Milwaukee, Wis. 53220; Margot Edwards, Communications: Dimensions in Childbirth Education, 1207 Presidio Blvd., Pacific Grove, Calif. 93950; The Lamaze method, Association of Psychoprophylaxis in Obstetrics, 1523 L St., N.W., Suite 410, Washington, D.C. 20005; and the Bradley method, "Have a Happy Birthday," American Association of Husband-Coached Childbirth, P.O. Box 5224, Sherman Oaks, Calif. 91413. The Red Cross, adult education centers, or community health agencies usually provide classes in childbirth and parenthood education. For additional information refer to the following sources: Bing, E. 1970. Six practical lessons for an easier childbirth. New York, Grosset & Dunlap, Inc.; and Goodwin, B. Psychoprophylaxis in childbirth. In Duffey, M., Anderson, E., Bergersen, B. S., Lohr, M., and Rose, M. H. (eds.). 1971. Current concepts in clinical nursing (vol. 3). St. Louis, The C. V. Mosby Co.

2. The mother gains the support of a partner who is trained to provide it.

3. There is opportunity to develop mechanisms for coping with pain or discomfort during labor and delivery (relaxation, diversion, disassociation) and thereby maintain self-controlling behaviors and control of one's environment.

4. Parent-craft activities are discussed and practiced.

SEXUAL COUNSELING DURING PREGNANCY

Nurses have many opportunities to counsel pregnant couples. Nurses offer expectant parent classes, work as nurse practitioners in clinics and physicians' offices, and make home visits as community health nurses. In addition, nurses provide around-the-clock care on hospital maternity units.

Counseling pregnant couples demands the same kind of self-assessment outlined in Chapter 4 plus a knowledge of the physical, social, and emotional responses to sex during pregnancy. Not all maternity nurses are comfortable dealing with the sexual concerns of their patients. The nurse who is aware of her personal strengths and limitations in dealing with sexual content is in a better position to make referrals when necessary.

The role of the maternity nurse in sex counseling is defined by the origin and severity of the sexual problem encountered. There are a significant number of patients who merely need *permission* to be sexual during pregnancy. An example would be to inform the couple that changes in libido are normal during pregnancy. Many other patients need *information* about the physiologic changes that occur during pregnancy and an opportunity to debunk myths associated with sex during pregnancy. Giving permission and providing information are within the purview of the maternity nurse and should be an integral component of patient care.

A smaller number of couples must be referred for either *sex therapy* or *family therapy.* Couples with sexual dysfunction problems of long-standing that may be intensified by the pregnancy should be referred for sex therapy. When a couple's sexual problem is a symptom of a more serious interactional problem, they would benefit from family therapy.

Sex counseling during pregnancy is the same three-part process described in Chapter 4: history taking, problem identification, and problem solving.

History taking

Following are the areas to be covered, as well as examples of questions to be asked:

A. Attitudes
   1. What has your family (partner, friends) told you about sex during pregnancy?
   2. What are your feelings about sex during pregnancy?
   3. Is it OK for married people to masturbate?
   4. How do your ideas and feelings about sex differ from those of your partner?
B. Sexual self-concept
   1. How do you feel about the changes in your appearance?
   2. How does your partner feel about your body now?
   3. Do maternity clothes make pregnant women attractive?
C. Marital relationships
   1. What will it be like to have a baby in the home?
   2. How is your life going to change by having a baby? Your partner's life?
   3. What plans do having a baby interrupt?
D. Physical status
   1. Tell me about your overall health? What is your energy level? When do you feel most alive?

History taking is an ongoing process. Receptivity to changes in attitudes, body image, marital relationships, and physical status has relevance throughout pregnancy. When changes occur, problems may develop that require unexpected interventions.

Problem identification

Sexual expression during pregnancy is affected by physical, emotional, and interactional factors. The couple's relationship is influenced by myths about sex during pregnancy, sexual dysfunctional problems, physical changes of the mother, and development of possible medical and obstetric problems.

Myths about how the body functions and fantasies about the influence of the fetus as a third party in lovemaking are frequently expressed. Anomalies and mental retardation, as well as other injuries to the mother and fetus, are often attributed to sexual relations at varying points during pregnancy. Many couples have fears that the woman's genitals will be drastically changed by the birth process. Magical thinking, embarrassment, and hesitancy because of not wanting to appear foolish often prevent couples from expressing these concerns to the health professional.

Changes in body shape, body image, and levels of discomfort influence the man and woman's desire for sexual expression as pregnancy progresses. Whether the pregnant body is perceived as beautiful or repulsive has

an impact on the couple's comfort and desire for sexual intimacy. During the first trimester, the woman is frequently plagued by nausea, fatigue, and sleepiness. However, as she progresses into the second trimester, her combined sense of well-being and increased pelvic congestion profoundly increase her desire for sexual release. Again in the third trimester, fatigue, fetal demands, and physical bulkiness increase her physical discomfort and lower her libidinal interests.

Partners who do not understand these seemingly rapid physiologic and emotional changes can become confused by the wife's erratic behavior. Unfortunately expectant fathers have received little attention in studies of sex during pregnancy. The health professional, however, cannot neglect the problems and concerns expressed by the father (Chapter 12).

Communication between the couple is important at this time. Since pregnancy is a developmental crisis, it is a time of emotional upheaval for both the man and woman. Talking to each other about the changes they are experiencing is of primary importance. When discussed and dealt with constructively, these changes can strengthen the relationship.

Dyspareunia (painful intercourse), differing sexual drives, and impotence are the three major dysfunctional problems experienced by pregnant couples. Dyspareunia may be caused by pressure on the pregnant abdomen or deep penile thrusting. In addition to pain during coitus, postcoital cramping and backache may occur. Severe breast tenderness has also been reported by multiparous women during the first trimester.

In addition to dyspareunia, differing sexual drives can create problems for both expectant parents. The father may become frustrated by his partner's sporadic lack of interest in sex. The mother may have difficulty when her partner becomes confused by her libidinal fluctuations. Changes in the father's level of sexual interest may disturb the mother.

The woman's expanding abdomen may become an object of ridicule and shame or a source of great pride for the couple. Some women resent losing their shape and wearing waistless maternity clothes, making derogatory comments about their abdomen. Frequently, these women begin wearing maternity clothes before they actually need to.

Men respond in a variety of ways to their wives' changing shape. Some say their wives are most beautiful when pregnant, whereas others make derisive comments about the pregnant contours and are repulsed by them.

For the man the pregnant state of his partner may mean freedom to engage in nurturing behavior. However, to other men, it represents a time of loneliness and alienation as the woman becomes physically and emotionally engrossed in her unborn child. He may find himself going outside of the home for comfort and understanding, becoming interested in a new hobby, or getting involved with his work. This also may be the time of the husband's first extramarital affair. Some men view pregnancy as a proof of their masculinity and as an outcome of their dominant role. To others, pregnancy as a result of their intercourse with a woman has no meaning in terms of feelings of responsibility to either mother or child. For most women and men, however, pregnancy functions as a time of preparation for the parental role, of fantasy, of great pleasure, and of intense learning.

Problem solving

Data collected through the history and identification of problems that may occur or are occurring during pregnancy and the postnatal period provide the framework for counseling the pregnant couple. Counseling includes countering misinformation, providing reassurance of normalcy, and suggesting alternative behaviors.

Countering misinformation. Many myths and much of the misinformation related to sex and pregnancy are masked behind seemingly unrelated issues. For example, a question about the baby's ability to hear and see in utero may be related to the baby's role as a third person in lovemaking. The counselor must be extremely sensitive to questions behind the question when counseling in this highly charged emotional area.

Fetal heart rates decrease during orgasm; however, fetal distress has not been noted. Although it has been suggested that premature delivery may be induced either by orgasmic contractions or by PG in the male ejaculate, researchers have not validated these hypotheses.

When possible, the couple should be counseled together. Expectant parent group education classes can also be an effective way to explore these kinds of concerns because of the support and sharing offered by the group.

Providing reassurance of normalcy. Couples are relieved to learn that their fears and concerns do not make them "weird" or "crazy." A breast-feeding mother may welcome the knowledge that her erotic response to suckling is normal. At the same time, the father may be relieved to know that many fathers are jealous of their suckling infants.

It is important for the counselor to view sexuality in its broadest sense. Kissing, hugging, massage, and petting are valid forms of sexual expression. Each of these behaviors is pleasurable in itself and is not always a secondary behavior leading to intercourse. When a couple cannot or chooses not to have intercourse, they can express their needs for closeness and intimacy in many other ways.

Suggesting alternative behaviors. The following discussion focuses on some suggested alternatives for sexual practice during pregnancy.

Safety of coitus. Coitus is not contraindicated at any time during pregnancy for the obstetrically and medically healthy woman. However, a history of more than one spontaneous abortion; a threatened abortion in the first trimester; impending miscarriage in the second trimester; and premature rupture of the membranes, bleeding, or pain during the third trimester warrant coital precaution. The patient should also be cautioned against masturbatory activities when orgasmic contractions are contraindicated. Studies have shown that orgasm is often more intense when induced by masturbation.

Alternatives to coitus. Solitary and mutual masturbation and oral-genital and anal intercourse may be alternatives to penile-vaginal intercourse. Couples who practice cunnilingus should be cautioned concerning the blowing of air into the vagina, particularly during the last few weeks of pregnancy. There have been cases reported of maternal death from air emboli due to forceful blowing of air into the vagina.

Coital positions. The female superior, side-by-side, and rear-entry positions are possible alternative positions to the traditional male superior position. The side-by-side position is the position of choice, especially during the third trimester, because it requires reduced energy and pressure on the pregnant abdomen.

Breast changes. Multiparous women have reported severe breast tenderness in the first trimester. A coital position that avoids direct pressure on the woman's breasts and decreased breast fondling during love play can be recommended. She should also be reassured that this condition is normal and temporary.

Lactating mothers lose milk in uncontrolled spurts in response to sexual stimulation. The mother can be counseled to wear a bra with breast pads if the couple finds the release of milk unpleasant.

Orgasmic changes. Some women complain of lower abdominal cramping and backache after orgasm during the first and third trimester. A backrub can often relieve some of this discomfort, as well as provide a pleasant experience.

A tonic contraction, often lasting up to a minute, replaces the rhythmic contractions of orgasm during the third trimester. Changes in fetal heart rates without fetal distress have been reported.

First postnatal intercourse. The couple can safely resume intercourse by the third to fourth postnatal week if bleeding has stopped and the episiotomy has healed. Vaginal lubrication is lessened due to inhibition of vasocongestive response by steroid starvation. A water-soluble gel or contraceptive cream or jelly may be recommended to increase lubrication. If there is some vaginal tenderness, the partner can be instructed to rotate one or two fingers around the vaginal os to help relax it and identify areas of possible discomfort. The side-by-side or female superior positions are recommended because the female has more control over depth of penile penetration.

Kegal exercises. The woman should be instructed to practice the Kegal exercises to strengthen her pubococcygeal muscle. As the master sphincter of the pelvis, the pubococcygeal muscle controls not only bowel and bladder function but also vaginal perception and response during intercourse. The exercise consists of the woman's tightening the anal sphincter, then the introitus, and then the meatal sphincter, holding for a count of ten, then relaxing. It may be repeated three or four times a day.

•   •   •

The history provides a baseline for identifying attitudes about sex during pregnancy, as well as perceptions of the pregnancy, the health status of the couple, and the quality of their marital relationship. Identification of the couple's subjective experience provides the direction and focus of sexual counseling. Sexual counseling includes countering misinformation, providing reassurance of normalcy and suggesting alternative behaviors. The uniqueness of each couple is considered within a biopsychosocial framework.

The well-informed nurse who is comfortable with her own sexuality and the sex counseling needs of pregnant couples can offer counseling in a valuable, often neglected area.

REFERENCES

Arms, S. 1975. Immaculate deception. Boston, Houghton Mifflin Co.

Benedict, T. 1959. Parenthood as a developmental phase: a contribution to the libido. J. Am. Psychoanal. Assoc. **7:**389.

Bobak, I. 1969. Self-image: a universal concern of women becoming mothers. CNA Bull. **9:**7, April.

Edwards, M. 1973. Communications: dimensions in childbirth education. Pacific Grove, Calif., M. Edwards, publisher.

Gordon, R., and Gordon, K. 1960. Social factors in prevention of postpartum emotional problems. Obstet. Gynecol. **15:** 453.

Grimm, E. 1967. Psychological and social factors in pregnancy, delivery and outcome. In Richardson, S. A., and Guttmacher, A. F. (eds.). Childbearing—its social and psychological aspects. Baltimore, The Williams & Wilkins Co.

Hazell, L. 1976. Common sense childbirth. Berkeley, Calif., Berkeley Publishing Co.

Larsen, V. L., Evans, T., and Martin, L. 1967. Differences between new mothers: psychiatric admissions vs. normals. J. Am. Med. Wom. Assoc. **22:**995.

Oehrtman, S. 1974. Assessment and crisis intervention: a model for the family. In Hall, J., and Weaver, B. (eds.). Nursing of families in crisis. Philadelphia, J. B. Lippincott Co.

Osipow, S., and Walsh, W. 1970. Strategies in counseling for behavioral change. New York, Appleton-Century-Crofts.

Steele, B., and Pollock, C. 1968. A psychiatric study of parents who abuse infants and small children. In Helfer, R., and Kempe, H. (eds.). The battered child. Chicago, University of Chicago Press.

CHAPTER 12

Fathers

In parent education classes, in labor units, at the nursery windows, wherever there is an expectant or new father, the complexity and urgency of his needs are dramatically evident. Nursing education once emphasized the mother, her needs, and her relationship to her child, and nursing literature supported this preoccupation. Cartoons, greeting cards, and popular literature perpetuate the image of the expectant father as a comic strip character too anxious and incompetent to remember to take his wife in his mad dash to the hospital when labor begins. While his wife labors, he paces with a day-old beard, droopy eyes, and dangling cigarette in the "Dads' Room" and later bungles his way through holding and diapering his child. He is a figure in the background whose task, aside from that of breadwinner, is to be patient with his wife's moods and bring her flowers. Gradually his existence and strategic position are being recognized; the importance of his true role is emerging.

In this chapter, *father* is defined as follows: the male who shares the pregnancy with the female in the psychosocial as well as the biologic sense. The relationship need not be legally sanctioned. Father is used interchangeably with husband, expectant father, or father of a newly born infant. This chapter will not deal with the man who shares the childbearing experience with a woman he knows is pregnant by another man or who was artificially inseminated. No studies have been done to provide data for comparing and contrasting the feelings and needs of these "social" fathers and those of "biologic" fathers.

THE COUVADE

Couvade (French, "to hatch") is a practice among some primitive peoples in which the man subjects himself to various behaviors and observes taboos associated with pregnancy and giving birth. By enacting the couvade through definite patterns of socially prescribed behaviors, the man's new status is recognized and endorsed. In addition, his responses are channeled into acceptable modes of expression. His behavior acknowl-

edges his psychosocial as well as biologic relationship to the mother and child.

Without a formally recognized and accepted couvade in our society, how do expectant fathers respond to their new status? How do expectant fathers make the transition to their new role with its demands and expectations?

BECOMING A FATHER

The observable behaviors and verbalized responses of fathers can be grouped into five identified time periods or phases. These phases are not mutually exclusive. Threads of each reaction, concern, and informational need span the entire experience but seem to be most salient in one phase over another. These phases are as follows:

Phase   I: Realization or confirmation of pregnancy
Phase II: Awareness of mother's increasing body size and fetal movements
Phase III: Anticipation of approaching labor
Phase IV: Involvement in the birthing process
Phase V: New parenthood

Phase I: Realization or confirmation of pregnancy

The expectant father: I am to become. In essence, the expectant father, like the expectant mother, has been preparing for parenthood for his entire life. Subconsciously he has given some thought to having a wife and children. During courtship and early marriage, the couple's discussion of future plans may even include the number, spacing, and names of their children-to-be. Yet pregnancy and the child remain in the realm of fantasy—illusions that can be savored, elaborated on, toyed with, or cast off at will. The first suspicion of pregnancy actualizes the need for facing role transition *now*. The presumptive signs of pregnancy initiate the first phase of transition from a childless married state to fatherhood.

"I couldn't believe it." "I felt inadequate and apprehensive." "I felt reassured, encouraged, and somewhat relieved that we could get pregnant.'' A sampling of the responses to news of confirmation of pregnancy, these spontaneous remarks voice an inner concern about one's virility, one's capacity to procreate, a basic human drive. They also reflect an anxiety and uncertainty that accompanies role transition. The initial glow (or concern) of confirmation of virility is rapidly followed by a tremendous burst of energy, which finds outlets in diverse activities.

Changing self-concept: provider role identity. The heightened concern for having enough money to meet needs is real. Many young married women are employed outside the home. Pregnancy eliminates one source of income and adds another demand on the budget. The loss of one income is often offset by a gain in a less tangible area, however. The wife may give up her employment at her husband's insistence: ''I can't see a wife of mine working beyond 8 weeks. For a while I wondered who was going to play the masculine role around here. I'll bring in the bread from now on.'' Some men try to compensate for their anticipated needs by keeping their present jobs even though they had anticipated a change prior to knowledge of conception, by putting more effort into work to earn rapid promotions, by working overtime, and by taking on an extra job.

The concern for making ends meet extends beyond the immediate future. Some men take out new insurance or extra coverage at this time, a fact well anticipated by insurance salesmen.

Even when budgets are tight, husbands may arrange for diaper service as early as the sixth month of pregnancy to ''help her out.'' Regardless of budgetary restrictions, husbands often provide for some sort of present for the expectant wife.

Many expectant fathers take an active role in arranging for the wife's medical care. Some search for free clinics. One husband visited the clinic and evaluated the care given before making an appointment for his wife. Those men who wish to participate actively in the event take special care to find physicians who are supportive of the couple's goals. On the other hand, some men think that choosing a physician is woman's work and that they need be responsible only for the bills.

Expectant fathers feel more confident during the middle trimester. This confidence is overtly expressed in decreased concern about the money matter. The initial flurry of activity ends.

Mitleiden: ''suffering along.'' Mitleiden, or psychosomatic symptoms of expectant fathers, has long been recognized as a phenomenon of expectant fatherhood. In 1627 Bacon observed, ''That loving and kinde Husbands, have a Sense of their Wives Breeding Childe,

by some Accident in their owne Body.'' Still in the 1600s, another commented, ''It often falls out, that when the woman is in good health, the husband is sick, yea sometimes being many miles off'' (Hunter and Macalpine, 1963).

During the discomforts such as nausea, lassitude, aches, and pains, the husband sympathizes or identifies with his pregnant wife. Frequently, he experiences these symptoms, although his wife is free of them. These behaviors can be a positive means of bringing the couple together and of helping the father become more responsive to his wife's and child's needs for love and care.

Inquiring about any symptoms validates their normalcy and conveys the nurse's understanding of and interest in the couple. Recognizing that the father may be experiencing ''pains'' brings his needs to the fore where they can be dealt with openly. This recognition seems to release his tensions and modify his need to express that tension in less overt ways such as nagging his wife, negating her discomforts, and engaging in potentially dangerous exploits. Before realizing this, the nurse may feel annoyed when fathers interrupt their wives to exhibit new wounds (burns, cuts, bruises), to talk of their gas pains and constipation, or to insist that they have bigger and better ''pot bellies.'' It quickly became apparent to one of us (I. M. B.) that fathers were not belittling their wives but were trying to convey their feelings in the only way open to them. Acknowledgment of their needs by encouraging open discussion of feelings seemed to result in more open acceptance of each other's feelings. This acceptance facilitated increased openness in other areas of communication between the spouses.

The nurse can cope with most of these problems of expectant fathers. Crisis intervention in most cases consists of discussing the very human problems and anticipations that surround the expectation of a new baby. Only in severe cases is psychiatric referral required.

Phase II: Awareness of mother's increasing body size and fetal movements

Sexuality. Evidence of increased abdominal size and palpable fetal movements heralds a new crisis situation. Men may struggle with feelings about the wife's changing body.*

Discussions on the pros and cons of husbands attending their wives during delivery uncover other areas of concern. Mental pictures of the woman's posture during

---

*The student is referred to psychoanalytic literature regarding revival of Oedipal conflicts, incestuous fantasies, and homosexual/heterosexual drives in the male during pregnancy.

delivery can be upsetting. After seeing a film on delivery, men described their uneasiness when listening to the grunting and groaning accompanying the last stage of labor.

In psychoanalytic literature, many aspects of the father's behavior are identified as indicators of rivalry. One example is a man's increased frustration and dissatisfaction with his present job—becoming bored with the work or irritated with what is perceived as internal politics and competition among the staff. When the husband is expressing these feelings, the tensions he feels seem to electrify the room. Wives are often amazed and unnerved that the husband is having this type of reaction when he was comfortable and secure in his job before. The couple can be forewarned to expect these feelings and discuss them openly when they occur.

Rivalry between the expectant father and his pregnant wife is not new. In Greek legend, Zeus, angered by his wife's superior wisdom after she conceived, swallowed her and later gave birth to Athena, who emerged full grown from his forehead. In the same instant, he both punished and replaced his wife.

Direct rivalry with the fetus may be evident, especially during sexual activity. Husbands may protest that fetal movements prevent sexual gratification, making comments such as "We can't have sex with 'that' kicking around in there."

The wife's increased introspection may be a source of anxiety to some men. He may experience a sense of uneasiness as she becomes preoccupied with thoughts of her mother and sister, with her growing attachment to her male physician, and with her reevaluation of him as her chosen mate and their relationship.

The nurse's role is evident. First, prepare the couple for these possible reactions to sexuality and sexual expression during pregnancy. Second, assist the couple in keeping open the lines of communication. Finally, when appropriate, involve the man in the pregnancy. It has been found that when the husband takes an active role during the pregnancy, the wife is less likely to develop such a strong attachment to the male physician.

Father-fetus relationship. Many fathers are actively and meaningfully involved in the pregnancy, but most find it difficult to relate to the fetus. The woman feels the fetal movements intimately and continuously. The man cannot share this intimacy in the same way, and he does have the option to step away physically, intellectually, or emotionally.

Frequently, during phase II there are attempts to ward off the inevitable with statements such as "It'll be a while yet" or "The baby isn't really a baby yet." Short excursions or second honeymoons occur during this period. Many wives confide concern about what they perceive to be their husbands' thwarted hopes and dreams. Many men fantasize openly, "If I were single now, I would be going to Australia . . . traveling around the world . . . living in the open with only a knapsack and bedroll . . . taking a chance with a new, exciting job."

In spite of remarks like these, the father becomes involved with the coming newborn by means of activities such as picking the child's name, anticipating the child's sex, and discussing the method of feeding the child.

What's in a name? As early as the first month, the name of the child may be selected. Family tradition, religious mandate, and continuation of one's own name or names of relatives and friends are important in the selection process. The names chosen are tried on for fit; for example, the father who emphatically states, "I just cannot picture myself as being a father to a boy named John." Some strive for originality in the name because "a common name just won't do." Armed with several names, one husband said he would hold out for his final choice until he saw the baby, pointing out that "To be named Eric, he *must* be blue-eyed and blond."

Concerns in this area center on disagreements between the couple and also between one of the expectant parents and one or both sets of the grandparents-to-be. Taking exception to the grandparents-to-be can bring the expectant couple together as a solid front or incite conflict between them. Asking the expectant couple how they arrived at a name can provide data for the nurse's decision to intervene.

Boy or girl? Cultural conditioning colors the couple's preference for the sex of the firstborn and subsequent children. Women frequently defer to their husband's stated preference. Cultural patterning alone cannot account for all the statements couching personal preference. Men more obviously than women work at finding an internal fit between the anticipated sex of the child and their own comfort with the imagined future relationship with that child.

Most men opt for a male child. Some refuse to voice a preference, fearing that verbalization would prevent its coming true. Some refuse to even consider girls' names and will not listen to their wives' prompting to be prepared for either sex.

At the time of birth, most parents are able to accept the sex born to them. Although disappointment is evident and often voiced, verbal acceptance is expressed to each other soon after the birth. Frequently, personnel assist parents in voicing their disappointment, then point out the positive attributes of the child as soon as it is appropriate. Normally there is a grief reaction and sense of loss at birth as the parents release the fantasized child and begin to accept the real child.

Occasionally the father (or mother) has a marked negative reaction to the "wrong" sex of the child. Disappointment at the birth of a girl prompted one husband to curse the nurses, the physician, his wife, and the wife's relatives. He refused to speak to his wife or even to see her or the child after delivery. There might have been clues to this problem area during the antenatal period that could have prompted intervention and modified this unfortunate outcome.

Breast or bottle? Deciding on the infant's feeding method is of concern when the partners' preferences differ or when one partner has intense reactions. Actual benefits and disadvantages of one method over another are irrelevant. Some expectant mothers are startled by the husband's strong insistence on one method or the other. Some men insist that the wife breast-feed; others are adamantly set against breast-feeding. Reasons given for this strong and sometimes vehement antinursing stance include its "animal-like" nature; competition for the wife's breast, concern that the breasts will sag later on, fear of effects on the baby (e.g., "It makes a sissy of a baby boy"), fear of being tied down, and inability to know (and perhaps control) how much the child receives.

When the husband refuses to take a stand, the wife experiences uneasiness. Inwardly she accuses him of disinterest or feels uncertain about choosing the right way. The wife seems to ask for his support for whatever choice is made. Many couples find it difficult to vent honest feelings without a supportive other, such as the nurse, to open up the subject or mediate the discussion.

Changing self-concept. During this time, men seem to become more introspective. There are many discussions about one's relationships with different family members and friends and about one's own philosophy of life, religion, and childbearing and child-rearing practices.

Just prior to phase III, noticeable changes and reactions occur in the father. During the last trimester, it is not unusual to find the clean-shaven expectant father growing a beard or mustache. Meanwhile his bearded counterpart suddenly decides to shave his face clean. Time, energy, and money are spent fixing up long-existent physical problems. Glasses are replaced with contact lenses. Weight reduction diets are usually successful if attempted. Old wardrobes are discarded and new ones acquired to show himself and others that he is indeed a new person. Wife, family, and friends are bewildered at this unexplained concentration on self at this

crucial time and often react with teasing or open hostility. A wife may believe he is withdrawing his attention from her. Anticipatory guidance for this eventuality can reassure and support the couple.

Creative activities. The urge to create appears in every human. Expressed biologically as the need to procreate, this drive is necessary for the survival of the species. For the female, a direct biologic mode of creative expression is available; for the male, other modes are possible. Whether or not the pregnancy was planned, many men express a profound feeling of awe or pride in being a part of the creation of a human being.

During the last 2 months of pregnancy, expectant fathers experience a surge of energy to create and to achieve in the home and on the job. These behaviors could be interpreted as tangible evidence of sharing the wife's creative experience while channeling the anxiety (or other feelings) of the final weeks before birth. Furthermore, these behaviors earn recognition and compliments from friends, relatives, and wives, and some may even dovetail with wives' nesting activities.

Rehearsing for fatherhood. Daydreaming is a form of role playing. This form of anticipatory psychologic preparation for the infant is most frequent in the last weeks before delivery. Rarely do men confide their daydreams unless they are reassured that daydreams are normal and fairly prevalent. Questions such as the following assist the nurse and the parent in identifying concerns and informational needs and allow for reality testing: What do you expect the child to look and act like? What do you think it will be like to be a father? Have you thought about the baby's crying? Changing diapers? Burping the baby? Being awakened at night? Sharing your wife with the baby? Occasionally just asking the questions suffices. The father may not wish to share his answers with the nurse at that moment but may need time to mull them over in his mind or with his spouse.

If an expectant father can imagine only an older child and has difficulty visualizing or talking about the infant, this area needs to be explored. Frequently, he only requires information. He may never have seen a newborn. He may need to talk about it, or he may benefit from early introduction to holding or handling the child. After delivery he may benefit from the chance to inspect his child inch by inch with a nurse or physician to become acquainted with it and to be reassured that his child's appearance and behavior are normal if they truly are.

Phase III: Anticipation of approaching labor

Changing self-concept. Dissatisfaction with present living space increases. The need to alter the present environment is acted on wherever possible. When a move into a new home or apartment is not possible, other changes are made to accommodate the new self-concept: furniture is rearranged; new furniture, appliances, or both are added; cats may be ousted; and acquisition of a new car may be considered.

Coping and defense activities. The days and weeks immediately preceeding the expected day of delivery are characterized by anticipation and anxiety. Many husbands (and couples) describe time as heavy, slowing down, and distorted. Boredom and restlessness are common. Expectant fathers and their wives focus on the birth process.

Fathers spend their heightened energies in diverse ways: conversing with others regarding their experiences; justifying fears of being with his wife in labor by basing these fears on past experiences with blood or needles; teasing and ridiculing the wife's ungainly bearing and movements; projecting hostilities toward homosexuals, landlords, fellow workers and those of other races, religions, and nationalities; ''copping out'' by stating refusal to think about the coming event or by planning to watch television or to go bowling during her labor; or sleeping and resting to the exclusion of all else.

The expectant mother's reactions to the observed behaviors in her mate vary. One prevailing reaction is concern about the possibility of being deserted physically or emotionally when she is feeling most vulnerable.

A primary concern of the father is his ability to get the mother to a medical facility on time. It is a convenient and acceptable focus for his fear and anxiety. Initially fathers fantasize several ridiculously humorous situations, then move on to plan what they will do. Many rehearse the routes to the hospital, timing each route at different times of the day. Suitcase, car, and essential telephone numbers are kept in readiness.

In addition, many fathers want to be able to recognize labor and to determine when it is appropriate to leave for the hospital (or call the physician or midwife). The concern here is twofold: getting to the hospital on time and not appearing ''stupid.''

Many fathers have questions about the labor suite's physical environment and staffing—furniture, nursing staff, location, and availability of physician and anesthesiologist. Others' interests lie in knowing what is expected of them when their wives are in labor.

Fathers have imagined the delivery room as containing ''10,000 lights'' with ''instruments everywhere and a delivery table like a slab.'' During delivery, men anticipate ''lots of blood'' and commotion and rushing about, with ''people everywhere, moving fast.''

The father has fears of mutilation and death for his wife and child. While he harbors these fears within, he is not free to listen to or to help his mate with her unspoken or overt apprehensions. Words such as ''dropped,'' ''rupture of bag of waters,'' ''bloody show,'' ''tears and stitches,'' and ''labor pains'' have violent overtones.

With the exception of parent education classes, there are few built-in means for a father to learn to be an involved, active, and needed partner in this rite of passage into parenthood. The unprepared, unsupported father may add to the mother's fears. Tensions and apprehensions are readily transmitted and may increase the mother's difficulties. His own self-doubt and fear of inadequacy may be realized if he is not supported. Self-confidence comes from achieving realistic self-goals and earning the approval of others.

Most men whose wives are about to go into labor may be reached through intervention before the event. Imaginings can be replaced by knowledge gained through activities such as the following:

1. A hospital tour to visualize the labor room and waiting areas so that he can begin to work out ways of using the environment when he arrives and to ''get the feel'' of the delivery room and see what is really there, where he will sit, and what his role will be
2. A demonstration of helping and supportive measures to comfort his wife during labor
3. A brief review of what to expect from his wife during the labor process if she has medication and/or anesthesia or if she delivers without medication and/or anesthesia (e.g., irritability, breathing, grunting)
4. A description of what to expect of the staff during his wife's labor

A realistic discussion of all known factors helps the father more rationally problem solve and plan for the event. These activities are ego strengthening, since they marshal one's energies toward more appropriate coping strategies and help alleviate anxieties emanating from that which still remains unknown: what his wife's labor will be like and whether the baby will be normal.

Father-fetus relationship. As the birth day approaches, questions regarding fetal and newborn behaviors increase: ''What do they do in there (in utero)?'' ''Is he hiccupping?'' ''Does he suck his thumb?'' ''How is he breathing?'' ''What does a newborn baby look like?'' Some express shock or amazement about the smallness of clothes and furniture received as gifts for the baby. Other fathers protest, ''He'll only be real to me when I can hold him in my arms.''

All these activities speak to his involvement and concerns in becoming a father to his own child. Throughout this pregnancy but to a heightened degree now, his memories emerge of being fathered as a child. These memories merge with his expectations of himself in the father role that is soon to be *his* role.

Phase IV: Involvement with the birthing process

Fatherhood with dignity. Miller (1966) remarked, "There is joy in having a baby, and joy is an experience worth sharing." Conception is a psychologic as well as a physiologic experience of a man and woman creating a new life; birth can be no less. Conception is the experience of two people; birth, the experience of three (or more) people.

Involving the father in the birth of his child dispels feelings of alienation, isolation, impotence, helpless inaction, and insignificance. Ethnic definition and role expectations govern the type and degree of the individual's involvement.

Individual preference for the kind of involvement spans a full spectrum of possibilities. One family, recent arrivals from Italy, is a case in point. The father absented himself to the waiting room while the female relatives took turns attending his wife and reporting her progress to him at intervals. After delivery, wife and son were wheeled back to the labor area. The father entered proudly as the female relatives stepped aside. He made what sounded like endearing comments to wife and son and kissed them both; then all relatives left. The new mother beamed. The students present expressed negative reactions about this father, whose participation in this event was perceived as tangential and unsupportive. One student was assigned to this mother's postnatal care and to make a home visit. Her report and discussion of her experience with the group clarified the situation as "right" for this family.

Other men seek a different type of involvement. What are his hopes and expectations for this experience for himself and for his wife? What is the nurse's role in relation to his decisions? These questions will be discussed in the following sections.

The birth process as seen through the father's eyes. The nurse should recall her feelings the first time she witnessed a woman in active labor. The father's experience can be no less intense. In addition, the woman in labor is not a patient to him; she is birthing their baby.

During the delivery he may see the following sights:
1. Her facial and physical expression of pain; grimace and effort written on her face while pushing

2. Blood, mucus, and watery drainage from her vagina
3. Fecal discharge
4. Bulging perineum just before birth
5. Episiotomy, if done, and repair
6. Delivery by forceps, if used
7. Her postures for vaginal examinations, for observations of the perineum, and for delivery
8. Dry heaves or vomiting

He may hear the following sounds:
1. Her moans and grunts (especially while pushing)
2. Dry heaves or efforts at vomiting
3. Hospital noises (e.g., call lights, page systems, clanging, sterilizer buzzers, fetal monitoring devices)
4. Silence when something is going wrong
5. Proclamations and defense of territorial rights by some staff
6. Extraneous, irrelevant social or business chatter among staff

He may smell the following:
1. Vaginal drainage
2. Fecal drainage
3. Vomitus (occasionally)
4. Cleaning solutions

With the emergence of the infant, the father will see and hear the following sights and sounds:
1. Small patch of scalp and hair at the introitus
2. Prolonged (usually) emergence of the molded fetal head (e.g., one father commented, "and then when all that kept coming out was head and more head and no eyes or ears, I wondered when they would come")
3. Blue-purple coloration of the fetal scalp and body along with blood, amniotic fluid, vernix, and, occasionally, meconium
4. Cord being loosened around the child's neck and/or being eased over his head or shoulders
5. Mucus draining from nose and mouth and the physician or nurse suctioning the infant
6. Sounds of suctioning
7. Cutting of the cord
8. Verbal communications between physician and nurse regarding position, cord, placement of episiotomy, and similar medical matters in terms often unfamiliar to him

The father in the labor suite. "He'll just be underfoot." "He'll add confusion and increase the chance of infections and the number of lawsuits." These typical statements for years kept the father apart from his wife and child. These fears proved largely unfounded when fathers were reunited with their laboring wives. Fathers

PLAN OF CARE: PHASES I, II, AND III—ANTENATAL PERIOD

NURSING INTERVENTIONS

Diagnostic	Therapeutic	Educational

1. Assess prospective or new father's self-concept as evidenced by following:
  a. Grooming, posture, walking, talking.
  b. Facial expressions.
  c. Body language (e.g., use of hands, feet).
2. Assess father's level of understanding and breadth and depth of knowledge he wishes to have.
3. Assess father's communication as follows:
  a. Is he listening, hearing, and taking in?
  b. Tune into his language.
4. Father's obstetric history:
  a. Age.
  b. Number of previous pregnancies and ages of other children.
  c. How have his partner's previous pregnancies been?
  d. What was his degree of involvement in previous pregnancies?
  e. How does he perceive his role in this pregnancy?
  f. Does he have questions regarding pregnancy, labor and delivery, or infant?
  g. How far along is this pregnancy?
  h. Was this pregnancy planned?
  i. What myths, "old wives tales," and other data has he heard regarding pregnancy?
  j. What pregnancy symptoms does his wife have? Do these upset him? Does he have any questions regarding them?
5. What is their life-style, i.e., foods and living arrangements that might affect her care, delivery, or other related matters?
	1. Call him (and wife) by name. Introduce yourself and your functions.
	2. Demonstrate interest in him by your manner and informed questions.
	3. Communicate.
	4. Acknowledge his feelings. Tune in to where he is at this moment. Does he have something else on his mind that prevents him from focusing on interview? Or does his cultural background find this type of involvement unnecessary or unmanly?
	5. Acknowledge his previous experiences.
	  a. Interaction with 16-year-old having his first baby may be different from interview with 42-year-old having his first or fifth baby in terms of education, past experiences, finances, career, and whether pregnancy is planned.
	  b. Previous experience with pregnancy, labor and delivery, and newborns color present experiences, although this experience may be different.
	  c. Gaps in knowledge are expected and mutually identified. Knowledge banishes ignorance, exposes unfounded beliefs, and will likely minimize fears and unnecessary anxieties.
	6. Do not pass judgment on his lifestyle. Work within what couple prefer or what they can manage. Many alternatives are possible and viable.
	7. Timing and pacing of interventions are important. (This takes practice and experience on nurse's part.) Talk about topic he is interested in *now*.
	8. Convey attitude of teamwork and of adult-to-adult relationship.
	9. Discuss symptoms of complications of pregnancy. Provide names and telephone numbers to use in case of emergency. Specify what and how to report problems. In addition to verbal instructions, all
		1. Feelings are involved for man and woman experiencing pregnancy.
		  a. There are physiologic and psychologic bases for emotional changes in woman, who needs support from significant others.
		  b. There is normal psychologic basis for changes in man. He may not be able to maintain supportive position if he does not receive support and relief too. He needs support if he is to meet woman's support needs.
		2. Starting from his questions and based on his background and stage of this pregnancy, consider following:
		  a. Normally expected changes (physiologic, anatomic, psychologic) of pregnancy; timing of changes; and their duration.
		  b. Possible areas of conflict—naming the baby, choice of feeding method, her introspection, and sexuality changes.
		  c. Types of supportive and comfort measures he can offer.
		  d. Clarification of misconceptions (e.g., eating cheese will not rot the uterus, crossing her legs will not make the baby's head pointed).
		  e. Signs and symptoms of complications of pregnancy.
		  f. Information regarding parent education classes designed for expectant parents.
		  g. Preparation for labor and delivery.
		3. Alert him to periods of greatest upset.
		  a. Confirmation of pregnancy. (Did he experience this?)
		  b. When he becomes aware of fetal movements and contours.
		  c. As delivery approaches.
		4. Parenthood is partnership. Sound medical care is based on teamwork between parents and staff.
		5. Information needs as delivery date approaches:
		  a. Getting to hospital—how to recognize true contractions and how to time them, timing of events of labor, when to have

---

PLAN OF CARE: PHASES I, II, AND III—ANTENATAL PERIOD—cont'd

NURSING INTERVENTIONS—cont'd

Diagnostic	Therapeutic	Educational
	this information should be on printed sheet for couple to have. 10. Provide information on types of parent education classes, times, and dates.	bags packed to go to hospital, practicing dry runs to hospital, telephone number of physician or labor unit. b. Hospital environment—suite, who will be with him, personnel, lay-out, accessibility of physician and anesthesiologist. c. Mechanics of getting permission to be in delivery room. d. Process of delivery—how labor works, birth canal and its stretchability, how baby looks when being born, how to deliver woman if he has to, forceps. e. If practicing prepared childbirth, how much responsibility is theirs.

---

proved helpful, comforting, and reassuring to their wives. There was no change in the incidence of infection or lawsuits. Furthermore, it was found that it was easier for the physician and parents to cope with the birth of a child with a defect when both parents were active participants on an adult-to-adult level with the physician.

The father may be an adjunct to the nurse-physician team in several ways. For example, he may assist with comfort measures such as pillows, ice chips, washcloths to forehead, and back rubs. He may provide almost constant companionship to offset the aloneness of labor and the anxiety it can foster. Should something occur when the nurse or physician is out of the room, the father can call for help. In addition, he is usually better equipped to interpret the mother's wishes and needs to the staff.

Participation in the birth is ego-building. The father *can* be of assistance; his presence *is* important. It is frequently observed that a caring person can be worth his (her) weight in Demerol (meperidine). Recently a 16-year-old unwed mother in labor with her first child thrashed about, moaning and screaming with each contraction. A nurse remained at her bedside, coaching and comforting to no avail. The unwed adolescent father arrived and was immediately escorted into her room. The young woman continued her labor calmly and unmedicated until delivery.

When the father is active and supportive, the mother turns to him; the physician remains the medical-surgical expert, without his taking on the father- or husband-surrogate role as well. The couple's future relationship and their relationship to their child may be positively influenced. Mutuality is fostered when the mother can turn to the father and say, "I could never have done it without you. You were my pillar of strength."

Supporting the father during labor. Supporting the father as well as the mother in labor elevates the nurse's role. It is another step forward from merely providing custodial care to enacting a therapeutic role.

Supporting the father reflects the nurse's orientation and commitment to the person, the family, and the community. Therapeutic nursing actions convey to the father several important concepts.

First, he is of value as a person. He is not a comic strip character, inept, bungling or idle, nervous, and inconsequential. Second, he can learn to be a partner in the mother's care. Finally, childbearing is a partnership.

Even if the father enters the labor unit without any parent education classes, he can be taught "on the job," and his choices can be supported. The nurse can support the father in the following ways:

1. Regardless of the degree of involvement desired, orient him to the maternity unit, including wife's labor room and what he can do there (sleep, telephone, smoke or not), restroom, cafeteria, Dads' Room, nursery, visiting hours, and names and functions of personnel present.

2. Respect his (or their) decisions as to his degree of involvement whether the decision is active participation

PLAN OF CARE: PHASE IV—PERINATAL PERIOD

NURSING INTERVENTIONS

Diagnostic	Therapeutic*	Educational

1. Assess father's behavior.
  a. Is he hesitant to go into labor room? Does he appear confident? Does he appear aggressive or hostile as he strides into labor room? (He may be asserting his felt need to be with his wife or just covering up his anxieties.)
  b. Is he sleepy, red-eyed, or glassy-eyed from fatigue? Is he worried-looking?
2. Assess his (and her) orientation to his participation.
  a. Is he prepared through classes? Which kind?
  b. Does he want to provide comfort measures? Which does he need to learn?
  c. Is he considering accompanying her to delivery room?
3. Has he been on hospital tour?
  a. Is he oriented to unit? To this hospital?
  b. What questions does he have regarding her room, delivery room, nursery, postnatal care?
	1. Establish adult-to-adult relationship.
	  a. Identify yourself and your function.
	  b. Call them by name.
	  c. Explore with them what father's involvement is to be; respect their position.
	2. Prepare him for what to expect of labor and delivery process, first appearance of newborn, and first hour postdelivery.
	3. Acknowledge his worth there by commenting on effectiveness of his comfort measures.
	  a. Involving him with comfort measures helps harness his energy and direct it toward mutually useful goal.
	  b. Help him see himself as adequate; increase his self-confidence.
	4. Offer to relieve him as necessary; offer food and fluids; offer blankets if he is to sleep in chair by bedside.
	5. Stay in room to assist them as necessary; leave if they are engrossed in Lamaze or other prepared childbirth method (if labor is progressing well and they need no assistance).
	6. Keep him (them) informed of progress.
	  a. What the nurse is monitoring and why.
	  b. Physician's examination. (Physician usually does this right after examination.)
	7. Keep him (them) informed of procedures to be done, what to expect from procedures, and what is expected of him.
	8. Ascertain how couple interprets information given them in classes (e.g., does "natural childbirth" mean woman is not to receive medication?)
	9. Determine if they have seen actual delivery or film of delivery and if so, how they felt about what they saw, especially, what he saw.
		1. Teach father comfort measures, i.e., tangible actions which serve to relieve discomfort directly or indirectly. Something can be done to make labor better experience for both mother and father.
		  a. Direct relief of cause—relieving leg cramps by forcing extension of affected muscles; relieving aches by change of position.
		  b. Indirect relief by flooding nerve pathways with impulses by doing or focusing on certain activity rather than leaving all pathways open for pain impulses and perception.
		  c. Nonverbal means of expressing concern and caring for another.
		2. Teach mother and father importance of mother's lying on side, especially left. Encourage breathing and relaxation techniques in side-lying position as well. Side-lying position for rest or sleep is physiologically healthier anytime (supports adequate perfusion of kidneys and prevents vena caval syndrome).
		3. Teach anatomy and physiology of birth process and birth canal, inform parents about skin and other changes that occur to accommodate pregnancy and labor and delivery. Depending on mother's phase of labor, parents' orientation, and time, many people are particularly receptive to this knowledge now.
		4. Explain anatomy and physiology of newborn: heart rate (especially if each has chance to hear it), breathing as it is in infant versus later in childhood; and maternal hormonal influences (linea nigra, breast enlargement) on infant. Newborn movements, color at birth, and head shape are also of great interest and prepare them for beginning relationship to own infant.
		5. Acknowledge stress of situation on each other and identify normal responses. Nonjudgmental attitude of staff helps father and mother accept own and other parent's behavior.

*These measures recognize parents' need for nurse to be psychologically as well as physically present. They may be accomplished by physician or nurse as situation warrants.

in the delivery room or just being kept informed. When appropriate, provide data on which he (or they) can base decisions; offer freedom of choice as opposed to coercion one way or another. This is *their* experience and *their* baby.

3. Indicate to him when his presence has been helpful.

4. Offer to teach him comfort measures to the degree he wants to know them. Reassure him that he is not assuming the responsibility for observation and management of his wife's labor. Supportive behavior can be classified into three categories:

    a. Physical care

    b. Nonverbal (e.g., holding her hand, smiling, kissing)

    c. Verbal (e.g., coaching, breathing, relaxation techniques, complimenting)

5. Communicate with him frequently regarding her progress and his needs.

6. Prepare him for changes in her behavior and physical appearance.

7. Remind him to eat; offer snacks and fluids if possible.

8. Relieve him as necessary.

9. Attempt to modify or eliminate unsettling stimuli (e.g., extra noise, extra light, chatter); keep the mother clean and dry.

A well-informed father can make a significant contribution to the health and well-being of the mother and child, their family interrelationship, and his self-esteem. It has been found that a significantly lower percentage of women suffered postnatal emotional upsets when their partners received support and assistance from antenatal classes, physicians (throughout the cycle), and public health nurses in the home.

Phase V: New parenthood

Father-newborn relationship. The baby is here, no longer fantasy but reality. What was once to be now is.

> Everybody is just fine! It's a girl! A beautiful, wonderful girl! (Wife) is just fine! Everything went perfect.

> When they wheeled her from the delivery room with the baby in her arms, all I could do was stare with my mouth open. The nurse told me to kiss (wife), so I did, then stared at my son again.

> I really got to feel she was mine in the hospital when I held her.

> Funny, not every day you have a son. It almost feels like we (wife, baby, self) are united, or the same even, a strange feeling.

Immediately after delivery, the father must distinguish the baby of fantasy from the baby of reality. His real infant has a sex, a definite size and weight, his own color of eyes, hair, skin, and his own body posture and posturing, reflexes, and activity patterns. Most parents quickly reconcile the differences between what was hoped for and what was realized. The process is facilitated by the nurse who verbalizes the naturalness of some disappointment, especially if she knew their hopes prior to the birth, allows the father to hold and fondle his offspring early and over protracted periods of time,* and examines the baby with the father from top of head to tip of toe. Each individual characteristic is described, including reflexes and sleep patterns.

Many feelings regarding newborn behaviors and dependency needs are uncovered and verbalized, and resolution regarding feelings may be begun. It is easier to perceive the infant's needs and learn appropriate responses if he is seen as an individual in his own right.

Newborn characteristics that evoke positive father responses include the following:

Male child	**Female child**
Large size (body, hands, feet)	Petite size
Lots of hair	Cute, little mouth
Vigorous sucking	Dimples
Loud burping	Bright eyes, long lashes
Loud, lusty cry	Soft cry
	Quiet personality

Fathers are sensitive to their children's behaviors. If the infant does not open his eyes and look at him or make some other contact, the father may feel hurt, although he knows the infant's responses are undifferentiated as yet. One father told of his first attempt to give his child a kiss. At that moment, the child turned her head. The father felt hurt even though he understood that the baby was totally unaware of her own movements. Another man commented on his son's grasp reflex, "I put my finger in his hand, and he grabbed right on. It is just a reflex I know, but it felt good anyway." After a woman described how hard her infant sucked on the breast, the father commented, "That's my little man."

If the birth occurs in a hospital, 12 hours to 3 days or more elapse before the child is taken home. Parents should be prepared for the ride home when the infant may awaken and become fussy. When the father is driving and the child is crying, the mother gets more frustrated in her efforts to quiet the child. For the first time no hospital attendant is nearby to take over. Knowledge of this possibility and having a bottle, breast, or pacifier ready may ease this distressing experience.

---

*This must be within the parents' own cultural prescription. For some, it is unmanly to be involved in this way with a baby.

Having a neighbor, friend, or family member in the home when the new family arrives home is helpful. The new parents may deal better with the situation if they have help with unpacking, meals, or other children or if someone just holds the baby for a few minutes while the parents get settled.

Soon the postbirth euphoria is gone. The job of incorporating the new family member begins in earnest. As one father reported:

I was euphoric for about 3 weeks. I wanted lots of kids. After 3 weeks, I found out what it's all about: it's expensive, your time isn't your own, she cries and leaves you frustrated. Now, I think one child is enough for a while at least.

By the sixth week, most fathers reflect that it is hard to remember when the baby was not there: "At first it was hard fitting him into our schedule, but now it seems he has been with us always. I can't imagine being without him."

Husband-wife relationship. Transition into new roles and responsibilities is seldom smooth. Readjustments and reorganization within the relationship may still be occurring at the end of 6 weeks.

Although the relationship remains dynamic, there are many possible unsettling experiences during this early postnatal period that stress the usual coping methods. Problems begun in pregnancy may continue with the same or different intensity now in areas such as sibling rivalry, breast-feeding, or self-concept, which is now mirrored by a real live baby.

One father seemed anxious to talk about "this weird dream I had about a month ago" (the baby was 4 weeks old):

I dreamed that we had a son and he was older already. Then I was preparing for a big wedding and I knew who was getting married . . . my son was marrying (my wife). All the people came and congratulated me and everyone was happy. Then I was running around trying to find my son and (my wife) after the wedding because I realized that I would never see them again. This dream really frightened me. I was very upset for about 3 days afterwards.

Other fathers experience a change of attitude toward the method of feeding. Some who originally believed that breast-feeding was the only good method subtly helped their wives to change to the bottle within a month.

Some new fathers appear to compete with their wives in mothering the infant. He tries to outdo her in feeding, comforting, and dressing the infant and points this out verbally to the mother and others. The mother's reactions vary from pleasure at his interest and skill to resentment.

The most frequent overtly expressed problem of the father is the wife's continuing fatigue and labile emotions, with him asking, "Shouldn't that be a thing of the past now?"

Nursing intervention during this first 6 weeks pays dividends. However, most couples are usually not in contact with health care professionals until a month postnatally when the baby visits the pediatrician and 6 weeks postdelivery when the mother visits the obstetrician. Couples without external sources of support may find this an extremely difficult period.

Couples also discover many new and exciting facets of the other's personality, such as finding the spouse to be a good parent, warm and goodhearted with baby and partner.

Common questions of new fathers. Closure of events surrounding the delivery is one important psychologic task after delivery. Questions that fathers ask immediately after delivery include the following:

1. If all this is so natural, why does it take so much time and so much pushing to deliver the baby?

2. Does it always take so long for the head to be born?

3. What happens where the cord is cut? When is the cord cut? Does it hurt the baby? Where is the cord attached inside of her?

4. Why was the baby turned with the forceps?

5. Why was she given an epidural?

6. When does the baby turn pink? Why is he so dark at first?

7. When is the baby able to breathe on his own?

These questions are asked even though the father may have read extensively during pregnancy, attended classes, and had some input during the labor and delivery. The need for repetition is natural and expected.

The father also has lingering thoughts regarding his behavior during labor. Many speak of having felt helpless even though they continued to stay with and coach or support the wife in other ways. Wives tend to be supportive of husbands who stay with them. The nurse, an objective bystander, can be helpful by filling all gaps in memory, pointing out what he did do and help him identify when he thought he was adequate or inadequate.

Fathers whose personal or cultural directives do not identify a role for him at the bedside of a laboring wife do not have this need to validate the labor and delivery experience.

The postnatal period also inspires questions by the new father. Regardless of the number of previous children one has, after each birth the person is in a unique position, since this situation and the existing configura-

PLAN OF CARE: PHASE V—POSTNATAL PERIOD (UNTIL END OF SIXTH WEEK)

NURSING INTERVENTIONS

Diagnostic	Therapeutic	Educational

1. Reaction to delivery:
  a. If father was in delivery room, ask following questions:
    1. What did you think of the delivery? Is it what you expected? Is there anything you would have liked to have known before you went in?
    2. Was there anything about delivery distressing for you? Episiotomy and its repair? Wife's position for delivery? Wife's behavior? Staff's actions or words? Appearance and care of your baby?
    3. What is your reaction to your newborn's appearance? Sex? Cry?
  b. If father was not in delivery room by his choice or the physician's, ask him how the waiting was for him.
  c. Assess nurse's or physician's observations of him (couple).
2. How does he behave? What does he say in following situations (in hospital and later at home)?
  a. Holding infant; staring at infant.
  b. Interacting with wife after delivery about labor, delivery, or newborn.
  c. At nursery window staring at infant. (Does he point out features or question characteristics of infant or his care?)
  d. When infant is crying.
  e. When he sees infant's bowel movement, wet diapers, regurgitations, and sleep habits.
3. Do gaps in knowledge exist regarding following?
  a. Labor, delivery, postnatal activities.
  b. Infant and his care.
  c. Mother's involution.
  d. Mother's resumption of activities of daily living.
	1. Allow father to hold and fondle baby immediately after delivery if possible. Holding baby and looking into his eyes early is essential for beginnings of attachment to infant. Also as soon as possible after birth, examine naked baby inch by inch with father and point out his individuality and characteristics.
	2. Inquire about his reactions and feelings and allow their expression to assist father to accomplish following:
	  a. Acknowledge that he has feelings and that they are all right.
	  b. Identify and verbalize areas of concern.
	  c. Process data in problem-solving format.
	  d. Fill in gaps as he (and wife) reconstruct events of birthing process.*
	3. Knowledge provides data base or reference points from which to function more effectively. It decreases possibility of misconceptions and misperceptions. Build on father's knowledge of following:
	  a. Newborn characteristics.
	  b. Postnatal involution—emotional and physical.
	  c. What to expect of himself.
	4. Identify and discuss universal concerns and problems of new parenthood: he is not alone in ambivalent feelings toward infant or wife-infant diad and forced change in life-style.
		1. Discuss common areas of concern or hurdles in new parenthood.
		  a. Physical care of infant.
		  b. Feelings about and dealing with crying, soiling, voiding, periods of irritability, altering one's daily schedule, and changed relationship with spouse and/or others.
		2. Discuss methods of coping with these concerns.
		3. Guided by his need and level of knowledge, teach regarding following:
		  a. Newborn.
		  b. Involution.
		  c. Reactions to becoming parent.
		  d. Continuing husband-wife relationship.

*This activity is essential for both to enable each to fit experience into their life-style, to see infant as individual in his own right, and for psychologic closure of event.

tion of social and emotional events have never been experienced before. Questions arise. Some questions that fathers ask are presented in the following list to help the nurse in devising individualized nursing care plans for postnatal interactions with families:

A. Siblings
   1. How does one prepare the older child or children at home?
B. Newborn
   1. How soon will it be all right to take the baby out, to fly out of state, to go camping, or to visit friends?
   2. When can the infant be left with a babysitter?
   3. What should we expect with regard to the baby's normal growth and development (even if there are one or more other children at home), smallness, fragility, cord, soft spot, acrocyanosis, smile, jaundice, circumcision, permanent eye and hair color, and other matters?
   4. How soon will we know what our infant is crying about?
   5. How do we take care of our baby, specifically holding, burping, dressing, temperature taking, and other activities?
C. Mother
   1. What should be expected with regard to the rate of healing (episiotomy and stitches), bleeding (amount, color, length of time), fatigue, and engorged breasts?
   2. When does her milk come in? How much milk? How do we know the baby is getting enough? What should the mother eat or not eat?
   3. When will she return to her prepregnant weight and shape?
   4. When can intercourse be started? What about contraceptives?

This last question is usually implied rather than asked directly. The nurse asks openly if the parents do not verbalize it. The nurse gives anticipatory guidance regarding first intercourse postnatally (pp. 150 and 151).

Reflections on fatherhood. What is it like after all the excitement of the pregnancy, birth, and new baby in the home dies down? Following are a few reactions of fathers:

With the first child, I was overwhelmed with the responsibility of it all. The second child, I can readily contend with the responsibility of fatherhood, although at times the responsibility is awesome.

Being a father feels good to me. It has exceeded my expectations. I realize more than ever, however, the tremendous amount of energy and commitment it requires. We have acquired different interests and friendships since we have had a child. I feel much closer to fathers now than I did before. Most importantly, I have come to appreciate the positive and negative aspects of domestic life in general. Consequently, I also feel that I understand women more as a result of this. Society has an obligation to support, in every way possible, mothers, fathers, and children.

My change in role from husband to father was marvelous. It gave me a much better perspective as a total person. Being a part of the lifegiving process, in my opinion, ranks close to, if not at, the top of all gifts bestowed on the human being. *Without it, there would be no me, no you.*

THE UNWED FATHER

Unwed fathers are also expectant parents. Including him along with the unwed mother in counseling provides an opportunity for learning and for growth in self-esteem and maturity for each partner. Consider the effects of commonly heard statements characterizing the unwed father such as, "He is just a boy sowing his wild oats," "He doesn't care what happens to her," "How would he know he's the father, anyhow?" and "Love 'em and leave 'em."

Statements such as these negate the existence of any positive interpersonal relationship between the couple. Furthermore, these comments infer clandestine, promiscuous relationships.

In the past, unwed pregnancy was* hidden away out of sight and out of mind. The unwed mother was assisted through the pregnancy and then was expected to forget the incident. The father was scarcely mentioned unless he was pressured into marriage or into accepting the financial responsibility. The complex social and emotional aspects of this unwed relationship were beclouded while the growth potential was overlooked.

Pannor and associates (1971) have demonstrated the feasibility of involving the unwed father in counseling and the benefits of this approach to him and the unwed mother. Male social workers, representing father figures, work with the unwed fathers. When Pannor and associates first introduced the idea of involving the unwed father in the counseling process, they found little support. Few believed that any unwed father wanted to be involved and that he actually had needs of his own. Another commonly believed myth was that the unwed mother would never reveal his name, if indeed she even knew who he was. Furthermore, it was believed that she wanted nothing more to do with him.

Who is the unwed father? What is he like? What type

---

*The past tense is used to signify a gradual shift in the public's values and definition of its own responsibility. However, "is" is still the appropriate tense in many situations.

of relationship is he likely to have with the unwed mother? How is he likely to relate to this pregnancy and child? Following are the data from the work of Pannor and co-workers:

1. Most women were willing and able to name the father. Most couples jointly participated in counseling.

2. The partners were usually close in age and social class.

3. The majority of unwed partners were from the middle class and had completed high school or above.

4. Ignorance of contraceptive methods was not a factor.

The Family Service Association of America, in cooperation with *Ladies' Home Journal,* conducted a study of unwed fathers (Robinson, 1969). Each affiliated agency in all parts of the United States was asked to analyze the case histories of the most recent unwed fathers. A detailed profile of 149 unwed fathers emerged as follows:

1. The men involved were not "philanderers" nor irresponsible.

2. The unwed father may be deeply involved with the unwed mother, the pregnancy, and the child. Sixty-one percent not only expressed an obligation to marry the woman but also *wanted* to marry her. In this study, it was the woman who frequently rejected the idea of marriage. Less than 20% of the fathers believed that the woman was trying to trap them into marriage. Only 1% described the woman as a "pickup."

3. Over 60% of the men visited their babies in the hospital and demonstrated strong paternal feelings. Seeing the baby and talking about it afterward completes the reality of the event and helps to integrate the experience into one's life pattern.

4. The Family Service Association study documents the case histories of several young men who were traumatized by having to release the child for adoption when the woman refused the offer of marriage and when he was refused the option of adopting the child himself. One young man, after his request to adopt his child was denied, lamented the loss of "his own flesh and blood."

Unwed parenthood: potentials for growth

Involvement of the unwed father with consideration and respect supports his ego and facilitates his psychologic and emotional growth. Active participation in decision making regarding the pregnancy and the infant improves problem-solving skills, moves the pregnancy and its outcome from the level of fantasy to that of reality, and may result in more maturity in approaching general problems of living.

The unwed adolescent father has special needs. Adolescence is characterized by struggles in achieving one's own identity and relating this identity to peers and meaningful adults in the situation. Being able to share the responsibility of deciding about this pregnancy and infant is therapeutic in that it can increase self-esteem and decrease guilt feelings. This process actually supports the unwed mother and her self-esteem as well. The couple chose each other. Each mirrors the other in "badness" and "goodness." The positive feelings engendered through counseling are likely to pave the way for improving their relationships with members of the other sex, those in authority (including their parents perhaps), and each other. Furthermore, the idea that parenthood is indeed a partnership situation is introduced and emphasized.

PSYCHIATRIC PROBLEMS DURING PREGNANCY AND POSTNATALLY

The experience of pregnancy and parenthood for the man is as crucial as it is for the woman. Extreme anxiety and even acute psychoses can be precipitated by the birth of a child. Many normal men exhibit some similar behaviors, but their difficulties are of a transitory nature. Few need referral for psychiatric treatment.

Some fathers suffering from depression and anxiety related to pregnancy and childbirth may never come to the attention of health care professionals. These casualties may carry long-term psychologic scars that may adversely affect their mental health and intrafamilial relationships.

The unwed father is also prone to the same subjective reactions as his wedded peers, with possible additional stresses such as the reaction of his family and society, his relationship with the unwed mother, and his ego strength.

Actual documented cases of mental illness in men due to pregnancy and early parenthood are limited. This may be a reflection of a tendency to view the problems of the father apart from the childbearing experience.

THE NURSE AS CHANGE AGENT
Problem-oriented patient care

The content of this chapter is designed to acquaint the student with available knowledge regarding the expectant and new father, to arouse curiosity, and to stimulate questions. However, shifting social emphasis and the passage of time may alter some of the core knowledge. The problem-oriented approach provides a framework for interaction with patients that helps identify new knowledge, new trends, and alterations in old knowledge. The organization of our present health care delivery system requires patients to interact with health professionals from many disciplines. The problem-oriented method pools these resources, eliminates fragmentation, and makes comprehensive care a realistic goal. Collaborative efforts recorded in on-going problem-oriented records (POR) stimulate the continuing education and self-directed learning of health professionals (Chapter 39). The patient benefits in many ways. Problem-oriented care allows him to set his own priorities for health (which may differ from the health professional's priorities). Energetic parent education enhances motivation to utilize medical know-how. The attitude of this approach promotes the idea of partnership in parenthood and in one's own health care. Problem-oriented care supports the health professional and the patient so that each may become more responsible and accountable for his behavior.

Involving the father

The stereotype of a bumbling, frantic, expectant father does little to reassure the mother that he can support and strengthen her. The husband can be helpful, useful, and involved. There is an important place for him. He does influence her physical and emotional well-being during pregnancy, childbirth, and postnatally. There are many ways of increasing the involvement of the father, including the following:

1. An informational brochure can be made available to expectant fathers. These brochures could be designed with sections such as the following: "Did you know. . . ."; "Fathers have needs too. . . ."; "Questions fathers ask. . . ."; and "For fathers only. . . ."

2. Those who provide medical supervision during childbearing could set up the expectation that the father would accompany the mother for her checkups at least once, preferably at the visit when pregnancy is confirmed or at the following one. Ample time needs to be allowed for a relaxed intake interview.

Confirmation of pregnancy usually brings a statement of "congratulations" to the woman without exploring with her the meaning of the pronouncement to her and to the father. Congratulations or counseling are inappropriate before all the facts are in. Do one or both partners want this pregnancy? What decisions regarding this pregnancy must be made, that is, carry to term, keep, adopt out, or abort? If the pregnancy test is negative, what does this mean to her, to him, and to them? What type of counseling is needed (e.g., contraception, family planning, infertility or sterility)?

If the test is positive and the couple wishes to maintain this pregnancy, antenatal care is begun. The data base

would include a brief narrative of their life-style, his intended involvement in the childbearing process, and their expectations of themselves and each other. Some anticipatory guidance can be started. Initial plans can be formulated to meet existing or anticipated needs. If possible, return visits should be planned: one during the middle of the pregnancy and one within a week or two of the due date. Both parents could benefit from a 6-week postnatal checkup in terms of their present situation and future pregnancies, if any.

3. Most nurses are female. Women may be able to answer many questions posed by expectant fathers, but fathers also need a man's perspective. Although male physicians can meet many needs of expectant and new fathers, the physician's role relationship is on a different level. However, experienced fathers can be taught to lead expectant and new parent group discussions. Perhaps the American Society for Psychoprophylaxis in Obstetrics or similar organizations could become involved in training men to lead such groups.

4. Nurses may have difficulty identifying and meeting the needs of expectant fathers of other races and from cultures other than the nurse's own. Bilingual and cross-cultural classes led by representatives of the respective groups are best able to communicate on a more personal basis. Furthermore, a person raised in a particular culture is more knowledgeable about the medical folklore and its role in that culture. Knowledge regarding needs of expectant fathers from other cultures must be identified, compiled, and written in the language, terminology, and context best suited to each population.

5. Delivery is a new beginning. New-parent rap sessions, discussions with the providers of health services, or "Helpful Hints to New Fathers" sections in newspapers and magazines can provide beneficial information and reassurance.

Pregnancy is more than a biologic destiny of women. It is a psychologic event of great import and potential for men and women. Although it depends on the birth of a child to give the event meaning, pregnancy is also a critical stage of development for both sexes.

REFERENCES

Bradley, R. A. 1974. Husband-coached childbirth. New York, Harper & Row, Publishers.

Bucove, A. 1964. Postpartum psychoses in the male. N.Y. Acad. Med., **40**:961.

Colman, A., and Colman, L. 1971. Pregnancy: the psychological experience. New York, Herder & Herder.

Hunter, R., and Macalpine, I. (eds.). 1963. Three hundred years of psychiatry, 1535-1860. London, Oxford University Press.

Josselyn, I. M. 1956. Psychology of fatherliness. Smith Coll. Stud. Soc. Work **26:**1, Feb.

Liebenberg, B. 1967. Expectant fathers. Paper presented at Conference of Pre-natal Counseling Project, Group Health Association, Inc., Oregon, March.

Miller, J. S. 1966. Return the joy of home delivery with fathers in the delivery room. Hosp. Top. **44:**105, Jan.

Neubardt, S. 1973. Brief guide to office counseling: coitus during pregnancy. Med. Asp. Hum. Sex., **7:**197, Sept.

Pannor, R., Massarik, F., and Evans, B. 1971. The unmarried father: new approaches for helping unmarried young parents. New York, Springer Publishing Co., Inc.

Robinson, D. 1969. Our surprising moral unwed fathers. Ladies Home Journal, pp. 49-50, Aug.

CHAPTER 13

Nutrition

Scientific research has identified the nutrient needs for optimal body function, growth, development, maintenance of body tissues, prevention of disease, and repair. Foods and their preparation to retain or enrich their nutrient value command a significant share of the scientific technology in North America. Yet many people are malnourished, undernourished, or obese. Dysfunctional nutrition prior to pregnancy may have long-term effects on the physical and mental development of the child and the subsequent health of the mother.

The nurse is in a strategic position. Nursing's orientation is to meet the health needs of individuals and groups. Among its tools are a sound knowledge of nutritional needs and the nursing process, and its function is based in the context of life's realities.

This chapter considers the following content areas: factors influencing the nutrition of individuals and groups, nutritional needs of pregnancy, specific nutrients and their food sources, basic four food groups, special concerns during pregnancy, lactation, nutrition and the pill, and nursing management.

FACTORS INFLUENCING NUTRITIONAL STATUS OF INDIVIDUALS AND GROUPS
Common misinformation about food

As with any significant aspect of human life, gradually myths have evolved around foods. Myths are beliefs that are taken for granted as truths and that usually uphold one's own preferences and practices. Several food myths have been identified by the United States Food and Drug Administration concerning health and disease. Examples of food myths that have persisted and are now assumed to be true by a significant segment of our society include the following:

1. A faulty diet is the basic etiology of all disease.
2. Soil depletion causes malnutrition. (Poor soil yields a small crop, but the nutritive content of each plant produced is unaffected.)
3. The nutritive value of food is destroyed by food processing. (Processing is rigidly controlled to preserve nutrients. Enrichment of certain products restores major natural vitamin and mineral content or adds a nutrient that is not found naturally such as vitamin D in milk.)
4. The population of the United States suffers from deficiencies that require vitamin and mineral supplements.
5. The combination of milk and fish at the same meal is harmful.
6. Citrus fruits produce ''acid stomach.''
7. Garlic and onion are effective in curing a cold and purifying the blood.
8. Wine, red beets, and tomatoes ''build'' blood; gelatin ''builds'' hair and fingernails.
9. Wonder foods such as blackstrap molasses, honey, and yogurt ensure good health. (Yogurt is an expensive form of milk, honey is the sugar fructose, and blackstrap molasses does contain vitamins and minerals, which are found in many other foods as well.)

Although food fads are usually short-lived, occasionally they persist and become incorporated into social custom. These popular fashions in food consumption are based on scientifically unsubstantiated beliefs about certain foods or combinations of foods. Many such fads are harmless; others may have serious implications for health. Examples of food faddism include the Atkins diet, Stillman diet, macrobiotic diet, and weight reduction regimens such as the bananas and skimmed milk diet, the eggs-only diet, and others.

Each nurse must be concerned about prevailing fads, myths, misinformation, and quackery surrounding foods. All have health, economic, and social ramifications. Self-diagnosis and treatment may seriously postpone appropriate attention by the physician and legitimate nutritionists. Many dollars are channeled into foods and drugs that may be harmless, as well as ineffectual, or that may be deleterious to the individual's health.

Psychosocial factors and food consumption

Hunger is a fundamental sensation; appetite is nature's way of ensuring food consumption to maintain life functions. Appetite and how it is satisfied are modified by the person's life experiences. Food behavior is influenced by one's emotional state, physical status, and environment (e.g., air of congeniality versus tension).

Each person has definite ideas about what to eat, how to eat, and which foods should be eaten when. These ideas and beliefs originate and are continually modified in the psychosocial and cultural milieu of each individual. Formal education about the types and quantities of essential nutrients may motivate one individual to modify personal dietary habits while remaining an academic exercise for another person.

Emotional needs of people play a significant role in the suboptimal utilization of sound nutrition data. Food and feeding or being fed has many emotional connotations for the average person; these special meanings go far beyond the physiologic need for food. Many feelings about food originate in infancy: food means love, security, comfort, and pleasure or the negative counterparts of these. During childhood, individuals may learn that some foods are used as bribes, rewards, and punishment or as a means of control by self or others. Eating with others signifies social acceptance, camaraderie, cultural and sometimes sexual identification, status, and position.

The nurse can analyze her own food behaviors by answering the following questions: What are your preferences? What types of foods do you like to eat? What time of day is appropriate (for you) to eat each type? Does your pattern vary during the week or at "special" times of the year? Where did you learn your preferences? When someone tells you to change your diet in some way because "it is good for you," how do you react? If possible, compare and contrast one day's diet and meal times with those of another person or persons and discuss the differences. Are any myths or food fads identified? Break down the foods into nutrients and calories and compare with the daily recommended requirements in Table 13-1.

Table 13-1. Daily dietary allowances of nonpregnant, pregnant, and lactating females*

	Nonpregnant females				Pregnancy	Lactation
	11 to 14 years†	15 to 18 years‡	19 to 22 years§	23 to 50 years§		
Energy (kcal)	2400	2100	2100	2000	+ 300	+ 500
Protein (gm)	44	48	46	46	+ 30	+ 20
Vitamin A (IU)	4000	4000	4000	4000	5000	6000
Vitamin D (IU)	400	400	400		400	400
Vitamin E (IU)	12	12	12	12	15	15
Ascorbic acid (mg)	45	45	45	45	60	80
Folacin (μg)	400	400	400	400	800	600
Niacin (mg)	16	14	14	13	+ 2	+ 4
Riboflavin (vitamin B_2) (mg)	1.3	1.4	1.4	1.2	+ 0.3	+ 0.5
Thiamin (vitamin B_1) (mg)	1.2	1.1	1.1	1.0	+ 0.3	+ 0.3
Vitamin B_6 (mg)	1.6	2.0	2.0	2.0	2.5	2.5
Vitamin B_{12} (μg)	3	3	3	3	4	4
Calcium (mg)	1200	1200	800	800	1200	1200
Phosphorus (mg)	1200	1200	800	800	1200	1200
Iodine (μg)	115	115	100	100	125	150
Iron (mg)	18	18	18	18	‖	18
Magnesium (mg)	300	300	300	300	450	450
Zinc (mg)	15	15	15	15	20	25

*From Food and Nutrition Board. 1974. Recommended dietary allowances (ed. 8). Washington, D.C., National Academy of Sciences–National Research Council.
†Weight 44 kg (97 pounds), height 155 cm (62 inches).
‡Weight 54 kg (119 pounds), height 162 cm (65 inches).
§Weight 58 kg (128 pounds), height 162 cm (65 inches).
‖The increased requirements of pregnancy cannot usually be met by ordinary diets; therefore the use of supplemental iron is recommended.

Adolescence and nutrition

Adolescence (ages 13 through 18 years) presents its own special nutritional and psychologic problems. Most adolescent girls attain physiologic maturity at 17 years of age; pregnancy prior to that age presents certain biologic hazards. Statistics for maternal and infant morbidity and mortality are discussed in Chapter 1. The course and outcome of pregnancy of women between 18 to 20 years of age are comparable to mature women 20 to 24 years of age.

The orderly sequence of growth and skeletal maturation is related to sexual maturation. Sexual maturity may be attained before musculoskeletal maturation is complete. Dietary surveys among adolescents have revealed that this group meets less than two thirds of the recommended daily intake for iron, calcium, and vitamins A and C (Committee on Maternal Nutrition, Food and Nutrition Board, 1970). About 1 in 10 adolescents who become pregnant is obese. ''Fat'' conscious adolescents may consume less than 2000 calories/day so that the recommended 18 mg/day of iron is deficient. Female adolescents who are anemic and underweight at a time when their bodily growth needs are at a peak (17 years of age or younger) are more vulnerable to skeletal problems, communicable diseases, and infections. Pregnancy at this time superimposes even greater metabolic demands for nutrients.

Working with the pregnant adolescent presents a challenge to one's ability to apply theory from the behavioral as well as physical sciences. The award for success is a physically healthy mother and infant and an emotionally more mature young mother, as well as the nurse's own personal and professional satisfaction.

Adolescence is a period of developing independence. Symbols of home—milk, fresh fruits and vegetables, and a ''square meal'' if these were present—are associated with dependency and as such may be threatening (e.g., ''peanut butter is for children''). Often there is the desire to ''be free,'' to choose ''forbidden'' foods. Peers congregate at the hamburger stand. Soda, hamburgers, and french fries may be supplemented with candy bars.

The young married adolescent may have just learned how to cook for her husband. This achievement plus her desire to please him and cater to his preferences must be considered in nutrition counseling. Supporting her inner desire to assert independence during nutrition counseling sessions lends support to the overall developmental task of this period: movement from the role of child to that of adult. Listen and allow her to talk. Build on what she and her family already know and practice. Reinforce sound dietary patterns and acknowledge willing adaptations that are made. Promote the idea that it is adult sometimes to do what one must, even if one does not wish to do so. When appropriate to meet the health needs of the mother and fetus, set some limits. Elicit help from the mother's parents or parent substitute in identifying these limits. In planning teaching strategy to meet the objectives of nutrition counseling the nurse must set realistic goals such as the following:

- To support the pregnant adolescent's psychosocial move toward independence
- To increase her knowledge of nutrients and daily allowances
- To teach her how to plan diets for self and family
- To teach her how to select foods to meet nutritional needs, personal preferences, budget, and seasonal availability
- To teach her how to prepare foods to ensure optimal nutritive value

Of necessity these goals go beyond the immediate objectives of a healthy pregnancy, an uneventful labor, and a full-term healthy infant whose weight and maturity are appropriate for gestational age and who subsequently grows and develops normally. Recent animal research has disclosed that it takes two generations to counteract the mental and physical retardation resulting from protein deficiency during pregnancy. The young mother who improves her own and her family's dietary patterns is building the foundation for a healthier beginning for generations to follow.

Another takeoff point in working with adolescents (and perhaps with older women as well) is calling attention to the relationship between sound nutrition and physical appearance. Frequently, the condition and appearance of the skin, hair, and nails are uppermost in the minds of adolescents. Body contours in both the male and female and muscular development in the male are selling points for good nutrition.

The following recommendations were drawn from the deliberations of the Committee on Maternal Nutrition, Food and Nutrition Board (1970):

1. Food programs for families with inadequate incomes should be implemented to recognize the top priority physiologic needs of infants and children, adolescents, and pregnant women.

2. One of the team providing comprehensive maternity care should be skilled in the psychosocial and physiologic needs of adolescents and be able to communicate effectively with them.

3. Family planning and antenatal care should be available to young girls, married or not.

4. Local statutes banning pregnant adolescents from staying in schools should be eliminated. Special school

programs should be developed in cooperation with health and social programs to ensure continuity of education, as well as maternity care for the pregnant adolescent.

5. Curricula of our schools should include instruction in personal and family living, nutrition, physiologic aspects of reproduction, importance and means of achieving responsible parenthood, and child care.

Socioeconomic status

Unfavorable outcomes of pregnancy are closely associated with the socioeconomic status of the mother, as well as other factors. Among the nutrition-related factors are biologic immaturity (17 years of age or younger), short stature (under 5 feet), prepregnancy weight that is 10% below normal for height, small weight gain during pregnancy, poor nutritional status prior to and during pregnancy, and chronic and infectious diseases.

It is difficult to make definitive statements regarding the relative importance of individual factors; empirical research on these factors would be difficult if not impossible. Some observations may be presented, however.

Persons who are most vulnerable are likely to have been raised in poor homes or in large families, in which access to medical care, food, and education for the children was inadequate. These conditions also favor poor food and health habits and the spread of disease. Frequently, young girls in these circumstances bear children early and tend to raise them in like surroundings.

Suboptimal health and nutritional status is not restricted to those raised in poverty. High educational and socioeconomic levels do not guarantee optimal health and nutrition. The current fashion for a slim figure, fad diets, and related health habits can result in inadequate stores and reserves to meet the metabolic needs of pregnancy.

Food habits of ethnic and religious groups

Nutrition counseling must be done within the cultural framework of the individual. Types and quantity of food, food selection and preparation, the number and spacing of meals, age, and special circumstances such as pregnancy, influence food patterns. The focus should be on the nutrient composition of foods, their preparation, and quantity consumed rather than the counselor's ideas of foods and meal number, type, and spacing. For example, the counselor should keep in mind that milk is not acceptable or possible for everyone to drink and that an order of ''iron tabs three times a day after meals'' will not fit a two- or four-meal-a-day pattern. Table 13-2 is included to alert counselors to possible variations between

ethnic groups. In addition, the following list contains useful nutrition vocabulary of various ethnic groups:

Japanese
Azuki—red beans
Denishoga—dried ginger
Konyaku—bean thread
Kuri—chestnuts
Mezashi—dried sardines
Miso—soybean paste
Shoga—ginger
Soba—whole wheat noodle
Taro—Japanese sweet potato
Tofu—soybean curd
Umeboshi—dried, pickled plums

Chinese
Dim sum—steamed dumpling filled with meat, fish, or sweet paste
Bok choy—green, leafy, stalklike vegetable

Black
Chitterlings—pork intestines, tripe

Mexican-Spanish
Arroz con leche—rice pudding
Chorizo—sausage
Flan—sweet custard
Frijoles refritos—refried beans
Guacamole—avocado, tomato, chilies, onion paste
Hoop—a Mexican cheese
Manteca—lard
Nopales—cactus leaf (prickly pear)
Pan dulce—sweet bread
Salsa—relish of tomato, pepper, onion
Sopapillas—fried bread
Sopas—soup
Tuna—cactus fruit (prickly pear)

Within all ethnic groups, various religions proscribe dietary patterns, with special observances for holidays and important life experiences (e.g., weddings, births). These too must be considered when planning menus if the counseling is to be accepted and implemented.

Vegetarian diets

Many people are turning to so-called health or natural foods. Some religions, including Buddhists and Seventh-Day Adventists, also adhere to vegetarian dietary regimens.

Several vegetarian variations are possible, but basic to all are vegetables, fruits, legumes, nuts, and grains. True vegetarians (vegans) eat only those items just listed. Lacto-ovovegetarians include milk, cheese, other dairy products, and eggs in their diets. Lactovegetarians exclude eggs but do consume milk, cheese, and other dairy products. Fruitarians restrict their diets to raw or dried fruits, nuts, honey, and oil.

The macrobiotic diet is most restrictive. The lowest of the ten levels of this regimen includes cereals, fruits,

Table 13-2. Dietary habits and acceptable foods

Ethnic group	Milk group	Meat group	Fruits and vegetables	Breads and cereals	Possible dietary problems
American Indian (many tribal variations; many "Americanized")	Fresh milk Evaporated milk for cooking Ice cream Cream pies	Pork, beef, lamb, rabbit Fowl, fish, eggs Legumes Sunflower seeds Nuts: walnut, acorn, pine, peanut butter	Green peas, beans Beets, turnips Leafy green and other vegetables Grapes, bananas, peaches, other fresh fruits	Refined bread Whole wheat Cornmeal Rice Dry cereals	In California major problems: obesity, diabetes, alcoholism, nutritional deficiencies expressed in dental problems and iron deficiency anemia Inadequate amounts of all nutrients Excessive use of sugar
Middle Eastern (Armenian, Greek, Syrian, Turkish)	Yogurt Little butter	Lamb Nuts Dried peas, beans, lentils	Peppers Tomatoes Cabbage Grape leaves Cucumbers Squash Dried apricots, raisins	Cracked wheat and dark bread	Fry many meats and vegetables Lack of fresh fruits Insufficient foods from milk group (use olive oil* in place of butter) Like sweetenings, lamb fat, and olive oil
Black	Milk Ice cream Puddings Cheese: longhorn, American	Pork: all cuts, plus organs, chitterlings Beef, lamb Chicken, giblets Eggs Nuts Legumes Fish, game	Leafy vegetables Green and yellow vegetables Potato: white, sweet Stewed fruit Bananas and other fruit	Cornmeal and hominy grits Rice Biscuits, pancakes, white breads Puddings: bread, rice Molasses†	Extensive use of frying, "smothering," or simmering Fats: salt pork, bacon drippings, lard, and gravies Like sweets Insufficient citrus and enriched breads Vegetables often boiled for long periods Limited amounts from milk group
Chinese (Cantonese most prevalent)	Cheese Milk: water buffalo; tofu	Pork sausage‡ Eggs and pigeon eggs Fish Lamb, beef, goat Fowl Nuts Legumes	Many vegetables Radish leaves Bean, bamboo sprouts	Rice/rice flour products Cereals, noodles Wheat, corn, millet seed	Tendency of northern China (Mandarin), coastal China (Shanghai), and inland China (Szechwan) emigrants to use more grease in cooking Limited use of milk and milk products Often low in protein, calories or both May wash rice before cooking
Filipino (Spanish-Chinese influence)	Flavored milk Milk in coffee Cheese: gouda, cheddar	Pork, beef, goat, deer, rabbit Chicken Fish Eggs Nuts Legumes	Many vegetables and fruits	Rice, cooked cereals Noodles: rice, wheat	Limited use of milk and milk products Tend to prewash rice May have only small portions of protein foods

*Olive oil is all fat, with no other nutrient value.
†Light molasses (first extraction): 1 tbsp = 50 calories, 33 mg of calcium, 0.9 mg of iron, 0.01 mg each of vitamins B_1 and B_2; dark molasses (third extraction): 1 tbsp = 45 calories, 137 mg of calcium, 3.2 mg of iron, 0.02 mg of vitamin B_1, 0.04 mg of vitamin B_2, 0.4 mg of niacin.
‡Lower in fat content than regular sausage.

Table 13-2. Dietary habits and acceptable foods—cont'd

Ethnic group	Milk group	Meat group	Fruits and vegetables	Breads and cereals	Possible dietary problems
Italian	Cheese Some ice cream	Meat Eggs Dried beans	Leafy vegetables Potatoes Eggplant Spinach Fruits	Macaroni White breads, some whole wheat Farina Cereals	Prefer expensive imported cheeses; reluctant to substitute less expensive domestic varieties Tendency to overcook vegetables Limited use of whole grains Enjoy sweets Extensive use of olive oil Insufficient servings from milk group
Japanese (Isei, more Japanese influence; Nisei, more westernized)	Increasing amounts being used by younger generations Tofu	Pork, beef, chicken Fish Eggs Legumes: soya, red, lima beans Nuts	Many vegetables and fruits Seaweed	Rice, rice cakes Wheat noodles Refined bread, noodles	Excessive salt: pickles, salty crisp seaweed Insufficient servings from milk group May use refined or prewashed rice
Mexican-Spanish	Milk Cheese Flan Ice cream	Beef, pork, lamb, chicken, tripe, hot sausage, beef intestines Fish Eggs Nuts Dry beans: pinto, chick peas	Spinach, wild greens, tomatoes, chilies, corn, cactus leaves, cabbage, avocado Pumpkin, zapote, peaches, guava, papaya, citrus	Rice, oats, cornmeal Sweet bread Tortilla Biscuits Fideo	Limited meats primarily due to economics Limited use of milk and milk products Some tendency toward increasing the use of flour tortillas over the more nutritious corn tortillas Large amounts of lard (manteca) Abundant use of sugar Tendency to boil vegetables for long periods
Polish	Milk Sour cream Cheese Butter	Pork (preferred) Chicken	Vegetables Cabbage Roots Fruits	Dark rye	Like sweets Tendency to overcook vegetables Limited fruits (especially citrus), raw vegetables, and meats
Puerto Rican	Limited use of milk products	Pork Poultry Eggs (Fridays) Dried codfish Beans	Avocado, okra Eggplant Sweet yams	Rice Cornmeal	Use small amounts of pork and poultry Use fat, lard, salt pork, and olive oil extensively Lack of butter and other milk products
Scandinavian: Danish, Finnish, Norwegian, Swedish	Cream Butter	Wild game Reindeer Fish Eggs	Fruit berries Dried fruit Vegetables: cole slaw, roots, avocado	Whole wheat, rye, barley, sweets (molasses for flavoring)	Insufficient fresh fruits and vegetables Like sweets, pickled salted meats, and fish

vegetables, and a few animal products. The highest level permits only brown rice. Little water or other fluids are included. Followers of the higher levels of the macrobiotic regimen are in danger of developing deleterious nutritional deficiencies.

If animal protein foods, eggs, or milk are absent or inadequate in the diet, the laboratory test for serum vitamin B_{12} should be done. If caloric as well as protein intake is minimal, serum albumin and total serum protein values should be obtained.

Vegetarian diets that include a variety of fruits and vegetables, including legumes, grains, nuts, and milk and milk products, can be nutritionally sound. However, certain plant foods must be eaten in combination with specific other plant foods to provide complete proteins. Incomplete proteins cannot be utilized to build and maintain body tissues. Information concerning complementary plant protein sources is available in publications such as *Diet for a Small Planet* by Frances Moore Lappé.

Advantages of a well-balanced, nutritionally sound, vegetarian regimen include the following:

- Low caloric intake with less chance of obesity
- High water and fiber content
- Low fat content
- Almost total absence of cholesterol

The vegetarian diet should be assessed so that appropriate measures can be taken as necessary:

1. If cow's milk is not consumed, vitamin B_{12} and iron should be supplemented to prevent anemia and eventual irreversible spinal cord degeneration. A deficiency of riboflavin may also occur. If four servings of cow's milk, goat's milk, or milk products are not included, calcium may need to be supplemented.

2. If cow's milk, soy milk fortified with vitamin D, or another vitamin D source is not in the diet, this vitamin should also be supplemented.

3. Iron supplementation may be needed even if enriched grain products are used.

4. The use of iodized table salt should be encouraged. Sea salt does not contain iodine.

5. An adequate amount of calories is necessary to utilize protein for growth and maintenance, rather than for energy needs.

NUTRITIONAL NEEDS DURING PREGNANCY

Nutritional assessment and follow-up are imperative for every pregnant woman. Certain physiologic, socioeconomic, and psychologic factors threaten the woman's nutritional status and classify her as high risk (Chapter 15).

Low prepregnancy weight, adolescence, high parity, and short intervals between pregnancies affect the physiologic preparedness for the nutritional demands imposed by pregnancy. Inadequate weight gain during pregnancy and reducing regimens diminish the available fuel and building blocks to meet maternal-fetal needs. In addition, metabolic changes from weight reduction diets (development of ketosis) during pregnancy have been associated with neuropsychologic problems in the infant.

Prior maternity complications should be assessed to determine the existence of any of the following nutrition-related conditions (e.g., inadequate weight gain, preeclampsia-eclampsia; low birth weight infant, small-for-date infant, anemia) and conditions depleting nutritional stores (e.g., multiple gestation, hemorrhage, age, short intervals between pregnancies).

Concurrent medical problems such as the following influence the pregnant woman's health and pregnancy outcome and may require thoughtful diet therapy:

1. Metabolic problems such as diabetes
2. Systemic disorders involving the heart, liver, or kidneys
3. Infections such as tuberculosis

Smoking to excess, alcoholism, and drug dependency may be responsible for diminished intake of essential nutrients, and altered metabolism of foods. Women who smoke more than six cigarettes a day or who are consistently exposed to smoke-filled environments have a greater chance of delivering a low birth weight infant. Alcohol consumed in large quantities may interfere with adequate dietary intake. Metabolism of alcohol requires additional thiamin, thus incurring a deficiency of this vitamin. Drug dependency affects dietary intake and usually leads to sporadic or total absence of antenatal medical supervision.

In general, the goals of reproductive nutrition are as follows:

1. Evidence of maternal health status
   a. Weight gain during pregnancy, laboratory results, and blood pressure within normal limits
   b. Pattern of weight gain during pregnancy
2. Correction of deficiencies, if present
3. Term delivery
4. Fetal maturity and size appropriate for gestational age
5. Improvement in the family's nutritional knowledge and status
6. Achievement of a sound nutritional base for the initiation and maintenance of lactation that meets nutritional needs of the infant and does not deplete maternal reserves

Physiology of pregnancy

During pregnancy, blood volume increases by 30% to 50% with a lag in production of hemoglobin, resulting in physiologic anemia. A lowered renal threshold is evidenced by the appearance of some amino acids and glucose (and later lactose) in the urine. Changes in circulation and a normal salt retention appear as generalized edema, a normal protective response of reproductive performance. Gastrointestinal tract changes include the following: reduction of hydrochloric acid in the stomach depresses calcium and iron absorption; ptyalism and a relaxed cardiac sphincter coupled with reverse peristalsis permit regurgitation into the esophagus with resulting heartburn, nausea, and aversion to foods; reduced motility of the tract delays emptying time in the stomach and favors constipation. Cravings and pica further stress the nutritional state during pregnancy. All these changes, which resemble pathologic conditions, are normal during pregnancy.

Fetoplacental nutritional needs

All stages of growth and development of the fetus and placenta are influenced by nutrition. The relationship between the diet prior to and during pregnancy and the physical condition of the infant has been well documented. Several factors influence the nutrition of the developing organism, including faulty implantation of the ovum, degeneration of the chorion, and alteration in the location and function of the placenta. Any of these factors can contribute to pregnancy failure (abortion), fetal malformation, or retarded fetal growth and development. Placental function correlates directly with the adequacy of the blood supply to that organ. Faulty dietary intake reduces the available building material for normal fetal cell proliferation and differentiation. Maternal dietary deficiencies from reduced total intake or amounts of specific nutrients produce fetal damage such as small weight for date, low birth weight, dysmaturity, and smaller brain weight. Early fetal development consists primarily of increasing cell numbers; later development consists of increasing cell size. Deficient nutrients during the period of rapid cell proliferation and differentiation are thought to cause fetal damage such as a significant deficit in the CNS.

Although organogenesis is occurring at a phenomenal rate during the first half of pregnancy, fetal weight gain is slow; at 12 weeks the fetus weighs 30 gm. Fetal size increases rapidly during the last half of pregnancy as follows: 24 weeks, 900 gm; 30 weeks, 1484 gm; 34 weeks, 2278 gm; 40 weeks, 3230 gm; and 42 weeks, 3310 gm. Growth of body tissues and the storage of fat and other nutrients account for the rapid weight gain.

The placenta regulates the flow of nutrients to the fetus. The placenta meets fetal demands of some nutrients (iron; vitamins B_6, B_{12}, and C; folic acid), even at the expense of depleting maternal stores. For other nutrients such as vitamins B_1, B_2, and D, the placenta allows maternal and fetal tissues to compete.

Caloric (energy) needs

The daily energy requirements of the average woman during the first part of pregnancy remain within the range for a nonpregnant, moderately active woman—about 2000 to 2100 calories a day for the 19- to 50-year-old. The Food and Nutrition Board of the National Academy of Sciences–National Research Council (1974) suggests an increase of 300 calories during the latter part of pregnancy and an increase of 500 more calories if lactating. Women who are extremely active or nutritionally deficient may need 3000 calories to meet energy and nutrient demands. Adequate calories also spare protein for tissue building. Weight gain reflects the physiologic consequences of pregnancy. Caloric intake, comprised of carefully selected nutritious foods, should be sufficient to support a weight gain of 25 to 30 pounds (Table 13-1).

Immediately after delivery about 8 pounds of weight gained during pregnancy remains; at 6 weeks after delivery, 4 pounds remain. All the weight gained during pregnancy is usually lost by 6 to 8 months after delivery.

The obese pregnant woman. Obesity is an indicator of dysfunctional nutrition prior to pregnancy. The diet of the obese expectant mother must be assessed to identify the nutritionally beneficial foodstuffs that are present and those that are excluded or limited. The focus is not on weight reduction per se. Weight reduction diets favor ketosis. Pregnancy makes the patient more prone to ketosis, to which the conceptus is highly susceptible. The focus is on eating the proper foods.

The obese woman may be able to "lose weight," that is, not gain the recommended 25 to 30 pounds (11.4 to 13.6 kg), without jeopardizing the health of the infant or herself by reworking her diet and increasing her intake of good sources of protein, vitamins, and minerals with only sufficient calories in the form of fats and sugars to protect her protein intake.

Excessive weight gain during pregnancy is discouraged. Occasionally one encounters the woman who gains 40 to 100 pounds (18.1 to 45.4 kg) or more during pregnancy. This type of weight gain, often based on quantity and not quality of foods, should be discouraged for the following reasons:

1. The risk factor in respiratory, operative, and diagnostic problems is increased.

2. Fetal growth may be excessive. Dystocia may result, which may compromise the infant's health and well-being.

3. Unnecessary pounds increase the work of back and leg muscles and result in added stress on posture. Backache, leg pains, increased fatigability, and aggravated varices are the result.

4. If the quality of food is poor (high fat and carbohydrate intake with low protein intake), the incidence of preeclampsia-eclampsia increases.

5. After delivery, the excess poundage may be difficult to lose. That permanent weight gain affects both health and figure is well known.

Helpful hints. In evaluating the adequacy of a diet, one must inquire about between-meal snacks or the "little extras." People frequently overlook these extras and are unaware of their caloric value. A few such foods are contained in the following list. Consider the nutritional value versus the caloric value:

Food	Amount	Calories
Cola (carbonated)	1 cup (240 ml)	100
Chocolate bar	2 ounces (60 gm)	300
Cocktail or highball	1	200
Cocoa	1 cup (240 ml)	235
Milk, whole	1 cup (240 ml)	160
Double-crust on pie without filling	$^1/_6$ of pie	265

Frying any product increases the caloric value without adding to the nutritive value.

Salad dressings add considerable calories without comparable nutritive value. However, dressings may make vegetables (raw and cooked) more inviting and palatable. Caloric value of 1-tablespoon portions: French, 60; Thousand Island, 75; blue cheese, 80; and mayonnaise, 110. Some people find that lemon juice or tarragon vinegar provides a tasty substitute for a high-calorie salad dressing.

One quart of milk provides protein of high biologic value, vitamins, minerals, and one fourth of daily energy needs. The daily milk requirement can be met in several ways. Five tablespoons of dried skim equals 1 pint (2 cups or 500 ml) fluid milk. Dried skim milk may be added to meatloaf, mashed potatoes, and baked goods. Fluid milk may be mixed with vanilla, nutmeg, instant coffee, or cinnamon to enhance its flavor. Skim milk or buttermilk may be substituted to decrease caloric intake of whole milk while maintaining nutritive value. One ounce of cheese equals an 8-ounce glass of whole milk.

Meat may be limited because of budgetary restrictions or taste. Liver may be ground and incorporated into meatloaf or hamburger to meet the recommended weekly intake of one serving. Braunschweiger may be substituted for liver. Meat expanders now available at meat counters may be mixed with hamburger or casseroles to help meet daily needs.

When preparing vegetables, one should avoid heavy salting, saucing, buttering, or rich dressings. Eating larger amounts of vegetables helps to curb the appetite. The fibrous network and bulk help to control constipation by stimulating the musculature and eliminative action of the intestines.

Fruits stimulate the appetite and have a laxative action. When substituting tomatoes for oranges and orange juice, twice the amount is needed to get the same amount of vitamin C. Prunes, raisins, and apricots are good sources of iron, copper, and other vitamins.

Coarse cereals and dark breads add to roughage to counteract constipation while ensuring an adequate supply of the B vitamins.

SPECIFIC NUTRIENTS AND THEIR FOOD SOURCES
Protein

Antenatal diet counseling should stress the importance of protein in the augmentation of maternal tissues, growth and development of the placenta and fetus, and production of breast milk. Nitrogen, the essential constituent of protein, is necessary for growth. Large amounts of nitrogen are used by both mother and fetus during pregnancy as follows: 55.9 gm are stored by the fetus in the last half of pregnancy, 17 gm are stored in the placenta, 1 gm in the amniotic fluid, 17 gm in the maternal breast tissue, 40 gm in uterine tissue, and 200 to 350 gm are stored by the mother to meet blood losses during labor and delivery (300 to 500 ml) and in preparation for lactation. In addition, the mother's own tissue requires protein for continuing repair and maintenance.

Protein deficiency is associated with increased incidence of abnormal bleeding, premature labor and delivery, preeclampsia-eclampsia, low hematocrit, and low IQ of infants.

The daily allowance for protein for a normal nonpregnant woman (19 to 50 years of age) is 46 gm; (pregnancy increases the daily requirement to 76 gm; lactation, to 96 gm).* For some high-risk or active women, the required amount increases to 100 gm or more per day.

Protein is an important food nutrient, since it contains all other nutrients except vitamins A, C, and D. Protein of high biologic value containing all essential amino

---

*Until 1968, the protein requirement for a nonpregnant woman was 55 gm; for a pregnant woman, 65 gm; and for a lactating woman, 75 gm.

Table 13-3. Sources of protein*

Servings	Foods
16 gm sources	
2 ounce	Beef, chicken, pork, fish, cheddar cheese
½ cup	Cottage cheese
1 cup	Dried beans (cooked)
½ cup	Peanuts
8 gm sources	
1 cup	Milk (whole, skim, dried)
2 tbsp	Peanut butter
1 large	Egg
½ cup	Peas (split, dry, cooked)
4 gm sources	
¾ cup	Macaroni, rice, oatmeal
¼ cup	Nuts: cashew, Brazil, pecans
1½ cup	Fresh, shredded coconut or 2 cups dried, shredded
2 slices	Bread

*Approximate values are listed.

Table 13-4. Sources of iron*

Servings	Foods
5 mg sources	
2 ounces	Liver, kidney
3 ounces	Beef heart
1 cup	Cooked dry beans
3 mg sources	
3 ounces	Beef, pork
½ cup	Spinach, greens
2 mg sources	
½ cup	Dried peaches or apricots, cooked; raisins; prunes; green peas
3 ounces	Chicken
1 mg sources	
1 medium	Egg, sweet potato
½ cup	Broccoli, oatmeal, enriched macaroni, winter squash
1 large	Orange
2 slices	Enriched bread

*Approximate values are listed.

acids in the right proportions is found in milk, meat, egg, and cheese. Protein-rich food contains other nutrients such as calcium, iron, and B vitamins. Legumes, whole grains, and nuts provide additional but incomplete protein. Sources of protein are shown in Table 13-3.

Iron

Iron is an essential constituent of hemoglobin, a protein substance that enables red blood cells to carry oxygen throughout the body. Iron is also a part of a variety of important enzymes. A daily intake of 18 mg of iron is needed during pregnancy to maintain hemoglobin levels, to maintain a reserve for use in the puerperium, to meet fetal developmental needs, and for storage reserve in the liver to supply the infant's needs for the first 3 to 4 months of extrauterine life.

The National Academy of Sciences–National Research Council suggests supplemental iron during pregnancy. It is difficult to meet the recommended intake of 18 mg plus the additional needs posed by pregnancy by dietary means alone. Teaching and encouragement are necessary to stimulate the use of foods high in iron. Sources of iron are shown in Table 13-4.

Calcium, phosphorus, and vitamin D

Vitamin D is predominantly associated with calcium and phosphorus; it influences their absorption, retention, and utilization in bones, teeth, blood, and other tissues. The interdependence of nutrients in total body function is further demonstrated by the role of vitamin D in citrate metabolism, which mobilizes minerals from bone tissue and removes calcium from blood, and in the movement of various divalent cations (e.g., ^{++}Mg) throughout the body.

Calcium occurs in large quantities in the human body, comprising about 1.5% to 2% of body weight. Most of this mineral (99%) is found in skeletal tissue, bones, and teeth. The remaining 1% is involved in important functions such as blood coagulation, neuromuscular irritability, muscular contractility and relaxation, and myocardial function. (Parathyroid hormone regulates serum calcium level. Although two thirds of fetal calcium are stored during the last months, the mother must store this mineral throughout pregnancy to meet fetal needs.) Recommended daily allowances are 800 mg for a nonpregnant woman and 1200 mg during adolescence, pregnancy, and lactation. Sources of calcium are shown in Table 13-5.

The pregnant woman in full body cast or in traction or otherwise immobilized must be observed for renal calculi formation due to shift of calcium out of bones into the blood. In these cases, it is especially important to avoid intake in excess of suggested daily requirements.

Table 13-5. Sources of calcium *

Servings	Foods
0.30 gm (300 mg)	
sources	
1 cup	Milk
1¼ ounce	Cheddar cheese
0.15 (150 mg)	
sources	
½ cup	Canned salmon (with bones), cottage cheese, broccoli
0.05 gm (50 mg)	
sources	
½ cup	Dried raisins, cooked beans: pinto, kidney
1 medium	Orange
1 medium	Sweet potato
2 slices	Enriched bread

*Approximate values are listed.

Phosphorus, which comprises about 1% of body weight, is known as the metabolic "twin" of calcium and is related closely to vitamin D. However, it also has some unique functions. Eighty percent to 90% of this mineral is compounded with calcium; the remaining 10% to 20% is distributed throughout each living cell and is intimately involved in energy production, building and repairing tissues, and buffering.

Vitamin D is acquired through exposure to sunlight and by ingestion. It is synthesized in the skin on exposure to sunlight (ultraviolet light), absorbed, and carried through the circulating blood to the liver and other organs to be stored and utilized.

Vitamin D is excreted in the bile. Main food sources of vitamin D include fortified milk, egg yolk, fish and fish oil, butter and fortified butter substitutes, and liver. Another good source is corn tortillas. Milk is an especially good source for this vitamin, since it also provides calcium and phosphorus in correct proportions and digestible form, permitting optimal utilization. The fetal tissues place a greater demand for these three nutrients. For recommended daily allowances, see Table 13-1.

One quart of milk, whole or skimmed, provides 1.2 gm of calcium and 100% of the daily requirement of vitamin D. Occasionally if the pregnant woman is drinking an excess of the recommended daily intake of milk, the phosphorus in the milk may depress ionizable calcium levels, resulting in muscular cramping. Furthermore, some people (notably ethnic groups such as Orien-

tal, Mexican-American, and black) lack the enzyme lactase necessary for the absorption and utilization of cow's milk. Lactose intolerance may be recognized by such manifestations as belching, flatulence, abdominal cramping, and watery diarrhea.

When supplementation is necessary, calcium preparations (calcium lactate) are prescribed, and protein foods should be increased in the diet. As with any drug during pregnancy, vitamin and mineral supplements should be taken only when prescribed and supervised by the physician.

Sodium

Sodium is crucially important to many metabolic activities. One third of the body's sodium is found in the skeleton; two thirds are in extracellular fluids, plasma, and nerve and muscle tissue. Its metabolic functions include fluid balance, acid-base balance, cell permeability, and normal muscle irritability (including cardiac muscle). The average North American diet includes an overabundance of this mineral (about ten times the daily need) (Williams, 1973). Some sources of sodium are table salt; milk; meat; eggs; vegetables such as carrots, beets, spinach, asparagus, celery, artichokes, and leafy greens; and carbonated beverages. Only 0.5 gm is needed, but the daily intake usually ranges between 2 and 6 gm.

Sodium is discussed further in the section on preeclampsia-eclampsia.

Iodine

Small amounts of iodine are needed for the health of mother and fetus. Readily available sources are seafoods, cod-liver oil, and iodized table salt. Supplementation with iodine is most essential in areas where the water and soil are iodine-poor (e.g., certain localities around the Great Lakes and in northwestern United States). In the 1920s and 1930s goiters were common among women who bore children in these areas; it was a sign of female maturity and motherhood, with no stigma attached. In the Ohio Valley it was not uncommon to lose infants who were born with goiters. The trace of iodine in iodized table salt is sufficient to meet dietary requirements.

When iodine levels are inadequate to meet the demands of pregnancy, goiters are apt to occur, especially among adolescents. When the mother develops a goiter, the chance of goiter in her offspring is increased ten times; the chance of cretinism (a severe form of iodine deficiency) also increases. In parts of the world where iodized salt used in cooking is the main source of this mineral, salt restriction adds insult to injury, making supplementation from other sources mandatory.

Table 13-6. Sources of vitamin A *

Servings	Foods
30,000 IU sources	
2 ounces	Beef or lamb liver
10,000 IU sources	
2 ounces	Chicken liver
1 medium	Sweet potato
½ cup servings	Spinach, carrots, turnip greens†
1 cup	Cooked collards
6000 IU sources	
½ melon	Cantaloupe
½ cup servings	Canned pumpkin, winter squash, dried apricots
¾ cup	Cooked kale
2000 IU sources	
½ cup servings	Papaya, broccoli, canned apricots
¾ cup	Tomato juice
500 IU sources	
½ cup servings	Prunes, green peas, peaches
1 medium	Egg (yolk)
1 tbsp	Butter or enriched margarine

*Approximate values are listed.
†Cooked short time, with small amount water.

Table 13-7. Sources of vitamin B_1 (thiamin) *

Servings	Foods
0.60 mg sources	
2 ounces	Pork
0.15 mg sources	
½ cup	Green peas
2 ounces	Liver
0.10 mg sources	
½ cup	Cooked oatmeal, enriched macaroni, orange juice
1 medium	Orange, potato, sweet potato
1 cup	Milk
2 slices	Enriched bread
0.06 mg sources	
½ cup	Cooked dry beans, spinach, tomato juice, broccoli
½ medium	Grapefruit
1 medium	Banana
1 medium	Egg

*Approximate values are listed.

Vitamins

During pregnancy, increased amounts of vitamins A, B, and C are recommended.

Vitamin A. The usual daily requirement of this fat-soluble vitamin is 4000 IU. An additional 1000 IU are needed during the last half of pregnancy, bringing the total to 5000 IU; another 1000 IU are necessary for lactation, bringing the total to 6000 IU. Vitamin A is an essential factor in cell growth and development and integrity of epithelial tissue, including the uterus, tooth formation, normal bone growth, and vision, and is also involved in fat metabolism. Changes in the absorptive tissues of intestinal mucosa or the presence of mineral oil in the intestinal tract prevents the absorption of fat-soluble vitamins. Sources of vitamin A are shown in Table 13-6. This vitamin is usually deficient in the newborn; however, colostrum is a great source of vitamin A.

B vitamins. A well-balanced diet usually meets the increased need for B vitamins during pregnancy and lactation. Supplements are prescribed if the physician thinks the increased demand is not being met. In general, B vitamins act as coenzyme factors in several metabolic processes, energy production, and muscle and nerve tissue functioning, all of which are especially important in the increased metabolic activities of pregnancy.

Thiamin (vitamin B_1). Daily allowance of thiamin rises by 0.3 mg in the last half of pregnancy and by 0.4 mg during lactation to accommodate the caloric intake increases. Thiamin assumes an essential role in carbohydrate metabolism. Required dietary allowances are as follows: adult, 1 to 1.1 mg; pregnancy, 1.3 to 1.4 mg; and lactation, 1.6 to 1.7 mg. Sources of vitamin B_1 are shown in Table 13-7.

Riboflavin (vitamin B_2). The nonpregnant woman needs 1.2 to 1.4 mg of vitamin B_2. Additional daily intakes of 0.3 mg during pregnancy and 0.5 mg during lactation are recommended for this vitamin, important for adequate tissue function. Tissue oxygenation and respiration and protein and energy metabolism are functions of this coenzyme. Riboflavin is excreted in breast milk, which accounts for the recommended daily allowance during lactation. Niacin has a close interrelationship with riboflavin in cell metabolism. Table 13-8 lists some sources of riboflavin.

Folacin or folic acid, (formerly B_9 or B_{10}). Folacin (Latin, *folium,* leaf) is a necessary coenzyme in the production of nucleoproteins (essential constituents of all living cells) basic to cell growth and reproduction and formation of heme (the iron-containing protein of hemoglobin). Therefore deficiencies of folic acid affect blood cell formation, resulting in a specific megaloblastic

Table 13-8. Sources of vitamin B₂ (riboflavin)*

Servings	Foods
2 mg sources	
2 ounces	Liver
0.40 mg sources	
1 cup	Milk
½ cup	Cottage cheese
0.20 mg sources	
3 ounces	Beef, pork
½ cup	Spinach, winter squash
2 slices	Enriched bread
1¼ ounces	Cheddar cheese
1 medium	Egg
½ cup	Nuts: cashew, peanuts
0.10 mg sources	
½ cup	Broccoli, green peas, asparagus (fresh)
1 cup	Enriched macaroni or spaghetti (cooked)
0.05 mg sources	
½ cup	Cooked dry beans, enriched macaroni, corn, prunes
1 medium	Sweet potato, banana
1	Hard roll

*Approximate values are listed.

Table 13-9. Sources of vitamin C*

Servings	Foods
75 mg sources	
1 medium	Orange
½ medium	Grapefruit
1 pod	Sweet red pepper
50 mg sources	
1 cup	Orange or grapefruit juice, broccoli, strawberries, papaya
½ melon	Cantaloupe
25 mg sources	
1 medium	Sweet potato, tomato, potato
½ cup	Cooked spinach, raw cabbage, tomato juice, mustard greens
2 ounces	Beef liver
12 mg sources	
½ cup	Green peas or beans, pineapple juice
1 medium	Banana

*Approximate values are listed.

anemia. Pregnancy increases the metabolic demand from the usual 400 μg to 800 μg and lactation, to 600 μg. Chronic hemolytic anemia and multiple pregnancy add a greater demand. Daily supplements may be needed to counter deficiency. Food sources of folacin are dark green, leafy vegetables such as spinach.

Niacin (nicotinic acid). Niacin is closely related to riboflavin in cell metabolism. Specific manifestations of deficiency involve the integumentary and nervous systems. Meat is a major source; fruits and vegetables are poor sources, except if fortified. For recommended daily intake, see Table 13-1.

Pyridoxine (vitamin B₆). Pyridoxine is an essential coenzyme with amino acids; the need for this vitamin increases with increased protein intake. Deficiency may result in hypochromic microcytic anemia and CNS disturbances.

Isoniazid (INH), a chemotherapeutic agent for tuberculosis, reacts as an antagonist for pyridoxine, necessitating large daily doses of 50 to 100 mg to offset neurologic involvement.

For recommended daily intake, refer to Table 13-1.

Cobalamin (vitamin B₁₂). Cobalamin is the antipernicious anemia factor and prevents the blood-forming defect and neurologic involvement of that anemia. (It receives its name from the peculiar characteristic of this vitamin: it contains cobalt.) Main food sources are animal meats and organs, eggs, and cheese. Some cobalamin is synthesized by intestinal bacteria in people. Natural deficiency is rarely seen; the only reported natural deficiencies have been in groups of true vegetarians living in Great Britain and India. Supplements are by injection only. Daily recommended intakes are found in Table 13-1.

Ascorbic acid (vitamin C). Many animal species are capable of manufacturing ascorbic acid; in humans this deficiency is an age-old genetic inborn error of metabolism. This water-soluble vitamin is not stored in the human body. Therefore daily supplementation of ascorbic acid is required. For required daily intake, see Table 13-1.

Vitamin C is essential for providing an intercellular cementing substance necessary for supporting the vascular system, bones, muscles, cartilage, and connective and other tissues. In general body metabolism, vitamin C plays an even broader role. Its presence in metabolically active tissue indicates a vital connection with protein and cell metabolic processes. Vitamin C functions in iron metabolism and therefore is influential in formation of

BASIC FOUR FOOD GROUPS

Milk group

Food value	Calcium, phosphorus, vitamin D, riboflavin, plus vitamins A, E, B_6, B_{12}, magnesium, and zinc; protein of high biologic value
Food sources	Milk: whole, skim, nonfat, buttermilk; goat; yogurt Cheese: cheddar, Swiss, cottage Ice cream
Single serving portions	1 cup (8 ounces or 240 ml) milk ½ cup evaporated or undiluted milk 3 to 4 tbsp dry milk 1¼ cups cottage cheese 1½ ounces (45 gm) cheddar or Swiss cheese 1½ cups (360 ml) ice cream
Recommended servings	Pregnancy: 4; lactation: 5 (1 cup of tofu can be exchanged for 1 serving)

Meat group

Food value	Protein of high biologic value; many sources supply considerable iron, vitamins B_1, B_2, niacin, and other vitamins and minerals
Food sources	Animal meats: beef, veal, lamb, pork, poultry Animal organ meats: liver, heart, kidney, tripe Fish, shellfish Eggs Dry beans and peas, lentils, nuts, and peanut butter
Single serving portions	2 ounces (60 gm) of meat, organs, fish (without bones): 2 frankfurters, 4 breaded fish sticks, 10 to 15 medium oysters 2 eggs 1 cup cooked dry beans, peas, lentils 4 tbsp peanut butter ½ cup nuts, sunflower seeds
Recommended servings	Pregnancy and lactation: 4

Vegetable and fruit group

Food value	Vitamins, especially C and A, and minerals
Food sources	Vitamin C: good sources—citrus fruits, juices, melons (cantaloupe, mango, papaya), peppers (green, red, chili), bok choy; fair sources—tomatoes, melons (honeydew, water) green vegetables (kale, asparagus tips, raw cabbage, collards, mustard and turnip greens, spinach), potatoes (white, sweet) Vitamin A: dark green and deep yellow vegetables (broccoli, carrots, chard), some fruits (apricots), other fruits and vegetables, potatoes Iron (significant sources): raisins, prunes
Single serving sources	½ to ¾ cup fruit or vegetable, 1 cup if raw 1 medium fruit ½ medium grapefruit, 2 tangerines or tomatoes 4 ounces orange or grapefruit juice, 12 ounces tomato or pineapple juice, 6 ounce drinks enriched with vitamin C

Recommended servings	Pregnancy and lactation: 4
	  1 serving vitamin C–rich fruit or vegetable
	  2 servings leafy green vegetables
	  1 serving other fruit or vegetable

Bread and cereal group

Food value	Fairly good sources of B_1 (thiamin) and niacin, iron, and lesser amounts of other vitamins and minerals
Food sources	Breads, cereals, baked goods: whole-grain, enriched, ready-to-eat (e.g., bagels, cornmeal, crackers, grits, macaroni, tortillas, rice, noodles, including spaghetti)
Single serving portions	1 slice bread, 1 large flour or 2 corn tortillas, 4 crackers 1 tbsp wheat germ 1 ounce (30 gm) ready-to-eat cereal, 1 waffle ½ to ¾ cup cooked cereal, grits, macaroni, rice, noodles, spaghetti
Recommended servings	Pregnancy and lactation: 3 1 serving should be a whole grain product to provide needed magnesium and zinc to diet

hemoglobin and maturation of red blood cells. The lack of hydrochloric acid during pregnancy hinders the absorption of this vitamin from the small intestine. Rapid growth periods, wound healing, smoking, fevers and infection, and stress situations also increase the required daily intake. Vitamin C supplement is occasionally prescribed during pregnancy to aid iron absorption, although there is no definitive evidence that supplemental vitamin C enhances the absorption or utilization of iron salts.

Main food sources are citrus fruits, strawberries, melon, potatoes, cabbage, and chili peppers (Table 13-9). It is also found in all green leafy vegetables with the exception of iceberg lettuce. Cooking destroys about half of this vitamin; exposing the food to air (e.g., leaving orange juice uncovered in the refrigerator) also destroys this vitamin.

Hypervitaminosis. Vitamins are vital but in small amounts. Excess amounts of some vitamins produce detrimental results. Symptoms of *hypervitaminosis A* are many: skeletal pain, thickening of long bones, loss of hair, and jaundice. The jaundice is the result of the breakdown of red blood cells due to the loss of hemoglobin and potassium. Permanent effects after cessation of consumption are rare.

Fat-soluble vitamin A is stored in the liver. Excessive intake over a period of time may lead to toxicity in a developing fetus, even if the mother shows no adverse symptoms. Single injections of this vitamin in pregnant animals has resulted in skeletal abnormalities in the young.

Public health personnel in the far north should be aware of the extremely high vitamin A potency in polar bear liver. Also all health personnel should be alert to possible cumulative amounts ingested from enriched foods plus vitamin A supplements of high potency and low cost that are available without prescription.

Hypervitaminosis D is of special concern in infant feeding. Many cereals and baby foods, including milk, are fortified with this vitamin. Overzealous consumption of vitamin supplements compound the dose well beyond the daily need of 400 IU. Symptoms of toxicity in children and adults from vitamin D–induced hypercalcemia include calcification of soft tissue (especially lungs and kidneys), bone fragility, and generally impaired bodily functions (e.g., loss of appetite, nausea, loss of weight, and failure to thrive in infants).

If large doses of vitamins A and D are taken concurrently, toxic symptoms tend to be reduced. The mechanism of this is unknown.

Possible toxic sequelae of excessive amounts of water-soluble vitamin C are also being studied.

Vitamin K taken in excessive amounts during pregnancy predisposes the newborn to hyperbilirubinemia.

Fluids

Fluids are as important to adequate nutrition and a state of well-being as the basic four food groups (p. 181). Six to eight glasses of water a day are recommended. Fluids aid in maintaining bodily functions such as distribution of mineral salts, elimination from intestines and kidneys, digestion and assimilation of foods, and body fluid balance.

If tea and coffee are not constipating or do not interfere with sleep, these fluids are acceptable. Alcohol when taken in moderation does not affect adversely the course of pregnancy or the developing fetus and may even perk up a lagging appetite. Alcohol does contain many nonnutritive calories, and if it interferes with adequate nutrition, it should be avoided.

SPECIAL CONCERNS DURING PREGNANCY
Diet and gastrointestinal discomforts in pregnancy

During pregnancy, hormonal changes and changes resulting from the increasing size of the uterus commonly result in one or more gastrointestinal difficulties such as nausea and vomiting, heartburn, constipation, and pica. Difficulties experienced are individual in form and extent. If symptoms are severe or persistent, the physician's attention may be required (Chapter 14).

Preeclampsia-eclampsia

Acute preeclampsia (toxemia of pregnancy) occurs after the twenty-fourth week of gestation. Many theories regarding its etiology have been postulated.

Brewer (1972) and other clinicians submit laboratory and clinical evidence that preeclampsia is a disease of malnutrition and that malnutrition affects the liver, adversely altering its metabolic activities. Historically, preeclampsia has been associated with poverty, occurring with greater frequency in women with inadequate diets and little if any medical care.

Preventive intervention encompasses a general state of good nutrition prior to conception and optimal nutrition throughout gestation.

Excess weight gain during pregnancy must be evaluated carefully. The pattern of weight gain is more significant than total weight gain. Weight gain due to excessive accumulation of fat has not been related to an increased tendency to develop preeclampsia. Weight gain due to edema is a characteristic feature of preeclampsia.

Treatment is determined by the individual patient's

symptoms and needs. Nutritional therapy is designed to correct and maintain metabolic balance and includes ample intake of protein foods of high biologic value and sources of vitamins and minerals. The Food and Nutrition Board of the National Academy of Sciences–National Research Council (1974) recommends that the generally accepted practice of stringent caloric and salt restriction be subjected to scientific scrutiny. Caloric and salt restricted diets necessitate the reduction of protein intake. The Council reports deleterious effects of salt restriction in pregnant rats and suggests that routine salt restriction and the use of diuretics during gestation be questioned.

Anemias complicating pregnancy and puerperium

A nutritionally adequate diet is required for normal hematopoiesis; an ample supply of protein, sufficient calories to protect protein from catabolism, iron and other minerals such as copper and zinc, and folic acid, vitamin B_{12}, and other vitamin coenzymes are needed in heme (iron) and globin (protein) synthesis. During pregnancy, maternal erythropoiesis, placental growth and development, and fetal growth and development add appreciably to the nutritional demands.

Hematologic values in anemia are as follows:

	Deficiency	Norm
Hct	$\leq 30\%$	3.0 to 3.5 gm/100 ml
Hgb	≤ 10 gm/100 ml	12 to 13 gm/100 ml (at sea level)
Serum folacin	≤ 3 μg/ml	6 μg/ml

If hematologic values suggest anemia, additional laboratory tests may be performed to obtain the following values:

	Deficiency	Norm
Serum albumin	≤ 2.5 mg/100 ml	3.0 to 3.5 mg/100 ml
Total serum protein	≤ 5.5 gm/100 ml	6.0 to 6.5 gm/100 ml
Serum vitamin B_{12}	≤ 80 μg/ml	200 μg/ml

Physiologic anemia of pregnancy. Maternal blood volume normally increases 30% to 50% late in the first trimester of pregnancy followed by a slower and relatively smaller increase in total volume of circulating red blood cells and hemoglobin. The changes reach a peak at 34 weeks' gestation then decrease toward term (40 weeks). Physiologic cost is 500 mg of iron.

Fetal needs. Most of the placental transfer of iron to the fetus occurs during the last half of pregnancy. Physiologic cost is 300 mg of iron. Iron needs are greater if there is more than one fetus.

Iron-deficiency anemia. This is by far the most common form of anemia in pregnancy. Iron utilization exceeds the available reserves in the average woman.

Iron intake of healthy young American women has been found to average about 300 mg per pregnancy, insufficient to meet pregnancy requirements.

Increased dietary intake and increased absorptive efficiency during pregnancy may supply the additional demands. Diets of pregnant women in the United States usually include only 12 to 15 mg of iron a day; at best only 10% to 20% of food iron is absorbed and utilized. Some women enter pregnancy with marginal stores insufficient to meet the augmented demand. When pregnancy needs exceed maternal intake and reserves, anemia results. In most instances, fetal needs will be met, but the mother suffers from the deficiency. Oral iron compound containing about 200 mg/day may be prescribed. Iron rich foods should also be encouraged. To replenish maternal reserves, oral therapy is advised for 3 to 6 months after the anemia has been corrected.

Ferrous sulfate or ferrous gluconate tablets are always taken in conjunction with meals for maximum absorption and tolerance. Persons on oral iron therapy should be alerted to possible problems with constipation (and how to alleviate these) and that the stool will appear black.

Hemorrhagic anemia. Blood loss may occur at any time during gestation. Abruptio placentae and placenta previa may occur during the latter part of pregnancy. Most blood loss occurs at the time of delivery and during the puerperium. Blood transfusions are given when indicated. To support hemoglobin formation, iron therapy may be instituted.

Megaloblastic anemia. Folic acid deficiency is the usual cause of megaloblastic anemia. Megaloblastic anemia is relatively uncommon in the United States but may occur late in pregnancy, especially among the poor. A diet low in animal protein and green, leafy vegetables is characteristic. Clinical manifestations include nausea, vomiting, and anorexia, which further compromise the nutritional status. Folic acid supplementation of 200 to 400 μg daily usually suffices to prevent deficiency in pregnant women. Supplementation is especially warranted in cases of chronic hemolytic anemia and multiple pregnancy.

LACTATION AND NUTRITION

During lactation, there is an increased need for nearly all nutrients; in fact, the physiologic stress of lactation surpasses that of pregnancy. Relative dietary needs posed by lactation as compared to gestation are seen in Table 13-1. (See Chapter 31.)

Nutritional needs

Basically the nutritional needs of pregnancy persist throughout lactation, with the following differences.

PLAN OF CARE: MATERNAL NUTRITION

NURSING INTERVENTIONS

Diagnostic	Therapeutic	Educational

Diagnostic

1. Maternal physiologic status is assessed for following:
   a. Age.
   b. Prepregnancy weight.
   c. Previous obstetric history (e.g., pregnancy intervals).
   d. Present physical examination and laboratory tests.
   e. Concurrent medical problems with nutritional base (e.g., diabetes, cystic fibrosis, PKU, anemia: hematologic values).
   f. Activity level (housewife, office worker, farm laborer).
2. Sociocultural assessment pertinent to nutrition:
   a. What is individual's life-style?
   b. If patient is not responsible for selection and preparation of food, who does it?
   c. How does religion, culture, or ethnic group influence dietary patterns day-to-day? During pregnancy?
   d. Does patient (and others in immediate environment) depend on welfare or food stamps? What is allotment?
   e. Are there other "special" circumstances (e.g., is patient a model or dancer)?
   f. How many people eat together for each meal? How many meals?
3. Dietary assessment:
   a. How many meals are served per day and how are they spaced?
   b. Typical daily menu: foods, quantities, preferences, dislikes?
   c. How are foods selected and cooked?
4. Identify her level of understanding.
5. Does she smoke, drink alcohol, or take drugs? Amount? Type of drugs?
6. Is she influenced by food fads?

Therapeutic

Involve patient as a participant in her own care.

1. Refer patient to physician and nutritionist* for special dietary and pharmaceutical prescriptions for unique circumstances (e.g., PKU, cystic fibrosis, diabetes, anemia). Confer with physician and nutritionist or refer to flow sheet regarding these therapies to ensure team approach to care.
2. Act as resource person for following:
   a. Dietary suggestions and alternatives.
   b. Channeling woman (and family) to appropriate community agencies for additional assistance as needed (school, welfare, public health nurse).
3. Acknowledge effort patient makes in altering and/or maintaining diet. Praise when appropriate.
4. Monitor weight gain throughout pregnancy. Weighing-in should be ego-building and psychologically unthreatening. (Many women "quiver in their shoes" waiting to hear disgust and condemnation for "gaining too much." Some starve evening before visit or take diuretics to avoid such unpleasant encounters; both alternatives are detrimental to health.)
5. Check to see how patient is managing her iron, vitamin, and mineral supplements.
6. Share with patient her laboratory results, weight, and BP. Discuss how these reflect her nutritional status.
7. Identify problems (e.g., situation present for more than 72 hours) and describe education accomplished and therapies begun or continuing. Note these in appropriate areas of POR flow sheet at each visit.

Educational

1. Any special diet patient may be following is reviewed (e.g., diabetes). Degree of knowledge is noted and praise given when appropriate. Changes in these diets to meet nutritional demands of pregnancy are discussed.
2. Identify nutrition-related folklore and myths with patient (e.g., "eating for two," "a tooth for every pregnancy," "if you eat green peppers, your baby will be hairy").
   a. Utilizing openings gained from identifying myths with patient, explore realities in myths and clarify or correct misconceptions without talking down to her.
   b. If some beliefs are firmly held (e.g., "green peppers . . ." myth), discuss foods of same nutritive value to substitute.
   c. Some physiologic demands on nutrition and body stores may be discussed in same context.
3. Briefly discuss physiologic demands (maternal and fetal) on bodily stores and daily intake.
4. Patient and her family's preferences, pocketbook, and other resources (cooking equipment, refrigeration, space) form context in which to review following:
   a. Her present weight.
   b. Current diet†: Divide into basic four groups. Compliment her on all nutritionally sound aspects of diet.
   c. Confer with her about types of food she would and could add or subtract from that diet. Discuss any possible problems she may encounter with other family members, purchasing, or preparing.
   d. Decide on alternatives to c. Set appointment at next visit to review successes or failures experienced in interim.
5. Discuss discomforts of pregnancy that can be managed by means of foods and fluids (e.g., nausea and vomiting, constipation, leg cramps, fatigue).
6. Make suggestions regarding best time and method to take iron pills if prescribed. Forewarn her regarding black color of stools and possible constipation while on iron therapy.

---

*In some rural and other areas, nutritionists may not be readily available. It then becomes nurse's and physician's responsibility to be thoroughly informed as to particular food habits in that community, that is, nutritive values, usual means of preparation, and other characteristics.

†Her menu plan is useful tool in clarifying and explaining. It also provides outline from which she could work.

Calories (energy). A minimum of 800 calories over that required for the average nonpregnant adult female every day is needed for lactation. About 120 calories are needed for every 100 ml of milk produced for the following reasons:

1. *Energy content of milk.* When lactation is well established, generally about 850 ml (30 ounces) are produced daily. Human milk contains about 20 calories/ounce for a total of 600 calories.

2. *Milk secretion.* Calories are expended in the production of milk: 400 to 420 calories are needed to produce 850 ml.

Allowing for individual differences, the nursing mother spends 800 to 1000 calories/day to meet the metabolic demands of lactation. The milk secreted in just a month's time burns more calories than the net energy cost of pregnancy.

Caring for a new baby also increases the new mother's energy requirement.

Protein. To the 76 gm of protein recommended for pregnancy is added another 20 gm bringing the total to 96 gm/day during lactation. Each 100 ml of milk contains 1.2 gm of protein.

Vitamins. The recommended daily allowance of vitamin A increases to 6000 IU and that of vitamin C increases to 80 mg, whereas that of vitamins D and E remain at gestation levels. Folic acid requirements drop below gestation levels but remain above nonpregnant requirements. Requirements for all B vitamins, except B_{12}, increase above levels for gestation. Augmentation of caloric intake necessitates higher levels of vitamin A, B_1, and B_2, since these act as coenzymes in cell respiration, glucose oxidation, and energy metabolism.

Minerals. The recommended daily allowance of most minerals remains at pregnancy levels. The high levels of calcium and phosphorus needed for fetal growth are now diverted into the mother's milk. Little iron is secreted into the milk so that maternal dietary requirements do not change. (What little iron is in breast milk is well utilized by the infant, however.)

Fluids. Increased amounts are needed for adequate milk production and urine formation. Decreased urinary output of highly concentrated urine results from inadequate intake. However, excessive fluid intake suppresses milk production by acting on the pituitary hormones.

Rest, moderate exercise, and relaxation are also significant in adequate milk production.

Incidental contaminants of breast milk

Recently concern has been expressed for the possible transfer of drugs, pesticides (DDT), herbicides, and other contaminants in human milk. Effects of these on the infant are either unknown or poorly understood.

Food patterns during lactation

The quantity of food consumed is increased, and the quality of food must be considered as well. The following additions to the daily diet are recommended: one extra serving each of meat, green and yellow fruits and vegetables, and citrus fruit and two cups of milk over normal requirements. This quantity of food may be more easily managed in four to six meals a day rather than three.

NUTRITION AND THE PILL

Oral contraceptive drugs have been approved for use in the United States since 1960. By the mid-sixties, publications began to appear reporting on effects of oral contraceptives on nutrition. Some data have been substantiated; much remains to be learned.

There is considerable evidence that oral contraceptives are implicated in deficiencies of vitamin B_6 (pyridoxine) (Rose and associates, 1973) and folic acid (Whitehead and others, 1973; DaCosta and Rothenberg, 1974) in about 20% to 30% of users.

Among some oral contraceptive users, symptoms such as headaches, nausea and vomiting, and emotional disturbance and depression have been alleviated by dietary supplementation of vitamin B_6.

Symptoms of folic acid deficiency are rarer, since folate is so plentiful in the North American diet. However, researchers postulate the possibility of folic acid deficiency in pregnancies that closely follow discontinuance of the oral contraceptives. Clinical symptoms of folic acid deficiency are those of megaloblastic anemia: increasing fatigue, pallor, moderate depapillation of tongue, and changes in peripheral blood and bone marrow. Symptoms are rapidly reversed with supplementation of folic acid or if the oral contraceptive is discontinued.

Some evidence exists in support of vitamin C (McLeroy and Schendel, 1973) and vitamin B_{12} (cobalamin) (Wertalik and others, 1972) deficiencies among users. No clinical effects of these deficiencies have been published as yet.

Vitamins whose metabolism is suspected of being altered by oral contraceptives are A (Wild and others, 1974), B_2 (Sanpitak and Chayutimonkul, 1974), D (Conney and Burns, 1972), and niacin (Rose and others, 1968). Early evidence suggests that users should increase daily intakes of vitamin A. The clinical significance of altered metabolism of these and other nutrients and of reduced (rather than deficient) levels of these nutrients is unknown at this time.

Metabolism of calcium does not seem to be affected by oral contraceptives.

Iron absorption from the gastrointestinal tract is enhanced. Increased absorption plus decreased loss of iron through diminished menstrual flow augments iron stores in oral contraceptive users.

REFERENCES

Brewer, T. H. 1972. Human maternal-fetal nutrition. Obstet. Gynecol. **40:**868.

Butterworth, C. E. 1973. Interactions of nutrients with oral contraceptives and other drugs. J. Am. Diet. Assoc. **62:**510.

Clausen, J., and others. 1976. Maternity nursing today. McGraw-Hill Book Co.

Conney, A. H., and Burns, J. J. 1972. Metabolic interactions among environmental chemicals and drugs. Science **178:**576.

Cross, A. T., and Walsh, H. E. 1971. Prenatal diet counseling. J. Reprod. Med. **7:**265, Dec.

DaCosta, M., and Rothenberg, S. P. 1974. Appearance of a folate binder in leukocytes and serum of women who are pregnant or taking oral contraceptives. J. Lab. Clin. Med. **83:**207.

Department of Health, Education, and Welfare. 1970. Maternal nutrition and the course of pregnancy: summary report. Pub no. (HSM) 72-5600. Washington, D.C., U.S. Government Printing Office.

Food and Nutrition Board. 1974. Recommended dietary allowances (ed. 8). Washington, D.C., National Academy of Sciences–National Research Council.

Guthrie, H. 1975. Introductory nutrition (ed. 3). St. Louis, The C. V. Mosby Co.

Iorio, J. 1975. Childbirth: family-centered nursing (ed. 3). St. Louis, The C. V. Mosby Co.

Jacobson, H. N. 1973. Nutrition in pregnancy: a critique. J.A.M.A. **225:**634.

Kaminetzky, H. A., and others. 1973. The effect of nutrition in teenage gravidas on pregnancy and the status of the neonate. 1. A nutritional profile. Am. J. Obstet. Gynecol. **115:**639.

King, A. 1970. Extension of guide to good eating: acceptable foods of some cultural and ethnic groups in California. Oakland, Calif., Dairy Council of California.

Kitay, D. A. 1971. Dysfunctional antepartum-nutrition. J. Reprod. Med. **7:**251, Dec.

McLeroy, V. J., and Schendel, H. E. 1973. Influence of oral contraceptives on ascorbic acid concentrations in healthy, sexually mature women. Am. J. Clin. Nutr. **26:**191.

Moustgaard, J. 1971. Nutritive influence upon reproduction. J. Reprod. Med. **7:**275, Dec.

Oakes, G. K., and Chez, R. A. 1974. Nutrition during pregnancy: with emphasis on overweight and underweight patients. Contemp. Obstet. Gynecol. **4:**147.

Pitkin, R. M., and others. 1972. Maternal nutrition: a selective review of clinical topics. Obstet. Gynecol. **40:**773.

Primrose, T., and Higgins, A. 1971. A study in human antepartum nutrition. J. Reprod. Med. **7:**257, Dec.

Rose, D. P., Brown, R. R., and Price, J. M. 1968. Metabolism of tryptophan to nicotinic acid derivatives by women taking oestrogen-progestogen preparations. Nature **219:**1259.

Rose, D. P., Strong, R., Folkard, J., and Adams, P. W. 1973. Erythrocyte aminotransferase activities in women using oral contraceptives and the effect of vitamin B_6 supplementation. Am. J. Clin. Nutr. **26:**48.

Ross, R. A. 1971. Nutrition and pregnancy: an invitational symposium. Part two: Nutrition in maternal and perinatal morbidity and mortality in a rural state: 1930-1950. J. Reprod. Med. **7:**264, Dec.

Sanpitak, N., and Chayutimonkul, L. 1974. Oral contraceptives and riboflavine nutrition. Lancet **1:**836.

Shank, R. E. 1970. The role of nutrition in the course of human pregnancy. Nutr. News **33:**11, Oct.

Wertalik, L. R., Metz, E. N., LoBuglio, A. F., and Balcerzak, S. P. 1972. Decreased serum B_{12} levels with oral contraceptive use. J.A.M.A. **221:**1371.

Whitehead, N., Reyner, F., and Lindenbaum, J. 1973. Megaloblastic changes in the cervical epithelium. Association with oral contraceptive therapy and reversal with folic acid. J.A.M.A. **226:**1421.

Wild, J., Schorah, C. J., and Smithells, R. W. 1974. Vitamin A, pregnancy, and oral contraceptives. Br. Med. J. **1:**57.

Williams, S. 1973. Nutrition and diet therapy (ed. 2). St. Louis, The C. V. Mosby Co.

Winik, M., Brasel, J., and Velasco, E. G. 1973. Effects of prenatal nutrition on pregnancy risk. Clin. Obstet. Gynecol. **16:**184.

Winston, F. 1973. Oral contraceptives, pyridoxine, and depression. Am. J. Psychiatry **130:**1217.

Zamenhof, S., and others. 1970. Pregnancy and proteins. U.C. News **46:**16, Nov. 24.

CHAPTER 14

Management of the antenatal period

The best method for ensuring the health of the expectant mother and her infant is proper antenatal care. During a woman's life, pregnancy is unique because only then does she seek ongoing health care. Regular antenatal visits, ideally beginning soon after the last menstrual period, offer opportunities to supervise the course of normal pregnancy, to reassure the patient and her family, and to teach parenting skills. Antenatal health supervision permits diagnosis and treatment of maternal disorders that may have been preexistent or may develop during the pregnancy and is designed to follow the growth and development of the fetus and to identify abnormalities such as pelvic tumors or imminent labor.

Before she has ever been pregnant, a woman is termed a *nulligravida*. A woman in her first pregnancy is termed a *primigravida*. A woman who is pregnant for the second or subsequent times is a *multigravida*. Before she has been delivered of a viable infant (legal definition: 24 to 28 weeks of gestational age), she is a *nullipara*. After she has been delivered of a viable infant, she is a *primipara*. After delivery of two or more babies, a woman is termed a *multipara*. This information is abbreviated as parity/gravidity. For example, 0/1 means a woman has not been delivered of a viable child (nullipara) and is pregnant for the first time (primigravida). Note that parity refers to the infant, gravidity to the uterus.

One obstetric abbreviation commonly employed in maternity centers is even more complete. It consists of four digits with dashes for separation. The first digit represents the total deliveries, the second indicates the number of premature babies, the third identifies the number of abortions, and the fourth is the number of children living at this time. If a woman pregnant only once with twins delivers at the thirty-fifth week and the babies survive, she is "para 1-2-0-2."

DIAGNOSIS AND DURATION OF PREGNANCY

The clinical diagnosis of pregnancy before the second missed period may be difficult in at least 25% to 30% of patients. Physical variability, lack of relaxation, obesity, or tumors, for example, may confound even the experienced obstetrician. Accuracy is most important, however, because social, medical, or legal consequences of an inaccurate diagnosis, either positive or negative, may be extremely serious. Unfortunately even laboratory tests are not invariably correct. A correct last menstrual period (LMP), date of intercourse, or basal body temperature (BBT) record may be of great value in the accurate diagnosis of pregnancy. Reexamination in 2 to 4 weeks may be required for certainty of diagnosis.

Great variability must be admitted in the subjective and objective symptomatology of pregnancy. Hence the diagnosis of pregnancy is classified as follows: presumptive, probable, and positive.

Presumptive symptomatology of pregnancy and differential diagnosis

Because all the presumptive signs and symptoms of pregnancy can be caused by conditions other than gestation, no one of the following can be relied on for a final impression, nor are combinations diagnostic.

SYMPTOMS

Amenorrhea. The majority of maternity patients have no periodic bleeding after the onset of pregnancy. However, at least 20% have some slight painless spotting during early gestation for unexplained reasons. A great majority of these continue to term and have normal infants.

Amenorrhea of the secondary type may also accompany emotional tension, any serious endocrine disorder, CNS abnormality, ovarian insufficiency or neoplasia, uterine disease, or cervical obstruction.

Nausea and vomiting. Digestive upsets, aversion to certain foods or cooking odors are common to many pregnant women, especially in the morning during the first trimester. Although the colloquialism "morning sickness'' is widely accepted as typical of a pregnant state, numerous expectant mothers have nausea later in the day or all day. Pregnancy nausea and vomiting may be of psychic origin.

Nausea and vomiting frequently are associated with gastrointestinal problems such as allergies, infection, obstruction, CNS disorders, or viremia.

Breast sensitivity. Breast engorgement in early pregnancy is assumed to be due to increased estrogen and progesterone stimulation.

Abnormal estrogen and progesterone stimulation may occur as a result of hormone therapy and mastalgia may be caused by estrogen excess associated with anovulatory menstrual cycles or ovarian tumors.

Urinary frequency and urgency. During pregnancy, the expanded production of estrogen and progesterone is responsible for an increased circulation to the pelvic viscera, including the bladder. Thus urinary frequency and urgency (without dysuria) frequently may be reported early in pregnancy.

Lassitude and easy fatigability. Listlessness and fatigue after only slight exertion are described by many women in early pregnancy, along with an increased need for sleep.

Ennui and fatigue may be psychologic or pathologic. One should also consider emotional disorders, anemia, infection, or malignant disease.

Quickening. The first recognition of fetal movements by the multiparous patient may be as early as the sixteenth week, but primiparas may not notice these sensations until the eighteenth week or later.

SIGNS

Skin pigmentation. *Facial melasma,* also called *chloasma,* or *mask of pregnancy,* is a blotchy, brownish hyperpigmentation of the skin over the malar prominences and the forehead, especially in dark-complexioned expectant women, beginning during the second trimester and increasing gradually to delivery. Chloasma usually fades after delivery. The *linea nigra* is a pigmented line extending from the symphysis pubis to the top of the fundus in the midline. The linea nigra and darkening of the skin about the nipples and over the vulva may occur concomitantly during pregnancy. This pigmentation is caused by the anterior pituitary hormone melanotropin, which is increased during pregnancy.

Hyperpigmentation of the skin in the nonpregnant woman may be due to local causes (e.g., excessive sunlight, tanning creams) or to systemic problems such as Addison's disease. Chloasma is commonly seen in women taking ''the pill'' because of the resulting in-

crease in the secretion of pregnancy-like hormones and may not fade after ''the pill'' is discontinued.

Epulis. Hypertrophy of the gingival papillae may develop during the last two trimesters of pregnancy. Estrogen may be responsible.

Gingival granulomas may develop as a result of dental calculus or infection in nongravid women.

Leukorrhea. Increased estrogen and progesterone stimulation of the cervix produces copious mucoid fluid that is whitish because of the presence of many exfoliated vaginal epithelial cells secondary to normal pregnancy hyperplasia. This vaginal discharge is never pruritic or blood stained.

Cervicitis or vaginitis may be responsible for leukorrhea in nonpregnant women. Irritation and discoloration finally develop in most of these cases.

Breast changes. Early pregnancy changes include enlargement, prominence of veins, and a secondary pinkish areola with prominence of the small sebaceous glands about the nipple (Montgomery's tubercles). This begins as early as the sixth week of gestation. Colostrum, a yellowish premilk secretion, may be expressed manually after the fourth to fifth month.

Nipple discharge may be the result of nonpregnancy problems, including breast stimulation, mammary neoplasia, or CNS disease.

Abdominal enlargement. The pregnancy may ''show'' after the fourteenth week, although this depends to some degree on the patient's height and weight.

Abdominal enlargement may be an expression of obesity, a sign of intra-abdominal neoplasm, or evidence of a hernia of the abdominal wall.

Changes in internal genitals. Following are typical changes in the internal genitals:

1. *Vagina.* Cyanosis, or bluish discoloration (Chadwick or Jacquemier's sign) may be noted as early as the sixth week of pregnancy.

2. *Cervix.* Softening of the tip may be observed about the fifth week in a normal unscarred cervix. Softening of the cervical-uterine junction (Ladin's sign) may be recorded about the fifth or sixth week (Fig. 14-1). The appearance of the cervix depends on the patient's parity (Fig. 14-2), as well as the hormones of pregnancy.

3. *Uterus.* About the seventh week, isthmic softening (Hegar's sign) may be noted (Fig. 14-3). Easy flexion of the fundus on the cervix (McDonald's sign) is likely by the seventh to eighth week. Softening and slight fullness of the fundus near the area of implantation (von Fernwald's sign) or a soft lateral bulge with cornual implantation (Piskacek's) may be noted by the eighth

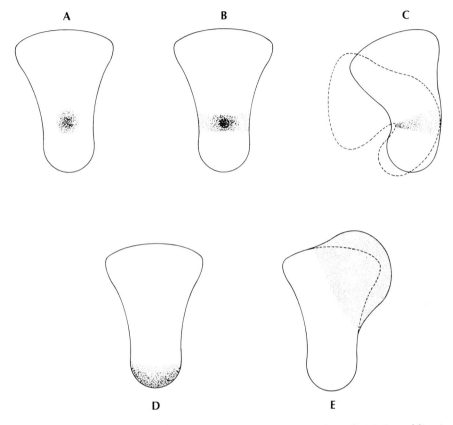

Fig. 14-1. Softening of uterus. **A,** Ladin's sign. **B,** Hegar's sign. **C,** McDonald's sign. **D,** Tip of cervix. **E,** Braun-von Fernwald's sign.

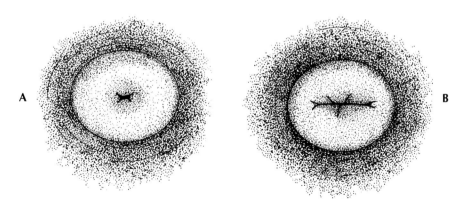

Fig. 14-2. External cervical os as seen through a speculum. **A,** Nonparous cervix. **B,** Parous cervix.

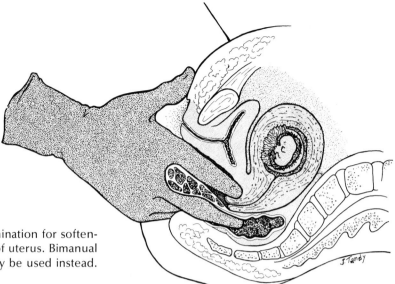

Fig. 14-3. Hegar's sign. Rectovaginal examination for softening of isthmus between cervix and body of uterus. Bimanual examination (vaginal and suprapubic) may be used instead.

week. After the eighth week, general enlargement and softening of the uterine corpus is likely.

In the nonpregnant woman, cervical and/or uterine anomalies, tumors, chronic passive congestion (with a retroflexed uterus), or the ''pelvic congestion syndrome'' may mimic the previous signs. A misinterpretation of findings in the obese or tense patient may lead to a false diagnosis of pregnancy.

Probable symptomatology of pregnancy
SYMPTOMS

These include all the symptoms considered previously under the presumptive symptomatology of pregnancy.

SIGNS

Uterine enlargement. A reasonably accurate correlation of uterine enlargement versus the duration of amenorrhea in weeks from the sixth week to term is possible in most normal pregnant patients. Variations in the positions of the fundus or the fetus, variations in the amount of amniotic fluid present, or the presence of more than one fetus reduces the accuracy of this estimation of the duration of pregnancy.

Uterine enlargement may be due to neoplasms or the normal-sized uterus may be displaced by a pelvic tumor (usually fibroid or myomata) of even larger size.

Uterine souffle or bruit. A swishing sound heard just above the symphysis and timed precisely with the mother's pulse is caused by augmented blood flow in the uterine arteries.

A souffle may be heard over a vascular tumor or aneurysm in the nonpregnant patient or may simply be abdominal aortic pulsation, particularly in a thin woman.

Uterine contractions (Braxton Hicks sign). Occasionally intermittent uterine contractions may be felt by the patient or observer almost any time after well-established pregnancy, but after the twenty-eighth week, contractions become much more definite, especially in slender patients.

Misinterpretation of contractions of muscles of the abdominal wall, intestinal peristalsis, and transmission of the abdominal pulse may be mistaken for the Braxton Hicks sign.

Laboratory tests for pregnancy. Most currently available laboratory tests for pregnancy (Appendix D), particularly those which test for the presence of HCG in serum or urine, are extremely accurate, simple, and inexpensive and available in kit form so that little practice is needed to perform them.

Improper collection of the specimen, hormone-producing tumors, drugs, or laboratory errors may be responsible for false reports of pregnancy.

Positive symptomatology of pregnancy
SYMPTOMS (NONE)

There are no particular symptoms that irrefutably indicate pregnancy.

SIGNS

Although rarely present until after the fifth to sixth month of pregnancy, any one of the following is both medical and legal proof of pregnancy.

Fetal heartbeat. Auscultatory or electronic verification of fetal heart activity requires the counting of the fetal heart tones (FHT) or impulse for 1 minute and a comparison with the mother's pulse rate for the same

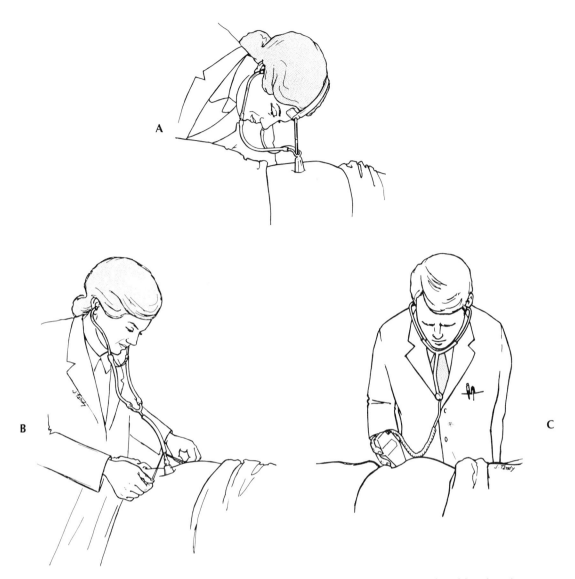

Fig. 14-4. Detecting fetal heartbeat. **A,** Fetoscope. **B,** Stethoscope with rubber band. **C,** Doppler principle.

period of time. Electronic devices employing the Doppler principle or fetal electrocardiography may pick up the fetal cardiac impulses by the tenth week (Fig. 14-4). Auscultation with a clinical stethoscope may not be successful until the seventeenth or eighteenth week under ideal circumstances.

Palpation of fetal outline. Palpation of the entire fetus, that is, head, back, and upper and lower small parts, may be outlined in most women, other than the obese patient, particularly after the twenty-fourth week.

Recognition of fetal movements. Active movements of the fetus by an observer other than the mother may be identified after the eighteenth week. When ascites or a tumor can be excluded, passive movements of the unengaged fetus (ballottement) generally can be identified at about the same time. This is done by gently palpating the fetus, which moves away and rebounds after a tap by the palpating fingers.

Ultrasonographic or radiographic demonstration of fetus. Ultrasonography has successfully identified an embryo as early as the sixth week; after the third month, this approach is most accurate. The fetal skeleton can be revealed by x-ray film as early as the twelfth week.

Ultrasound is safe to use at any time, even repeatedly,

during gestation. X-ray diagnosis should be used only when absolutely necessary to avoid fetal or ovarian damage and subsequent genetic alteration.

• • •

The definite diagnosis of an early pregnancy or its exclusion requires cautious interpretation of the signs, symptoms, and the commonly available laboratory tests. Although these tests are helpful, they are not entirely diagnostic. However, when radioactive immune antibody tests for HCG become available commercially, positive diagnosis will be possible even as early as 1 to 2 weeks' gestation.

ESTIMATED DATE OF CONFINEMENT AND GESTATIONAL AGE

A term pregnancy is a gestation of 38 to 42 weeks. Occasionally patients will be certain of their LMP, date of coitus on or just prior to ovulation, or both. Hence the duration of pregnancy can be assessed with certainty. More often, however, patients will have none of these essential data, and estimates of the length of gestation by the physician will be necessary.

In pregnancy, numerous indices of gestational age may be employed. No one of these is infallible, but a combination of the results of two or three of the following is accurate.

Indirect noninvasive methods

Because the precise date of conception must remain conjectural, many formulas or rules-of-thumb have been suggested to calculate the estimated date of confinement (EDC). None of these is accurate, but the following approximations are helpful.

Naegele's rule. Naegele's rule is as follows: add 7 days to the first day of the LMP, subtract 3 months, and add 1 year, or EDC = LMP + 7 days − 3 months + 1 year. An example is as follows: if the first day of the last menstrual period (LMP) was July 10, 1976, the EDC is April 17, 1977.

Naegele's rule assumes that the patient has a 28-day cycle and that the pregnancy occurred on the fourteenth day. Hence an adjustment is in order if the cycle is longer or shorter than 28 days.

Using Naegele's rule, only about 4% of patients will deliver spontaneously on the EDC. The majority of patients will deliver during the period extending from 7 days before to 7 days after the EDC.

Fundal height. During the first two trimesters of pregnancy, the fundal height, as measured on the anterior abdominal wall, affords a gross estimate of the duration of pregnancy. The anteverted uterus often can

be palpated slightly above the symphysis pubis at 8 to 10 weeks. The fundus should be half the distance from the symphysis to the umbilicus at 16 weeks and at the umbilicus at 20 to 22 weeks.

McDonald's rule. McDonald's rule adds precision to the measurement of fundal height during the second and third trimester (Fig. 14-5).

With a flexible (no stretch) tape, measure the height of the fundus from the notch of the symphysis pubis over the top of the fundus without tipping the corpus back. Then calculate as follows:

Height of fundus (in centimeters) $\times$ $^2/_7$ (or $\div$ 3.5) = Duration of pregnancy in lunar months

Height of fundus (in centimeters) $\times$ $^8/_7$ = Duration of pregnancy in weeks

McDonald's method may aid in identification of such high-risk factors as intrauterine growth retardation (IUGR), multiple gestation, and polyhydramnios.

Estriol levels in maternal urine (p. 196). Correct estimates are unlikely with obesity, multiple pregnancy, or pelvic tumors because the EDC will often be an early estimate. Growth retardation of the fetus, oligohydramnios, or fetal death may suggest a false later EDC.

Direct invasive methods

The following direct invasive methods are useful in determining gestational age.

Ultrasonography. An A-scan fetal biparietal diameter at 36 weeks should be approximately 8.7 cm. Term pregnancy can be diagnosed with considerable confidence if the biparietal cephalometry by ultrasonography is greater than 9.8 cm. (See Fig. 14-6.)

Radiography. The presence of distal femoral ossification centers indicates a fetal age of 36 weeks. If the proximal tibial centers are present, the fetus is 40 weeks' gestational age. X-ray visualization of the distal femoral and proximal tibial epiphyseal centers also indicates term pregnancy.

Amniocentesis. Greater accuracy in estimating the duration of an advanced pregnancy is now possible utilizing amniotic fluid or its exfoliated cellular content (Fig. 14-7). Technically, term has been reached if more than one of the following is properly demonstrated by laboratory studies:

1. L/S ratio that is greater than 2 indicates adequate lung maturity for extrauterine life. This will be achieved if the fetus is older than 36 weeks' gestational age. A practical variation of the L/S ratio is the rapid surfactant test, also known as the shake test or "bubble test." Equal parts of fresh amniotic fluid and normal saline are added to two parts of 95% ethyl alcohol. The mixture is

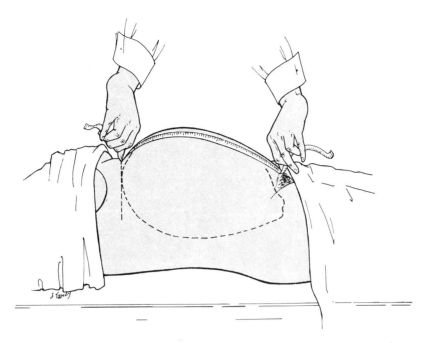

Fig. 14-5. Measurement of fundal height from symphysis (McDonald's method).

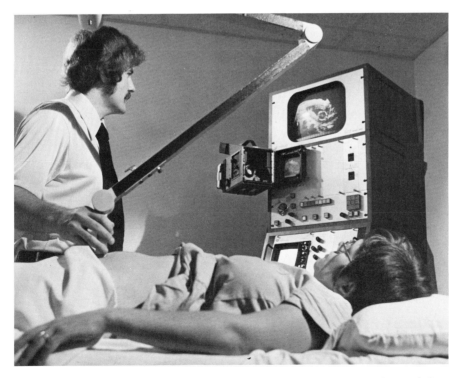

Fig. 14-6. Ultrasonography is safe, painless method of scanning mother's abdomen with high-frequency sound waves to follow fetal growth and development. (Courtesy March of Dimes.)

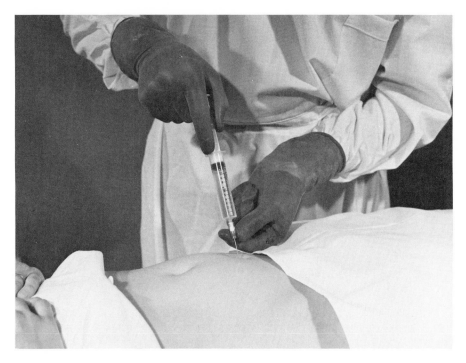

Fig. 14-7. Transabdominal amniocentesis. (Courtesy March of Dimes.)

shaken vigorously for 30 seconds. If bubbles are still present at the meniscus 15 minutes after shaking, the fetal lung is judged to be mature.

2. When the optical density of bilirubinoid pigments is 450 nm = <0.01, this indicates a gestational age of greater than 38 weeks.

3. When the creatinine (estimate of renal maturity) value is greater than 1.8 mg/100 ml, gestational age is greater than 36 weeks in the absence of maternal renal disease, dehydration, or fetal anomaly. At term an amniotic fluid osmotic pressure of about 250 mOsm/ℓ can be expected.

4. After staining fetal lipid-containing exfoliated cells with Nile blue sulfate, a finding of more than 20% orange-staining cells indicates a gestational age of greater than 35 weeks.

Prolonged or postdate pregnancy

About 10% of all pregnancies continue for at least 2 weeks beyond the EDC (280 days + 14 = 294 days). Pregnancies are considered prolonged if they continue beyond the forty-second week. Most postdate gestations are normal, but the morbidity and mortality rates for the infant are increased by three times because of the increased incidence of meconium aspiration pneumonia. Large babies, fetopelvic disproportion, malpresen-

tation, malposition, and so-called placental insufficiency or dysfunction are problems of prolonged pregnancy.

In cases suspected of being greater than 2 weeks overdue, one should recalculate the EDC, utilizing assists such as the time of quickening (midpregnancy ± 2 weeks), early uterine size versus the supposed duration of pregnancy at the examination, and others. One should repeat the pelvic measurements, examine for fetal engagement, and assess the character of the cervix such as dilatation and effacement. The patient's medical status should be reappraised. Diabetic or gestational diabetic mothers have large babies, which may confuse the estimate of gestational age. Amniocentesis to ascertain the true gestational age is also advised. Preterm delivery of large babies should be avoided.

A decision should be made regarding vaginal delivery (assuming no medical problems or obstetric complications) or cesarean section. Postdate pregnancy per se is not an indication for cesarean section. A reasonably accurate estimation of the gestational age is most important when elective induction of labor or elective repeat cesarean section is chosen.

The calculated duration of pregnancy (from the LMP or other indices) may require adjustment. For example, if the dates are accurate but the uterus is larger than

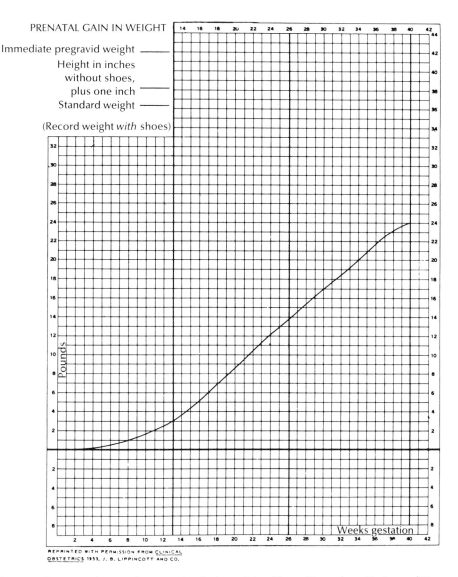

Fig. 14-8. Pattern of normal prenatal gain in weight. (From Hunscher, H. A., and Tompkins, W. T. 1953. Clinical obstetrics. Philadelphia, J. B. Lippincott Co.)

expected for the duration of pregnancy, hydramnios or multiple pregnancy may be the cause. If the dates seem correct but the size of the fetus is disparate, fetal compromise such as IUGR, may be the problem, particularly in association with preeclampsia or cardiovascular-renal disease.

If the gestational age of the fetus thought to be 37 weeks is actually only 33 weeks at delivery, early delivery reduces chance for survival, even with the best of care, from about 95% to approximately 60%. In contrast, if the fetus is undergrown because of, for example, placental insufficiency, delivery may be imperative, assuming the fetus is mature enough (older than 33 to 34 weeks' gestational age) to survive with good pediatric care.

SCHEDULE OF CARE

The patient should be seen once each month until the thirty-second week, every 2 weeks until the thirty-sixth week, and each week thereafter until delivery. More frequent visits may be required if complications ensue.

At each visit, the following should be completed and recorded in the patient's history:

1. Inquire regarding the patient's general well-being, her complaints, or problems.

2. Weigh the patient and determine whether the gain (or loss) is compatible with the overall plan for weight gain (Fig. 14-8).

3. Do a gross urinalysis on a first-voided morning urine specimen. Note the degree (1-4 +) of protein and glucose.

4. Obtain the blood pressure (right arm, patient sitting).

5. Proceed with abdominal palpation as follows:

   a. Measure the height of the fundus above the symphysis pubis (with tape). Identify unusual tenderness, masses, herniation, and other important details.

   b. After the twenty-fourth week, determine the fetal presentation; auscultate and count the FHT. (These may be heard from the tenth week using the Doppler method.)

   c. Beginning at the thirty-second week, the examiner or nurse identifies the fetal presentation, position, and station (engagement) and assesses uterine measurements and size (weight) of the fetus versus the supposed duration of pregnancy. Thus possible growth retardation of the fetus, multiple pregnancy, or inaccuracy of the EDC may be disclosed.

6. Vaginal or rectal examination may be done at any time (unless the patient is bleeding) to investigate leukorrhea, confirm the presenting part, corroborate the station, and determine cervical dilatation and effacement. This may be especially important if labor is impending or induction is anticipated.

7. Obtain a specimen of venous blood for repeat hematocrit or hemoglobin to diagnose and treat possible anemia. Repeat anti-Rh titer also if there is a reasonable chance that isoimmunization may have developed.

8. Complete and concise problem-oriented records are essential for the documentation of maternal progress. Many standard printed record forms are available (Appendix J). The best records incorporate medical, laboratory, nursing, and dietary data in an easily readable arrangement from the first through subsequent office or clinic visits.

FETAL HEALTH

Maternal urinary (24-hour specimen) or plasma estriol. This is an indicator of the normalcy of the fetoplacental unit. Estriol levels are elevated in multiple pregnancy, but they are extremely low in the presence of a failing pregnancy, anencephaly, and fetal death. Estriol levels fall in dysmaturity, preeclampsia-eclampsia, complicated diabetes mellitus, and partial separation of the placenta. Serial estriol determinations (never a single estimate) are essential to establish a trend to justify delivery of the fetus.

Amnioscopy. Fetal hypoxia is known to result in meconium passage by the mature fetus. Transcervical visualization of greenish amniotic fluid through the intact membranes indicates fetal asphyxia. Unfortunately the cervix must be more than 1 cm dilated, and special equipment (amnioscope with tungsten lamp) is needed.

Oxytocin stress or challenge test (OCT). Cautious uterine stimulation with careful external FHT electronic monitoring is a simulated test of the fetoplacental functional reserve (pp. 304 and 305).

FHT. Using the traditional clinical stethoscope, the FHT can first be heard between the eighteenth and twenty-second weeks of gestation. Because bone conduction increases hearing, the fetoscope is a preferred instrument. The fetal heart rate, rapid in early pregnancy, slows to about 120 to 140 beats/min at term. The rate is not a reliable index of the length of gestation. If the Doppler principle (Dopptone) is used, FHT can be heard at the tenth week or later.

Fetal presentation, position, and station (pp. 281 to 286). Early in the second half of pregnancy, careful palpation of the uterus should reveal the fetal lie, the presenting part, its position, and possible entry of the lower pole into the birth canal. This is done by accomplishing the four maneuvers of Leopold (p. 282).

The fetal axis, or lie, may be vertical or parallel with the maternal vertebral column or it may be transverse, or perpendicular to the vertebral column. If vertical, it may be possible to identify the larger, firmer head and smaller, softer breech. It is important also to determine whether the fetal back is directed to the mother's right or left side or whether it is anterior or posterior. Fetal small parts will be opposite the back, and FHT will be heard best through the back in most cases. Suspicion of multiple gestation, breech presentation, hydramnios, or other abnormality may require confirmation by x-ray examination or ultrasonography.

MATERNAL HEALTH
Minor discomforts of pregnancy

Abdominal discomfort. Abdominal discomfort (rarely pain) may be due to pressure. This sense of heaviness or weight of the pregnant uterus is most notable when the woman is standing or walking. Relief is afforded by frequent rest periods when the woman can

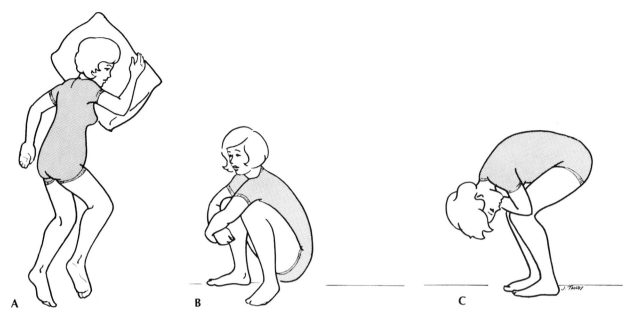

Fig. 14-9. A, Relaxed position. Some women prefer upper leg to be supported by pillow also. **B,** Squatting helps to relax pelvic floor and is preferred to bending over at waist. (Bending over at waist causes or aggravates heartburn from reflux of gastric contents into esophagus.) **C,** Rising in this manner aids in maintaining balance.

actually lie down or assume relaxing positions (Fig. 14-9). With considerable abdominal distention, as with multiple pregnancy, an elevating maternity girdle may afford relief.

Uterine contractions (Braxton Hicks contractions). These irregular contractions are normal. However, occasionally sharp twinges may develop during late pregnancy, disturbing the patient particularly when she is quiet or lying down. Rest, a change in position or activity, analgesics, or even alcohol may be beneficial.

Tension on the round ligaments (especially on the left due to the usual dextrorotation and displacement of the uterus) may cause pain in the groin during the last trimester. To reduce this tension while getting out of bed, the patient should be instructed to (1) roll to a side-lying position, (2) push with hands and arms to a sitting position, and (3) swing legs over the edge of the bed.

Inflammatory disorders such as urinary tract infections or appendicitis, torsion of the adnexa, and intestinal obstruction are other causes of abdominal distress that must be considered and treated appropriately.

Backache. Lumbosacral backache due to the increased spinal curvatures is secondary to the altered posture of the pregnant woman. Better posture (with the pelvis tilted forward and under the fetus to straighten the back), exercise (Fig. 14-10), medium-height heels, a firm mattress, rest, and analgesics are helpful. Orthopedic problems such as arthritis or neurologic disorders such as a herniated intervertebral disc must also be considered. Fig. 14-11 shows various positions for rest and relaxation.

Breast soreness. A well-fitting, supportive brassiere with wide nonstretch straps is effective in relieving mastalgia during pregnancy. Cool compresses may give temporary relief. Breast tumors or infection must be excluded. Normal nipple hygiene using warm water and minimal soap is recommended, but ointments and creams are unnecessary and may cause dermatitis.

Headache. Tension headaches are common during pregnancy. Emotional and physical stresses generally are responsible, and explanation, reassurance, and relaxation are beneficial. Physical causes of headache (e.g., sinusitis, eye strain, neurologic problems) must be sought and treated.

Constipation. Poor food choice, lack of fluids, questionable bowel habits, and iron supplementation may be responsible for constipation during pregnancy, as at other times. Hemorrhoids and diverticulosis may be aggravated by constipation. Intrinsic bowel problems such as intestinal obstruction, usually are acute and not persistent disorders. Good bowel habits, bulk foods, laxative fruits and vegetables, exercise, and a generous fluid

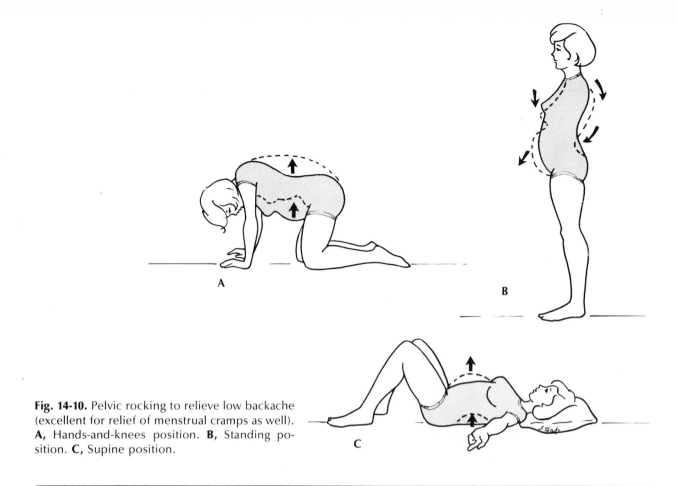

Fig. 14-10. Pelvic rocking to relieve low backache (excellent for relief of menstrual cramps as well). **A,** Hands-and-knees position. **B,** Standing position. **C,** Supine position.

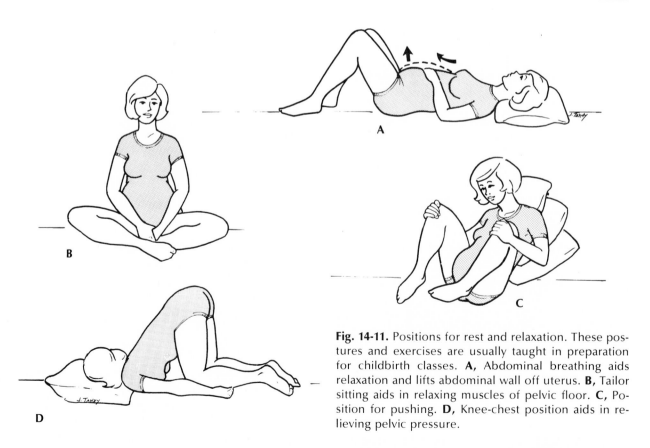

Fig. 14-11. Positions for rest and relaxation. These postures and exercises are usually taught in preparation for childbirth classes. **A,** Abdominal breathing aids relaxation and lifts abdominal wall off uterus. **B,** Tailor sitting aids in relaxing muscles of pelvic floor. **C,** Position for pushing. **D,** Knee-chest position aids in relieving pelvic pressure.

intake are recommended. Stool softeners may be prescribed, but enemas or extended use of laxatives are contraindicated.

Faintness. Faintness is generally due to vasomotor lability or postural hypotension and is reported by many pregnant women. Sudden changes of position, often in a warm crowded area, may precipitate this unpleasant sensation. Actual syncope is rare, however. Slow, deliberate movements, a cool environment, and elastic hose are helpful. Hypoglycemia or neurologic disorders should be considered in serious cases.

Heartburn, pyrosis, or "acid indigestion." Heartburn is symptomatic of gastroesophageal regurgitation. Heartburn may be associated with tension, nausea, and vomiting in early pregnancy; displacement of the stomach by the enlarged uterus may be responsible in late pregnancy. Neostigmine (Prostigmine) or acidifying agents such as glutamic acid hydrochloride to increase the progress of food or fluid through the stomach may be welcomed. Hot tea or chewing gum are common remedies. Antacids such as aluminum hydroxide gel preparations between meals may often afford relief, but the patient should be cautioned to avoid sodium bicarbonate preparations. A hiatus hernia or peptic ulcer should be considered in patients with persistent symptoms.

Hemorrhoids or piles. These are anal varices. Hemorrhoids are painful and often bleed during pregnancy when pelvic congestion develops. Constipation and straining at stool or bearing down during the second stage of labor frequently precipitate the appearance of hemorrhoids. Outlet forceps delivery may prevent enlargement of hemorrhoids.

Conservative treatment is recommended during gestation because resolution generally follows delivery. Regulation of bowel habits, proper posture on the toilet seat, stool softeners, rectal suppositories, and mild laxatives may be prescribed. A thrombosed hemorrhoid may be evacuated within 24 hours of its occurrence. Excision or injection of hemorrhoids is contraindicated because of the threat of infection or thrombosis of pelvic veins.

Leg cramps. Sudden spasms of muscles of the calf, thigh, or buttock may occur after the pregnant patient has been lying down. Leg cramps are common during the first 3 months and the last month of pregnancy from pressure on the nerves supplying the lower extremities. Poor peripheral circulation or fatigue seem to contribute to the problem. The calcium intake should be increased; calcium lactate 0.6 Gm three times a day before meals is beneficial. Excessive phosphorus intake can be prevented by limiting meat to one serving and milk to one pint daily. Phosphorus can be eliminated by absorption with aluminum hydroxide gel, 1 Gm orally with each meal.

Nausea and vomiting. Nausea and vomiting affect the majority of pregnant women during the first trimester. Altered hormone levels and metabolic changes may be precipitating factors. Tense, ambivalent women seem prone to this problem, which may occur at any time of day. Rarely intractable nausea and vomiting (hyperemesis gravidarum) develops (pp. 268 and 269).

Nausea and vomiting of pregnancy may be relieved with small (salt-free) snacks of dry crackers, toast, or popcorn before arising; small feedings of bland food; milk; sedative or antiemetic drugs; avoidance of offen-

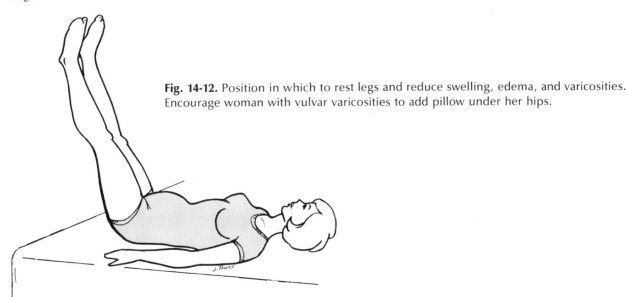

Fig. 14-12. Position in which to rest legs and reduce swelling, edema, and varicosities. Encourage woman with vulvar varicosities to add pillow under her hips.

sive odors; reassurance; and general supportive measures. Other common causes for gastrointestinal upset, for example, food poisoning or infectious diseases, should be considered.

Swelling of the ankles. Edema of the ankles and lower extremities affects the majority of women during late pregnancy. Edema often is associated with varicose veins and is augmented by prolonged sitting or standing and warm weather.

In the absence of hypertension or proteinuria, edema of the lower portion of the body only is not a sign of impending preeclampsia. Rest periods with the patient lying down or sitting with elevation of the legs and hips (Fig. 14-12), avoidance of tight garters, support stockings applied prior to arising, and ample fluids by mouth should suffice. Diuretic therapy should be avoided.

Urinary frequency and urgency. Urinary frequency and urgency are described by virtually every pregnant patient, especially early or late in pregnancy. In the absence of other symptoms of urinary tract infection, reassurance, practicing Kegal's exercises, and wearing a perineal pad for stress incontinence may be the only measures possible.

Varicose veins. Varicose veins usually are a problem of the older, multiparous patient or the obese pregnant woman with poor muscular tone. A hereditary tendency to varices has been noted. These unsightly veins may occur in the legs or the vulva and often are associated with aching of the legs and tenderness.

Phlebothrombosis and thrombophlebitis rarely complicate the antenatal period unless local injury and infection ensue. Clotting problems increase after delivery, with possible embolism formation; also superficial or deep thrombosis may develop.

Elastic support stockings or leotards are recommended. Vascular surgery or injection treatment of varices during pregnancy should be avoided because of possible sepsis, and the wide collateral venous circulation may doom these procedures to failure.

Spider nevi. Spider nevi or telangiectases sometimes appear over the face, upper trunk, or thighs. They are believed to be the result of the increased concentration of estrogen and usually disappear after the pregnancy terminates. Palmar erythema may also appear during pregnancy.

Frequent questions

Alcohol. Occasional alcoholic beverages are not harmful to the mother or her infant. Excesses must be avoided; chronic alcoholics often have small-for-gestational age (SGA) babies (Chapter 34). On the other hand, a glass of wine at bedtime may aid sleep. Alcohol should be avoided by those on weight control diets because of the nutritionally empty calories in the alcohol and because of the tendency to eat more.

Bathing. Tub bathing is permitted even late in pregnancy because water does not enter the vagina unless under pressure. Physical maneuverability presents a problem (increased chance of falling) late in pregnancy. Tub bathing is contraindicated after rupture of the membranes.

Clothing. Comfortable, loose clothing is best. Tight belts, stretch pants, garters, panty girdles, and other constrictive clothing should be avoided. A well-fitted maternity girdle, frequently readjusted, may be welcomed by obese women or those with multiple pregnancy for backache. Elastic hose or leotards may give considerable comfort to women with large varicose veins or swelling of the legs.

Dental problems. Nausea during pregnancy may lead to poor oral hygiene, and dental caries may develop. Hence dental care during pregnancy is especially important. Calcium and phosphorus in the teeth are fixed in enamel. No physiologic alteration during gestation can cause dental caries. The old adage "for every child a tooth" need not be true therefore.

There is no scientific evidence that filling of teeth or even dental extraction using local or nitrous oxide–oxygen anesthesia causes abortion or premature labor. Antibacterial therapy should be considered for sepsis, however, especially in patients who have had rheumatic heart disease or nephritis. Extensive dental surgery should be postponed until after delivery for the patient's comfort, if possible.

Drugs (medications). Although much has been learned in recent years about drug toxicity for the fetus (Table 31-1), the possible teratogenicity of many drugs is still unknown. This is especially true for new medications and combinations of drugs. Moreover, certain subclinical errors or deficiencies in intermediate metabolism in the fetus may convert an otherwise harmless drug into a hazardous one. The greatest danger of causing developmental defects in the fetus from drugs exists from fertilization through the first trimester (e.g., the period of organogenesis). Self-treatment must be discouraged. All drugs, including aspirin, should be limited, and a careful record of therapeutic agents used should be kept.

Employment. Many women continue to work during pregnancy. Whether the expectant mother can or should work and for how long depend on the physical activity involved, industrial hazards, fetotoxic environment (e.g., chemical dust particles, gases such as inhalation anesthesia*), medical or obstetric complications, and employment regulations of the company. Activities dependent on a good sense of balance should be discouraged, especially during the last half of pregnancy. Frequently, excessive fatigue is the deciding factor in the termination of employment.

Immunization. Immunization against poliomyelitis (Salk, not Sabin) and killed-virus immunizations such as influenza are advisable during gestation because of the increased susceptibility to these infections. In contrast, attenuated live virus immunizations such as rubella (German measles), rubeola (measles), and epidemic parotitis (mumps) and vaccinia vaccination against variola (smallpox) are contraindicated during pregnancy because of the teratogenicity of the viruses. Smallpox vaccination should be accomplished only during an epidemic.

Nursing. Every pregnant woman should be encouraged to nurse her infant. Good rapport and an explanation of the advantages of breast-feeding for mother and child may spell the success of lactation for many women. Immaturity of the infant, deep-seated aversion to nursing by mother or father, and certain medical complications such as pulmonary tuberculosis are contraindications to nursing. Women desiring to breast-feed may determine nipple formation (retracted, flat, normal) by the pinch test. Place the thumb and forefinger on the areola and squeeze. This causes the nipple to stand erect or flatten (i.e., retract or invert). If retraction occurs, nipple preparation can be started in the last 6 weeks of pregnancy; beginning earlier does not add to success. After bathing, nipples are dried with a rough towel and gently rolled between the fingers. A nipple shield may be worn for increasing lengths of time each day. This process may have to persist during the early nursing period.

Pregnancy and the female figure. Many women actually appear more beautiful during pregnancy. True, the altered silhouette and posture differ from the nonpregnant woman, but this is temporary and a gradual return to normal after the puerperium is likely. Concern for personal appearance, proper nutrition for her individual needs, proper breast support, and regular exercise will do much to maintain the figure. Personal neglect, not pregnancy, generally is the cause of a poor figure.

Smoking. Heavy cigarette smoking (more than six cigarettes a day) or continued exposure to a smoke-filled environment (even if the mother does not smoke) is associated with fetal growth retardation and an increase in perinatal and infant mortality. Laboratory studies indicate a lowered Po_2 and an elevated Pco_2 in both mother and fetus when exposed to cigarette smoke. Smoking is deleterious to patients with asthma, chronic respiratory infections, and allergy to pollen, dust, or dander. Smoking does not deter the success of lactation, nor are harmful substances transferred to the fetus in the milk.

Travel. Travel is neither a cause of abortion nor of premature labor. In high altitude regions, lowered oxygen may cause fetal hypoxia. Patients who travel widely expose themselves to the risk of serious accidents and/or may find themselves far removed from good maternity care. In addition, fatigue or tension, as well as altered regular personal habits and diet during arduous travel, may be detrimental. If long distance travel is necessary, the trip should be made by air. Perhaps fortuitously, flight regulations do not permit pregnant women aboard during the last month of pregnancy without a statement from an obstetrician.

Antenatal examination procedures

The examination procedures used during the antenatal period are relatively few in number and are common to many clinical areas.

PELVIC EXAMINATION

Purpose. A pelvic examination is done to permit visual and digital examination of the external and internal genitals and pelvic contours.

Procedure

1. Have patient void.

2. Equipment is selected and readied for use (Fig. 14-13). The speculum is warmed before inserting.

3. Assist the patient into lithotomy position. Drape and explain the procedures to follow.

4. Help patient to relax by having her pant-breathe; distract her with touch and conversation before the insertion of the speculum and as the vaginal examination is made.

5. When the examination is complete, assist the patient into a sitting position and then to stand. Provide wipes for removal of lubricant.

CLEAN-CATCH URINE SPECIMEN

Purpose. A specimen of urine is needed for examination at the initial visit (for routine urinalysis and test for pregnancy, if indicated) and at routine visits (for evaluation for glucose and protein).

Procedure. The specimen is obtained ideally on first arising in the morning. A clean container must be used. The woman should be instructed as follows:

1. Spread labia and wipe from front to back using moistened toilet paper.

2. Begin voiding and then obtain the specimen during

---

*Operating room personnel who are pregnant should be aware of the dangers of their working environment to the fetus.

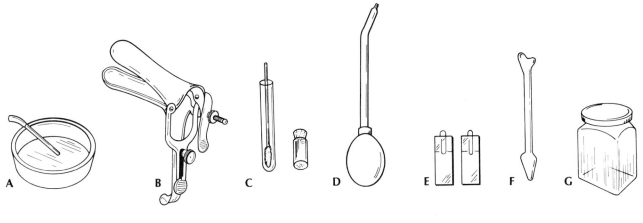

Fig. 14-13. Equipment used for pelvic examination during antenatal care. **A,** Petri dish with media for cultures. **B,** Vaginal speculum. **C,** Swab for cultures. **D,** Vaginal pipette with rubber bulb. **E,** Slides. **F,** Spatula for Pap smear and cytology. **G,** Preservative. **H,** Slide for hanging drop preparation. **I,** Cotton pledgets. **J,** Forceps. **K,** Uterine sound. **L,** Sterile lubricant. May be antiseptic. **M,** Sterile glove for vaginal examination (clean for rectal examination).

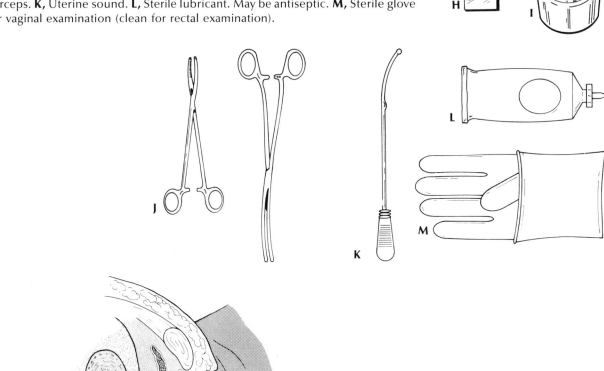

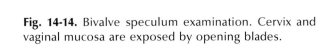

Fig. 14-14. Bivalve speculum examination. Cervix and vaginal mucosa are exposed by opening blades.

midstream in a clean container. Thirty to sixty milliliters or 1 to 2 ounces of urine are sufficient.

3. Bring the specimen for analysis (it does not have to be kept cool).

PAPANICOLAOU (PAP) SMEAR

Purpose. A smear is taken to detect abnormalities of cell growth by examining secretions and cells from the squamocolumnar junction, the cervix, and the vagina.

Procedure. Smears should be obtained at the first opportunity, although bleeding or douching within 12 hours of taking smears may result in a higher percentage of unsatisfactory or negative specimens. Patients should be advised routinely that repeat smears may be necessary so that they will not be unduly anxious if asked to return for this purpose.

The examiner will require a vaginal speculum sized according to patient's gravidity, spatula for removal of specimen, clean glass slides, and cytology fixatives such as Spray-Cyte or its equivalent, hairspray (Aqua-Net).

No digital examination should be employed prior to obtaining the cytologic specimens because the findings may be distorted. The speculum must be introduced with *no* lubricant. Warm tap water or vaginal fluid may be used to moisten the speculum and assist its introduction.

The cervix should not be wiped nor endocervical bacteriologic specimens taken with cotton swabs prior to taking the spatula scraping of the cervix. The mucus may contain the best carcinoma cells. If gross exudate or mucus is present, the excess is gently pushed away from the os with the end of the spatula. The specimen is taken by placing the S-shaped end of the cervical spatula just within the cervical canal at the external os. The blade is rotated 360 degrees, thus firmly scraping the surface at the squamocolumnar junction. The mucus is spread on a slide without allowing drying or rubbing, sprayed lightly with fixative, and then allowed to dry.

Some mucus is obtained from the posterior fornix (vaginal pool) with the rounded end of the spatula, spread on another slide, sprayed, and dried.

The first slide will contain mainly cells from the endocervix and ectocervix in the area where cervical cancer is most often found. The second slide may reveal cells from the endometrium, endocervix, ectocervix, and vagina. Generally, it is not necessary to identify the slides as to sites but by name of patient.

The patient's name, age, parity, chief complaint, or reason for taking the cytologic specimens must be recorded on a form to accompany the slides. They should be sent to the pathology laboratory promptly for staining, evaluation, and a written report, with special reference to abnormal elements, including cancer cells.

EVALUATION OF VAGINAL DISCHARGES (OTHER THAN BLOOD)

Any irritating vaginal discharge should be evaluated promptly and appropriate treatment initiated immediately for maternal and fetal well-being.

Normal discharge: leukorrhea. *Leukorrhea* is a whitish discharge, consisting of mucus and exfoliated vaginal epithelial cells, secondary to hyperplasia of vaginal mucosa such as occurs during pregnancy, at the time of ovulation, and just before menstruation. If it is copious, it can cause discomfort from excoriation.

Abnormal discharge: vaginal infections

Simple vaginitis. Infectious organisms such as *Escherichia coli,* staphylococci, and streptococci change the normal acidity of the vagina. A pH of 3.5 to 4.5 is needed to support the Döderlein bacilli, the vagina's main line of defense. The proximity of the urethra to the vagina predisposes to a concurrent urethritis.

Burning, pruritus (itching), redness, and edema of surrounding tissues are characteristics. These symptoms are particularly discomforting during voiding and defecating.

Objectives of management are to relieve discomfort, to foster growth of Döderlein's bacilli, to eradicate offending organisms, and to prevent recurrence. Interventions include the following:

1. Maintain scrupulous cleanliness, especially after elimination.

2. Douche with a weak acid solution such as 15 ml (1 tbsp) white vinegar to 1000 ml (1 qt) water (e.g., Massengill, Nylmerate).

3. Insert a beta-lactose suppository (to enhance growth of Döderlein's bacilli).

4. Administer chemotherapy specific for organism by inserting into the vagina with an applicator or applying cream locally to the area as directed.

Trichomonas vaginitis. *Trichomonas vaginalis* is a hearty protozoan that thrives in an alkaline milieu. Of all pregnant women, 20% to 30% harbor this organism, usually with no symptoms. The profuse, bubbly, white leukorrhea characteristic of this infection causes irritation, hyperemia, edema of the vulva, and dyspareunia. Urinary frequency and dysuria may occur. In the male partner, the protozoan may be harbored in the urogenital tract (without symptoms) and remain a source of reinfection for his mate.

Objectives of management are the same as for simple vaginitis. Interventions include the following:

1. Maintain scrupulous cleanliness, especially after elimination.

2. Douche with a weak acid solution (same as simple vaginitis).

3. Administer chemotherapy as follows:
   a. Metronidazole (Flagyl) 250 mg orally three times a day for 10 days. (Flagyl is contraindicated during the first half of gestation even though there is no evidence of fetotoxicity.)
   b. If Flagyl is not well tolerated by mouth, insert vaginal suppositories such as furazolidone (Tricofuron) or Vagisec.
   c. Treat male partner with metronidazole and inform him that intercourse should be avoided until the infection is cured.

Relief should be noted in 1 to 2 weeks. Rarely is a second course of treatment necessary.

Monilial vaginitis. Candida albicans, a fungus (yeast) normally found in the intestinal tract, contaminates and infects the vagina. (It is present in about 1 out of 4 women at term.) This infection is commonly seen in women with poorly controlled diabetes, since the organism thrives in a carbohydrate-rich milieu. Antibiotic or steroid therapy may be causative factors by reducing the numbers of Döderlein bacilli.

The thick vaginal discharge is irritating and pruritic. Frequently, dysuria and dyspareunia are common complaints. Speculum examination reveals thick, white, tenacious cheeselike patches adhering to the pale, dry, and sometimes cyanotic vaginal mucosa.

Objectives of treatment are the same as for simple vaginitis with one exception: women with recurrent infection should be checked for diabetes and/or control of diabetes should be instituted.

Interventions are as follows:

1. Maintain scrupulous cleanliness, especially after elimination.
2. Administer chemotherapy as follows:
   a. Gentian violet (2%) swabs should be administered to vaginal mucosa with applicator every 2 to 3 days until cured. (Patient should wear perineal pad to prevent permanent staining of clothing.)
   b. Nystatin (Mycostatin) vaginal tablets, 100,000 units twice each day for 14 days, or suppositories, 0.5 Gm twice each day for 10 days, should be inserted.
3. Abstain from intercourse until the infection is cured.
4. Local application of K-Y jelly or gentle bathing of the vulva with a weak solution of sodium bicarbonate relieves discomfort.

This organism also causes thrush in the newborn. Infection may occur by direct contact with an infected birth canal and from the contaminated hands of those who take care of him (p. 607).

Other infections. Neisseria gonorrhoeae infection causes a profuse purulent discharge. This infection is treated with penicillin (p. 606). Fetal and neonatal infection is discussed on pp. 602 to 607.

Herpesvirus may cause a sudden onset of vaginal discharge. The management of the woman infected with herpesvirus type 2 during pregnancy and labor and the care of the infant are discussed on pp. 604 and 605. After

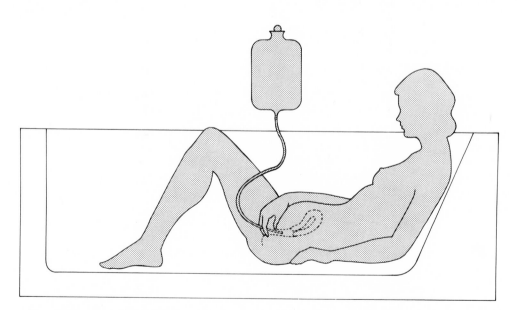

Fig. 14-15. Vaginal douche should be taken while lying in bathtub. Douche pan may be placed under patient in tub if desired.

herpetic infection, women should be monitored closely using cytologic smears for early detection of cervical carcinoma.

Management of vaginal infections becomes more complicated if more than one organism or agent is involved. Pediculosis pubis, threadworm, varicosities, and allergic response to perineal deodorants may compound the differential diagnosis and management. The discomforts imposed by these conditions challenge the woman's emotional as well as her physical well-being.

Vaginal douche procedure

Purpose. A vaginal douche is used to cleanse the vagina and to apply local medication and/or heat.

Procedure. The patient is instructed as follows:

1. Void and wash hands before douching.
2. Position:
   a. The optimal positon is semirecumbent in a clean tub (after a bath) or in bed (Fig. 14-15). A douche pan may be used in the tub as well.
   b. One can douche while seated on the toilet; however, the labia should be held together to permit solution to fill the entire vaginal vault.
3. Prepare solution. The temperature should be 40° to 43° C (105° to 110° F), comfortably warm to the inner aspect of the wrist. Allow some solution to flow out of nozzle to lubricate tip, or lubricate with K-Y jelly or other water-soluble lubricant.
4. Hold or place solution container 2 feet above the hips (avoid greater heights, which increase the pressure of the flow). *Do not* use a bulb syringe; air embolus followed by death may ensue.
5. Insert nozzle upward and backward for 3 inches.
   a. Rotate nozzle so that fluid flushes entire mucosa, including that of the posterior fornix. Rotation of nozzle also reduces the chance of forcing fluid into the cervix.
   b. When douching seated on a toilet, hold labia together to fill vaginal vault, then allow fluid to exit rapidly to flush out debris. Repeat until solution is used up.
   c. Hold labia together for specified period of time if the objective of the douche is to expose the mucosa to medication or moist heat.
6. If the woman is in the semirecumbent position for douching, sitting up and leaning forward aid in emptying the vagina.
7. Wash douche equipment with warm soap and water, dry, and store in well-ventilated place away from extremes of temperature.
8. Wash hands!

PLAN OF CARE: ANTENATAL PERIOD—INITIAL CONTACT WITH PATIENT

PATIENT CARE OBJECTIVES

1. Patient, staff, and family establish a therapeutic relationship.
2. Examination of patient confirms the diagnosis of pregnancy, reveals maternal reproductive capabilities and the possibilities of bearing a healthy child, and establishes an EDC.
3. Patient is advised of findings and is given an opportunity to express her feelings about the pregnancy.
4. Information regarding the options of continuing or discontinuing the pregnancy is given if warranted.
5. Patient makes decision as to continuing the pregnancy or arranging for an abortion with awareness of the implications such a decision has for her and her family.
6. On the basis of the decision, medical and nursing care plans are instituted for the following situations:
   a. Projected normal pregnancy, delivery of a healthy newborn, an uneventful puerperium, and acceptance of the parental role.
   b. Projected pregnancy, delivery, or puerperium complicated by known maternal or fetal deficiencies or complicated by adverse social conditions.
   c. Abortion.
7. Data base is recorded, including medical and nursing assessments.

NURSING INTERVENTIONS

Diagnostic	Therapeutic	Educational
Patient interview		
1. Physical data:	1. Establish a relationship with patient.	1. Review plan of care with woman and her family:
a. Family history:	a. Attitudes of personnel reflect interest in patient, that is, greet by name, use eye contact, show consideration for personal belongings. Touch should be gen-	a. Schedule: Check for convenience of timing, problems in transportation, and care of other children, and provide a written copy of schedule for patient.
(1) Health status of parents and siblings (if deceased, note cause of death).		
(2) History of tuberculosis, cancer, diabetes, vascular dis-		

Continued.

NURSING INTERVENTIONS—cont'd

Diagnostic	Therapeutic	Educational

Patient interview—cont'd

ease, neuromuscular disease, allergies, other serious illnesses, or multiple gestation.
  b. Past medical history:
    (1) Age.
    (2) Racial origin (Sickle cell anemia—black).
    (3) Ethnic background (Tay-Sachs syndrome—Jewish).
    (4) Childhood diseases and other serious diseases (e.g., venereal disease, operations, injuries, transfusions).
    (5) Problems related to body systems: eye, ear, nose, and throat; cardiovascular; gastrointestinal; urinary.
    (6) Menstrual history: menarche and present interval, amount of flow, pain.
  c. Past obstetric history:
    (1) Gravidity, parity, abortions, stillborns, living children.
    (2) If multigravida, description of previous pregnancies, hours of labor, type of delivery, antenatal, intranatal, and postnatal complications.
  d. Present pregnancy:
    (1) Date of LMP and one prior to that.
    (2) Any abnormal symptoms noted.
    (3) Medications, prescription or nonprescription (e.g., aspirin), including alcohol, tobacco, and caffeine. X-ray examinations if any.
2. Patient's profile (initial and subsequent visits):
  a. Identification: birthplace, marital status or history, education, occupation, employment history.
  b. Situational supports: family composition and/or availability of friends, living arrangements, sources of income, health of family members, ages of other children, how family perceives this pregnancy and how family supports or frustrates patient, health care concepts, particularly for pregnancy.
  c. Perception of this pregnancy: wanted or not, planned or not, pleased, displeased, accepting, nonaccepting, problems engen-

tle, instructions must be willingly repeated, and manner is warm and friendly.
  b. Organization and physical facilities are geared to patient's needs (e.g., appointment system may be used to minimize waiting for care; seating arrangements should be comfortable). Play area should be provided for children, bathrooms are clean and readily accessible, pertinent reading matter is available in language native to patients. Privacy is provided for interviewing, counseling, and examining.
  c. Reasons for procedures and review of plans for care are given.
2. Develop a plan of care for continuing assessment of maternal and fetal well-being.
  a. Schedule regular office or clinic visits every 4 weeks for 32 weeks, every 2 weeks for between thirty-second and thirty-sixth weeks, and then every week until term or labor begins.
  b. Establish routines:
    (1) For obtaining medical care if abnormal symptoms or incidences occur.
    (2) For treatment of ongoing problems common to pregnancy.
    (3) For preparation of patient for childbirth and child care activities.
3. Treat current problems, for example, profuse vaginal discharge with pruritis. Microscopic examination of hanging drop preparation reveals infection, and physician institutes therapy.

  b. Need for continuity of care: Check for understanding of reasons for periodic reassessment.
  c. Describe routine physical examinations, including instructions for obtaining clean-catch urine specimen for routine analysis.
  d. Provide written directions as to procedure for obtaining medical care if abnormal symptoms occur. List danger signals (e.g., vaginal bleeding, physical trauma, persistent depression).
2. Instruct regarding general health care:
  a. Personal hygiene (e.g., an increase in perspiration and mucoid vaginal discharge are normal and necessitate frequent bathing; cotton panties may be more comfortable). If vaginal discharge causes itching, is bloody, frothy, or has a foul odor, report immediately.
  b. Diet.
  c. Rest and exercise: Normal participation in sports need not be curtailed, except those creating sudden changes in pressure, such as diving. Walking is excellent exercise. Sleep patterns may change, and taking naps if tired is advised.
  d. Dental care may be undertaken during pregnancy.
  e. Instruct regarding prescription drugs, douches, general hygiene, etc.
3. Discuss current problems.
  a. Physical symptoms she may be experiencing: Give physical basis for discomfort in terms of physical changes occurring during pregnancy; be specific as to outcome and treatment and use terminology patient can understand.
    (1) Urgency and frequency of urination: "These symptoms are the result of the enlarging uterus pressing on the bladder. By about the twelfth week, these symptoms will disappear as the enlarging uterus moves upward into the abdominal cavity. These are normal symptoms. However, if pain or burning is ex-

NURSING INTERVENTIONS—cont'd

Diagnostic	Therapeutic	Educational

Patient interview—cont'd

dered by pregnancy, financial, career, living accommodations.

d. Coping mechanisms: knowledge of pregnancy, maternal changes, fetal growth, care of self, and care of newborns; knowledge of parent craft classes available; decision-making ability; use of significant others and use of community affiliations (church, clubs) as supports; living habits (e.g., exercise, sleep, diet, diversional interests).

Physical examination

1. Describe techniques to be used for examinations, general and pelvic, and instruct patient how to relax to facilitate process.
2. Check temperature, pulse, respirations, BP, height, and weight (usual and present).
3. Have patient undress completely and don hospital gown, position for examination, and drape as necessary.
4. Assist physician or midwife with examinations.
   a. General:
      (1) General appearance, body type, skin, lymph nodes.
      (2) Head and neck, eyes, ears, nose, throat, mouth, thyroid.
      (3) Chest, lungs, heart, breasts.
      (4) Abdomen, hernia, scars, striae, tenderness.
      (5) Extremities, edema, varicosities.
      (6) Neuromuscular reflexes.
   b. Pelvic:
      (1) Vulva, perineum, vaginal discharge.
      (2) Uterus, cervix, adnexa, cystocele, rectocele, height of fundus.
      (3) Rectovaginal examination.
      (4) Assessment of bony pelvis.
   c. Laboratory tests:
      (1) Minifilm of chest or tine test (for tuberculosis).
      (2) Cervical smears: one for cancer (Pap smear) and one for gonorrhea.
      (3) Blood: VDRL, Hct, blood type, Rh, sickle cell.
      (4) Urinalysis, including glucose, albumin, and culture and sensitivity if necessary.

perienced on urination, let the physician know right away."

(2) Languor and malaise: "Many women experience this. It disappears once the pregnancy is well established. Some women feel better than ever before in their lives."

(3) Nausea and vomiting: "It is thought that this occurs because of intense hunger—a drop in available carbohydrates. Try eating some crackers just before getting out of bed in the morning. If it happens in the afternoon, a light snack—milk and a cookie—can be helpful. By the end of the third month, it usually disappears."

b. Emotional responses to diagnosis of pregnancy: Acceptance of individual's feelings as normal, continued support, and provision of opportunities for ventilation of feelings serve to help patients explore methods of coping with pressures with view to retaining successful methods, rejecting unsuitable ones, and eventually discovering new techniques.

PLAN OF CARE: ANTENATAL PERIOD—FIRST AND SECOND TRIMESTERS

PATIENT CARE OBJECTIVES

1. Physical findings are indicative of a normal physical response of the maternal organism to pregnancy and normal growth and development of the fetus.
   a. Weight gain:
      (1) 3 to 4 pounds—first trimester.
      (2) 12 to 14 pounds—second trimester.
      (3) 8 to 10 pounds—third trimester.
   b. Urinalysis: ideally negative for albumin and no greater than 1+ glucose.
   c. Blood pressure: normal range with rise of less than +15 systolic +15 diastolic over baseline.
   d. Edema: Dependent edema is not uncommon, but puffiness of the face, especially eyelids, and hands is not normal (e.g., rings tight).
   e. Uterus: Progressive enlargement of the uterus and fundal height from the symphysis pubis is consonant with estimated gestational age.
   f. FHT can be detected by the tenth week and are regular in rhythm, with a rate of 120 to 160 beats/min.
   g. Fetal movements (quickening) often are felt by the mother between the sixteenth and eighteenth weeks and felt consistently thereafter. It is good to have the patient record the first time she is aware of this.
2. Emotional assessment is indicative of a normal psychologic response to pregnancy, including the birth process and parenthood.
   a. During the first trimester, patient may be self-centered and concerned with her own adjustment to the idea of pregnancy and the eventual responsibilities of parenthood, as well as the physical symptoms being experienced.
   b. During the second trimester, the woman usually is reasonably free of symptoms. She should be tranquil and at ease. The reality of the child is now recognized, and most women come to accept their state.
3. Abnormal findings are followed by additional assessment and modification of the plan of care.
4. Mother is aware of the cause, treatment, and prognosis of the symptoms common to pregnancy that she is experiencing.
5. Mother should be aware of the methods for infant feeding (breast or bottle) and the advantages or disadvantages of each; if she chooses to breast-feed, she begins preparation of breasts.
6. Mother (father) participates in educational programs for childbirth and parenthood that meet her (his) needs.
7. Record findings, therapies, and add these to the data base.

NURSING INTERVENTIONS

Diagnostic	Therapeutic and educational
1. Patient is weighed, BP taken, and urinalysis for glucose and albumin obtained on sample brought by patient.	1. Abnormal symptoms or laboratory test results require initiation of additional therapy.
2. Patient is asked to remove outer clothing; she may keep her panties on if pelvic examination is not necessary.	a. Nausea and vomiting: If persisting beyond twelfth week, these may be indicative of hyperemesis gravidarum, and specific medical therapy is indicated.
3. Nurse assists physician (nursing practitioner) with physical examination.	b. Common cold: Discuss need for increased rest, fluid intake, hot or cold steam inhalations, increased head elevation when reclining.
a. Check height of fundus.	c. Gastroenteritis: If severe, physician may request stool sample in addition to encouraging increased fluid intake, instruct in careful personal hygiene, and plan protection for other family members (diarrhea in newborn can be anticipated problem in families with little understanding of control of infections).
b. Determine amount of participation parents desire in childbirth and whether parent craft classes are appropriate.	d. Anemia: If Hct is >30%, physician may prescribe a type of iron preparation; if <30%, physician may order additional blood test for reticulocytes, corpuscular volume, Hgb, hemoconcentration, and cell pattern determination (if patient is black) as a basis for further treatment.
c. Consider current family happenings and their effect on patient.	e. Positive serologic tests: Physician institutes specific therapy.
d. Appraise patient's knowledge of infant care, including methods of feeding.	2. Problems common to first and second trimester require treatment.
e. Identify problems that patient may be experiencing.	a. Constipation:
	(1) Physician may order laxative (e.g., milk of magnesia, 30 ml hs prn), suppository to be inserted rectally at usual time of bowel movement, e.g., visacodyl (Dulcolax), or stool softener, e.g., dioctyl sodium sulfosuccinate (Colace) tablets, 2 hs prn.

PLAN OF CARE: ANTENATAL PERIOD—FIRST AND SECOND TRIMESTERS—cont'd

NURSING INTERVENTIONS—cont'd

Diagnostic	Therapeutic and educational
	(2) Review physical basis of problem (e.g., steroid sex hormones reduce motility of bowel, faulty bowel habits, faulty dietary and fluid intake practices).
	(3) Instruct patient regarding bowel habits (privacy, timing), diet (including fluids), and exercise.
	b. Heartburn:
	(1) Physician may order antacid (e.g., aluminum hydroxide gel). (NOTE: Tums contain sodium; therefore caution patient regarding excessive use of this or other sodium preparations.)
	(2) Review physical basis (e.g., steroid sex hormones cause lessened motility of stomach and relaxation of cardiac sphincter).
	(3) Instruct about diet, i.e., small, more frequent meals and decreased intake of fatty foods.
	c. Increased skin pigmentation:
	(1) Review physical basis (e.g., increased production of anterior pituitary hormone melanotropin causes increased brownish pigmentation of skin).
	(2) Inform patient about prognosis for "mask of pregnancy" (facial melasma, chloasma), which fades after delivery.
	3. Care of breasts and nipples if breast-feeding is contemplated:
	a. After regular bathing using minimum of soap, dry with rough towel. This usually will be all nipples will require.
	b. If woman has flat or inverted nipples, she may pull nipple out until it stands erect twice daily (pull only until it is uncomfortable, not painful). Pure lanolin ointment (e.g., baby oil) can be massaged into nipple as lubricant.
	4. Counseling for emotional tension should be related to problem involved.
	a. Sexual relationships with spouse: Normalcy of changes in sexuality must be emphasized. Give information about safe and unsafe sexual practices and provide patient with pertinent reference materials. Freedom to discuss these problems openly must be encouraged.
	b. Changes in self-image: As body contours change, doubts as to attractiveness may occur. Listening, complimenting patients on their appearance, instruction in antenatal exercises aimed at figure control, diet, and weight gain can be tried for effectiveness; concern over ability to be a "good mother" can begin in second trimester. Discuss with patient her concepts regarding "mothering." Note her expectations and how realistic they are.
	c. Complaints of "nervousness": Assess what she means by this term. Emphasize naturalness of anxiety and stress response in all life situations; determine how she has coped with her nervousness previously.

PLAN OF CARE: ANTENATAL PERIOD—THIRD TRIMESTER

PATIENT CARE OBJECTIVES
1. Physical findings, maternal and fetal, are indicative of normal progress.
    a. Maternal findings:
        (1) Temperature: normal range.
        (2) Pulse: gradual rise to +8 to +10 by thirty-fifth week.
        (3) Respirations: 18 to 20/min; may be difficult in prone position.
        (4) Blood pressure: systolic and diastolic no greater than +15 over baseline, which is normally higher (+6 to +10) as term approaches.
        (5) Weight gain: no more than 1 pound/wk.
        (6) Urinalysis: no albumin; no greater than 1+ glucose; lactose present as hormone prolactin increases.
        (7) Readiness for labor:
            (a) Patient may be conscious of Braxton Hicks contractions by thirty-fourth week.
            (b) Cervix becomes softened as term approaches.
            (c) In multiparous patient, external os of cervix may be about 3 cm dilated by thirty-fifth week.
            (d) Engagement occurs about 2 weeks prior to term in a primigravida; may not occur until labor is well established in multigravida.
    b. Fetal findings:
        (1) Gestational age and growth: Height of fundus, abdominal growth, and estimation of weight are within normal limits for estimated gestational age.
        (2) Presentation and size of infant permit vaginal delivery.
        (3) FHT, rate, and rhythm are normal (120 to 160 beats/min and regular).
2. Assessment of emotional responses to pregnancy and those relating to self-image, relationship with significant others, and relationship with child to be born indicates normal responses typical of pregnancy.
3. Medical and nursing care has been increased to permit detection of normal response, maternal or fetal. The patient is examined every 2 weeks between 32 and 36 weeks and every week between 36 and 40 weeks; if indicated, plan of care is modified.
4. Patient is aware of what abnormal symptoms might occur, to whom to report findings, and measures that she can institute.
5. Patient is aware of cause, treatment, and prognosis of problems common to third trimester of pregnancy.
6. Preparations for delivery have been made by thirty-sixth week. Patient is aware of process of labor, what care is needed, and types of pain relief available; knows symptoms of impending labor, whom to contact, and what information to give; and has made arrangements for either hospital or home delivery.
7. Records are completed and made available to personnel responsible for labor and delivery.

NURSING INTERVENTIONS

Diagnostic	Therapeutic and educational

1. Physical assessment by physician and nurse.
  a. Maternal: Procedures and examinations used in first and second trimesters are continued. Pelvic examination is also made on weekly visits from thirty-eighth week to term to permit evaluation of amount of cervical softening, effacement, and dilatation and station of presenting part.
  b. Fetal:
    (1) Additional measures other than palpation may be employed to determine presentation, position, and size of infant (e.g., ultrasonography, radiography, and area of maximum density of fetal heartbeat).
	1. If maternal or fetal complications are detected that preclude normal labor and delivery, modifications of original plan of care are necessary. Patient and fetus are in jeopardy, and specific remedial interventions are indicated.
	2. Patient should be instructed in second trimester to report following symptoms immediately:
	  a. Vaginal bleeding:
	    (1) Rule out brownish spotting occurring 48 hours after vaginal examination.
	    (2) Rule out "show" of pinkish stained mucus. Patient to come to emergency area of hospital immediately for diagnosis and treatment if not one of above.
	  b. Persistent headache, with epigastric pain, double vision, edema of face and fingers, and sudden gain in weight (more than 2 pounds in 1 week). Patient to come to clinic or physician's office for evaluation.
	  c. Cessation or noticeable dimunition in amount of fetal movement. Patient to come to clinic or physician's office for evaluation.
	  d. Rupture of membranes. Patient to come to hospital for evaluation and to rule out prolapse of cord.
	  e. Burning or pain on urination. Patient to come to clinic or physician's office for evaluation and bring urine sample for analysis.

PLAN OF CARE: ANTENATAL PERIOD—THIRD TRIMESTER—cont'd

NURSING INTERVENTIONS—cont'd

| Diagnostic | Therapeutic and educational |

(2) Precise calculations of fetal age may be made by using various techniques.
2. Nursing assessment of patient in following areas:
    a. Emotional status, e.g., anxiety about labor and control of pain.
    b. Knowledge and understanding of labor process and symptoms of beginning labor.
    c. Understanding of responsibilities related to preparing for hospital or home delivery.
    d. Preparation for care of family at home. Report to physician.
    e. Plans for postnatal care of infant.

f. Chills and/or elevated temperature. Report to physician.
g. Abdominal pain. Report to physician.
h. Persistent nausea and vomiting. Report to physician.
3. Instructions are given concerning preparation for delivery.
    a. Symptoms of impending labor and what information to report are reviewed and are as follows:
        (1) Uterine contractions: Report frequency, duration, and intensity. Primigravidas are usually counseled to remain at home until contractions are regular and 5 minutes apart. Multigravidas are counseled to remain at home until contractions are regular and 10 minutes apart. If woman lives more than 20 minutes from hospital or has history of rapid labors, these instructions are modified accordingly.
        (2) Rupture of membranes (see opposite page).
        (3) Bloody "show" or a mucous plug is noted early in labor. "Show" is scant, pink in color, and sticky (contains mucus).
    b. If patient is not attending classes in preparation for parenthood, clinic or office nurse assumes responsibility for instruction in process of labor and what care to expect; methods to control pain, e.g., analgesia and anesthesia and breathing-relaxing techniques; responsibilities of patient's spouse, family member, or friend who will be accompanying her through labor and delivery; and the care of newborn, i.e., clothing, feeding, and daily hygienic care.
    c. If hospital delivery is planned, patient is required to register at hospital of choice. Most hospitals now provide pamphlets containing information such as where to report when labor begins, policies pertaining to visitors, and visiting hours and also conduct tours of facilities to be used.
4. Treatment of problems common to third trimester:
    a. Hemorrhoids: Review physical basis and instruct in avoiding constipation, use of sitz baths, cold witch hazel compresses, or Tucks.
    b. Varicosities: Review physical basis and discuss prognosis for varicosities remaining after birth of child, i.e., if familial problem may remain; if not, possibility of disappearance good. Instruct in use of support hose and avoiding use of round garters, knee-highs, or anklets with tight tops; suggest raising foot of bed at night, resting during day with legs elevated, and avoiding sitting with knees crossed.
    c. Leg cramps: Review physical basis and instruct in alternating rest and activity; use of support hose (when at home, three ordinary weight stockings can be worn simultaneously as effective support hose); how to perform dorsiflexion of foot, remembering *not* to stretch leg with toe pointing downward; suggest standing on cold surface. If pain is decreased by measures just noted, massage and local heat may speed relief. If pain intensifies (Homan sign), woman should not massage or knead muscle but refer to her physician immediately, since pain may be due to thrombophlebitis or thrombus formation.
    d. Hypermobility of joints: Review physical basis and instruct in use of well-fitted girdle that supports fetus from below and does not restrict breathing.
    e. Backache: Review physical basis and instruct in pelvic tilting and rocking to relieve strain (Fig. 14-10), careful attention to posture (most individuals stand with their body weight unevenly distributed on favored foot, resulting in distortion of spine, which compounds problem), care in using good body mechanics when lifting or moving objects (e.g., 2-year-old child).
5. Instruct about care of breasts and nipples if breast-feeding is contemplated.

Continued.

PLAN OF CARE: ANTENATAL PERIOD—THIRD TRIMESTER—cont'd

NURSING INTERVENTIONS—cont'd

Diagnostic	Therapeutic and educational

	6. Counseling for emotional tensions:
	  a. These often relate directly to childbirth experience (e.g., anxiety about pain or possible delivery of child before reaching hospital). Nursing strategies include providing opportunity for discussing specific fears or anxieties, helping patient make definite plans for what she will do when labor starts, repeating instructions willingly, and having "sharing sessions" with recently delivered mothers. If possible, involve significant others in preparation for birth and arrange to have them participate in supportive way during labor and delivery; this may be effective in allaying or diffusing anxiety.
	  b. Other tensions relate to responsibilities of soon-to-be-assumed role of parent. Promote discussions with other mothers, help patients to have reasonable and attainable expectations of their role, involve other family members as prospective child-care aides, give anticipatory guidance regarding possible conflicts of new mother to minimize problems in postnatal period.
	  c. Husband-wife relationships.

REFERENCES

Clark, A. L., and Affonso, D. 1976. Childbearing: a nursing perspective. Philadelphia, F. A. Davis Co.

Curtis, F. 1974. Observations of unwed pregnant adolescents. Am. J. Nurs. **74**:101.

Ernst, E. K., and Forde, M. P. 1975. Maternity care: an attempt at an alternative. Nurs. Clin. North Am. **10**:241.

Grimm, E. 1967. Psychological and social factors in pregnancy, delivery and outcome. In Richardson, S. A., and Guttmacher, A. F. (eds.). Childbearing: its social and psychological aspects. Baltimore, The Williams & Wilkins Co.

Haycel, L. 1974. Ethnography of home birth in the San Francisco Bay area. Unpublished master's thesis, California State University, Hayward, Calif.

Huttel, F. 1972. A qualitative evaluation of psychoprophylaxis in childbirth. J. Psychosom. Res. **16**:81.

Reud, D. F., and others. 1972. Principles and management of human reproduction. Philadelphia, W. B. Saunders Co.

Tanzer, D., and Black, J. 1972. Why natural childbirth? Garden City, N.Y., Doubleday & Co., Inc.

UNIT FIVE

Interferences

CHAPTER 15

High-risk pregnancy

A high-risk pregnancy is one in which the mother or fetus has a significantly increased chance of morbidity, mortality, or both before, during, or until 29 days after birth or an increased chance of subsequent disability. The infant may be threatened by a host of maternal and perinatal problems. Maternal death or serious sequelae usually occur within a month of delivery because of obstetric complications but morbidity or mortality of the child may ensue months or years after birth.

A better understanding of human reproduction has greatly reduced maternal morbidity and mortality, although there is still much to be done. In contrast, fetal and neonatal morbidity and mortality have not shown this dramatic decrease, since knowledge of fetal and neonatal disorders has lagged far behind. The full significance and impact of these problems are only now being recognized.

Of the 5 to 10 million pregnancies that occur in North America each year, 2 to 3 million terminate as spontaneous abortions. Many of these are due to genetic faults or infection. Purposeful interruption of about 1 million early gestations add to the attrition. Approximately 3.5 million pregnancies reach viability (24 to 25 weeks' gestational age), but of these at least 45,000 fetuses fail to survive. About the same number of infants die during the first month of life. Another 40,000 babies have severe but perhaps correctable congenital anomalies. Pregnancy and delivery complications are responsible in part at least for approximately 90,000 mentally retarded individuals. These complications have partially handicapped another more than 150,000 persons who have difficulty coping in our complex society.

Even considering fetuses who have reached viability, perinatal mortality exceeds that of all other causes of death combined until 65 years of age. When viewed in this perspective, high-risk pregnancy presents one of the most critical and urgent problems of modern medicine.

A new social emphasis on the quality rather than the quantity of life has developed. Family planning has reduced family size and unwanted pregnancy. With these

trends, the wanted child has become increasingly important. As a consequence, constant periodic maternal and perinatal assessment is essential to emphasize safe delivery of normal infants who may develop to their maximal potential.

PSYCHOSOCIAL FACTORS
Emotional aspects of pregnancy

Pregnancy and delivery are anxious periods for many women because of ill-founded fear and misinformation, and many disorders of maternity patients are aggravated by anxiety. Although pregnancy may be complicated, with proper counsel and good natal care, serious problems are uncommon. For example, to facilitate bonding or attachment to a prematurely born infant, the mother may be enlisted for partial care of her baby, even though the infant is in an isolette.

Race

Small parents usually have small babies, evidenced by people in Southeast Asia as contrasted with larger individuals in Scandinavia. Moreover, black mothers as a group have smaller newborns than whites. Although race has some bearing on the problem of the underweight infant, socioeconomic differences may be even more important in consideration of prematurity (birth at less than 36 weeks' gestational age or a birth weight of less than 2500 gm). When opportunities are equalized, race becomes a lesser factor.

Occupation and income

Occupation of the father particularly relates to the incidence of abnormally early birth and low birth weight infants. Specifically these problems are increased in individuals with menial occupations and limited income. Maternity ward patients have a 50% higher incidence of low birth weight infants than do private patients. Moreover, women with only a grade school education have twice as many growth-retarded newborns as college women. Lack of money to purchase the necessities of life is a factor in poor general health and thus in poor maternal performance. However, it is difficult to incriminate insufficient funds per se because lack of education and lower socioeconomic status are usually notable also. Educational and socioeconomic advantages tend to be equated with a healthier life and progeny.

Teenage mothers

The age of first pregnancy is decreasing, and many new mothers are teenagers. The adolescent girl, married or not, suffers from lack of emotional, intellectual, and physical maturity and all that this implies. For these reasons, she and her partner may be incapable of properly responding and adjusting to the complex problems of pregnancy, the establishment of a home, and the development of self-sufficiency required to rear a family. Thus teenage unions, even for those who are married, often end in abandonment or divorce.

Frequently, pregnancy signals the beginning of a "syndrome of defeat" for the teenager: failure to complete high school education, failure to achieve economic independence, failure to establish a stable family unit, and failure to exploit available contraceptive methods.

As a result, the pregnant teenager has many more problems than the average married woman. Inadequate antenatal nutrition is a documented problem in the adolescent. One must expect an increase in the incidence of anemia, vaginitis, gonorrhea, urinary tract infection, and poor weight gain during gestation.

The duration of labor is about average for the pregnant adolescent, but babies generally are slightly smaller than those of older women. Twice as many infants weighing less than 1500 gm are born of teenage mothers as to older mothers. Unmarried mothers have many more low birth weight infants than married mothers. Moreover, the perinatal mortality of children born to married women is about half that of unmarried women.

An adolescent mother has many problems, especially when she is unsupported. These include lack of knowledge about how to care for the baby at home, how the baby will change her life-style, and what she must do for herself as a new mother. Therefore it is important to help adolescents think through the problems and seek assistance for them through social agencies. In keeping with the precept that there is an ideal time for every function, with few exceptions, teenage pregnancy is a serious personal, social, and medical misadventure.

MATERNAL FACTORS

Serious biologic handicaps, health problems, obstetric disorders, and social deprivation may compromise the infant in subtle or more obvious ways. Early or late fetal damage may occur. The baby may be small for gestational age (SGA), preterm, or postterm. Occasionally the infant may be preterm but of excessive size. In other instances, the postterm infant may be large. Such hazards and their management constitute unique perinatal problems.

One must identify early those who may have a greater likelihood of pregnancy complications. Careful continuing evaluation during pregnancy will minimize completely unexpected serious complications. If abnormal trends develop, disorders can be anticipated, and prompt treatment may eliminate or reduce the difficulty. Everyone in the health care delivery system should complement the physician's efforts in the promotion of maternal and fetal health, particularly in stressful social situations or during illness that may compromise mother and infant.

High-risk factors that contribute to perinatal morbidity and mortality are numerous. Some categorizations are unduly complex. The following is a reasonably inclusive list of associations that should aid in the identification of high-risk patients:

1. History of any of the following:
   a. Hereditary abnormality (e.g., osteogenesis imperfecta, Down's syndrome)
   b. Premature or small-for-dates infant (most recent delivery)
   c. Congenital anomaly, anemia, blood dyscrasia, preeclampsia, and other conditions
   d. Severe social problem (e.g., teenage pregnancy, drug addiction)
   e. Long-delayed or absent antenatal care
   f. Younger than 18 or older than 35 years
   g. Teratogenic viral illness or dangerous drug administration in the first trimester
   h. Fifth or subsequent pregnancy, especially when the woman is 35 years of age or older
   i. Prolonged infertility or sequential drug or hormone treatment
   j. Significant stressful or dangerous events in the present pregnancy (e.g., critical accident, excessive exposure to irradiation)
   k. Heavy cigarette smoking
   l. Conception within 2 months of a previous delivery
2. Diagnosis of any of the following:
   a. Height under 60 inches or a prepregnant weight of 20% less than or over the standard for height and age
   b. Minimal or no weight gain
   c. Obstetric complications (e.g., preeclampsia-eclampsia, multiple pregnancy, hydramnios)

d. Abnormal presentation (e.g., breech, presenting part unengaged at term)

e. Fetus that fails to grow normally or is disparate in size from that expected

f. Fetus of more than 42 weeks' gestation*

Almost 20% of all maternity patients fall into the categories in the previous list. These high-risk conditions account for 50% of all perinatal deaths. However, most perinatal deaths are associated with only six obstetric complications:

1. Breech presentation
2. Premature separation of the normally implanted placenta
3. Preeclampsia-eclampsia
4. Multiple pregnancy
5. Pyelonephritis
6. Hydramnios

Harmful drugs, viral infections, and irradiation are pregnancy hazards also. Although difficult to estimate, personal or social problems, for example, lack of knowledge, poverty, or unwanted pregnancy, may be potent factors that compromise pregnancy and its outcome.

PATERNAL FACTORS

The father's influences on early birth and other manifestations of high-risk pregnancy are largely speculative. What genetic damage is sustained by chronic alcoholism or other drug abuse is unknown, for example. Small-for-dates infants are often reported, and the incidence of congenital anomalies may be slightly elevated when the father has diabetes mellitus or is a drug addict. Admittedly the mother may suffer some impairment also so that the responsibility may not be clear-cut.

Certain inheritable disorders such as Rh-D isoimmunization are traceable to the father.

FETAL FACTORS

Fetal factors that may jeopardize the infant include congenital anomalies, short cord, cord entanglement or compression, hydramnios, abnormal presentation or position, immaturity, prematurity, and fetal infection.

NEONATAL FACTORS

The period after delivery, especially the first hour, may be critical for the infant who must quickly and effectively adapt to extrauterine life. Problems of resuscitation, especially the establishment of a patent airway, and the reversal of undesirable drug effects, for example, those which occur after the administration of nalorphine

*Modified from Wigglesworth, R. 1968. "At risk" registers. Dev. Med. Child. Neurol. **10:**679, 1968.

(Nalline) or its equivalent as an antidote for narcotic overdosage, are particularly important. The early diagnosis and proper management of congenital anomalies such as tracheoesophageal fistula and myelomeningocele may be important also. The incidence of cerebral palsy, mental retardation, and other neurologic disorders depends in large measure on the skillful management of the intranatal and immediate neonatal period.

The following associations identified before and immediately after birth place the infant at increased risk and demand special observation and treatment of the child:

1. History in the mother of previously listed pregnancy factors, particularly the following:
   a. Prolonged rupture of membranes
   b. Abnormal presentation and delivery
   c. Prolonged, difficult labor or precipitous labor
   d. Prolapsed cord
2. Birth asphyxia as suggested by the following:
   a. Fetal heart rate fluctuations
   b. Meconium staining, particularly aspiration
   c. Fetal acidosis (pH below 7.2)
   d. Apgar scores less than 7, particularly if present at 5 minutes
3. Preterm birth (less than 38 weeks' gestation)
4. Postterm birth (more than 42 weeks' gestation) with evidence of fetal wasting
5. Small-for-dates infants (less than fifth percentile)
6. Large-for-dates infants (greater than ninety-fifth percentile), especially the large preterm infant
7. Any respiratory distress or apnea
8. Obvious congenital anomalies
9. Convulsions, limpness, or difficulty in sucking or swallowing
10. Distention, vomiting, or both
11. Anemia (less than 45% hemoglobin) or bleeding tendency
12. Jaundice in first 24 hours or bilirubin levels above 15 mg/100 ml

OTHER FACTORS

High altitude and poor obstetric performance together with other less well-understood high-risk factors must play a part in increased perinatal morbidity and mortality.

MANAGEMENT

Antenatal care is necessary to prevent, detect, and treat threatening maternal and fetal disorders. Hence antenatal care screens those patients who are jeopardized (high risk) from those who are not endangered (low risk). The system is only effective when it imposes a relentless search for problems that may threaten the pregnancy.

Individualized antenatal care for the identification of risk factors requires as a minimum the following:

- A carefully detailed history
- A thorough general physical examination
- Urinalysis and hematologic and other major diagnostic laboratory tests
- Frequent periodic fetal assessment
- Appropriate studies to appraise fetal well-being or fetal maturity

Once a diagnosis of high-risk pregnancy has been made, the following considerations are most important:

1. The obstetrician must anticipate the worst possible eventuality and prepare for this in the hope that this serious turn of events may not ensue.

2. All aspects of the case must be appraised with the realization that the studies must be appropriate in the overall management. No single test report must justify sudden conclusive action.

3. Intranatal monitoring, preferably the direct method, should be available and used to appraise fetal cardiac function, intrauterine pressure changes, and other functions. Fetal scalp sampling for a determination of blood pH should also be available when fetal hypoxic states develop.

4. Transfer of the patient to a maternity center should be arranged if a maternal-fetal intensive care unit is not available in the physician's local community. In most instances, the referring physician may continue as one of the patient's physicians, a member of the obstetric "team."

IDENTIFICATION OF HIGH-RISK FACTORS
Laboratory tests

Laboratory tests are essential for the detection or confirmation of abnormal or disease processes (risk factors). The following laboratory screening studies should be obtained as early as possible in pregnancy:

1. Hematocrit and hemoglobin
2. WBC
3. Differential blood count
4. Urinalysis
5. Culture of the urine (with bacterial sensitivities if 10^5 bacteria/ml is reported)
6. Serologic tests for pregnancy
7. Rubella antibody titer
8. Toxoplasmosis antibody titer
9. Blood grouping and Rh determination
10. Screening test for isoimmunization antibodies (Hemantigen or equivalent screening test)
11. Papanicolaou cervical and vaginal smears
12. Cervical and anal culture for *N. gonorrhoeae*

13. Test for sickle cell trait or disease, when appropriate

Pregnant patients 35 years of age or older have an increased incidence of bearing children with Down's syndrome (mongolism). For this reason, an amniocentesis should be performed at the fourteenth to sixteenth week of pregnancy to identify or exclude this genetic problem by tissue culture of fetal cells and chromosomal analysis. If Down's syndrome is diagnosed, the couple should be given the option of therapeutic abortion.

In a complicated pregnancy (e.g., diabetes mellitus), hormonal assessment of the pregnancy may be required. Environmental tests such as quantitative estriol levels in 24-hour urine specimens or in serum, human placental lactogen determinations, or amnioscopy may help to determine whether continuation of the pregnancy is reasonable. The OCT may be employed also to determine the fetal response to the simulated stress of labor (p. 304).

Other studies including maternal renal tests, Rh sensitization, and placental scanning may be necessary in specific cases.

Fetal maturity studies should also be done to determine when the infant at risk can survive extrauterine existence. In poorly controlled diabetes mellitus or in moderately severe isoimmunization, one may have to rescue the fetus because it may not survive if allowed to remain undelivered. (For diagnostic studies to indicate probable maturity, see Chapter 14.)

It is important to repeat the hematocrit or hemoglobin and the Rh-D antibody screening test at the twenty-eighth and the thirty-fourth week of pregnancy to note any significant change. Other tests may be obtained or repeated as indicated. Special studies for comprehensive fetal assessment are also required.

Periodic screening

A maternity patient with *any* significant problem is termed *high risk* in common parlance. To be logical and practical, however, it is apparent that the infant may be at greater risk because of certain factors as contrasted with others. Only those threatened by the most critical factors can really be called *high risk;* others of lesser magnitude then will be *moderate risk*.

To make these judgments, certain checkpoints during the continuum of maternity care should be identified to ensure that all serious risks will be identified for proper evaluation and treatment. The following timing may be employed.

1. Initial pregnancy screening examination
2. Antenatal screening at the time of office or clinic visits

3. Intranatal screening when the patient is admitted to the hospital or to the maternity intensive care area
4. Delivery evaluation, maternal and infant
5. Postnatal appraisal, maternal and infant

Patients at risk are then identified by established criteria at each checkpoint. The criteria for diagnosis of high-risk pregnancy are as follows:

I. Initial screening
   A. Biologic and maternal factors
      1. High risk
         a. Maternal age of 15 years or younger
         b. Maternal age of 35 years or older
         c. Massive obesity
      2. Moderate risk
         a. Maternal age of 15 to 19 years
         b. Maternal age of 30 to 34 years
         c. Nonwhite
         d. Single
         e. Obesity (more than 20% of standard weight for height)
         f. Malnutrition (less than 100 pounds)
         g. Short stature (60 inches or less)
   B. Obstetric history
      1. High risk
         a. Previously diagnosed genital tract anomalies
            (1) Incompetent cervix
            (2) Cervical malformation
            (3) Uterine malformation
         b. Two or more previous abortions
         c. Previous stillborn or neonatal loss
         d. Two previous premature labors or low birth weight infants (less than 2500 gm)
         e. Two excessively large previous infants (greater than 4000 gm)
         f. Maternal malignancy
         g. Uterine leiomyomata (5 cm or more or submucous)
         h. Ovarian mass
         i. Parity of eight or more
         j. Previous infant with isoimmunization
         k. History of eclampsia
         l. Previous infant with
            (1) Known or suspected genetic or familial disorders
            (2) Congenital anomaly
         m. Previous history of need for special neonatal-infant care or birth-damaged infant
         n. Medical indications for termination of previous pregnancy

      2. Moderate risk
         a. Previous premature labor or low birth weight infant (less than 2500 gm)
         b. One excessively large infant (more than 4000 gm)
         c. Previous operative deliveries
            (1) Cesarean section
            (2) Midforceps delivery
            (3) Breech extraction
         d. Previous prolonged labor or significant dystocia
         e. Borderline pelvis
         f. Previous severe emotional problems associated with pregnancy or delivery
         g. Previous uterine or cervical operations
         h. Primigravida
         i. Parity of five to eight
         j. Involuntary sterility
         k. Prior ABO incompatibility
         l. Prior fetal malpresentation
         m. Previous history of endometriosis
         n. Pregnancy occurring 3 months or less after last delivery
   C. Medical and surgical history
      1. High risk
         a. Moderate to severe chronic hypertension
         b. Moderate to severe renal disease
         c. Severe heart disease (class II to IV or a history of congestive heart failure)
         d. Diabetes (class B to F)
         e. Previous endocrine ablation
         f. Abnormal cervical cytology
         g. Sickle cell disease
         h. Drug addiction or alcoholism
         i. History of tuberculosis or PPD test reaction more than 1 cm diameter
         j. Pulmonary disease
         k. Malignancy
         l. Gastrointestinal or liver disease
      2. Moderate risk
         a. Mild chronic hypertension
         b. Mild renal disease
         c. Mild heart disease (class I)
         d. History of mild hypertensive states of pregnancy
         e. History of pyelitis
         f. Diabetes (class A)
         g. Family history of diabetes
         h. Thyroid disease
         i. Positive serology
         j. Excessive use of drugs

k. Emotional problems
l. Sickle cell trait
m. Epilepsy
II. Antenatal visit screening
  A. Early pregnancy
    1. High risk
      a. Failure of uterine growth or disproportionate uterine growth
      b. Exposure to teratogens
        (1) Radiation
        (2) Infection
        (3) Chemicals
      c. Pregnancy complicated by isoimmunization
      d. Need for antenatal genetic diagnosis
      e. Severe anemia (9 gm/100 ml or less Hgb) at sea level
    2. Moderate risk
      a. Unresponsive urinary tract infection
      b. Suspected ectopic pregnancy
      c. Suspected missed abortion
      d. Severe hyperemesis gravidarum
      e. Positive VDRL
      f. Positive gonorrhea screening
      g. Anemia not responsive to iron treatment
      h. Viral illness
      i. Vaginal bleeding
      j. Mild anemia (9 to 10.9 gm/100 ml Hgb) at sea level
  B. Late pregnancy
    1. High risk
      a. Failure of uterine growth or disproportionate uterine growth
      b. Severe anemia (9 gm/100 ml Hgb or less) at sea level
      c. Longer than 42½ weeks' gestation
      d. Severe preeclampsia
      e. Eclampsia
      f. Breech if vaginal delivery is planned
      g. Moderate to severe isoimmunization (necessitating intrauterine transfusion or neonatal exchange transfusion)
      h. Placenta previa
      i. Hydramnios or oligohydramnios
      j. Antenatal fetal death
      k. Thromboembolic disease
      l. Premature labor (less than 37 weeks' gestation)
      m. Premature rupture of bag of waters (less than 38 weeks' gestation)
      n. Tumor or other obstruction of birth canal

      o. Abruptio placenta
      p. Chronic or acute pyelonephritis
      q. Multiple gestation
      r. Abnormal OCT
      s. Falling urinary estriol levels
    2. Moderate risk
      a. Hypertensive states of pregnancy (mild)
      b. Breech if cesarean section is planned
      c. Uncertain presentations
      d. Need for fetal maturity studies
      e. Postdate pregnancy (41 to 42½ weeks)
      f. Premature rupture of the membranes (more than 12 hours without labor if gestation longer than 38 weeks)
      g. Induction of labor
      h. Suspected fetopelvic disproportion at term
      i. Floating presentations 2 weeks or less from EDC
III. Intranatal screening (on admission to the hospital or on admission to a maternity intensive care area)
  A. High risk
    1. Previous factors indicative of high-risk category
    2. Severe preeclampsia or eclampsia
    3. Hydramnios or oligohydramnios
    4. Amnionitis
    5. Premature rupture of membranes more than 24 hours before labor
    6. Uterine rupture
    7. Placenta previa
    8. Abruptio placenta
    9. Meconium staining of amniotic fluid
    10. Abnormal presentation
    11. Multiple gestation
    12. Fetal weight less than 2000 gm
    13. Fetal weight greater than 4000 gm
    14. Fetal bradycardia (longer than 30 minutes)
    15. Breech delivery
    16. Prolapsed cord
    17. Fetal acidosis (pH 7.25 or less in first stage of labor)
    18. Fetal tachycardia (longer than 30 minutes)
    19. Shoulder dystocia
    20. Fetal presenting part not descending with labor
    21. Evidence of maternal distress
    22. Abnormal OCT
    23. Falling urinary estriol levels
    24. Immature or intermediate L/S ratio or rapid surfactant test

B. Moderate risk
 1. Mild hypertensive states of pregnancy
 2. Premature rupture of membranes more than 12 hours before labor
 3. Primary dysfunctional labor
 4. Secondary arrest of dilatation
 5. Meperidine (Demerol), more than 200 mg
 6. Magnesium sulfate, more than 25 Gm
 7. Labor longer than 20 hours
 8. Second stage of labor longer than 1 hour
 9. Clinically small pelvis
 10. Medical induction of labor
 11. Precipitous labor (less than 3 hours)
 12. Elective induction
 13. Prolonged latent phase
 14. Uterine tetany
 15. Oxytocin (Pitocin) augmentation
 16. Marginal separation of the placenta
 17. Operative forceps
 18. Vacuum extraction
 19. General anesthesia
 20. Any abnormality of maternal vital signs
 21. Abnormal uterine contractions

IV. Postnatal criteria for risk

Postnatally mothers are closely observed in the delivery room for a brief interval before transfer to the postnatal recovery room where the vital signs, lochia, and other responses are observed carefully for the first 1 to 4 hours (fourth stage of labor).

 A. Specific factors that make mother high risk
  1. Hemorrhage
  2. Infection
  3. Abnormal vital signs
  4. A traumatic delivery

The infant is observed briefly in the delivery room, and an initial screening physical exam is completed. He is then transferred to the transitional nursery where all infants are admitted temporarily for transition care in incubators or under radiant warmers. Approximately 5% of infants born are of sufficient risk to transfer to a neonatal intensive care unit. Another 20% are at medium risk and receive special care. These include those who are disproportionate in weight, height, and gestational indices, light for length (ponderal index less than 2.25), or have bilirubin over 10 mg/100 ml. The following criteria are used to select high-risk infants for admission to neonatal intensive care units:

 A. Specific factors that make infant high risk
  1. Infants continuing or developing signs of RDS

  2. Asphyxiated infants (Apgar score of less than 6 at 5 minutes)
  3. Preterm infants (less than 33 weeks' gestation)
  4. Infants weighing less than 1600 gm
  5. Infants with cyanosis or suspected cardiovascular disease
  6. Infants with major congenital malformations requiring surgery
  7. Infants with convulsions, sepsis, hemorrhagic diathesis, or shock
  8. Meconium aspiration syndrome

 B. Additional factors indicating high risk
  1. Prematurity (weight of less than 2000 gm)
  2. Resuscitation required at birth
  3. Fetal anomalies
  4. RDS
  5. Dysmature infants with meconium staining
  6. Congenital pneumonia
  7. Anomalies of the respiratory system
  8. Neonatal apnea
  9. Other respiratory distress
  10. Hypoglycemia
  11. Hypocalcemia
  12. Major congenital heart anomalies that require immediate catheterization
  13. Congestive heart failure
  14. Hyperbilirubinemia
  15. Hemorrhagic diathesis
  16. Chromosomal anomalies
  17. Sepsis
  18. CNS depression for longer than 24 hours
  19. Seizures
  20. Persistent cyanosis

 C. Factors indicating moderate risk
  1. Dysmaturity
  2. Prematurity (weight between 2000 and 2500 gm)
  3. Apgar score at 1 minute less than 5
  4. Feeding problems
  5. Multiple birth
  6. Transient tachypnea
  7. Hypomagnesemia or hypermagnesemia
  8. Hypoparathyroidism
  9. Failure to gain weight
  10. Jitteriness or hyperactivity
  11. Cardiac anomalies not requiring immediate catheterization
  12. Heart murmur
  13. Anemia
  14. CNS depression for less than 24 hours

Research and experience have led to the identification of factors that jeopardize the pregnant and postnatal woman and the infant. This knowledge has permitted the development of increasingly effective preventive and therapeutic measures that could minimize the incidence of morbidity, disability, and death of the mother or infant. Frequently, it is the alert nurse, conversant and familiar with deviations from normal, who notes and reports potential or real high-risk factors. Nurses and physicians are in a position to be instrumental in education of the general populace in good health habits and good nutrition, which could reduce significantly the incidence of high-risk pregnancy.

REFERENCES

Anderson, J. M. 1965. High risk 'groups—definitions and identifications. N. Engl. J. Med. **272**:309.

Hall, M. H. 1974. Blood and neoplastic diseases: pregnancy anemia. Br. Med. J. **2**:661.

Hurley, R. 1974. Contemporary obstetrics and gynecology: viral diseases in pregnancy. Br. J. Hosp. Med. **12**:86.

Kazazian, H. H., Jr. 1972. Antenatal detection of sickle cell anemia. N. Engl. J. Med. **287**:41.

Lindheimer, M. D., and Katz, A. I. 1974. Managing the patient with renal disease. Contemp. Obstet. Gynecol. **3**:49.

Lynch, G. A. 1969. Breast cancer associated with pregnancy. Ulster Med. J. **38**:34.

Mabatoff, R. A., and Pincus, J. A. 1970. Management of varicose veins during pregnancy. Obstet. Gynecol. **36**:928.

McCorriston, C. C. 1973. Non-obstetrical abdominal surgery required during pregnancy. J. Abdom. Surg. **15**:85.

Messer, J. V. 1973. Heart disease in pregnancy. J. Reprod. Med. **10**:102.

Weisman, S. A., and others. 1973. Nephrotic syndrome in pregnancy. Am. J. Obstet. Gynecol. **117**:867.

White, K. C. 1973. Ovarian tumors in pregnancy: a private hospital 10-year survey. Am. J. Obstet. Gynecol. **116**:544.

Wilson, E. A., Dilts, P. V., Jr., and Simpson, T. J. 1973. Appendectomy incidental to postpartum sterilization procedures. Am. J. Obstet. Gynecol. **116**:76.

Wilson, E. A., Thelin, T. J., and Dilts, P. V., Jr. 1973. Tuberculosis complicating pregnancy. Am. J. Obstet. Gynecol. **115**:526.

CHAPTER 16

Hemorrhagic disorders

Hemorrhagic disorders in pregnancy represent one of three leading causes of both maternal and fetal death. These medical emergencies require expert teamwork on the part of physician and nurse to minimize the deleterious effects. The goals of therapy are as follows:

1. To prevent and/or control severe hemorrhage
2. To establish a diagnosis
3. To sustain the pregnancy if possible or feasible
4. To provide emergency care
   a. Replace blood loss
   b. Perform cesarean section
   c. Treat compromised infant, premature or full-term
5. To manage grief resulting from the loss of the infant or mother and/or loss of positive self-concept of mother

The nurse must be alert to the symptoms of hemorrhage and shock and be prepared to obtain necessary blood replacement and complete laboratory orders. (If there is not time for typing and matching of blood, group O Rh-negative blood may be ordered.) The patient and her family need much supportive care during these times of stress, including prompt attention to needs, competent technical care, and information regarding the rationale for care and the progress of treatment. The woman's inability to carry a pregnancy to term or to maintain a normal sequence of development to delivery often causes her to question her femininity and capabilities as a woman.

Early in pregnancy, abortion or ectopic pregnancy are the most common causes of excessive bleeding. Later, premature separation of the normally implanted placenta or placenta previa may cause hemorrhage.

EARLY PREGNANCY
Spontaneous abortion

General considerations. Abortion is the termination of pregnancy before viability of the fetus. The abortion may be spontaneous, resulting from natural causes, or the pregnancy may be interrupted deliberately for medi-cal reasons (therapeutic abortion) or for social reasons (elective abortion).

Viability is reached at about the twenty-fourth week of gestation, when the fetus weighs 600 gm or more. With excellent neonatal care, such an infant has at least a chance to survive. An early spontaneous abortion or miscarriage is one that occurs prior to 16 weeks' gestation; a late abortion is one occurring between 16 and 24 weeks' gestation. About three fourths of abortions occur before the sixteenth week of pregnancy, and the majority of these take place prior to the eighth week.

Pathogenesis. Recurrent (habitual) abortion is the loss of three or more previable pregnancies. More than half of all spontaneous abortions, which account for an attrition of at least 15% of all pregnancies, are due to fetoplacental developmental defects. Approximately 15% are due to maternal causes; the reasons for the remainder are speculative. Many very early pregnancies are lost for reasons unknown before the diagnosis of pregnancy is made.

Admittedly the exact cause(s) of spontaneous abortion may be difficult to ascertain, but the possibilities include the following:

1. *Fetoplacental*—chromosomal anomalies, abnormal placental implantation, and premature separation
2. *Maternal*—endocrine disorders, uterine maldevelopment, uterine tumors, sepsis, cervical incompetence, and trauma
3. *Other*—drug ingestion and irradiation

Clinical classification of abortion. A threatened abortion is a jeopardized pregnancy associated with cramps, bleeding, or both. Nonetheless, the pregnancy persists for a time at least.

Spontaneous abortion may be characterized as follows:

1. *Incomplete abortion*. Uterine bleeding and cramps develop and portions of the products of conception are passed. The flow of blood and pain persist, however. Slight patulousness of the cervix and irregular softening

of the slightly enlarged uterus suggest retained products of conception.

2. *Inevitable abortion*. Uterine hemorrhage, pain, dilatation, and effacement of the cervix persist, suggesting impending evacuation of the products of conception.

3. *Complete abortion*. The entire products of conception are expelled.

4. *Missed abortion*. After death in utero, the products of conception are retained for longer than a month. Loss of symptoms of pregnancy occur, discomfort is denied, and a brownish discharge may develop but no actual bleeding ensues. The cervix remains slightly patulous but firmer than before. The uterus shrinks in size and becomes irregularly firm. The adnexa are normal on examination.

An odorous discharge, fever, persistent bleeding, and a dilated cervix together with a soft boggy uterine corpus and adnexal pain or tenderness indicate infection.

Complications of abortion include the following:

1. *Uterine lithopedion, or ''womb stone.''* A missed abortion is retained for months or years during which time the products of conception have calcified.

2. *Carneous or blood mole*. The separated conceptus is surrounded by partially organized blood clot.

3. *Placental polyp*. Retained placental fragments are surrounded with fibrin and blood clot.

4. *Hemorrhage and/or sepsis*. Hemorrhage and sepsis (e.g., salpingitis, peritonitis) occur especially in induced (criminal) abortion and in neglected cases. Death may follow instrumentation and perforation of the soft, slightly enlarged uterus, or septicemia or septic emboli, may follow spontaneous incomplete abortion. Even mild infection may be followed by tubal occlusion and infertility.

Three stages of abortion are recognized, depending on the character of the implantation site:

1. *Early or decidual stage*. Until the sixth week of pregnancy, the conceptus, which is virtually surrounded by decidua, is poorly attached to the uterus.

2. *Intermediate or attachment stage*. From the sixth to twelfth week of pregnancy, the anchor villi in the chorion frondosum (area of the basal plate) become moderately well attached to the myometrium.

3. *Late or placental stage*. The placenta is fully formed after the twelfth week and is firmly attached to the uterus.

Frequently, the pregnancy will have been terminated for a week or so before signs or symptoms of abortion become definite. For this reason, it may be difficult to date the actual termination of pregnancy.

Clinical findings

Symptomatology. Persistent uterine bleeding and cramplike pain characterize abortion in progress. In the early or decidual stage of abortion, the symptomatology is only worrisome. During the intermediate or attachment stage of abortion, however, moderate discomfort and blood loss are expected because of the larger conceptus and adherence of portions of the placenta. The late or placental stage of abortion is typified by severe pain similar to that of labor because the fetus must be expelled. Bleeding is less than that of patients with an intermediate stage abortion because the placenta does not separate completely until after the fetus has been delivered. At this point, uterine contractions generally are strong, checking any brisk bleeding.

Laboratory findings

1. *Urine*. A negative or weakly positive urine pregnancy test is characteristic of abortion.

2. *Blood*. With considerable or persistent blood loss, anemia is likely (Hgb is less than 10.5 gm/100 ml). Sepsis may develop with incomplete or missed abortion. Temperature is greater than 100.4° F (38° C), and WBC is greater than 12,000/mm^3. An increased sedimentation rate is the rule with pregnancy, anemia, or infection.

Serum or plasma HCG pregnancy tests usually are equivocal in abortion.

3. *Endocrine studies*. HCG, estrogen, and progesterone titers are minimal or absent in established abortions.

4. *Vaginal cytology*. The diagnosis of a failing or terminated pregnancy often can be determined from vaginal smears taken from the lateral vaginal wall, then fixed and stained by the Papanicolaou or comparable method. Unfortunately this test is of only ancillary value.

X-ray findings. X-ray findings are not helpful in early abortion. In late, missed abortion, disordered skeletal continuity may be observed. Increased calcific density of the pregnancy should be expected in lithopedion.

Differential diagnosis. Abortion may be an obvious conclusion in pregnant women who are bleeding and in pain. In complicated cases or in those without accurate menstrual background information, however, the diagnosis may be obscure.

Ectopic pregnancy classically involves amenorrhea or menstrual changes, unilateral pelvic pain, uterine bleeding, and a sensitive adnexal mass. Decidua but no placental villi may be found on curettage.

In membranous dysmenorrhea, the patient suffers pain, uterine bleeding, and the passage of tissue, but none of the usual symptoms of pregnancy can be identified. Moreover, the cast will contain secretory endometrium but no pregnancy decidua or chorionic villi.

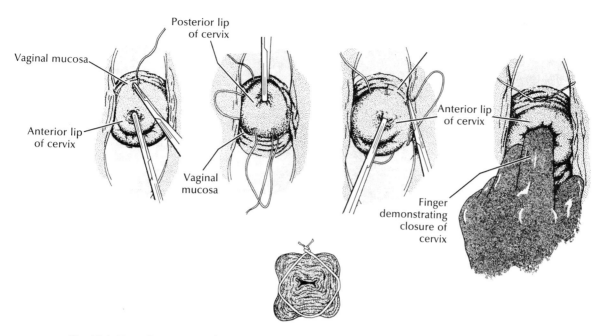

Fig. 16-1. *Top,* Correction of incompetent internal cervical os: McDonald operation. *Bottom,* View of closed internal os (cross section).

Prevention. Although little can be done to avoid genetic causes of pregnancy loss, prepregnancy correction of maternal disorders, immunization against infectious diseases, proper early antenatal care, and treatment of pregnancy complications will do much to prevent abortion.

Cervical incompetency, a cause of second trimester abortion, can be surgically corrected before or even during pregnancy in the majority of cases (Fig. 16-1).

Management. An early, accurate diagnosis is vital. In threatened abortion, bed rest, sedation, and avoidance of stress and orgasm are recommended. Further treatment will depend on the patient's course. There is no convincing evidence that estrogen and/or progestogen therapy is beneficial in threatened abortion. Actually the incidence of missed abortion is increased by such endocrine therapy.

Dilatation and curettage (scraping) are performed for incomplete abortion or to assure that all the decidua has been passed. For a discussion of dilatation and curettage see Chapter 6.

Hemorrhage and pain as a complication of first or second trimester pregnancy suggest an inevitable abortion, and prompt termination of the pregnancy is in order. A full history and a general and pelvic examination should be performed. Laboratory tests should include a complete blood count (CBC), blood-typing, and cross matching as well as urinalysis. Cervical cultures and sensitivity studies are important if sepsis is suggested. The passage of the entire product of conception or the recovery of all portions usually will alleviate discomfort and check heavy bleeding. Three or four doses of ergonovine, 0.2 mg orally or intramuscularly every 4 hours, should be given. If brisk bleeding resumes, the diagnosis probably is incomplete abortion rather than complete abortion, and surgical dilatation and curettage should be accomplished.

Patients who are more than 2 months' pregnant, who have had bleeding and cramping, and who have passed fragments of tissue (not an organized blood clot) should be hospitalized. Prompt medical evacuation of the uterus and limitation of blood loss may follow the administration of oxytocin, 1 ml (10 units) in 500 ml of 5% dextrose in water intravenously. Ergot products such as ergonovine, which contract the uterus and cervix, are contraindicated until the uterus is emptied.

If the entire product of pregnancy does not pass, a surgical dilatation and curettage should be accomplished using general or regional anesthesia. Then ergonovine, 0.2 mg intramuscularly or orally should be administered every 4 hours for three or four doses.

Broad-spectrum antibiotic therapy (e.g., ampicillin) should be given if infection seems likely. Transfusion may be required for shock or anemia.

Perforation of the uterus may require laparotomy. Septic thromboembolization may necessitate intensive anti-

PLAN OF CARE: SPONTANEOUS ABORTION

PATIENT CARE OBJECTIVES

1. Prevent or control severe hemorrhage. Replace blood loss, if any.
2. Prevent infection.
3. Maintain reproductive function.
4. Prevent Rh isoimmunization.
5. Manage grief resulting from loss.

NURSING INTERVENTIONS

Diagnostic	Therapeutic	Educational
Antenatal		
1. Observe for signs of abortion: vaginal discharge or bleeding, abdominal cramps. Note time of onset. 2. Observe for additional symptoms: shock, amount and location of pain. 3. Observe patient's response to treatment. 4. Note previous obstetric history. 5. Take history of this patient since last visit: drugs, activities, infections, etc.	1. Refer patient to physician stat; alert physician. 2. Save all tissue or clots passed so physician can institute appropriate treatment. 3. Give medications per order: sedatives, tranquilizers. 4. Order lab tests. 5. Facilitate rest: physical rest by pain medication; emotional rest by encouraging expression of feelings, answering questions. 6. Avoid accusatory responses: verbal, nonverbal.	1. Patient should know signs and symptoms and whom to call should they occur. 2. Teach patient regarding saving clots and tissue and bringing to physician. 3. If patient to be treated at home, teach about rest, diet, and avoidance of coitus or straining at stool.
Intranatal		

1. Note past obstetric history.
 2. Note progress and duration of this pregnancy.
 3. Observe current symptoms: vital signs; character of uterine consistency, cramping, vaginal discharge (save all bloodied material, keep pad count, save all vaginal discharge for physician to evaluate); note Rh.
 4. Note if patient had cerclage for incompetent cervix.
 5. Note patient's religious preference:
   a. Ask regarding baptism of products of conception.
   b. Ask regarding feelings about blood transfusions.
	1. Maintain calm, confident, sympathetic manner.
	 2. Alert physician if cerclage had been done earlier.
	 3. Avoid accusatory verbal responses (e.g., "You and your man been fooling around, eh?") or nonverbal responses.
	 4. Stay with patient and provide comfort measures used with women in labor.
	 5. Comfort family members.
	 6. Assist with treatments and procedures (e.g., blood transfusion, antibiotic therapy).
	 7. Prepare patient and family if D and C are contemplated.
	 8. Have products of conception baptized or have clergy there.
		1. Acquaint regarding treatments, procedures (e.g., what to expect during D and C).
		 2. Answer questions.

Postnatal		
1. Monitor physiologic responses: vital signs, bleeding, lab reports; response to blood transfusion, etc. 2. Assess patient and family's emotional responses to loss, medical-surgical care, and nursing management.	1. Administer physician-ordered medications and treatments. 2. Assist patient and family with emotional reactions (p. 243). 3. Give anti-D immune globulin within 72 hours if appropriate. 4. Notify clergy to visit if patient and family desire.	1. Acquaint patient regarding what to expect during recovery. 2. Teach patient regarding danger signs: fever, cramping, pain. 3. Provide information regarding contraceptives as appropriate.

biotic therapy, anticoagulation, and even ligation of the internal iliac veins or vena cava.

Missed abortion is best treated expectantly. If spontaneous evacuation of the uterus does not occur after 2 to 3 months, however, dilatation and curettage should be considered for pregnancies up to 3 months in duration. After this, intrauterine injection of hypertonic saline solution or $PGF_{2\alpha}$ and oxytocin intramuscularly or intravenously probably will be necessary. In unresponsive cases, anterior vaginal hysterotomy may be required to empty the uterus.

Disseminated intravascular coagulation and incoagulability of the blood with uncontrolled hemorrhage may develop in cases of fetal death after the twelfth week if the products of conception are retained for longer than 6 weeks. Plasma fibrinogen determination should be secured. If the level is 100 mg/100 ml or less and the patient is bleeding, heparin therapy to correct the coagulation defect may be necessary for several days prior to oxytocin stimulation and uterine evacuation. The coagulopathy should respond also to the administration of human fibrinogen intravenously. The incidence of serum hepatitis is high with this medication, however. Hence it is used now only in an emergency.

Late (second trimester) abortion may be chronic, even habitual. In many instances, this is due to a prior traumatic delivery or forceful dilatation and curettage of the cervix, with resultant occult laceration and *cervical incompetence*. Other instances may be due to a congenitally short cervix or anomalous uterus. In most of these cases, painless dilatation and effacement of the cervix and spontaneous rupture of the membranes without bleeding initiate labor. An immature fetus soon is delivered, but it generally does not survive. Correction of the weakened cervix is possible by wedge trachelorrhaphy in the nonpregnant patient. During gestation, a cerclage, band of homologous fascia, or nonabsorbable ribbon (Mersilene) may be placed around the cervix beneath the mucosa to constrict the cervix. Successful continuation of the pregnancy to viability or beyond occurs in the great majority of patients, provided the membranes remain intact and that the cervix is not more than 3 cm dilated or more than 50% effaced at the time of correction.

Prognosis. Correction of maternal disorders that may cause abortion usually is followed by a normal pregnancy.

Ectopic pregnancy

General considerations. Ectopic pregnancy is a gestation implanted outside the normal uterine cavity. Fully 90% of ectopic pregnancies occur in the fallopian tube, most of these on the right side, for undetermined reasons. Partial tubal obstruction or anomalies of the generative organs are major causes, and many women with ectopic pregnancy have infertility problems. Approximately 1 of every 200 pregnancies are ectopic and at least three fourths of these become symptomatic and are diagnosed during the first trimester. Ectopic pregnancy is a significant cause of maternal morbidity and mortality even in developed countries.

Pathogenesis. The majority of extrauterine pregnancies result from abnormalities that impede or prevent the transit of the fertilized ovum through the fallopian tube such as peritubal adhesions. Delayed implantation of the fertilized ovum after transmigration to one tube from the opposite ovary may be a cause of tubal pregnancy (Fig. 16-2). Nonetheless, ectopic gestations may be due to retention of the zygote within the ovary after fertilization of an unextruded ovum such as occurs in ovarian pregnancy. A rare fertilized ovum may be accommodated outside the uterine cavity, resulting in cervical or abdominal pregnancy (Fig. 16-3). Nidation has occurred despite almost insurmountable odds: more than thirty gestations have been described after hysterectomy and in the most unlikely sites, even in the lesser peritoneal cavity.

Pathology. The uterus is the only organ capable of containing and sustaining a term pregnancy. In the uterus, the trophoblast, which normally invades to the depths of the endometrium, is finally held in check by a fibrinoid zone, which forms to limit the eventual placenta. Meanwhile hypertrophy and hyperplasia of the myometrium allow increasing capacity of the uterus. A greatly augmented vasculature can maintain the pregnancy. Nitabuch's layer, a layer of fibrinoid material at the level of contact between the trophoblast and decidua, is either absent or deficient in organs like the fallopian tube or ovary, where the trophoblastic cells erode blood vessels and weaken the contiguous tissue to the point at which hemorrhage and/or rupture of the organ soon occurs. Moreover, the capacity of organs like a vestigial uterine horn is drastically limited. Hence advanced ectopic pregnancy is rare, and the delivery of a viable fetus that survives is exceptional. In tubal abortion after local hemorrhage, for example, subsequent implantation elsewhere in the abdominal cavity (secondary abdominal pregnancy) may occur, but proof that this occurs is still awaited.

Syncytotrophoblast cells produce HCG, and this hormone stimulates the early corpus luteum of pregnancy to produce progesterone. When abortion occurs, endometrial bleeding ensues secondary to progesterone with-

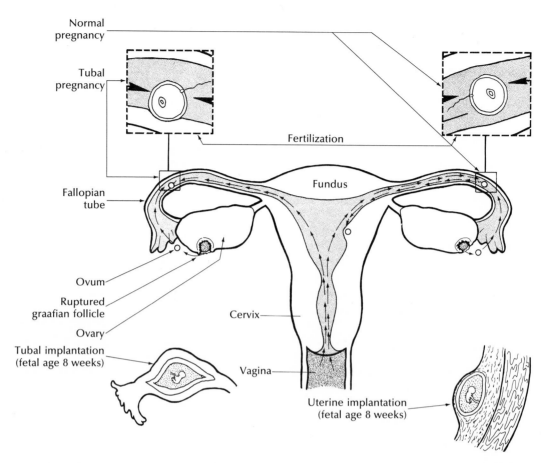

Fig. 16-2. Fertilization of ovum followed by normal implantation *(bottom right)* or abnormal implantation (ectopic) *(bottom left)*.

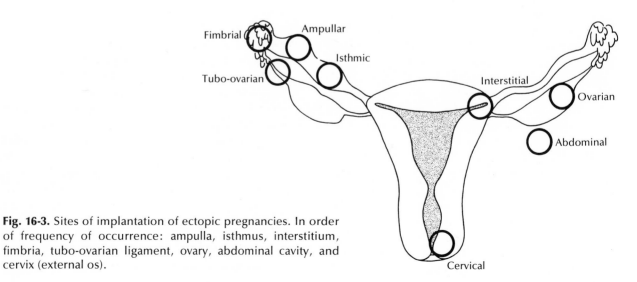

Fig. 16-3. Sites of implantation of ectopic pregnancies. In order of frequency of occurrence: ampulla, isthmus, interstitium, fimbria, tubo-ovarian ligament, ovary, abdominal cavity, and cervix (external os).

drawal. Vaginal bleeding associated with an aborting ectopic pregnancy is due to endometrial slough, a step in uterine involution. At times a decidual cast of the endometrial cavity may be passed, but because the pregnancy is extrauterine, no trophoblastic villi will be present—confirming an ectopic pregnancy. Only in a bleeding interstitial ectopic pregnancy can blood drain from the tube back through the uterus.

The sequel to a tubal pregnancy may be rupture through the wall of the tube and hematoperitoneum. Occasionally an early pregnancy may be extruded into the peritoneal cavity through the fimbriated extremity, and this may limit internal bleeding. An interstitial pregnancy may burst into the uterine cavity. An unusual abdominal pregnancy may rupture retroperitoneally, or even into a viscus such as the bowel or bladder.

Death of a more advanced fetus may be followed by mummification; if it calcifies, a lithopedion is the result. On rare occasions, an abdominal pregnancy may be diagnosed, and a living fetus is delivered by laparotomy. Far more often, however, the diagnosis is inaccurate, and the fetus dies because of abnormality, restriction, and/or placental insufficiency.

The unusual combination of intrauterine and extrauterine pregnancy (dizygous twinning) has been reported. Generally, the uterine gestation continues, but the ectopic pregnancy succumbs.

Clinical findings. There are no signs or symptoms diagnostic of early ectopic pregnancy. A missed period, adnexal fullness, and tenderness may suggest an unruptured tubal pregnancy. In contrast, the following triad is associated with early ruptured extrauterine pregnancy in almost 50% of cases:

- Amenorrhea or an abnormal menstrual period followed by slight uterine bleeding
- Adnexal or cul-de-sac mass
- Unilateral pelvic pain over the mass

Additional details may include shock, shoulder pain, or evidence of acute blood loss in chronic ruptured tubal pregnancy.

Hysterosalpingography is contraindicated in suspected tubal pregnancy because it may initiate tubal rupture or hemorrhage. In possible advanced abdominal pregnancy, x-ray films showing a fetus high out of the pelvis, often in abnormal presentation, may be diagnostic.

In chronic ruptured tubal pregnancy, which represents slightly more than half the total of ectopic pregnancies, internal bleeding usually has been slow and the symptomatology atypical or unconclusive. In addition to slight dark vaginal bleeding, a sense of pelvic pressure or fullness, lower abdominal tenderness, flatulence, and a tense, sensitive, semicystic, perhaps crepitant, cul-de-

sac mass may be felt. Slight fever, leukocytosis, and a falling hematocrit or hemoglobin level may be noted. An ecchymotic blueness of the umbilicus (Cullen's sign), indicative of hematoperitoneum, may develop in neglected ruptured intra-abdominal ectopic pregnancy.

Diagnosis. The following procedures are useful in the diagnosis of ectopic pregnancy:

1. A careful history with identification of a late LMP or an actual missed period followed by slight vaginal bleeding may be indicative.

2. Careful pelvic examination, under anesthesia, if necessary, reveals an adnexal or cul-de-sac mass.

3. Culdocentesis may yield free blood that will not clot (already clotted).

4. Culdotomy may release gross clotted blood, perhaps including the aborted products of an extrauterine pregnancy.

5. Laparoscopy may disclose an extrauterine pregnancy.

6. Dilatation and curettage will produce pregnancy endometrium, without chorionic villi in ectopic pregnancy. However, a uterine pregnancy or perhaps a threatened or incomplete abortion may be encountered.

7. Laparotomy will reveal the correct diagnosis and provide the best opportunity for treatment.

Differential diagnosis. The differential diagnosis of ectopic pregnancy involves a consideration of numerous disorders that share many, perhaps all, of the same signs and symptoms. One must consider uterine abortion (pp. 223 and 224), ruptured corpus luteum cyst, appendicitis, salpingitis, ovarian cysts, or torsion of the ovary, and urinary tract infection.

The diagnosis of salpingitis is as follows: A few days after sexual contact, perhaps just prior to a period, leukorrhea and dysurea are noted. Cervical or rectal smears or cultures for *N. gonorrheoea* may be positive. Pelvic pain that generally is bilateral develops. A tender adnexal mass (or masses) is poorly circumscribed, but the uterus is neither enlarged nor softened.

Appendicitis occurs without menstrual abnormality. Gastrointestinal complaints are notable. No pelvic mass will be felt unless an appendiceal abscess has developed.

Ovarian cysts or tumors are discreet, nonadherent, nontender, and generally larger than an asymptomatic tubal pregnancy. The mass of a ruptured tubal or ovarian pregnancy is adherent and painful.

An interstitial pregnancy results in an enlarged asymmetric, softened uterus. A myoma in the same area is firm as are the cervix and the uterus, and other nodules often are palpable.

Prevention. Prevention of ectopic pregnancy per se is

impossible. Early vigorous treatment of gonorrhea should prevent salpingitis or limit tubal disease. Prolonged bleeding or fever after supposed complete abortion should be treated by dilatation and curettage and antibiotic therapy to reduce the likelihood of postabortal salpingitis.

Management. The major problem in ectopic pregnancy is hemorrhage; bleeding must be quickly and effectively controlled. The physician must consider blood loss and impending shock. Blood transfusions must be available. Laparotomy may be effected immediately after the diagnosis of ectopic pregnancy is made. Blood and clots are evacuated, and bleeding vessels are controlled. Excision of the cornua and fallopian tube is rec-

ommended if the tube is grossly involved. The ovary should be conserved if possible. Hysterectomy usually is necessary for ruptured cornual or interstitial pregnancy.

Linear incision of the tube, salpingostomy, and evacuation of a small tubal pregnancy may be feasible in rare instances.

Ovarian pregnancy always requires sacrifice of the ovary, and the tube if the latter is densely adherent.

Prophylactic appendectomy or other elective procedures are permissible only if the patient's general condition is good, the procedure is not difficult, and the patient has given consent.

Chronic or advanced ectopic pregnancy requires

PLAN OF CARE: ECTOPIC PREGNANCY

PATIENT CARE OBJECTIVES
1. Patient's physiologic functions are restored.
2. Patient understands the anatomic and physiologic alterations resulting from the surgical intervention.
3. Patient retains a positive sense of self-esteem and self-worth.

NURSING INTERVENTIONS

Diagnostic	Therapeutic	Educational
Antenatal		
1. Observe for symptoms: colicky pain on affected side, severe pain and shock (with rupture).	1. Refer to physician stat; alert physician that patient is coming in to hospital.	1. Inform patient briefly of happenings.
2. Note significant data on past medical, surgical, and obstetric history: treatment for gonorrhea or other pelvic inflammatory disease, abdominal surgeries, previous spontaneous or voluntary abortions, previous ectopic pregnancies.	2. Alert lab and request blood work; type, cross match.	2. Reexplain (clarify, simplify) physician explanations regarding cause, management, and postoperative recovery, including chances for subsequent pregnancies.
3. Note patient's religious preference: ask patient (and/or family) regarding baptism of products of conception; blood transfusions.	3. Set up for administration of IV fluids (use large bore needle to accommodate blood if necessary), O_2, and emergency medications, with appropriate equipment. (Frequently, patients are admitted directly to surgery by way of emergency room.) Carry out preoperative procedures.	
4. Note patient's Rh to assess if candidate for anti-D immune globulin.		
Postnatal		
1. Assess physiologic response: vital signs, bleeding, reaction to therapy, elimination, etc.	1. Give anti-D immune globulin, if indicated.	1. Acquaint patient with what to expect during recovery.
2. Assess patient's and family's emotional reactions to experience.	2. Facilitate grieving process (p. 243).	2. Alert her to symptoms to report to physician immediately.
	3. Administer and monitor fluids, medications, treatments, and diet per physician order, patient preference, and tolerance.	3. Reinform patient regarding physician's explanations.
	4. Inform patient and family if baptism was done (also appears on nurses' notes).	
	5. Notify clergyman to visit if patient and family desire this.	

laparotomy as soon as the patient is fit for surgery. If the placenta of a second or third trimester abdominal pregnancy is attached to a vital organ, for example, the liver, no attempt at separation and removal should be made. The cord should be cut flush with the placenta and the afterbirth left in situ. Degeneration and absorption of the placenta usually occur without complications.

Prognosis. Maternal death due to ectopic pregnancy is now about 1 in 800 in North America. Maternal morbidity and second surgery is high, however, principally because of inaccurate or delayed diagnosis of ectopic pregnancy.

The perinatal mortality in ectopic pregnancy is virtually 100%.

Ectopic pregnancy recurs in approximately 10% of patients, but more than 50% of women who have had an ectopic pregnancy achieve at least one normal gestation thereafter.

Hydatidiform mole (hydatid mole)

Pathogenesis. Hydatidiform mole is a developmental anomaly of the placenta. The fertilized ovum deteriorates, and the chorionic villi convert into a mass of clear, grapelike vesicles of tapioca consistency.

Incidence. Hydatidiform mole occurs in 1 out of every 2000 spontaneous pregnancies; its highest incidence occurs with maternal aging (45 years of age or older). When clomiphene citrate (Clomid) has been used to stimulate ovulation, the risk of hydatidiform mole is increased to about 1 in every 650 pregnancies. This increased rate also may be related to maternal age, since the mean age of infertile women seeking this therapy is higher than the mean age of women having spontaneous pregnancies.

Clinical findings and diagnosis. The uterus becomes enlarged out of proportion to the duration of pregnancy; at 3 months, it may be the size of a 5-month pregnancy (Fig. 16-4). About the twelfth week, an intermittent or continuous brownish discharge is common.

No FHT can be heard nor can fetal parts be discerned on abdominal palpation. Ultrasonography reveals no fetal skeleton.

Hyperemesis gravidarum is encountered frequently. In addition, symptoms of true preeclampsia-eclampsia may

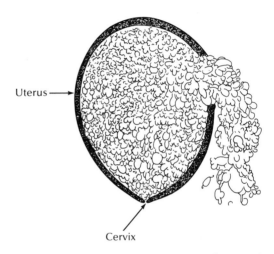

Fig. 16-4. Uterine rupture with hydatidiform mole.

PLAN OF CARE: HYDATIDIFORM MOLE

PATIENT CARE OBJECTIVES
1. Patient attains physiologic recovery from the molar pregnancy with an intact uterus, no choriocarcinoma, or both.
2. Patient retains a positive sense of self-esteem and self-worth.

NURSING INTERVENTIONS

Diagnostic	Therapeutic and educational
1. Observe for symptoms: excessive vomiting, hypertension, continuous or intermittent brown spotting or passage of grapelike vesicles, unusually rapid uterine enlargement.	1. Refer patient immediately to physician; alert physician of findings.
2. Observe patient's response to medical induction or surgical intervention: vital signs, pain, etc.	2. Prepare patient for diagnostic activities: sonography, serum HCG, induced abortion, possible D and C and/or hysterectomy.
3. Observe for signs of grief and grieving by patient and family. Assess patient's support system.	3. Assist physician with induction or other procedures.
	4. Facilitate patient and family's grief and grieving.
	5. Reinforce (clarify, simplify) physician's explanations regarding cause, management, and postdelivery long-term supervision. (Assist patient and spouse in deciding on contraceptive method suitable for them if patient retains uterus.)

occur even though it is well before the twentieth week of pregnancy.

HCG serum levels are high 100 days or more after the LMP.

Management. The uterus is evacuated by careful induced abortion, or hysterectomy is performed. Induced abortion may be followed by dilatation and curettage in a few days after the friable uterine wall becomes firmer. Curetted tissue is examined for residual or proliferative trophoblastic tissue. Hysterectomy is often the procedure of choice, especially if the woman is 45 years of age or older or if the uterus appears to be ready to rupture. Blood loss is replaced.

Follow-up supervision for 1 year includes cautioning the patient against conception for a year and measuring HCG at intervals. After termination of normal pregnancy, HCG is measured within 1 week; after hydatidiform mole, it is measured within 60 days.

Continued high titers or rising titers of HCG are pathologic. Dilatation and curettage are done if the uterus is intact, and the tissue is examined. If malignant cells are found, chemotherapy for choriocarcinoma is begun: methotrexate and dactinomycin are the drugs of choice. If chemotherapy is ineffective, the choriocarcinoma has a tendency toward rapid and widespread metastasis.

If HCG levels remain within normal limits for a year, the physician may assure the woman or couple that normal spontaneous pregnancy can be anticipated, with low probability of recurrence of hydatidiform mole if the woman is 40 years of age or younger.

LATE PREGNANCY
Premature separation of the placenta

Premature separation of the placenta is also termed *abruptio placentae, placental apoplexy, ablatio placentae,* and *accidental hemorrhage.*

General considerations. Premature separation of the placenta is that which occurs before the third stage of labor. Bleeding, apparent or concealed, always accompanies placental ablation. The source of bleeding is the maternal circulation from the uterine surface. Abruptio placentae is considered extensive separation, with retroplacental hemorrhage the most serious type of premature separation.

Certain individuals seem predisposed to premature separation of the placenta. This problem is much more common in women with hypertension of any cause and is found in greater numbers in deprived socioeconomic groups. Premature separation of the placenta occurs about once in 115 late gestations; about 80% are multiparas. The incidence is three times greater in women

with a gravidity of more than five than in primigravidas. Women with a history of reproductive wastage (abortion, premature labor, antenatal hemorrhage, stillbirth, or neonatal death) experience premature separation of the placenta more than twice as often as the average population at risk. Between 15% to 20% of women who have had a previous premature separation of the placenta will have a recurrence. If the patient has had two prior premature separations, the chance in the next pregnancy is at least 25%.

About 50% of patients suffer placental separation in the late third trimester prior to the onset of labor. Another 10% have a separation in the second stage of labor.

Premature separation of the placenta is a serious disorder and accounts for about 15% of all perinatal deaths. Approximately one third of infants of women with premature separation of the placenta will die. More than 50% of these succumb as a result of preterm delivery, and many die of hypoxia.

Pathogenesis. The pathogenesis for premature separation of the placenta is unknown in most cases, but a sudden increase or decrease in uterine size (as can occur with rupture of the membranes) may be responsible. Precipitating factors include vascular engorgement during the vena caval syndrome and sudden uteroplacental vasodilatation. Abdominal trauma is a factor in less than 5% of cases, and short cord is identified in less than 1%.

It has been suggested that anemia, defective folate metabolism, or folate deficiency may play a major role in the etiology of this condition; however, this is no longer accepted.

Pathology and pathophysiology. Gross examination of the placenta generally will reveal a retroplacental blood clot. Microscopic examination often discloses considerable intravillous thrombosis and degeneration of the syncytial trophoblast if preeclampsia-eclampsia is present also. In abruptio placentae, the extreme form, renal cortical necrosis, or cor pulmonale may occur.

Bleeding with premature separation of the placenta continues until the blood clots, the blood pressure falls to shock levels, the blood escapes internally into the amniotic cavity (the filling intrauterine cavity tamponades the bleeding surface), or the placenta separates completely and the uterus contracts to close the vessels beneath the placental site.

Confined (concealed) subplacental bleeding discharges into the endometrium. If this is extensive, the uterus loses its ability to contract, becomes ecchymotic, copper-colored, and ligneous (Couvelaire uterus). Concomitantly, disseminated intravascular coagulation occurs, whereupon the patient's blood becomes incoagulable. This defibrination syndrome also occurs with amniotic fluid embolism or septic abortion and after prolonged retention of a dead fetus.

Two types of premature separation of the placenta may be identified:

1. Marginal separation of the placenta with drainage of blood behind the membranes down through the cervix. (This so-called external bleeding generally is painless.)

2. Central separation of the placenta, with blood trapped behind the placenta and no external evidence of bleeding. (This is painful, concealed bleeding of abruptio placentae. Failure of blood coagulation occurs in 5% to 8% of serious cases of concealed bleeding.) The sequence is as follows:

   a. Bleeding with disruption of the retroplacental vascular bed results in necrosis of the decidua and gross localized clotting.

   b. Depletion of fibrinogen from the general circulation follows fixation of fibrinogen in clotted blood behind the placenta.

   c. If the peripheral blood fibrinogen falls to less than 100 mg/100 ml, free bleeding from all mucosal surfaces occurs. Extravasation of this blood into the myometrium causes a *Couvelaire uterus*. Couvelaire uterus is tetanic, ligneous, tender, and severely painful. Dysrhythmic or arrested labor occurs. Maternal shock out of proportion to the estimated blood loss is the rule, and fetal death is certain.

Degrees of placental separation and their clinical features are as follows:

1. *Grade 0 (approximately 30%).* No specific symptomatology is present. The diagnosis of premature separation is made after delivery when the placenta is examined, and a dark, adherent clot is found over a segment of placenta.

2. *Grade 1 (approximately 45%).* External bleeding often is present, but uterine tetany and tenderness may or may not be noted. No shock or fetal distress occurs. Grade 1 rarely progresses to grade 2.

3. *Grade 2 (approximately 15%).* External bleeding may be observed together with uterine tetany and tenderness. Fetal distress always is present, and fetal death may occur.

4. *Grade 3 (approximately 10%).* External bleeding may or may not be evident. Uterine tetany, maternal shock, fetal death, and a coagulopathy are typical.

Clinical findings

Symptomatology. Painless vaginal hemorrhage suggests unrestricted bleeding from the edge or a portion of the placenta.

Severe uterine pain, backache, regional tenderness, or fetal distress occurring prior to or during labor may indicate retroplacental hemorrhage. Shock; bleeding from the mouth, nose, or needle puncture sites; and loss of FHT indicate severe abruptio placentae and hypofibrinogenemia. The uterus may enlarge if the bleeding is concealed.

Occasionally patients with partial separation of the placenta will present the classic symptomatology described.

Laboratory findings. Hemoconcentration is likely. Anemia, particularly in concealed hemorrhage, may be noted later.

Hypofibrinogenemia may be confirmed by the following:

1. Failure of the blood to clot or a fragile clot after 1 hour in a Lee-White tube at 37° to 38° C

2. Poor coagulation or no clot with Fibrindex test after 1 minute (1 drop of reconstituted human thrombin added to 1 drop of the patient's plasma)

3. Fibrinogen determination (e.g., gravimetric test), 100 mg/100 ml of blood

X-ray findings. Radiography will not diagnose premature separation, but it may reveal placenta previa.

Differential diagnosis. The differential diagnosis of premature separation involves a number of disorders. Nonplacental disorders include cancer, varices, vaginitis or cervicitis, cervical polyps, blood dyscrasias, trauma, bloody show, or ruptured uterus. One must also eliminate the placental abnormalities of placenta previa and vasoprevia.

Prevention. If folate deficiency can be established as a cause of premature separation of the placenta, better nutrition and prevention of hypertension may be appropriate intervention. One must also include under prophylaxis careful rupture of the membranes (avoidance of sudden reduction in the size of the uterus) and early recognition of a short cord.

Management. Management must be aimed primarily at correcting blood loss and shock and preventing or ameliorating blood-clotting defects. *No matter how the patient is to be delivered, the membranes should be needled and gradual drainage of the amniotic fluid accomplished.* This decreases intrauterine tension, reduces the extravasation of blood into the myometrium if retroplacental hemorrhage has occurred, and lessens the possibility of amniotic fluid emboli. It may also reduce the total length of labor.

Following is the suggested management for the various grades of placental separation.

Grade 0. Management of labor and delivery is routine.

PLAN OF CARE: PREMATURE SEPARATION OF PLACENTA

PATIENT CARE OBJECTIVES
1. Blood loss is minimized and replaced.
2. Hypofibrinogenemia is prevented or successfully treated.
3. Normal reproductive functioning is retained.
4. The fetus is safely delivered.
5. Patient retains a positive sense of self-esteem and self-worth.

NURSING INTERVENTIONS

Diagnostic	Therapeutic	Educational
Antenatal		

1. Assess all women for predisposing factors: hypertension, multiple gestation, vena caval syndrome, diabetes, short cord, multiparity, advanced maternal age.
2. Observe for signs of premature separation (may occur during labor):
  a. Vaginal bleeding or port-wine colored amniotic fluid.
  b. Shock: drop in BP, increase in pulse, dyspnea, pallor, syncope. Symptoms are often out of proportion to amount of bleeding seen.
  c. Pain: may be severe and sudden (if retroplacental) or painless (if separation is marginal and blood drains out through vagina).
  d. Uterine contractions: during labor, uterus may not contract evenly or relax between contractions.
  e. Abdomen: may or may not be rigid (if bleeding can exit, uterus is not rigid); myometrium becomes boardlike (Couvelaire).
  f. Hyperactivity of fetus with onset of pain may be followed by loss of FHT. Use electronic monitor if available.
3. Observe for complications: shock, pulmonary emboli, hypofibrinogenemia, puerperal infection, hemorrhage, Couvelaire uterus, acute renal failure.
	1. Encourage side-lying position during labor to avoid pressure on vena cava. Instruct regarding breathing and other techniques while in side-lying position.
	2. If symptoms are noted:
	  a. Send for physician.
	  b. Turn patient onto her side; administer O$_2$ per face mask; start IV or increase flow (if IV does not have oxytocin in it!); raise legs, avoiding Trendelenberg position (p. 241).
	  c. Do not leave patient.
	  d. Have someone request lab work: type, cross match.
	  e. Prepare for abdominal surgery (cesarean section, hysterectomy) or for immediate vaginal delivery, if cervix is dilated and presenting part is low.
	3. Alert pediatrician to be present for delivery. Infant may require attention for prematurity, hypoxia, birth injury due to interventions.
	4. Allow no rectal or vaginal examinations after any suspicious symptoms occur. No enema!
		1. Teach patient regarding benefits of side-lying position.
		2. Briefly explain to mother's family what is occurring.

Postnatal		

1. Ascertain following:
  a. If hysterectomy was performed.
  b. If fetus succumbed.
  c. If neonate is alive, its condition.
2. Assess physiologic response: amount of bleeding, vital signs, gastrointestinal functioning, urinary function. If uterus was retained, check height of fundus and contractility. Observe for reaction to fibrinogen if this was given.
3. Assess patient and family's emotional response to experience.
	1. Administer medications per order for discomfort, infection, anemia, uterine atony. Monitor IV fluids.
	2. Report oliguria or hematuria so that therapy for acute renal tubular necrosis (may be reversible) or bilateral renal cortical necrosis (may be fatal) can be started promptly if either of these diagnoses is made.
	3. Assist patient and family with grieving.
		1. Reinforce physician's explanation regarding cause, management, prognosis.

Grade 1. If the patient is not at term and not in labor, observe for further bleeding, fetal distress, and other problems. Have blood typed and cross matched, ready for possible transfusion. If the patient is in mild labor, allow labor to proceed. Stimulate cautiously if necessary. Monitor FHT during labor. If fetal distress develops, cesarean section may be performed. If labor progresses satisfactorily and no fetal distress is noted, the patient may be permitted to deliver from below, assuming normal pelvic measurements.

In patients with abruptio placentae, central venous pressure (CVP) monitoring, shock therapy, continuous oxygen administration, and even digitalis may be necessary. Forceps delivery for the shortening of the second stage of labor may be helpful. Narcotics may be given for severe pain.

With hypofibrinogenemia, correction of any coagulopathy will be necessary before surgery. Otherwise uncontrollable bleeding may ensue and exsanguination may result. Cryoprecipitate may be administered in amounts sufficient to restore coagulation mechanisms. Cryoprecipitate contains both fibrinogen and factor VIII. Therefore it is more effective in restoring normal coagulation than lyophilized fibrinogen. Additionally cryoprecipitate has the advantage of minimizing the transmission of serum hepatitis (about 20% of patients who receive fibrinogen acquire homologous serum hepatitis). If cryoprecipitate is unavailable, fresh frozen plasma, platelets, or both may be given. Occasionally, when the uterus cannot be emptied or when there is continued disseminated intravascular coagulation, heparin therapy will be necessary. Heparin should be administered only after appropriate investigative studies, however, and usually in consultation with a hematologist.

Grade 2. Cesarean section is indicated if the fetus does not seem to be seriously jeopardized. If the fetus is dead, vaginal delivery may be allowed if rapid labor is likely. If not, a cesarean section may be necessary.

Grade 3. These patients should be delivered as quickly and as safely as possible.

Prognosis. Maternal mortality approaches 1% in premature separation of the placenta; this condition remains a leading cause of maternal death. The mother's prognosis depends on the extent of the placental detachment, overall blood loss, degree of hypofibrinogenemia, degree of disseminated intravascular clotting, and time between the placental "accident" and delivery. Fortunately 80% to 90% of all premature separations of the placenta only involve two or three cotyledons, and therefore, the prognosis generally is not grave.

Fetal prognosis is poor. At least 25% of babies die before, during, or soon after birth. Of those who survive, there is an increase in the absolute numbers of neurologically damaged infants. Fetal depression occurs with at least twice the normal frequency. If the Apgar score at 5 minutes is less than 7, there is about one chance in three that the child will be normal neurologically. If the 5 minute Apgar score is 7 or greater, there is about a 90% chance of normal growth and development. Infants with premature separation of the placenta who weigh more than 2500 gm and who have good Apgar scores usually develop normally. About 60% of infants with premature separation of the placenta who weigh less than 2500 gm at birth develop normally.

Placenta previa

General considerations. In placenta previa the placenta is implanted in the lower uterine segment where it encroaches on the internal os. All or a portion of the placenta may cover the internal os. Under these circumstances, the placenta precedes the fetus in vaginal delivery.

Pathogenesis. The cause of placenta previa is speculative. Reduced vascularity of the upper segment due to scarring or tumor necessitating lower implantation of the placenta is a plausible theory. If this be the case, it should not be surprising that placenta previa is far more common in multiparas; the frequency does increase with parity. The incidence of placenta previa is about 1 in every 200 pregnancies. The placenta completely covers the internal os in slightly more than 10% of the cases.

Persistent excessive antenatal bleeding may seriously threaten the mother. The maternal (not fetal) circulation is the source of bleeding. Vaginal or rectal examination or attempts to deliver from below may lacerate or separate the placenta, and as a consequence, exsanguinating maternal (or fetal) hemorrhage may occur. Certainly placenta previa is a major cause of maternal and perinatal morbidity and mortality.

The site of implantation and size of the placenta are related. Specifically, because the circulation of the lower uterine segment is less favorable than the fundus, placenta previa may have to cover a larger area for adequate efficiency. In placenta previa the surface area may be at least 30% greater than the average placenta implanted in the fundus. Twice as many placenta previas involve the anterior uterine wall than in normal implantation, and the probability is even greater after a cesarean section (scarring).

Classification. Placenta previa often is described as *complete, total,* or *central* if the internal os is entirely covered by the placenta, when the cervix is fully dilated. *Partial placenta previa* implies incomplete coverage. Nonetheless, complete placenta previa may be partial

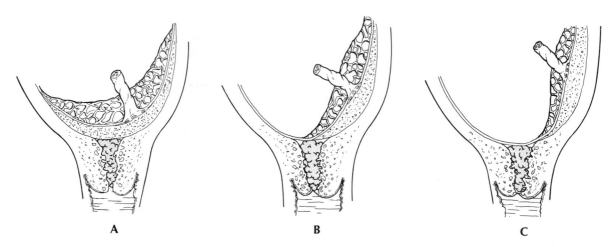

Fig. 16-5. Types of placenta previa prior to onset of labor. **A,** Complete or total. **B,** Incomplete or partial. **C,** Marginal or low-lying.

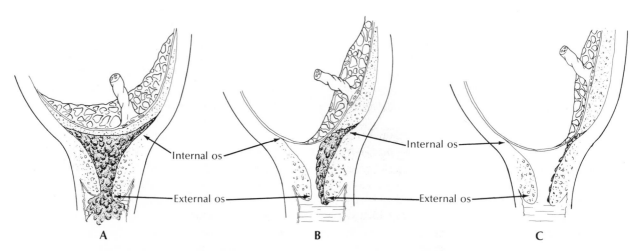

Fig. 16-6. Types of placenta previa after onset of labor. **A,** Complete or total. **B,** Incomplete or partial. **C,** Marginal or low-lying.

after dilatation of the internal os, and marginal previa may become partial. Hence with this terminology, true comparisons are impossible.

Marginal placenta previa indicates that only an edge of the placenta approaches the internal os. The term *low-lying* or *low implantation* is used when the placenta is situated in the lower uterine segment but away from the os (Fig. 16-5).

A better classification of placenta previa is the estimation of percentage coverage of the internal os *at full dilatation,* the diameter required for delivery of a mature fetus through the cervix (Fig. 16-6).

To assess the proportionate (percentage) coverage, the obstetrician should note whether on gentle vaginal exam-

ination the placental edge can be felt at or near the center of the internal os. Then consider how much of the os would be covered were the cervix fully dilated. If about half of the area would be covered by the placenta were the cervix at full dilatation, this would be a 50% placenta previa (Fig. 16-7). Although this is admittedly an estimate, and one should not pursue the examination too vigorously or hemorrhage may ensue, a patient with a placenta previa less than 30% probably can be delivered safely vaginally, whereas one with a placenta previa greater than 30% is better delivered by cesarean section. The nurse should never perform a vaginal or rectal examination on a patient with vaginal bleeding.

Pathology and pathophysiology. Bleeding from

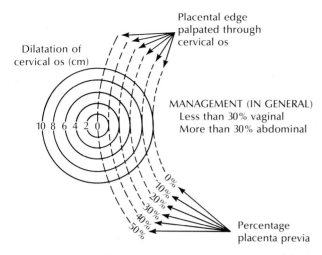

Fig. 16-7. Classification of placenta previa. (Modified from Tatum, H. J., and Mule, J. G. 1965. Am. J. Obstet. Gynecol. **93:**768.)

placenta previa may be due initially to retraction of the lower segment and concomitant separation of the placenta. The lower segment is relatively noncontractile, and bleeding can be considerable from open sinusoids. Placentitis, especially in the area of exposure at or over the os, may be responsible also.

Placenta previa or low-lying placenta may encourage breech or transverse presentation and may prevent engagement of either fetal part.

Clinical findings

Symptomatology. Painless uterine bleeding, especially during the third trimester, characterizes placenta previa. Obviously placenta previa may occur in the first or second trimester also, but abortion generally occurs without knowledge of the site of placentation.

The bleeding may be intermittent, in gushes, or, more rarely, continuous. Fortunately exsanguination almost never occurs unless examination or manipulation initiates the bleeding before or during early labor.

Vaginal examinations. Sterile vaginal examination by the physician will diagnose placenta previa, but examination should be postponed, if possible, until viability has been reached (preferably after the thirty-fourth week). Moreover, the examination should be a so-called double-setup procedure.

A double setup is a sterile vaginal examination that is performed in an operating room with staff and equipment ready to effect an immediate vaginal delivery or cesarean section. Since manipulation of the lower uterine segment or cervix may result in profound hemorrhage, preparation for immediate delivery is essential. Readiness im-

plies an intravenous unit in place with needle large enough to accommodate blood transfusion, two units of matched blood for the mother, sterile tables set up and open, anesthetist present, at least one physician and one nurse scrubbed and pediatrician present. Amniotomy for anticipated vaginal delivery (if placenta is low-lying, cervix is favorable, and presenting part is low) or cesarean section (if placenta encroaches on or covers the cervical os or fetus is in oblique or transverse lie) should be performed.

The examination should be performed as follows:

1. Inspect the vagina and cervix for varices or bleeding ulcerations.

2. Palpate about the cervix for a thicker area (placenta). Ballottement should be performed to the presenting part to identify a zone of soft tissue, possibly placenta, between the vertex or breech and the cervix.

3. Note the dilatation and effacement of the cervix and the intactness of the membranes, and feel for spongy placental tissue partially or totally covering the os.

4. Observe for bleeding or loss of amniotic fluid.

Laboratory findings. Laboratory findings are not diagnostic of placenta previa. Blood clots and blood may contain fetal red blood cells.

Special examinations

1. X-ray studies
   a. Soft tissue radiography may outline the placenta in the fundus, thereby ruling out low-lying placenta or placenta previa.
   b. Vesicouterine contrast involves the following procedure: If the head is presenting, a radiopaque solution is introduced into the bladder, and an anteroposterior film is obtained with the patient standing. If the distance from the fetal skull and the bladder is greater than 4 cm, placenta previa may be present.
   c. Amniography, or x-ray films obtained after amniocentesis and the injection of an iodine solution such as diatrizoate sodium (Hypaque-M), may outline the placenta.
   d. Percutaneous transfemoral aortography generally will reveal a forelying placenta but not the degree of previa.

2. Ultrasonography is useful in that the two dimensional B-scan can reveal the presence of a low-lying placenta, but whether the placenta overlays the cervix cannot be determined by this modality.

3. Radioisotope localization involves injection of minute amounts of ^{125}I bound to serum albumin (RISA), red blood cells tagged with ^{51}Cr, or other substances. These will localize in vascular areas (including the placenta), which can be identified by scintillation scan-

PLAN OF CARE: PLACENTA PREVIA

PATIENT CARE OBJECTIVES

1. A viable neonate is delivered.
2. Patient sustains minimal hemorrhage or hypovolemia, and anemia is rectified.
3. Patient and family understand the cause of, management of, and expected recovery from the experience.
4. Patient maintains a positive sense of self-worth and self-esteem.

NURSING INTERVENTIONS

Diagnostic	Therapeutic	Educational
Antenatal		
1. Observe for and assess external blood loss: count pads, weigh pads, and linen. Ask patient if bleeding ran down legs, amounted to "cupful" or "tablespoonful." Bleeding is usually red (as opposed to dark as in abruptio).	Position of placenta and amount of bleeding guide management.	1. Explain what is happening—that location of placenta and dilatation of cervix is causing bleeding and not anything she or they did.
2. Assess pain, if present. Bleeding is generally painless, but patient may be experiencing labor as well, or previa may be complicated by abruptio.	1. Keep NPO.	2. Explain procedures; answer questions.
3. Assess uterine contractibility. Uterus should relax completely between contractions if not complicated by abruptio.	2. Allow no rectal or vaginal examinations; no enemas.	
4. Monitor FHT with cardiotocograph or corometric monitor.	3. Institute bed rest with head of bed elevated 20 to 30 degrees (semi-Fowler's). (This encourages fetal body to act as tamponade.)	
5. Monitor vital signs, CVP.	4. Start IV (lactated Ringer's solution is better volume expander than 5% dextrose in water). Monitor drip rate.	
6. Assess fetal lie; transverse or oblique lie is frequent. Placental placement also hinders engagement of presenting part.	5. Throughout encourage verbalization of concerns, questions. If FHT are being monitored electronically and are good, turn audio on so parents can listen if they wish.	
7. Check chart for EDC, Rh, history of this pregnancy. (Was there spotting earlier?)	6. Explain procedures to patient and family. Assist with delivery if cervix is favorable, presenting part is low, and bleeding is minimal or contained. Not possible if previa is complete.	
8. Request lab work: Hgb, Hct, Rh, urinalysis.	7. Prepare patient for double-setup examination (p. 237). Prepare patient for surgery: shave, Foley catheter, IV, consent form.	
9. Request one of following to locate placenta: a. Ultrasonography. b. Placenta scan.	8. Alert pediatrician to be present for delivery.	
10. Prepare patient for double-setup examination.		
Postnatal		
1. Monitor height of fundus, uterine contractility, and amount of bleeding. (Lower uterine segment does not contract well; myometrial trauma may predispose to atony.)	1. Postvaginal delivery: usual postnatal care plus monitor blood transfusion, give antibiotics, oxytocics, analgesics as ordered.	1. Reaffirm physician's explanations about cause, management, expected recovery.
2. Observe for signs of infection. Patient is at increased risk for infection because abnormal placental site is slower to heal and hemorrhage predisposes to infection.	2. Postcesarean section: give postoperative care.	
	3. If infant has died or is ill, provide emotional support.	
	4. Encourage verbalization and questions about this experience.	

ning. Unfortunately one cannot distinguish a marginal from a partial or complete placenta previa by RISA studies because lateral scanning cannot be accomplished through the bones of the pelvic girdle.

Differential diagnosis. The differential diagnosis of cervical or uterine bleeding requires inspection and palpation. Biopsy of suspicious areas should be done. Bleeding from a marginal or partial separation of a normally implanted placenta may be painless also. Occasionally bleeding due to a placenta previa may not begin until labor starts. In such instances, the discomfort reported may confuse the diagnosis.

Unfortunately the cause of slight to moderate antenatal bleeding is never accurately diagnosed in 20% to 25% of patients.

Management. Delivery by the most conservative means is the treatment of placenta previa. When fetal maturity is not too far off, conservative management is usually possible because initial spontaneous critical bleeding almost never occurs in placenta previa. When fetal survival is likely, then elective termination of pregnancy can be carried out.

After the diagnosis of placenta previa has been made, the patient should remain in the hospital. At least two units of blood, typed and cross matched, must be available for emergency use. The duration of pregnancy should be confirmed and, except in emergency, delivery postponed until after the thirty-sixth week.

If the patient has greater than a 30% placenta previa or if bleeding is excessive, cesarean section is indicated, preferably with the patient under light general inhalation anesthesia.

If hemorrhage is in progress and vaginal delivery is planned, the membranes are ruptured, if it is easy, to permit the presenting part to tamponade the edge of an incomplete placenta previa to check brisk bleeding. Assuming less than a 30% placenta previa, cautious stimulation of labor by continuous intravenous oxytocin drip is permissible unless bleeding is aggravated. If labor does not ensue within about 6 hours and if progress is not rapid, cesarean section is indicated. The fetus may have bled through the placenta; hence the cord is clamped early at cesarean section.

Bipolar or Braxton Hicks version or internal podalic version should not be employed because of the serious risk of rupture of the lower uterine segment, cervical laceration, or hemorrhage.

Blood loss may not cease with the delivery of the infant. The large vascular channels in the lower uterine segment may continue to bleed, and uterine packing, ligation of the internal iliac arteries, or even hysterectomy may be necessary.

Treat hemorrhage and shock effectively. Generally, at least twice the estimate of the volume of blood lost will be required to replace blood loss.

Prevention. Placenta previa cannot be prevented. The problem can be detected early, however, and with the avoidance of aggressive diagnostic methods, safe delivery after viability has been reached usually is possible.

Prognosis. Placenta previa and placenta previa accreta are more common after uterine surgery (e.g., cesarean section or myomectomy).

Maternal mortality in placenta previa has dropped almost 50% to about 0.6% during the past decade in larger centers in North America because of conservative therapy. Regrettably, however, the perinatal mortality still approaches 20% in most hospitals. This figure undoubtedly can be reduced by half with better management. Currently, placenta previa increases the likelihood of death of the neonate by about ten times.

MANAGEMENT OF SHOCK

Hemorrhage is a major threat to the mother during the childbearing cycle. Shock may result. Shock is an emergency situation in which the perfusion of body organs may become severely compromised and death may ensue. A brief explanation of the physiologic mechanism involved is provided to assist the nurse in implementing appropriate actions.

Physiologic mechanisms

Physiologic compensatory mechanisms are activated in response to hemorrhage (or other trauma such as cardiac arrest). The adrenals release catecholamines, causing arterioles and venules in the skin, lungs, gastrointestinal tract, liver, and kidney to constrict, thus diverting available blood flow to the brain and heart. If shock is prolonged, the continued reduction in cellular oxygenation results in an accumulation of lactic acid and acidosis (from anaerobic glucose metabolism). Acidosis (lowered serum pH) causes arteriole vasodilatation; venule vasoconstriction persists. A circular pattern is established: decreased perfusion, increased tissue anoxia and acidosis, edema formation, and pooling of blood further decrease the perfusion (Fig. 16-8). Cellular death occurs. Table 16-1 is an assessment guide to assist the nurse in the observation and evaluation of the degree of shock.

Assessment and interventions

The following nursing interventions for the patient in shock should be considered (Royce, 1973):

1. Stay with the patient. Send others to alert the physician and to obtain needed equipment. An emergency

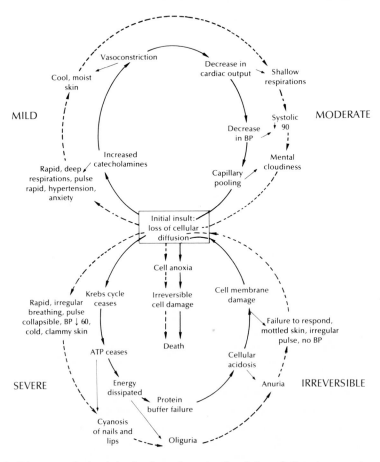

Fig. 16-8. Diagram of physiologic alterations in shock in relation to symptoms. (From Royce, J. A. 1973. Nurs. Clin. North Am. **8:**377.)

Table 16-1. Symptoms of shock*

	Mild	Moderate	Severe	Irreversible
Respirations	Rapid, deep	Rapid, becoming shallow	Rapid, shallow, may be irregular	Irregular, or barely perceptible
Pulse	Rapid, tone normal	Rapid, tone may be normal but is becoming weaker	Very rapid, easily collapsible, may be irregular	Irregular apical pulse
Blood pressure	Normal or hypertensive	60 to 90 mm Hg systolic	Below 60 mm Hg systolic	None palpable
Skin	Cool and pale	Cool, pale, moist, knees cyanotic	Cold, clammy, cyanosis of lips and fingernails	Cold, clammy, cyanotic
Urine output	No change	Decreasing to 10 to 22 cc/hr (adult)	Oliguric (less than 10 cc) to anuria	Anuric
Level of consciousness	Alert, oriented, diffuse anxiety	Oriented, mental cloudiness or increasing restlessness	Lethargy, reacts to noxious stimuli, comatose	Does not respond to noxious stimuli
CVP	May be normal	3 cm H$_2$O	0 to 3 cm H$_2$O	

*From Royce, J. A. 1973. Shock: emergency nursing implications. Nurs. Clin. North Am. **8:**377; Wagner, M. M. Clinical Nursing Specialist, University of Iowa Hospitals and Clinics.

cart should be well supplied, available at all times, and include equipment to start intravenous fluids and to give oxygen, suction, retention catheter with urinometer, and blood pressure and CVP apparatus.

Nurses should have standing orders to start intravenous fluids and know the type of infusion fluid to use and laboratory tests to order.

2. While waiting for the physician, the following should be performed:

    a. Insert an airway to facilitate oxygen administration (at 2 to 3ℓ/min) and suction.

    b. Start intravenous administration of 5% dextrose and water to maintain peripheral vascular circulation.

    c. Elevate the right hip (if patient cannot be in side-lying position) to avoid vena caval syndrome. The Trendelenberg position (with head down and feet elevated) is not advised. This position may interfere with cardiac function. Use this position on physician request only.

3. Assist physician to institute and monitor measures to increase tissue perfusion. Monitor intravenous fluids. Too slow a rate (caused by slowing of drip rate, kinking, or occlusion of tubing) may be inadequate to dilute blood viscosity or to maintain peripheral circulation. Too rapid a rate may result in fluid overload and pulmonary edema.

Fluids to increase blood volume include whole fresh blood, plasma, and albumin. Fluids to dilute hemoconcentration (viscosity) are dextrose in water and lactated Ringer's solution.

4. Monitor, assess, and record respirations, pulse, blood pressure, skin condition, urine output, level of consciousness, and CVP to evaluate effectiveness of management (Table 16-1):

    a. *Respirations.* The body rids itself of excess acids by increasing respiratory rate. Ventilatory assistance with oxygen, respirator, or both may be needed.

    b. *Pulse.* The pulse rate increases and becomes irregular as shock progresses in severity.

    c. *Blood pressure.* In later stages of shock, the systolic pressure decreases.

    d. *Skin.* Perfusion of the skin is sacrificed in the body's attempt to maintain blood flow to the heart and brain. Therefore the condition of the skin is a valuable index to the severity of shock. The nurse assesses the degree of ischemia and/or cyanosis of the nailbeds, eyelids, and inside the mouth (buccal mucosa, gums, tongue). The nurse notes the degree of coolness and clamminess.

    e. *Urine output.* Measure hourly output. Oliguria (50 ml/hr) may indicate worsening of shock or inadequate fluid therapy; an increased output indicates improvement in the patient's condition.

    f. *Level of consciousness.* The adequacy of cerebral perfusion may be estimated by an evaluation of the patient's level of consciousness. In the early stages of decreased blood flow, the patient may complain of "seeing stars," feeling dizzy, or feeling nauseous. She may become restless and orthopneic. As cerebral hypoxia increases, the patient may become confused and react slowly or not at all to stimuli. An improved sensorium is an indicator of improvement.

    g. *CVP.* CVP readings measure the contractility of the heart and the adequacy of the blood volume. Normal values range between 6 and 12 mm H_2O. Low or falling value indicates inadequate blood volume or hypovolemia. High or rising value indicates impaired contractility of the heart.

Anxiety is contagious. The nurse's calm, confident manner, coupled with brief, simple explanations, is an important adjunct to the interventions just discussed.

CVP. The CVP provides critical data if the urinary output decreases despite adequate infusion. To obtain the CVP, a catheter must be inserted through a major vein in the antecubital area and threaded into the right atrium. The tubing is kept open with a slow drip of 5% dextrose in water. The procedure is as follows (Fig. 16-9):

1. Mark the patient's chest at the midright atrium level (in line with the midaxillary plane).

2. Place the patient in the supine position. All readings should be made with the patient in the same position (e.g., supine, sitting).

3. With the manometer at the level of the right atrium, set at the zero point.

4. Open the stopcock to the manometer to fill with fluid (without bubbles!) from the intravenous fluid bottle (or bag) (Fig. 16-9, *A*).

5. Turn the stopcock to allow the fluid to flow from the manometer to the patient (Fig. 16-9, *B*).

6. Fluid level in the manometer fluctuates with each respiration. Take the reading when the fluid level stabilizes. If the patient is on a respirator, turn it off during readings for accuracy, since a false high reading occurs otherwise.

7. Turn the stopcock so that the fluid flows from the bottle to patient (Fig. 16-9, *C*), at a drip rate ordered by the physician.

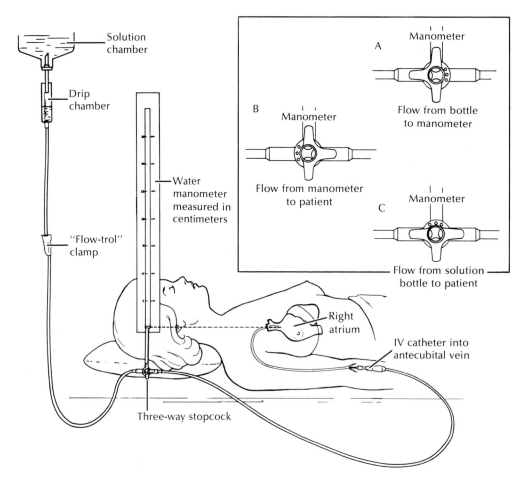

Fig. 16-9. Measurement of CVP using manometer.

8. Record the reading and patient's position (supine).

9. Scrupulously clean the insertion site daily, and reapply bactericidal ointment and sterile dressing.

10. Hazards of the procedure are phlebitis, infection at the insertion site, bacteremia, or septicemia; and air embolus.

Hazards of therapy

The 24 hours after the shock period is critical. Patients should be observed for fluid overload, shock lung, and oxygen toxicity. *Fluid overload* results in pulmonary and peripheral edema. Alert the physician and decrease the drip rate if moist respirations, stridor, or dyspnea occur. *Shock lung* may develop after the patient receives mechanical ventilatory assistance, especially if the ventilator is not maintained between 50 and 70 mm Hg. Tachypnea, dyspnea, anxiety, a rise in blood pressure,

cyanosis, and harsh loud breaths follow alveolar capillary damage. *High concentrations of oxygen are toxic* to the adult, as well as to the neonate. Irritation of mucous membranes of the upper respiratory tract, substernal pain, and cough may occur. The first sign may be muscular twitching about the face, followed by convulsions resembling grand mal seizures. Later neurologic symptomatology includes tinnitus, euphoria, confusion, and respiratory arrest.

The nurse-physician team's quick response and coordinated efforts are essential to institute, monitor, and continuously readjust therapy to the patient's changing needs. This collaboration, given the essential emergency apparatus and supportive services (e.g., laboratory testing) is requisite to meeting the following patient care objective: The patient recovers from shock without adverse sequelae (e.g., cellular death, fluid overload, shock lung, and oxygen toxicity).

PLAN OF CARE: SPONTANEOUS ABORTION AND ECTOPIC PREGNANCY

PATIENT CARE OBJECTIVES
1. Patient retains a positive sense of self-esteem and self-worth.
2. Patient appraises the situation realistically (e.g., her ambivalent or negative feelings toward pregnancy did not cause the abortion).

NURSING INTERVENTIONS

Diagnostic	Therapeutic	Educational

1. Assess patient's behavior:
  a. Euphoric, talkative.
  b. Quiet, nonverbal.
  c. Denial or acknowledgment.
2. Review her obstetric history:
  a. Was there difficulty conceiving?
  b. Any previous abortions?
3. Was anything done to initiate abortion?
	1. Make yourself available to patient and indicate your willingness to listen and sit with her.
	2. Encourage and assist her to verbalize:
	  a. Feelings of loss, of being cheated.
	  b. Fear of not being able to ever carry to term; fear of having something wrong with her.
	  c. Any feelings, actions, or lack of action that she may believe caused this.
	  d. Reflections on previous pregnancies, labors, etc.
	3. Act as her advocate to physician regarding her questions of cause and her biologic functioning capacity.
	4. Make appropriate referrals: family planning, psychiatric social worker, genetic counselor, etc.
		1. Verbal repetition of experience helps one to cope with situation and integrate experience into one's perception of self in nonthreatening manner.
		2. People experiencing loss may need to ask same questions repeatedly from same and/or other people. Answers may need to be given frequently, with patience and understanding.
		3. People experiencing grief feel alienated from others, lonely, and helpless and may exhibit anger even in presence of accepting, understanding, and caring other.

GRIEF RESPONSE IN PREGNANCY
Spontaneous abortion and ectopic pregnancy

Conception affirms the woman's ability to initiate her biologic role. Spontaneous abortion or ectopic pregnancy that occurs after the woman is aware of conception may be an assault to her self-concept and self-worth. The woman questions her biologic intactness and ability to carry a normal pregnancy. She may feel cheated. Many women experience ambivalent feelings toward the idea of pregnancy; many harbor thoughts of self-abortion. Coincident loss of the pregnancy may precipitate a guilt reaction for real or imagined negative thoughts or actions.

For the woman who has a history of difficulty in conceiving and carrying a pregnancy to viability, negative feelings about herself as a complete woman may be expected. Nursing care of such a woman should focus on helping her verbalize her feelings openly and honestly. Sympathetic, active listening by the nurse may assist the woman in retaining or regaining her self-esteem and feelings of self-worth.

Antenatal fetal death

Fetal movements cease. The mother may deny a lack of fetal activity, "Maybe he's just asleep . . . he's quiet sometimes." She may call the physician for reassurance that everything is all right. Subsequently she may be admitted to the hospital for tests of fetal status. Even in light of evidence from the tests and clinical symptoms, some women cling tenaciously to the hope that the infant will be born alive and well.

Other women acknowledge fetal death by a change in their behavior. One woman arrived on a maternity unit in active labor. A check of her chart showed that she had kept all her clinic appointments until 4 weeks prior to labor. She stated she was feeling well and described her labor so far. She said nothing as the nurse checked for the FHTs. When none were heard, the nurse inquired about fetal activity. Quietly and unemotionally, the mother replied, "They stopped a month ago."

PLAN OF CARE: ANTENATAL FETAL DEATH

PATIENT CARE OBJECTIVES

1. Patient retains a positive sense of self-esteem and self-worth.
2. Patient appraises the situation realistically (e.g., her ambivalent or negative feelings toward pregnancy did not cause the fetus to die).

NURSING INTERVENTIONS

Diagnostic	Therapeutic	Educational
Antenatal		

1. Detection by patient:
  a. Time interval between first suspicion of cessation of fetal movements and calling physician.
  b. Note time when she stopped keeping appointments.
2. Detection by physician:
  a. Pattern of increase in fundal height; weight gain not consistant with normal pregnancy.
  b. Tests for fetal status: estriol levels, sonography, amniocentesis, others.
  c. Test for maternal fibrinogen levels.
3. Past obstetric history:
  a. Previous spontaneous abortion or fetal loss?
  b. Was she in high-risk category?
  c. Did she have any recent experiences with or is she now experiencing loss (other than this fetus)?
	1. Arrange for immediate appointment:
	  a. Call patients who miss appointments.
	  b. Schedule sufficient time to meet with physician or nurse, if situation is suspicious.
	2. Assist patient to ventilate feelings of guilt or self-blame for acts of commission or omission.
	  a. "Many women are unhappy when they first learn they are pregnant and wish they were not pregnant."
	  b. "Are you thinking you may have done something to cause this?"
	  c. "You are trying to find reasons. . . ."
	3. Assist patient to express her feelings about carrying dead baby:
	  a. "It isn't easy to know the baby is dead."
	  b. "Do you wonder if you can stand it until delivery?"
	  c. "Do you wonder if you will be hurt somehow?"
	  d. "Are you wondering how to tell the other children, husband, grandparents, etc?"
	4. Fill in gaps in information, and clarify misconceptions. Help her formulate questions for physician; help her understand what physician tells her.
	5. Prepare her (and spouse or family) for procedures, tests for fetal status.
		1. After mother feels life, or quickening, most mothers begin to relate differently to child. Child is now real; there is, at least in fantasy, promise of child.
		2. Generally, people feel uneasy about death. It is difficult to realize that one is carrying within her something that is dead.
		3. When medical and nursing staff are able to communicate comfortably and openly about fetal death and patient's possible reactions and feelings, patient may be better able to face and cope with situation.
		4. Knowledge about any situation helps dispel fear of unknown, misconceptions, fantasy. Knowledge supports ego strength. She needs to know following:
		  a. When to expect labor and delivery. (Will it be induced, and when, how?)
		  b. What to expect of her labor.
		  c. What physiologic effect this may have on her.
		  d. What may have caused fetal death. She has had sole responsibility for care and nurturance of embryo-fetus. She needs to be advised of possible causes well beyond her control.
		  e. How to tell other children at home.
		  f. What reactions she may expect from others and some help on how to handle these.

Intranatal		

1. Assess maternal emotional response:
  a. Quiet, composed.
  b. Denial: "I just don't believe it," euphoric, animated.
  c. Overtly upset, crying.
  d. Angry toward staff, others: "Why do I have to feel anything. Give me something now"; "If
	1. Do not do Leopold's maneuvers or listen for FHT. Focus on her (and family).
	2. Introduce yourself and immediately indicate your awareness of situation:
	  a. "This is a very difficult and sad time for you."
	  b. If possible, keep father close by;
		1. Open communication and making yourself available physically and psychologically helps in following ways:
		  a. Fosters open communication between mother and her significant others and with staff. Energy does not have to be diverted to keeping up "front."

PLAN OF CARE: ANTENATAL FETAL DEATH—cont'd

NURSING INTERVENTIONS—cont'd

Diagnostic	Therapeutic	Educational

Intranatal—cont'd
the doctor had only . . ."; "If I had only . . ."
  e. Sad, tearful.
2. Assess patient's external support system:
  a. Relatives present.
  b. Behavior of relatives. (Does patient seem reassured by their presence and actions?)
  c. Assess family's interest and ability to stay with her, to provide comfort measures, etc.
3. Assess patient and family's desires regarding seeing and holding infant.
	he may feel awkward in "Dad's Room." "This is hard for you, too. One feels so helpless. Can I help you?"
	3. Respect her choice of anesthesia. If she wishes to be awake or if couple wishes father to be present at birth, prepare them for following:
	  a. Silence and tension at delivery.
	  b. Sight of still, pale, or reddish infant, infant's peeling skin, and markedly molded head.
	4. If mother, spouse, or relatives wish to see, hold infant:
	  a. Prepare family for sight of infant and tell them you will stay with them.
	  b. Prepare infant: bathe, wrap.
	  c. Provide private space; physician, clergy, nurse, or other may stay close by for support.
	  d. Give permission to cry by your actions, by giving tissues, by saying, "It's worth crying over."
	5. Be cognizant of your own nonverbal messages.
		b. Gives permission to grieve. Validates appropriateness of grieving here and now in a manner acceptable to them. Gives permission to speak of death.
		2. General anesthesia may keep experience unreal, dreamlike, thereby complicating efficient grieving.
		3. Seeing and holding infant is useful in following ways:
		  a. Validates reality of event.
		  b. Allows identification of real infant and eliminates fantasy of what woman or couple thought infant looked like (fantasy is frequently more horrifying than reality).
		  c. Permits grieving process to begin. Even if event was anticipated, reality reactivates entire grief process. Steps in grieving process usually take less time when death has been diagnosed prior to beginning of labor.

Occasionally it is the nurse who responds with denial. The nurse may rationalize the absence of FHT and funic and uterine souffles as "positional," "too much noise in the room," "defective fetoscope," and the like. The nurse may choose to avoid the patient or to avoid open communication on the subject. The nurse has several therapeutic alternatives available, however.

After removal of hydatidiform mole

The aberrant pregnancy resulting in an hydatidiform mole poses psychologic as well as physical threats:

Psychologic hazards
1. An assault on one's femininity, womanhood, and self-esteem (some women verbalize, "I feel like some sort of freak")
2. A threat to one's intactness and life

Physical hazards
1. Preeclampsia-eclampsia
2. Hyperemesis gravidarum with dehydration and starvation
3. Hemorrhage
4. Perforation of the uterus
5. Sepsis
6. Highly malignant and rapidly metastasizing choriocarcinoma

Many of the nursing interventions discussed through-

out this chapter are pertinent in this situation as well. A brief summary of the psychosocial aspects of nursing interventions follows:

1. Provide simple, cogent explanations to the patient and her family, reemphasizing or repeating what the physician has told her (them), regarding the following:
   a. Etiology.
   b. Course of treatment for hydatidiform mole and any of the coexisting problems (e.g., hemorrhage, dilatation and curettage, hysterectomy).
   c. Follow-up supervision for 1 year:
      (1) Need for repeated urinalysis for HCG.
      (2) Need for strict contraception.
2. Encourage the patient and her family to grieve by assisting them in the following ways:
   a. To cry and act out their grief.
   b. To identify and explore feelings (inadequacy, guilt) regarding this event, one's responsibility for it, or delay in seeking treatment (should this exist).
   c. To talk of fears for future childbearing, possible surgery, and death from cancer.

Pathologic mourning

The critical period for intervention is in the immediate crisis period. Appropriate mourning has been described previously. The goal of crisis intervention is to assist the mother and her family to begin to mourn appropriately and *now*. The following signs may signal pathologic mourning:

1. Cheerfulness
2. Avoidance of the topic
3. Marked and/or persistent hostility toward the staff, husband, or maternal or paternal family
4. Marked and/or persistent guilt feelings regarding the event
5. Viewing the sick and/or premature infant or infant with a disorder as normal or as deceased

The nurse must be aware of possible cultural prescriptions for mourning and the expression of grief when assessing the appropriateness of a grief response.

• • •

The nurse's role in the management of complications such as hemorrhagic disorders extends beyond support of physiologic functioning of the mother and the fetus or infant. The mother and her family need assistance in coping effectively with the grief and grieving engendered.

REFERENCES

Aladjem, S. (ed.). 1975. Risks in the practice of modern obstetrics (vol. 2). St. Louis, The C. V. Mosby Co.

Boyce, J., and Hales, J. 1974. Problems in the management of patients who have abortions. Drug Ther. **4:**59, Feb.

Brotherton, J., and Craft, I. L. 1972. A clinical and pathologic survey of 91 cases of spontaneous abortion. Fertil. Steril. **23:**289.

Connally, W. J., and Breen, J. L. 1972. Aggressive management of septic abortion: report of 262 cases. South. Med. J. **65:**1480.

Franklin, E. W., III, and Zeiderman, A. M. 1973. Tubal ectopic pregnancy: etiology and obstetric and gynecologic sequelae. Am. J. Obstet. Gynecol. **117:**220.

Hammond, H. 1972. Death from obstetrical hemorrhage. Calif. Med. **117:**16, Aug.

Harralson, J. D., and others. 1973. Operative management of ruptured tubal pregnancy. Am. J. Obstet. Gynecol. **115:**995.

Jones, W. B., and Lewis, J. L., Jr. 1974. Treatment of gestational trophoblastic disease. Am. J. Obstet. Gynecol. **120:**14.

Kuptsow, P. 1973. Cerclage in the treatment of incompetent cervix. J. Am. Osteopath. Assoc. **72:**1094.

Little, H. M., Jr. 1974. Managing incomplete abortion. Am. Fam. Physician **9:**136.

Lunan, C. B. 1973. The management of abruptio placentae. J. Obstet. Gynaecol. Br. Commonw. **80:**120.

McLaren, H. C. 1972. Management of recurring abortion. Practitioner **209:**661.

Murray, J., and Smallwood, J. 1977. CVP monitoring: side stepping potential perils. Nursing 77 **7:**42, Jan.

Rao, S., and others. 1974. Hydatidiform mole. Clinician **38:**129.

Royce, J. A. 1973. Shock: emergency nursing implications. Nurs. Clin. North Am. **8:**377.

Scheer, K. 1973. Ultrasonic diagnosis of placenta previa. Obstet. Gynecol. **42:**707.

Semmens, J. P. 1968. A second look at expectant management of placenta previa. Postgrad. Med. **44:**207.

Van Iddekinge, B. 1972. Ectopic pregnancy: a review. South African Med. J. **46:**1844.

Varma, T. R. 1973. Fetal growth and placental function in patients with placenta previa. J. Obstet. Gynaecol. Br. Commonw. **80:**311.

Wallner, H. J. 1974. The fate of the child after threatened abortion. J. Perin. Med. **2:**54.

CHAPTER 17

Hypertensive states in pregnancy

PREECLAMPSIA-ECLAMPSIA

Hypertension, usually of vasospastic origin, often complicates pregnancy. Multiple metabolic aberrations are involved. Occasionally the vascular disorder may antedate the pregnancy; in other instances it develops during gestation or soon after delivery. Except perhaps for the surgically correctable abnormalities that may cause hypertension, for example, pheochromocytoma or renal artery stenosis, the cause of most of the hypertension syndromes diagnosed during pregnancy is unknown.

Hypertension predating pregnancy may be a manifestation of cardiovascular or renal disease. In contrast, hypertensive disorders that first appear during well-established pregnancy are largely preeclampsia-eclampsia (heretofore termed *toxemia of pregnancy* or *eclamptogenic toxemia*). Other current synonyms are edema-proteinuria–hypertension complex and gestosis. Multiple pregnancy, hydramnios, diabetes, placental disorders such as hydatidiform mole, and dietary deficiency predispose to preeclampsia-eclampsia. Primigravidas and women who have developed chronic cardiovascular or renal disease are prone to preeclampsia-eclampsia.

About 5% of pregnant women in North America suffer from preeclampsia, and approximately 5% of these develop eclampsia. In lower socioeconomic groups here and abroad, the incidence figures may be three to five times as high.

Preeclampsia-eclampsia is a major cause of maternal morbidity and mortality. Almost 15% of eclamptics die of the disease or its complications. Moreover, perinatal morbidity is high because most patients with preeclampsia-eclampsia deliver prior to the thirty-seventh week of gestation. A single maternal convulsion increases the prospect of perinatal death at least fivefold.

Definitions

Hypertension in pregnancy is a rise in the systolic and diastolic pressures of 15/15 mm Hg or more after rest in a sitting position. Pressures in excess of 125/75 prior to 32 weeks' gestation have been found to be associated with increases in fetal risk, as have pressures of over 125/85 at term. The previously accepted level of 140/90 is not meaningful in pregnancy, since blood pressure readings are normally low. Hypertension has developed when the mean arterial pressure is 105 mm Hg or more or when there is a rise of 15 mm Hg or more on two occasions at least 6 hours apart, as compared with previously recorded blood pressure determinations.

Gestational hypertension is the development of hypertension during pregnancy or within the first 24 hours postdelivery when the previous blood pressure determinations were normal. The blood pressure in gestational hypertension usually returns to normal within 10 days after delivery.

Chronic hypertensive disease is the presence of persistent hypertension of any cause before pregnancy or before the twentieth week of gestation or a persistent hypertension after the forty-second postnatal day.

When insufficient information is available for diagnosis, hypertensive disease must be termed *unclassified,* or *atypical.* If the physician is diligent, however, the unclassified hypertensive states observed during pregnancy are few.

Gestational edema is a generalized accumulation of fluid (a value of greater than 1+ is diagnostic of pitting edema) after 12 hours of bed rest or a weight gain of more than 3 pounds/wk in the second trimester or more than 1 pound/wk in the third trimester.

Gestational proteinuria is the occurrence of proteinuria during pregnancy or the early puerperium in the absence of hypertension, edema, urinary tract infection, or identifiable intrinsic vascular-renal disease. The protein must be in amounts greater than 0.3 gm/ℓ in a 24-hour specimen or greater than 1 gm/ℓ (1+ to 2+) by standard turbidimetric methods in a random urine collection on two or more occasions at least 6 hours apart. The urine must be midstream clean-catch or catheter-derived specimens.

Preeclampsia

Preeclampsia is the syndrome of hypertension with proteinuria or edema or both during pregnancy or within 48 hours of delivery. Preeclampsia-eclampsia is a catabolic disease with associated altered vascular reactivity, compromised metabolic function, notable sodium retention, and reduced renal function, together with alterations in vascular volume and increased CNS activity. Preeclampsia develops after the twentieth week of gestation, but it may occur earlier in the presence of hydatidiform mole or choriocarcinoma. Preeclampsia may be divided into mild or severe degrees for treatment purposes.

Mild preeclampsia implies the following:

1. Hypertension with a rise in blood pressure 15/15 mm Hg or more on two occasions at least 6 hours apart
2. Weight gain of more than 3 pounds/wk during the second trimester or more than 1 pound/wk during the third trimester
3. Slight generalized edema
4. Proteinuria of 0.3 gm/ℓ on a random specimen or on two occasions 6 hours apart

Severe preeclampsia includes the symptoms just listed, as well as the following:

1. Hypertension with a blood pressure of 160/110 mm Hg or more on two separate occasions 6 hours apart with the pregnant patient at bed rest
2. Proteinuria of 5 gm/24 hr or more
3. Oliguria of 400 ml/24 hr or less
4. Other signs or symptoms noted earlier and becoming more serious
   a. Severe generalized headache
   b. Visual problems
      (1) Blurred vision or other visual changes
      (2) Retinal arteriolar spasm on funduscopy
   c. Epigastric pain or nausea, vomiting
   d. Irritability, emotional tension
   e. Other

Eclampsia

Eclampsia includes the symptoms of severe preeclampsia and one or more of the following:

1. Tonic and clonic convulsions or coma, with the coma possibly following an unobserved seizure unrelated to other seizure disorders
2. Hypertensive crisis or shock

Pathogenesis

Preeclampsia-eclampsia is defined in empirical clinical terms because its cause and pathogenesis are unknown. Preeclampsia-eclampsia has always been a subject of much speculation. One current theory is that of uterine ischemia, which proposes impaired uteroplacental circulation secondary to uterine distension. High myometrial tone in primigravidas, multiple pregnancy, hydramnios, even a hydatidiform mole pregnancy may be responsible. As a consequence of slight relative hypoxia, placental or decidual metabolic products capable of causing sodium and water retention and vascular constriction may be released into the maternal circulation. It is hypothesized that this causes the development of preeclampsia-eclampsia in a sensitive or reactive patient. Be this as it may, none of the catabolites per se are toxic substances, and no "toxin" has ever been identified. Hence it is illogical to refer to the hypertensive syndromes of pregnancy as *toxemias*.

A more recent theory stresses the concept that pregnancy is a salt-losing state and that inadequate sodium intake in the face of increased loss leads to hypovolemia, which in turn results in compensatory vasospasm. According to this theory, salt intake should not be restricted and should in fact be increased.

Another concept that is also gaining increased acceptance is that preeclampsia-eclampsia is a function of poor nutrition, especially of diets poor in protein. Proponents of this theory prescribe high-protein diets without caloric or sodium restriction in prevention and treatment of this disorder. Refer to references at the end of this chapter.

Chronic glomerular nephritis, renal artery stenosis, pyelonephritis, or coarctation of the aorta are common causes of hypertensive cardiovascular disease in young people. Even when there is no evidence of these disorders (essential hypertension), a uniform pattern of regulation probably does not exist in all patients. Certain individuals may have increased sympathetic nervous system responses or a fault in the renin-angiotensin-aldosterone system. Unfortunately the physiology of even normal pregnancy so complicates the picture that the diagnosis of a primary defect is virtually impossible.

Pathology

In preeclampsia a renal lesion has been described consisting of cloudy swelling of the capillary endothelial cells and the deposit of amorphous material between these cells and the basement membrane. The vascular lumen is thus diminished. This alteration is temporary, and the kidney changes resolve after delivery.

Patients who die as a consequence of eclampsia disclose edema of the brain and lungs particularly. Many microfocal hemorrhages in the brain may be noted. Numerous small thrombi are present in the lungs. Slight enlargement of the blanched kidneys is common. Cut sections usually disclose ischemic glomerular capillaries adherent to the thickened basement membrane. Degeneration of the endothelial cells is apparent. The tubular cells generally show hyaline degeneration. The dilated tubules contain protein and casts together with occasional red blood cells and white blood cells.

Frequently, the placenta is smaller than normal for the duration of pregnancy. Premature aging is apparent with numerous areas of broken syncytium. Ischemic necrosis (white infarcts) are numerous, and intervillous fibrin deposition (red infarcts) may be recorded.

Sustained hypertension causes the initially reversible "functional" arteriolar narrowing to become permanent *(structural)* as a result of intimal thickening, hypertrophy of the muscular coats, and hyaline degeneration. Hypertension accelerates the development of coronary and cerebral artery atherosclerosis; myocardial infarction and cerebral hemorrhage or thrombosis often are sequelae.

Pathophysiology

General arteriolar spasm is characteristic of preeclampsia-eclampsia. Whether this is a primary or secondary reaction is uncertain, however. In any event, the arterial system becomes hyperresponsive to vasopressor drugs such as vasopressin and angiotensin II. Nonetheless, the vascular tone is not well maintained. With this liability of the vascular system, shock states may be rapid and profound.

Blood chemistry changes include elevated serum uric acid, urea nitrogen, and creatinine. Low serum albumin and globulin and reduced carbon dioxide combining power (particularly after convulsions) are notable in preeclampsia-eclampsia.

The glomerular filtration rate is reduced in preeclampsia-eclampsia. With the small volume of urine produced in this disorder, however, tubular reabsorption of sodium is more efficient. Sodium and water retention is also augmented by the increased secretion of antidiuretic hormone, corticosteroids, and aldosterone in many patients. The albumin/globulin (A/G) ratio is altered, even reversed, secondary to hypoproteinemia, which, despite hemoconcentration, aggravates edema.

Because of degenerative changes in the glomeruli, serum protein, largely albumin, is lost in the urine. Actually, tubular changes account for only minor leakage of protein. Be this as it may, oliguria concentrates the protein. As much as 4 gm of protein per 100 ml urine (4+) may be passed by the preeclamptic-eclamptic patient.

Eclampsia is an awesome, frightening sequence to observe. Increased hypertension preceeds the tonic-clonic convulsions; hypotension and collapse follow. Stertor-

---

> ### CONVULSIONS
>
> **Description**
>
> *Stage of invasion:* 2 to 3 seconds; eyes fixed; twitching of facial muscles.
>
> *Stage of contraction:* 15 to 20 seconds; eyes protrude and bloodshot; all body muscles in tonic contraction, e.g., arms flexed, hands clenched, legs inverted.
>
> *Stage of convulsion:* Muscles relax, contract alternatively. Respirations are halted, then begin again with long, deep, stertorous inhalation. Coma ensues (2 to 3 minutes to hours).
>
> **Occurrence:** During antenatal, natal, or postnatal period.
>
> **Recurrence:** Within minutes of first convulsion or never.

---

ous breathing and coma are the aftermath of a seizure. Nystagmus and muscular twitching persist for a time. Disorientation and amnesia cloud the immediate recovery. Oliguria and anuria are notable. (A more detailed description of tonic-clonic convulsions is shown above.)

At least 20% of patients with chronic hypertension develop superimposed preeclampsia-eclampsia.

Hypertension greatly increases the incidence of cardiac failure, myocardial infarction, hemorrhagic and thrombotic stroke, and renal failure.

Renal artery stenosis causes an arterial bruit in the left or right epigastrium transmitted to the abnormal renal artery. Characteristically this bruit can be traced to the flank and the costovertebral angle.

Differential diagnosis

In the differential diagnosis of preeclampsia, the physician considers arteriolar hypertension, adrenocortical tumor or hyperplasia, coarctation of the aorta, glomerulonephritis, pyelonephritis, renal arterial disorder, hyperaldosteronism, or pheochromocytoma.

The differential diagnosis of eclampsia requires a consideration of all the causes of seizures, including CNS tumor, fluid intoxication, drug overdosage, hyperglycemia, and porphyria. A woman in advanced pregnancy who has had preeclampsia and who develops tonic-clonic convulsions must be presumed to have eclampsia. Subsequent tests may disprove this impression, however, and the diagnosis should be reclassified.

Abnormal signs indicative of the cardiovascular origin of hypertension include moderate to marked retinal changes, such as arteriovenous nicking, flame-shaped hemorrhages, and cotton-wool exudates, and heart sound changes, such as a loud aortic second sound and an early systolic ejection click. Left ventricular enlargement or presystolic gallop rhythm may be noted. Bruits over the large vessels may be heard in hypertensive cardiovascular disease.

Signs of Cushing's disease, an endocrinologic cause of hypertension, include trunk obesity, hirsutism, acne, purple striae, and perhaps evidence of an adrenal tumor.

The diagnosis of coarctation of the aorta requires a weak or delayed femoral pulse and basal systolic murmur transmitted to the intrascapular area.

The development of hypertensive renal or neurologic findings in a previously normal pregnant patient should distinguish preeclampsia-eclampsia from primary hypertensive cardiovascular-renal or neurologic disease.

Primary aldosteronism involves muscular weakness and absence of tendon reflexes or diminished vasomotor circulatory reflexes. Endocrine tests may confirm a pheochromocytoma.

Renal parenchymal disease often has its onset in glomerular nephritis or recurrent pyelonephritis. Polycystic kidneys are large and easily palpable.

Prognosis

Maternal. Eclampsia, together with hemorrhage and infection, has been among the three leading causes of maternal death for years in North America. Women with preeclampsia almost never die of this disorder, but in eclampsia the maternal mortality may be 10% to 15%. Should convulsions develop, one woman in about fifteen will die of an intracranial hemorrhage, aspiration pneumonia, or cardiac failure or from hemorrhage, shock, or lower nephron nephrosis caused by premature separation of the placenta.

In addition, patients who sustain eclamptic convulsions may bite their tongue or lips. They often fracture ribs or vertebrae. Retinal detachments may ensue. With good therapy, most patients improve significantly in 24 to 48 hours. Rapid improvement follows early termination of pregnancy.

Except for patients with malignant hypertension who should be aborted, most women with hypertension of cerebrovascular origin tolerate pregnancy without critical complications. The fetal outcome is more questionable, however, because of placental insufficiency. Generally, the fetus is small for gestational age and may even die before delivery can be effected.

Fetal. In many parts of North America the perinatal mortality is at least 20% with eclampsia. This is due mainly to the effects of hypoxia, prematurity, and/or acidosis during maternal convulsions.

With correct intensive therapy, the need for early delivery will reduce the perinatal death rate to about 10%.

Infants of mothers with preeclampsia-eclampsia are small for their gestational age, presumably the result of placental malfunction. However, they do better generally than preterm babies of the same weight and gestational age born of nonhypertensive mothers.

Management

The management of mild preeclampsia is directed principally toward preventing further increase in severity of the disease and fetal death. The management of severe preeclampsia is largely maternal (to prevent convulsions). The goals of therapy are as follows:

- To prevent or control convulsions
- To ensure survival of the mother with minimal morbidity
- To secure an infant as mature as possible without significant postnatal complications

Coordinated, vigorous symptomatic treatment of preeclampsia-eclampsia is required. Monitoring of the pregnant woman is important for the following reasons:

1. Early adequate antenatal care, including good nutrition, will protect against preeclampsia-eclampsia.

2. Prompt intensive therapy of preeclampsia will drastically reduce the incidence of eclampsia and the severity of its complications.

3. Proper definitive therapy of eclamptic convulsions will considerably reduce maternal and perinatal morbidity and mortality.

Pregnant women who do not receive regular antenatal care and consequent monitoring of their unborn child's condition are particularly vulnerable to the complications of preeclampsia-eclampsia. The first requisite of a successful health service is to make contact with childbearing families. Preventive measures include educational programs directed toward alerting pregnant women about (1) the symptomatology of the disease, (2) maternal and fetal nutritional requirements, and (3) when and where to go for treatment and advice.

Ultimate therapy is the termination of pregnancy by the easiest method that will be the least harmful to the mother and fetus. If the patient is not a good subject for induction, cesarean section, preferably after the thirty-sixth week of pregnancy, may be required. A delay of more than 2 weeks in severe preeclampsia is poor policy because fetal death may ensue. If delivery is still awaited 4 weeks or more after fetal death, disseminated intravascular coagulation may result. If there is no improvement after 48 hours of treatment at home, the woman should be admitted to a hospital.

PLAN OF CARE: SEVERE PREECLAMPSIA OR ECLAMPSIA

PATIENT CARE OBJECTIVES

1. Within 24 to 48 hours the following is achieved:
   a. Blood pressure: within normal limits.
   b. Urine: output >700 ml/24 hr. Protein: <+2.
   c. Blood within normal limits: BUN, CO_2 combining power, serum electrolytes. Serum protein >5 mg/100 ml.
   d. Symptoms have disappeared: edema, weight gain, headache, midepigastric pain, double vision.
2. If uncontrolled, vaginal delivery is effected.
3. If vaginal delivery is not possible, delivery by cesarean section is effected.
4. Patient and family are aware of the need for care, the cause of symptoms, and prognosis.
5. Emergency management is available at all times for convulsions, anuria, fetal distress, etc.
6. Records are complete at all times.

NURSING INTERVENTIONS

Diagnostic

1. Physical examination:
   a. Check BP frequently during acute phase and every 2 to 4 hours thereafter.
   b. Auscultate FHT when BP is obtained, if fetal monitor not used.
   c. Examine face and extremities, especially sacrum (dependent area when patient is in bed), for edema.
   d. Record 24-hour fluid intake and urine output.
   e. If labor begins, assess progress carefully (Chapter 20).
   f. Record results of daily funduscopic examination.
   g. Assess patient's affect.
2. Laboratory evaluation:
   a. Determine amount, character, and protein content of each 24-hour urine specimen until fourth to fifth postnatal day.
   b. Order serum BUN, CO_2 combining power and content, serum electrolytes, and serum protein as often as severity and progression of disorder indicate. If serum protein is <5 gm/100 ml, notify physician.

Therapeutic and educational

1. Admit patient to single darkened room. Place on absolute bed rest on her side with side rails up. Permit no visitors. Do not disturb patient for unnecessary procedures (e.g., baths, enemas) and leave BP cuff on arm. IV fluids are started and monitored to "keep open" or to maintain drug therapy. Foley catheter is inserted, and amount of urine is recorded at 1- to 4-hour intervals. Emergency equipment and drugs are kept in patient's room, including plastic airway, padded tongue blade, O_2 and suction equipment, and medications such as magnesium sulfate, calcium gluconate, cardiac stimulants, and hypertensive controls such as hydralazine, 50% glucose. Emergency delivery pack is kept in room. Attitude and approach of personnel should be matter-of-fact and calm; rationale of treatment is given briefly.
   NOTE: Plastic airway is preferred over padded tongue blade. Airway permits passage of tubes for suction and for administration of O_2.
2. Emergency care of convulsions:
   a. If convulsions occur, turn patient on her side to avoid aspiration of vomitus and to prevent vena caval syndrome.
   b. Insert folded towel, plastic airway, or tongue (padded) blade into side of mouth to prevent biting of lips or tongue and to maintain airway. Do not put your fingers into her mouth.
   c. Aspirate food and fluid from glottis or trachea.
   d. Administer O_2 by face cone or tent (masks and nasal catheters cause excessive stimulation).
   e. Give magnesium sulfate as ordered.
   f. Record time, duration, and description of convulsion (p. 249).
3. Have patient typed and matched. Keep blood available for emergency transfusion. (Patients with eclampsia often develop premature separation of placenta, hemorrhage, and shock.)
4. Diet and fluids: Give as directed; record time, amount, and patient's response.
   a. Permit nothing by mouth if patient is convulsing.
   b. Insert retention catheter for accurate measurement of urinary output. If urine output is >700 ml/24 hr, replace output, plus other fluid loss, with salt-free fluid (including parenteral) each day. If output is <700 ml/24 hr, allow no more fluid than 2000 ml/24 hr, including IV fluid. If patient can eat, give low-salt (<1 Gm NaCl/24 hr), high-carbohydrate, low-fat, moderate-protein diet. Give potassium chloride as salt substitute.
   c. Assist physician with infusion of 200 to 300 ml of 20% solution of dextrose in water IV, two to three times a day during critical period to support liver function, aid nutrition, and replace fluid. Note and record patient response. Avoid 50% glucose, which often will sclerose veins. Sodium-containing fluids, such as Ringer's solution, are contraindicated. If patient is oliguric or if serum protein is low, the physician may order salt-poor albumin (25 to 50 ml) or 250 to 500 ml of plasma or serum to be administered IV.

Continued.

PLAN OF CARE: SEVERE PREECLAMPSIA OR ECLAMPSIA—cont'd

NURSING INTERVENTIONS—cont'd

Diagnostic	Therapeutic and educational

	5. Medications: Give as directed; monitor and record patient response. Record drugs, dosages, times given.
	  a. Diuretics such as chlorohydrothiazide, 25 to 50 mg orally or well-diluted IV, may promote diuresis (in patients who are not anuric or severely oliguric).
	  b. Sedatives such as phenobarbital, 0.05 Gm, are given orally or IM on admission to hospital and repeated to maintain moderate sedation until patient is improved.
	  c. Magnesium sulfate IV or IM as necessary (see above) may be ordered.
	6. Physician and/or nurse explains procedures briefly and quietly to patient. Patient is never left alone if condition is severe. Family is also kept informed of management, rationale, and patient's progress. Family is encouraged to express concerns.
	7. Delivery: Preeclampsia-eclampsia and severe hypertensive or renal disease are intensified by continuing pregnancy. Termination of gestation is only practical treatment. Fetus may therefore be premature or otherwise compromised (Chapter 36).
	  a. Eclampsia is controlled before attempting induction of labor, then labor is induced by amniotomy (Chapter 20).
	  b. Oxytocin may be used cautiously to stimulate labor (Chapter 20).
	  c. Nitrous oxide (70%) and oxygen (30%) may be given with contractions, but 100% oxygen should be given between contractions.
	  d. Vaginal delivery under pudendal block anesthesia is preferred. However, if patient cannot be induced readily, if she is bleeding, if there is fetal distress, cesarean section will be performed, preferably under procaine or equivalent local infiltration of abdominal wall. Thiopental (Pentothal) may be given after delivery of baby for incisional closure (Chapter 36).
	  e. Pediatrician is present for delivery.
	8. Postnatal:
	  a. BP is checked every 4 hours for 48 hours or more frequently as patient's condition warrants.
	  b. Patient is asked to report headaches, blurred vision, etc. Nurse assesses her affect, alert or dull. BP is checked before giving analgesic for headache.
	  c. Patient is given information as to (a) prognosis, i.e., preeclampsia-eclampsia does not necessarily recur in subsequent pregnancies, but careful antenatal care is essential; (b) necessity for careful evaluation at sixth postnatal week check to rule out chronic hypertension; and (c) family planning information; i.e., pregnancy should be delayed 2 years.
	  d. Opportunity to discuss emotional response to having this complication is provided.

Medical directives will include the following:
1. Absolute bed rest (without visitors); quiet room; minimal stimulation
2. Blood pressure, serum electrolytes, urine protein determinations, and plasma or urinary estriols at frequent intervals
3. Funduscopic examination daily to note arteriolar spasm, edema, hemorrhages, and exudates
4. High-carbohydrate, low-fat, moderate- or high-protein diet with low or moderate salt
5. A zero fluid balance if the urine output is more than 500 ml/24 hr
6. Sedatives, diuretics, and antihypertensive and anticonvulsant drugs to be given as indicated
7. Monitoring for signs of labor and FHT

Magnesium sulfate is an excellent anticonvulsant for the prevention or control of eclampsia. The drug may be given intravenously by intravenous push (20 ml of a 10% aqueous solution), injected slowly (5 ml every 30 seconds), and repeated after 1 or more hours. The drug may also be administered by volutrol (4 mg in 100 ml of 5% dextrose in water) over a 30-minute period, followed by intravenous infusion (10 mg in 900 ml of 5% dextrose in water) at 100 drops/min. No more than 20 to 25 Gm should be given over 24 hours, however, or toxic effects may develop. Magnesium sulfate may be given intramuscularly also (10 ml of a 50% solution), injected slowly into each buttock, followed by a single injection of 10 ml/6 hr. In this instance, the recommended maximum dose is 50 ml/24 hr.

Magnesium sulfate has a CNS-depressant effect, and it reduces blood pressure by splanchnic vasodilatation. Therefore the blood pressure should be monitored continuously while the drug is being administered intravenously and every 15 minutes at other times. The drug also augments urine flow. (Do not repeat the drug if the urinary output is less than 100 ml/hr.) Magnesium salts cross the placenta and may not be well tolerated by the fetus.

Maternal (and fetal) toxicity has been reached when the respirations are fewer than 16/min or when the knee jerks are no longer present. The antidote is a calcium salt such as calcium gluconate, with 20 ml of a 10% aqueous solution given intravenously slowly and repeated every hour until the respiratory, urinary, and neurologic depression has been alleviated. The maximum number of injections of a calcium salt is 8/24 hr.

HYPERTENSIVE CARDIOVASCULAR DISEASE

Hypertension is considered to be present in women during the childbearing years when the blood pressure is maintained at above 140/80 at rest. Hypertensive disorders during pregnancy comprise an extremely important group that accounts for a high maternal and perinatal morbidity and mortality.

The vascular complications of hypertension, such as intracranial hemorrhage, are the consequence of increased arterial pressure and related atherosclerosis.

Hypertension without apparent impairment of the heart is termed *hypertensive vascular disease,* in contrast with *hypertensive cardiovascular disease,* in which left ventricular hypertrophy, coronary artery disease, or heart failure has developed.

Primary (essential) hypertensive disease in which no cause can be determined for the hypertension is the diagnosis in about 85% of nonpregnant premenopausal hypertensive women. The remaining 15% of hypertensives will have secondary hypertensive vascular disease caused by disorders such as chronic pyelonephritis or glomerulonephritis, renal artery stenosis, or coarctation of the aorta.

Why hypertension occurs in the primary variety is still undetermined, but abnormalities in the regulation of blood pressure, including increased vascular resistance or activity of the sympathetic nervous system, may be responsible, at least in part. Moreover, hypertension may be produced in ways difficult to explain by adrenal glucocorticoids, aldosterone, desoxycorticosterone, or other hormones.

The cardiac output and blood volume continue to be maintained until heart failure or severe edema develop. Obviously the increased "load" associated with even normal pregnancy increases the work of the heart and adds to the stress on the vasculature. When obstetric complications such as preeclampsia-eclampsia, diabetes mellitus, or multiple pregnancy ensue, vascular complications, even heart failure, may develop.

When hypertension is sustained for years, the initially reversible arteriolar constriction becomes permanent as a result of intimal thickening, hypertrophy of vascular muscular coats, and hyaline degeneration. Left ventricular hypertrophy follows eventually. Coronary and cerebral artery atherosclerosis usually develop, often leading to myocardial infarction, cerebral hemorrhage, or infarction.

The patient with mild to moderate essential hypertensive vascular disease may enjoy apparently normal health for years. Sooner or later, complaints typical of progressive, now symptomatic, disease may include suboccipital headaches, especially those which occur in the early morning but subside during the day, lightheadedness, tinnitus, and palpation of the heart. With more progressive disease, signs of heart failure, renal incompetency, or CNS complications develop.

Management

With chronic hypertensive disease, the physician treats the symptomatology during pregnancy. The pregnancy is usually permitted to continue if the patient responds to therapy. Frequent estriol determinations after the thirty-second week will be ordered in an attempt to carry the fetus to 34 to 36 weeks. Protracted therapy is futile if the patient is unresponsive. Fetal death or maternal CNS, cardiac, or renal complications may develop. If the blood pressure reaches 200/110, immediate medical attention is necessary. The physician will usually order antihypertensive drugs, for example, hydralazine (Apresoline), and assess the need for a prompt delivery.

REFERENCES

Baskett, T. F., and Bradford, C. R. 1975. Active management of severe preeclampsia. Can. Med. Assoc. J. **109:**1209.

Ferris, T. 1975. Toxemia and hypertension. In Medical complications during pregnancy. Burrow, G., and Ferris, T. (eds.). Philadelphia, W. B. Saunders Co.

Friedman, E. A. 1975. Effect of blood pressure on perinatal mortality. In International Workshop on the Clinical Criteria of Toxemia. Vollman, R. (ed.). Springfield, Ill., Charles C Thomas, Publishers.

Lopez-Leera, M., and Hernandez-Horta, J. L. 1974. Pregnancy after eclampsia. Am. J. Obstet. Gynecol. **119:**193.

Macgillivray, I., and others. 1969. Blood pressure in pregnancy. Clin. Sci. **37:**395.

Pahe, E. W. 1972. On the pathogenesis of preeclampsia and eclampsia. J. Obstet. Gynaecol. Br. Commonw. **79:**883.

Roach, C. J. 1973. Renovascular hypertension in pregnancy. Obstet. Gynecol. **42:**856.

Sullivan, M. 1974. Blood pressure elevation in pregnancy. Prog. Cardiovasc. Dis. **16:**375.

Wilber, J. A. 1972. The management of hypertension during pregnancy. J. Reprod. Med. **8:**53.

Wiser, W. L. and others. 1972. Laboratory characteristics in toxemia. Obstet. Gynecol. **39:**866.

CHAPTER 18

Medical-surgical diseases complicating pregnancy

MAJOR MEDICAL COMPLICATIONS

Pregnancy confers no immunity against infectious disorders. In fact, certain contagious diseases such as poliomyelitis or other infectious conditions such as appendicitis may be more severe or their complications more serious in pregnant women as compared with nonpregnant women. Both mother and fetus must be considered when the pregnant woman contracts an infection. In some disorders, for example, tuberculosis, the fetus is almost always spared, even though the mother may be dying. In other diseases such as rubella, the fetus may be critically compromised, whereas the mother may be only slightly ill.

What is the effect of the disease on pregnancy, and what is the effect of pregnancy on the disease? These are two basic questions that invariably require answers in maternity care. If the probable risk to the fetus is too great such as in the case of rubella, interruption of the pregnancy may be justified on a fetal indication. On the other hand, therapeutic abortion for maternal reasons (e.g., diabetic retinitis) may also be warranted.

Preventive medicine is particularly important in obstetrics, since many tragedies can be averted by informed anticipation. For example, vaccination against rubella before pregnancy currently is the only means to control this disorder because no cure has yet been developed. Similarly, women should be given contraceptive advice so that pregnancy will not occur until they have either recovered or have reached a phase in a chronic disorder when the mother or fetus may not be seriously jeopardized. Progressive chronic diseases for which treatment is still sought and that may be aggravated by pregnancy, such as Marfan's syndrome, may be an indication for sterilization.

Acute infectious diseases

Rubella (German measles). Rubella is extremely teratogenic especially during the first trimester (pp. 606

and 607). Vaccination of pregnant women is contraindicated, however, and pregnancy should be prevented for 2 months after vaccination. Nonetheless, hemagglutinin-inhibition antigen–negative parturients can be safely vaccinated after delivery.

Variola (smallpox). Variola now is extremely rare, thanks to worldwide vaccination. The virus responsible for smallpox often causes abortion or premature delivery, and postnatal hemorrhage is common. Maternal mortality is greatly increased. The child may be born with the pox and may die in severe cases.

Vaccination during pregnancy is so hazardous for the fetus, however, that such treatment should be employed only during smallpox epidemics.

Rubeola (measles). Rubeola is uncommon during pregnancy because most women have had the disease and are immune. When it does occur as a complication of gestation, measles may cause abortion or premature labor, but maternal death is rare due to the exanthem. The fetus may be born with a rash but generally survives without developmental anomalies. Prophylactic gamma globulin may prevent the disease. Measles vaccination of susceptible women prior to (but never during) pregnancy is recommended.

Varicella (chickenpox). The virus responsible for varicella is also the cause of herpes zoster (shingles). The severe disseminated epidemic type of varicella during pregnancy may be fatal for the mother (and fetus) because of necrotizing angiitis. In milder cases, growth retardation or fetal deformity such as skin or muscle anomalies, chorioretinitis, or hydrocephalus may develop. These abnormalities are rare, however, so that therapeutic abortion generally is not recommended. Whether gamma globulin will prevent varicella is still undecided. A vaccine for varicella has not yet been developed.

Influenza. Pregnant women may have an increased incidence of influenza. The influenza virus, antigen types A and B, which are clinically indistinguishable, may cause severe, even critical illness in the mother, particularly when viral pneumonia develops. Type C influenza ordinarily is a minor malaise. Conclusive proof that influenza causes congenital anomalies is lacking. Polyvalent influenza virus (attenuated live virus) vaccine is contraindicated for pregnant patients.

Infectious hepatitis. *Viral hepatitis,* one of several causes of liver failure during pregnancy, usually is spread by droplet or hand contact, especially by culinary workers. Another specific type is *serum hepatitis,* generally passed by contaminated needles, syringes, or blood transfusions. Serum hepatitis can also be transmitted orally or by coitus, however, but the incubation period is longer. Transmission of the virus to the infant occurs during birth, not transplacentally as was previously thought. Hepatitis is not an indication for abdominal delivery, however, because the virus is not limited to the lower genital tract.

Viral hepatitis is not an indication for interruption of pregnancy because most mothers and their children do well with supportive therapy, but premature delivery may occur in severe cases. Gamma globulin can be given as prophylaxis for infectious hepatitis but not for serum hepatitis.

The differential diagnosis includes fatty metamorphosis of the liver, tetracycline liver toxicity, anesthetic (halothane, methoxyflurane) toxicity, and obstetric hepatosis.

Mumps (epidemic parotitis). The viremia of mumps, rarely a severe maternal complication of pregnancy, may cause fetal maldevelopment. Microcephaly and hepatomegaly have been reported, and abortion, as well as premature labor, may occur. Prophylaxis of epidemic parotitis is possible with the administration of hyperimmune mumps gamma globulin.

Herpesvirus hominis infections. Genital herpesvirus hominis infections are caused by herpes simplex type 2 virus. The external genitals, vagina and cervix, may be involved. Painful vesicles develop, then drain, and superficial ulceration develops. Scrapings of the open lesions stained by Giemsa or other appropriate stain reveal intranuclear inclusion bodies (virus aggregations). Symptomatic therapy alone is available; no specific cure has been identified.

The virus, lethal for the fetus, inoculates the neonate during vaginal delivery. Hence if the mother has genital herpes, cesarean section should be recommended. If premature rupture of the membranes occurs before term but after viability, cesarean section within 3 hours of release of amniotic fluid usually will prevent neonatal infection (p. 604).

Cytomegalic inclusion disease. The cytomegalovirus, which occasionally infects the lower female genital tract without symptomatology, is extremely teratogenic for the fetus. It probably reaches the fetus by invasion through the membranes or placenta. Microcephaly, chorioretinitis, periventricular necrosis, and calcification and sclerosis of cranial bones may be identified at birth. In the neonatal period, early jaundice, melena, hematemesis, and hematuria may develop. Cytomegalic inclusion cells in the gastric washings, fetal cerebrospinal fluid, or fresh urine are diagnostic. Neonatal death or the survival of a severely handicapped infant is likely. No medical treatment is effective. Diagnosis prior to delivery is impossible so that therapeutic abortion is not feasible.

Toxoplasmosis. Toxoplasmosis, caused by the *Toxoplasma gondii,* is found in cat feces and may be responsible for repeated abortion, premature delivery, and perinatal death. The mother may be asymptomatic, but the fetus is affected by transplacental parasitemia. A positive Savin-Feldman serotest or positive Westphal complement fixation reaction may identify maternal toxoplasmosis. Unfortunately this will not establish whether it is an old (cured) infection or a recent infectious state. Cats may be dangerous pets for pregnant women if they come in contact with the feces because no effective treatment is available. Therapeutic abortion, sterilization or both are not justified for toxoplasmosis under the circumstances.

Listeriosis. The small gram-negative coccus *Listeria monocytogenes* occasionally may cause abortion or later termination of pregnancy. Leukorrhea, urinary frequency or dysurea, and enteritis may be the only symptoms recalled by the pregnant woman.

Amnionitis or placentitis may initiate fetal infection, or the disease may be acquired by contamination during the birth process. Septicemia and localization of the disease is the rule, but abnormal development has not been described. The diagnosis may be made by culture or complement fixation tests.

Treatment with penicillin or erythromycin usually is successful. The organism is sensitive to tetracycline also, but this drug may cause dysplasia of the dental enamel and discoloration of the teeth of the infant. Unfortunately the diagnosis of listeriosis often is obscure or delayed; hence the prognosis for the fetus generally is poor, but maternal death due to this disorder is exceptional.

Malaria. Acute febrile disorders including fulminating attacks of malaria may cause abortion or premature labor. In general, however, pregnancy termination by malaria is most uncommon. The plasmodia of malaria are not responsible for anomalous fetal development, although the parasite can be identified in the cord blood occasionally. Quinine may be harmful to the fetus (nerve deafness), but it will not induce abortion or early labor. Nonetheless, chloroquine phosphate (Aralen) may be fetotoxic. In severe cases of malaria, however, the employment of appropriate medications may be an acceptable calculated risk.

Gonorrhea. Gonorrhea is the most common contagious bacterial disease in North America. Gonorrhea often is only mildly symptomatic in women, or the diplococci may persist unsuspected in the lower genital tract. After the third month of pregnancy, gonorrheal salpingitis rarely occurs, perhaps because with progressive pregnancy, the chorion laeve fuses with the decidua parietalis, thus obliterating the endometrial cavity.

Gonorrhea during pregnancy must be treated adequately, or the sexual partner may be infected or reinfected after treatment. Moreover, gonococcal ophthalmia neonatorum may be contracted by the neonate during delivery. Postnatal maternal complications of untreated gonorrhea include acute salpingitis, dermatitis, or arthritis. (For further discussion of gonorrheal infection of the neonate, refer to p. 606.)

Penicillin G, 4.8 million units intramuscularly, is the therapy recommended by the Federal Drug Administration for the treatment of gonorrhea in women. It is interesting and important that this dosage is the same for the treatment of both gonorrhea and syphilis.

Erythromycin, tetracycline, the cephalosporins, and kanamycin (in adequate doses) can be given to women sensitive to penicillin.

Syphilis (lues). Syphilis probably continues to be the major cause of late abortion throughout the world, despite the widespread success of diagnosis and treatment of this disease. Congenital syphilis still occurs, even in developed countries, since it may be acquired in early pregnancy after the initial obstetric examination and negative serum test for syphilis (STS) has been obtained.

Because the chancre of syphilis may be transient, asymptomatic, or obscure (e.g., on the cervix) in pregnant women, the diagnosis of primary lues may be delayed or overlooked. On the other hand, secondary luetic lesions such as condylomata lata may be more extensive in pregnant than in nonpregnant patients. Serum from such lesions should be subjected to dark-field study to identify *Treponema pallidum,* the cause of syphilis. When the diagnosis is in doubt or when the woman is exposed to the disease during the course of gestation, a repeat STS during the second or third trimester is recommended.

Pregnancy may reduce the severity of syphilis. On the

other hand, the pathology and pathophysiology of syphilis for the pregnant woman depends on whether the maternal lues was contracted before pregnancy, at conception, or later in gestation.

If syphilis is acquired before or at the time of conception, midtrimester abortion or fetal death may ensue, but early abortion due to the disease rarely, if ever, occurs. Frequently, untreated syphilis that begins during pregnancy can cause the untimely delivery of a deformed fetus with congenital syphilis. Such an infant may suffer growth retardation, rhagades, or other stigmata of syphilis. If stillborn or if neonatal death occurs, autopsy may disclose abnormally wide osteochondritic epiphyses, luetic hepatitis, or CNS lesions. The placenta often is larger than normal for the gestational age and is thick and pallid (fibrotic). In contrast, if the diagnosis is made early and treatment is completed by the fifth month of gestation, congenital syphilis probably will not occur.

One should obtain an STS at the patient's first obstetric visit, and ideally it should be repeated again late in pregnancy. A positive STS is not proof of syphilis; positive STS reactions may be reported in collagenous diseases and viral or other spirochetal diseases. A negative STS is not a guarantee of the absence of this disease either, since a negative STS may be obtained in very early syphilis (before a positive STS can result). If the STS is positive, a presumptive diagnosis of syphilis must be made. A fluorescent treponemal antibody (FTA) test and a *T. pallidum* immobilization (TPI) test should determine the specificity of a persistently positive STS. This sequence should be followed also when the STS is equivocal in patients who have no history or symptomatology of syphilis, assuming they are not on antiluetic therapy.

A successful treatment regimen for syphilis during pregnancy requires the administration of procaine penicillin G with 2% aluminum monostearate (PAM) intramuscularly, 4.8 million units total usually given as 2.4 million units initially (as noted), then 1.2 million units at each of two subsequent injections 3 days apart.

The patient with untreated syphilis in labor should receive 3 million units intramuscularly and 2 million units every other day for a total of 6 million units. The infant should be treated also.

If the mother is allergic to penicillin, erythromycin should be administered 2.4 Gm orally over a 2-week period of therapy.

All cases of syphilis must be reported to the health authorities, and contacts should be treated.

The infant suspected of having congenital syphilis should be isolated until the correct diagnosis can be established. If confirmed, the newborn should receive 50,000 units/kg of procaine penicillin G with 2% aluminum monostearate intramuscularly, and this dose should be repeated 2 days later. (For further discussion of syphilitic infection of the neonate, refer to pp. 602 to 604.)

Monthly examinations of the pregnant woman and a quantitative blood STS should be done once each month until delivery and for 1 month after delivery. If there is evidence of relapse or if the STS titer remains high, penicillin treatment should be repeated.

Yaws. Yaws, a nonvenereal, highly contagious disease, is caused by the spirochete *Treponema pertenue,* closely related to the causative organism of syphilis. Both syphilis and yaws give a positive result in the Wasserman test. Yaws is a common disease in equatorial Africa, Hawaii, South America, and the East and West Indies. It is effectively treated with antibiotics, especially penicillin.

Poliomyelitis (polio). Prophylaxis for poliomyelitis has almost eradicated this disorder in some countries. Polio is still prevalent and potentially devastating in parts of Asia and Africa.

Poliomyelitis exerts a serious, even critical, effect on pregnancy, and pregnancy increases the severity of poliomyelitis. Bulbar poliomyelitis and paralysis of the diaphragm are especially dread complications. However, therapeutic abortion is rarely indicated. Early delivery, often by cesarean section, may be important to the life or health of the paralyzed mother or growth-retarded fetus.

The incidences of abortion, premature delivery, and fetal death are increased in poliomyelitis. Moreover, occasional birth defects have been ascribed to polio. A fetal viremia may occur or the infant may be inoculated by the organism during the birth process. Surviving infants have been born with flaccid paralysis.

Prophylaxis for pregnant women is possible with Salk vaccine (killed virus) but *not* Sabin vaccine (attenuated live virus). The first confers an immunity of about 2 years; the Sabin vaccination is followed by permanent immunization.

Tuberculosis. Pulmonary tuberculosis does not jeopardize pregnancy, although urinary and CNS tuberculosis may. Congenital tuberculosis is extremely rare, but infection of the infant by its mother with active disease may occur during nursing or newborn care, with serious consequences.

Chemotherapy of tuberculosis, using drugs such as streptomycin, para-aminosalicylic acid, and isoniazid, has been extremely effective and is safe for the fetus in the dosages recommended. Ancillary procedures such as pneumothorax or lobectomy are not contraindicated

by pregnancy. Therapeutic abortion rarely is indicated for tuberculosis. Cesarean section is warranted only for obstetric indications in tuberculous patients.

Once the infant has been delivered, it should have no intimate contact with the mother or others who may have the disease until contagion is no longer a problem.

Contraception is most important for women with active tuberculosis. All pregnant women should be evaluated for tuberculosis (tine test), early in pregnancy and later if suspicion exists.

The prognosis for the tuberculous mother depends on the stage of the disease, her resistance, and the success of therapy. Sterilization may be elected but is rarely indicated for the tuberculous patient. Nonetheless, pregnancy is contraindicated until the patient has been free of the disease for 1½ to 2 years.

Bacteremic shock (septic shock)

Critical infections particularly by bacteria that liberate endotoxin, for example, enteric gram-negative bacilli, may cause septic shock. Pregnant patients, especially those with diabetes mellitus, or women who are receiving immunosuppressive drugs are at increased risk of having this disorder.

Decreased capillary resistance, activation of arteriovenous shunts, leakage of plasma into the interstitial tissues, reduced blood volume, and diminished cardiac output are important factors in the development of this type of shock. Disseminated intravascular coagulation (DIC) may develop to cause abnormal bleeding. Hypoxia is the major problem, however, and this is especially noxious to the CNS, myocardium, and lungs.

High spiking fever and chills are evidence of serious sepsis. Anxiety, then apathy ensue. Concomitantly, the temperature often falls to slightly subnormal levels. The skin then becomes pale, cool, and moist. The pulse will be rapid and thready. Marked hypotension and peripheral cyanosis develop. Oliguria ensues.

Laboratory studies should reveal marked evidence of infection. (Blood culture may reveal bacteremia later.) Hemoconcentration, acidosis, and consumption coagulopathy may develop. CVP generally is low; ECG may reveal changes indicative of myocardial insufficiency. Evidence of cardiac, pulmonary, and renal failure will be notable.

The physician will initiate antishock therapy. Massive doses of antibiotics and corticosteroids are given intravenously if possible. The patient is digitalized. Heart function and urinary output are monitored closely. The infected area is drained or the focus of infection is removed, for example, by hysterectomy or infected abortion if the patient's condition will permit.

PLAN OF CARE: INFECTIONS DURING PREGNANCY

PATIENT CARE OBJECTIVES
  1. Infection is prevented.
  2. Infection is treated promptly with no or minimal sequelae for mother and infant.

NURSING INTERVENTIONS

Diagnostic	Therapeutic	Educational
	Educate the general public regarding immunization for nonimmune people. Many states are introducing or passing laws requiring screening for rubella titer. Tests for exposure to syphilis are routine. Easily accessible and person-oriented (nonjudgmental) clinics should be available to all so that people are encouraged to use them for diagnosis and treatment.	

Antenatal

Diagnostic	Therapeutic	Educational
1. Observe for any signs of infection: rash, fever, gland enlargement. 2. Viral studies: culture and sensitivity studies of exudates, blood, urine; microscopic (fluoroscopic) examination for causative agents.	1. Viral infections are treated symptomatically. Prophylactic antibiotic therapy may be instituted to prevent secondary infection. 2. If patient is to be treated at home, assist her and family in planning how she will implement prescribed care. 3. Assist physician and support patient and family during tests and when hearing results. 4. Assist with counseling prior to proposed therapeutic abortion. 5. If genital lesions are found (herpesvirus type 2), prepare patient for elective cesarean section. 6. Isolation techniques (institute and prepare patient for this situation).	1. Reinforce physician's explanations of cause, management, possible outcomes. 2. General care: a. Adequate hydration. b. Rest. c. Adhere to medication regimen (if on oral antibiotics, woman may prevent gastrointestinal upset by taking Lactinex or eating yogurt between doses). d. Keep temperature down with acetaminophen (Tylenol), fluids, cool sponge baths.

Postnatal

Diagnostic	Therapeutic	Educational
1. Assess effects on fetus or neonate. 2. Obtain cultures from mother and infant; send specimens. 3. Monitor vital signs. 4. General postnatal care: evaluate findings.	1. Provide nursing-medical care for high-risk infant. 2. Isolate infant and mother if indicated. 3. Assist patient and family with grieving if indicated. 4. Bed rest, diet.	1. Answer questions regarding infection, cause, management, expected prognosis.

Prompt diagnosis and intensive treatment afford a fairly good prognosis. Encouraging signs include increasing alertness and the establishment of good urine flow.

Diabetes mellitus

Diabetes mellitus is a recessive inheritable metabolic disorder in which glucose is poorly utilized because of a deficiency of insulin. Consequently glucose is elevated in the blood and excreted in the urine. Since glucose is lost with large amounts of water in the urine, dehydration results. The glucose deficit is partially restored from protein and fat, but acidosis and muscle wasting may ensue. Most metabolic defects are correctable by diet or the administration of insulin.

Many consider diabetes mellitus to be the most important of all endocrine diseases. About 4% of females (2% of males) are or will become diabetic. Diabetes complicates at least 1 of every 300 pregnancies in North America. This disorder is a major cause of increased maternal morbidity and of perinatal morbidity and mortality.

Definitions. Numerous definitions involving insulin-dependent and noninsulin dependent states seek to clarify the problem of diagnosis of diabetes during pregnancy:

1. *Prediabetes* is a latent phase of diabetes that may exist prior to the diagnosis of actual diabetes mellitus. Because this is only a concept, it is not a clinical entity and is an inappropriate term in patient management.

2. *Chemical diabetes* refers to a metabolic disorder typified by an abnormally high glucose tolerance test (GTT) in asymptomatic patients. Treatment usually is diet except in severe cases and during pregnancy when insulin may be required.

3. *Gestational diabetes* is diabetes diagnosed during pregnancy but subclinical and unidentifiable by standard tests in nonpregnant women. Diet usually is adequate for the control of this disorder.

4. *Manifest diabetes mellitus* is frank diabetes and insulin dependent except in mild cases.

White's commonly used *Classification of Pregnant Diabetics* relates the duration and severity of the disease to treatment and prognosis.

1. *Class A*—abnormal GTT due to diabetes mellitus
2. *Class B*—frank diabetes with onset over age 20 years; duration 0 to 9 years; no vascular disease
3. *Class C*—onset of diabetes between 10 to 19 years of age; duration of disease 10 to 19 years; no vascular disease
4. *Class D*—onset under age 10 years; duration 20 years or more; vascular disease (retinitis, calcification in leg muscles)
5. *Class E*—diabetes with calcified pelvic vessels
6. *Class F*—same as class E plus retinopathy and nephropathy (often Kemmelstiel-Wilson intercapillary nephrosclerosis)

Although even milder forms of diabetes pose a threat to mother and infant, the incidence of perinatal death increases with the presence and degree of vascular or renal pathology (classes D, E, and F).

Effects of diabetes mellitus on pregnancy. Perinatal and neonatal mortality increases in about 25% of patients (gestational diabetes and those with insulin-dependent diabetes). Ketoacidosis presents the greatest fetal risk. In addition, there is a higher incidence (three to four times) of preeclampsia-eclampsia, especially if vascular complications exist.

There is a greater likelihood of large fetuses associated with dystocia, often requiring operative vaginal delivery and fetomaternal trauma or cesarean section.

Hydramnios occurs about ten times as often in diabetic pregnancies as in nondiabetic pregnancies, and major congenital anomalies (all types) are diagnosed approximately four times as often as with normal pregnancy.

Fetal-neonatal hypoglycemia is more common in insulin-dependent diabetics (p. 599).

Effects of pregnancy on diabetes mellitus. One effect is hyperemesis during early pregnancy. With complications such as gastrointestinal disorders, dietary control of diabetes is reduced, and the development of acidosis is increased.

Hypertrophy of pancreatic islets of Langerhans occurs; hyperinsulinemia may develop, but there is a reduced utilization of insulin by peripheral tissues.

In addition, there is an increased need for exogenous insulin in women on insulin in most cases as pregnancy progresses.

The occurrence of acidosis, hypoxia, and fetal death is increased. There is also a greater incidence of hypoglycemia after the "work" of labor in both mother and neonate.

Infections are much more common and serious in diabetic women who are pregnant (e.g., pyelonephritis, monilial vaginitis).

Headache is manifested by about 10% of diabetic women, beginning in the latter half of pregnancy.

Diagnosis. Diabetes mellitus should be considered when there is a family history of diabetes, recurrent preeclampsia-eclampsia, a previously large fetus (4000 gm or more), polyhydramnios, unexplained fetal death or anomaly, obesity, or glycosuria.

Glycosuria can be diagnosed with Tes-Tape or Clinistix, which depends on enzyme reactions specific for glucose, without confusion with fructosuria or lactosuria.

Patients with insulin-dependent diabetes diagnosed prior to pregnancy will not need a GTT. In contrast, pregnant women suspected of having diabetes, especially those with glycosuria, should be screened after a standard meal by a 2-hour blood sugar determination. If the blood glucose value is 120 mg/100 ml or more, the patient should then have a complete GTT. Retesting during pregnancy may be necessary in borderline cases.

An intravenous GTT frequently is done, since gastrointestinal motility and therefore absorption is delayed during pregnancy. Some physicians prefer the 5-hour oral test, however.

Normal blood sugar values for the GTT in most institutions are as follows: fasting level, 100 mg/100 ml; 1 hour, 160 mg/100 ml; 2 hours, 120 mg/100 ml; and 3 hours, a return to a normal fasting level.

PLAN OF CARE: DIABETES AND PREGNANCY

PATIENT CARE OBJECTIVES

1. Family and patient understand the disease process and are informed about and willing to participate actively in its management.
2. Patient suffers no sequelae of diabetes (e.g., nephropathy, retinopathy).
3. Patient suffers no related complication of pregnancy: hyperemesis gravidarum, preeclampsia-eclampsia.
4. Fetus is not exposed to maternal acidosis.
5. Infection (maternal) is prevented or treated promptly with no sequelae for mother or infant.

NURSING INTERVENTIONS

Diagnostic	Therapeutic	Educational
Antenatal: early pregnancy	Severity of disease determines management.	Nurse's prime role is to elicit patient's and her family's cooperation in management of diabetes and pregnancy: keeping all appointments, daily urine tests, strict dietary control, early treatment for infection, etc.
1. Identify woman at risk by thorough intake history. 2. Assess patient's knowledge regarding disease, diet, urine, and blood tests.	1. Diet (must be individualized): a. Calories: 30 to 40 calories/kg. b. Carbohydrates: 150 to 250 gm. c. Protein: 60 to 80 gm. d. Fats: 80 to 90 gm. 2. Hospitalize patient to assess physical and disease status and management (diet, insulin type, dosage).	
Antenatal: last trimester	1. Encourage visits every week to supervise management.	1. Insulin needs are usually higher during third trimester.
1. Observe for hypoglycemia or hyperglycemia, preeclampsia, etc. 2. Urine: Tes-Tape, Diastix, Clinistix for glucose. 3. Patient may be hospitalized for following: a. IV GTT. b. OCT. c. 24-hour determinations of urine estriols, proteins. d. Amniocentesis for L/S ratio, creatinine levels. e. Sonography A scan for gestational age. f. Assessment of vital signs, FHT, signs of onset of labor, weight, output, dietary intake, and insulin requirements. 4. Assess patient and family's need for referral to social services (housekeeping aid, financial assistance, etc.). 5. Assess patient and family's reaction to situation; assess patient's support system. 6. Assess mother's knowledge of her diabetes, its management, etc.	2. Hospitalize patient for following reasons: a. To control diabetes, readjust insulin. (Oral medications to control diabetes are contraindicated.) b. To treat infection. c. To estimate fetal age, maturity, and placental sufficiency; to plan delivery by induction or cesarean section, usually at 37 weeks' gestation. 3. Encourage expression of feelings regarding self and baby. 4. Provide diversional activities if hospitalized.	a. Maintenance: NPH until delivery. b. Fractional urines are tested qid as necessary 2. Diet. 3. Prepare for tests. 4. Keep patient informed; reinforce physician's explanations. 5. Fill in gaps in mother's knowledge regarding diabetes and its care.
Intranatal	1. Keep NPO. Monitor IV:	1. Keep patient informed regarding treatments, fetal status.
1. Observe for hypoglycemia: palpitation, tachycardia, hunger, weakness, sweating, tremor, pallor. Observe for preeclampsia. 2. Check urine: protein, glucose.	a. For induction (with Pitocin). b. 10% dextran in water and insulin to meet mother's calorie and insulin needs for work of labor.	

Continued.

PLAN OF CARE: DIABETES AND PREGNANCY—cont'd

NURSING INTERVENTIONS—cont'd

Diagnostic	Therapeutic	Educational

Intranatal—cont'd
3. Monitor labor:
  a. Monitor induction: maternal and fetal responses.
  b. Use fetal monitor, if available.
  c. Assess amount and character of amniotic fluid.
	2. Supportive labor nursing is especially important to prevent hypoglycemia from anxiety.
	3. Prepare for induction or cesarean section (fetal distress, fetopelvic disproportion, lack of response to induction).
	4. Alert pediatrician and nursery personnel.	

Postnatal
1. During first 24 to 48 hours, there is rapid insulin requirement fluctuation. Termination of pregnancy reverses gestation-induced endocrine changes: high serum blood sugar, elevated HGH and its potentiator, human placental lactogen (HPL).
  a. Frequent fractional urines.
  b. Monitor foods and fluids taken.
  c. Assess for clinical manifestations of high or low serum glucose levels.
2. Assess patient and family's reaction to experience, especially if fetal-neonatal death occurs or infant is malformed or at risk.
3. Monitor vital signs, amount of bleeding, uterine contractility, output, etc., as per usual postnatal routine.
	1. Adjust insulin (usually regular insulin). Patient may need no insulin for the first 24 to 48 hours. Progress to NPH per physician order. Allow patient to take over insulin injections when she desires.
	2. Provide postnatal nursing care (after vaginal or cesarean section delivery) per routine. (For nursing care of infant, see p. 600.)
	3. Provide care for patient and family after fetal-neonatal death or if neonate is malformed or at risk (pp. 243 to 245).
		1. Keep patient and family informed of her status and infant's condition.
		2. Infant will not necessarily have the disease during his lifetime.

Management. The overall management of the diabetic pregnant woman is directly related to associated problems: changes in glucose tolerance, alterations in insulin metabolism and utilization, and increased tendency to ketosis.

Therapeutic abortion may be justified for patients with class F diabetes.

Management is complicated by hyperemesis gravidarum, dietary indiscretion, nutritional imbalance, pyelonephritis, and preeclampsia-eclampsia. Diabetic pregnant headache may require hospitalization for narcotics, parenteral fluids, and bed rest therapy.

Ideally collaborative management of the diabetic patient should be accomplished by the obstetrician and internist. More frequent antenatal visits, for example, every 2 weeks until the thirty-second week and then every week thereafter, are desirable to avoid significant hypoglycemic and hyperglycemic states or sepsis. Dietary or insulin management must be based on blood glucose (not urine glucose) values. Oral hypoglycemics are contraindicated, since they may be fetotoxic and provide poor control of diabetes.

Delivery. The infants of class A diabetic women generally do well, and these mothers may be allowed to go to term unless complications develop.

Because fetal death is much more prevalent with diabetes classes B through F, planned delivery about the thirty-seventh week has become accepted policy in most maternity centers.

If adequate maturity (gestational age 37 weeks or more) can be established by ultrasound or x-ray examination, induction of labor may be initiated. Careful electronic monitoring of the fetus should be carried out. If strong labor and good progress do not ensue within 6 to 8 hours, cesarean section should be carried out. Poorly controlled diabetes or obstetric indications such as fetopelvic disproportion, positive OCT, change in estriol levels, or preeclampsia-eclampsia are also indications for a cesarean section. A pediatrician should be present at delivery to initiate proper neonatal care.

Prognosis. Proper medical-obstetric care, assuming good cooperation of the patient, should prevent serious complications and maternal death. Under the best of circumstances, the death rate of perinates of mothers with class A diabetes should be 5% or less, and in classes B through D, a 10% loss must be anticipated. At least a 50% perinatal mortality is likely even under optimal conditions in the presence of classes E and F diabetes.

Heart disease

Every pregnancy taxes the cardiovascular system. The heart rate is accelerated, and the blood volume and the cardiac output increase 30% to 50%. The normal heart can compensate for these and associated burdens so that pregnancy and delivery are generally well tolerated. If myocardial or valvular disease develops or if a congenital heart defect is large, cardiac decompensation is likely.

Symptoms of cardiac decompensation may appear abruptly or gradually. Medical intervention must be instituted immediately to correct cardiac status.

The patient notes the following symptoms: increasing fatigue, dyspnea, or both with her usual exertion; a feeling of smothering or difficulty in breathing; the need to cough frequently (coughing may be accompanied by hemoptysis); and periods of palpitation and tachycardia.

The examiner notes the following:

- Progressive, generalized edema
- Rales at the bases of the lungs
- Pulse irregularity

Heart disease affects 0.5% to 2% of pregnant women. In North America, rheumatic heart disease is responsible for 90% to 95% of cases and congenital heart disease, about 3% of problems. Syphilis and arteriosclerosis, as well as pulmonary and renal disorders, are responsible for cardiac complications, and some of these develop during pregnancy. Heart disease is of considerable importance for the expectant woman because a maternal mortality of 1% to 3% is likely with severe heart disease, and a perinatal mortality of up to 50% must be expected with persistent cardiac decompensation.

Rheumatic fever attacks the mitral, aortic, or tricuspid valves. Congenital maldevelopment involves the septa, valves, and conduction system, and persistently patent fetal cardiovascular communications may reduce the efficiency of the heart. Syphilis and arteriosclerosis alter the aortic valves and the conduction system principally.

The effects of pregnancy on heart disease involve an altered heart rate, blood pressure, cardiac output, blood volume, and other changes during pregnancy, labor, and postnatal readjustments.

One effect of heart disease on pregnancy is chorea gravidarum, ascribed to rheumatic fever often associated with rheumatic heart disease. In addition, spontaneous abortion is increased, and premature labor and delivery are more prevalent with heart disease. A growth-retarded fetus is typical of the cardiac patient.

The differential diagnosis involves respiratory problems, primarily arrhythmias.

The diagnosis of heart disease depends on the history, physical examination, x-ray films, and ultrasonograms when required.

The degree of dysfunction (disability) of the cardiac patient is often more important in the treatment and prognosis of heart disease complicating pregnancy than the diagnosis of the valvular lesion per se. The New York Heart Association's functional classification of organic heart disease, a widely accepted standard, is as follows:

1. *Class I*—patients with cardiac disease who have no limitation of physical activity
2. *Class II*—slight limitation of physical activity
3. *Class III*—considerable limitation of activity, with even ordinary activity producing symptoms
4. *Class IV*—patients unable to undertake any physical activity without discomfort; symptoms of cardiac insufficiency occurring even at rest

No classification of heart disease can be considered rigid or absolute, but this one offers a basic practical guide for treatment, assuming frequent antenatal visits, good patient cooperation, and proper medical-obstetric care.

Obstetric management

Class I. Patient should limit stress to protect against cardiac decompensation. Additional rest at night and after meals, frequent evaluations, and the early and effective treatment of respiratory and other infections should be stressed. Therapeutic abortion is never medically warranted. Assuming no obstetric problems, vaginal delivery using pudendal block anesthesia with prophylactic forceps for shortening of the second stage is recommended.

Class II. A program similar to class I should be followed. However, the patient should be admitted to the hospital near term (if signs of cardiac overload or arrhythmia develop) for evaluation and treatment often including subdigitalization.

Penicillin prophylaxis of nonsensitized patients against bacterial endocarditis in labor and during the early puerperium is good policy. Mask oxygen and pudendal block anesthesia are important. Ergot products should be avoided because of increases in blood pressure, but dilute intravenous oxytocin immediately after delivery may be employed to prevent postnatal hemorrhage. Tubal sterilization may be carried out, but surgery should be delayed several days at least to ensure homeostasis. If sterilization is not accomplished, effective contraception must be provided.

Class III. Bed rest for a full day each week should be a requisite. Cardiac decompensation occurs during pregnancy in about 30% of class III patients. With this possibility, hospitalization of the patient for the remainder of pregnancy and the early puerperium is advised. Early therapeutic abortion may be warranted, particularly after a previous episode of cardiac failure. Therapeutic abortion and elective sterilization may be feasible. Breast-feeding is contraindicated. Sterilization should be postponed until a later date, but explicit contraceptive advice must be given.

Class IV. Because these patients are decompensated even at rest, a major initial effort must be made to improve the cardiac status. Soon, early therapeutic abortion, although not innocuous, may be feasible under regional anesthesia in some cases. Prophylactic antibiotic therapy should cover the procedure. Vaginal delivery of patients with class IV lesions is the safest approach if abortion is not effected. The maternal mortality approaches 50% in class IV heart disease, and the perinatal mortality is even higher.

Postnatal adjustments. The immediate postnatal period is hazardous for a patient with a compromised heart. Cardiac output increases rapidly as extravascular fluid is remobilized into the vascular compartment.

At the moment of delivery, intra-abdominal pressure is reduced drastically; pressure on veins is removed, the splanchnic vessels engorge, and blood flow to the heart is increased. Fluid begins to move from extravascular spaces into the bloodstream. Some physicians favor the application of an abdominal binder or alternating tourniquets on the extremities to minimize the effects of this rapid change in intra-abdominal pressure.

Ergonovine (Ergotrate) and related oxytocics are contraindicated. Estrogen-containing compounds are contraindicated for the suppression of lactation, since these foster fluid retention and thromboembolization.

The patient's hospital stay is extended to 7 days or more for the following reasons:

1. Cardiac decompensation may occur as late as the sixth postnatal day.

2. Cardiac and respiratory function must be carefully supported. Support is achieved by the following measures:

   a. Proper positioning in bed with same position as for labor.

   b. Bed rest with bathroom privileges as tolerated. The nurse meets the patient's grooming and hygiene needs and may even assist her with turning in bed, eating, and other activities.

   c. Frequent opportunities to see and hold the baby but not to provide newborn care. The mother may nurse if her condition warrants.

   d. Progressive ambulation as tolerated. The nurse assesses her pulse, skin, and affect prior to and after walking.

   e. Bowel movements without stress or strain. Stool softeners, diet, and fluids plus mild analgesia and local anesthetic spray applied to the episiotomy may facilitate the process.

3. Hemorrhage or infection must be prevented or treated promptly and energetically.

4. Preparation for discharge home must be carefully planned with the patient and her family as follows:

   a. The mother will need help in the home from relatives, friends, social services, and others whether or not she plans to keep the newborn.

   b. The mother must plan rest and sleep periods, activity, and diet.

   c. The couple may need information regarding reestablishment of sexual relations, contraception, or sterilization (male, female) and medical supervision.

Surgery for heart disorders. Operations for the correction of congenital or acquired heart disease should be done prior to pregnancy, if possible.

Closed cardiac surgery such as release of stenotic mitral orifice can be accomplished with little risk to mother or fetus. Open heart surgery, on the other hand, requires extracorporeal circulation, and under these circumstances, hypoxia may develop. As a consequence, the risk of fetal damage or loss rises to almost 30%. If anticoagulant therapy is required during pregnancy, heparin should be used because this large molecular drug does not cross the placenta. Oral anticoagulants such as warfarin (Coumadin) compounds cross to the fetus and may cause anomalies or hemorrhage in the infant. Valvuloplasty patients should receive penicillin or other antibiotic prophylaxis against bacterial endocarditis during gestation, however.

PLAN OF CARE: HEART DISEASE

PATIENT CARE OBJECTIVES
1. Patient is able to tolerate the stresses imposed by pregnancy.
2. Congestive heart failure (the primary cause of maternal mortality in cardiac patients) is prevented.

NURSING INTERVENTIONS

Diagnostic	Therapeutic	Educational
Antenatal		
1. Observe for signs of cardiac decompensation.	1. Schedule a weekly patient contact; hospitalize to stabilize cardiac status as necessary.	1. Reinforce physician's explanation for need for close medical supervision.
2. Assess for additional factors that would increase stress on the heart: a. Anemia. b. Infection. c. Home situation including responsibility for house, other children, extended family members.	2. Medical mangement in hospital. 3. Support cardiac function: a. Promote rest. b. Restrict activity. c. Maintain adequate diet. d. Avoid infection.	2. Review with patient and family symptoms of cardiac decompensation. 3. Promote rest: sleep 8 to 10 hours every day and ½ hour after meals. Alleviate anxiety whenever possible.
3. Routine monitoring for antenatal period: weight gain and pattern of weight gain, edema, vital signs, discomforts of pregnancy, urine analysis, blood work.	4. Anticoagulation therapy. If patient is taking dicumarol, change to heparin. (Dicumarol causes fetal hemorrhage.)	4. Restrict activities: no housework, no shopping, no laundry; restrict climbing.
4. Note medications patient is taking.		5. Maintain adequate nutrition (especially difficult when someone else shops and cooks): diet high in iron and protein; adequate calories to gain 24 pounds during pregnancy.
		6. Avoid infection: avoid large crowds; notify physician at first sign of infection or when exposed to infection.
		7. Teach patient to give herself heparin.
		8. Provide anticipatory guidance for management of her labor and early postnatal period.
Intranatal		
1. Note medications patient is taking.	1. Stop heparin if patient is taking it. Give prophylactic antibiotics to prevent further valvular damage from infection.	1. Keep patient and family informed.
2. Assess for cardiac decompensation: a. Vital signs every 10 to 30 minutes, at least. Alert physician if pulse $\geq$100/min, respirations $\geq$25/min. b. Respiratory status: color and temperature of skin; presence of dyspnea, coughing, rales at base of lungs.	2. Promote cardiac function: a. Alleviate anxiety: calm atmosphere, keep patient informed. b. Position: side-lying and with head and shoulders elevated and body parts supported (with pillows, etc.).	
3. Assess emotional reaction to experience of labor.	c. Medicate for discomfort; sedate as needed. d. Anesthesia: saddle block (low spinal), caudal, or lumbar epidural to minimize discomfort, eliminate bearing-down reflex, and decrease peripheral resistance, venous return, and cardiac output. (NOTE: prevent hypotension, which may follow anesthesia.)	

Continued.

PLAN OF CARE: HEART DISEASE—cont'd

NURSING INTERVENTIONS—cont'd

Diagnostic	Therapeutic	Educational
Intranatal—cont'd		
	3. Treat cardiac decompensation (pulse ≥115/min, respirations ≥28/min, dyspnea).	
	a. Digitalize. Deslanoside (Cedilanid-D) is fast acting.	
	b. Oxygen by intermittent positive pressure. (Decreases chance of pulmonary edema.)	
	c. Diuretics. (Lasix is potent and fast acting.)	
	4. Alert pediatrician and nursery personnel.	
	5. Delivery should be accomplished in side-lying position or supine with legs down (not in stirrups). Episiotomy and outlet forceps also decrease work of heart.	
Postnatal		
1. Assess for cardiac decompensation.	1. Head of bed is elevated; patient is encouraged to lie on her side.	1. Keep patient and family informed regarding rationale for management, her progress, expected course of recovery.
2. Monitor vital signs, bleeding, uterine contractility, output, pain, rest, diet, daily weight.	2. Bed rest and bathroom privileges as tolerated.	2. Teach patient and family regarding rest, activity, diet, as necessary.
3. Assess laboratory results: Hgb, Hct, urinalysis, other.	3. Frequent contact with infant as desired (with no caretaking).	
4. Assess patient and family's reactions to experience and to infant.	4. Progressive ambulation as tolerated and with assistance.	
5. Assess patient's support system.	5. Promote bowel movements without stress and strain or discomfort.	
	6. Avoid overdistention of bladder followed by rapid emptying (≥1000 ml), since this results in too rapid drop in intra-abdominal pressure and causes uterine relaxation.	
	7. Isolate patient from sources of infection: people, objects, etc.	
	8. Assist with grieving process if infant has died or is at risk.	

OTHER MEDICAL PROBLEMS COMPLICATING PREGNANCY
Anemia

Anemia, the most common medical disorder of pregnancy, affects at least 20% of pregnant women. Anemic maternal patients have a higher incidence of puerperal complications such as infection than patients with normal hematologic values.

Anemia results in reduction of the oxygen-carrying capacity of the blood. An indirect index of the oxygen-carrying capacity is the packed red blood cell volume or hematocrit. The normal hematocrit range in nonpregnant women is 38% to 45%. However, normal values for pregnant women with adequate iron stores may be as low as 34%. This has been explained by hydremia, or the *physiologic anemia of pregnancy*.

About 90% of cases of anemia in pregnancy are of the iron-deficiency type. The remaining 10% of cases embrace a considerable variety of acquired and hereditary anemias, including folic acid deficiency and hemoglobinopathies.

Normal and abnormal changes confuse the hematologic profile during pregnancy. The blood values of pregnant patients differ significantly from those of nonpregnant women. All the constituents of blood normally increase during pregnancy: plasma volume, by 30% to 35%; red cell volume, by 20% to 30%; and hemoglobin mass, by 12% to 15%. The dilution of red blood cells and hemoglobin resulting from the relatively greater increase in plasma volume does not significantly change cell indices such as the mean corpuscular volume. However, this dilution does affect RBC, hemoglobin, and hematocrit values; laboratory values drop progressively to a low between the thirtieth and thirty-fourth weeks of pregnancy. At or near sea level, during the first trimester, the patient is anemic when her Hgb is less than 11 gm/100 ml or her Hct falls below 37%. She is anemic in the second trimester when the Hgb is less than 10.5 gm/100 ml or the Hct is under 35% and in the third trimester when the Hgb is less than 10 gm/100 ml and the Hct is less than 33%. Much higher values are indicative of anemia in areas of higher altitude; for example, at 5000 feet above sea level, an Hgb less than 14 gm/100 ml indicates anemia.

Iron-deficiency anemia. The demand for iron during pregnancy is about 1000 mg (250 mg for the fetus and 750 mg for the mother). Maternal needs are approximately as follows: placenta, 150 mg; blood volume increases, 300 mg; and blood loss at delivery and during the puerperium, 300 mg. If the demand for iron were constant throughout pregnancy, the average daily requirement (18 mg) would have to be increased by at least 3 mg. Actually the demand is not constant. During the first half of pregnancy, the additional demand for iron is small and usually met by iron conserved because menstruation has ceased, but during the last 20 weeks, a serious deficiency is likely.

In response to the increased requirements, the maternal organism adjusts to increased daily absorption by improved iron binding, from about 1.5 mg in the first trimester to approximately 3 mg in the second and to less than 4 mg in the third trimester. Despite this improvement, the balance is tenuous. If iron-deficiency anemia mars the onset of pregnancy and iron supplement is not given, anemia usually ensues.

Even the normal pregnant woman who has enjoyed excellent nutrition will conclude pregnancy with a deficit in iron storage. Inadequate nutrition will most certainly mean iron-deficiency anemia during late pregnancy and the puerperium. A woman cannot replace gestational iron losses merely from dietary sources.

Successful iron therapy during pregnancy can be carried out in the vast majority of cases with oral iron supplements (e.g., ferrous sulfate 0.3 Gm three times a day). Some pregnant women are intolerant or fail to take the prescribed oral iron. In such cases, the patient should receive parenteral iron such as iron-dextran (Imferon).

Folic acid–deficiency anemia. Folic acid–deficiency anemia occurs in at least 2% of pregnant patients in North America, an incidence much higher than suspected even 5 years ago. Many of these women suffer from preeclampsia-eclampsia or urinary tract infection because of their anemia.

Poor diet, cooking with large volumes of water, or canning of food may lead to folate deficiency. Also malabsorption or increased folate utilization may play a part in the development of anemia due to lack of folic acid.

Macrocytic (megalobastic) anemia, hypersegmentation (multinucleate) neutrophils, thrombocytopenia, markedly elevated lactic dehydrogenase (LDH), or low–serum folate levels are diagnostic of folate deficiency anemia. Many of these patients also show abnormalities in vaginal or cervical cytology that may suggest folate lack.

It is important to recall that iron-deficiency or hemoglobinopathy anemia may be associated with folate deficiency.

During pregnancy the recommended daily intake is 150 μg of folic acid. In folate deficiency, a dosage of about 5 mg/24 hr orally for several weeks should ensure a remission. A generous maintenance dose each day should prevent a relapse. Because iron-deficiency anemia may also accompany folate deficiency, augmented iron intake should also be provided.

Sickle cell hemoglobinopathy. Sickle cell trait (SA hemoglobin pattern) is sickling of the red blood cells but with a normal RBC and life span. Maternity patients with sickle cell trait are susceptible to urinary tract infection. Hematuria is common.

With the sickle cell test, induced sickling of abnormal hemoglobin-containing red blood cells, which occurs at a low Po_2, especially at a low pH, may be demonstrated by observing a sealed drop of blood under the microscope after constriction of the finger by a rubber band or by adding a drop of 2% sodium bisulfite to the blood and viewing the sealed, moist preparation.

Sickle cell anemia (sickle cell disease) is a recessive, hereditary, familial hemolytic anemia peculiar to those of black or Mediterranean ancestry. These individuals usually have abnormal hemoglobin types (SS or SC). Sickle cell anemia patients have recurrent attacks (crises) of fever and pain in the abdomen or extremities beginning in childhood. These attacks are attributed to vascular occlusion (due to abnormal cells), tissue hypoxia, edema, and red blood cell destruction. Crises are associated with normochromic anemia, jaundice, reticulocytosis, positive sickle cell test, and the demonstration of abnormal hemoglobin (usually SS or SC).

Almost 10% of blacks in North America have the sickle cell trait, but less than 1% have sickle cell anemia, often complicated by iron and folic acid deficiency.

Pregnant women with sickle cell anemia are prone to pyelonephritis, leg ulcers, bone infarction, and cardiopathy. (Oral contraceptives are contraindicated postnatally.) An aplastic crisis may follow serious infection. Medical therapy is essential but cesarean section is warranted only on obstetric indications.

Pregnancy may impose critical complications in sickle cell disease. Maternal mortality often ranges between 5% to 10% and the perinatal mortality may reach 30%. Therapeutic abortion is not medically indicated, but the limitation of pregnancy, often by sterilization, will be beneficial.

Urinary problems

Urinary tract infection. Urinary tract infection affects about 10% of maternity patients, most of these in the antenatal period. Those who have had previous urinary tract infections are especially prone. Cervicitis, vaginitis, obstruction of the flaccid ureters (particularly on the right due to pressure by the pregnant uterus against the slightly dilated flaccid ureters), vesicoureteral reflux, and the trauma of delivery predispose to urinary tract infection, generally due to *E. coli.* Asymptomatic bacteriuria (100 colonies/ml or more) occurs in about 5% of all pregnant patients. If untreated, pyelonephritis during gestation will develop in approximately 30% of these women. Premature labor and delivery may be more frequent also.

Urine culture and sensitivity tests should be obtained early in pregnancy, preferably at the first visit, from a clean-catch urine specimen. Catheterization should be avoided if possible. If infection is diagnosed, treatment with an appropriate antibiotic drug for 2 to 3 weeks, together with forced fluids and urinary sedatives, is recommended. Infections due to the colon aerogenes organisms generally respond well to sulfisoxazole or nitrofurantoin. Treatment should be continued for 2 to 3 weeks until two negative cultures are obtained.* Retreatment may be necessary if there is a recurrence. Acute pyelonephritis may be confused with appendicitis, cholecystitis, or premature labor.

If persistent or recurrent infection is noted, urologic investigation will be necessary to identify contributory causes such as urinary tract obstruction, stone, diverticulum, tuberculosis, or poor personal hygiene.

Glomerulonephritis. Acute glomerulonephritis, generally caused by a respiratory infection due to group A streptococcus, is a rare complication of pregnancy. The disorder is characterized by hematuria, edema, and hypertension. Treatment requires antibiotic therapy, bed rest (in side-lying or semi- to high-Fowler's position to facilitate renal perfusion), and fluid-electrolyte and dietary control. Pregnancy does not seriously affect acute early glomerulonephritis. Severe or prolonged glomerulonephritis may be an indication for therapeutic abortion during the first trimester.

Women with mild, inactive glomerulonephritis generally can go through pregnancy safely. Women with progressive, chronic glomerulonephritis, severe renal damage associated with proteinuria, hypertension, and elevated blood urea nitrogen (BUN) do not tolerate pregnancy well. If pregnancy is not interrupted, spontaneous abortion is likely; preeclampsia-eclampsia often supervenes, and fetal death may result. Cardiac or renal failure generally is the cause of maternal death.

Nephroureterolithiasis. Pregnancy causes dilatation of the renal hilum and calyces so that small stones often are dislodged, and most of these pass painfully. Occasionally a stone impacted in the ureter may require recovery from below or, if this is impossible, extraperitoneal ureterolithotomy. Whether urinary stones form more readily during pregnancy because of urinary stasis, hypercholesterolemia, or increased calciuria and vitamin D is still debated.

Gastrointestinal problems

Compromise of gastrointestinal function during pregnancy is apparent to all concerned. There is a large psychogenic overlay generally admitted in nausea and vomiting of pregnancy. However, a capricious food choice is observed in many women during pregnancy. In addition, obvious physiologic alterations such as the greatly enlarged uterus and less apparent changes such as hypochlorhydria require understanding for proper diagnosis and treatment.

Hyperemesis gravidarum (pernicious vomiting of pregnancy). Many pregnant women suffer nausea and vomiting at some time during early gestation. The indisposition is mild in most cases, but in about 1 of every 1000 maternity patients, severe intractable emesis will require hospitalization and perhaps even therapeutic abortion.

The cause of hyperemesis during pregnancy is still debated. Psychologically unstable women whose established reaction patterns to stress involve gastrointestinal

---

*The infant should be observed for hyperbilirubinemia (p. 593).

disturbances often are affected. In extreme cases, dehydration leads to fluid-electrolyte complications, particularly acidosis. Starvation causes hypoproteinemia and hypovitaminosis. Degenerative changes produce characteristic symptomatology. Jaundice and hemorrhage secondary to vitamins C and B—complex deficiency and hypothrombinemia lead to bleeding from mucosal surfaces. The embryo or fetus may die, and the mother may succumb to irreversible metabolic alterations.

The differential diagnosis may involve infectious diseases such as viral hepatitis or encephalitis or peptic ulcer, intestinal obstruction, or molar pregnancy.

Psychotherapy, parenteral fluids, electrolytes, sedatives, and vitamins will be required. Cautious resumption of a dry diet in six small feedings with clear liquids an hour after meals generally is acceptable. In most cases, hyperemesis will respond to therapy; hence the prognosis is good.

Peptic ulcer. Peptic ulcer is more infrequent in women than men, and this problem is even more uncommon during pregnancy. Moreover, patients with a diagnosed peptic ulcer generally improve during gestation. Therefore hemorrhage and perforation are unlikely. Fortunately emergency surgery for peptic ulcer complications rarely jeopardizes the pregnancy. Postnatal reactivation of the ulcer may occur. Medical therapy is similar to that recommended for nonpregnant individuals.

Cholelithiasis and cholecystitis. Women are more likely to have cholelithiasis than men, and pregnancy seems to play a part in its development. Certainly gallstones are more frequently diagnosed in women of advanced parity as compared with nulliparas of the same age and background. Increased biliary cholesterol and biliary stasis are probably causes. Cholecystitis does not commonly occur during pregnancy.

Generally, gallbladder surgery should be postponed until the puerperium but impaction of a stone in the cystic or common duct during pregnancy may require cholelithotomy or cholecystectomy.

Meperidine (Demerol) or atropine alleviates ductal spasm and pain. Morphine may be given also. It does not contract the sphincter of Oddi (hepatic-pancreatic ampulla) as claimed previously.

Ulcerative colitis. The cause of ulcerative colitis is unknown, but its effect on pregnancy is minimal unless there is marked debilitation, whereupon spontaneous abortion, fetal death, or premature delivery may occur. In general, when pregnancy coincides with active ulcerative colitis, the great majority of patients will suffer a severe exacerbation of the disease. When pregnancy occurs during a period of inactivity of the disorder, a flare-up is unlikely.

No specific therapy is known, but adrenocorticosteroids and antibiotics may be beneficial. Therapeutic abortion is justified in fulminating cases, and limitation of pregnancy is important because of chronic invalidism.

Dermatologic problems

Major physiologic changes that occur during normal pregnancy are mirrored in the skin as follows:

1. The skin thickens, and subdermal fat is increased.
2. Hyperpigmentation develops due to increased sensitivity of the skin to light.
3. Increased hair and nail growth is notable in many women.
4. Sweat and sebaceous gland activity is accelerated.
5. There is greater fragility of cutaneous elastic tissues noted as striae gravidarum or stretch marks.
6. Increased circulation and vasomotor activity and dermagraphism are evident.
7. Cutaneous allergic responses are enhanced.
8. Vascular permeability is increased.

Dermatologic disorders induced by pregnancy include melasma (chloasma), herpes gestationis, noninflammatory pruritus of pregnancy, vascular spiders, palmar erythema, and pregnancy granulomas (including epulis).

Skin problems generally aggravated by pregnancy are acne vulgaris (in the first trimester), erythema multiforme, herpetiform dermatitis, granuloma inguinali, condylomata accuminata, neurofibromatosis, and pemphigus. Dermatologic disorders usually improved by pregnancy include acne vulgaris (in the third trimester), seborrhea dermatitis, and psoriasis.

An unpredictable course during pregnancy may be expected in atopic dermatitis, lupus erythematosus, and herpes simplex.

Therapeutic abortion or early delivery may be justified if the following dermatologic conditions occur: herpes gestationis, disseminated lupus erythematosus, and neurofibromatosis (von Recklinghausen's disease).

Management. Explanation, reassurance, and common sense measures should suffice for normal skin changes. In contrast, disease processes during and soon after pregnancy may be extremely difficult to diagnose and treat.

Thyroid disorders

Hypothyroidism. Hypothyroidism may be responsible for anovulation in the infertile woman. Moreover, thyroid deficiency may cause spontaneous abortion, fetal maldevelopment, or fetal goiter.

Mild degrees of hypothyroidism in women may go unrecognized or may suggest a disease process of another system, for example, menorrhagia. Then diagnosis depends largely on laboratory tests.

Simple goiter generally is due to iodine lack, and the patient is only slightly thyroid deficient.

Clinical early hypothyroidism is characterized by easy fatigability, cold intolerance, lethargy, constipation, dry skin, or headache. Thin, brittle nails, dry skin, alopecia, poor skin turgor, and delayed deep tendon reflexes are typical.

During pregnancy, normal or reduced protein-bound iodine (PBI), reduced thyroxin (T_4) (column or D), reduced triiodothyronine (T_3) (resin), and a reduced T_4 index will aid in the confirmation of hypothyroidism.

Thyroid replacement during pregnancy is not increased over that needed before pregnancy, but it must be adequate for fetal growth and development. Adequate replacement may be determined by the plasma-free T_4 index (normal range is 0.75 to 2.5 units if T_4 by column is used; 1.3 to 5 units if T_4 [D] is used with resin T_3 uptake).

Hyperthyroidism. Hyperthyroidism, which affects about 1 of every 1500 pregnant women, may seriously complicate gestation or endanger the fetus. Hyperthyroidism may be responsible for anovulation and amenorrhea, but the disease is not a cause of abortion or fetal anomaly. Hyperthyroidism is associated with an increased incidence of premature labor and delivery. Symptoms include weakness, sweating, weight loss (or poor gain), nervousness, loose stools, and heat intolerance. Warm, soft, moist skin, tachycardia, stare with exophthalmos, tremor, and goiter with a bruit are characteristic. Laboratory findings, particularly the free T_4 index, will be elevated.

Radioactive iodine must not be used in testing or in therapy because it may destroy or compromise the fetal thyroid. Other antithyroid drugs such as iodine or the thiouracils may be employed to control the overactive maternal thyroid, provided the free T_4 index remains normal and that leukopenia does not develop.

Partial thyroidectomy, also an acceptable treatment for toxic goiter, requires preoperative preparation by antithyroid medication, usually Lugol's solution. Hypothyroidism, which occurs in at least 20% of patients postoperatively, must be treated promptly to spare the fetus. A free T_4 index determination on the cord blood at birth should be run to aid in determining the status of the infant.

Adrenal disorders

Hypoadrenocorticism (Addison's disease). Hypoadrenocorticism, idiopathic in less than 50% of cases and the remainder due to tuberculosis, is an uncommon complication of pregnancy. These patients whose fluid-electrolyte balance may be precarious, especially after pernicious nausea and vomiting of pregnancy, are susceptible to infection and especially to shock. Low plasma sodium chloride, reduced 17-potassium sulfur and 17-hydroxide, low or absent plasma cortisol, together with eosinophilia and lymphocytosis, are diagnostic laboratory findings in Addison's disease. With cortisone replacement therapy, electrolyte supplementation, and the avoidance of hemorrhage, the patient usually can be carried through successfully. Therapeutic abortion rarely is indicated; vaginal delivery is desirable. Cortisone may be teratogenic in humans.

Patients with Addison's disease display easy fatigability, anorexia, and frequent episodes of nausea, vomiting, and diarrhea; have sparse axillary hair and increased skin pigmentation; and suffer hypotension.

Hyperadrenocorticism. Hyperfunction of the adrenal cortex occurs in Cushing's syndrome, Cushing's disease, adrenogenital syndrome, hyperaldosteronism, and pheochromocytoma. The patient's principal problem in all these disorders is hypertension and its related complications. Pregnancy is not easily achieved in such patients because of amenorrhea and anovulation. A tumor (e.g., pituitary, adrenal) should be identified if present and removed if feasible. Adrenocortical hyperplasia and hyperfunction may be controlled with one of the cortisones. Preclampsia-eclampsia, infection, osteoporosis, and shock may be associated problems. The frequency of fetal anomaly is not increased in hyperadrenocorticism, but there is risk of premature delivery.

Epilepsy

Epilepsy may result from developmental abnormalities or injury. Epilepsy seriously complicates about 1 of every 1000 gestations. Convulsive seizures may be more frequent or severe during complications of pregnancy such as edema, alkylosis, fluid-electrolyte imbalance, cerebral hypoxia, hypoglycemia, and hypocalcemia. On the other hand, the effects of pregnancy on epilepsy are unpredictable.

The differential diagnosis of epilepsy versus eclampsia may pose a problem. Certainly epilepsy and eclampsia can coexist, but a past history of seizures, the absence of hypertension, generalized edema or proteinuria, and a normal plasma uric acid point to epilepsy. Retinal vasospasm is notable in epilepsy only. Electroencephalography (EEG) rarely is diagnostic.

Grand mal seizures can be controlled by intravenous sodium amobarbital or magnesium sulfate. Diphenylhydantoin (Dilantin) and its analogues may be fetotoxic, but diazepam (Valium) or chlordiazepoxide (Librium) are safe analeptic drugs. Epilepsy is not an indication for therapeutic abortion or cesarean section. Diazepam and chlordiazepoxide both affect the newly delivered infant.

Multiple sclerosis

Multiple sclerosis, a patchy demyelinization of the spinal cord and CNS, may be a viral disorder. Multiple sclerosis frequently develops initially after a pregnancy and is more common during the childbearing years. Multiple sclerosis may occasionally complicate pregnancy, but exacerbations and remissions are unrelated to the pregnant state. For this reason, medically indicated therapeutic abortion is illogical. Nonetheless, the burden of pregnancy and subsequent care of the child may warrant early interruption of pregnancy and sterilization in extreme cases. Patients occasionally may have an almost painless labor. The character of uterine contractions are unaffected by multiple sclerosis, however.

Disseminated lupus erythematosus

As with other collagen disorders, when lupus erythematosus is not severe, pregnancy usually can be undertaken without great risk to the mother or fetus, especially if the patient is in remission. Cortisone therapy may or may not be required. If renal or vascular complications develop or the disorder is active, pregnancy usually worsens the disease, and early therapeutic abortion may be warranted. Fortunately disseminated lupus erythematosus does not affect the fetus.

Psychiatric disorders

Serious psychotic illness occurs in about 0.2% of maternity patients. The major breakdown occurs in about 15% of these patients during pregnancy. For almost half of these patients, the breakdown occurs in the early puerperium. The remainder occur in the late puerperium. The two principal categories are manic-depressive and schizophrenic psychoses, with the incidence of both about equal. Pregnancy per se is not an etiologic factor in mental illness, but stresses may precipitate a psychotic episode in susceptible patients.

Therapeutic abortion may be warranted, particularly in serious recurrent psychoses. Hospitalization, temporary separation of the mother from the infant (if the patient has delivered), electroshock, ataractics, and psychotherapy are essential.

The prognosis for the mother cannot be generalized but must be determined on an individual patient basis. Although hereditary tendencies have been suggested, there is no convincing evidence that the infant is affected by maternal psychoses.

Nursing management of medical complications

A careful intake history and assessment of the patient's symptomatology at each antenatal contact provide the data base needed to initiate a diagnostic workup. After diagnosis, the nurse assists the patient in the following ways:

- To understand the disorder, its management, and probable outcome
- To understand her role in the management including when and how to take medication, diet, and preparation for and participation in treatment
- To cope with the emotional reactions to a pregnancy and infant at risk

If the patient is hospitalized, nursing care is governed by the medical problem diagnosed. In addition, the nurse must consider the patient's pregnancy, including FHT and fetal activity, uterine activity, vaginal discharge, and discomforts of pregnancy. Tests for fetal maturity and placental sufficiency may be necessary. The public health nurse, social worker, and pediatrician are some of the resource people whose services may need to be incorporated into the plan of care.

SURGICAL CONDITIONS COINCIDENT WITH PREGNANCY

The acute surgical abdomen occurs as frequently among pregnant as among nonpregnant women of comparable age. Diagnosis is more difficult in the pregnant woman, however. An enlarged uterus and displaced internal organs may prevent adequate palpation and alter the position of the acute surgical process.

Differential diagnosis includes consideration of obstetric complications, such as ectopic pregnancy and premature separation of the placenta, and the onset of labor.

Mild leukocytosis and increased serum values of alkaline phosphatase and amylase are characteristic of pregnancy, as well as an acute surgical intraperitoneal process. Rising or abnormally high laboratory values are suspect, however. X-ray evaluation, a valuable adjunct to diagnosis, is contraindicated particularly in the first trimester, except in extreme cases. The surgeon is confronted with both a surgical and an obstetric problem.

Laparotomy or laparoscopy may be required. Hazards of these procedures include abortion and premature labor. Surgical or anesthetic intervention does not affect the incidence of congenital malformations, however.

Appendicitis

Acute suppurative appendicitis complicates about 1 in every 1000 pregnancies. This disorder poses the following special problems during gestation:

1. Appendicitis is more difficult to diagnose during pregnancy. The appendix is carried high and to the right away from McBurney's point by the enlarging uterus.

2. Appendiceal rupture and peritonitis occur two to three times more often than in nonpregnant individuals.

3. Maternal and perinatal morbidity and mortality are greatly increased when appendicitis occurs during pregnancy.

Most cases of acute appendicitis occur during the first 6 months of gestation, with decreasing frequency through the third trimester, labor, and puerperium.

The differential diagnosis of appendicitis during pregnancy is also difficult because of gastrointestinal or genitourinary problems that may be confused with appendicitis. A high level of suspicion is important in the diagnosis of appendicitis.

Management. Appendectomy before rupture is extremely important. Antibiotic therapy before rupture is of questionable value; after rupture it may be lifesaving. Therapeutic abortion is never indicated in appendicitis. Cesarean section at or near term may be justified in association with appendectomy.

Prognosis. Maternal mortality increases to about 10% in the third trimester and is about 15% when appendicitis develops during labor. Perinatal mortality is approximately 10% with unruptured appendicitis but is at least 35% with peritonitis.

Genital problems

Ovarian cysts and twisting of ovarian cysts or adnexal tissues may occur. Pregnancy predisposes to ovarian pathology especially during the first trimester. Pathology may include retained or enlarged cystic corpus luteum of pregnancy, ovarian cyst, and bacterial invasion of reproductive or other intraperitoneal organs.

Laparotomy or laparoscopy is required to discriminate between ovarian pathology and early ectopic pregnancy, appendicitis, or other infectious processes.

See p. 203 for common vaginitis.

Abdominal hernias

The incidence of abdominal hernias and related incarceration of the bowel is reduced during pregnancy despite permanent enlargement of umbilical or incisional hernial rings. Displacement of nonadherent bowel by the enlarging uterus and its shielding of so-called weak areas of the abdominal wall are fortuitous. In fact, temporary spontaneous reduction of some abdominal wall hernias occurs during gestation. In contrast, however, the uncommon irreducible or adherent hernias may become incarcerated as pregnancy progresses.

Patients with hernias should not strain or bear down during the second stage of labor. Therefore low forceps delivery should be planned. Abdominal hernia is not an indication for cesarean section; herniorrhaphy should be done as an interval procedure (i.e., between pregnancies).

Carcinoma of the breast

The obstetrician should carefully check for breast tumors. Although breast cancer is an uncommon complication of pregnancy or the puerperium, a malignant neoplasm may develop to considerable size, obscured by the increased breast fullness during childbearing. Contrary to popular belief, however, pregnancy does not accelerate the progress of breast cancer. Hence therapeutic abortion is not medically indicated. If breast cancer is diagnosed during gestation, prompt radical mastectomy should be effected. The 5-year arrest of stage I breast cancer (cancer confined to the breast without nodal spread) diagnosed and surgically treated during pregnancy is about 65%. In stage II (cancer confined to the breast but with metastases to the axillary nodes on the same side), the likelihood of 5-year arrest with radical surgery and irradiation therapy is only about 10%.

Intestinal obstruction (dynamic ileus)

Although intestinal obstruction is not common during pregnancy, any patient with a laparotomy scar is more likely to suffer intestinal obstruction during gestation because of adhesions, an enlarging uterus, and displacement of the intestines. A dynamic ileus can also occur with incarcerated hernia, volvulus, or intussusception, but such cases are seen rarely by the obstetrician.

Persistent abdominal cramplike pain, vomiting, auscultatory rushes within the abdomen, and "laddering" of the intestinal shadows on x-ray films aid in the diagnosis of intestinal obstruction. Immediate operation is required for release of the obstruction. Pregnancy is rarely affected by the surgery, assuming the absence of complications such as peritonitis. Cesarean section is not indicated in intestinal obstruction.

Varices and hemorrhoids

See pp. 199 and 200 for discussion of varices and hemorrhoids complicating pregnancy.

Thromboembolization

Thromboembolization is the term applied to vascular occlusive processes (e.g., thrombophlebitis, phlebothrombosis, dissemination of venous clot to the lungs). The incidence of thrombophlebitis in parturients delivered vaginally is about 0.5%, but 1% to 2% of cesarean section patients have this complication. At least 50% of emboli originate in the pelvic vessels. Other sites are the veins of the lower extremities.

Thromboembolization results from circulatory stasis, vascular abnormality, infection, and the increased postnatal coagulability of blood. Obesity, varices, heart disease, preeclampsia-eclampsia, prolonged labor, anemia, and hemorrhage predispose to thromboembolization. Abortion, operative delivery, particularly cesarean section, and postnatal pelvic infection may initiate the process.

Phlebothrombosis is a development of a noninflammatory venous clot that often does not completely occlude the vein. Venous stasis is responsible. Dislodgment of the clot may cause a small or massive pulmonary embolization during the puerperium.

Suppurative emboli, usually from thrombophlebitis in the uterine or ovarian veins, always involve the lung, but secondary abscesses may develop almost anywhere in the body. If the saphenous or femoral vessels are involved, the leg will be swollen, red, painful, and tender. Neglected thrombophlebitis of the leg leaves the extremity permanently swollen and pallid (phlegmasia alba dolens or "milk leg").

Management includes oxygen, sedation, treatment for shock, and anticoagulation therapy. Occasionally thrombectomy may be feasible in nonseptic embolization.

Antibiotic therapy and even ligation (or clipping) of the vena cava and ovarian veins may be necessary for septic embolization of thrombophlebitis.

The prognosis is grave with massive pulmonary embolization, but early successful treatment of other thromboembolism should be anticipated.

Nursing management of surgical complications

Principles of maternity nursing are added to those of nursing care of the surgical patient. The preoperative and postoperative plan of care incorporates consideration for the woman's concern for her infant as well as for herself, fetal vital signs and activity, uterine contractility (labor may have begun), and constant vigilance for symptoms of impending obstetric complications. The woman and her family may have heightened concerns regarding effects of the procedure and medications on fetal well-being and the course of pregnancy.

REFERENCES

Ayromlovi, J., and others. 1973. Thyrotoxicosis in pregnancy. Am. J. Obstet. Gynecol. **117:**818.

Bates, G. W. 1974. Management of gestational diabetes. Postgrad. Med. **55:**55.

Bellingham, F. R. 1973. Syphilis in pregnancy: transplacental infection. Med. J. Aust. **2:**647.

Bobeck, S., and Schasten, B. 1974. Detection and diagnosis of bacteriuria in pregnancy: a study from general practice. Practitioner **212:**257.

Cabaniss, C. D. 1972. Management of heart disease in pregnancy. J. Reprod. Med. **8:**51.

Caldwell, J. G. 1971. Masking of syphilis (leading article). Br. Med. J. **3:**206.

Fairbanks, W. L., and Loomis, G. W. 1972. Nephrotic syndrome in pregnancy. Nebraska Med. J. **57:**432.

Caselnova, D. A. 1974. Hyperemesis gravidarum with retinal hemorrhage. Int. J. Gynaecol. Obstet. **12:**19.

Friedrich, E. G., Jr. 1973. Relief of herpes vulvitis. Obstet. Gynecol. **41:**74.

Gaither, D., and Clark, J. F. J. 1973. Pregnancy and latent diabetes. J. Natl. Med. Assoc. **65:**139.

Goluboff, L. G., and others. 1974. Hyperthyroidism associated with pregnancy. Obstet. Gynecol. **44:**107.

UNIT SIX

Labor

CHAPTER 19

Normal labor

Labor (parturition, childbirth) is the process by which the products of conception are expelled from the uterus and the vagina into the external environment. For the infant the repetitive stress of labor culminates in delivery and the necessity for successful transition from a dependent to an independent biologic state. For the mother, an essentially normal process carries a potential risk of disability for herself and the child she bears. For the mother and father, childbirth marks the time when each assumes the role of parent with its personal and social connotations.

The goal of the health team is the safe delivery of mother and child and the promotion of this critical process as one of emotional fulfillment for the parents.

ESSENTIAL FACTORS IN LABOR

Every health care professional involved in maternity care should recognize that few factors will shorten labor but many will prolong the process. In every labor five essential factors affect the process:

1. The size, presentation, and position of the passenger
2. The passage
   a. The configuration and diameters of the pelvis
   b. The distensibility of the lower uterine segment, cervical dilatation and effacement, and distensibility of the vaginal canal and introitus
3. The strength, duration, and frequency of uterine contractions, the so-called primary powers of labor
4. The site of insertion of the placenta
5. The psychologic state of the woman

Variation in any of these factors may alter the character and course of labor. For example, the baby may be large and the pelvis normal in size, but the uterine contractions may be weak; hence labor may not be successful. In contrast, given the same fetal and pelvic factors, together with good labor, safe vaginal delivery may ensue.

In a sense, labor is a contest among these factors, and the prognosis in each labor is dependent on a careful and consistent evaluation of their effects.

The passenger

The passage of the fetus through the birth canal is influenced by the size of its head, shoulders, and hips and by its presentation and position.

FETAL HEAD

Because of its size and relative rigidity, the fetal head has a major effect on the birth process. The bony skull is comprised of the larger and more compressible cranial vault and the smaller, incompressible face and base of the skull. The bones of the cranial vault are not firmly united, and slight overlapping of the bones or *molding* of the shape of the head, occurs during labor (Figs. 19-1 and 19-2). This malleability permits adaptation to the various diameters of the pelvis. Molding can be extensive, but with most neonates, the head assumes its normal shape within 2 days after birth.

The cranial vault is composed of two parietal, two temporal, and the occipital bones. These are united by membranous sutures: the sagittal, lambdoidal, and coronal. At the points of intersection, these sutures become enlarged to form the fontanels ("soft spots") (Figs. 19-3 and 19-4), the two most important being the anterior and posterior fontanels. The anterior fontanel is found at the intersection of the sutures of the two parietal and two frontal bones, is diamond shaped, and is the larger of the two. It closes at about 18 months of age. The posterior fontanel is at the junction of the sutures of the two parietal and one occipital bones and is therefore triangular in shape. It is smaller than the anterior fontanel and closes by about the twelfth week of life.

The fetal head can move on the neck about 45 degrees in flexion or extension and approximately 180 degrees during rotation. This permits smaller diameters of the fetal head to present as it descends through the birth canal.

Principal measurements of the fetal skull are shown

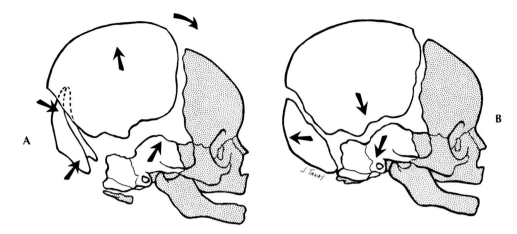

Fig. 19-1. Molding during birth process. Shaded area indicates stationary noncompressible portions of skull. **A,** Overlapping (molding) of cranial bones during labor. **B,** Realignment of cranial bones by third day of life to normal position.

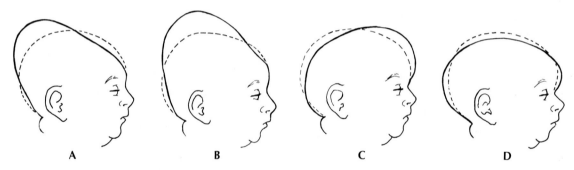

Fig. 19-2. Molding of head in cephalic presentations. **A,** Occipitoanterior. **B,** Occipitoposterior. **C,** Brow. **D,** Face.

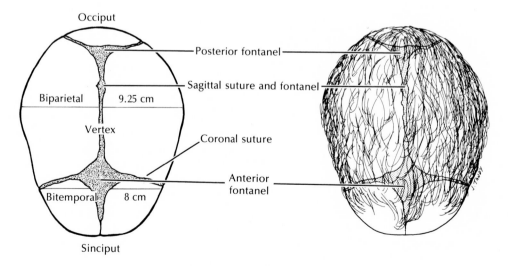

Fig. 19-3. Newborn infant's head.

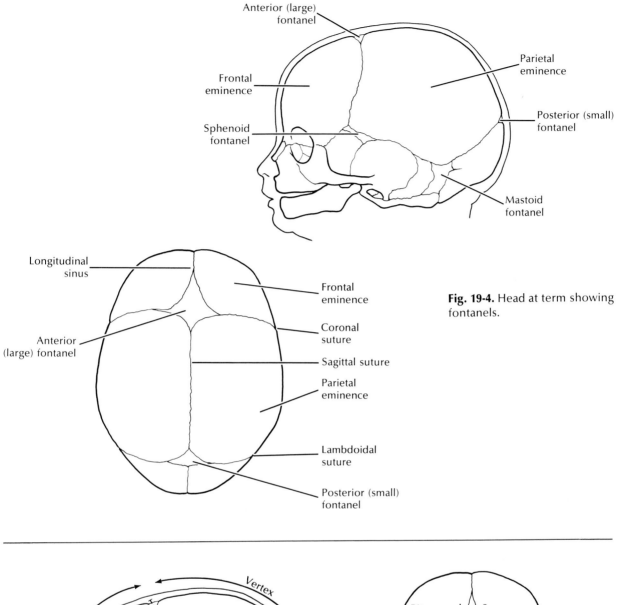

Fig. 19-4. Head at term showing fontanels.

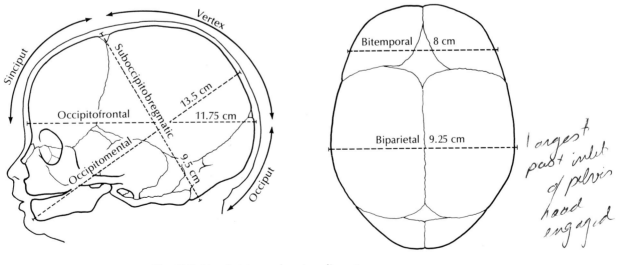

Fig. 19-5. Head at term showing diameters.

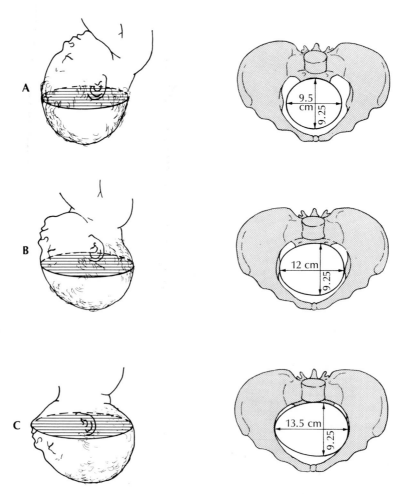

Fig. 19-6. Head entering pelvis. **A,** Suboccipitobregmatic diameter: complete flexion so smallest diameter enters. **B,** Occipitofrontal diameter: moderate extension (military attitude) so large diameter enters. **C,** Occipitomental diameter: excessive extension (deflexion) so largest diameter is presenting, which is too large to permit head to enter pelvis.

in Figs. 19-5 and 19-6 and are as follows (in centimeters):

Anteroposterior diameters

Occipitomental (OM)	13.5
Occipitofrontal (OF)	11.75
Suboccipitofrontal (SOF)	10.5
Suboccipitobregmatic (SOB)	9.5
Tracheobregmatic (TB)	9.5

Transverse diameters

Biparietal (Bip)	9.25
Bitemporal (Bit)	8.0
Bimastoid (Bim)	7.0

The biparietal diameter is the largest of the transverse diameters. When the biparietal diameter has descended past the inlet of the pelvis, the head becomes fixed in the pelvis (is said to be *engaged*) and is no longer freely movable.

Of the anteroposterior diameters shown in Fig. 19-6, it can be seen that the attitudes of flexion, moderate flexion, and hyperextension cause diameters of different sizes to enter the pelvis. The smallest diameter to present is with the head in complete flexion, and this can enter easily, whereas the largest diameter with hyperextension is too large to enter the average pelvis, and the birth process will not progress.

SHOULDER AND HIPS

Because of their mobility, the position of the shoulders can be altered during labor, so that one shoulder occupies a lower level than the other. This permits a

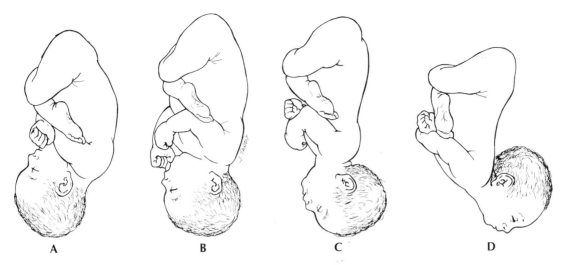

Fig. 19-7. Differences in attitude cause different presentations. **A,** Complete flexion: vertex presentation. **B,** Moderate flexion (military attitude): sinciput presentation. **C,** Marked extension (deflexion): brow presentation. **D,** Excessive extension (deflexion): face presentation.

smaller diameter to negotiate the passage. The circumference of the hips is usually small enough not to create problems.

FETAL LIE, PRESENTATION, AND ATTITUDE

Lie is the relationship of the long axis of the fetus to the long axis of the mother. There are two lies: *longitudinal* (when the long axis of the fetus is parallel with the long axis of the mother) or *transverse* (when the long axis of the fetus is at right angles to that of the mother).

Longitudinal lies are either cephalic (head) or pelvic (breech) presentations, depending on the fetal structure that first enters the mother's pelvis.

The *presenting part* is that portion of the fetus that enters the pelvis first and covers the internal os of the cervix. In cephalic (head) presentations, the presenting part varies with the attitude of the infant. *Attitude* is the relationship of the fetal body parts to each other. This is responsible for three different cephalic presentations:

1. If the head is flexed on the chest, the occiput (vertex) presents first, and this is termed an *occipital or vertex presentation* (Fig. 19-7, *A*).

2. If the head is midway between flexion and extension, the brow is the presenting part and is termed a *brow presentation* (Fig. 19-7, *C*).

3. If the head is hyperextended, the chin (mentum) is the presenting part and is termed a *face* or *chin presentation* (Fig. 19-7, *D*).

In pelvic (breech) presentation, the thighs may be flexed on the abdomen and the legs extended (frank breech presentation), the legs may be flexed on the thighs so that buttocks and feet present (complete breech), or one or both feet may extend downward (single or double footling breech).

Transverse lies are referred to as *shoulder presentations*. Unless the fetus rotates or is rotated to a longitudinal presentation, birth is only possible by cesarean section.

Position is the relationship of the point of direction on the presenting part to one of the four quadrants of the mother's pelvis; that is, the most prominent portion of the presenting part is related to one of the four quadrants of the mother's pelvis. These quadrants are formed by drawing an imaginary line from the sacral promontory to the upper edge of the symphysis pubis and bisecting it transversely with a line from one side to the other. These are termed *right posterior and anterior quadrants* and *left posterior and anterior quadrants* (Appendix E). In a vertex presentation, if the occiput is the most prominent portion of the presenting part and is located in the right anterior quadrant, the position is noted as *right occiput anterior (ROA)*. Additional examples are given in Table 19-1 and Appendix E.

The most common presentations are vertex (96%) and then breech (3%). The others are rarely encountered and act to slow or prevent the birth process.

Fetal presentation, position, and descent may be provisionally determined by external palpation after the sixth month of pregnancy, by identifying the maximal density of FHT through auscultation, and by vaginal

Table 19-1. Fetal lie and position

Longitudinal lie	Prominent part	Example of position
Cephalic		
Vertex	Occiput	LOP Left occiput posterior
Face (rare)	Mentum	RMP Right mentum posterior
Brow	Brow	LBA Left brow anterior
Pelvic		
Breech	Sacrum	RSA Right sacrum anterior
Transverse lie		
Shoulder	Scapula	RScA Right scapula anterior

examination. The vaginal examination yields more precise information once cervical dilatation has progressed to 5 cm (Appendix E).

Certain confirmation of fetal presentation or position is possible with ultrasound or radiography in the obese woman or one with multiple pregnancy. Either method will add accurate data about pelvic architecture and actual fetopelvic diameters. Ultrasound is harmless and may be repeated often without jeopardy. X-ray films should be ordered only in emergency situations, however, to avoid posssible injury to mother or infant.

Abdominal palpation. The use of the four maneuvers of Leopold provides for a systematic examination. Proficiency in determining presentation and position by abdominal palpation requires considerable practice so every learning opportunity needs to be utilized. Gross maternal obesity or excessive amniotic fluid (hydramnios) may obscure fetal contours.

The patient empties her bladder before the examination is begun and lies on her back with one pillow under her head. The examiner's hands should be warm. The examiner stands facing the patient on the right of the patient if right-handed (and vice versa if left-handed). The examiner keeps the following assessment in mind while carrying out the procedure (Towler and Butler-Manuel, 1973):

1. Is there one fetus or more than one?
2. What is the presentation (lie)?
3. What is the position?
4. Is the presenting part engaged?
5. Is there fetal movement?
6. Do the uterine size and fundal height correspond with due dates? (McDonald's rule)?
7. Is there any indication of uterine, pelvic, or fetal abnormality?

Leopold's maneuvers are as follows:

1. The fetal part that occupies the fundus of the uterus is identified first. The head will be round, firm, and ballotteable; the breech will be less regular and softer (Fig. 19-8, *A*).

2. The back is then identified by feeling a smooth convex contour anteriorly or to one side using the palmar surface of the hand. The fetal ventral (front) surface is concave and soft, and the small parts (feet, hands, elbows) are irregularities felt on the side opposite the back (Fig. 19-8, *B*).

3. The examiner should next determine with the right hand which fetal part is lying over the inlet. This is done by gently grasping the lower pole of the uterus between the thumb and fingers and pressing in slightly. If the head presents and is not engaged, it may be rocked gently from side to side (Fig. 19-8, *C*).

4. Finally, the degree of descent is estimated. To do this, the examiner faces the patient's feet and uses both hands (Fig. 19-8, *D*). When the presenting part has descended deeply, only a small portion of the presenting part may be outlined. If the vertex is presenting, the cephalic prominences—those portions of the head that are most easily palpated—may be identified. The prominences will be opposite the back if the head is flexed or on the side of the back with deflexion of the head, save when the face is directed posteriorly. Palpation of the anterior shoulder will aid in assessment of descent of the vertex.

Auscultation. The area of maximum intensity of the FHT is an ancillary aid in determining the fetal position. For example, in vertex and breech presentations, FHT are best heard through the back of the fetus. In face presentation, however, FHT generally are loudest when transmitted through the chest.

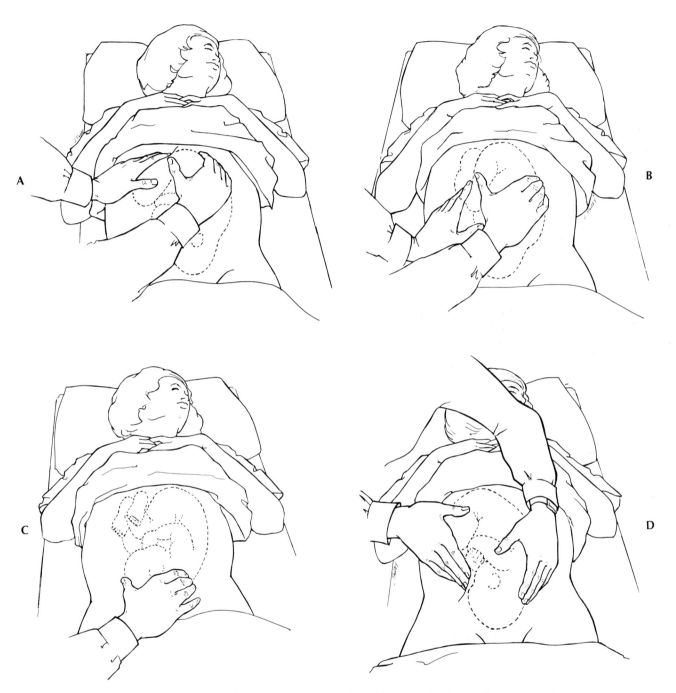

Fig. 19-8. Palpation of fetal presentation and position. For **A, B,** and **C,** examiner faces patient's head. For **D,** examiner faces her feet. **A,** Palpation of fundus. **B,** Palpation of fetal back and small parts. **C,** Checking for engagement of presenting part. **D,** Palpation of cephalic prominence.

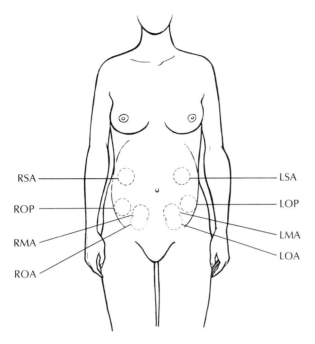

Fig. 19-9. Areas of maximum density of FHT for differing positions: *RSA,* right sacrum anterior; *ROP,* right occiput posterior; *RMA,* right mentum anterior; *ROA,* right occiput anterior; *LSA,* left sacrum anterior; *LOP,* left occiput posterior; *LMA,* left mentum anterior; and *LOA,* left occiput anterior.

In vertex presentations, FHT commonly are heard below the mother's umbilicus in a lower quadrant of the abdomen but above the level of the umbilicus in breech presentations.

The site of the best FHT audibility generally confirms anterior positions but is misleading in posterior positions because of poor flexion of the head or displacement of the uterus (Fig. 19-9).

Vaginal examination. The vaginal examination has almost replaced the rectal examination, since clinical studies have indicated that there is no significant increase in infection with vaginal examinations. It is more accurate in determining the condition, effacement, and dilatation of the cervix. It is less painful and requires less manipulation. Prolapse of the cord can be detected more readily as can compound presentations.

The examination must be done carefully, gently, and under aseptic conditions. The use of sterile gloves is recommended, as well as an antiseptic solution. For the first examination in labor, sterile water can be used as a solution to lubricate the fingers, since lubricants can alter the response of the Nitrazine paper used to diagnose rupture of membranes.

Vaginal examinations must never be performed by a nurse if bleeding (as distinguished from bloody show) is present. If bleeding is copious, the physician may do the vaginal examination in the operating room so that, if necessary, a cesarean section can be immediately performed (Chapter 10).

The patient lies in a supine position with one pillow under her head and knees flexed and separated (the lithotomy position) and suitably draped. While the patient is being positioned, she should be told that she is to be examined internally to assess her progress and that although the procedure may be uncomfortable, it should not be painful.

The examining hand is then gloved, and the other hand may be placed on the abdomen to steady the fetus and to exert a gentle downward pressure, which applies the presenting part more closely to the cervix. The index and middle fingers are introduced into the vagina. Discomfort is less if the fingers are directed with the palmar surface downward so that the initial pressure is directed toward the less sensitive posterior vaginal wall. Then they may be rotated. The following should be assessed:

1. Is the cervix soft or hard? What is the degree of effacement and dilatation of the os?

2. Are the membranes intact? If so, are they bulging through the os?

3. What is the presentation: vertex, breech, or other (e.g., hand, face)?

4. What is the position? If the vertex presents, the sagittal suture is located and traced to the posterior fontanel (triangle) if the head is well flexed or to the anterior fontanel (diamond) if the head is extended (Fig. 19-10). Once the fontanel is located, determine its position in relation to the quadrants of the mother's pelvis. The most common position will be LOA.

5. What is the station?

To accomplish the foregoing assessment the student must understand the following terms in addition to those related to presentation and position.

Effacement of the cervix. Effacement of the cervix means the shortening and thinning of the cervical canal during the course of labor. The cervix, normally 2 to 3 cm in length and 1 cm thick, is obliterated or "taken up" by a shortening of the uterine muscle bundles during the enlargement of the lower uterine segment in advancing labor. Eventually only a thin edge of the cervix can be palpated when effacement is complete. Effacement generally is advanced in primigravidas at term before more than slight dilatation occurs. In multiparas, effacement and dilatation of the cervix tend to progress together. Degree of effacement is expressed in percentages (e.g., a cervix that is 50% effaced) (Fig. 19-11 and Appendix E).

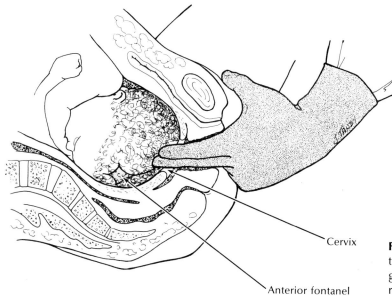

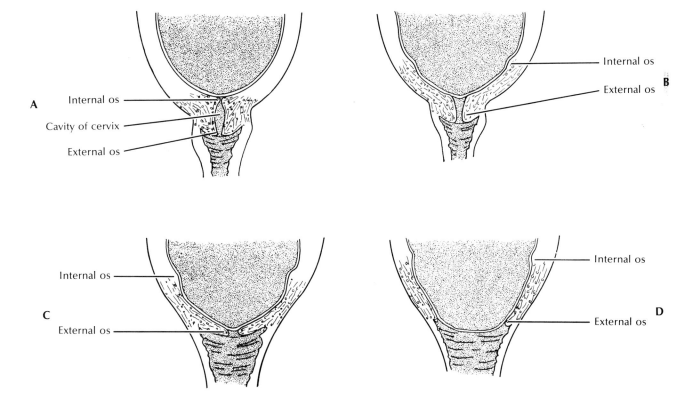

Fig. 19-10. Vaginal palpation of sagittal suture line. Note position of hand: two fingers are introduced into vagina and thumb rests on pubis externally.

Cervix

Anterior fontanel

A

Internal os

Cavity of cervix

External os

B

Internal os

External os

C

Internal os

External os

D

Internal os

External os

Fig. 19-11. Cervical effacement and dilatation. Note how cervix is drawn up around presenting part (internal os). **A,** Before labor. **B,** Early effacement. **C,** Complete effacement (100%). **D,** Complete dilatation (10 cm).

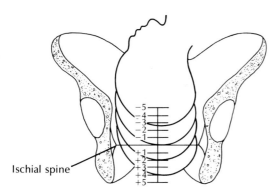

Ischial spine

−5
−4
−3
−2
−1
0
+1
+2
+3
+4
+5

Fig. 19-12. Stations of presenting part (degree of engagement). Location of presenting part in relation to level of ischial spines is designated station and indicates degree of advancement of presenting part through pelvis. Stations are expressed in centimeters above (minus) and below (plus) level of ischial spines (zero). Head is usually engaged when it reaches level of ischial spines.

Dilatation of the cervix. Dilatation of the cervix is the enlargement or widening of the cervical os and the cervical canal during the course of labor. The diameter increases from perhaps less than a centimeter to approximately 10 cm to allow delivery of a term fetus. When the cervix is fully dilated (and completely retracted), it can no longer be palpated (Fig. 19-11).

Dilatation of the cervix is involuntary and occurs by the drawing upward of the musculofascial components of the cervix with strong uterine contractions. Pressure exerted by the amniotic fluid while the membranes are intact or force applied by the presenting part also encourages cervical dilatation. Scarring of the cervix as a result of infection or surgery may retard cervical dilatation.

Voluntary bearing-down efforts by the patient are counterproductive to cervical dilatation. Straining will exhaust the patient, and cervical edema may develop because of chronic passive congestion.

Station. Progress in the descent of the presenting part is determined by vaginal examination until the presenting part can be seen at the introitus. The level of the tip of the ischial spines is considered to be station zero, and the position of the head (the bony prominence, not the edematous scalp or caput) or the fetal ischial tuberosities with a breech is described in centimeters minus (above the spines) or plus (below the spines) (Fig. 19-12). In a vertex position the presenting part is definitely engaged when the biparietal diameter of the fetal skull has passed the level of the inlet. At this time, the presenting part is usually at the level of the spines.

The passage (birth canal)

The birth canal is composed of the rigid bony pelvis and the soft tissues of the cervix, vagina, and introitus.

Numerous constrictions and changing contours characterize the birth canal (Fig. 19-13). Therefore the passage is not like a smooth bent tube; instead it resembles a curved pipe with baffles. The baffles direct the presenting part, and the narrower portions require the head, for example, to turn, seeking the easiest way through. Both bony and soft parts serve to restrict or deflect the presenting part, but the fetus always is a passive participant, propelled by the forces of labor.

PELVIS

In Chapter 3 the anatomy of the pelvis was reviewed. A further discussion of the significance of pelvic configurations to labor is necessary.

Pelvic configurations. The _gynecoid pelvis_ is the most favorable for normal delivery. Engagement usually is in the transverse or oblique diameter, descent is rapid, rotation occurs in the midpelvis, and delivery of the vertex as an occiput anterior position often occurs spontaneously.

The _anthropoid pelvis_ is also favorable obstetrically. Descent occurs without hindrance, but because the bispinous diameter is smaller than normal, rotation in the midpelvis cannot occur, and the head must pass to the outlet as it entered the pelvis. The outlet is not far enough below the midplane, however, and the arch may be narrow. Hence delivery as an OP may be required. If an OA is the original position, delivery generally is rapid and uncomplicated.

The _platypelloid pelvis_ offers delay only at the inlet. The presenting part must enter the superior strait in the transverse, and to do this one may have to wait until the cervix is considerably dilated and effaced to make room. The platypelloid pelvis is shallow and the spines blunted. The presenting part rotates at or below the spines, and delivery is rapid because the arch is wide and the outlet usually is ample.

The _android pelvis_ is the least favorable obstetrically. Lack of engagement or delayed entry of the presenting part occurs; the oblique diameter may be selected. Slow descent of the head, often as an OP, may be expected, and arrest at the spines often occurs. A difficult forceps rotation and extraction, possibly as an OP, may be necessary. Cesarean section commonly is required.

Regrettably a shortened diagonal conjugate will identify only patients with a flat pelvis. Therefore other clinical evidence of pelvic type such as the character of the sacrum, the subpubic arch, and other characteristics must be considered. Moreover delayed engagement and

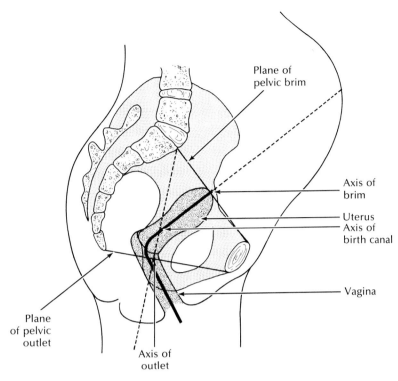

Fig. 19-13. Contours of birth canal. Infant navigates canal by steps in mechanism of labor.

poor progress in labor should indicate the need for x-ray (or ultrasonographic) pelvimetry.

Pelvic abnormalities may be due to rickets, osteomalacia, spinal deformity, abnormalities of the legs, pelvic neoplasm, or poorly aligned pelvic fracture. Most abnormalities can be suspected because of history or abnormal physical findings. Other rare pelvic variations include congenital anomalies such as Naegele's pelvis, in which an abnormally narrow sacrum is fused with the ilium on each side.

The pelvic type occasionally may be suspected from the patient's body build. Small women of slight stature generally have small, rounded, generally contracted gynecoid pelves. Fortunately most of these women will have small babies, despite the fact that their husbands may be appreciably larger.

In contrast, the short, fat, or thick-set woman with broad shoulders is a poor obstetric performer. Her pelvis may be predominantly android, and she may personify the "dystocia-dystrophy syndrome." However, hirsutism, male physique, or other characteristics do not indicate an android pelvis.

By and large, the tall, slender woman, perhaps with wide shoulders, often has a favorable long, oval (anthropoid) pelvis. She does well in labor and usually delivers without difficulty. No general body index exists that will accurately predict the type of pelvis and suggest the obstetric prognosis.

Major gynecoid features can be expected in about one half of all maternity patients: significant anthropoid tendencies will be present in slightly less than one fourth of patients, android configuration will affect almost one fifth of pregnant women, and the small remainder will have platypelloid pelves.

Pelvic appraisal. One should evaluate the fetopelvic relationships close to term if possible. Pelvic capacity, relative size of the fetus, and its presentation and position must be considered with reference to possible fetopelvic disproportion.

A useful formula to follow is the "rule of threes," which indicates that there are three parts of the pelvis to examine and three components to each part (Fig. 19-14):

1. Inlet
   a. Diagonal conjugate
   b. Posterior surface of the symphysis pubis
   c. Iliopectineal line
2. Pelvic cavity or midplane
   a. Sacral curve, shape, and length

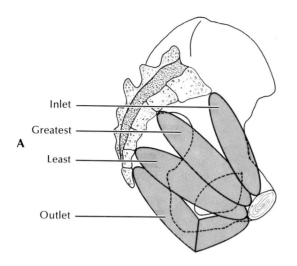

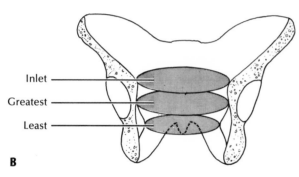

Fig. 19-14. Planes of true pelvis. **A,** Sagittal section. **B,** Coronal section.

    b. Ischial spines
    c. Sacrospinous ligaments
  3. Outlet
    a. Subpubic angle and arch
    b. Intertuberous diameter
    c. Sacrococcygeal joint

The diagonal conjugate is the most important clinical measurement relative to the pelvic inlet. One should record whether the sacral promontory is reached with ease or difficulty or if it is not reached. Palpation of the posterior symphysis pubis may reveal a normal, smooth, rounded curve or an abnormal angulation or beaking. Prominence of the iliopectineal line (if palpable) suggests pelvic abnormality.

Palpation of the pelvic cavity should include its curve, shape, and length and any tumors or abnormalities that might reduce the pelvic capacity. The length of the sacrospinous ligaments (the width of the sacrosciatic notch) should be about 5 to 6 cm (three fingerbreadths). The bluntness of the spines and their angulation and the concavity of the sacrum should be noted.

The pelvic outlet is the easiest area to evaluate. The subpubic arch should be about 4 to 5 cm wide and rounded. The inferior pubic rami should be short, and the intertuberous diameter should be 8.5 cm or more (admitting the knuckles of a man's clenched fist). Commonly the prominence of the terminal sacrum and the direction and mobility of the coccyx must be determined.

SOFT TISSUES

The soft tissues of the passage include the distensible lower uterine segment, cervix, and vaginal canal.

Before labor begins, the uterus is composed of the uterine body (corpus) and cervix. After labor has begun, the uterine contractions cause the uterine body to differentiate into an upper segment, thick and muscular; a lower segment, a thin-walled passive muscular tube; and a physiologic retraction ring that separates the two (Fig. 19-15). The lower uterine segment gradually distends to accommodate the intrauterine contents as the walls of the upper segment become thicker and its content reduced.

The downward pressure caused by contraction of the fundus is transmitted to the cervix, and it effaces and dilates sufficiently to allow descent of the presenting part into the vagina.

The vagina in turn distends to permit passage of the fetus into the external world. As noted earlier, the soft tissues of the vagina develop throughout pregnancy until at term the vagina can dilate to accommodate the fetus. Women who do not realize the extent of this distensibility may be fearful of the fetus "tearing them" to emerge. It may relieve her apprehension to remind the patient how much the vagina has expanded since her initial examination from a size that only just accommodated the speculum to one that will accommodate the examiner's entire hand. The rugae of the vagina become smooth, and the surface enlarges, just like spreading out a piece of corrugated paper.

A full bladder or rectum can impinge on the vaginal canal and act to block the descent of the fetus. Therefore during labor the patient is encouraged to void at least every 2 hours, or if the bladder becomes distended and she is unable to void, a catheterization will have to be done. Similarly, an enema may be given early in labor to clear the lower bowel of feces.

The powers

The forces acting to expel the fetus and placenta are derived from three sources:
- The involuntary uterine contractions
- The voluntary bearing-down efforts
- The contraction of the levator ani muscles

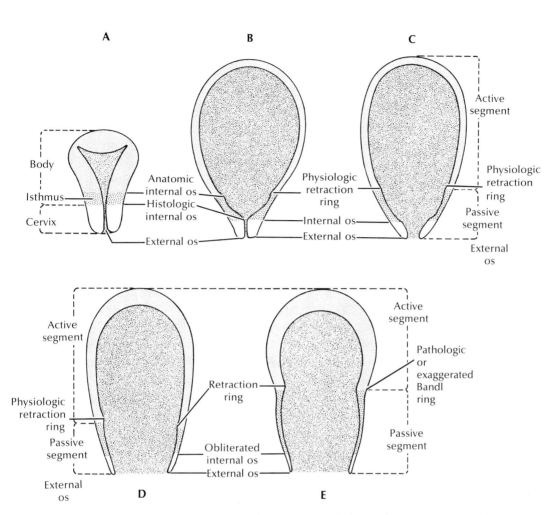

Fig. 19-15. Progressive development of segments and rings of uterus at term. Note comparison between nonpregnant uterus, **A,** uterus at term, **B,** and uterus in normal labor in early first stage, **C,** and second stage, **D.** Passive segment is derived from lower uterine segment (isthmus) and cervix and physiologic retraction ring, from anatomic internal os. **E,** Uterus in abnormal labor in second stage dystocia. Pathologic retraction ring that forms under abnormal conditions develops from physiologic ring. (Modified from Willson, J. R., Beecham, C. T., and Carrington, E. R. 1975. Obstetrics and gynecology [ed. 5]. St. Louis, The C. V. Mosby Co.)

Uterine contractions (primary powers). These operate independently of the CNS; that is, they are involuntary. This is attested to by the observations that paraplegics can deliver vaginally, and uterine action is not stopped by use of spinal anesthesia. However, certain events act to inhibit them. For example, patients in active labor find that once admitted to the hospital, the labor ceases for a short time or that active labor can be interrupted transitorily by analgesia or anesthesia.

In describing a uterine contraction (Fig. 19-16), reference is made to the following characteristics:

1. *Frequency.* Contractions occur intermittently throughout labor. The interval between contractions gradually diminishes as labor progresses. They begin about 20 to 30 minutes apart and become closer together until, at the height of the expulsive efforts, they recur as often as 2 to 3 minutes.

2. *Regularity.* Contractions become more and more regular in occurrence as labor becomes well established.

3. *Duration.* The length of time a contraction lasts increases from 30 seconds to 60 to 90 seconds nearing full dilatation of the cervix, and then the duration becomes about 60 seconds until delivery of the fetus is accomplished.

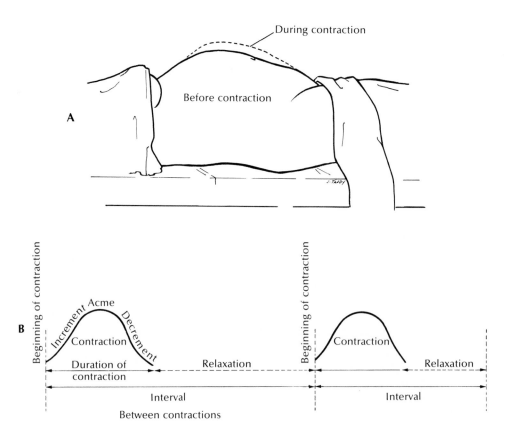

Fig. 19-16. A, Changes in abdominal contour before and during uterine contraction. **B,** Assessing contractions: frequency in minutes—interval between contractions (time from beginning of one to beginning of next); duration in seconds—how long contraction lasts (e.g., 45 seconds); regularity—whether intervals are same length or uneven lengths (e.g., 4 minutes); intensity—how strong contraction is (e.g., strong, moderate, weak).

4. _Intensity_. The strength of the contraction also increases as labor progresses from weak contractions noted early in labor to strong expulsive contractions evidenced near the time of delivery.

A contraction exhibits a wavelike pattern; it begins slowly, gradually reaches a peak, and then rather rapidly diminishes. There is an interval of rest, and then the next contraction begins. Contractions that have been augmented by administration of oxytocin tend to increase more rapidly, hold the acme (peak) longer, and diminish rapidly. Patients describe them as sharper, harder contractions.

There are three methods of assessing contractions. The first is the subjective description given by the mother; the second, palpation and timing by a nurse or physician; and the third, use of electronic monitoring devices.

When the mother reports that contractions have begun, she is asked, "When did they start?" "How often are they coming?" "Are they coming regularly?" "Would you say they were weak or strong?" Depending on the mother's knowledge, her answers can be definite or vague, but they serve as a basis for deciding whether the mother should be admitted to hospital.

The second method is used routinely throughout labor by the attending nurse. Palpations are done by using the fingertips, not the palmar surface, and the fingers must be kept moving. The uterus begins to contract in the fundal portion, and as the contraction proceeds, the uterus is less easily indented, until at the height of the contraction, the uterus feels very firm and hard. Then as the contraction diminishes, the fingers can again indent the uterine surface. The mother is not aware of the sensation of the uterus contracting until the contraction is fairly well established. Frequently, her description of the end of the contraction is related to the end of the pain sensation (felt in the lower portion of the uterus, not the fundus), and this can remain after the contraction is completed. Therefore her description may not be as accurate as that obtained by the nurse.

Monitoring devices measure frequency, duration, and strength of the contractions. The findings are automatically recorded by the machine.

Voluntary bearing-down efforts (secondary powers). As soon as the presenting part reaches the pelvic floor, the patient experiences an urge to "push," a voluntary bearing-down effort similar to that used in the process of defecation. The patient takes a deep breath, holds it, and contracts her diaphragm and abdominal muscles. (See Chapter 21 for additional patient instruction.) This results in increased intra-abdominal pressure. This pressure compresses the uterus on all sides and adds to the power of the expulsive forces.

This reflex needs to be held in check until the presenting part can emerge from the cervix at full dilatation (10 cm). Otherwise the cervix can be bruised and traumatized as it is forced against the pubis. The woman can control the urge to push by panting breaths. These reflexes are lost with spinal anesthesia; however, the woman can be coached when to push with a contraction so that labor is not impeded.

Contractions of the levator ani muscles. As the presenting part is being forced through the introitus by the expulsive power, contraction of the levator ani muscles in the rest interval between uterine contractions causes the part to recede and permits a temporary restoration of circulation. Extension of the presenting part also is aided by contractions of these muscles as is the birth of the placenta.

The placenta

Since the ovum usually implants in the fundal portion of the uterus, the developed placenta rarely acts as an impediment to labor. When implantation takes place in the lower uterine segment, the placenta may cover part or all of the internal cervical os and act as a barrier to birth of the fetus. This condition is known as a *placenta previa* and necessitates medical intervention (pp. 235 to 239).

Psychologic response

Patients who are relaxed, knowledgeable, and capable of actively participating in the control of the birth process usually experience shorter, less intense labors. Preparation in childbirth classes is based on such premises.

PROCESS OF LABOR
Changes preliminary to onset of labor

The head descends into the pelvis in most primigravidas 2 to 3 weeks before delivery. With this descent (lightening), some increased pelvic pressure is noted, but the mother can breathe more easily. In multigravidas, descent and the onset of labor coincide.

Prior to the onset of labor, the vaginal mucus is more profuse, and a brownish or blood-tinged cervical mucous plug may be passed. Streaks of blood or brownish secretion ("bloody show") may be noted. Frequently, this type of discharge is noted within 48 hours after a vaginal examination or coitus.

Persistent low backache may be described, and occasionally strong, frequent, but irregular uterine contractions may be identified by the patient.

The cervix becomes soft, partially effaced, or dilated. The membranes may rupture spontaneously.

Onset of labor

The onset of labor cannot be ascribed to a single cause; multiple factors, including changes in the maternal uterus, cervix, and pituitary, are involved. The integrity of the fetal hypothalamus, pituitary, and adrenal cortex probably is essential to the initiation of labor. Progressive uterine distention, increasing intrauterine pressure, and aging of the placenta seem to be associated with increasing myometrial irritability. In actuality, a convergence or compounding of numerous changes and their mutually coordinated effects result in strong, regular, rhythmic uterine contractions, which normally terminate in the birth of the fetus and the placenta. How certain alterations trigger others and how proper checks and balances are maintained are still not completely understood.

Afferent and efferent nerve impulses to and from the uterus alter its contractility. Although nerve impulses to the uterus will stimulate contractions, the denervated uterus still contracts well during labor because oxytocin is the regulator of labor.

During the course of pregnancy, one part of the fetus generally becomes directed toward the pelvic inlet, in large measure due to the uterus changing from a spheroid to an elliptoid contour after about the sixth month of gestation. The uterine tone increases, and the presenting part descends. Uterine activity increases, and the lower uterine segment, which is poorly contractile, thins, whereas the fundus, the strongly contractile portion, thickens (Fig. 19-15). Concomitantly uterine capacity becomes slightly but progressively reduced and an optimal uterine tension reached. At about this time the myometrial and placental circulation peak, and pregnancy apparently terminates when nutritional supplies to the fetus become insufficient.

Perhaps even more important, changes in the ratio of the concentration of estrogens and progesterone alter the contractility of the uterine musculature. Estrogens increase intermittent contractions, whereas progesterone relaxes smooth muscle, reducing uterine contractility. Progesterone, produced largely by the placenta after the third month, is present in greater concentration in the subplacental area than elsewhere in the uterus. It is theorized that with the proper estrogen-progesterone concentration, labor will not ensue. Moreover, it is believed that with adequate progesterone present in the myometrium beneath the placenta, this area will not contract excessively even during labor. Thus the placenta is permitted to remain attached and functional until the fetus has been delivered.

Unfortunately for this theory, there is no significant identifiable drop in progesterone production with the onset of labor, although both estrogen and progesterone excretion diminish slightly in the days prior to labor. In any event, the myometrium becomes increasingly sensitive to oxytocin prior to and during labor.

Physiologic uterine contractions can be initiated by oxytocin even early in established pregnancy if administered in considerable amounts. As pregnancy progresses, decreasing dosages of this hormone are required so that at term minute amounts of oxytocin will induce strong labor.

Fetal factors in initiation of labor. Another theory postulates that the increasing fetal secretion of hypophyseal and adrenocortical hormones acts to trigger the onset of labor. This is an important concept because adequate development is essential for the survival of the infant after birth.

Evidence from studies in sheep, in many ways comparable to the human, suggests that a steady rise in adrenocortical function and cortisol production occurs during the last trimester of pregnancy. This aids pulmonary (surfactant) maturation particularly.

Moreover, glucocorticoids probably play a role in the initiation of labor at term. It is hypothesized that 17-estradiol, produced by the fetoplacental unit, may initiate labor by stimulating the biosynthesis of PG. In sheep, at least, the level of 17-estradiol in the maternal plasma is low until about 24 hours prior to labor. PG biosynthesis in the placenta and myometrium is low while the uterus is quiescent and the cervix is uneffaced and closed, or "unripe." However, during the last 24 hours, there is a marked increase in estrogen production and a concomitant increase in PG release. Uterine activ-

ity is augmented, and the cervix begins to efface. The administration of large amounts of progesterone appears to block PG release to prevent cervical effacement and later dilatation. Smaller amounts of progesterone allow incomplete effacement and dilatation of the cervix and often result in prolonged labor. Hence the steady rise in circulating 17-estradiol seems to cause a proportional increase in myometrial and, theoretically, in decidual production of PG, which is responsible for the uterine activity (Braxton Hicks contractions) during the last month of pregnancy at least.

Mechanism of labor

The female pelvis has varied contours and diameters at different levels, and the presenting part of the passenger is large in proportion to the passage. For delivery to occur therefore the fetus must adapt to the birth canal during its descent. The turns and other adjustments that are necessary in the human birth process are called the *mechanism of labor.*

PHASES OF THE MECHANISM OF LABOR IN VERTEX PRESENTATION

Descent is a continuing process through the superior strait due mainly to uterine contractions. Engagement can be expected in the majority of patients near term or shortly after the onset of labor. The vertex usually enters the superior strait in the oblique or anteroposterior diameter (Fig. 19-17).

Flexion. Flexion is due to uterine contractions and the force of gravity exerted through the fetal body to the head. The skull may be compared to a lever, the short arm being the forward portion (e.g., the face and mandible) and the long arm being the posterior portion (e.g., the head). The fulcrum is the articulation between the occipital bone and the atlas (first cervical vertebra). With labor, flexion of the head usually occurs.

Descent. Descent of the vertex progresses more rapidly when complete dilatation and effacement of the cervix have occurred. Descent depends on the size and shape of the pelvic planes, the size and malleability of the head, and the forces of labor.

Internal rotation. When the vertex reaches the troughlike pelvic floor, made up largely by the levator musculature, the head usually rotates to the anteroposterior diameter to pass between the ischial spines. Arrest of the head in midpelvis, a frequent occurrence in primigravidas, may be due to cephalopelvic disproportion or irregular and/or weak contractions. The head often will have rotated to the anterior by the time it reaches the midpelvis, or the head, originally in a posterior position, may rotate the long way to the sym-

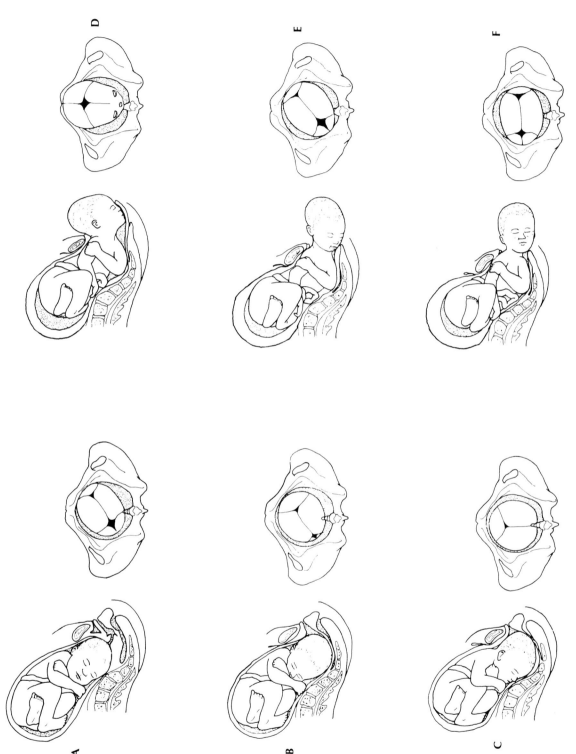

Fig. 19-17. Mechanism of labor in LOA presentation. **A,** Onset. **B,** Flexion. **C,** Internal rotation. **D,** Extension. **E,** Restitution. **F,** External rotation. (Courtesy Ross Laboratories, Columbus, Ohio.)

physis pubis rather than the short distance to the sacrum for reasons unknown.

Extension. When the fetal head reaches the perineum to be born, it is deflected anteriorly by the perineum. The occiput acts as the fulcrum as it passes under the lower border of the symphysis pubis. As a result, the occiput is born first, then the remainder of the head, then the face, and finally, the chin is born.

External rotation or restitution. After delivery of the head, it rotates briefly to the position that it occupied when it engaged in the inlet. Concomitantly the shoulders engage and descend in a manner similar to the head. The shoulders rotate anteroposteriorly for delivery, usually the posterior shoulder first, then the anterior shoulder. At this point, the head rotates back to its original position at delivery, and the body and extremities of the infant deliver. When the entire infant has emerged from the mother, birth is said to be complete. This is the time noted on the records.

PERSISTENT OCCIPUT POSTERIOR OR OCCIPUT TRANSVERSE POSITION

Prolongation of the first or second stage of labor may be due to persistent occiput posterior or occiput transverse position. During the normal mechanism of labor, the occiput may be directed posteriorly, particularly in an anthroid pelvis. In any event, dilatation of the cervix may be delayed because the head does not fit the pelvis

well or because the head does not press with equal firmness around the internal os. As a consequence, labor may be slowed by either cause or effect. Midpelvic or outlet contracture as a cause of cephalopelvic disproportion must be sought, usually by x-ray pelvimetry. If adequate measurements are noted, treatment requires stimulation of labor and/or forceps rotation and extraction of the fetus after full dilatation of the cervix. If a difficult midforceps delivery is likely, however, cesarean section is indicated.

DURATION OF LABOR

Normal labor (eutocia) is recorded when the patient is at or near term, without complications, when a single fetus presents by vertex, and when labor is completed by the mother (or by elective outlet forceps) within 24 hours. Its course is remarkably constant. Four stages of labor are recognized; the mean duration of the first three stages is approximately 13 hours for primigravidas and 8 hours for multigravidas.

A description of the labor experience of a significant number of parturients is described in Fig. 19-18. Friedman and Sachtleben (1965) utilized the information to predict the duration of normal labor for the first and second stages.

First stage of labor. The first stage is considered to be from the onset of regular contractions to full dilatation of the cervix (Fig. 19-19). Frequently, the onset of labor is

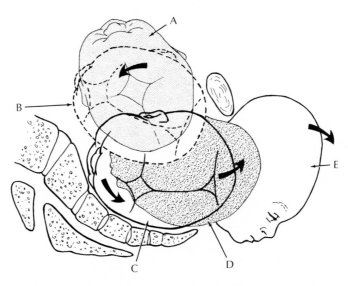

Fig. 19-18. Steps in normal mechanism of labor (head passing through birth canal): *A,* increased flexion; *B,* descent and engagement; *C,* internal rotation; *D,* internal rotation and beginning of extension; and *E,* extension (external rotation not shown). (Courtesy Ross Laboratories, Columbus, Ohio.)

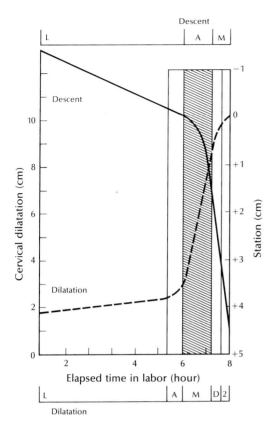

Fig. 19-19. Composite mean curves for descent and dilatation. (Modified from Friedman, E. A., and Sachtleben, M. R. 1965. Am. J. Obstet. Gynecol. **93:**522.)

difficult to establish; the patient may be admitted to the labor floor just before delivery so that the beginning of labor may be only an estimate. The first stage is much longer than the two others combined, averaging about 12 hours for primigravidas and approximately 6 hours for multigravidas. Great variability is the rule, however, depending on the essential factors discussed earlier. Some multigravidas may become fully dilated in less than an hour, or infrequently, a primigravida may not be completely dilated in 24 hours.

Second stage of labor. This stage lasts from full dilatation of the cervix to delivery of the fetus. The mean duration of the second stage of labor is 20 minutes for multigravidas, and 1 hour for primigravidas. Up to 2 hours is considered within the normal range.

Third stage of labor. This is from delivery of the fetus to delivery of the placenta. The placenta normally separates after the third or fourth strong uterine contraction after the infant has been delivered. The placenta should be removed with the next uterine contraction after separation, but unusual adherence of the placenta or mismanagement of the third stage of labor may result in placental retention. The actual duration of the third stage of labor depends on how this stage of labor is managed by the physician, since manual removal or expression of the placenta may be necessary.

The third stage of labor is about 3 to 4 minutes long for primigravidas and 4 to 5 minutes for multigravid women.

Fourth stage of labor. This lasts 1 to 4 hours after delivery of the placenta. It is the period of recovery when homeostasis is reestablished.

REFERENCES

Brackbill, Y., and others. 1974. Obstetric premedication and infant outcome. Am. J. Obstet. Gynecol. **118:**377.

Friedman, E. A., and Sachtleben, M. R. 1965. Station of the fetal presenting part. Am. J. Obstet. Gynecol. **93:**522.

Gunther, R. E., and Harer, W. B. 1964. Vaginal examinations during late pregnancy and labor. Obstet. Gynecol. **24:**695.

McLennan, C. E., and Sandberg, E. C. 1974. Synopsis of obstetrics. St. Louis, The C. V. Mosby Co.

Peterson, W. F., and others. 1965. Routine vagination examinations during labor. Obstet. Gynecol. **92:**310.

Reeder, S., and others. 1976. Maternity nursing. Philadelphia, J. B. Lippincott Co.

Towler, J., and Butler-Manuel, R. 1973. Modern obstetrics for student midwives. London, Lloyd-Luke, Ltd.

Walker, P. A. 1973. Drugs used in labour: an obstetrician's view. Br. J. Anaesth. **45:**787.

CHAPTER 20

First stage of labor

GENERAL CONSIDERATIONS

The first stage of labor begins with the onset of regular contractions and is complete when the cervix is fully dilated. The symptoms the expectant mother has been prepared to recognize herald the beginning of labor. The waiting period of pregnancy is at an end. The time to be born has come.

The forces at work during this stage are the uterine contractions. These act to retract and dilate the cervix. They are involuntary and as such are outside the patient's direct control. No amount of maternal effort, that is, bearing down or pushing, will hasten the process.

MANAGEMENT

Care of the patient in labor begins with the patient's report of the following:
1. The onset of progressive, strong, frequent, sustained uterine contractions
2. Rupture of the membranes
3. Vaginal bleeding (bloody show)

She is usually instructed to report to her physician or midwife and then to the hospital if she is to have a hospital delivery. (See Chapter 23 if patient is to have a home delivery.) On admission, the questions to be answered are the following:

1. *Is she in labor* (Table 20-1)? False labor may be experienced from the thirty-eighth week on. It is frustrating for the patient to find that the labor she was experiencing was not "true" and that she must return home until more definite symptoms are present. For those who experience this two or three times, the onset of "true" labor comes as an anticlimax, and only attentive care can eradicate the feelings of disappointment and even anger.

2. *How far has she progressed* (Table 20-2)? The nullipara, because of eagerness to have labor over and done, may come to the hospital very early in the first stage. If she lives near the hospital, she may be asked to return home and wait for further progress either in frequency and strength of contractions or amount of show. She is encouraged to walk about but to restrict her intake to clear fluids. If she lives a distance from the hospital, she may be admitted and the same care given.

3. *Have the membranes ruptured?* Labor is initiated by spontaneous rupture of the membranes (SRM) in almost 25% of maternity patients. A lag period, rarely exceeding 24 hours, precedes the onset of labor. The length of uterine inactivity is directly related to the duration of pregnancy. If the woman is only 32 weeks' pregnant, for example, several days may pass before labor begins. If she is at term, labor usually ensues within 12 hours of rupture of the membranes. After a delay of 24 hours, the woman is said to have premature or prolonged rupture of the membranes (PROM). Rupture of membranes is discussed further in the following section.

4. *Are there complications that may require treatment?* Although some complications of labor are anticipated, others appear only in the clinical course of labor (Chapter 24). Knowledge of the pregnancy, careful initial assessment, and follow-up of progress are necessary during normal labor and essential if some abnormality intervenes.

Assessing progress in labor

Progress in normal labor is a constant entity, although for some women it may be more rapid than for others. The symptomatology of progress is well defined, and careful assessment provides the cues for selection and institution of modes of care. The nurse assumes much of the responsibility for making the assessment of progress and for keeping the physician informed as to progress and any deviations from normal. Tables 20-1 and 20-2 summarize the symptomatology, and Table 20-3 provides a plan for assessment.

Rupture of membranes
TESTS FOR RUPTURE OF MEMBRANES

Drainage of amniotic fluid may be an obvious prelude to labor. Questionable leakage of amniotic fluid usually

Table 20-1. Comparison of labors

True labor	False labor	Complicated labor (examples)
Show: usually present; pinkish mucus, may be mucous plug from cervix	Show: usually none or brownish-stained mucus (inquire if she had vaginal examination within last 48 hours)	Hemorrhage: patient reports blood trickling down legs as she stands or has soaked perineal pad with bright red blood
Contractions: occur regularly; interval between has shortened; intensity has gradually increased; located in lower back (may feel like gastrointestinal upset with some diarrhea); intensified by walking	Contractions: occur irregularly; intervals remain long; intensity unchanged; located in abdomen; relief with walking or no effect	Contractions: suddenly intensify, then cease; abdomen becomes rigid and boardlike; feels very ill, nervous, shocked
Cervix: becomes effaced and dilates progressively	Cervix: no change	Cervix: excessive vaginal bleeding precludes vaginal examination
Fetal movement: no significant change	Fetal movement: intensifies (for a short period) or remains the same	Fetal movement: intensifies then ceases altogether

Table 20-2. Maternal progress in first stage of labor within normal limits*

	Early phase	Midphase	Transition phase
Duration	About 8 to 10 hours	About 3 hours	About 1 to 2 hours
Cervix Dilatation Effacement	0 to 5 cm	6 to 7 cm Nullipara: often complete before dilatation begins Multipara: occurs simultaneously with dilatation	8 to 10 cm
Contractions Magnitude Rhythm Frequency Duration	Mild Irregular 5 to 30 minutes apart 10 to 30 seconds	Moderate More regular 3 to 5 minutes apart 30 to 45 seconds	Strong to expulsive Regular 2 to 3 minutes apart 45 to 60 seconds (few to 90 seconds)
Descent Station of presenting part	Nulliparous: 0 Multiparous: 0 to −2 cm	About +1 cm to +2 cm About +1 cm to +2 cm	+2 cm to +3 cm +2 cm to +3 cm
Show Color Amount	Brownish discharge, mucous plug Scant	Pink to bloody mucus Scant to moderate	Bloody mucus Copious
Behavior and appearance	Excited; thoughts center on self, labor, and baby; may be talkative or mute, calm or tense; some apprehension, pain controlled fairly well; alert, follows directions readily; open to instructions	Becoming more serious, doubtful of control of pain, more apprehensive; desires companionship and encouragement; attention more inner directed; fatigue evidenced; malar flush; has some difficulty following directions	Pain described as severe, backache common; feelings of frustration, fear of loss of control, and irritability surface; vague in communications; amnesia between contractions; writhing with contractions; nausea and vomiting, especially if hyperventilating; hyperesthesia; circumoral pallor, perspiration on forehead and upper lip; shaking, tremor of thighs; feeling of need to defecate, pressure on anus

*The pace of progress in cervical dilatation (according to Friedman and Sachtleben, 1965) varies as follows: from 0 to 2 cm (latent phase), progress is slow; from 2 to 4 cm (phase of acceleration), pace quickens; from 4 to 9 cm (phase of maximum acceleration), pace is most rapid; and from 9 to 10 cm (phase of deceleration), pace slows again.

Table 20-3. Minimum reassessment of progress of first stage of labor

	Cervical dilatation		
	0 to 5 cm	**6 to 7 cm**	**8 to 10 cm**
Vital signs*	Every 4 hours	Every 4 hours	Every 4 hours
Blood pressure	Every 60 minutes	Every 60 minutes	Every 60 minutes
Contractions	Every 30 minutes to 1 hour	Every 15 minutes	Every 5 to 10 minutes
FHT	Every 30 minutes	Every 15 minutes	Every 5 minutes
Show	Every 60 minutes	Every 30 minutes	Every 10 to 15 minutes
Behavior, appearance, energy level	Every 30 minutes	Every 15 minutes	Every 5 minutes
Vaginal examination	To be done only for following reasons: 1. To confirm diagnosis when symptoms indicate change (e.g., strength, duration, or frequency of contractions; increase in amount of bloody show; membranes rupture; or patient feels pressure on her rectum) 2. To determine if dilatation (and descent) are sufficient for administration of anesthetic 3. To reassess progress if labor takes longer than expected 4. To determine station of presenting part		

*If membranes have ruptured, check temperature every 2 hours.

is not an indication for the induction of labor. If obvious loss of fluid does not persist, one probably should await the onset of uterine contractions in pregnancies of doubtful viability. Loss of urine by the incontinent patient or leukorrhea in the woman with vaginitis must be differentiated from amniotic fluid for proper maternity management.

The following simple procedures are useful in the diagnosis of ruptured membranes:

1. Spread a drop of the fluid on a clean slide. Allow the fluid to dry. Dried amniotic fluid (in the absence of blood or gross infection) will show a frondlike crystalline pattern when viewed under the microscope. This result is known as a *positive fern test*. It should not be confused with the cervical mucous test (p. 65), which also shows fernlike formation. Urine, vaginal discharge, or blood will not show a crystalline pattern.

2. Determine the pH of the vaginal fluid. Amniotic fluid is slightly alkaline; urine or pus is acid. Nitrazine paper moistened with amniotic fluid will turn dark blue in the alkaline range and yellow in the acid.

3. Fetal lanugo hairs or fetal squamous cells may be noted under the microscope if amniotic fluid is the test material. Moreover, some of the squamous cells, presumably derived from skin sebaceous glands, contain lipids that stain yellow after the addition of aqueous Nile blue stain. Other squamae and hairs stain blue.

COMPLICATIONS ASSOCIATED WITH RUPTURED MEMBRANES

Infection. Once the membranes have ruptured, the "clock of infection" begins to tick. The frequency of chorioamnionitis follows a progressive linear course after a prodromal period of about 4 hours. Fulminating, clinically evident sepsis often is notable after 72 hours. Hence it is good practice to stimulate labor with dilute oxytocin solution intravenously when the lag period exceeds 6 to 8 hours, assuming a definitely viable fetus (weight 2000 gm and gestational age 34 weeks or more). If the survival of the fetus is doubtful because of immaturity, watchful expectancy is the better policy. Once clinical amnionitis supervenes, induction of labor is indicated (p. 305). If induction is unsuccessful, cesarean section may be required.

Prophylactic antibiotic therapy rarely will protect against amnionitis. In most cases, such treatment often results in the development of antibiotic-resistant strains of many pathogenic organisms.

Prolapsed cord. Prolapse of the umbilical cord is displacement of the cord downward, often below the presenting part (Fig. 20-1). Occasionally the cord may even slip through the cervix into the vagina or beyond. A long, loose cord and an unengaged presenting part, frequently associated with rupture of the membranes, may allow prolapse of the cord because, with a sudden gush

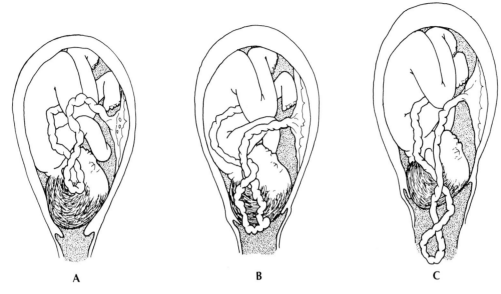

Fig. 20-1. Prolapse of cord. Note pressure of head on cord, which endangers fetal circulation. **A,** Occult prolapse of umbilical cord. **B,** Forelying umbilical cord. **C,** Complete prolapse of umbilical cord.

of fluid, the cord may be carried downward. Prolapse of the cord, which occurs in 1 of every 400 late pregnancies and more often in immature gestations, is important because the cord may be compressed after its displacement; fetal hypoxia and death of the infant may occur. Prompt delivery in the manner least harmful to mother and baby is imperative.

The maternity patient may feel the cord slither into the vagina when the membranes rupture. More often, vaginal examination by an alert nurse or physician immediately after a sudden gush of fluid may lead to the diagnosis of prolapsed cord.

Upward pressure against the presenting part by the examining hand vaginally may protect the cord from obstruction until delivery can be accomplished. Another effective emergency measure requires the mother to assume the knee-chest position, which should carry the presenting part away from the cervix, thus easing compression of the cord. Immediate cesarean section is indicated unless the cervix is fully dilated, in which case forceps delivery of a vertex or extraction of a breech presentation may be feasible.

Prolonged cord compression, that is, more than 5 minutes, usually causes CNS damage or death of the neonate. Fetal or maternal trauma may follow inexpert or ill-advised delivery from below.

Meconium-stained amniotic fluid. The fluid is normally pale straw colored. Greenish brown color indicates that the fetus has probably undergone stress, causing a passage of meconium from the bowel. Yellow-stained fluid may indicate fetal hypoxia that occurred 36 hours or more prior to rupture of membranes or to fetal hemolytic disease (Rh or ABO incompatibility, intrauterine infection). It is a normal finding in breech presentations. If an iodine preparation is used as a vaginal disinfectant during vaginal examinations, it can be difficult to differentiate iodine staining from meconium staining.

Although meconium-stained fluid is found with fetal asphyxia, its presence is not always diagnostic of prospective fetal distress. It should be promptly reported and recorded, however.

Monitoring fetus during labor

The fetal oxygen supply must be maintained during labor to prevent severe debilitating conditions after birth or even death in utero or shortly after birth. The fetal oxygen supply can be reduced in a number of ways:

1. Reduction in blood flow through the maternal vessels as a result of maternal hypertension or hypotension (systolic blood pressure of 60 mm Hg)
2. Reduction of the oxygen content of the maternal blood as a result of hemorrhage or severe anemia
3. Alterations in fetal circulation as might occur with compression of the cord, placental separation, or head compression, which causes increased intra-

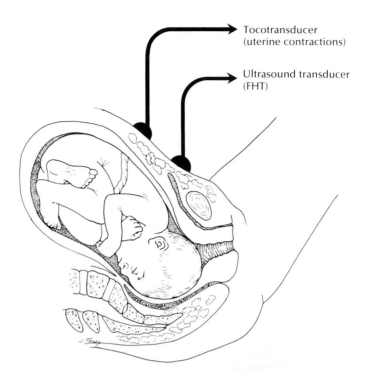

Tocotransducer
(uterine contractions)

Ultrasound transducer
(FHT)

Fig. 20-2. External noninvasive fetal monitoring.

cranial pressure and vagal nerve stimulation with slowing of the heart rate

Following are methods of determining the degree of fetal distress throughout labor:

- Assess the rate and rhythm of the fetal heart
- Sample fetal blood pH and concentrations of oxygen and carbon dioxide (PO_2 and PCO_2)
- The oxytocin challenge (stress) test
- The presence of meconium-stained amniotic fluid (Fetal hypoxia causes relaxation of the anal sphincter and a bowel movement.)

Fetal heart rate monitoring. *Periodic auscultation of the fetal heart,* a time-honored method of assessment of fetal status, may reveal tachycardia, bradycardia, or arrhythmia that may occur during the brief examinations. Serious, even critical jeopardy interspersed or not recurring during the periods of auscultation may pass unrecognized by the examiner. Hence only marked degrees of fetal distress can usually be identified by listening to the FHT periodically. An improved method that is more likely to diagnose fetal compromise is the counting of FHT during sequential contractions and for a full 3 minutes thereafter. Persistent, postcontraction bradycardia (e.g., FHT, 100 beats/min or a persistent drop of 20 beats/min or more below baseline) or gross irregularity indicates fetal distress.

Naturally the patient becomes anxious if the examiner cannot hear the FHT. For the inexperienced listener, it often takes time to locate the heartbeat and find the area of maximum density. For a vertex presentation, it is suggested that the student start at the umbilicus and move in a widening half circle below the umbilicus until the beat can be heard. The mother can be told that the nurse is "finding the spot where the sounds are loudest." If it takes considerable time to locate them, offer to let the mother hear them too, to reassure her. Use a portable Doppler apparatus. If the examiner cannot locate the FHT, an experienced nurse should be asked for assistance, and the spot can be marked with an **X**.

Continuous beat-to-beat fetal heart auscultation by the use of an abdominal transducer and amplification of the cardiac impulses or augmented Doppler principle impulses is a better method of fetal monitoring. Unfortunately a clear sound is difficult to achieve using this modality, especially during the second stage of labor. Moreover, the interpretation of important frequency and regularity differences in relation to the uterine contraction pattern may be impractical or impossible.

External electronic monitoring of FHT and uterine contractions is a good, indirect, noninvasive method of fetal monitoring (Fig. 20-2). Phonocardiographic or Doppler pickup of FHT through the maternal abdominal

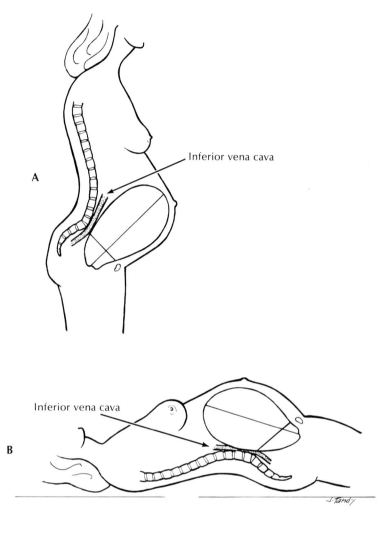

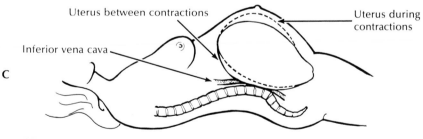

Fig. 20-3. Vena cava syndrome. Note relationship of gravid uterus to ascending vena cava in standing posture **(A)** and in supine posture **(B)**. Note how enlarged uterus compresses vena cava, particularly during contraction **(C)**, reducing return of blood to heart. Reduced cardiac output causes maternal hypotension and reduced flow of blood to placenta with consequent fetal distress.

wall, together with tocodynamometer impulses displayed on an oscilloscope, or a multigraph recording may be employed. This method is especially valuable during the first stage of labor in patients with intact membranes. This equipment can neither record the intensity of the uterine contractions nor the intra-amniotic pressure, however.

The equipment is easily applied by the nurse but must be repositioned as the mother or fetus changes position. It should be removed periodically to permit washing the applicator sites and giving backrubs. Although the equipment is recommended for use in the supine position, this position can cause maternal hypotension and consequent fetal hypoxia through compression of the vena cava by the weight of the uterus and a resultant decrease in return of blood to the right ventricle and thus a decrease in cardiac output (Fig. 20-3). Also, many women find the supine position uncomfortable, particularly during a contraction.

The use of any "machine" may be frightening to the patient and her family. Careful explanation of the reasons for use, what actions will be required of the patient, and whether pain will result is necessary to allay fears and suspicions. The patient tends to assume that all is not well with her baby; if this is the case, honesty is the best policy because the more sophisticated patient and her husband are capable of "reading the results."

Continuous internal fetal monitoring affords the most

accurate appraisal of fetal well-being during labor (Fig. 20-4). For this type of monitoring, the membranes must have ruptured and the presenting part be low enough for placement of the electrode. A small electrode is attached to the fetal scalp and yields a continuous rate on a graph and a visual report of the fetal cardiograph on the oscilloscope.* A catheter filled with saline is introduced into the uterine cavity. The fluid acts as a transmitter of changes in uterine pressure to a transducer. This converts the pressures into millimeters of mercury (75 mm Hg is normal).

Early deceleration (slowing of heart rate) in response to compression of the fetal head is normal, and does not indicate fetal distress (Fig. 20-5). It is characterized by a uniform shape and an early onset in relation to the rise in amniotic fluid pressure as the uterus contracts. Transient bradycardia during a contraction is normal.

Late deceleration is also uniform in shape but begins after the contraction is established (Fig. 20-6). When persistent or recurrent, this usually indicates fetal hypoxia because of deficient placental perfusion. Bradycardia (below 100 beats/min) is not a requirement here because

---

*Before this method is used, the possibility of hemophilia or other coagulation disorder in the infant must be ruled out by careful questioning of the mother, for example, "Have any of your relatives had trouble with bleeding?" A fetal death due to exsanguination from the puncture wounds in the scalp can occur.

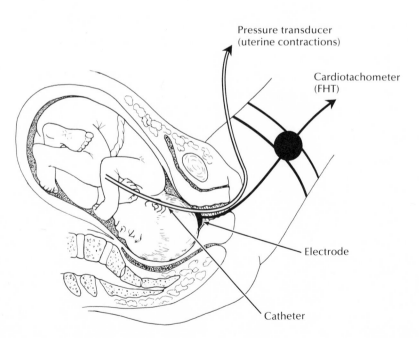

Pressure transducer
(uterine contractions)

Cardiotachometer
(FHT)

Electrode

Catheter

Fig. 20-4. Internal invasive fetal monitoring (membranes ruptured and cervix dilated).

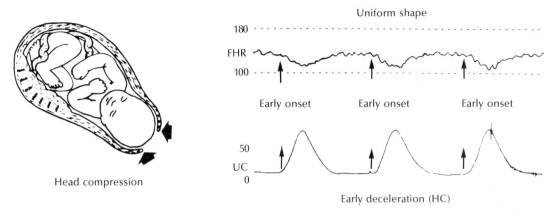

Fig. 20-5. Early deceleration pattern. (From Hon, E. H. 1968. An atlas of fetal heart rate patterns. New Haven, Harty Press.)

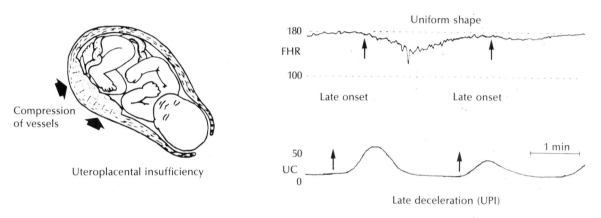

Fig. 20-6. Late deceleration pattern. (From Hon, E. H. 1968. An atlas of fetal heart rate patterns. New Haven, Harty Press.)

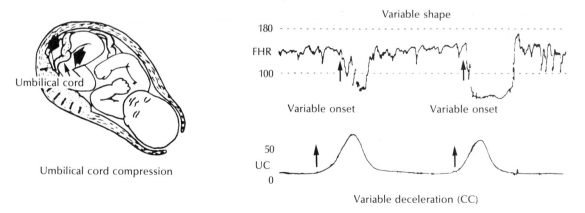

Fig. 20-7. Variable deceleration pattern. (From Hon, E. H. 1968. An atlas of fetal heart rate patterns, New Haven, Harty Press.)

a drop in the fetal heart rate from 160 to 120 beats/min, for example, is sufficient for the diagnosis of late deceleration. Only constant recording may identify this abnormality.

Variable deceleration indicates a transient reduction in the fetal heart rate before, during, or after a uterine contraction (Fig. 20-7). There is no uniformity in the pattern here, but the range generally is 140 to 160 beats/min. Variable deceleration may be related to partial, brief, cord compression. This abnormal pattern usually is eliminated by change of the mother's position such as from back to side or one side to the other. Variable deceleration is associated with neonatal depression only when severe or prolonged.

Persistent bradycardia (FHT of 100 beats/min or less) is an ominous sign, especially when it follows a uterine contraction. Bradycardia during several contractions may indicate cord compression or separation of the placenta. Turning the patient on her other side and administering oxygen may improve the FHT pattern. If no benefit results, however, emergency delivery, usually by cesarean section, is indicated.

Tachycardia when continued for an hour or more or when accompanied by late deceleration is an indication of fetal distress.

A loss of minimal irregularity of the baseline (loss of beat-to-beat variation) or "smoothing out" of the baseline (not induced by drugs such as diazepam or atropine) is a serious development, often a prelude to infant death.

Normal fetal heart rate patterns correlate with high Apgar scores and low neonatal morbidity. An abnormal pattern is equated with fetal hypoxia, low Apgar scores, and high neonatal morbidity in many but by no means all cases. More investigation and clarification of the factors and findings involved will be necessary to perfect fetal monitoring.

If an abnormal tracing appears, the nurse immediately effects the following measures:

1. Changes the patient's position from supine to side or from one side to another
2. Administers oxygen by mask (6 to 7 ℓ/min)
3. Stops oxytocin administration; changes to bottle of lactated Ringer's solution or 5% dextrose in water and increases drip rate to 20 drops/min (adult flow)
4. Notifies the physician of the tracing and the effect of repositioning and oxygen administration
5. Completes preparation for cesarean section if the pattern persists (pp. 403 and 404)

Fetal blood sampling. The blood sample is obtained from the fetal scalp transcervically after rupture of the membranes. The scalp is swabbed with a disinfecting solution before the puncture is made. Fetal acidosis follows fetal hypoxia, and some perinatologists believe that true fetal distress can only be diagnosed when serious FHT changes can be correlated with fetal blood acidosis (pH 7.20).

Most infants who have low Apgar scores have scalp blood readings of pH 7.15 or less. If there are consecutive blood samples with a pH below 7.20 that show a continuing decrease, the need for prompt delivery of the infant should be assessed. Because of the difficulty of measuring scalp blood Po_2, it has been largely supplanted by determination of the pH and base excess (BE).

Maternal respiratory alkalosis and a subsequent decrease in cardiac output, occurring as a result of the hyperventilation passively induced during anesthesia, can cause paradoxical fetal acidosis and depression of the neonate. However, hyperventilation in the conscious adult is self-limiting (patients will complain of tingling in hands and feet and a "whoosy" feeling), can be readily controlled by having the patient breathe into a brown paper bag, and is probably without noxious effects on the fetus.

Oxytocin challenge (stress) test. The OCT is designed to assess the circulatory-respiratory reserve of the fetoplacental unit. It is employed in the evaluation of high-risk pregnancy. The exact value of the OCT is still debated, and for the present, directors of maternity services must evaluate the test according to their own experience.

An abdominal-fetal ECG (noninvasive external monitor) system is employed together with an external tokodynamometer. The output from the fetal heart rate and uterine contraction transducers is registered by a two-channel strip recorder. An accurate infusion pump is required for administration of intravenous oxytocin solution.

Relative contraindications include previous classic cesarean section, placenta previa, prematurity, multiple pregnancy, incompetent cervix, ruptured membranes, or pregnancy of less than 33 to 34 weeks.

The patient is admitted to the labor unit in the hospital because the care requires specific judgments by experienced health professionals, and all facilities for immediate operative delivery by cesarean section may be required.

The patient is placed in semi-Fowler's position and tilted slightly to one side to avoid vena caval compression by the enlarged uterus. The blood pressure is taken and recorded every 10 minutes during the OCT. Monitors are placed on the abdomen at sites for the best pickup of FHT, and recording is tested. The baseline

FHT rate and uterine activity are obtained before oxytocin is administered.

If spontaneous uterine activity is less than three contractions every 10 minutes, the patient is stimulated with intravenous oxytocin. If three or more contractions every 10 minutes are noted, this spontaneous uterine activity is adequate for the OCT. Mist oxygen should be available in case fetal distress develops.

If there is no spontaneous activity, oxytocin is administered as an intravenous infusion. The usual dosage is 10 units of Pitocin in 1000 ml of 5% dextrose in water without medication. The initial drip rate is 5 drops/min. If the contraction frequency remains less than three contractions every 10 minutes, oxytocin administration is increased by doubling the rate every 15 to 20 minutes until a maximum rate of 20 to 30 drops/min is reached. Adequate uterine activity to induce fetoplacental stress is three contractions of 40 to 60 seconds' duration in a 10-minute period. If late deceleration occurs, the test must be terminated immediately. The infusion with the oxytocin is closed off, and the infusion containing no medication is opened.

Once the mother has developed a contraction frequency of three contractions every 10 minutes, the oxytocin is discontinued. The recording of FHT and uterine contractions should be continued until uterine activity returns to prestimulation levels.

Persistent late deceleration occurring with at least three contractions is a *positive OCT,* but three contractions in a 10-minute period without late deceleration is a *negative OCT.* Occasional or several nonpersistent decelerations constitute a *suspicious OCT.* If the fetal heart decelerations occur with excessive uterine activity, the test is termed *hyperstimulation OCT* and is not interpretable. Poor quality recording or a frequency of contractions less than three every 10 minutes renders the study an *unreliable OCT,* and a repeat test within 24 to 36 hours is in order.

A negative OCT generally rules out the need for intervention. A positive OCT correlates well but not absolutely with uteroplacental insufficiency. In cases of serious jeopardy, such as diabetes mellitus, low estriol excretion, or intrauterine growth retardation, prompt delivery, probably by cesarean section, is warranted.

The test may be repeated at weekly or biweekly intervals from the thirty-fourth week of gestation until delivery. Such a regimen is extremely tiring and anxiety provoking for the mother and father. These patients require much supportive nurturing care. Although intellectually they may accept these tests as necessary for the infant's health, the interruption in the normal progress of the pregnancy may be disquieting.

Induction of labor

Induction of labor may be used to either begin the labor process or to augment a labor that is progressing slowly because of inadequate uterine contractions. The indication for induction may be medical or elective (social).

Medical indications include the following:
- Management of abortion, to stimulate the uterus to pass the conceptus
- Prolonged rupture of the membranes
- Prolonged pregnancy (42 to 43 weeks)
- Preterm delivery in diabetic mother or infants with severe isoimmunization
- Severe preeclampsia, placenta abruptio, or fetal death necessitating termination of the pregnancy artificially
- Uterine inertia (p. 359)

Elective indications are as follows:
- Multigravidas with a history of precipitate labor
- Patients who live long distances from the hospital

Methods used are surgical (rupture of the membranes) or medical (use of labor-inducing drugs).

Intravenous drip method. Natural oxytocin (Pitocin) or synthetic oxytocin (Syntocinon) are added to an intravenous infusion of 5% dextrose in water. The usual dose is 10 units/1000 ml 5% dextrose in water. A piggyback setup with 500 ml 5% dextrose in water is used so that the induction solution can be turned off and the vein kept open with the second solution. A pump for steady flow administration is desirable or a very slow drip, beginning at 5 adult drops/min and gradually increasing (or decreasing), depending on the strength, duration, and frequency of contractions.

If fetal monitors are available, they are used during an induction. If not available, the FHT are assessed using a fetoscope every hour until contractions begin and then every 15 to 30 minutes, depending on the quality of the contractions. If excessive uterine contractions occur (over 40 to 50 seconds' duration or more often than every 2 to 3 minutes) or if there is fetal bradycardia, tachycardia, or heart irregularity, the oxytocin is stopped and 5% dextrose in water infused.

Continuous and careful assessment is necessary to safeguard mother and fetus as the danger of uterine rupture, placental separation, and fetal asphyxia may result from too frequent and prolonged uterine contractions. Record the time the contractions begin or intensify, and then record concomitantly with assessment.

Transcervical amniotomy or artificial rupture of membranes. The cervix should be soft, partially effaced, and slightly dilated, preferably with the presenting part engaged or engaging. Simple rupture of the membranes using a hook or other sharp instrument passed over a finger into the cervix will allow the drainage of amniotic fluid. The mother can be assured that neither she nor the infant will feel any pain. Within 6 to 8 hours, labor may be under way. Some obstetricians prefer to first stimulate the uterus with intravenous oxytocin and as soon as good contractions are evident, rupture the membranes. Others prefer merely to rupture the membranes, knowing that oxytocin stimulation is often unnecessary.

Methods not recommended

1. Intramuscular or intranasal oxytocin are condemned because of the physician's inability to control the effects of the drug, which may suddenly cause tetanic, prolonged uterine contractions.

2. "Stripping of the membranes" before or instead of rupture of the membranes is a dangerous procedure. It consists of the physician inserting a finger through the soft, dilatable cervix at term and stripping the fetal membranes off the uterine wall in and around the internal os. It may cause rupture of membranes, displacement of the presenting part, prolapse of the cord, or initiate bleeding or sepsis. In the rare instance, it may predispose to amniotic fluid embolism.

3. Insertion of a bougie or packing in the cervix may eventuate in labor. However, these procedures are condemned because of the dangers of trauma, bleeding, and infection.

4. Intravenous administration of PG is effectual for the induction of labor, but cost and unpleasant side effects are deterrents to its use (Chapter 6).

5. Intra-amniotic injection of hypertonic sodium chloride is lethal for the infant and cannot be employed for induction of labor unless the fetus is dead or grossly abnormal (Chapter 6).

Control of discomfort and pain

The alleviation of pain is important, although discomfort and pain are a natural protective mechanism for the individual. The pain associated with parturition was accepted as a necessary part of childbirth until the discovery of the first anesthetics, nitrous oxide and ethyl ether.

Since that time, much research has gone into the development of methods of pain control that can bring effective relief for the mother without harm to the child. The perfect solution is yet to be found; thus at times the safety of the child must take precedence over the comfort of the mother.

Pain results in both reflex motor and psychic reactions. The quality of physical pain has been described as pricking, burning, aching, throbbing, sharp, nauseating,

or cramping. These differences arise apparently from different body locations or by stimulation of pain receptors and other types of receptors simultaneously. The reaction to pain arises as a result of the transmission of pain impulses through the nervous system.

Whatever pain relief modality or combination of modalities is used in the best interests of the mother and child, indications for its use are evidenced in the behavior of the patient. Pain in childbirth gives rise to symptoms that are measurable. It may cause increased activity of the sympathetic nervous system with resultant changes in blood pressure, pulse, respirations, and skin color. Bouts of nausea and vomiting and excessive perspiration are also commonplace. Certain affective expressions of suffering are familiar to all and include increasing anxiety with a lessened perceptual field, writhing, crying, groaning, gestures (hand clenching, wringing), and excessive muscular excitability throughout the body. Baselines for these symptoms need to be established early in labor.

NURSE-PATIENT INTERACTION

The quality of the nurse-patient relationship is a factor in patients' ability to cope with the pain or discomfort experienced as part of the labor process. An understanding, competent nurse acts as a protective agent for the patient. Through coaching and encouraging the patient to make best use of the expulsive forces, suggesting various breathing, relaxation, or postural techniques to counter the effects of pain sensations, and *judicious* recommendation of analgesia or anesthesia when indicated are all appropriate nursing interventions in the control of pain. The responsibility for initiating and maintaining such a therapeutic relationship rests with the nurse. Awareness of the points given in Table 20-4 can assist in this process.

Individuals perceive comparable degrees of pain stimuli in a like manner; that is, thresholds for pain are remarkably similar in all persons, regardless of sexual, social, ethnic, or cultural differences.

Although the concepts just discussed are employed as the basis for the use of analgesia and anesthesia in obstetrics, they do not explain all the phenomena that make up the human pain experience. The reasons for the effects of such factors as one's culture, use of counterstimuli, and distraction in causing radically different reactions to pain stimuli are still incompletely understood. The meaning of pain and the verbal and nonverbal expression given to pain are apparently learned from interactions within the primary social group and personalized for each individual. As pain is experienced, people develop types of coping mechanisms to deal with it. Pain or the possibility

Table 20-4. Significance of pain experience

	Patient	Nurse
Perception of meaning	*Origin:* Cultural concept of and personal experience with pain; for example: Pain in childbirth is inevitable, something to be borne Pain in childbirth can be avoided completely Pain in childbirth is punishment for sin Pain in childbirth can be controlled	*Origin:* Cultural concept of and personal experience with pain; in addition, nurse becomes accustomed to working with certain "expected" pain trajectories. For example: in obstetrics, pain is expected to increase as labor progresses, be intermittent in character, and have end point; relief can be derived from drugs once labor is well established and fetus or newborn can cope with amount and elimination of drug; relief can also come from patient's knowledge and attitude and support from family or friends.
Coping mechanisms	Patient may: Be traditionally vocal or nonvocal; crying out and/or groaning may be part of ritual of her response to pain Use counterstimulation to minimize pain; for example, rubbing, applying heat, or counterpressure Have learned to use relaxation, distraction, autosuggestion as pain-countering techniques Resist any use of "needles" as modes of administering pain relief	Nurse may: Have learned to use self effectively; for example, tone of voice, closeness in space, touch, etc., as media for message of interest and caring Use avoidance, belittling, or other distancing actions as protective device for self Use pharmacologic resources at hand judiciously Be skilled in use of comfort measures Assume accountability for control and management of pain
Expectations of others	Nurse may be seen as someone who will accept patient's statement of pain and act as her advocate Medical personnel may be expected to relieve patient of all pain sensations Nurse may be expected to be interested, gentle, kindly, and accepting of behavior exhibited	Nurse may accept only certain verbal or nonverbal behaviors as responses to pain Nurse may expect couple who are prepared for childbirth to refuse medication and to wish to "do everything on their own" Nurse may find it difficult to accept patient's definition of pain; that is, patient may wish to experience and participate in controlling pain or may not be able to accept any pain as reasonable

of pain that has unknown qualities can induce fear states in which anxiety borders on panic. At times, pain stimuli that are particularly noxious can be ignored. Malzack and Wall (1968) have postulated that certain nerve cell groupings within the spinal cord, brain stem, and cerebral cortex have the ability to modulate the pain impulse through a blocking mechanism. These blocking mechanisms can arise from internal or external stimuli and act to modify the individual's reaction to pain. This *gate control theory,* as it is known, is helpful in understanding the approaches used in education for childbirth programs or the use of hypnosis in labor.

Pain during labor and delivery is caused by the following:

* *Emotional tension*—anxiety, fear
* *Traction*—on the peritoneum, uterocervical supports during contractions, or with expulsive efforts
* *Pressure*—by the presenting part on the bladder, bowel, or other sensitive pelvic structures
* *Hypoxia*—circulatory stasis in the myometrium and adjacent tissues, during and immediately after strong uterine contraction may cause a local oxygen deficit (the pain has been compared to angina pectoris associated with myocardial hypoxia)

Pain may be *local,* with cramplike uterine pain and a "tearing" or a "bursting" sensation due to distention and laceration of the cervix, vagina, or perineal tissues; or *referred,* with the discomfort felt in the back, flanks, or thighs.

Pain impulses during the first stage of labor are transmitted through the spinal nerve segment of T11-12 and

Table 20-5. Breathing and relaxation techniques

	Breathing	Coaching	Distraction	Relaxation
Early phase Contractions 10 to 30 seconds long, 30 to 5 minutes apart, mild to moderate, cervix dilatation 0 to 3 cm	Begin contraction with deep breath in through the nose and out through pursed lips Slow chest breathing, 6 to 9/min through contraction End contraction with deep breath in and out	Contraction starts Time called out at 15 seconds, 30 seconds, etc. Contraction ends	Concentrate on fixed point in room Listen to me and follow my breathing Watch my face Concentrate on breathing technique	Position most comfortable for patient Use comfort measures Keep aware of progress, explain procedures and routines Give praise Offer ataractics as ordered
Midphase Contractions 30 to 45 seconds long, 5 to 3 minutes apart, moderate to strong, cervix dilatation 6 to 7 cm	Begin contraction with deep breath in and out Slow chest breathing until contraction intensifies Shallow, effortless breathing, moderate pace, high in chest through peaking of contraction Slow chest breathing as contraction subsides End contraction with deep breath in and out	May need encouragement to maintain breathing techniques Use same instructions	Use same devices as in preliminary phase	Position on side to minimize pressure of uterus on vena cava Use comfort measures: voluntary relaxation of muscles of back, buttocks, thighs, and perineum; effleurage (gentle stroking of abdomen, use both hands, begin at pubes and stroke upward and outward) Use counterpressure to sacrococcygeal area Encourage and praise Keep aware of progress Offer analgesics and anesthetics as ordered
Transition phase Contractions 45 to 60 to 90 seconds long, 2 to 3 minutes apart, strong, cervix dilatation 8 to 10 cm	Same as in accelerated phase One pant, one blow to overcome urge to push	Probably will need to remind, reassure, and encourage to reestablish breathing pattern and concentration If sedated or drowsy, needs warning to begin breathing pattern before contraction becomes too intense Use same instructions—one-pant, one-blow breathing	Difficult in this phase, needs reassurance regarding end point of first stage	Encourage, but accept inability to comply with instructions Accept irritable response to helping, such as counterpressure Support patient who has nausea and vomiting, give mouth care as needed Use countertension techniques (effleurage and voluntary relaxation) Keep aware of progress, tell when ready to push

accessory lower thoracic and upper lumbar sympathetic nerves.

Pain impulses during the second stage of labor are carried through S1-4 and the parasympathetic system. Pain experienced during the third stage, as well as so-called afterpains, is uterine, similar to that described early in the first stage of labor.

Fetopelvic disproportion, dysrhythmic uterine activity, and other causes of dystocia cause even greater pain than might be expected in normal labor.

The pain described by poorly prepared, tense, anxious, or fearful patients even during normal labor is far worse than that reported by well prepared, calm, self-reliant patients. Psychoprophylaxis and the beneficial presence of an understanding, helpful nurse often may be as effective as pain medication to relieve the distress of labor and delivery.

TECHNIQUES FOR CONTROL

Breathing and relaxation techniques. The use of breathing and relaxation techniques helps the parturient participate actively in the control of pain and conservation of her energies. Experience with informed and relaxed women in labor indicates that the birth process is viewed by many as exciting and rewarding. Those couples who have attended childbirth education programs using the psychoprophylactic approach will have knowledge of the labor process, coaching techniques, and comfort measures. However, the staff should be supportive and should keep them informed of progress. Even if husband and wife have not attended such classes, the various techniques may be taught to a degree during the preliminary phase of labor; the nurse will be expected to do more of the coaching and give some supportive care. If the woman is alone, the nursing staff acts as the substitute family, coaching and supporting her. (See Table 20-5.)

Obstetric analgesia and anesthesia. A totally painless labor is rarely possible. However, a reasonably comfortable labor is feasible. In the final appraisal, the success of pain relief must be judged by an obvious index: the patient's response to the stimuli of labor.

All the drugs and procedures used to alleviate the discomforts of birth have some advantage or desirable characteristic, but none is perfect. In fact, widespread reappraisal of medications and methods used to relieve pain in obstetrics is important because at least 10% of maternal deaths are now due to anesthesia problems, mainly aspiration of vomitus and high spinal anesthesia. Moreover, perinatal morbidity and mortality are greatly dependent on the analgesia and anesthesia employed, although the specific effects of drugs on the fetus during labor and delivery are not easily interpreted.

Pain relief in use today may be classified as follows:
1. *Education*—positive conditioning, psychoprophylaxis, suggestion (including hypnosis) to limit fear and tension
2. *Analgesics*—to increase the threshold of pain
3. *Amnesics*—to dull the memory of experiences, including pain
4. *Regional anesthesia*—to interrupt afferent pain pathways
5. *General anesthesia*—to eliminate CNS pain perception

A number of these approaches to pain relief are applicable to home as well as hospital delivery.

Anesthesia embraces analgesia, amnesia, relaxation, and reflex activity. Hence analgesia is a component of anesthesia. Analgesia is best reserved, then, to describe only those states in which there is elimination of the sensation of pain. Anesthesia, in contrast, should be used to describe the loss of other faculties also, particularly that of awareness.

Analgesia can be induced by (1) positive conditioning and (2) analgesic drugs. A basic understanding of the normal course of labor and delivery and proper physical and psychologic preparation by the maternity patient will reduce pain during childbirth. Especially important is good antenatal care in its broadest sense; reassurance and suggestion are beneficial. Participation in childbirth preparation classes such as those proposed by Grantly Dick Read or psychoprophylaxis by Lamaze should do much to alleviate distress.

Sedative drugs. Sedatives such as barbiturates, meprobamate, or alcohol relieve anxiety and induce sleep. In large doses, they may cause unsteadiness, excitement, or even partial anesthesia. Undesirable side effects include respiratory and vasomotor depression of mother and neonate. Sedatives do not cause amnesia but may confuse or distort recollection.

Sedative drugs may be short-acting, such as pentobarbital sodium (Nembutal), moderate or intermediate-acting, such as amobarbital (Amytal), or long-acting, such as phenobarbital (Luminal Sodium). Each of these drugs can be given orally, 100 to 150 mg, three or four times a day or they may be administered parenterally in half this dose.

Useful in early labor to ally apprehension, these drugs should not be employed late in the first or early in the second stage because the neonate may exhibit severe CNS depression. Sedatives should not be administered if delivery within 1 to 2 hours is likely. Immaturity, long labor, infection, or trauma enhance narcosis of the neonate.

Barbiturates do not lessen the strength or frequency of uterine contractions appreciably. With the establishment of good labor (after the cervix is dilated more than 3 cm and partially effaced) 100 to 200 mg of pentobarbital may be given orally, or half this dose intramuscularly. Repeated smaller doses may be given about 2 to 3 hours apart until the approach of full dilatation of the cervix, after which this type of sedation should be avoided or neonatal respiratory depression may result.

Narcotic analgesic drugs. Narcotic, opium-related drugs are especially effective for the relief of severe, persistent, or recurrent pain. They provide solace from anxiety and suppress the cough reflex and diarrhea. The maximal effect of most narcotic analgesics occurs about 15 minutes after an intramuscular injection, and the duration is approximately 2 hours. They have no amnesic effect. These medications, for example, morphine, meperidine (Demerol), pentazocine (Talwin), oxycodone (Percodan), or codeine, may be addictive if given regularly for a prolonged period of time, but labor does not fall into this category. They may have other undesirable side effects for the maternity patient. Nausea and vomiting, respiratory depression, constipation, or urinary retention may develop. The fetus is also depressed, and resuscitation of the neonate may be difficult if sizable doses of narcotics are given within 1 to 2 hours of delivery. Narcotics should not be given after full dilatation in a primigravida or after 7 to 8 cm dilatation in a multipara, assuming good labor.

The most potent narcotic in general use is morphine, which usually is administered subcutaneously in 8 to 15 mg doses, 4 to 6 hours apart. Meperidine (Demerol), a synthetic opiate drug of intermediate potency, can be given intramuscularly or orally in doses of 50 to 100 mg. It overcomes inhibitory factors in labor and may even relax the cervix. Codeine is the least potent of the narcotics and can be administered subcutaneously, intramuscularly, or orally, 30 to 65 mg, every 3 to 4 hours.

Narcotic antagonist drugs. Narcotic antagonist drugs have been produced chemically by varying one of the theoretical opium alkaloid receptors. By themselves, commonly used narcotic antagonists such as nalorphine (Nalline), levallorphan (Lorfan), or naloxone (Narcan) provide potent narcotic properties. If a traditional narcotic has been administered to a maternity patient, these drugs promptly reverse the narcotic effects, including respiratory depression of the neonate. Therefore narcotic antagonists are especially valuable if labor is more rapid than expected. If given to the mother about 10 to 15 minutes before delivery, 2.5 to 5 mg of nalorphine

intravenously or 1 mg of levallorphan intravenously will counteract maternal and neonatal narcotic effects. Narcotic antagonists will intensify the effects of sedative drugs, however. If there is insufficient time for reversal of maternal-fetal effects of a narcotic drug, nalorphine or levallorphan can be given, well diluted, into the umbilical vein of the newborn in doses of 0.05 mg or 0.1 mg, respectively.

Analgesic-potentiating drugs (ataractics). Phenothiazines, so-called tranquilizer or antipsychotic drugs such as promazine (Sparine) and hydroxyzine pamoate (Vistaril), have the property of augmenting most of the desirable but few of the undesirable effects of analgesics or general anesthetics. As little as 50 mg of meperidine can be effective for the relief of pain during labor when given intramuscularly with, for example, 50 mg of promazine. Fetal or neonatal problems rarely develop with these doses, and the combination can be administered safely about every 2 hours up until the end of the first stage of labor.

Amnesic drugs. Scopolamine, a parasympathetic drug, causes misinterpretation of stimuli and delirium—even hallucinations—when given parenterally in large doses. Such patients have almost no recall of recent events. Doses of 0.2 to 0.4 mg of scopolamine hydrobromide must be given slowly intravenously or intramuscularly to achieve amnesia or forgetfulness. Fortunately, scopolamine in these doses has no serious effect on the fetus. However, scopolamine has no analgesic effect, and a narcotic drug such as meperidine must be given concomitantly. Even so, the patient may become very excitable. The management of such women is often difficult because they may require constant attendance, even restraint to prevent injury to themselves and others. Various degrees of excitement, physical and vocal activity, hallucinations, and even delirium can occur. Fetal apnea may occur, so intensive fetal monitoring is essential. Today, most mothers-to-be wish to experience their labor and delivery; therefore scopolamine has declined in popularity.

Regional anesthetic drugs. Regional anesthetics, most of which are synthetically produced, are related chemically to cocaine and carry the suffix *caine.* This helps identify a local anesthetic, but it does not distinguish the chemical group to which the drug belongs.

The principal pharmacologic effect of local anesthetics is the temporary interruption of the conduction of nerve impulses, notably pain. The local anesthetic drug must reach the plasma membrane of the axon of the nerve to be blocked before it can act. Hence, in the relief of pain of labor or delivery, drugs like procaine, the standard of reference, must be injected in well-diluted

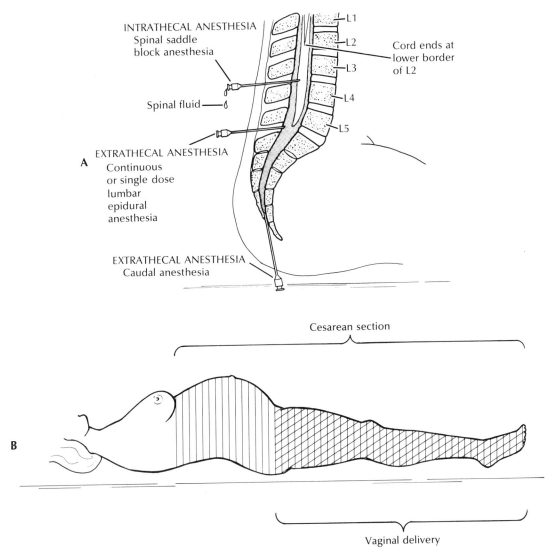

INTRATHECAL ANESTHESIA
Spinal saddle
block anesthesia

Spinal fluid

EXTRATHECAL ANESTHESIA
Continuous
or single dose
lumbar
epidural
anesthesia

A

L1
L2
L3
L4
L5

Cord ends at
lower border
of L2

EXTRATHECAL ANESTHESIA
Caudal anesthesia

Cesarean section

B

Vaginal delivery

Fig. 20-8. A, Regional anesthesia in obstetrics. **B,** Level of anesthesia necessary for cesarean section and vaginal delivery. (Courtesy Ross Laboratories, Columbus, Ohio.)

aqueous solution (0.5% to 2%) for epidural or caudal anesthesia (Fig. 20-8). Some local anesthetic drugs such as tetracaine (Pontocaine), chloroprocaine (Nesacaine), bupivacaine (Marcaine), or lidocaine (Xylocaine) have much longer effectiveness than procaine. These drugs can also reach pain nerves by diffusion if injected in the area of nerves to be blocked (e.g., pudendal block). Some local anesthetic drugs such as cocaine or dibucaine (Nupercaine) can be absorbed through the mucous membrane or skin to yield superficial local anesthesia.

Rarely individuals are sensitive to one or more local anesthetic drugs and develop tachycardia, syncope, or convulsions, usually associated with intravenous or rapid takeup of the medication. Testing with minute amounts of the drug may determine such sensitivity. When excessive amounts of a regional anesthetic drug are injected, CNS stimulation followed by depression, hypotension, and other serious adverse effects can be expected. Atropine, antihistaminic drugs, oxygen, and supportive measures should bring relief.

Inhalation analgesics such as nitrous oxide or trichloroethylene (Trilene) are nontoxic when adminis-

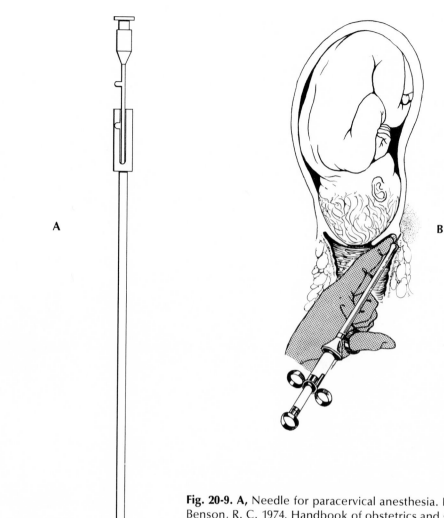

A

B

= <0.5 cm

Fig. 20-9. A, Needle for paracervical anesthesia. **B,** Paracervical block. (**B** from Benson, R. C. 1974. Handbook of obstetrics and gynecology [ed. 5]. Los Altos, Calif., Lange Medical Publications.)

tered with ample air or oxygen. Self-administration of these gases may be most helpful, especially during the second stage of labor.

Potentiating drugs (e.g., tranquilizers) augment the effect of analgesics or sedatives. Unfortunately they may also prolong the effect of these drugs unduly because tranquilizers also cross the placental barrier to the fetus. Therefore potentiating drugs should be used in small doses.

PARACERVICAL (UTEROSACRAL) BLOCK. Paracervical anesthesia is the injection of a dilute local anesthetic drug (e.g., 5 ml of 1% procaine), just beneath the muco-

sa in each fornix posterolateral to the cervix (9 and 3 o'clock) after the cervix is more than 5 cm dilated. This results in excellent pain relief for at least 1 hour. Anesthesia extends from the lower uterine segment and cervix to the upper one third of the vagina; there is no perineal anesthesia. Although there may be a transient depression of contractions, there is little or no effect on the labor. Repeat injections may be given until the cervix is dilated to 8 cm, whereupon another method such as pudendal block will be necessary. A needle guide (e.g., the "Iowa trumpet") is useful but not indispensable in facilitating the paracervical block (Fig. 20-9, *A*).

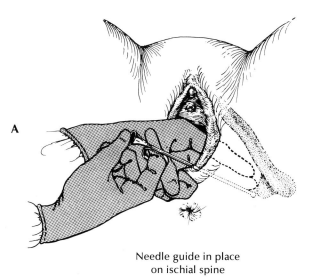

A

Needle guide in place
on ischial spine

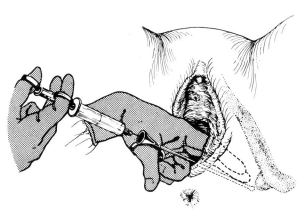

Needle inserted
through needle guide

Fig. 20-10. A, Use of needle guide ("Iowa trumpet") in pudendal anesthetic block. **B,** Pudendal block technique. Superficial and deep innervations on both sides are injected through only two skin wheals. Dotted lines show paths of needle infiltrating both pudendal and ilioinguinal nerves. (**A** from Benson, R. C. 1974. Handbook of obstetrics and gynecology [ed. 5]. Los Altos, Calif., Lange Medical Publications; **B** from McLennan, C. E., and Sandberg, E. C. 1974. Synopsis of obstetrics [ed. 9]. St. Louis, The C. V. Mosby Co.)

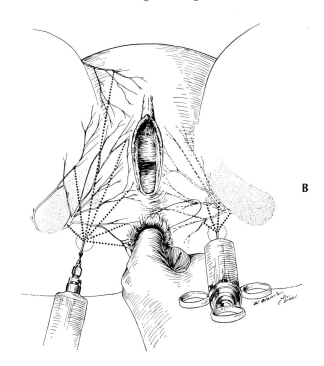

B

Paracervical block anesthesia may cause fetal intoxication because of rapid absorption of the drug. When the anesthetic is injected into the tissues lateral to the cervix, it is picked up by the circulation, which quickly involves the uterus and placenta. When overdosage occurs, the fetus may exhibit bradycardia because of the quinidine-like effect of the anesthetic on the myocardium. CNS medullary depression may develop, and the neonate may show vascular collapse and apnea at delivery. Amide-linkage drugs, including lidocaine, mepivacaine, and prilocaine, are more likely to cause these perinatal complications than are anesthetics with an ester bond, such

as procaine and tetracaine, which are better metabolized by the placenta with less transfer of the drug to the fetus. Proper selection of the anesthetic agent and limitation of the dosage as well as the drug concentration should protect both mother and fetus.

The procedure needs to be explained to the patient. The patient is asked to void if bladder is full. Maternal vital signs and FHT are taken and recorded. The sight of the long needle used to reach the site may be frightening (Fig. 20-9, *B*). The patient can be reassured that only the tip of the needle will be inserted. FHT are rechecked and recorded after the procedure. A transient slowing of the fetal heart rate may be noted. Bradycardia due to paracervical block cannot be reversed by turning the mother to her side or by administering oxygen. If it persists, report it immediately; the anesthetic solution may have been injected into the fetal scalp. Relief from discomfort is noticed within about 5 minutes. This is a sterile procedure, and the anesthesiologist will need the nurse's assistance in positioning the patient (dorsal recumbent position with knees flexed), handling supplies, and helping the mother to remain still while the injection is made.

PUDENDAL BLOCK. Once the presenting part descends through the cervix, vaginal and soon pudendal distention occur. Under these circumstances, vaginal and perineal pain can be eliminated by an anesthetic block of the pudendal and posterior femoral cutaneous and hemorrhoidal nerves (Fig. 20-10). The bearing-down reflex is lessened or lost completely.

The pudendal nerve traverses the sacrosciatic notch just medial to the tip of the ischial spine on each side. Injection of an anesthetic solution at or near these points will anesthetize the pudendal nerves peripherally. Anesthetic block of the posterior femoral cutaneous nerves can be effected by depositing a small amount of the drug beneath the inferior median border of the ischial tuberosity. Infiltration of the anesthetic solution subcutaneously around the anus should block the hemorrhoidal nerves.

SPINAL ANESTHESIA (SADDLE BLOCK). Spinal or intrathecal injection of a dilute, usually hyperbaric, solution of an anesthetic drug such as procaine (Novocain) or tetracaine (Pontocaine), generally at L3-4 or L4-5, should effect sensory and motor anesthesia in 5 to 10 minutes. Used mainly for delivery, spinal anesthesia can be employed to alleviate pain during the late first and entire second stage of labor, since it produces effective anesthesia for 1 to 2 hours.

Advantages of spinal anesthesia include ease of administration and absence of fetal hypoxia with maintenance of normotension; also, maternal consciousness is maintained, excellent muscular relaxation is achieved, blood loss is not excessive, and no other anesthetic agents (e.g., inhalation drugs) are required.

Disadvantages of spinal anesthesia embrace drug reactions, rare chemical myelitis or infection, hypotension, high spinal anesthesia with respiratory paralysis, increased need for operative delivery (episiotomy, low forceps extraction) because of elimination of voluntary expulsive efforts, increased tendency for bladder and uterine atony, and headache.

A minimal amount of drug should be employed, for example, 40 to 50 mg of procaine (0.8 ml of a 0.5% solution or its equivalent). The injection is made with the patient in a sitting position with her legs over the side of the delivery table and her feet supported on a stool. The nurse stands in front of her. The patient rests her chin on her chest, arches her back, and leans on the nurse for support. The nurse comforts and coaches her. This posture is assumed to widen the intervertebral space for ease in inserting the spinal needle and to allow the heavy anesthetic solution to gravitate downward. The injection is made between contractions. Once the anesthetic has been injected, the patient is assisted to a supine position. The patient must remain supine with the head elevated slightly. The table can be tilted appropriately to "fix" the drug so that the level of anesthesia is at or below the umbilicus. A very low spinal ("saddle") block anesthetizes the nerves L1-5 and S1-4, supplying the area over the low back, pudendum, and symphysis pubis, as well as the pelvic viscera. The blood pressure, pulse, respirations, and FHT must be taken and recorded every 5 to 10 minutes. If signs of serious hypotension or fetal distress develop, oxygen should be given by mask. Vasopressors such as epinephrine intravenously or intramuscularly and 5% glucose intravenously may be given if marked hypotension develops. Since the patient is not able to sense her contractions, she must be instructed when to bear down. Low outlet forceps will be required to complete the delivery. After delivery of the placenta, the patient will need assistance to move back to her recovery bed. She must remain in a supine position for a minimum of 8 hours to prevent spinal headache.

EPIDURAL, INCLUDING CAUDAL, ANESTHESIA. Extrathecal injection of a dilute anesthetic solution between a lumbar interspace or caudally (through the sacral hiatus) results in excellent analgesia-anesthesia. This modality may be employed during well-established first and subsequent stages of labor.

Advantages are numerous: fetal distress is rare, but this may occur with rapid absorption or marked hypotension; the mother maintains consciousness, and only partial motor paralysis develops; good relaxation is achieved; blood loss is not excessive; and headache almost never occurs. Continuous, prolonged analgesia-anesthesia is feasible in many cases.

Disadvantages include the following: special training and experience are required; a considerable amount of the drug must be used, hence reactions or rapid absorption of the anesthetic agent may result in hypotension, convulsions, or paresthesia; the incidence of operative delivery is increased because the patient cannot bear down effectively; and occasional accidental high spinal anesthesia may follow inadvertent perforation of the thecal membrane.

For introduction of epidural anesthesia, the patient

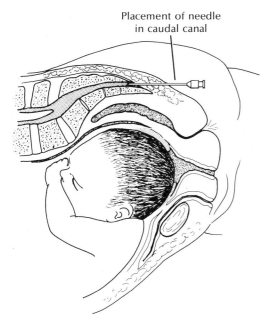

Placement of needle
in caudal canal

Fig. 20-11. Patient assumes modified knee-chest position to permit access to sacral hiatus. Once needle and catheter are in place, she may assume side-lying position. Note cervix is approximately 5 cm dilated. (Courtesy Ross Laboratories, Columbus, Ohio.)

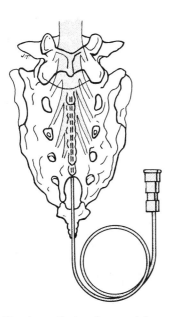

Fig. 20-12. Plastic catheter in caudal canal through sacral hiatus. (Courtesy Ross Laboratories, Columbus, Ohio.)

is positioned as for a spinal or in a modified Sims position. For introduction of caudal anesthesia, the patient is placed in a modified knee-chest or Sims position, with the upper leg well flexed at the hip and knee and the lower leg extended. The injection site is cleansed and draped. The procedure is a sterile technique. Once the needle (Fig. 20-11) and fine plastic catheter have been inserted into the caudal canal, a test dose is given. After 5 minutes, the anesthesiologist checks the anal sphincter for relaxation and the temperature of the lower extremities. Relaxation of the anal sphincter and increased warmth of the feet indicate proper placement of the catheter in the caudal canal (Fig. 20-12). The remainder of the dose is then given. Relief is experienced in a few minutes, and repeated doses may be administered as the effect wears off. The catheter and syringe are taped securely in position so that the patient is free to move about in bed. The blood pressure, pulse, respirations, and FHT must be measured and recorded every 15 minutes. If hypotension develops, summon assistance, turn the patient on her side, and administer oxygen.

As with a spinal anesthetic, progress in labor must be monitored carefully, since the patient will not be aware of changes in strength of uterine contractions or descent of the presenting part. Occasionally depression of contractions may result, necessitating augmentation with oxytocin. She will need coaching to push, and low forceps will be required to complete delivery. After the third stage, she will need assistance to move to the recovery bed.

General anesthetic drugs

INTRAVENOUS ANESTHETIC DRUGS. Intravenous anesthetics such as thiopental (Pentothal) and thiamylal (Surital), although widely used in general and dental surgery, are usually not suitable for obstetric delivery because of the rapid transit of the drug across the placenta to the fetus. Within 5 to 10 minutes, the fetomaternal plasma concentration will have equalized and the infant, if not already delivered, may be at least as narcotized as the mother. Frequently, resuscitation of the neonate may be difficult or impossible with delayed delivery. However, these agents are useful in controlling convulsions such as those occurring in eclampsia or epilepsy. Full intravenous anesthesia is therefore not considered safe for obstetrical use. Small sedative doses of thiopental or its equivalent are often given for so-called balanced anesthesia (thiopental, succinylcholine chloride, and nitrous oxide) for cesarean section without undue risk.

INHALATION ANESTHETIC DRUGS. Ethyl ether is a low-cost, volatile, portable anesthetic that is easy to administer and has a wide margin of safety. The disadvantages include its objectionable odor, its explosive nature, irritation of the respiratory passages, maternal agitation during contractions, and prolonged narcosis and nausea of the mother and neonate. In addition, ether induces marked uterine atony, which encourages postnatal hemorrhage. Once employed for version and extraction, now regarded as a hazardous and all but outmoded operation, ether is rarely used in obstetrics today except in an emergency. It is contraindicated in the delivery of a premature or immature infant because of prolonged respiratory suppression.

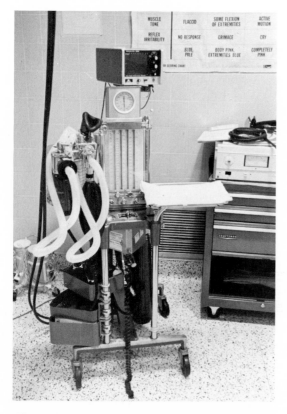

Fig. 20-13. Anesthetic machine in delivery room.

Cyclopropane, a not unpleasant gas, causes rapid anesthesia and relaxation. It must be administered with a high percentage of oxygen (75% to 80%) by an experienced anesthetist because its safety range is narrow. Unfortunately cyclopropane is explosive; it also may cause cardiac arrhythmia or nausea and vomiting. Cyclopropane is an acceptable brief anesthetic for normal or premature delivery (Fig. 20-13).

Halothane (Fluothane) is a volatile nonflammable hydrocarbon related to chloroform. Halothane is the most potent inhalation anesthetic drug. It has a short induction time and causes deep anesthesia, but recovery is rapid. A calibrated vaporizer is generally used to avoid overdosage. Halothane must be administered by an anesthesiologist because of its cardiotoxicity and hepatotoxicity. This anesthetic is contraindicated in patients with liver disease, and it should not be given to the same person a second time within 6 months to avoid toxic hepatitis. Brief halothane anesthesia is useful when prompt delivery is required for fetal distress. Marked uterine relaxation with halothane predisposes to postnatal hemorrhage. Nevertheless, premature and other high-risk infants usually tolerate halothane well.

Combination anesthesia for cesarean section. Light general anesthesia, considered by many to be ideal for cesarean section, is a combination of thiopental, nitrous oxide–oxygen, and succinylcholine. An individual experienced in anesthesiology is required, however.

Thiopental, 200 to 300 mg in solution, is administered intravenously for induction just before the skin incision is made. When the patient is somnolent, nitrous oxide–oxygen, 75%:25%, is given (Fig. 20-13). After about 3 minutes, the mixture is reduced to equal volumes. Then a skeletal muscle relaxant (succinylcholine, or Anectine) is administered.

Excellent tolerance of the anesthetic and rapid resuscitation of the mother and even SGA or growth-retarded infants are widely reported.

PLAN OF CARE: NORMAL LABOR—FIRST STAGE

PATIENT CARE OBJECTIVES
1. Patient, family, and personnel establish a therapeutic relationship.
2. Maternal response indicates continued well-being.
   a. Maternal progress in labor is within normal limits.
   b. Rupture of membranes may occur at any time. Amniotic fluid is pale straw-colored. FHT remain stable; cord does not prolapse.
   c. Temperature: 37.2° C (99° F); increase from dehydration and labor. Pulse: as in antenatal period. Respirations: change with use of breathing techniques and pain. Blood pressure: may be elevated during a contraction or with excitement.
   d. Voiding: voids qs every 2 hours.

PLAN OF CARE: NORMAL LABOR—FIRST STAGE—cont'd

PATIENT CARE OBJECTIVES—cont'd

    e. Gastrointestinal tract: motility of stomach decreases; motility of bowels decreases.

    f. Mother accepts her responses to the labor process.

  3. Fetal response through the first stage indicates continued well-being.

    a. FHT (auscultation).

      (1) Rate: between 120 and 160/min, recorded between contractions.

      (2) Normal baseline variability.

      (3) No periodic changes.

    b. No meconium staining of amniotic fluid.

  4. Husband or substitute participates in supporting relaxation during contractions and in providing comforting measures; husband or substitute meets self-expectations.

  5. Recordings in Labor Record are done concurrently with interventions.

  6. Preparations for delivery are completed.

NURSING INTERVENTIONS

Diagnostic	**Therapeutic and educational**

1. Review data base prior to admission if possible.
  a. Obstetric history:
    (1) Age and EDC.
    (2) Para, gravida, previous obstetric history (problems, type of labor, abortions, stillbirths).
    (3) Maternal vital signs, BP.
    (4) FHT.
    (5) Results of lab tests—urinalysis (albumin, glucose) and blood tests (Hct, Rh, blood group, VDRL).
    (6) Type of analgesia and/or anesthesia requested.
    (7) Note problems listed and treatment.
  b. Patient profile: preparation for childbirth; problems (e.g., no supportive people available, anxieties about pain, fear of injections and needles).
  c. General history: any pertinent notations.
2. Initial assessment on admission:
  a. General appearance and behavior:
    (1) Verbal interactions, overtalkative, mute.
    (2) Body posture and set, relaxed or tense.
    (3) Perceptual acuity.
    (4) Energy level.
    (5) Amount of pain patient relates she is experiencing.
  b. Vital signs and BP (if elevated, repeat 30 minutes after patient has relaxed to obtain true reading).
  c. FHT: rate, regularity; mark area of maximum density.
	1. Admit patient to labor unit.
	  a. Welcome patient, address by name. Determine whether patient wishes husband to stay through examinations. If not, direct husband to waiting area.
	  b. Have patient undress and get into bed; care for her personal belongings. Check for understanding of use of call bell and inform patient whether bathroom privileges are permitted (if membranes have ruptured, have patient remain in bed until medical directive is obtained).
	  c. Review routine of care, which techniques will be used to assess progress, reasons for these, and how patient may assist in reporting her progress.
	  d. Have patient sign necessary permit-for-care papers for self and newborn (if circumcision is not desired, bring to attention of physician), and put on patient's identification bracelet.
	2. Follow medical directives for preparation of vulva, administration of enema and use of bathroom privileges.
	3. Encourage patient to void frequently. Although it may be necessary to catheterize patient if full bladder blocks descent of presenting part, catheterization during labor almost invariably results in symptomatic or asymptomatic bacteriuria.
	4. Limit dietary intake to clear fluids as ordered by physician. Intravenous fluids may be ordered to counteract dehydration and provide available energy.
	5. Have patient lie on her side whenever possible to minimize compressing effect heavy uterus has on ascending vena cava.
	6. Rupture of membranes:
	  a. Note time, color, and odor of amniotic fluid. If fluid is meconium stained or has foul odor, report immediately.
	  b. Examine for prolapse of cord:
	    (1) Frank prolapse: examine perineum for presence of cord. If it is not visible, patient is examined vaginally to feel for cord in vagina (pulsates).
	    (2) Occult prolapse: If neither of above, check FHT at 30-minute intervals for decreasing rate and irregularity.
	    (3) Notify physician immediately if prolapse occurs. Tilt pelvis upward with pillow under hips (or raise foot of bed) and exert upward pressure manually on presenting part to ease it out of pelvis and reduce constriction of cord. (For further details, see p. 299.)
	7. Comfort measures:
	  a. Control of anxiety and pain
	    (1) Work through number of contractions with patient and husband, noting effectiveness of their method of relaxation, breathing, and other supportive techniques. If none are used, introduce techniques and coach husband in their use. Breathing techniques, counterpres-

Continued.

PLAN OF CARE: NORMAL LABOR—FIRST STAGE—cont'd

NURSING INTERVENTIONS—cont'd

Diagnostic | **Therapeutic and educational**

d. Contractions:
  (1) Have patient describe when they began; what they are like now.
  (2) Nurse assesses duration, intensity, frequency, regularity.
e. Amount of "show": assess amount, color, character.
f. Rupture of membranes (bag of waters): if ruptured, ask time of rupture and check vaginal discharge with Nitrazine paper for pH (positive = dark blue).
g. Inquire regarding symptoms of infection (e.g., diarrhea, colds, coughs, sore throats).
h. Recheck for allergies: mention names of drugs routinely used such as meperidine (Demerol) or mepivacaine (Carbocaine).
i. Check for edema: legs, face, hands.
j. Obtain specimen of urine for routine analysis and presence of albumin and glucose.
k. Check patient's dietary intake for last 4 hours.
l. Recheck preparation for childbirth.
3. Assist physician or midwife with general and obstetric examinations to determine:
  a. General health of body systems.
  b. Presentation and position of fetus.
  c. Station of presenting part.
  d. Diagnosis of true labor.
4. Establish routine for reassessing patient's progress on basis of phase of labor and rapidity of progress, as shown in Table 20-3.
5. Check for bladder distention every 2 hours.
6. If discomfort or pain increases, ask patient if there is change from her earlier wishes regarding use of analgesia and/or anesthesia.

sure against sacrum during contraction, effleurage, and letting patient assume position most comfortable for her may contribute to comfort. If patient is alone, nurse provides supportive care early to minimize later stress.
  (2) Analgesia may be ordered on admission or soon thereafter to allay anxiety and enhance relaxation.
  (3) Anesthesia will be delayed until active labor is established, that is, until strong and regular contractions are coming every 5 minutes and the cervix is dilated 4 to 6 cm. Patient may not wish to use any type of analgesia or anesthesia.
b. General hygiene of patient: Showers or bed baths may be taken, depending on progress of labor. Frequent washing of vulva is indicated. Mouthwash and mouth care are given as necessary.
c. Although most patients feel very warm as result of labor, a number complain of feeling cold. One warm blanket placed over patient and another wrapped around her feet is comforting. Many wish to wear bedsocks.
d. Nurse's attitude toward patient and husband: Help patient use her energy constructively in relaxing and "working" with contractions. Calm manner, gentleness in carrying out necessary procedures, and acceptance of patient's definition of pain and desires for alleviation of discomfort need to be coupled with willingness to repeat instructions and to stay with patient having unavoidable pain, giving as much support as possible.
8. Preparations for delivery are completed.
a. Scrubbing facilities, scrub brushes, cleansing agent, and masks are available.
b. (1) Sterile gowns and gloves for physician or nurse-midwife, sterile drapes and towels for draping patient, and sterile instruments and other supplies (e.g., sutures, anesthetic solutions) are arranged for convenience in use on sterile table.
  (2) Sterile basin and water for hand-washing during delivery process are readied for use.
  (3) Supplies for cleansing vulva are available (e.g., sterile basin, sterile water, and cleansing solution).
  (4) Infant receiving blanket and heated crib are readied. Material for prophylactic care of infant's eyes is available (e.g., $AgNO_3$ capsules and sterile water to flush out eyes).
c. Equipment is in working order: delivery table, overhead lights, and mirror.
d. Emergency equipment and supplies are available and in working order, if needed for control of maternal hemorrhage or fetal respiratory distress.
e. Additional supplies (anesthetics, oxytoxics, forceps) are available.
f. Patient's record is up-to-date, ready for use in delivery area. In areas such as labor unit, recordings are made concomitantly as care is given, symptoms noted, or assessments made. Patient's condition can change quickly, so it is imperative to have recordings complete at all times.

REFERENCES

Behrman, R. E. (ed.). 1973. Neonatology: diseases of the fetus and infant. St. Louis, The C. V. Mosby Co.

Bradley, R. A. 1974. Husband-coached childbirth. New York, Harper & Row, Publishers.

Cassidy, J. E. 1974. A nurse looks at childbirth anxiety. J. Obstet. Gynecol. Nurs. **3:**52.

Friedman, E. A., and Sachtleben, M. R. 1965. Station of the presenting part. Am. J. Obstet. Gynecol. **93:**522.

Gabert, H. A., and Stenchever, M. A. 1974. Electronic fetal monitoring as a routine practice in an obstetric service: a progress report. Am. J. Obstet. Gynecol. **118:**534.

Hon, E. H. 1968. An atlas of fetal heart rate patterns. New Haven, Harty Press.

Hon, E. H. 1972. The present status of electronic monitoring of the human fetal heart. Int. J. Gynecol. Obstet. **10:**191.

Karmel, M. 1965. Thank you, Dr. Lamaze. New York, Doubleday & Co., Inc.

Lamaze, F. 1972. Painless childbirth. New York, Pocket Books.

Liston, W. A., and Campbell, A. J. 1974. Dangers of oxytocin-induced labor to the fetus. Br. Med. J. **3:**606.

McCaffery, M. 1972. Nursing management of the patient with pain. Philadelphia, J. B. Lippincott Co.

Melzack, R., and Wall, P. D. 1968. Gate control theory of pain. In Soulairac, A., and others (eds.). Pain. Proceedings of the International Symposium on Pain organized by the Laboratory of Psychophysiology, Faculty of Science, Paris, 1967. London, Academic Press.

Modamlou, H., and others. 1973. Fetal and neonatal biochemistry and Apgar scores. Am. J. Obstet. Gynecol. **117:**942.

Mosler, K. H., and others. 1974. Tocolytic therapy in obstetrics. J. Perinatal Med. **2:**3.

Sturrock, E. W., and Yeomans, S. A. 1973. Management and supportive care during labor and delivery. In Maternity nursing today. New York, McGraw-Hill Book Co.

Vellay, P. 1971. Childbirth without pain. New York, E. P. Dutton & Co., Inc.

CHAPTER 21

Second stage of labor

GENERAL CONSIDERATIONS

When the cervix is fully dilated, the second stage of labor begins, and it ends with the delivery of the baby. As noted earlier, the transition period between the first and second stages is marked by more frequent contractions and often severe pain. One indication of the beginning of the second stage is lessening of this discomfort. Other symptoms are an increase in bloody show and a feeling of pressure on the rectum, accompanied by a desire to defecate and an urge to bear down with each contraction. A definitive diagnosis is made by vaginal examination to confirm dilatation of the cervix and station of the presenting part. The *forces* at work in this stage are (1) uterine contractions, which occur every 2 to 3 minutes and last 50 to 60 seconds, and (2) the contractions of the diaphragm and abdominal musculature, which exert a downward pressure on the fetus, as well as decrease the size of the abdominal cavity. These latter forces can be voluntarily controlled, and efficient use of them expedites descent, crowning, and delivery of the head. The combined forces overcome the resistance of the soft tissues of the vagina and introitus, and the baby is born.

The *emotional responses* to entering the second stage of labor are usually excitement at the prospect of the imminent birth of the baby and eagerness to participate actively in the expulsion of the child. Even if parents have not attended preparation for childbirth classes, they are most amenable to suggestions as to how they may cooperate and share in this important event in their lives.

The *duration* of the second stage for a multipara is about 20 minutes and for a nullipara, approximately 50 minutes. Once the head reaches the pelvic floor (the outlet), fewer than ten contractions probably will be required for delivery if the patient previously has given birth to a full-term infant. For a first delivery, about twenty contractions will be necessary. Many labors are considerably shorter, however; hence one must be ready for the delivery when the head reaches the introitus.

MANAGEMENT

Continuous care is required during the second stage to check for progress in descent of the head, to monitor the quality and rate of contractions and the rate and regularity of FHT, and to assist the patient in controlling the voluntary bearing-down efforts.

If the woman assumes a dorsal position with the upper part of the body elevated about 30 degrees, she approximates the squatting position, which enables her to bear down more efficiently. FHT must be checked after every contraction. If the rate begins to drop, the woman can be turned on her side to reduce the pressure of the uterus against the ascending vena cava, and oxygen can be administered by mask. This is often all that is required to restore the normal rate. If it does not, report this immediately, since medical intervention to hasten the birth may be indicated.

Bearing-down efforts

The natural urge to push is coupled with breathing and relaxation techniques to make effective use of the patient's expulsive efforts. Amnesia between contractions is pronounced in the second stage, and the woman may have to be roused to cooperate in the bearing-down process. The husband, friend, or nurse may act as coach. Parents who have attended preparation for childbirth classes devise a set of verbal cues for the parturient to follow. It is helpful if they print these on a card that may be attached to the head of the bed so the nurse can better substitute as coach if the partner has to leave.

Care in delivery room

The nullipara is transferred to the delivery room when the caput is seen at the introitus and the multipara, when the cervix is 10 cm dilated and the head is at +2 station. Both will need assistance to move from the labor bed to the delivery table. If this is done between contractions, the patient can help, but because of her awkwardness, she cannot be rushed.

The delivery room tables are specifically designed to

facilitate care during delivery (Figs. 21-1 and 21-2). Once the patient is positioned and the physician is ready to assist with the delivery, the lower portion of the table may be dropped down and rolled back under the top. It is equipped with stirrups for supporting the legs and handle grips to aid in bearing down. A bolster wedge can be inserted under the top of the mattress to raise it slightly or the head of the table can be raised. The husband or coach helps the mother to remember not to touch the sterile drapes.

The position assumed for delivery may be (1) modified Sims position (if this is the case, the attendant will need to support the upper leg), (2) a dorsal position, or (3) a lithotomy position (Fig. 21-3). The lithotomy position is used most often in hospitals because it is the ideal position for the physician to deal with any complications that may arise. For this position, the buttocks are brought to the edge of the table, and the legs are placed in stirrups. Care must be taken to pad the stirrups, raise and place both legs simultaneously, and adjust the shank of

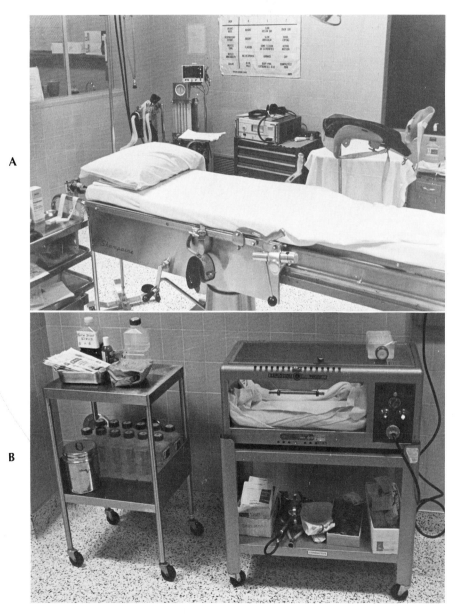

A

B

Fig. 21-1. A, Delivery room. **B,** Table for extra equipment and supplies and infant receiving crib (warmed) in delivery room.

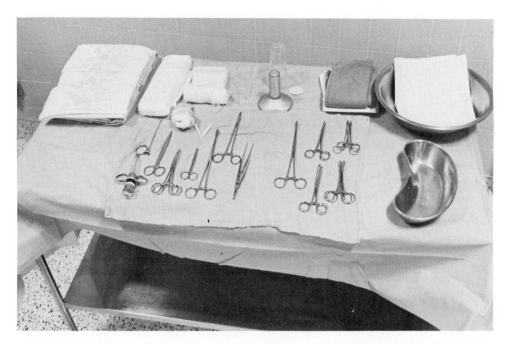

Fig. 21-2. Instrument table (all equipment sterile). *Top, left to right:* Receiving blanket, perineal pad, vaginal roll, medicine glasses (for anesthetic agent), hand cover for spotlight, urine specimen bottle, towels, and placenta bowl and paper towel for covering scales. *Bottom, left to right:* Syringe (anesthetic) needle guard, episiotomy scissors, bulb syringe (covered with gauze for aspirating newborn), two artery forceps, scissors, cord clamp, uterine forceps needle holder, thumb forceps (for repair of episiotomy), extra instruments (uterine forceps, small artery forceps, toothed forceps, draping forceps), and kidney basin.

the stirrups so that the calf of the leg is supported and there is no pressure on the popliteal space. If the stirrups are uneven in height, the woman can develop strained ligaments in her back as she bears down. This strain causes considerable discomfort in the postnatal period.

Once the patient is positioned for delivery, the vulva is washed thoroughly with soap and water or a surgical disinfectant (Fig. 21-4). Meanwhile the physician dons cap and mask, scrubs hands, and puts on the sterile gown and gloves. The patient is then draped with sterile towels and sheets.

The circulating nurse will continue to coach and encourage the patient. Once the patient's legs are in stirrups, the handle grips can be used to pull against, keeping the elbows bent as before. The nurse will check FHT after every contraction and notify the physician as to the rate and regularity. The equipment for taking the blood pressure should be readied for instant use if signs of shock develop. However, the readings are distorted by the increase in thoracic and abdominal pressures as the

woman pushes. A reading will be taken after delivery before transferring the patient to the recovery room. The oxytocic medication may be prepared for administration after delivery, supplies for the infant organized, and observations and procedures recorded on the chart.

Increasingly, fathers are present at the birth of their babies. This promotes the psychologic closeness of the family unit and permits the fathers to continue the supportive care given in labor.

DELIVERY

There are three phases to a spontaneous, noninstrument delivery of the fetus in vertex presentation:

- Delivery of the head
- Delivery of the shoulders
- Delivery of the body and legs

The presenting part, in this instance the vertex, advances with each contraction and recedes slightly as the contraction wanes; descent is constant, and late in the second stage the head reaches the pelvic floor. The occiput generally rotates anteriorly, and with voluntary

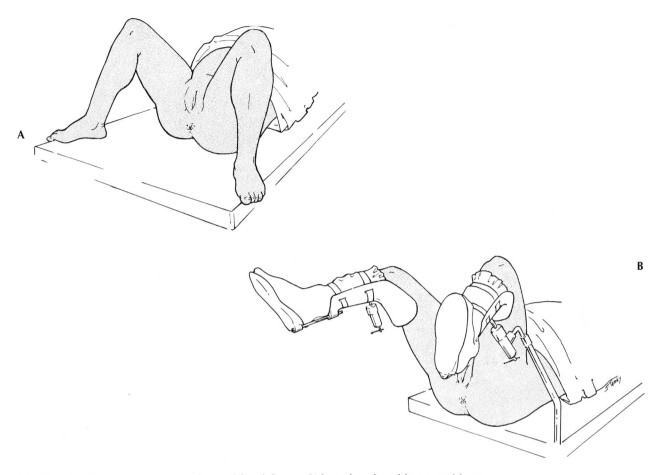

Fig. 21-3. Positions most frequently used for delivery. Side or hand-and-knee positions may be used in home delivery. **A,** Dorsal recumbent position. **B,** Lithotomy position.

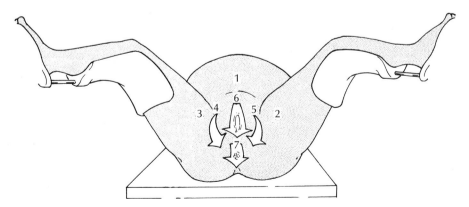

Fig. 21-4. Steps in perineal cleansing. Use cotton swabs or gauze squares well moistened with disinfectant solution. Discard swab after each step. Finish cleansing with wash of sterile water.

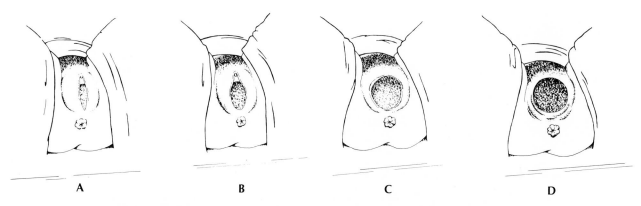

Fig. 21-5. Changes in shape of introitus as dilatation of introitus occurs. **A,** Slitlike. **B,** Oval. **C,** Round. **D,** Crowning of head.

bearing-down efforts, the head distends the introitus. Although more and more caput may be seen with each push, the head "crowns" when its widest part (the biparietal diameter) distends the vulva just before birth (Fig. 21-5). Immediately prior to delivery, the perineal musculature becomes greatly distended. This is the time when an episiotomy should be done to reduce soft tissue damage.

Delivery of head

The vertex first appears, followed by the forehead, face, chin, and neck (Fig. 21-6). The speed of delivery of the head must be controlled, or sudden extrusion of the head may cause severe lacerations through the anal sphincter or even into the rectum. This may be done by (1) applying pressure against the rectum, drawing it downward to aid in flexing the head as the back of the neck catches under the symphysis; (2) then applying upward pressure from the coccygeal region (modified Ritgen's maneuver) to extend the head during the actual delivery, thereby protecting the musculature of the perineum (Fig. 21-7); and (3) controlling the bearing-down efforts and panting. Gradual delivery is imperative to prevent fetal intracranial injury.

The cord often encircles the neck—rarely so tight as to cause critical hypoxia. The cord should be slipped gently over the head. If there is a tight or second loop, the cord is clamped twice and severed between the clamps, and then the delivery is continued. Mucus, blood, or meconium in the nasal or oral passages may prevent the newborn from breathing. Moist gauze sponges are used to wipe the nose and mouth. A bulb syringe is inserted into the mouth and throat (oral pharynx) to aspirate contents. The nares are cleared similarly while the head is being supported to establish a patent airway. After the head is delivered and an airway has been established, haste is unnecessary. The baby can breathe even before his complete birth.

Delivery of shoulders

Before the shoulders can be delivered, they must engage in the pelvic inlet. For this to occur, the head is drawn back slightly toward the perineum, and external rotation of the head or restitution must occur. Then the shoulders pass through the bony strait.

Now the head is drawn downward and backward to aid the anterior shoulder to impinge against the symphysis and slide beneath the arch. If the head is then lifted upward, the posterior shoulder may be seen to distend the perineum. Several fingers gently inserted into the vagina allows delivery of the posterior arm. Slight downward traction is applied to the head to deliver the anterior shoulder and arm. On occasion, it may be easier to deliver the anterior shoulder first, however.

If spontaneous rotation does not occur, the shoulders are rotated slowly to the anteroposterior diameter of the outlet.

Occasionally, a hand may present with or after the head. If this occurs, the hand and arm are swept out gently before delivery of the shoulder. Traction and pressure must be limited to avoid damage to the brachial plexus or the neck vessels.

Delivery of body and extremities

Easy, gradual traction should now deliver the baby. Slight rotation to the right or left may facilitate the birth. The "time to be born" has come. The infant, with all his potential, is now part of this world.

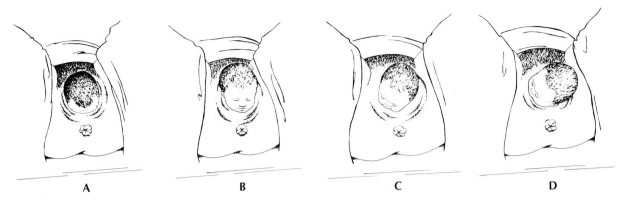

A   B   C   D

Fig. 21-6. Delivery of head (compare with Fig. 19-18). **A,** Extension. **B,** Delivery. **C,** Restitution. **D,** External rotation.

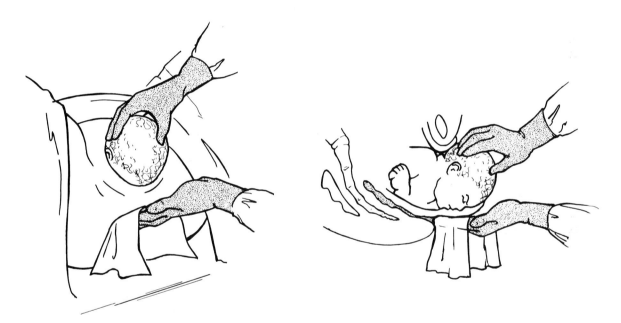

Fig. 21-7. Delivery of head by modified Ritgen maneuver. Note control to prevent rapid delivery of head.

IMMEDIATE CARE OF NEONATE

After delivery of the infant, the following measures must be effected immediately:

1. Ensure a clear airway. The newborn baby is held with the head lowered (10 to 15 degrees) to expedite drainage or aspiration of amniotic fluid, mucus, and blood. Suction the oral pharynx with a small bulb syringe as soon as the head is delivered; next, aspirate the nares. It should be noted that if the sequence is reversed, the infant may aspirate. Do not deep suction the nasal passages with a catheter lest bradycardia and laryngospasm occur.

2. When breathing is unimpeded, the neonate is held at about the same level as the uterus, until pulsations of the cord cease. If higher, for example, on the mother's abdomen, fetal blood may drain to the placenta; if lower, excessive blood may flow to the neonate prior to cessation of cord pulsations. Cord pulsations usually cease within seconds after respiration is initiated.

3. The cord is occluded close to the umbilicus with a

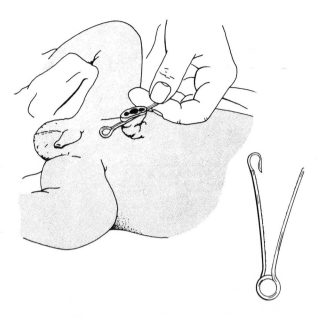

Fig. 21-8. Hesseltine cord clamp.

plastic or other cord clamp in approximately 30 seconds after delivery when cord pulsations cease, assuming a normal mature newborn (Figs. 21-8 to 21-10). However, if the need for transfusion is likely such as in erythroblastosis, an 8 to 10 cm proximal length of cord should be left. The cord is examined for two arteries and one vein (normal) and other cord abnormalities are noted. Ordinarily it is unwise to strip the cord prior to clamping and cutting because postdelivery red blood cell destruction, which normally occurs neonatally, will be increased and hyperbilirubinemia may ensue. In addition, polycythemia increases blood viscosity, leading to cardiopulmonary problems in the neonate (p. 520).

Early clamping of the cord to limit excessive breakdown of red blood cells is desirable if the infant is premature or if isoimmunization is likely. Immediate resuscitation of the newborn because of respiratory or circulatory problems is preceeded by rapid clamping and tying of the cord.

At cesarean section, the cord is clamped prior to the delivery of the fetus from the uterus to prevent retrograde flow of blood into the placenta.

4. The neonate is dried immediately and the infant's warmth is maintained and ensured by use of warm blankets, infrared heat lamps, or a heated bassinet. This avoids chilling and subsequent increased cardiac output and dissipation of glycogen stores.

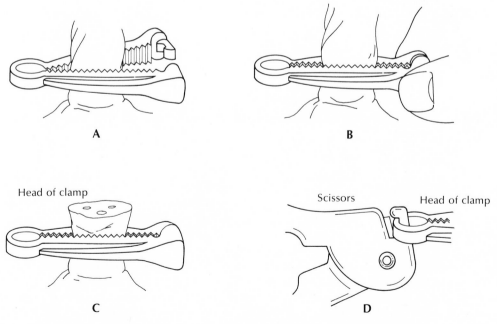

Fig. 21-9. Hollister cord clamp. **A,** Position clamp close to umbilicus. **B,** Secure cord. **C,** Cut cord. **D,** Remove clamp using scissors.

5. The condition of the neonate is appraised at 1 minute and again at 5 minutes. The scoring method of Apgar is the simplest and most practical method clinically available. The Apgar score permits a rapid and semiquantitative assessment based on five signs indicative of the physiologic state of the neonate (Fig. 21-11): heartbeat (auscultatory), respiration from observed movement of the chest wall, color (pallid, cyanotic, or pink), muscle tone from movement of the extremities, and reflexes from slaps on the soles of the feet. The 5-minute score correlates with neonatal mortality and morbidity.

6. If the infant fails to breathe normally after delivery, immediate resuscitative measures (e.g., aspiration of the trachea through an infant laryngoscope, administration of oxygen by mask) are initiated. Obtain immediate pediatric assistance if needed. Transfer the critical or seriously compromised infant to the pediatric neonatal intensive care unit as soon as possible.

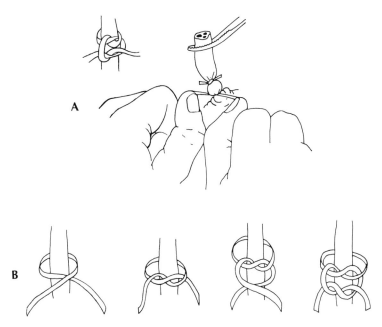

Fig. 21-10. Technique of tying off umbilical cord using (**A**) soft flat tie to prevent cutting through cord as it is drawn tight and (**B**) square knot to prevent slippage.

SIGN	0	1	2
Heart rate	Absent	Slow (below 100)	Over 100
Respiratory effort	Absent	Slow, irregular	Good, crying
Muscle tone	Flaccid	Some flexion of extremities	Active motion
Reflex irritability	No response	Cry	Vigorous cry
Color	Blue, pale	Body pink, extremities blue	Completely pink

Fig. 21-11. Apgar scoring chart.

7. It is a legal requirement for all newborns to have treatment to prevent gonococcal or pneumococcal infection in the conjunctiva. Such infections, or ophthalmia neonatorum, can lead to blindness. Currently a 1% solution of silver nitrate is used. This may be prepared as a fresh solution, or a commercial product may be obtained. Instill 1 or 2 drops of 1% aqueous silver nitrate in each eye, and after 15 to 30 seconds, the eyes may be irrigated with sterile water (Fig. 21-12).

8. The baby is weighed and measured.

9. Although rare, an occasional mixup in the identity of newborns occurs, causing much anxiety and legal complications. As a precaution, newborns are identified by one of a number of techniques before leaving the delivery area. One technique uses ''identibands,'' one to be attached to the mother's wrist, two others to the infant's wrist and ankle. Some hospitals take handprints and footprints of the baby. Others make up bead necklaces spelling out the infant's name. Most hospitals have policies that require the mother to acknowledge the identity of her baby before discharge from the delivery room.

Minimal physical examination and assessment of neonate

External. Note the skin color, staining, peeling, or wasting (dysmaturity). Consider the length of the nails and the development of the creases on the soles of the

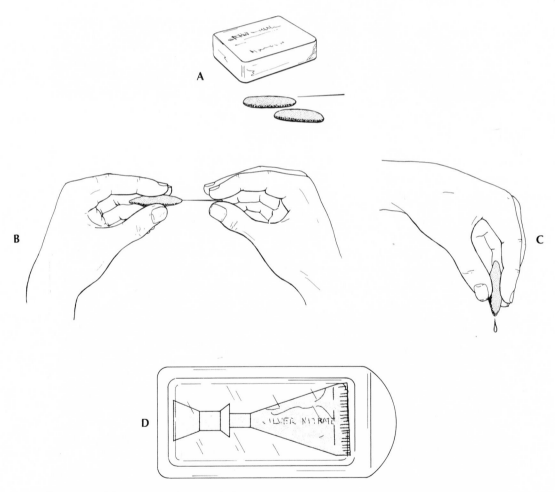

Fig. 21-12. Silver nitrate for prophylactic eye care of newborn. **A,** Silver nitrate 1% in wax containers. **B,** Puncture wax containers with needle. **C,** Squeeze to release drops. Administer by placing 1 or 2 drops in lower conjunctival sac of lower lid and close eye to spread medication. Leave 15 to 30 seconds. Open eye and flush thoroughly with sterile water. **D,** New style container for silver nitrate.

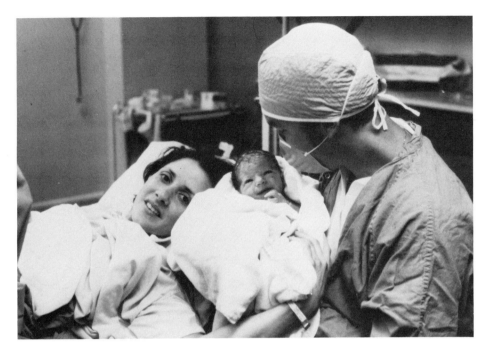

Fig. 21-13. Mother-infant-father: initiating family relationship.

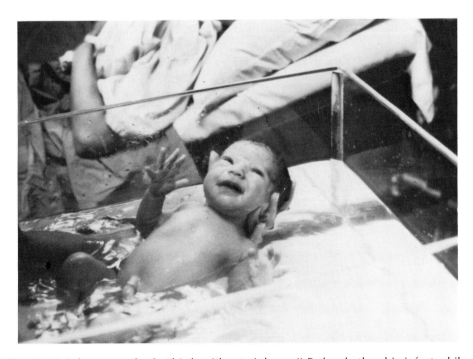

Fig. 21-14. Leboyer method: "birth without violence." Father bathes his infant while mother watches.

feet (Fig. 30-12). Check the presence or absence of breast tissue. Assess nasal patency by closing one nostril at a time while observing the infant's respirations and color.

Chest. Palpate for the site of maximal cardiac impulse and auscultate for the rate and quality of heart tones. Compare and note the character of respirations and the presence of rales or rhonchi by holding the stethoscope in each axilla. Contrast the percussion resonance of the chest posteriorly right and left with the index finger.

Abdomen. Palpate and percuss the liver for consistency and enlargement (3 cm or more below the costal margin). The causes of hepatomegaly include infection, pneumothorax with depression of the diaphragm, and erythroblastosis fetalis.

Neurologic. Check muscle tone and reflex reaction, and appraise the Moro reflex (at 1 and 5 minutes) (Fig. 21-11). Palpate the large fontanel for fullness or bulge. Note by palpation the degree of approximation of the edges of parietal bones as evidence of CNS abnormality.

Other observations. Gross structural malformations are obvious at birth. Describe these in general terms and record them on the delivery room record. Note the following, which are frequently associated with malformations:

1. Polyhydramnios and oligohydramnios
2. Two-vessel cord
3. Monozygotic twinning
4. SGA (or small-for-dates) neonates
5. Placental size and confirmation

For further discussion of the infant at risk, refer to Chapters 32 to 37.

PARENT-CHILD RELATIONSHIPS

The mother's reaction to the sight of her newborn may extend from excited outbursts of laughing, talking, and even crying to apparent apathy. A polite smile and nod acknowledge the comments of nurses and physicians. Occasionally the reaction is one of anger or indifference; the mother turns away from the baby, concentrates on her own pain, and sometimes makes hostile comments. These varying reactions can arise from pleasure, exhaustion, or deep disappointment. Whatever the reaction and cause may be, the mother needs continuing acceptance and support from all the staff.

Most parents enjoy being able to handle, hold, and examine the baby right after birth (Figs. 21-13 and 21-14). The nurse needs to make sure the baby is kept warm and is in no danger of slipping from the parent's grasp. Some mothers wish to begin breast-feeding the infant as soon as possible.

Parents are responsive to praise of their newborn. Many require reassurance that the blue appearance of the baby after delivery is normal until respirations are well established. The reason for the molding of the baby's head must be reviewed with parents. Information about hospital routine as to future parent-child contacts can be repeated. The hospital staff, by their interest and concern, can do much to make this a satisfying experience for both parents.

TRANSFER TO NURSERY

When the newborn's immediate response to birth has been accomplished satisfactorily and his parents have had an opportunity to see and touch him, the infant is transferred to the nursery. In some areas, he is transported in a covered warm crib unit; in others he is wrapped warmly in blankets. The nurse who receives him will check the name and identification with that on the record and be informed about any significant happenings during pregnancy or labor, such as whether the cord was around the neck, meconium had been passed, or voiding had taken place since delivery.

PLAN OF CARE: NORMAL LABOR—SECOND STAGE

PATIENT CARE OBJECTIVES

1. Maternal progress through the second stage is within normal limits.
   a. Contractions: magnitude, expulsively powerful; frequency, 2 to 3 minutes; duration, 60 seconds; rhythm, regular.
   b. Descent is constant:
      (1) For primigravidas, it takes ½ to 1 hour for descent from station +1 cm to +4 cm. From station +4 cm to birth of infant, approximately twenty contractions.
      (2) For multigravidas, it takes 10 minutes to ½ hour for descent from station 0 cm to +4 cm. From station +4 cm to birth of infant, approximately ten contractions.
   c. Show: Copious amount of blood and mucus are mixed.
   d. Behavior and appearance: Pain sensations lessen in the early phases of the second stage. Urge to push can only be controlled by panting. Eager to cooperate and give birth to infant. Fretful and irritable if progress not deemed fast enough. Needs coaching to work with contractions. Amnesia between contractions. Fatigue becomes ap-

PATIENT CARE OBJECTIVES—cont'd

parent, especially in primigravidas. Can follow simple clear directions. Often comments with surprise at sensation of birth.

2. Fetal well-being continues.
   a. FHT remain within normal limits (rate 120 to 160 beats/min).
   b. No evidence of meconium staining of amniotic fluid.
3. Neonate is in good health.
   a. Apgar rating 7 to 10 (at birth and in 5 minutes), respirations present, color dusky to pink, muscle tone good, cry strong, reflexes present.
   b. Examination by physician reveals no immediately discernible abnormalities, e.g., two vessels in the cord, clubfeet, imperforate anus.
4. Immediate maternal response to her infant is within normal limits (e.g., open expression of concern for infant's health, joy or disappointment tempered by her physical state, amount of pain or fatigue experienced). Reactions vary from euphoria to sleepy exhaustion, with unawareness of surroundings.
5. Recording of findings is done concomitantly with care.

NURSING INTERVENTIONS

Diagnostic

1. Before birth:
   a. Contractions are monitored constantly.
   b. FHT are checked after every contraction or every 5 minutes.
   c. Descent is confirmed by vaginal examination until presenting part can be seen at introitus.
   d. Show is checked for evidence of excessive bleeding.
   e. Amniotic fluid is checked for meconium staining and amount.
   f. Vital signs, including BP, are checked (must be taken between contractions).
2. At birth, physician and/or nurse does following:
   a. Assesses respirations.
   b. Estimates infant's health status using Apgar rating at 1 and 5 minutes of age.
   c. Examines cord.
   d. Completes physical examination.
   e. Assesses parent's response to newborn.
   f. Confirms position (e.g., LOA) for medical records.
   g. Collects cord blood for analysis (RH factor, blood grouping, and Hct).

Therapeutic and educational

1. Assist patient to use her expulsive powers to expedite descent and birth of infant:
   a. Patient is encouraged to push with contractions until vertex "crowns."
      (1) Patient assumes a semi-Fowler position with support to her back.
      (2) Patient is instructed to "work" with contractions.
         (a) She draws her knees up toward abdomen, spreads them apart, and grasps her thighs above popliteal space.
         (b) She then takes deep cleansing breath and one short breath, in and out. Then she takes another breath, holds it, and pushes for 6 seconds. She releases breath, takes one short breath in, holds it, and pushes for 6 seconds.
         (c) She continues until contraction ceases and then relaxes completely.
   b. When presenting part crowns, patient is instructed to control urge to push by panting, thereby permitting slow delivery of head and eventually of complete infant.
   c. Patient needs simple, clear directions.
2. Care for delivery:
   a. Patient is transferred to delivery area for completion of birth process.
      (1) Multiparous patient: at end of first stage if presenting part is +1 or +2.
      (2) Nulliparous patient: when vertex can be seen at introitus with each contraction.
   b. Patient is moved to delivery table between contractions, placed in lithotomy position, and vulva is cleansed with antiseptic solution.
   c. Sterile equipment, solutions, and supplies are readied for physician's use.
   d. Physician or nurse-midwife is assisted with donning sterile cover gown and gloves, and any extra supplies or equipment are obtained as necessary (e.g., if any episiotomy is to be done, add anesthetic solution and sutures to equipment on table).
   e. Crib and equipment are readied for receiving infant.
   f. Contact with patient is maintained by touch and verbal comforting, instructions as to reasons for care, assistance with coaching during contractions, and sharing in parents' joy at birth of their child.
   g. If father is to attend delivery, he is given instructions as to donning cover gown, mask, hat, and shoes and then shown where to sit during delivery; he is advised as to areas wherein he has freedom to move and what support he can give his wife (some are prepared to do coaching for pushing and panting).
   h. Note and record time of birth (i.e., when infant is born completely).
   i. When physician or nurse has completed care of newborn (assists infant to establish and maintain respirations by clearing air passages and applying tactile stimulation, clamps and cuts cord), nurse takes infant, wraps him in warm blanket, and places him in crib. Nurse then proceeds with initial neonatal care (pp. 325 to 328).
3. Nurse shows infant to parents and confirms sex and health status. Parents are allowed to hold infant when appropriate.

REFERENCES

Hellman, L. M., and Pritchard, J. A. 1971. Williams obstetrics (ed. 14). New York, Appleton-Century-Crofts.

Klaus, M., and Kennell, J. 1976. Maternal-infant bonding. St. Louis, The C. V. Mosby Co.

Kopp, L. M. 1971. Ordeal or ideal—the second stage of labor. Am. J. Nurs. **71:**1140.

Leboyer, F. 1975. Birth without violence. New York, Alfred Knopf, Inc.

Oxorn, H., and Foote, W. 1968. Human labor in birth (ed. 2). New York, Appleton-Century-Crofts.

Reed, B., and others. 1971. Management of the infant during labor, delivery, and in the immediate neonatal period. Nurs. Clin. North Am. **6:**3.

CHAPTER 22

Third and fourth stages of labor

THIRD STAGE

The third stage of labor extends from the birth of the baby until the delivery of the placenta. The goal in the management of the third stage of labor is the prompt separation and recovery of the placenta, achieved in the easiest, safest manner. Outmoded procedures such as kneading the corpus (Credé's maneuver), pushing the fundus downward, and others have been abandoned because of the serious hazards of uterine bleeding, retention of the placenta, contamination of the cervix outside the introitus, and possible inversion of the uterus.

Separation and delivery of placenta

The placenta is attached to the myometrium beneath the extremely thin endometrium of the basal plate by numerous, randomized, fibrous anchor villi—much like a postage stamp is attached to a sheet of postage stamps. After the fetus is delivered, assuming strong uterine contractions, the placental site is markedly reduced in size. This constriction breaks the anchor villi, and the placenta severs from its attachments. Normally the first few strong contractions 5 to 7 minutes after the birth of the baby shear the placenta from the myometrium. Logically a placenta will not be easily freed from a flaccid uterus. Moreover, although manipulation of the fundus may cause fundal contractions, the irritation may also cause the cervix to contract. Thus the placenta, after being partially separated, may be trapped within the uterus, and bleeding may be dangerously profuse.

Placental separation is indicated by the following, in sequence (Fig. 22-1):
1. A firmly contracting, rising fundus
2. A change in configuration of the fundus from discoid to globular shape
3. A visible and palpable rounded prominence above the symphysis (the placenta), assuming an empty bladder
4. A slight gush of dark blood from the introitus
5. Lengthening of the umbilical cord
6. A vaginal fullness (the placenta) noted on vaginal or rectal examination

Misinterpretation of the signs of placental separation is uncommon, but confusion may result because of a uterine neoplasm or anomaly, an undelivered fetus, a vaginal tumor, or even retained feces.

Whether the placenta presents by the shiny fetal surface (Schultze mechanism) or whether it turns to first show its dark roughened maternal surface (Duncan mechanism) is of no clinical importance. At one time, it was believed that the Duncan mechanism was associated with a significantly greater blood loss, but this has been disproved. After delivery of the placenta, it should be examined for intactness to be certain that no portion of it remains in the uterine cavity.

Immediate care of mother

Immediately after delivery of the placenta and before repair of the episiotomy, the physician or midwife completes a thorough examination. The gloved hands should be rinsed in sterile solution and the introitus swabbed with wet sponges. It is unnecessary to change the drapes. The perineum, vagina, and cervix should be inspected for lacerations, extensions of the episiotomy, or hematomas.

The cupped hand should be inserted into the vagina and, if possible, through the cervix. The other hand on the patient's abdomen steadies the uterus and pushes it downward gently. Thus the uterine cavity can be examined and the placental site identified. Any retained placental fragments may be removed manually and any membrane strands grasped with an appropriate forceps for removal.

To examine the vaginal canal, the vaginal retractors are positioned, the cervix is grasped with sponge forceps, and the entire circumference is systematically inspected. The nurse assists by repositioning the light if

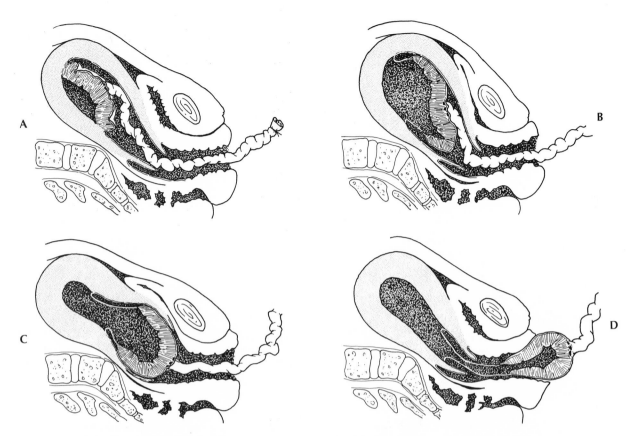

Fig. 22-1. Third stage of labor. **A,** Placenta begins by separating in central portion with retroplacental bleeding. Uterus changes from discoid to globular shape. **B,** Placenta completes separation and enters lower uterine segment. Uterus is globular in shape. **C,** Placenta enters vagina, cord is seen to lengthen, and there may be increase in bleeding. **D,** Expression (birth) of placenta and completion of third stage.

necessary and by elevating the fundus. This is done by dipping the fingers down behind the patient's symphysis pubis and elevating the uterine body, thus opening and tenting the vaginal fornices. The lateral and posterior fornices can then be examined together with the areas beneath the bladder and over the ischial spines (p. 407). Pudendal block or light inhalation anesthesia is entirely adequate for examination and repair of most lacerations.

In routine postnatal examinations of the uterus and vaginal canal, unsuspected cervical lacerations 2.5 cm long may be found in 5% to 7% of patients. Retained membranes may be identified in almost 5% of cases, and vaginal lacerations, including an episiotomy extension, may be identified in about the same percentage of patients. Retained placental tissue may be expected in about 2% to 4% of cases. Uterine anomalies and pelvic tumors are occasionally identified for the first time during this appraisal.

Excessive blood loss during the third stage of labor or within the first hour thereafter may be due to uterine atony, often associated with one or more of the following: excessive analgesia or anesthesia, traumatic delivery, multiple pregnancy, polyhydramnios, uterine neoplasm, or hypertensive cardiovascular renal disease. A poor labor, especially when due to uterine inertia, may be followed by postnatal uterine hypotonia, faulty placental separation (p. 408), and hemorrhage. Thus if an early problem such as uterine hypotonia can be anticipated and properly treated, it may be possible to avoid a later complication such as postnatal hemorrhage.

Ergot causes firm contraction of the uterus. For this reason, ergot products such as ergonovine (Ergometrine), 0.2 mg, or methylergonovine (Methergine), 0.2 mg, are useful after the placenta has separated to prevent or control postabortal or postnatal bleeding. One parenteral dose or repeated oral doses may be given. Ergot is a

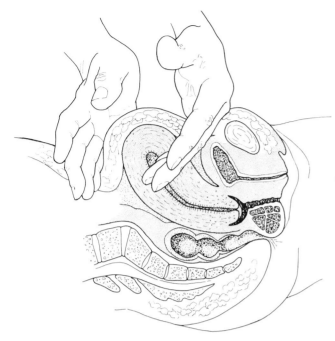

Fig. 22-2. Palpating fundus of uterus during first hour postdelivery. Note that upper hand is placed over fundus; lower hand dips in above pubis and supports uterus while it is gently massaged.

vasoconstrictor also. Hence hypertension may be a side effect of parenterally administered ergot medications and is avoided in patients with elevated blood pressure.

Synthetic oxytocin (Syntocinon, 10 units, or Pitocin, 10 units) may be administered either intramuscularly or intravenously to accomplish the same purpose. The effect lasts about 30 minutes. If excessive bleeding continues, an intravenous infusion of 1000 ml of Ringer's lactate solution with 10 to 20 units of oxytocin may be ordered.

FOURTH STAGE

This period is a critical one for the mother. During the next 2 hours the maternal organism makes its initial readjustment to the nonpregnant state, and body systems begin to stabilize; therefore the immediate reaction of the mother to the birth process is kept under careful scrutiny.

Management

When the delivery of the placenta is complete and the episiotomy is sutured, the vulva is gently cleansed with sterile water, a sterile perineal pad is applied, the drapes are removed, and the patient is dressed in a clean gown and covered with a warm blanket. The bottom of the delivery table is repositioned, and the mother's legs are lowered simultaneously from the stirrups. Assistance will be needed to effect the transfer from the delivery table to her bed. Although some are able to move readily

by themselves, others, for example, those who have had a spinal anesthetic, will need to be correctly positioned and rolled from one surface to the other. These patients will remain supine in bed with the head raised not more than 6 to 8 inches to prevent development of a spinal headache. The patient is then taken to the recovery room or back to her labor room.

The pattern of care includes routine checking for hemorrhage; significant increases or decreases in blood pressure and pulse rate; and tension, pain, or thirst states that prevent rest. The techniques used are as follows:

1. Patients are to remain in a supine position at bed rest for 2 hours. The head of the bed may be raised to a 45-degree angle unless a spinal anesthetic has been used. No bathroom privileges are allowed until patient recovers from effects of analgesics and/or anesthetics.

2. Check for evidence of hemorrhage every 10 minutes, or more often if indicated, for the first hour and every 30 minutes for the second hour.

Palpate the fundus to note consistency and position (Fig. 22-2). Immediately after delivery, the fundus is located in the midline about 2 cm below the umbilicus. Within an hour it has risen slightly above the level of the umbilicus and remains there for the next 12 hours. Normally the fundus remains firm or may be returned to a state of firmness with intermittent gentle massage. As noted earlier, atony of the uterine musculature may occur, and as the relaxed uterus distends with blood and clots, blood vessels in the placental site are not clamped off by the "living ligature," and hemorrhage results. It is necessary to gently express the accumulated blood and clots before the uterus can again contract. If the atony is not controlled by such treatment, medical intervention must be instituted (p. 364).

A distended bladder may also contribute to postnatal hemorrhage. The full bladder forces the uterus upward and to the right of the midline. Such a position interferes with the contractability of the uterine muscle, and hemorrhage results. The patient is encouraged to void, or if necessary, an order for catheterization is obtained. Palpation to determine the amount of bladder distention accompanies the palpation of the fundus.

Note the amount of lochia. This may be described as scant, moderate, or marked. As the effect of the oxytocic medication administered after delivery wears off, the amount will increase. Always check under the patient's buttocks, as well as on the perineal pad. If a perineal pad is soaked through (100 ml) in 15 minutes or blood is found to be pooling under the buttocks, continuous observation is indicated. If marked bleeding persists, immediate medical intervention will be necessary. If bleeding is in the form of a continuous trickle or is seen to come in spurts, lacerations of the vagina or cervix or the presence of an unligated vessel in the episiotomy is suspected. The patient is returned to the delivery area to permit visualization of the site and correction.

3. The blood pressure and pulse rate are checked every 15 minutes during the first hour, then every 30 minutes during the second hour.

4. Some patients experience intense tremors after delivery that resemble the shivering of a chill. This chilling may be related to the sudden release of pressure on pelvic nerves. According to another theory, chilling may be symptomatic of a fetus-to-mother transfusion that occurs during placental separation. Warm blankets relax the patient even if the shaking is not relieved.

5. Because of the restrictions on fluid intake and the loss of fluids (blood, perspiration, or emesis) during labor, most women are thirsty and request fluids. Any clear fluids may be offered in moderate amounts, and the woman is instructed to drink slowly. Excessive fluids or drinking too quickly often precipitates bouts of nausea and vomiting. After the first hour, a light diet may be offered.

6. Pain may originate in the episiotomy or from the strong contractions of the uterus as they act to expel blood, decidual debris, and clots. These contractions are called *afterpains* and are particularly noticeable in multiparous patients. A covered ice pack may be applied to the episiotomy to minimize edema and numb the area. Analgesics may be administered. The sedating effect of these analgesics necessitates such protective care as raising side rails, placing the call bell within reach, and cautioning about remaining in bed. Patients must be warned about the "head-spinning" effect of the medications.

7. Psychic states range from euphoria, a feeling of well-being, to a sleepy state marked by an unawareness of surroundings. As noted earlier, first reactions of mothers and fathers to their newborns may vary widely.

Table 22-1. Assessment during fourth stage

	Minimal assessment	Findings
Fundus	Every 15 minutes	Firm: midline, at umbilicus Soft: massage until firm and express clots until contracted to midlevel Right of midline: check bladder for distention
Lochia	Every 15 minutes (in conjunction with assessment of fundus)	Moderate flow: normal; if flow comes in spurts, suspect cervical tear Heavy flow: recheck in 3 to 5 minutes and report
Perineum	Check in conjunction with assessment of lochia	Condition of episiotomy and perineum: clean, edematous, discolored, stitches intact
Blood pressure	Every 15 minutes for 1 hour, then every 30 minutes during second hour	Slightly accelerated from excitement and effort of delivery; returns to normal within 1 hour
Pulse	Every 15 minutes	Normal rate for individual within 1 hour

These reactions give the medical team cues to use in individualizing plans of care. Patients who have experienced long, difficult labors or are in pain are frequently too exhausted to extend interest to the child. After sufficient rest, their attitudes can be surprisingly different. The child unwanted for diverse reasons may continue to be rejected or given only mild interest. The attitude of the husband is often reflected in the mother. His pleasure arouses a responsive pleasure, or his disappointment arouses corresponding disappointment.

Ethnic or cultural origins dictate behaviors that are deemed appropriate for special occasions. Some parents may not be able to express their delight openly; others wish to welcome the newcomer noisily. The unwed mother may think that she is not expected to express joy or pleasure in her baby, and indeed, she may not wish to see or touch the child. Some mothers, particularly with their firstborn, are surprised and disturbed by the passivity or disinterest they experience on seeing their long-awaited infant. They need reassurance of the normalcy of these feelings. The idealized mother love does not necessarily come into being right after delivery. The gradual growth of such love comes to some as they assume the care of and responsibility for their child.

8. At the end of the second hour, the patient is examined thoroughly and if her physical state has stabilized, she is ready for transfer to the postnatal area. A verbal report of her condition is given to the ward staff even though her completed labor record accompanies her.

Table 22-1 summarizes the routine assessment procedures performed during the fourth stage of labor.

See references for Chapters 20 and 21.

PLAN OF CARE: NORMAL LABOR—THIRD AND FOURTH STAGES

PATIENT CARE OBJECTIVES
1. Placenta is delivered intact with membranes within 30 minutes (usually 3 to 5 minutes).
2. Uterine muscles contract sufficiently to limit loss of blood from the placental site.
3. Bleeding from cervical tears is within normal limits or controlled by ligation of torn vessels.
4. Repair of episiotomy eliminates bleeding from vessels within the incised area.
5. Patient voids sufficiently to prevent bladder distention.
6. Uterus remains firm. Position in midline:
   a. At birth midway between pubis and umbilicus
   b. 2 hours after birth rises to slightly above umbilicus.
7. Vital signs and blood pressure remain within her normal range.
8. Behavior and appearance are within normal limits:
   a. The initial excitement is replaced with drowsy satisfaction.
   b. The desire to rest is not curtailed because of discomfort from pain, thirst, or hunger.
9. Initial mother (father)-child interactions are enough to satisfy the need to touch, hold, and examine the infant; to reassure as to the normalcy of the infant's appearance and behavior; to provide eye contact with the infant (if possible); and to initiate breast-feeding of the infant (if desired).
10. Recordings of findings done concomitantly with care.

NURSING INTERVENTIONS

Diagnostic	Therapeutic and educational
Third stage	
1. Note symptoms of placental separation and time of delivery. Uterus changes from discoid to globular shape as placenta is extruded. Cord protrudes further from vagina and there is gush of blood prior to birth of placenta.	1. Instruct patient to push as contractions are felt and thereby assist in delivering placenta.
2. Physician checks placenta and membranes for intactness.	2. Administer oxytocin as ordered.
3. Fundus is palpated, and its degree of firmness and position in relation to midline are checked.	3. Remove legs from stirrups; put perineal pad and binder in place. Cover with warm blanket and change gown.
4. Mother's level of anxiety, excitement, or restlessness is noted.	4. Help patient to move from delivery table to bed or stretcher (if epidural or spinal anesthetic has been used, patient will need to be lifted or rolled into position on her bed).
	5. Administer antilactogenic hormones if mother chooses to bottle-feed.
	6. Facilitate mother-father-child bonding.
	7. Transfer patient to recovery area.

Continued.

PLAN OF CARE: NORMAL LABOR—THIRD AND FOURTH STAGES—cont'd

NURSING INTERVENTIONS—cont'd

Diagnostic	Therapeutic and educational
Fourth stage 1. Assess routinely and record findings (Table 22-1). 2. Note amount of discomfort: 　a. "Afterpains" in multiparous patients. 　b. Pain from site of episiotomy. 3. Note evidence of fatigue or exhaustion, hunger, thirst. 4. Note response to excitement of birth; drowsiness and urge to sleep usually come within hour. 5. Note any response from either mother or father that may be indicative of future parent-child relationship.	1. Settle patient comfortably in bed. 2. Share in excitement and joy over birth. Facilitate mother-father-child bonding. Accept any expressions of disappointment from parents and reassure them that such feelings are normal. Reassure mother that her behavior during labor was acceptable if she appears worried about it. 3. Change perineal pads as necessary; wash vulva with soap and water. 4. Encourage to void qs. If distention occurs and patient is unable to void, catheterize and record amount, character, and type. Send specimen if indicated. 5. Teach regarding afterpains, lochia, reason for checking fundus and expressing clots, return of sensation to legs after regional anesthesia, and need to keep bladder empty. 6. Provide fluids and nourishment. Record amounts and types. 7. Give medication for pain if ordered and desired. 8. Check record for completeness and prepare record for transfer to postnatal unit. 9. Transfer patient to postnatal unit when her condition has stabilized. 　a. Assist patient into bed; introduce her to nurse on postnatal unit and to other patients sharing room. 　b. Give report to nurse as to type of labor and delivery and any problems encountered in antenatal period; state of fundus, amount of lochia, vital signs, and BP; whether episiotomy was done; whether medication for pain has been given, what it was, dosage, and time of administration; condition and sex of infant; whether breast- or bottle-feeding of infant is desired; whether patient voided and IV fluids given.

CHAPTER 23

Home delivery

GENERAL CONSIDERATIONS

Home delivery has always been popular in certain advanced countries such as Great Britain, Sweden, and the Netherlands. It is rapidly gaining popularity in the United States and Canada. In developing countries, hospitals or adequate lying-in facilities often are unavailable to most pregnant women, and home delivery is a necessity.

Selective home delivery of uncomplicated patients is feasible, provided elimination of those women at high risk can be accomplished during good antenatal care and assuming that a transport system is available for transfer of suddenly complicated labors to a nearby adequate medical facility. Another acceptable plan provides for specialist care to be brought to the home by means of a so-called flying squad service, which is utilized in Great Britain, for example.

Collaboration with and supervision of midwives are the obstetrician's duty in many countries. Moreover, obstetric nurse practitioners or nurse midwives have proved to be invaluable components of the health care team. Thus nurse specialists, general practitioners, and obstetric specialist consultants have become incorporated into home delivery units. A midwife or general practitioner can call on or refer women or infants to numerous essential backup services for study or specialty care during pregnancy and the early puerperium.

When a woman is to be delivered by a midwife, it is the practice in many areas for the general practitioner to supervise her; meanwhile, both are under the direction of the obstetric specialist.

Advantages of home delivery

One advantage is that delivery may be more "natural" or physiologic in familiar surroundings. The mother may be more relaxed and less tense than she might be in the impersonal, sterile environment of a hospital. The family can assist in and be a part of the happy event, and mother-father-infant contact is sustained and immediate.

In addition, home delivery may be less expensive than a hospital confinement.

Finally, serious infection may be less likely, assuming strict aseptic principles are followed. People generally are relatively immune to their own home bacteria.

Contraindications to home delivery

Hospital, not home delivery, is indicated for the following:
1. High-risk patients (fetal or maternal jeopardy)
2. Patients with a history of premature or postdate delivery in their last gestation
3. Women suffering serious medical or surgical complications in this or prior pregnancies
4. Women who cannot be transferred easily to a hospital should the need arise unexpectedly
5. Women who are opposed to home delivery
6. Patients with inadequate home facilities.

Basic requirements for home delivery

Maternity patients with physical and/or obstetric or emotional complications, those with an uncertain prognosis, and those opposed to home delivery must be eliminated as candidates for home confinement. Couples opting for home delivery should be apprised of the potential risks involved and be willing to take responsibility for the health and well-being of their unborn child and the mother.

Women qualified for home delivery must be examined at monthly intervals until the thirty-second week, then bimonthly until the thirty-sixth week, and at least weekly thereafter. If a nurse practitioner, nurse midwife, or physician's assistant is assigned to do antenatal evaluations, a physician must see the woman with the other examiner initially, regularly during each trimester, or when unusual symptomatology is noted.

An evaluation of each pregnant woman tentatively scheduled for home confinement should be made by an obstetric specialist at the thirty-fourth to thirty-sixth week. Pelvic mensuration, fetal size, presentation, laboratory studies, nutritional status, and other factors must be appraised. The generalist and midwife should be present so that there is no misunderstanding regarding the woman's status and the plan of action. Then if a midwife is scheduled to deliver her, the physician examines the patient with the midwife regularly during the third trimester.

The home facilities are assessed and preparations for the confinement completed by the twenty-fourth week before easy fatigue or complications, such as premature labor, are likely. The names, addresses, and telephone numbers of the generalist, midwife, and hospital to be used for emergency admission should be prominently posted in the patient's home to avoid delay or confusion. (If the telephone call is to be made from a pay telephone booth, have the correct change taped to the list of telephone numbers.)

Even with primitive facilities of lighting and home conveniences, improvisations usually are possible and safe delivery feasible. Good obstetric principles are the same regardless of the locale.

When the woman goes into labor, the midwife who is to deliver the patient contacts the physician with whom she is associated. The physician must remain available until successful delivery has been accomplished.

FAMILY'S PREPARATION FOR HOME DELIVERY

If a home delivery is planned, it will usually be possible to obtain and store the necessary articles in advance for childbirth. In contrast, if delivery in the home or elsewhere is an emergency or is determined by circumstances beyond control, considerable improvisation may be necessary.

Facilities and supplies can approximate those available in hospitals. The family will work closely with the physician or nurse to complete preparations well in advance of delivery. If possible, attendance by both parents-to-be at some type of preparation for childbirth classes adds to the pleasure and competence of the parents. Detailed descriptions for preparation are required and may be obtained from either the physician's office or from local health agencies. The agencies may provide some of the equipment and supplies.

A visit to the home by the public health nurse is recommended well before the expected date of delivery. At that time, the process of delivery can be discussed so that all are aware of the characteristics of normal labor and delivery and the newborn, deviations from normal, and the plan of care for each.

Supplies

The family may wish to supply and prepare some of the sterile linen or paper items used. To sterilize linen, paper, and laundered cloth items in the home, place items in paper bags or wrap in newspaper and secure with masking tape and label. Set oven at 200° F (use an oven thermometer to double-check setting). Place a pan of water on the bottom shelf to help prevent scorching. Bake for 3 hours. If there is no thermometer or oven setting, bake a 1-pound potato with the linens. When it is done, so are the packages.

Following is a list of supplies necessary for the home delivery:

1. Bedding:
   a. A minimum of two sets of linen and blankets. Supply should be sufficient for mother's and baby's needs during and after labor.
   b. A rubber or plastic sheet or dropcloth to protect the mattress.
   c. Substantial supply of newspapers for padding and for wrapping wastes.
   d. Disposable or cloth underpads to use after delivery.
2. Laundered and packaged gowns or other washable clothing of choice for the mother to wear during and immediately after delivery.
3. Toilet articles:
   a. Four laundered, bagged or wrapped, and baked washcloths.
   b. One pound roll of absorbent cotton or soft toilet paper and a bedpan.
   c. Three basins, sterilized by boiling. These will be used by the assistant for handwashing during delivery, for preparing the mother, and for the placenta.
   d. Lotion or powder for backrubs and effleurage.
   e. Supplies of choice for mouth care such as mouthwashes, glycerin and lemon swabs, Chapstick, etc.
   f. One new, unopened box of large sanitary pads.
   g. One new, unopened sanitary belt (or improvise).
4. Sterile water:
   Water may be purchased, or tap water may be boiled and put into bottles that have been boiled or run through a dishwasher with a "sani" cycle.
   a. Warmed sterile water is used for preparing the mother and for handwashing by the attendant who is gloved.
   b. Cool sterile water is used for irrigating the baby's eyes after instilling the silver nitrate.
5. An ironing board or sheet of plywood that may be put under the mattress on a bed at hip level to provide a firm surface. The mother may wish to labor and deliver on pillows and a mattress placed on a draft-free floor, however.

6. Miscellaneous:
   a. Waste collection bags.
   b. Cold water soap for soaking soiled linens.
   c. Lighting, with extra new bulbs.
7. Baby's kit or layette:
   a. Clothing, including receiving blankets, T-shirts, gowns, diapers.
   b. A rubber or plastic pad to cover the mattress.
   c. Washcloths and towels, the latter large enough to wrap around the baby after a bath. (NOTE: Cotton or synthetic fiber clothing and blankets are better than wool, which often shrinks and may cause allergy. Storage of laundered layette articles should be in plastic bags, clean sheets, pillowcases, or even clean paper bags. Newly ironed or "sterilized" newspapers may also be used to wrap and protect clothing.)
   d. A new bulb (ear) syringe to suction mucus from the baby's mouth and nose.
   e. Alcohol or thimerosal (Merthiolate) with cotton or cotton swabs for cord care.

Facilities

Labor area. A clean, light, well-ventilated room with adjacent toilet facilities is desirable. The labor area should be large enough to serve as a delivery area in an emergency. A bed (or mattress on the floor), two chairs, and a small table or stand are recommended, although furnishings may vary with the family's preferences and individuality.

Delivery area. The kitchen may be used as a delivery room because a stove, water, good light, a large table, and a tub or sink generally are available. If such facilities are not included, delivery in the mother's own bed may be feasible. The area to be used for delivery is organized, clean, draft-free, and cleared of unnecessary furniture. It needs to be screened against flies and other insect vectors. In addition, family members with contagious diseases should be excluded from the area.

Baby's area. The new baby may have his own clean, quiet room. A sink or bath with running water nearby is desirable. If the mother must or wants to keep the new baby in her room, fewer requirements will be necessary.

The baby's crib can be a bassinet, basket, or dresser drawer, as long as it is scrubbed and clean. One useful arrangement that provides warmth as well is a box within a box, lined on both sides and the foot with hot water bottles. (*Do not* place hot water bottles at the head or in direct contact with the baby.)

A bureau or cabinet for clothing and a stand or shelf for toiletries will be needed. A small table or bathinette for changing or bathing is suggested. A closet with hooks for clothing is desirable. A low, armless chair or rocker may be helpful for nursing or feeding the baby. A covered diaper pail or refuse container lined with plastic bags should be provided. Cheerful, light hangings and decorations are appropriate if desired.

HEALTH CARE TEAM'S PREPARATIONS

The woman's antenatal record, including blood pressure readings, urinalysis, pattern of weight gain, serology, Rh, blood type, hemoglobin, and other laboratory reports should be available for reference.

The obstetrician and the maternity nurse usually can carry the medications, instruments, and other necessities in two large kits.

Physician's or midwife's kit

1. Medications:
   a. Hypnotics (e.g., meperidine, 1 ml ampules) for pain
   b. Sedatives (e.g., phenobarbital, 0.03 mg tablets) for tension and anxiety
   c. Oxytocics (e.g., Pitocin, 10-unit ampule) and ergonovine maleate (0.2 mg tablets); the first to augment ineffective labor; both for postnatal bleeding
   d. Magnesium sulfate, 10 ml of 25% solution, as antihypertensive analeptic drug
   e. Calcium carbonate, 1 Gm in 10 ml solution (10%), to counteract respiratory depression caused by magnesium sulfate
   f. Mercuric chloride, 0.475 Gm, for preparation of antiseptic solution; two tablets per quart of water equals 1:1000 concentration
   g. Procaine hydrochloride 1%, 120 ml, for paracervical or pudendal block anesthesia
   h. Silver nitrate, 1% solution, in wax plastules or individual plastic dispensors for instillation into baby's eyes to prevent ophthalmia neonatorum
   i. Dehydrated plasma, distilled water, needles, and tubing for intravenous administration
2. Instruments:
   a. One needle holder and round and cutting needles
   b. Catgut in sterile packets, chromic and plain, sizes 00 and 000
   c. One tissue and one suture scissors
   d. One scalpel handle and blades
   e. One posterior and one lateral vaginal retractor
   f. One smooth and one toothed forceps
   g. Three ring or uterine forceps

h. Four artery forceps
i. One uterine packing forceps
j. One sterile DeLee mucous trap with catheter
k. One sterile No. 16 soft rubber catheter
l. One pelvimeter (Breisky type or its equivalent)
m. One sterile measuring tape
n. One cord clamp or sterile ties
o. One obstetric forceps (Simpson's)
p. Sterile 6-inch gauze roll for uterine and vaginal packing

3. Other materials:
   a. Two pairs of sterile gloves
   b. Two sterile hand brushes and germicidal detergent or soap
   c. One sterile gown, face mask, and cap
   d. One package of 10 sterile 4 × 4 inches gauze sponges
   e. One plastic or rubberized apron
   f. Labor record and birth certificate
   g. Clinistix or Uristix for urine glucose and protein determination

Nurse's kit

1. One plastic or rubberized half sheet to place beneath the parturient
2. One sterile large and one half sheet for draping the mother during delivery
3. Four sterile towels
4. Two packages of 10 sterile 4 × 4 inches gauze sponges
5. Two sterile hand brushes and germicidal detergent or soap
6. One oral and one rectal thermometer and water-soluble lubricant such as K-Y jelly or Lubrafax
7. Two pairs of sterile gloves
8. One stethoscope and one blood pressure manometer
9. One safety razor and blades to shave the parturient if necessary
10. One Fleet or similar enema
11. One flashlight with extra batteries and bulb
12. Baby scales
13. Plastic bags for placenta and refuse
14. One lifting forceps to remove hot sterile instruments
15. One sterile 5 ml hypodermic syringe with long and short No. 22 and No. 24 needles
16. One 1 ml ampule each of oxytocin and ergonovine maleate
17. One plastic or rubberized apron
18. One sterile gown, mask, and cap

LABOR AND DELIVERY
Identification of high-risk problem

Should untoward signs and symptoms appear, the nurse-physician team is notified, and the preplanned arrangements for transfer to a medical facility are initiated immediately. These signs and symptoms include the following:

1. Onset of true labor 2 weeks prior to EDC or earlier
2. Bleeding more than spotting anytime, even at start of true labor at term
3. Sudden pain in abdomen
4. Chills and fever
5. Symptoms of preeclampsia-eclampsia
6. Meconium-stained amniotic fluid
7. Failure of labor to progress
8. Prolapse of cord

Onset of normal labor

The prepared couple is able to distinguish true from false labor with some degree of accuracy. At the first signs of approaching labor (p. 297), the couple alerts the nurse-physician team. Once in labor, the parturient is never left alone.

The father or coach takes command of the situation: arranging for the care of the other children, coaching and making the mother comfortable as appropriate for the phase of labor, noting the progress of the labor, and similar activities.

Preparation of the parturient. The following activities may be done by the father-coach or nurse:

1. Enema and perineal clip or shave may be given if necessary.

2. Permit the mother to take a shower if desired or available. Otherwise cleanse her lower abdomen, upper legs, and perineum with germicidal soap or detergent.

3. Clothe the mother in a clean nightgown or slip. She may wish to wear a pair of warm socks.

Initial examination and assessment of labor status. Abdominal and sterile vaginal examination by the nurse or physician is required to determine the following:

- The character of uterine contractions
- The dilatation and effacement of the cervix
- The position, presentation, and station of the presenting part
- Rupture of membranes, bleeding, or unusual discharge

Organization of facilities, supplies, and equipment. Gather and assemble supplies and equipment. Put clean sheets on the bed over plastic mattress cover or newspapers. Cover the patient with a clean sheet and a blanket as necessary.

Ensure good light. Eliminate any clutter. Make the area pleasant.

If not previously done and if time and facilities permit, sterilize diapers, newspapers, and other linens by first sprinkling with water and then baking in an oven for 45 to 60 minutes at 375° F or follow procedure on p. 340.

Determine whether to deliver the woman in her bed or in another room and set up for the delivery.

Conduct of labor and delivery

Normal labor and delivery. In the absence of hospital facilities, all but the operative field is considered contaminated. The operator conducts the labor and delivery in a manner similar to that followed in the hospital (p. 322). Hospital record forms are used for documenting events. Customary analgesia, local anesthesia, episiotomy, and suture of the incision or lacerations are no different than that offered in a maternity center.

An actual home delivery is depicted in Figs. 23-1 to 23-9.

The extent of father-coach participation is governed by individual or couple preference and degree of preparation and is mutually determined with the nurse-physician team.

The placenta and membranes are inspected for intactness; count the vessels in the cord and record. Weigh the placenta and place it into a plastic bag for pathology study or disposal. Show to the parents if they wish to view it.

Deviations from normal progress. Signs and symptoms that may herald imminent complications requiring treatment in an appropriate medical facility include the following:

1. Leakage of amniotic fluid 24 hours or more prior to delivery
2. Foul-smelling or greenish drainage from the vagina
3. Regular, strong contractions for 18 hours or longer or inadequate uterine relaxation between contractions
4. Lack of cervical dilatation or progress of presenting part with adequate contractions
5. Transition of 2 hours' duration or longer
6. Second stage (mother pushing) 2 hours or longer
7. Drop of 20 beats/min in fetal heart rate or 100 beats/min or less

Text continued on p. 348.

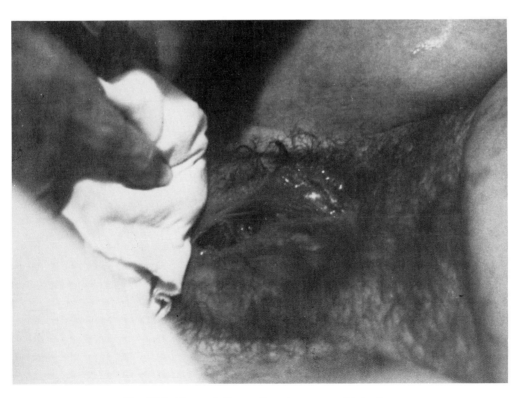

Fig. 23-1. Home delivery. Caput appears at introitus.

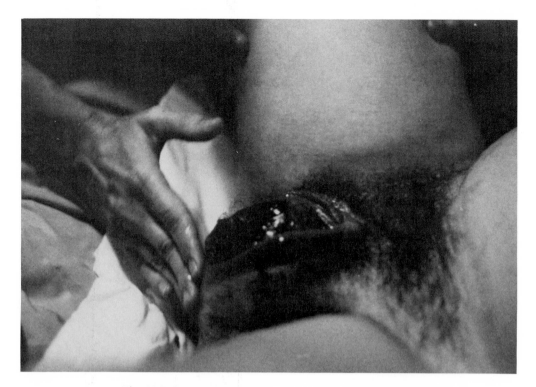

Fig. 23-2. Supporting perineum to control birth of head.

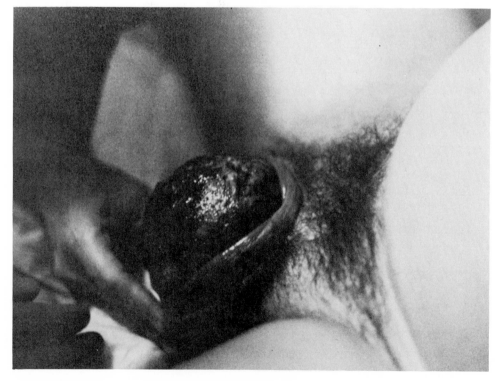

Fig. 23-3. Crowning.

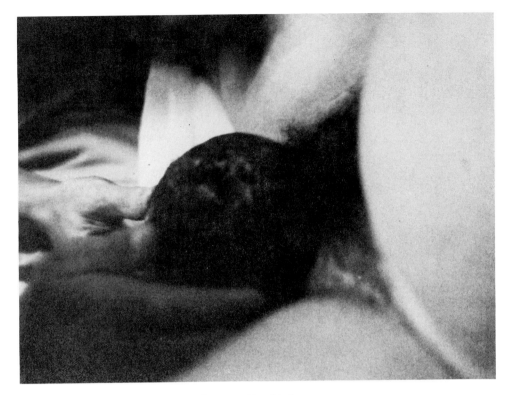

Fig. 23-4. Head is born.

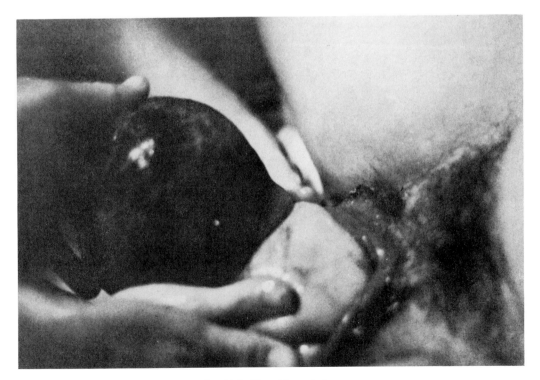

Fig. 23-5. Shoulders deliver.

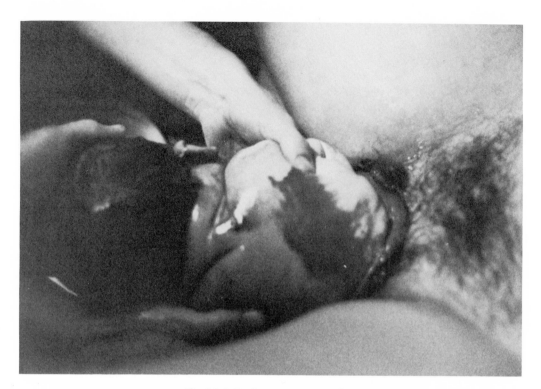

Fig. 23-6. Body emerges rapidly.

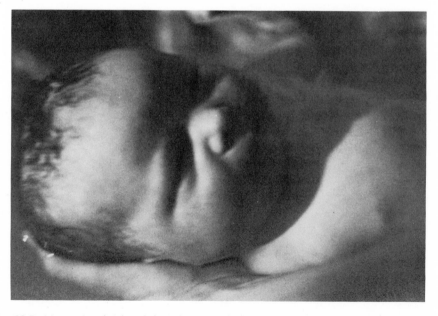

Fig. 23-7. Massaging body while infant is submerged in tub of warm water. Note relaxed, contented expression.

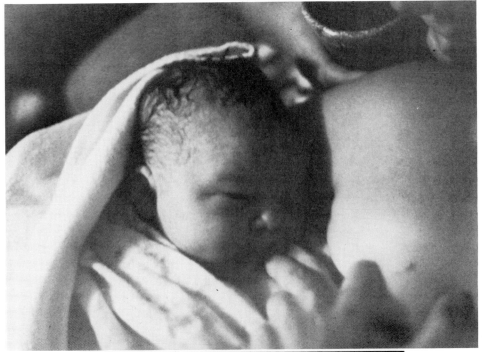

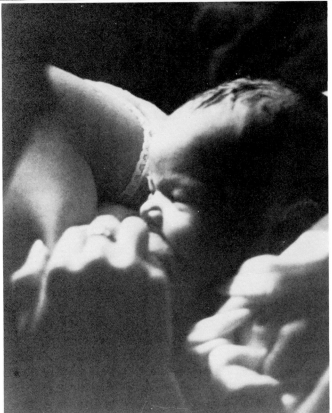

Fig. 23-8. Infant at breast.

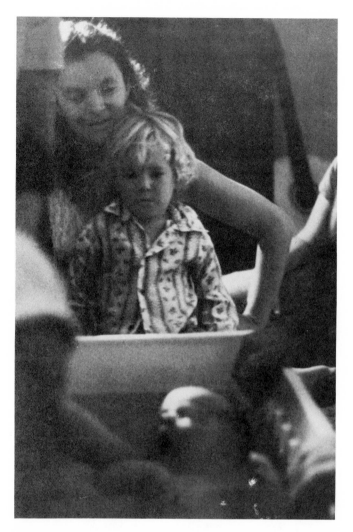

Fig. 23-9. While being held by mother, older child catches first glimpse of baby brother.

8. Third stage 2 hours or more
9. Blood loss more than spotting during first stage; 500 ml (2 cups) or more lost during second, third, or fourth stages
10. Placenta that does not appear intact
11. Uterine atony during fourth stage or continued bleeding in spite of firm uterus, lacerations, or beginning development of hematomas
12. Infant in distress: a sick infant, infant who "doesn't look well," very small infant

After delivery

Immediate postnatal care of the mother. Her care is similar to that provided in the hospital (pp. 335 to 337).

Immediate postnatal care of the neonate. The care of the neonate is similar to that provided in the hospital (pp. 325 to 328). In the event that undiagnosed twins or triplets are delivered in the home or the singleton is SGA or in jeopardy, prompt transfer to the hospital should be effected. (For resuscitation of the mildly depressed neonate, see p. 372.)

After pulsation ceases and the infant is breathing well, tie and cut the cord. Keep the umbilicus and cord stump dry.

The infant may then be wiped clean of blood, dried, and wrapped in a warm blanket. He may be placed on his mother's abdomen or in her arms or may be breast-fed. This contact with the mother is physiologically helpful in stimulating uterine contractions and placental separation and emotionally helpful in initiating the bonding between them.

Instill a drop of 1% aqueous silver nitrate solution and flush the eyes with cool sterile water.

Weigh and measure the infant. Assess the infant's status (pp. 328 and 330).

The infant may be positioned on his side in the crib (or in bed with his mother) to facilitate drainage of mucus and should be covered with a blanket for warmth. Although the family will want to hold him, undue handling is not reasonable. The infant has just completed the process of birth, and adjustment to extrauterine existence requires gentle nurturing care, with rest and quiet.

At one home delivery, after the care of the newborn was completed, the infant was taken to the living room where the three older siblings were seated in a row on the sofa, the eldest in the center. The baby was placed in the eldest's arms, and it was announced that she was theirs as much as the mother's and father's. Their delight, awe, and excitement augured well for the introduction of this child into the home and the family.

Resuscitation of mildly depressed baby. For the planned home delivery, supplies and equipment, at least one trained person, and a means of rapid transport of the mother or infant to a medical facility are essential for the serious unpredictable complication. During emergency delivery these essentials may be lacking. The following measures may be sufficient to resuscitate or sustain the neonate until medical assistance and equipment are available:

1. Hold the infant's head down to drain mucus. Place him on his left side on a firm surface, with his head lower and turned slightly laterally.

2. Dry first and then wrap him quickly to prevent heat loss and its sequelae (e.g., metabolic acidosis and increased need for oxygen).

3. Clear mucus and debris from his mouth with your finger.

4. *Gently* rub his back and flick the soles of his feet.

5. If gentle stimulation is ineffectual, place your mouth over his mouth and nose and exhale a short puff, forming the sound "ho."

> NOTE: Do not waste time by milking the trachea, jackknifing his body, or slapping him. These measures are ineffective and potentially traumatizing.

6. Feel his heartbeat through the chest wall. If the heartbeat stops, initiate cardiopulmonary resuscitation (p. 367).

EMERGENCY DELIVERY

Whether a home delivery is planned or not, the expectant mother and adults in general should know the basic points in birthing a baby. Some women, after "silent" labor, awaken in the middle of the night well into the second stage of labor. For others, an unexpected or fast labor surprises them and the immediate family in the home or anywhere else! Finally, when major disasters occur, the woman and adults near her may be called on to deliver the child. The procedure for labor, delivery, and care of the newborn varies little, although the circumstances under which they occur vary considerably.

Emergency delivery of fetus in vertex presentation

The following measures are necessary for the emergency delivery of a fetus in the vertex position:

1. Position the woman comfortably. She will usually assume the position most suitable for her delivery.

2. Reassure her. If there is someone else available (e.g., the father), that person could help support her in position, assist with coaching, and compliment her on her efforts.

3. Wash your hands with soap and water or "wash-and-dry" pledgets if possible.

4. Place under her buttocks whatever clean material or clean newspapers are available.

5. Avoid touching the vaginal area to decrease possibility of infection. (If there is time, scrub your hands for 5 minutes before touching the parturient.)

6. As the head begins to crown:
   a. Tear the amniotic membrane *(caul)* if it is still intact.
   b. Instruct her to pant, thus avoiding the urge to push.
   c. Place two fingers on the fetal head and apply *gentle* back pressure to prevent the head from "popping out." The mother may participate by placing her hand under yours on the emerging fetal head.
   > NOTE: Rapid delivery of the fetal head must be prevented because (1) rapid emergence of the fetal head is followed by a rapid change of pressure within the molded fetal skull, which may result in dural or subdural tears, and (2) may cause vaginal and/or perineal lacerations.

7. Instruct the mother to pant as you check for an umbilical cord. If the cord is around the neck, try to slip it up over the baby's head or down over the shoulders.

8. After restitution, with one hand on each side of the baby's head, exert gentle pressure so that the an-

terior shoulder emerges under the symphysis pubis and acts as a fulcrum; then as *gentle* pressure is exerted in the opposite direction, the posterior shoulder, which has passed over the sacrum and coccyx, delivers.

9. Be alert! Hold the baby securely because the rest of his body may deliver quickly. He will be slippery!

10. Hold the baby over your hand and arm with his head down to drain away the mucus.

NOTE: Do not hold baby upside down by his ankles because (1) it hyperextends the spine, which has been flexed since conception, (2) it increases intracranial pressure and the danger of capillary rupture, (3) it may cause direct tissue trauma to his ankles, and (4) it is easier to drop a wet, slippery baby.

11. Dry the baby rapidly (to prevent rapid heat loss), keeping him at the same level as the mother's uterus.

NOTE: Keep the baby at the same level to prevent gravity flow of baby's blood to or from the placenta and the resultant hypovolemia or hypervolemia. In addition, do not "milk" the cord: hypervolemia can cause respiratory distress initially and/or hyperbilirubinemia subsequently; and if isoimmunization has occurred, the baby may receive an additional inoculation of harmful antibodies (e.g., anti-Rh positive or anti-A or anti-B antibodies).

12. As soon as he is crying, place baby on mother's abdomen, cover him with her clothing, and have her cuddle him. Compliment her (them) on a job well done and on the baby if appropriate. (If something appears to be the matter with the baby, do not lie!)

NOTE: Soon after the Wharton's jelly in the cord is exposed to cool air and expands and the infant cries, the umbilical vessels stop pulsating, and the blood flow ceases. The baby's presence on the mother's abdomen stimulates uterine contraction, which aids in placental separation.

13. *Wait* for the placenta to separate; *do not* tug on the cord.

NOTE: Injudicious traction may tear the cord, separate the placenta, or invert the uterus. Signs of placental separation include (1) a slight gush of dark blood from the introitus, (2) lengthening of the cord, and (3) change in uterine contour from discoid to globular shape.

14. Instruct the mother to push to deliver the separated placenta: (a) do not cut the cord without proper clamps or ties and a sterile cutting tool, and (b) inspect the placenta for intactness. Place the baby on the placenta and wrap together for warmth.

NOTE: There is no hurry to cut the cord. The infant will not lose blood through the placenta because the cord circulation ceases (clots) within minutes of birth.

15. Check the firmness of the uterus. Gently massage the uterus and demonstrate to the mother how she can properly massage her own uterus.

16. Clean the area under the mother's buttocks.

17. Prevent or minimize hemorrhage as follows:
   a. From uterine atony:
   (1) *Gently* massage fundus to stimulate uterine musculature to contract.
   NOTE: Overstimulation may fatigue the myometrium and cause atony.
   (2) Put the baby to breast as soon as possible.
   NOTE: If baby does not suckle, manually stimulate the mother's breasts.
   (3) If medical assistance is delayed, do not allow the mother's bladder to become distended.
   (4) Expel any clots from her uterus.
   NOTE: The fundus should be firm to prevent accidental inversion during this procedure. While holding the bottom of the uterus just above the symphysis pubis, apply gentle pressure on the firm fundus downward toward the vagina.
   b. From perineal lacerations:
   (1) Apply a clean pad to the perineum.
   (2) Instruct the mother to press her thighs together.

18. Comfort or reassure the mother and her family or friends. Keep her and the baby warm. Give her fluids if available and tolerated.

19. If this is a multiple birth, identify the infants in order of birth.

20. Make notations regarding the birth:
   a. Fetal presentation and position.
   b. Presence of the cord around the neck or other parts and number of times cord encircles the part.
   c. Color, character, and amount of amniotic fluid.
   d. Time of delivery.
   e. Estimate of Apgar score, resuscitation, and ultimate condition of baby.
   f. Sex of baby.
   g. Approximate time of placental expulsion, its appearance, and completeness.
   h. Maternal condition: affect, amount of bleeding, and status of uterine contractions.

Emergency delivery of fetus in breech presentation

The voluntary home delivery of the fetus presenting in the breech position is strongly discouraged.

Should it become necessary for an individual to deliver a breech baby, one should consider the following points:

1. Elevate the infant's body during the birth process.
2. Avoid traction and compression to prevent the arms from being swept upward above the head, thus blocking delivery.
3. Bring the body upward as head is being born to ensure a patent airway.

Delivery and management of preterm baby

The actual process of delivering the preterm infant does not vary from that of the term infant. However, the care of the infant after delivery requires some modification as follows:

1. Warmth is essential.
2. Minimize handling, maintain a clear airway, and feed and change him.
3. Nutrition may be a problem if a medical facility is not available. Although the neonate may be unable to nurse at the breast, slow feeding is important, using a medicine dropper, for example.
4. Urge the preterm infant to breathe by stimulating him *gently* when he "forgets."
5. Transport the newborn to a medical facility equipped to handle the preterm infant as early as possible.

• • •

Home delivery is a selected alternative to hospital delivery for some women and a necessity for many. A physically and emotionally safe outcome can be anticipated for most women and their babies, especially if parents are prepared and have adequate health care support and backup.

Emergency delivery also can be physically safe and emotionally gratifying for parents and those who assist in the birthing process. In most instances, birth, whether in a structured or emergency situation, is a normal process. Consequently, with knowledge of a few basic measures, a potentially frightening and dangerous incident can be transformed into a self-fulfilling experience for all the participants.

REFERENCES

Edwards, M. 1973. Unattended home birth. Am. J. Nurs. **73:** 1332.

Enkin, M. 1975-1976. The family in labour. Birth Fam. J. **2:** 133, Fall-Winter.

Hazell, L. D. 1974-1975. A study of 300 elective home births. Birth Fam. J. **2:**11, Fall-Winter.

Hazell, L. D. 1976. Commonsense childbirth. Berkeley, Calif., Berkeley Windhover Books.

Lang, R. 1972. Birth book. Ben Lomand, Calif., Genesis Press.

Mehl, L. E., and others. 1975-1976. Complications of home birth. Birth Fam. J. **2:**123, Fall-Winter.

Myles, M. 1971. A textbook for midwives (ed. 7). Edinburgh, Churchill Livingstone.

Ritchie, C. A., and Swanson, L. A. 1976. Childbirth outside the hospital—the resurgence of home and clinic deliveries. MCN Am. J. Mat. Child Nurs. **1:**372.

Towler, J., and Butler-Manuel, R. 1973. Modern obstetrics for student midwives. London, Lloyd-Luke, Ltd.

UNIT SEVEN

Complications of labor

CHAPTER 24

Dystocia

Complications of labor can cause death or injury to both mother and infant. Prevention and detection of complications and consequent institution of remedial measures require the concerted efforts of the obstetric team. Many of the complications can be diagnosed prior to the beginning of labor, and preparation can limit their effects. Others arise suddenly, and only the critical judgment of those present safeguards the mother and/or the fetus. The goal is the safe delivery of mother and infant, and the care afforded the expectant mother through normal labor must be adjusted to meet additional needs. The nurse needs to utilize all assessment skills (observation, interviewing, and physical examination) to determine conditions hazardous to the mother, fetus, and/or family unit. The reaction of parents as they face threats to concepts of themselves as capable childbearing individuals is in essence a grief reaction and will require much supportive care.

Patient problems that the nurse will be concerned with are as follows:

1. *Prolonged labor.* Most women and families have definite ideas about how long the labor process should be. Any deviation in this time causes the anxiety level to rise, doubts as to the attending staff's interest and ability, and doubts as to their own capacity to cope. The nursing interventions will need to include the following:

   a. Clear and repeated descriptions of progress and explanations for delay, for example, "The baby's head needs to flex more on the chest (demonstrates with self) so that the head can fit through the pelvis." "The baby's head needs to turn from the side position (sutures transverse) until he is facing to the back, then the head can come down and the back of the neck can come under the pubic bone" (show on patient).

   b. Careful assessment for maternal exhaustion, including circumoral pallor, sunken eyes, and listless response. Report to physician, give bed bath, backrubs, change in position, cool cloth to forehead, and breathing and relaxation instructions. Stay with patient; do not abandon her.

   c. Acceptance of patient's frustration and hostility. "Yes, I know it's hard to take." "I'll try a backrub—tell me if it helps a little." "If the doctor gives medication now, it will slow up the labor even more."

2. *Unexpected pain sensations.* The uterine contractions can give rise to colicky, sharp pains if they are related to uterine dystocia (pp. 359 to 361). The contractions of induced labor are often more painful because they increase in intensity more rapidly, maintain the acme (peak) longer, and decrease rapidly. Women often say, "It hits me so fast I can't control it." Low back pain is increased in posterior positions of the fetal head. The hard back of the head (occiput) is forced against the soft tissue of the sacrum and compresses the sensitive tissue against the sacral bone, thus intensifying pain.

Women who have attended preparation for childbirth classes and who are desirous of controlling their responses to pain and/or experiencing a drug-free labor can develop feelings of failure or anger because of the conflict between expectations and reality. (Some men become disappointed in their wives' inability to cope and can turn from being supportive to being actively hostile.) The nurse needs to keep complimenting the woman on any effort she is able to make and to help her with her coaching. Also the staff should offer analgesia and/or anesthesia as though it were an expected result of a change in the labor pattern and openly discuss what this may mean to the mother, for example, "Some women are very distressed when they feel more pain than expected; they feel somehow they have failed."

3. *Fear for her own or the baby's safety.* A frank and detailed discussion of what operative procedures entail should be given, depending on the amount of time available. From a psychologic standpoint, surgery constitutes a stress situation wherein the patient fears a combination

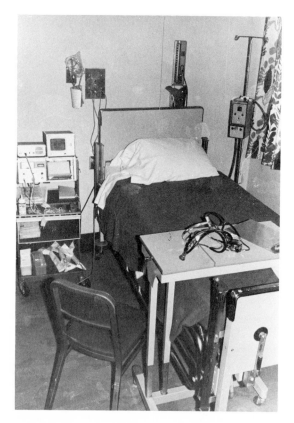

Fig. 24-1. Labor room. Equipment necessary for high-risk pregnancy: labor bed with side rails, oxygen flowmeter, call bell, blood pressure apparatus on wall behind bed, fetal monitoring equipment to left of bed, intravenous stand and drip meter to right of bed, and stethoscopes on overhead table. Parents need careful explanation of use of this equipment to reduce anxiety on seeing it for first time.

of three major imminent dangers: (a) the possibility of suffering acute pain, (b) the possibility of undergoing serious bodily damage, and (c) the possibility of death. Since presurgical anxiety is rooted in fear of the unknown, relief from this anxiety may stem in part from the information given as part of supportive care (Saylor, 1975). The emergency nature of some conditions precludes any but the physical priorities of care, and this situation needs to be recognized. One nurse described such a situation: "As I was wheeling her down the corridor to the OR, I said, 'I can't explain much just now, but tomorrow I'll come up and go over all the things we've been doing so you'll understand.' "

The nurse can use gentle touch, soft voice tones, attention to details, and explanations to convey interest and concern while carrying out procedures. The patient and her husband expect competent and efficient care.

There is no way to guarantee the infant's safety, and the nurse should indicate acceptance of parental concern: "I can appreciate how worried you must be." Again, the nurse's tone of voice, touch, and attitude convey the sincerity of her feelings to the patient and family.

The complications reviewed in this chapter and the next have been grouped into (1) those in which the mother's response and safety are in jeopardy (realizing, of course, that what affects the mother also affects the infant) and (2) those in which the baby's health is the primary concern. The labor unit is designed to facilitate assessment of maternal or fetal problems (Fig. 24-1).

PELVIC DYSTOCIA

The size of the pelvis is more important than its architecture so far as the *outcome* of labor is concerned. However, the *mechanism* of labor depends on the configuration of the interior of the pelvis (Chapter 3).

Pelvic dystocia may occur with significant shortening of one or more of the internal diameters of the bony pelvis. Such diminution in capacity is termed *pelvic contraction* (or *contracture*).

Pelvic contraction generally is congenital, but malnutrition, neoplasms, or disorders of the spine or lower extremities may be responsible. Small pelvic measurements capable of causing dystocia are recorded in at least 15% of women in North America. Racial characteristics may vary the size and architecture of the pelvis greatly; for example, small pelvic measurements are common to the natives of Southeast Asia. The size of the bony pelvis is not complete until maturity at approximately age 20 years. Hence young teenagers may have dystocia, whereas several years later normal delivery of similar- or even larger-sized babies may be possible. Disease such as rickets or osteomalacia may cause serious bony deformity and narrowing of pelvic diameters—often disastrous obstetrically. Increased maternal and perinatal jeopardy is due directly (or indirectly) to obstructed labor.

The diagnosis of pelvic contraction requires accurate mensuration of the major pelvic diameters. There are three principal levels or planes of concern: the pelvic inlet, the midpelvis, and the pelvic outlet (pp. 287 and 288).

A limited number of important internal pelvic diameters, as well as the major outlet dimensions, can be determined clinically. Other necessary measurements and, perhaps equally important, the architecture of the bony pelvis require radiography or ultrasonography for elucidation.

If one considers normal fetal cephalic and pelvic measurements in their relation to pelvic architecture, the cause and treatment of pelvic dystocia can be elicited.

X-ray films have revealed four pelvic types: gynecoid, platypelloid, anthropoid, and android. Actually, features of several types may be present, for example, a gynecoid posterior segment and an android anterior segment (Fig. 3-14).

Each pelvic type has a favorable diameter, often varying considerably from another type. The pelvic girdle is rigid, and the fetal head is only slightly malleable (moldable); hence one must deal with relatively fixed diameters.

Good flexion of the head is usual in uncomplicated vertex presentations, and this allows the "best" diameter of the fetal head, the biparietal diameter, to negotiate the birth canal. When malposition occurs, however, wider diameters of the fetal skull, such as the suboccipitobregmatic or occipitofrontal diameter, must pass through the pelvis. This requires significantly more room. If additional space is not available, pelvic arrest will occur.

Management

Anticipation of possible pelvic dystocia and proper planning are far more important than the immediate management of the patient. Accurate clinical measurement of the bituberous (BT) and posterior sagittal (PS) diameters of the outlet should be obtained at the initial antenatal visit.

An experienced physician can predict accurately by clinical pelvimetry alone the course of labor in about two thirds of patients before or early in labor. The remainder will require consultation, trial of labor, or x-ray or ultrasonographic study.

Previous successful performance is no guarantee of safe delivery. A woman who has been delivered of one or more average-sized babies without difficulty may produce one equal in size or larger or one smaller that may present abnormally. The head may fail to engage or may arrest deep in the pelvis because of malposition or failure to rotate.

The diagnosis of pelvic *adequacy* generally is easy and accurate; the diagnosis of pelvic *inadequacy* is difficult and inaccurate. The cost of error in both is increased fetal and maternal morbidity and mortality.

Trial of labor. A trial of labor is a reasonable period (4 to 6 hours) of observation of the patient, preferably with the membranes ruptured, to demonstrate engagement of the presenting part and continued descent. During this period, it is essential to assess carefully the following:

- Strength, frequency, and character of uterine contractions
- Progressive effacement and dilatation of the cervix
- Descent of the head
- Fetal well-being

Trial of labor is seldom induced artificially. Once spontaneous labor has begun, heavy analgesia is avoided because it slows progress. Membranes are ruptured only when the cervix nears complete dilatation. If advancement of the fetal head fails to occur within 4 to 6 hours of strong labor (or 6 to 8 hours of moderate labor), cesarean section is indicated. Any signs of significant maternal or fetal distress also make cesarean section mandatory.

Indications. A trial of labor should be justified by clinical and often radiologic consultation. With rare exceptions, the radiologist cannot predict whether the woman will deliver vaginally because he cannot forecast the quality of labor or how much the head will mold.

In vertex presentations, when the radiologist reports pelvimetry values below average with a "small" fetus, one that is 3000 gm or less (6 pounds 10 ounces), a trial of labor should be permitted. If pelvimetry results are above the mean and the infant is not excessive in size, the physician should probably allow a trial of labor; even with slow progress, pelvic dystocia will be unlikely.

Contraindications. If any of the following conditions are diagnosed, cesarean section is performed (p. 400).

- A diagonal conjugate (DC) less than 8.5 cm, assuming a full-term infant
- A breech or face presentation
- A contracted outlet, that is, when the sum of the BT and PS is less than 12 cm (Thom's rule)

Inlet contraction

Inlet contracture occurs in 1% to 2% of maternity patients at term. The DC determined in the antenatal period helps to detect only *marked* contraction. Inlet contraction exists when the anteroposterior diameter (AP) of the inlet is 10 cm or less, or when the transverse diameter is 12 cm or less. Moreover, if the DC is less than 11.5 cm, the AP probably is less than 10 cm. Therefore, when the DC is less than 10.5 cm, the pelvis must be considered foreshortened. The transverse diameter of the inlet can only be measured by x-ray studies or ultrasonography.

Pseudo-overriding of the head above the inlet may be caused by acute flexion of the uterus, a pendulous abdomen, a low-lying placenta, and/or malpresentation or anomaly of the fetus. Therefore an attempt should be made to impress the presenting part into the pelvis (the DeLee-Hillis maneuver); the physician may allow a trial of labor but probably will order internal pelvimetry.

A contracted pelvic inlet often prevents descent and engagement of the presenting part. Lack of pelvic accommodation of the fetus frequently results in malpresentation or position and prolapse of the cord.

The type and degree of pelvic inlet contraction, as determined by pelvic measurements, are the major factors pertaining to the mechanism of labor. The size and moldability of the head, as well as the contractile forces, also are important but less easily determined factors of the process.

Anteroposterior inlet contraction will require the fetal head to enter the flattened pelvis in the transverse diameter. If the DC exceeds the biparietal only slightly, the bitemporal or forehead (average diameter = 8 cm) may enter the inlet first. Deflexion is inevitable at this point, and a face presentation may develop. If the fit is not too snug and strong contractions prevail, the head may mold, allowing it to descend through the inlet.

Another mechanism in a contracted inlet permits entry of the head by lateral flexion when the anterior parietal bone presents (anterior asynclitism). Thus the head escapes the prominent sacral promontory while pressing against the symphysis pubis. The head may then slip downward, describing a slight lateral curve. Less frequently, the posterior parietal bone presents (posterior asynclitism); as the head is propelled past the symphysis, it glides posteriorly below the promontory and the sacrum, and unless disproportion exists, it may pass through the superior strait.

Breech presentation involves special problems when the pelvic inlet is contracted. Prolapse of the cord, an extremity, or both may occur because of delayed or poor engagement. If the body does deliver, the aftercoming head may arrest. Serious trauma or death may result from attempts at delivery of the aftercoming head. Hence perinatal morbidity and mortality are greatly increased in a contracted inlet with breech presentation.

Midpelvic contraction

The hallmark of good maternity care is the recognition of midpelvic contracture. This is the real challenge—not inlet or outlet problems.

Midpelvic dystocia occurs three to four times as frequently as isolated inlet contraction.

The capacity of the midpelvis may be reduced in the following ways:

1. Narrowing of the interspinous or transverse diameter of the midpelvis (normal = 10.5 cm)

2. Shortening of the AP of the midpelvis: the distance from the subsymphysis to the juncture of S4-5 (normal = 11.5 cm)

3. Reduction of the PS of the midpelvis: the distance from the interspinous of the midpelvis to the juncture of S4-5 (normal = 5 cm)

Midpelvic dystocia probably will occur at term with a normal-sized fetus when the midspinous measurement is less than 9 cm and the posterior sagittal diameter is less than 4 cm.

Although accurate measurement of the interspinous diameter is possible with the little-used Hanson pelvimeter, the PS of the midpelvis can only be obtained from x-ray films. For patients with a reduced interspinous diameter, prominent spines, or a contracted intertuberous diameter (TI) (8 cm or less), x-ray pelvimetry is mandatory.

No specific duration of labor or set of circumstances can determine whether safe delivery will occur in borderline midpelvic contracture. If the head descends past the spines to distend the perineum, the problem may be solved. If the head is arrested at the spines, however, a midforceps delivery must be considered. This may entail rotation (OT or OP to OA) or delivery as a molded OP, and the operation may or may not be complicated. A difficult midforceps delivery often is especially traumatic for the infant. An alternative is the vacuum extractor, assuming there is no need for rotation. The vacuum extractor does not occupy space laterally in contrast to the forceps, and it maintains flexion of the head, which is desirable. In any event, if satisfactory progress after engagement is not forthcoming, cesarean section is a far better alternative than a difficult forceps extraction.

Outlet contraction

Because the plane of the outlet is only 3 to 4 cm below the plane of the midpelvis, an isolated outlet contraction with a normal midpelvis must be exceptional. The usual cause of a contracted pelvic outlet is a long, narrow pubic arch. Rare exostoses, bony tumors, or acute beaking of the terminal sacrum (not a jutting coccyx that is movable) may cause outlet contracture. Most patients who have midpelvic narrowing have outlet constriction also, the best examples being an android or so-called funnel pelvis (Fig. 3-14).

The two major outlet dimensions that determine the available space at the pelvic outlet are the TI (normal = 10 to 11 cm) and PS of the outlet, or the distance from the center of the BT to the inner aspect of the sacral coccygeal articulation (normal = 7 to 8 cm).

Ideally the subpubic arch should be rounded, low, and

wide. This permits the fetal head to utilize the anterior pelvis and to come readily beneath the arch. Here a short PS may not compromise delivery. However, if the arch is narrow and long, the head must pass further posteriorly toward the tip of the sacrum and be propelled downward for delivery. Thus a longer PS will be required.

The outlet is seriously contracted when the TI is 8 cm or less or when the PS of the outlet is less than 7 cm.

Both these measurements can be obtained with the Thoms pelvimeter. The TI alone can be taken with a Williams or Breisky pelvimeter, and a direct PS measurement can be taken on the rectal finger, measuring from the plane of the intertuberous to the sacral coccygeal articulation.

A generally reliable index of adequacy of the pelvic outlet is *Thoms' rule:* If the sum of the transverse diameter and PS of the outlet is 15 cm or more, the head of the mature fetus probably will pass through the outlet.

Maternal complications with contracted pelvis

Frequently, premature rupture of the membranes and slow dilatation of the cervix are due to the lack of engagement of the presenting part. Prolonged, often obstructed labor may give rise to secondary uterine inertia (Fig. 24-2) (p. 362). Infection may develop. If strong labor persists, rupture of the uterus, perhaps after the development of a pathologic retraction ring, may ensue. Vaginal fistulas occur when impaction of the presenting part persists. Trauma, hemorrhage, and sepsis may occur, especially after attempts at delivery.

Fetal complications with contracted pelvis

Premature and often prolonged rupture of the membranes may result in amnionitis, omphalitis, placentitis, septicemia, or congenital pneumonia. Prolapse of the umbilical cord will cause hypoxia if occlusion develops. Severe molding of the head, often with excessive overlapping of the bones at the suture lines, may result in intracranial hemorrhage. Difficult forceps delivery can be critically traumatic.

UTERINE DYSTOCIA

Uterine dystocia is the inefficient action of the uterine musculature during the birth process. The uterine contractions may be too weak, too short, irregular, or infrequent. Hence progressive cervical dilatation and effacement and descent of the presenting part do not occur.

Uterine dystocia complicates almost 5% of all labors at term, and about 90% of these patients are primigravidas. Uterine dystocia is responsible for increased maternal and perinatal morbidity and mortality, resulting mainly from infection, hemorrhage, or trauma.

In primary uterine inertia, inefficient contractions persist from the onset of labor. The latent phase of the first stage of labor is usually prolonged, but inefficient contractions may continue into and even through the subsequent stages of labor (Fig. 24-3).

Inefficient uterine contractions may be characterized as hypertonic, hypotonic, or dystonic.

Although the periodic uterine contractions are of special significance, the resting tone or degree of uterine

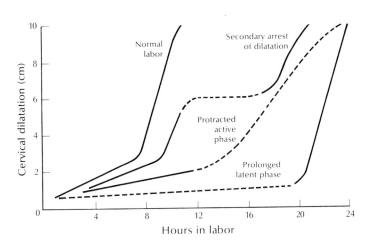

Fig. 24-2. Three major aberrations may be detected by comparing progress of dilatation with normal curve.

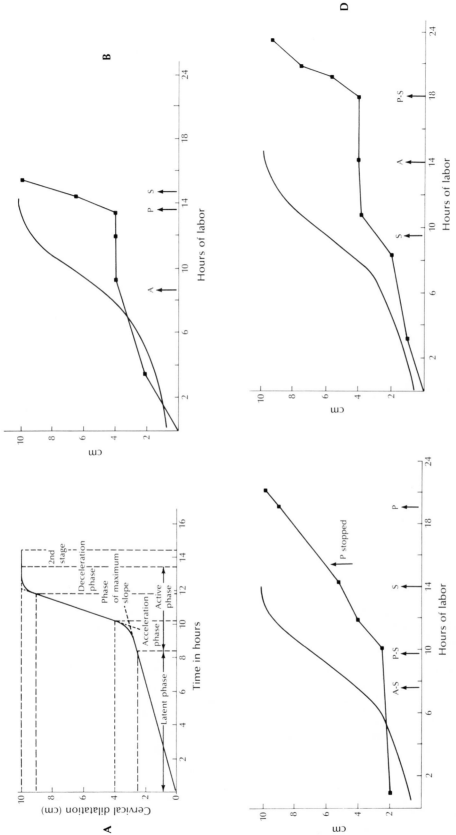

Fig. 24-3. A, Graphic appraisal of time factor in labor. *Latent phase* includes that portion of first stage between onset of labor contractions and acceleration in rate of cervical dilatation. Upswing in curve denotes onset of *active phase* of first stage of labor, which includes *acceleration phase, phase of maximum slope,* and *deceleration phase.* **B,** Labor graph of primigravida with prolonged latent phase of labor. Sedation was given at 9 hours, and amniotomy was performed at fourteenth hour. Latent phase persisted until oxytocin (Pitocin) was given. Position was ROP; infant weighed 2405 gm. *S* = sedation, *P* = Pitocin, *A* = amniotomy. **C,** Labor graph of primigravida with dysfunctional latent and slow slope active phase of labor. Notice that amniotomy and sedation did not terminate latent phase but Pitocin did. Pitocin did not influence slope of active phase. Position was LOT; the infant weighed 3543 gm. **D,** Anxious primigravida with tense, restless latent phase of labor. Amniotomy at 9 hours did not terminate latent phase. Sparteine sulfate was given at tenth, eleventh, and twelfth hours, but latent phase continued. Intravenous Pitocin was started at thirteenth hour, and perfectly normal active phase ensued. Position was LOA; infant weighed 3293 gm. (Modified from Friedman, E. A. 1955. Bull. Sloane Hosp. Wom. **1:**42.)

relaxation between contractions also is of great importance. When strong contractions are noted but with poor relaxation between, the pattern is hypertonic. Moreover, a uterus that is flaccid between contractions rarely contracts strongly. Here the pattern is hypotonic. Occasionally one encounters a patient whose uterus contracts irregularly, with one portion of the corpus more firm than the opposite side, for example. This is a dystonic pattern. Each of these abnormal sequences is inefficient, and if persistent, dystocia will result.

Normally a labor contraction is initiated in the myometrium near one cornu. It spreads rapidly over the uterus and to the lower segment, which has a low resting tone and is poorly contractile. In hypertonic uterine dystocia, the contractions may begin in the lower uterine segment and from there may spread upward (reversed polarity).

Occasionally there is general irritability of the uterus so that numerous ectopic contractions develop (colicky uterus). These dysrhythmic uterine contractions are not productive, and progress of labor is poor.

Hypertonic uterine contractions are extremely painful, and if due to reversed polarity, uterine discomfort and low backache are reported before the observer can palpate a contraction. Moreover, uterine irritability may be apparent, and one may observe an irregular firmness to the uterus as the uterus tightens. Increased tone often prevails even during the phase of relaxation. Another type of hypertonic uterine contraction pattern involves well-coordinated but extremely strong, prolonged contractions but with good relaxation between. A hypertonic contraction pattern may develop during oxytocin stimulation of labor. Fetal and maternal distress may develop.

Hypertonic uterine contractions endanger mother and fetus because of their violence and rapid recurrence. Moreover, if there is reversed polarity, the lack of uterine relaxation also reduces placental perfusion, and fetal hypoxia results.

Hypotonic uterine contractions display a normal gradient from fundus to cervix, but the contractions are weak, brief, or irregular. Severe pain is not a problem, and fetal distress is rare.

Hypotonic uterine contractions, often indistinguishable from prodromal labor, increase the likelihood of the patient having prolonged labor, sepsis, and the need for operative intervention.

Hypotonic uterine dystocia occurs in the following conditions:

1. False labor or the prodromal stage of true labor
2. Multiple pregnancy or hydramnios (uterine wall thinned or overstretched)
3. Missed or delayed labor, often after fetal death (? altered hormonal status)
4. Uterine abnormality (scarring, tumor anomaly)
5. Excessive analgesia (uterine contractions dulled)
6. High anxiety levels

Hypotonic and dystonic uterine dysfunction often recurs in subsequent labors.

Brief, weak (hypotonic) contractions may indicate that the woman is not yet in true labor or that she is only in the prodromal stage of labor. In other cases, such poor performance may be the result of inanition (a pathologic state of the body resulting from lack of food and water) due to debilitating systemic disease.

No abnormality of the uterus usually can be identified with uterine dystocia. However, anomalies of the uterus, such as bicornuate uterus, or tumors, such as myomata, occasionally may be present.

Hypertonic labor may terminate in abrupt, precipitate delivery. Unless this eventuality is anticipated and preparations made, delivery may be unattended, and maternal lacerations and excessive bleeding may result. If delivery is not controlled, fetal injury may occur.

The development of amnionitis is directly related to the length of labor and is more rapid and severe after rupture of the membranes. The incidence of instrument delivery is also increased in uterine inertia. If uterine atony complicates the third stage of labor, postnatal hemorrhage may further jeopardize the mother.

Hypertonic uterine dysfunction demands heavy sedation and expectant management. Uterine stimulation is absolutely contraindicated. After morphine, 15 mg intramuscularly, and glucose, 5 to 10% intravenously, tumultuous or dystonic labor usually will subside. After a period of sleep, a more normal pattern of labor may evolve.

Because the factors involved in primary uterine inertia are relative, the decision to intervene, for example, stimulate labor, depends on good clinical judgment rather than the passage of an arbitrary period of time.

Hypotonic uterine dysfunction may really be false labor. Mild sedation, for example, using phenobarbital (3 grains or 200 mg intramuscularly) or equivalent, may permit a period of rest after which a normal pattern of labor may be established. Occasionally, after fetal death, labor may be ineffectual, presumably because of hormonal deficiencies. Assuming a prolonged latent phase of labor, stimulation of uterine activity is required (p. 305).

In any case, fluid-electrolyte imbalance must be avoided and emotional support ensured.

Secondary uterine inertia

Secondary uterine inertia results when well-established, effectual uterine contractions become weak, brief or cease altogether. Secondary uterine inertia may occur as a result of one of the following:

- Fetopelvic disproportion (e.g., contracted pelvis)
- Excessive analgesia or anesthesia (e.g., epidural block)
- Overdistention of the uterus (e.g., multiple pregnancy)
- Maternal exhaustion or extreme emotional tension

Although secondary inertia may be serious in one pregnancy, it need not recur in a subsequent normal gestation.

The treatment of secondary uterine inertia depends on the cause. Ultrasonographic or radiographic studies must be obtained to rule out disproportion. Overdistention of the uterus may be relieved by rupture of the membranes, provided the cervix is at least 3 to 4 cm dilated and the presenting part is at least beginning to engage. The effects of excessive analgesia-anesthesia will dissipate with time. Heavy sedation (sleep) restores the tense or tired mother.

Oxytocin stimulation of labor, after assurance of no obstructive pathology and resolution of temporary difficulties, is in order. If, after a reasonable time, vaginal delivery seems unlikely or unduly hazardous, cesarean section must be accomplished. Generally, a low cervical cesarean section is most appropriate.

Annular uterine strictures

In normal labor, the cervix and rather passive lower uterine segment are drawn upward by the strongly contracting uterine fundus. The juncture between the two segments blends evenly. With neglected, obstructed labor, however, a narrow depressed *pathologic retraction ring (Bandl's ring)* develops and rises as labor wears on (Fig. 19-15). Bandl's ring, which holds the fetus in a powerful unrelenting grip even under anesthesia, is a sign of impending uterine rupture, and fetal distress often is recorded. Bandl's ring may be felt from above if the patient is thin, but generally, the ring is too high to be palpated vaginally. The treatment is immediate cesarean section.

In dysrhythmic uterine dystocia, perhaps initiated or aggravated by ill-advised oxytocin administration, the lower uterine segment fails to retract normally but tightens about the narrower parts of the fetus in one or more spastic *constriction rings*. After a constriction ring forms, the fetus cannot descend. Occasionally a ring may be felt from below through the partially dilated cervix, but the stricture will not rise or dissipate with continued labor.

Assuming the cervix to be fully dilated, deep inhalation anesthesia may relax the rings and operative vaginal delivery performed. In most instances, however, cesarean section may be necessary.

DYSTOCIA OF FETAL ORIGIN

Dystocia may be caused by fetal anomalies, excessive size, or malpresentation or malposition of the fetus. Although these are uncommon, they constitute obstetric emergencies.

Fetopelvic disproportion due to excessive size, abnormal development, and unusual presentation or position of the fetus almost always results in nonengagement. In vertex presentations, a large head (e.g., hydrocephalus) may never enter the superior strait. The same applies to malpresentation due to any fetal cause. In other instances, the head or breech may engage but obstructive labor follows because of gross abdominal enlargement (e.g., polycystic kidneys) or because the aftercoming head is large and deformed. The type of arrest will depend on (1) the presentation and the type and degree of pelvic deformity and (2) the mother's pelvic architecture and pelvic diameters.

Fetal dystocia may be classified in accordance with the cause of the abnormality as follows:

1. *Large fetus.* Excessive fetal size is arbitrarily 4000 gm (8 pounds 13½ ounces or more) in North America. Such large fetuses represent about 5% of term births. Frequently, excessive size is a result of diabetes mellitus, obesity, maternal multiparity, or large size of one or both parents.
2. *Fetal anomaly* (e.g., hydrocephalus, conjoined twins, gross ascites or abdominal tumor, myelomeningocele).
3. *Fetal malpresentation or position* (e.g., compound presentation or mentum posterior).

Lack of engagement or poor progress invariably leads to prolonged labor. Maternal distress may impress the observer. With a transverse lie, a floating vertex, or breech, rupture of the membranes often permits prolapse of the cord, whereupon fetal distress becomes an acute problem. Extended labor, multiple examinations, and the need for operative intervention increase the likelihood of sepsis—a threat to both mother and baby.

Unusual size or contour of the uterus may be noted with a fetal anomaly. Polyhydramnios often accompanies fetal maldevelopment. Moreover, an abnormal lie may be diagnosed, or the presenting part may fail to engage if anomalous cranial or sacral development pertains. A fetus with an abdominal tumor, for example, may deliver partially, only to arrest because of its protuberant abdomen. Breech birth of a fetus with hydrocephalus may proceed normally until the head must enter the inlet where obstruction occurs.

X-ray films may disclose fetal skeletal maldevelopment. Soft tissue films or amniography may disclose unusual fetal contours. Maternal pelvimetry and fetometry should be obtained if disproportion or anomaly is suspected. Moreover, an abnormal lie or position may be revealed.

One considers malpresentation or malposition of a normal fetus when engagement fails to occur. Abdominal tumors such as an ovarian cyst or a low-lying placenta may arrest the fetal presenting part above the inlet.

Management

X-ray pelvimetry and, if feasible, fetal cephalometry are done if the fetus is clinically "large" and at term or postdue. Assuming no demonstrable disproportion, a trial of labor is in order when the cervix is favorable (p. 357).

Shoulder dystocia is a serious complication, particularly in the delivery of a large postdate fetus. In shoulder dystocia, the head delivers to the neck, but the shoulders fail to engage or they jam in the inlet. If the posterior arm of the fetus is manually swept down and into the vagina, the shoulders may come through and the delivery can be completed. In another maneuver to encourage engagement of the shoulder girdle, the operator may "rock" the anterior fetal shoulders from side to side using an exterior hand placed over the lower uterine segment. A third solution may be internal rotation of the most accessible shoulder around 180 degrees. Thus, with the addition of traction, the fetus is "rotated out" of the birth canal. Cleidotomy may be employed for delivery of a dead fetus with shoulder dystocia.

Persistent, compound transverse lie generally will require cesarean section because elective podalic version is a hazardous procedure, even when the membranes are intact.

Breech delivery of an unrecognized hydrocephalic fetus will require decompression of the head. This can be accomplished by the insertion of a trocar passed vaginally through the foramen magnum of the fetus. Severe damage to the neonate is likely, but cesarean section could never be accomplished in time to save the abnormal infant.

Early recognition and elective vaginal delivery (if feasible) of a fetus that cannot survive are best. A long labor or traumatic delivery should be avoided in the best interests of the mother, fetus, and family. The prognosis for an anomalous infant depends on the seriousness and extent of the abnormality. A large infant may require special neonatal care. Moreover, investigation of the mother for possible diabetes mellitus within 24 hours of delivery is important.

COMPLICATIONS OF THIRD STAGE OF LABOR
Postnatal hemorrhage

Hemorrhage is a leading cause of maternal death the world over. Postnatal hemorrhage, traditionally the loss of 500 ml of blood or more after delivery, is the most common and most serious type of excessive obstetric blood loss. At least 5% of maternity patients suffer postnatal hemorrhage. Approximately 2% of these receive blood replacement, but fully twice this number should be transfused. Frequently, blood is unavailable or it is not considered an urgent need. Generally, an estimate is given, but many women lose at least 500 ml during the birth process and the first 24 hours after delivery. Hemorrhage of 1000 ml of blood or more is rare today.

A small woman can withstand the loss of blood less than a large one. It has been noted that the average maternity patient can lose up to 1% of her blood volume without immediate critical consequence. Therefore a more meaningful definition of postnatal hemorrhage is the loss of 1% or more of body weight, a figure easily referable to blood volume because 1 ml of blood weighs 1 gm.

Postnatal hemorrhage may be sudden, even exsanguinating, or moderate but persistent bleeding, with a significant total. This may continue for days or weeks. Postnatal hemorrhage may be early, within the first 24 hours after delivery, or late, from the 24 hours after delivery until the twenty-eighth day.

Control of bleeding from the placental site is accomplished by prolonged contraction and retraction of interlacing myometrial muscle strands. A firm or contracted uterus does not bleed postnatally. Therefore careful assessment of uterine tone and the maintenance of uterine contractions through manual or chemical stimulation are important parts of postnatal care.

Etiology. The causes in approximate order of frequency are as follows:

1. Mismanagement of the third stage of labor (e.g., incomplete placental separation)
2. Uterine atony due to excessive analgesia or anesthesia, prolonged labor, overdistention of the uterus

3. Lacerations of the birth canal
4. Hematologic disorders (e.g., defibrination syndrome)
5. Complications of pregnancy (e.g., inversion of the uterus, placenta accreta)
6. Tumors of the cervix or uterus
7. Medical complications of pregnancy (e.g., hyperthyroidism, vitamin K deficiency)
8. Infections of the genital tract (e.g., endometritis)

Early postnatal hemorrhage almost invariably is due to uterine atony, lacerations of the birth canal, or coagulopathy. Late postnatal hemorrhage most commonly is the result of subinvolution of the placental site, retained placental tissue, or infection.

Clinical findings. It is helpful to consider the problem of excessive bleeding with reference to the stages of labor. From delivery of the fetus until the separation of the placenta, the character and quantity of the blood passed may suggest the cause of excessive bleeding. For example, dark blood is probably of venous origin, perhaps from varices or superficial lacerations of the birth canal. Bright blood is arterial and indicates, for example, deep lacerations of the cervix. Spurts of blood with clots may indicate partial placental separation; the failure of blood to clot or remain clotted is indicative of a coagulopathy.

The period from the separation of the placenta to its delivery may be when excessive bleeding occurs. Frequently, this is the result of incomplete placental separation, often due to poor management of the third stage of labor (e.g., undue manipulation of the fundus, failure to elevate the corpus, a separated placenta trapped by partial closure of the cervix).

After the placenta has been recovered, persistent or excessive blood loss usually is the result of atony of the uterus (e.g., its failure to contract well or maintain its contraction) or prolapse of the uterus into the pelvis.

Late hemorrhage may be the result of partial involution of the uterus and unrecognized lacerations of the birth canal.

Complications of postnatal hemorrhage are immediate or delayed. Hypovolemic shock (pp. 239 to 242) and death may occur from sudden exsanguinating hemorrhage. Delayed complications provoked by postnatal hemorrhage include anemia, puerperal infection, and thromboembolization.

Prevention. Correct management of labor and delivery, particularly the third stage of labor, is vital for the control of bleeding during the third stage and for the period immediately after delivery. One must anticipate possible complications and plan to avoid postnatal hemorrhage. The following may be of great value in support of the patient:

1. Intravenous fluids are administered prior to delivery, and the rapid administration of 5% glucose in normal saline, for example, should replace fluids and electrolytes, especially after a long labor.
2. Analgesia is limited and anesthetics that provoke hypotension (e.g., spinal anesthesia) and that relax the uterus (e.g., halothane, ether) are avoided.
3. Dilute oxytocin is administered after delivery, 5 units in 500 ml of 5% dextrose in water "piggy-back" or with a "Y" adapter joined to the original intravenous started earlier.
4. Ergonovine, 0.2 mg, is given intramuscularly, immediately after the recovery of the placenta.
5. The fundus is elevated and gently massaged for at least 15 minutes after completion of the third stage of labor.
6. The patient is observed for at least an hour in the delivery room or in the postnatal recovery room until all vital signs are normal and bleeding is minimal.

Management. See hemorrhagic disorders (pp. 232 to 242) and fourth stage of labor (pp. 335 to 338).

1. Emergency measures (performed by physician)
   a. Inspect and repair the episiotomy and lacerations, including those involving the cervix, in *all* postnatal patients.
   b. Attempt placental expression only when signs of separation are notable.
   c. With incomplete separation of the placenta and marked bleeding, do not delay—manually separate and extract the placenta. (Additional anesthesia probably will not be necessary.)
   d. Treat uterine atony by elevation of the uterus and the intravenous administration of oxytocin, 5 units well diluted.
   e. Compress the uterus with the fist if necessary.
   f. Pack the uterus if additional assistance or subsequent surgery is necessary, as for repair or removal of a ruptured uterus. (Packing is poor primary treatment for uterine bleeding because often the uterus will not remain tightly packed and the patient will bleed around the pack.)
   g. Transfuse the patient early, administer oxygen by face mask, and apply additional antishock therapy—do not wait for collapse.
2. Specific therapy
   This depends on the problem. For example, partial inversion of the uterus may require replacement of the fundus and temporary packing; late bleeding may require dilatation and curettage.

Prognosis. The cause of the bleeding, the amount and rapidity of the blood loss, and the success of correction determine the patient's prognosis in large measure. One must consider also the patient's general health and other obstetric problems such as preeclampsia-eclampsia with respect to her likely recovery. Maternal mortality and morbidity are directly related to the amount of blood lost by postnatal hemorrhage. Moreover, a febrile puerperium is likely if blood loss is not replaced promptly.

Puerperal inversion of the uterus

Inversion of the uterus (turning inside-out) after delivery is a critical obstetric complication. The inversion may be complete or partial. Traction applied to the fundus, especially when the uterus is flaccid, may result in inversion. More specifically the causes include straining (Valsalva's maneuver); traction on the cord before the placenta has separated; the Credé maneuver, that is, kneading the uterine fundus in an attempt to separate an adherent placenta; and placental extraction under deep relaxing anesthesia. Occasionally a large uterine tumor may be responsible for inversion.

Profound shock follows complete inversion; postnatal hemorrhage accompanies partial uterine inversion. Prompt assistance is imperative because the maternal mortality may reach 30% without immediate correct therapy.

Prevention, always the easiest, cheapest, and most effective therapy, is especially appropriate in the avoidance of puerperal uterine inversion. One must not pull on the umbilical cord unless the placenta has definitely separated. The fundus should never be used as a piston to "push the placenta out." The Credé maneuver is not used; it is harmful and not useful. Regional anesthesia is employed when feasible. A responsible attendant remains with the patient until the uterus is firm and rounded.

Physical findings. Complete inversion of the uterus is obvious; a large, red, rounded mass (perhaps with the placenta attached) protrudes 20 to 30 cm outside the introitus. Incomplete inversion cannot be seen but must be felt; a smooth mass will be palpated through the dilated cervix, reducing the size of the uterine cavity by at least half.

Treatment

1. Combat shock, which invariably is out of proportion to the blood loss. Give oxytocin intravenously to contract the uterus. (Ergot products are strictly contraindicated because the cervix, as well as the uterus, will contract, and replacement may be difficult unless the cervix is severed.)

2. Replace the uterus under deep ether or halothane anesthesia by inserting and "working" first the lower uterine segment, then finally, the fundus upward while applying traction to the cervix. Leave the placenta attached if it has not yet separated, then manually free the placenta. Give ergonovine maleate (Ergotrate) intramuscularly, and as the uterus and cervix contract, withdraw the placenta with the hand. Pack the uterus if inversion seems about to recur.

3. Abdominal or vaginal surgery may be necessary to reposition the uterus if successful manual replacement fails.

4. Transfuse the patient; initiate broad-spectrum antibiotic therapy; and insert a nasogastric tube to decompress the stomach and to minimize adynamic or paralytic ileus, a frequent sequel.

Prognosis. Successful prompt vaginal replacement is likely in about 75% of patients. Uterine inversion may recur in a subsequent delivery occasionally, despite the usual precautions.

Retained placenta

See Chapter 26.

REFERENCES

Aladjem, S. 1975. Risks in the practice of modern obstetrics (ed. 2). St. Louis, The C. V. Mosby Co.

Babson, S. G., Benson, R. C., Pernoll, M. L., Benda, G. I. 1975. Management of high-risk pregnancy and intensive care of the neonate (ed. 3). St. Louis, The C. V. Mosby Co.

Beazley, J. M., and others. 1975. Maintenance of labor. Br. Med. J. **2**:248.

Crinkshank, D. P., and White, C. A. 1973. Obstetric malpresentations: twenty years' experience. Am. J. Obstet. Gynecol. **116**:1097.

Edington, P. T., and others. 1975. Influence on practice of routine intrapartum fetal monitoring. Br. Med. J. **3**:341.

Fujikara, T., and Klionsky, B. 1975. The significance of meconium staining. Am. J. Obstet. Gynecol. **121**:45.

Gabert, H. A., and Stenchever, M. A. 1973. Continuous electronic monitoring of fetal heart rate during labor. Am. J. Obstet. Gynecol. **115**:919.

Greenhill, J. 1974. Biologic principles and modern practice of obstetrics. Philadelphia, W. B. Saunders Co.

Hellman, L., and Pritchard, J. 1971. Williams obstetrics (ed. 14). New York, Appleton-Century-Crofts.

Jacob, S. J. 1971. Rupture of the uterus: a study of 52 cases. J. Obstet. Gynaecol. India **21**:22.

Joyce, D. N., and others. 1975. Role of pelvimetry in the active management of labour. Br. Med. J. **4**:505.

Kalyanikutty, C., and Rajagopalam, C. K. 1973. Engaged–unengaged head in primiparas getting into labor: graphic appraisal utilizing Friedman curve. J. Obstet. Gynaecol. India **23**:259.

Natelson, I. E., and Sayers, M. P. 1973. Fate of children sustaining severe head trauma during birth. Pediatrics **51**:169.

O'Driscoll, K., and Stronge, J. M. 1975. Active management of labour and occipito posterior position. Aust. N.Z. J. Obstet. Gynaecol. **15:**1.

Oxorn, H., and Foote, W. 1968. Human labor in birth (ed. 2). New York. Appleton-Century-Crofts.

Persianinov, L. S. 1973. Effect of normal and abnormal labor on the fetus: a survey. Acta Obstet. Gynecol. Scand. **52:**29.

Saylor, D. E. 1975. Understanding presurgical anxiety. AORN J. **22:**624.

Southerst, J. R., and Case, B. D. 1975. Caesarean section and its place in the active approach to delivery. Clin. Obstet. Gynecol. **2:**241.

Specht, E. E. 1975. Brachial plexus palsy in the newborn: incidence and prognosis. Clin. Orthop. **110:**32.

Stookey, R. A., and others. 1973. Abnormal contraction patterns in patients monitored during labor. Obstet. Gynecol. **42:**359.

Tan, K. L. 1973. Brachial palsy. J. Obstet. Gynaecol. Br. Commonw. **80:**60.

CHAPTER 25

Fetal-neonatal complications

CARE OF HIGH-RISK OR COMPROMISED NEONATE AT BIRTH

Because only about 60% of potential neonatal problems can be diagnosed prior to delivery, every maternity service must have proper facilities and experienced personnel available to care for any distressed neonate until its vital signs are stable or until it can be transferred to a neonatal special care center by a capable transport team.

RESUSCITATION OF DEPRESSED NEONATE

The life or health of an individual depends on early adequate pulmonary ventilation at birth. Spontaneous breathing by most newborns will occur within 1 minute. Respiratory delay, usually the result of predelivery asphyxia or respiratory depression after heavy maternal analgesia or anesthesia, may complicate the process. If resuscitation is delayed or ineffectual, permanent neurologic deficiency or death may result. Therefore at every delivery the attending physician, nurse midwife, or nurse practitioner should be experienced in resuscitation techniques to effectively treat the likely or occasionally unsuspected depressed infant. Moreover, a specially trained physician-nurse team should be available in addition to the obstetrician, who may be too occupied in the treatment of a serious obstetric problem, for example, eclampsia, to resuscitate the depressed neonate.

Resuscitation equipment and medications needed in delivery room

A resuscitation console, cart, or trolley in the delivery room (Fig. 25-1) should be adjacent to oxygen and vacuum outlets and provide the following:
1. Well-lighted area of sufficient height for easy infant intubation
2. Radiant heat source for prevention of cold stress
3. Battery-powered heart rate monitor
4. Stethoscope

5. Ambu bag (or equivalent) and infant masks of varied sizes
6. Pharyngeal airways (Nos. 00, 0, and 1)
7. Infant laryngoscopes with Nos. 1 and 0 blades, together with spare batteries and bulbs
8. Endotracheal tubes attached to adaptors
9. Umbilical vessel catheterization equipment
10. Appropriate syringes and needles
11. Intravenous tubing and arm board

Medications needed in the delivery room include the following:
1. Sodium bicarbonate solution (1 ml = 0.9 mEq)
2. Glucose, 10% and 50% solutions
3. Distilled water
4. Epinephrine (1:1000 in 1 ml ampules)
5. Calcium gluconate, 10% solution
6. Isoproterenol (Isuprel)
7. Digitoxin (0.1 mg/ml)
8. Nalorphine, levallorphan, or naloxone
9. Dexamethasone (Decadron)
10. Plasma protein fraction (human) plasmanate
11. Furosemide (Lasix)

The physician member of the resuscitation team will be expected to know the dosage, mode of administration, and other information concerning the drugs just listed. The nurse anticipates the need for solutions and equipment and has them ready for use.

Severely depressed infants (Apgar score 0 to 3)

Severely depressed infants require immediate resuscitation. Pathophysiology involves hypoxia and significant acidosis. Most severely depressed neonates are flaccid, pale, grossly apneic, and either only slightly reactive or unresponsive to stimulation. In most cases, the heart rate will be 80 beats/min or less. Speed and skill are of the utmost importance.

Most severely depressed neonates will require the treatment measures listed on p. 370.

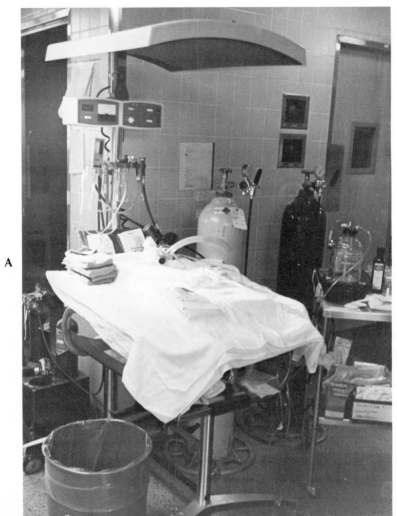

A

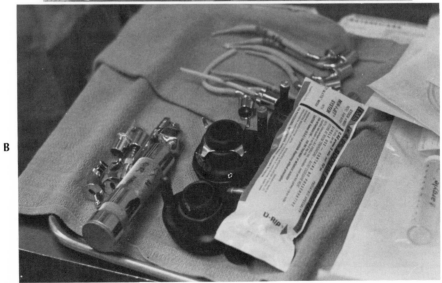

B

Fig. 25-1. A, Resuscitation or treatment console for neonate at risk: radiant overhead heater, suction, oxygen by mask or CPAP, and bronchoscope. **B,** Resuscitation equipment for newborn.

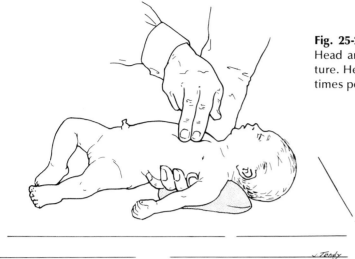

Fig. 25-2. Technique for closed chest heart massage. Head and shoulders are supported in "sniffing" posture. Heart is compressed 100 to 120 times/min, or two times per second.

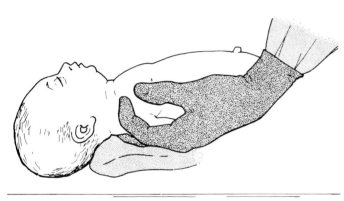

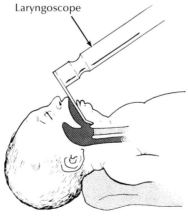

Laryngoscope

B

Fig. 25-3. Technique of intubation and resuscitation. **A,** Neonate's shoulders are supported so that head is in "sniffing" posture. **B,** Laryngoscope supports tongue to permit view of nasopharynx and introduction of suction tube.

Continued.

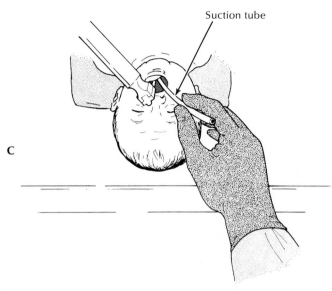

Suction tube

C

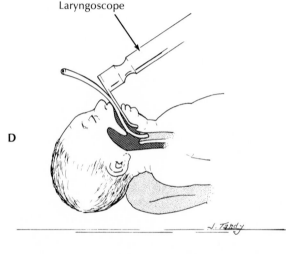

Laryngoscope

D

Fig. 25-3, cont'd. **C,** View from above of laryngoscope in place and suction tube. **D,** Tracheal suctioning with laryngoscope in place. (Modified from Benson, R. C. 1974. Handbook of obstetrics and gynecology [ed. 5]. Los Altos, Calif., Lange Medical Publications.)

1. Laryngoscopy and suction of the airway, particularly if thick mucus or meconium is present
2. External cardiac massage to augment the circulation if the heart rate is 80 beats/min or less (Fig. 25-2)
3. Sodium bicarbonate solution via an intraumbilical vein catheter to reduce acidosis
4. Support of metabolism by glucose and calcium gluconate solution intravenously
5. Epinephrine solution via the umbilical vein catheter or in critical cases by intracardiac administration
6. Levallorphan (Lorfan) or nalorphine (Nalline) intravenously (preferably) or intramuscularly if depression is due to a narcotic administered to the mother (Naloxone [Narcan], a pure narcotic antagonist, may be given, since it does not depress respiration or cause sedation in the individual whose depressed state may *not* be narcotic induced.)

7. Chest x-ray studies if persistent cyanosis or other marked respiratory difficulty is noted, but with continuing ventilatory support provided (consider diaphragmatic hernia or another congenital anomaly or massive collapse of the lung due to complications of resuscitation) in such cases

The technique of intubation and resuscitation is as follows (Fig. 25-3):

1. After placing the infant on a flat surface, elevate the shoulders with a folded towel.
2. Introduce the infant laryngoscope with the left hand through the right angle of the neonate's mouth.
3. Advance the blade gently about 2 cm while bringing it to the midline and while pushing the tongue to the left.
4. Visualize the pharynx and epiglottis, and by lifting the tip of the blades, expose the vocal cords.
5. Suction the trachea free of mucus, blood, and meconium.
6. Insert an endotracheal tube (Cole Fr 14 or 16 or

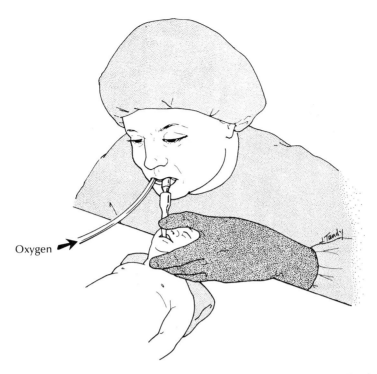

Fig. 25-4. Operator puffs oxygen-enriched air into neonate's endotracheal tube.

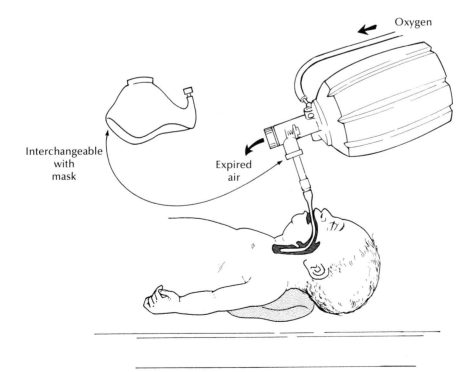

Fig. 25-5. Methods of administering oxygen through endotracheal tube.

equivalent for term infants; use a smaller size for preterm infants). Advance the tip about 1.5 cm beyond vocal cords. (Stylets may be traumatic and are rarely essential.)

7. Withdraw the laryngoscope; give a few short oxygen (or air) insufflations while auscultating the chest to assure proper tubal placement (in the trachea, not in the esophagus) (Figs. 25-4 and 25-5).

Methods of artificial ventilation include mouth-to-mouth ventilation, mouth-to-tube intratracheal ventilation, and resuscitators (e.g., Kreiselman, Ambu, Hope, Penlon).

Moderately depressed infants (Apgar score 4 to 6)

Moderately depressed neonates will be cyanotic or pale. Irregular or absent respiration will be apparent, together with diminished muscle tone and reflex responsiveness. Generally, the heart rate will not be increased.

The resuscitation procedure for these infants is as follows:

1. Apply gentle peripheral stimulation.

2. Administer air or oxygen by mask ventilation if the infant does not breathe spontaneously after several inflations of the lungs or if bradycardia develops (Fig. 25-6).

3. Laryngoscope the infant, suction the airway, and insert an intratracheal tube.

4. Administer oxygen in puffs every 5 to 10 seconds. If not promptly responsive, the infant should be treated as severely depressed.

Mildly depressed infants (Apgar score 7 to 8)

Infants who are mildly depressed may be slightly cyanotic, and their respirations often are irregular. Muscle tone usually is reduced. Vigorous resuscitation measures rarely are required. In addition to keeping the infant warm and clearing the airway, the following may be effective:

1. Stimulate the infant gently by rubbing the back or slapping the soles of the feet.

2. Apply thermostimulation by blowing oxygen from a mask or funnel into the infant's face. If these measures do not evoke a prompt respiratory response, treat as a moderately depressed infant.

INTRANATAL FETAL DEATH

FHT may be lost late in the first stage of labor or during the second stage. The atmosphere in the labor unit becomes tense and subdued. There is a sudden change from joyful anticipation to dread. Silence accompanies the birth. Resuscitative measures are attempted. All focus on the newborn. Shock and disbelief are experienced by parent and staff alike.

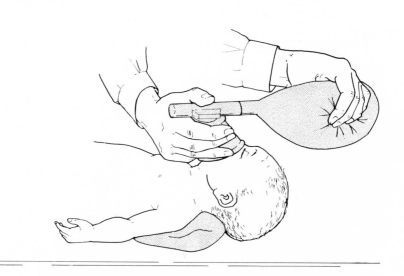

Fig. 25-6. Portable resuscitator. Method of administering room air under positive pressure. Mask fits over nose and mouth snugly but does not encroach on eyes. Some portable resuscitators may be connected to oxygen sources.

Stillbirth, neonatal death, and the nurse

The nurse may be unaware that she is struggling with her reactions to grief. She may resort to reassuring and comforting the grieving individual(s) in a manner that does not foster a healthy grieving response. Some commonly heard responses given by physicians, nurses, and well-meaning friends are as follows:

- "There was a reason why God wanted this baby. Have faith."
- "It's God's will. We have to have faith that it was for the best."
- "It's probably better this way. This often happens when the baby has something wrong with it."
- "You are so young. There's time for more."
- "Be thankful you have those other lovely children at home. They'll be a solace and comfort to you."

Other such behaviors give the message that to face grief is "bad" for a person and to avoid facing it is better for all concerned. The following behaviors by nurses and physicians are examples:

1. Transferring the mother to another ward
2. Telling the mother to stay in her room (usually single) room when the babies are out with the other mothers
3. Avoiding talking about the infant, quelling tears, and forbidding her to see and hold the infant

Somehow it is thought that to avoid an issue is the healthiest and easiest way. It does prevent "scenes." Out of sight is out of mind. But out of sight is not out of the mother's mind. The mother has felt life. She has developed a relationship with the infant through shared internal physical sensation and fantasy. If the child lives for a few hours or days after birth, the mother's relationship to the child has progressed even further. Even after delivery, the hormones that sustain an attachment between mother and child are still present, as are the physical signs and discomforts that a delivery has occurred. At home are the baby clothes and furniture, family, and friends, awaiting the hoped-for new arrival. Resolution of grief is important *now*. Resolution of grief can be a healthy growth-inducing process.

Mothers and family look to the hospital staff to meet their needs. Having had an unfortunate maternity experience, these mothers may suffer a severe blow to their sense of worth associated with the ability to give life and to their role concept, self-esteem, and femininity. Nursing interventions that may assist the grieving family in coping with this ego-threatening experience may foster a healthy mourning process and can be incorporated easily within the busiest nursing assignment. Death is often equated with powerlessness, an end, and failure. However, the nurse need not be professionally and personally helpless. Preventive mental health measures are well within the scope of the nurse. Some therapeutic reactions and actions by the nurse are as follows:

1. Parents need an objective listener, one who is genuinely interested and willing to face true feelings and will not try to "talk them out of it."
2. Parents need to feel that those around them know that it is natural for them to feel sad, weepy, and easily distracted.
3. Nurses should convey to parents that grieving takes time and that they may never really "get over it," although the pain does ease with time; good memories then tend to persist.
4. Nurses should be prepared for the anger and self-blame parents may feel and assist the parents to identify these feelings: "You may be wondering if you did or did not do something to cause this." Parents may not be able to work through their anger before discharge; some parents return or write many months later to apologize for their behavior and to thank those who were able to see beyond their anger and help them with their needs.
5. Coping with grief and recovering from childbirth exact a heavy toll on the mother's resources. Although the grieving process often makes sleep difficult and appetite nonexistent, adequate rest and diet must be assured to replenish the mother's vitality. Thoughtful nursing actions (e.g., backrubs, just sitting quietly with her) can meet very real, critical needs.
6. The nurse should prepare the parents for returning home, for example, what to expect of themselves emotionally and physically and what they can expect from the older children. People frequently express the fear of "going crazy" when they experience reactions that they do not expect or understand.

Physical symptoms that parents may experience include sleep problems with fatigue, anorexia, muscle aches and "knots," gastrointestinal symptoms, and palpitations.

Psychologic or emotional symptoms that parents may experience include an inability to concentrate for long on any one activity (i.e., their minds may wander or they may feel everything is whirling around in their heads) and pressure in the head. The mother may hold her abdomen and state she feels "empty" and that her arms "ache to hold a baby." Parents may fear being alone, wish to go away somewhere, or become overconcerned about or disinterested in their other children. Irritability with or disinterest in the other children may compound guilt feelings.

Reactions of the older children are discussed on pp. 570 and 571.

PLAN OF CARE: STILLBIRTH AND EARLY NEONATAL DEATH

PATIENT CARE OBJECTIVES
1. Mother (and family) begins the grieving process.
2. Mother (and family) receives anticipatory guidance regarding components of grief process and possible reactions of family and friends.
3. Mother retains feelings of self-worth.

NURSING INTERVENTIONS

Diagnostic	Therapeutic	Educational

1. Assess mother's response: Does she show appropriate signs and symptoms of grieving process?
  a. Shock, disbelief, and anger.
  b. Developing awareness.
  c. Resolution or acceptance (this may not be seen during short hospital stay).
2. Assess mother's support system: husband, family, friends.
3. Note mother's age—adolescent's needs are different from middle-aged woman.
4. Are there definite cultural (or religious) influences that help mother define death and direct her grieving process?
	1. Provide physical care and meet dependency needs in thoughtful and unhurried manner.
	2. Arrange for time for mother to talk over labor and delivery:
	  a. To validate and assimilate experience.
	  b. To work through shock and disbelief.
	  c. To clarify events.
	  d. To ease her need to search for reasons.
	3. Assist her to identify and verbalize feelings:
	  a. "You must feel like you were cheated."
	  b. "Somehow it just doesn't seem fair."
	  c. "You seem so angry. I wonder if you're thinking that someone may have done something."
	  d. "One feels so helpless, so powerless, in this type of situation."
	  e. "There are times when your feelings may seem strange to you."
	  f. "How do you feel when you see the babies in the nursery, in another mother's arms, or when someone asks you about your baby?"
	4. *Do not* minimize event with comments like "You are still young," "You have others," etc.
	5. Let mother share her feelings without giving scientific reasons, referring to logic, etc.
		1. Mother's postnatal physical needs must be met:
		  a. To revitalize after pregnancy and labor.
		  b. To release energy for emotional work.
		2. In her search for causes, mother reviews and rehashes events leading up to stillbirth.
		  a. It is normal to look for answers. Nurse should not feel she must have all answers on her fingertips.
		  b. Focusing in on event to exclusion of all other activities of daily living and interaction with other family members is normal now.
		  c. It is normal to feel confused, indecisive, and a sense of unreality. Some grieving persons fearfully confide, "I think I must be going crazy."
		3. Adolescent needs:
		  a. Reassurance of her femininity. Adolescent who is unwed may have become pregnant to prove to herself her femininity and reproductive capacity.
		  b. Reassurance that her conversations with nurse are confidential.
		  c. "Safe" authority figure to whom to vent angry feelings. Bravado, defensiveness, and withdrawal may be signs of immaturity and struggles with autonomy.
		  d. Support and empathy. Self-esteem and a sense of worth can be generated by including her in planning for her care after discharge, providing information regarding her body after delivery, referring her to teenage rap sessions at family planning and adolescent clinics or other groups in area.
		  e. Role modeling in facing grief, open communication, feeling safe and comfortable in dealing with unpleasant situation.

PLAN OF CARE: STILLBIRTH AND EARLY NEONATAL DEATH—cont'd

NURSING INTERVENTIONS—cont'd

Diagnostic	Therapeutic	Educational
		4. *This* baby is important *now*. Mother needs to talk about *this* baby. She does not want or need to focus on her other children or any suggestions for substitutes for her loss.
		5. Occasionally mother must withdraw for short while as if to take experience a small piece at a time. Signs that she is withdrawing are closing her eyes, drawing curtains around her bed (or shutting door), changing subject.

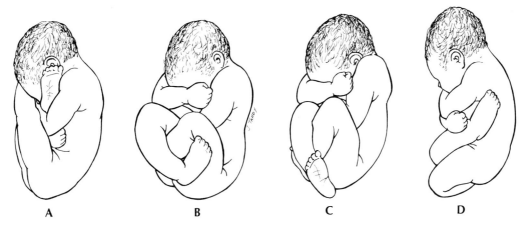

Fig. 25-7. Types of breech presentation. **A,** Frank breech. **B,** Complete breech. **C,** Incomplete breech. Foot extends below buttocks. **D,** Incomplete breech. Knee extends below buttocks.

DELIVERY OF FETUS IN BREECH PRESENTATION
Mechanism of labor in breech presentation

The mechanism of labor in breech presentation is comparable to that in vertex presentation, only the polarity is reversed. The bitrochanteric diameter, the greatest breech dimension, must be related to pelvic diameters just as the biparietal of the vertex, which is the largest diameter of the well-flexed vertex. The types of breech presentation are shown in Fig. 25-7. The steps in the passage of the frank breech through the pelvis are as follows (Fig. 25-8):

1. *Engagement* generally occurs in the longest diameter, for example, an oblique diameter of the pelvic inlet of the gynecoid pelvis.

2. *Lateral flexion* (rather than anteroposterior flexion in a vertex presentation) is not great, but it is important. The anterior hip usually descends more rapidly than the posterior at the pelvic inlet and outlet.

3. *Internal rotation* can be expected to occur when the breech reaches the pelvic floor (levator musculature). The bitrochanteric diameter then rotates to the AP of the pelvis.

4. *Lateral flexion* (rather than extension in vertex presentations) occurs when the anterior hip pivots beneath the symphysis pubis to allow delivery of the posterior hip, which appears first.

5. *External rotation* or *restitution* occurs after delivery of the breech and the legs. The baby's body turns toward the mother's side to which its back was directed when engagement occurred.

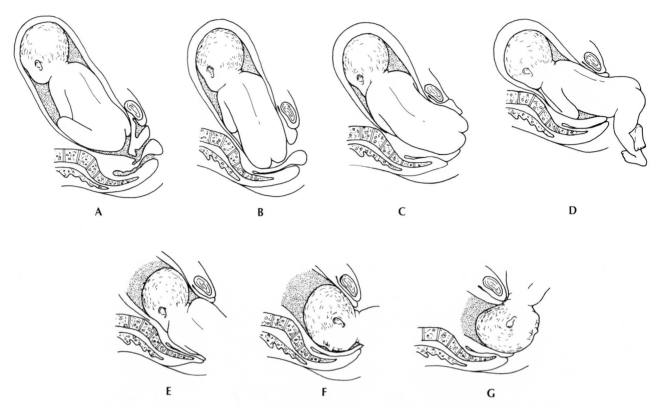

Fig. 25-8. Mechanism of labor in breech position. **A,** Breech before onset of labor. **B,** Engagement and internal rotation. **C,** Lateral flexion. **D,** External rotation or restitution. **E,** Internal rotation of head. **F,** Face rotates to sacrum when occiput is anterior. **G,** Head delivers by gradual flexion during elevation of fetal body.

With this sequence, the bisacromial diameter of the shoulders engages in the same diameter as the breech. Progressive descent occurs, and the anterior shoulder rotates to bring the shoulders into the AP of the pelvic inlet. Like the posterior hip, the posterior shoulder in breech presentation is delivered first while the body is supported.

The head engages in the identical diameter as the shoulders. Flexion occurs when the head enters the pelvic inlet, and the biparietal diameter occupies the oblique diameter accepted by the shoulders. The head descends in the same manner as the shoulders. The occiput, if posterior, rotates to the hollow of the sacrum; or the face will rotate to the sacrum when the occiput is anterior on engagement. Hence the presenting part is brought to the AP of the outlet. Here the neck or chin stems beneath the symphysis pubis, and the head delivers by gradual flexion during elevation of the body by the attendant.

Breech delivery

Delivery of the fetus presenting as a breech is accomplished by one of the following methods:

- *Spontaneous breech delivery*—usually occurs when the mother is unattended and/or if the fetus is small
- *Assisted breech delivery*—support of the fetus only
- *Partial breech extraction*—extraction of the fetus after its expulsion to the umbilicus
- *Complete breech extraction*—the entire fetus delivered by the attendant
- *Cesarean section*—selected for delivery of high-risk breech presentations

The *spontaneous breech delivery* is in essence an emergency situation or one of neglect. Common in premature labor, the mother may deliver the breech at home without assistance or enroute to the hospital.

Assisted breech delivery is an "easy" birth, often of an infant smaller than average. The mother may be a multipara in strong labor who has made rapid progress. The attendant may have time only to elevate the fetus as it is quickly expelled.

Partial breech extraction requires knowledge of the mechanism of labor in breech presentation and procedures commonly used in the delivery of the shoulders and head. The following describes the actions of the physician conducting the delivery:

1. The cord is drawn down as soon as the umbilicus appears after delivery of the legs and trunk to avoid cord compression. If there is a short cord or one tightly wrapped about the trunk, neck, or other fetal part, the cord should be doubly clamped and cut.

2. A deep mediolateral episiotomy should be done at this point to minimize resistance of the muscles of the introitus.

3. Traction on the trunk of the infant wrapped in a towel to avoid slippage and provide warmth, together with slight rotation, should carry the bisacromial diameter into the AP of the pelvis. At this point, two fingers can be inserted into the vaginal canal to deliver the posterior shoulder first. This may be done by elevating the fetus upward and toward the mother's inguinal region to the side opposite its back. Thus the posterior shoulder is brought to the perineum, and the arm and shoulder can be brought out easily. Then the anterior arm can be delivered digitally.

If an arm is extended beside or above the head, two fingers passed over the shoulder usually can carry the arm downward across the chest for delivery as described in the previous step. The shoulder or arm must never be "hooked" with the operator's finger for the application of traction because neurologic or other injury may occur.

4. The aftercoming head may be delivered by the Mauriceau-Smellie Veit maneuver, the Bracht maneuver, or with forceps (Piper) application to the aftercoming head.

   a. The Mauriceau-Smellie-Veit maneuver

     (1) The fetus is placed astride the operator's left arm who then places two fingers of the left hand tightly over the mandible to flex the head.

     (2) He next places his right hand over the back, with two fingers curved over the shoulders, to guide the delivery with the right hand, using no traction, until the chin is visible.

     (3) An assistant standing to the patient's side applies firm, steady suprapubic pressure to bring the infant's head further into the pelvis.

     (4) The body is elevated slowly, and delivery gradually is accomplished without shoulder traction.

     (5) While flexion of the head is maintained by maxillary pressure, the occiput should deliver beneath the symphysis pubis.

   b. The Bracht maneuver

     (1) As soon as both scapula become visible, the back is gently lifted in an arch (without extension to avoid spinal injury) to the mother's abdomen. Generally, the arms will emerge spontaneously.

     (2) Suprapubic pressure is next applied to guide the head into the pelvis.

     (3) The suspended body is slowly brought closer toward the mother's abdomen, whereupon the chin, mouth, nose, and brow should deliver spontaneously.

     Bracht's maneuver is simple and effective. No intravaginal manipulation, traction, or rotation is required. However, this procedure cannot be employed if labor is desultory, the patient is uncooperative, the infant's position is posterior, the arms are extended, or the perineum is rigid. If the infant tries to breathe before it is delivered, Bracht's maneuver is abandoned and forceps extraction effected.

   c. Forceps delivery of the aftercoming head (p. 400).

Complete breech extraction often is called *breaking up a breech*. This may be necessary when a frank breech presents and progress ceases, with prolapse of the cord or when fetal distress is diagnosed. The feet are brought down for traction in a frank breech by Pinard's maneuver as follows:

1. The attendant inserts the right hand into the vagina if the fetal back is on the mother's right (or opposite if this applies), and the breech is displaced upward slightly. The anterior fetal thigh is identified, and the hand is slipped upward to the knee. The thigh is slightly abducted, which causes the knee to flex; the foot is grasped; and the foot and leg are brought out through the introitus.

2. Traction is applied downward in the axis of the vagina. If the breech descends readily, one should proceed with delivery.

3. If the breech is impacted, it will be necessary to bring the other leg down and extract the breech.

Neither forceps nor the vacuum extractor can be used to deliver a frank breech.

Traction by the fingers in the groin is never warranted unless the baby is dead.

The optimal size for a breech baby is between 2720 and 3410 gm (between 6 and 7 pounds 8 ounces). Those smaller or larger are at greater risk during delivery.

Average analgesia should not harm even the small breech fetus. A vaginal examination is performed at the

Table 25-1. Criteria for scoring*

	Points		
	0	**1**	**2**
Parity	Primigravida	Multipara	
Gestational age	39 weeks or more	38 weeks	37 weeks or less
Estimated fetal weight	More than 8 pounds (3630 gm)	7 pounds to 7 pounds 15 ounces (3175 to 3600 gm)	Less than 7 pounds (3175 gm)
Previous breech†	None	1	2 or more
Dilatation‡	2 cm	3 cm	4 cm or more
Station‡	−3 or higher	−2	−1 or lower

*From Zatuchni, G. I., and Andros, G. J. 1967. Am. J. Obstet. Gynecol. **98:**855.
†Greater than 2500 gm.
‡Determined by vaginal examination on admission.

time of rupture of the membranes to rule out prolapse of the cord. The patient is coached not to bear down until the cervix is definitely fully dilated. An experienced obstetrician and an assistant are scrubbed for every breech delivery. Pudendal block anesthesia is preferred for breech delivery, but this is delayed until the breech is crowning.

Prognostic scoring is a valuable approach toward planning for breech delivery (Table 25-1). A score of 3 or less generally justifies cesarean section, although it may be weighted slightly against the primigravida. A score of 4 requires further observation and reevaluation. If labor is strong, vaginal delivery is likely. With a score of 5, a successful vaginal delivery usually can be expected. Consultation and more liberal use of cesarean section in borderline cases are necessary to improve the salvage in breech presentation.

An ultraconservative attitude has gradually developed because the gross fetal mortality is 5% to 8% in breech delivery of infants over 2050 gm, even in large well-staffed hospitals. Now in numerous maternity centers, breech presentation is an indication for cesarean section at or near term in primigravidas and in multiparas with fetuses larger than 7½ pounds (estimate) when labor is ineffective or when hazardous complications arise.

The nursing care needed for a breech delivery is as follows:

1. *Prebirth labor of a term breech presentation.* The nursing care is unchanged from that of a vertex presentation because the complications arise as part of the delivery of the infant. However, the FHT are located above the umbilicus (Fig. 19-9). The labor may be prolonged

because the presenting part is soft and therefore does not help to dilate the cervix as efficiently.

The breech does not fill the pelvic cavity as completely as does the larger head; therefore the danger of prolapsed cord occurring with rupture of the membranes is increased. Frank meconium draining from the introitus is a normal finding in breech presentations, since the pressure on the abdomen forces the meconium from the bowel. Its appearance thus is not an indication of fetal distress.

Parents are more anxious if they are aware of the dangers to the fetus associated with the delivery and need support from attending nurses and physicians. The use of cesarean section as the mode of delivery for questionable fetopelvic disproportion has lessened the fear for infant survival. Mothers in this situation will need the care outlined for cesarean section (p. 400).

2. *Delivery.* Extra sterile towels and Piper forceps are added to the routine supplies and equipment on the delivery table.

Resuscitation equipment and supplies (p. 367) are readied for use. The resuscitation team and the operating room staff* should be notified and present for the delivery.

3. *Puerperium.* The care will depend on the method of delivery. For example, in the event of vaginal delivery, care is the same as for all mothers (Chapter 27) (for cesarean section, see p. 404).

The infant has little molding of the head, but his rest-

---

*In some areas the labor unit staff are responsible for care of patients undergoing cesarean sections.

ing posture, being that of a breech (if frank, the legs are straight up over the abdomen), must be explained to the parents.

VERSION

Version is a maneuver applied to change the presentation of the fetus within the uterus to one more favorable for delivery. Version is most often accomplished to convert a transverse lie to a vertex or breech presentation.

Three types of version are recognized:

* *External or cephalic version*—the change of a transverse or breech presentation to a vertex by external means
* *Podalic version*—breech presentation accomplished by internal manipulation
* *Combined version*—simultaneous external and internal manipulations employed

External or cephalic version

External version should reduce the perinatal mortality from about 15% (for all breech presentations) to approximately 3% for all vertex presentations. Actually, with external version, considerable improvement in perinatal morbidity and mortality is possible. Risks are involved such as cord accidents and premature separation of the placenta. Some frank breech presentations cannot be turned because of the fetal configuration or the situation of the placenta. Others, after being converted to a vertex presentation, often revert. However, some breeches spontaneously turn to vertex during the last trimester.

Gentle external version may be employed during the ninth month, since despite occasional need for repeated turning, many breech presentations can be converted to vertex for easier, safer delivery. The procedure is usually done in the physician's office or clinic. The patient is told what the procedure entails and also that it is not always successful (Fig. 25-9).

Requirements for external version. External version can be attempted in the following circumstances:

1. *An unengaged breech presentation.* The breech must not be "fixed" in the pelvis.

2. *No fetopelvic disproportion.* There is a good likelihood of vaginal delivery.

3. *No oligohydramnios or rupture of the membranes.* Adequate amniotic fluid must be present to allow unrestricted turning of the fetus.

4. *Uterine relaxation.* A tight or contracting uterus will prevent external version.

Procedures for external version

1. The nurse places the patient in slight Trendelenburg position to "float" the presenting part.

2. The physician identifies the presentation and position using Leopold's maneuvers (p. 282). (Ocasionally the breech may have already converted to a vertex presentation.)

3. Then with one hand over each pole, the physician gently displaces the breech laterally out of the pelvis while guiding the head in the opposite direction (Fig. 25-9). Frequently, the fetus will "somersault" or roll into the vertex presentation. Manipulations are stopped during a uterine contraction. If turning is not possible

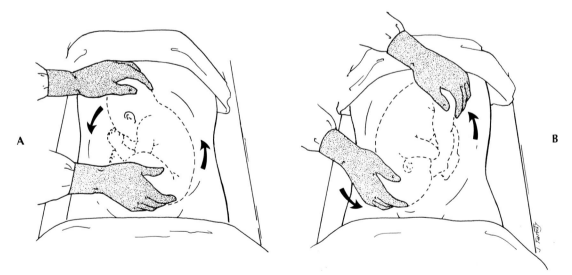

Fig. 25-9. External version of fetus from breech to vertex presentation. This must be achieved without force. **A,** Breech is pushed up out of pelvic inlet while head is pulled toward inlet. **B,** Head is pushed toward inlet while breech is pulled upward.

one way, an attempt is made to turn the fetus in the opposite direction.

4. The vertex is held in the new presentation for a time to permit the head to "settle-in."

5. The nurse checks FHT frequently.

6. External version is discontinued if fetal or maternal distress develops or turning is difficult.

7. The procedure is repeated in a week if necessary.

Internal or podalic version

Internal version is a technique for turning a fetus from vertex or transverse to breech presentation during the second stage of labor by internal (and often external) manipulation. The operator grasps one, or better still, both feet of the fetus and turns the fetal body within the uterus to complete the delivery by breech extraction.

Podalic version and extraction is the most hazardous obstetric operation for the fetus, whether undersized or mature. The procedure must be reserved for use when fetal distress, such as prolapsed cord; maternal difficulty, such as eclampsia; or other critical conditions require immediate delivery. Deep surgical anesthesia (fluothane or ether) is essential for adequate uterine relaxation during internal version. If time permits, delivery by cesarean section is used.

Internal or podalic version is contraindicated when the cervix is not fully dilated, when a contracted pelvis has been diagnosed, when the uterus is abnormally contracted (e.g., Bandl's contraction ring), or after uterine operations such as myomectomy or cesarean section in a previous pregnancy.

Procedures for internal version

1. The physician reassesses the presentation, auscultates the FHT, and reappraises the size of the pelvis relative to the fetus.

2. Full dilatation of the cervix is confirmed.

3. The patient is transferred to the delivery unit and positioned, the vulva cleansed, drapes applied, and other preparations made as for a normal delivery.

4. The anesthetist administers the anesthetic agent.

5. The physician inserts a hand through the cervix toward the feet after rupturing the membranes. If in transverse presentation, the back is anterior, and the lower foot is grasped; if the back is posterior, the upper foot is grasped. If possible, both feet are grasped and drawn downward, rotating the back anteriorly. Concomitantly the head is pushed upward with the external hand on the abdomen (combined version). When the knees are delivered, the version is complete.

6. The fetus is then delivered by breech extraction (p. 377).

These emergency procedures require close teamwork on the part of all concerned. The patient is kept informed of what is happening, and if possible, someone is assigned to explain the procedure to the husband and/or family. The need to change plans concerning the husband's participation during the birth or the possible need for a cesarean section or for the mother having to forego participation in the birth process because of anesthesia will necessitate additional postnatal support.

MULTIPLE PREGNANCY

Multiple pregnancy is the gestation of twins, triplets, quadruplets, or any other number. Twins produced from a single ovum are termed *monozygotic,* or *identical,* and the sibling is always of the same sex (Fig. 25-10). Those produced from separate ova are *dizygotic,* or *fraternal,* and may be of the same or opposite sex (Fig. 25-11). Monozygotic twinning is a random occurrence. Dizygotic twinning (multiple ovulation), on the other hand, is a recessive autosomal trait carried by the daughters of mothers of twins and occurs more frequently as maternal age at conception increases. Triplets can develop from one, two, or three ova (Fig. 25-12).

Infants of multiple pregnancies account for 2% to 3% of all viable births. Of twins, more than 15% weigh less than 2500 gm, and most of these are preterm. Twins occur about once in 99 conceptions, triplets approximately once in 99^2, and quadruplets about once in 99^3 in North America. Multiple pregnancy is most common in blacks, least common in orientals, and of intermediate occurrence in whites. Almost 30% of twins are monozygotic; nearly 70% are dizygotic. Fewer males are born in multiple pregnancies than as singletons. Maternal morbidity and perinatal morbidity and mortality are greatly increased in multiple pregnancy by comparison with single pregnancy because of medical and obstetric complications. The antenatal diagnosis of multiple pregnancy is made in only about 75% of cases and often late in gestation. This is regrettable, since much can be done for the mother and her infants if treatment is established early.

Pathophysiology of multiple pregnancy

Multiple pregnancy is a high-risk problem because of the increased frequency of maternal anemia (40% to 50%), preeclampsia-eclampsia (25%), hemorrhage (before, during, and after delivery, 20%), and uterine inertia (10%). The fetuses may be jeopardized by the higher frequency of hydramnios (5% to 7%), premature delivery (50%), and abnormal presentation and position (10%).

Monozygotic twins are smaller, have a higher incidence of congenital abnormalities (especially when they are of disparate weight), and succumb more often in utero and in the neonatal period than dizygotic twins. Restriction, cord compression and entanglement, growth retardation, and operative delivery are responsible for a significant part of perinatal morbidity and mortality in multiple pregnancy.

A single (monochorionic) placenta probably is less competent than a fused (dichorionic) placenta. As a consequence, more problems occur with the single than with the fused placenta. Most of these are placental vascular disorders. Partial infarction or thinning or inequities of the placental circulation may deprive or destroy one fetus, although the other thrives.

The most serious problem with monochorionic placentas is local shunting of blood—so-called twin-to-twin transfusion syndrome, cross-transfusion, the "third circulation," or intrauterine parabiosis. This occurs because of vascular anastomoses to each twin, established early in embryonic life probably by random growth. The possible communications are artery to artery, vein to vein, artery to vein, and combinations of these. Artery-to-vein communication is the most serious by far; it is most likely to cause twin-to-twin transfusion (if not relieved by a rare vein-to-artery return). In uncompensated cases, the twins, although genetically identical, differ greatly in size and appearance.

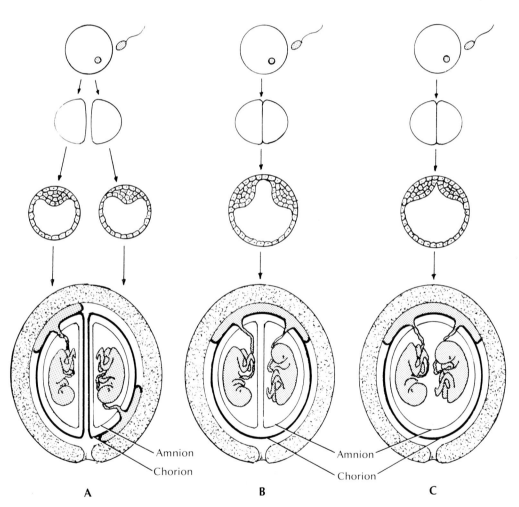

Fig. 25-10. Formation of monozygotic twins. **A,** One fertilization, blastomeres separate, resulting in two implantations, two placentas, and two sets of membranes. **B,** One blastomere with two inner cell masses, one fused placenta, one chorion, separate amnions. **C,** Later separation of inner cell masses, with fused placenta and single amnion and chorion. (From Whaley, L. F. 1974. Understanding inherited disorders. St. Louis, The C. V. Mosby Co.)

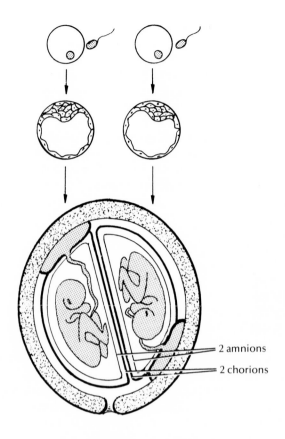

Fig. 25-11. Formation of dizygotic twins. There is fertilization of two ova, two implantations, two placentas, two chorions, and two amnions. (From Whaley, L. F. 1974. Understanding inherited disorders. St. Louis, The C. V. Mosby Co.)

2 amnions

2 chorions

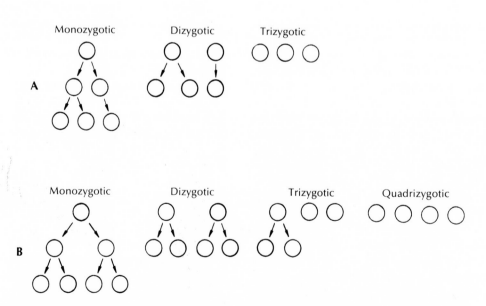

Fig. 25-12. Formation of triplets and quadruplets, indicating variety of mechanisms that can produce multiple births. **A,** Triplets can be formed from one, two, or three ova. **B,** Quadruplets can be formed from one to four ova. (From Whaley, L. F. 1974. Understanding inherited disorders. St. Louis, The C. V. Mosby Co.)

The *recipient* twin will be plethoric, edematous, and hypertensive. Ascites and kernicterus are most likely. Its heart, liver, and kidneys will be enlarged (glomerular-tubal hypertrophy). Hydramnios is associated with fetal polyuria. Although ruddy and apparently healthy, the recipient twin may die of congenital heart failure during the first 24 hours after birth.

The donor twin will be small, pallid, dehydrated, malnourished, and hypovolemic. Oligohydramnios will be present. Severe anemia due to chronic blood loss to the other twin may lead to hydrops and cardiac decompensation.

Maternal problems

Anemia often develops because of greater demand for iron by the fetuses.

Marked uterine distention and increased pressure on the adjacent viscera and pelvic vasculature occur in multiple pregnancy. Diastasis of the two recti abdominis muscles (in the midline) may occur.

Lutein cysts and even ascites may be the result of abnormally high levels of HCG in occasional multiple pregnancies.

Placenta previa develops more frequently in multiple pregnancies because of the large size of the placentas. Premature separation of the placenta may occur before the second and subsequent fetuses are born.

Fetal problems

Each twin and its placenta usually weigh less than the infant and placenta of a singleton pregnancy after the thirtieth week, but the aggregate weight is almost twice that of a singleton near term. The mean weight of twins in the United States is more than 5 pounds (2270 gm).

At delivery, the membranous T septum, or dividing membranes of the placenta between the twins, is inspected and sectioned for evidence of the probable type of twinning. Monozygous twins usually have a transparent (thin) septum made of two amniotic membranes only (no chorion and no decidua). Dizygous twins have an opaque (thick) septum made of two chorions, two amnions, and intervening decidua.

Placentation is of help only in zygosity determinations in twins with monochorionic placentas, since these are always monozygotic. In this group, single ovum twinning can be determined in about two thirds of cases. Placental forms (single, fused, or double) will not aid in determining zygosity in individual twin pairs because any of these forms may be found in monozygous or dizygous twins.

Congenital malformations are twice as frequent in monozygotic twins as in singletons, but there is no in-

crease in the incidence of congenital anomalies in dizygotic twins. Velamentous insertion of the cord and vasa previa occur in about 7% of twin placentas.

Two-vessel cords occur more often in twins than in singletons, and this abnormality is most common in monozygotic twins for unknown reasons.

Diagnosis

Clinical diagnosis of multiple pregnancy is accurate in only about three fourths of cases. With a high degree of suspicion and careful examination, a correct diagnosis of twins may be possible in most instances by the twenty-fourth to twenty-sixth week based on the following:

1. History of dizygous twins in the female lineage
2. Abnormally large maternal weight gain (inconsistent with diet or edema)
3. Polyhydramnios
4. Palpation of excessive number of small or large parts
5. Asynchronous fetal heart beats or more than one fetal ECG tracing
6. Radiographic or ultrasonographic (B-scan) evidence of more than one fetus

In twin pregnancy, both fetuses will present by the vertex in about one half of cases; one will be present by the vertex and one by the breech in approximately one third of the total. Other combinations are uncommon.

Management

Antenatal. Antenatal visits by the patient with multiple pregnancy are scheduled no less than every 2 weeks in the second trimester and weekly thereafter.

The physician supervises the patient's diet and weight control to allow a weight gain of about 50% more than the average woman with a singleton pregnancy (as much as 40 pounds above the patient's ideal nonpregnant weight). Iron and vitamin supplementation is desirable. Attempts are made to prevent preeclampsia-eclampsia and vaginitis; if they do develop, they are treated early and properly.

Because of considerable uterine distention and, perhaps, backache, a well-fitted maternity girdle may be welcomed. Elastic stockings or leotards may control leg varices.

The patient with multiple pregnancy may go into premature labor; the couple is advised to abstain from coitus (orgasm) during the last trimester. Enforced rest periods, with the patient lying down on her side, begun as soon as pregnancy is diagnosed and continued throughout the pregnancy may help to avoid untimely early labor; delivery after the thirty-sixth week increases the likelihood of survival of the neonates.

Natal. Delivery of the patient in a maternity center where specialty care is always available is advisable.

The patient is typed and cross matched, and several units of bank blood are kept available in the delivery room for emergency transfusion. An assistant-nurse team for each neonate is scrubbed, gowned, and gloved for the delivery of a patient with multiple pregnancy. Parenteral infusion of 5% dextrose in water is started through a No. 16 or 18 needle (which can accommodate blood if needed) in the first stage of labor and continued until the fourth stage is completed. Blood or drugs, if indicated, are administered intravenously slowly.

Cesarean section is done only for accepted obstetric reasons. Multiple pregnancy itself is not an indication, but disproportion (e.g., conjoined twins), fetal distress, or monoamnionic twins (diagnosed by amniography) are.

The following delivery procedure is recommended:

1. The patient is admitted to the hospital at the first sign of labor.

2. Analgesia must be limited drastically. Infants often are premature, and operative intervention may be necessary. Pudendal block anesthesia is highly desirable. Supplementary general anesthesia for delivery of the second twin or manual removal of the placenta may be unnecessary.

3. If the first fetus presents by vertex or breech, it is delivered in the usual manner as an assisted breech. If the first fetus is in transverse presentation, an external version is effected and slow, gentle delivery of the fetus accomplished when the cervix is almost fully dilated. A deep episiotomy is worthwhile.

4. The cord must be clamped promptly to prevent the second twin of a monozygotic pregnancy from partially exsanguinating through the first cord. The twins and the cords attached to the placentas are labeled *A* and *B*.

5. Oxytocin or ergot products are not given after the birth of the first twin. Reduction of the uteroplacental circulation will jeopardize the second twin.

6. Vaginal examination of the patient immediately after delivery of the first infant will ascertain the presentation of the second infant. If there is a second sac, the possibility of cord prolapse or entanglement must be considered.

7. Within minutes after the birth of twin A, twin B is brought into a longitudinal presentation (preferably vertex) by abdominovaginal manipulation. The membranes are cautiously ruptured, allowing a slow loss of fluid while the presenting part is being impressed into the inlet by an assistant.

If there is no second amniotic sac (monoamnionic monozygotic twins), twin B is delivered at once to pre-

vent cord entanglement, asphyxia, or premature separation of the placenta. Almost 50% of such second twins die if prompt delivery is not accomplished.

A vertex presentation is encouraged to progress with the next few contractions toward spontaneous delivery or prophylactic forceps delivery. If the breech is presenting, the physician proceeds with an assisted breech delivery. If descent is delayed, version and gradual extraction are better than procrastination or a difficult forceps delivery.

Dilute oxytocin may be administered intravenously to stimulate contractions when uterine inertia becomes a problem.

8. The third stage of labor must be managed with care. Excessive blood loss is common to multiple pregnancy. Oxytocin (Pitocin) is administered, 1 ml intravenously, immediately after delivery of the second twin; the intravenous oxytocin drip is continued. The fundus is elevated but not massaged until after the uterus contracts and expels the separated placenta; then an ergot preparation is given such as ergonovine (Ergotrate), 0.1 mg intravenously, if the patient is not hypertensive. Gentle massage and elevation of the fundus is continued for 15 to 30 minutes. If separation of the placenta is delayed or bleeding is brisk, the physician manually separates and extracts the placenta.

Puerperium. The mother requires the same physical care as any other parturient. She is more prone to develop postnatal hemorrhage because of excessive uterine distension and therefore must be carefully assessed.

Psychologically, however, even the most willing of mothers can find their coping mechanisms overwhelmed by both the idea and reality of caring for two or more infants. Parents must organize simplified and flexible plans of care. The almost constant attention required until the infants' schedule of care can be synchronized may prove exhausting. If possible, help is obtained, particularly to guarantee sufficient rest for the mother. The added expense can also be burdensome to a young family. One mother expressed anger at the surprise birth of twins. The explanation of such errors did not placate her. She needed time to vent these feelings before she could be helped with changing her anticipated plan of care.

If the infants are born prematurely or are SGA, their prolonged hospital stay can cause parental separation anxiety (Chapter 34). If this is the case, the mother may be encouraged to visit and/or care for the infants in the hospital and to utilize this waiting time to recover as much physical strength as possible, as well as to prepare for the infants' homecoming. Introduction of multiple siblings into a family can also result in intense rivalry as all children compete for the mother's attention. Substitute mothering by interested relatives can do much to ease the strain.

Treatment of complications

Preeclampsia-eclampsia, premature labor, and delivery are managed appropriately. If dystocia occurs, obtain x-ray films to rule out malpresentation or conjoined twins. Explore the cervical canal and lower uterine segment vaginally for soft-tissue dystocia.

Prognosis for mother

Maternal morbidity with multiple pregnancy is seven to eight times that for patients who deliver a singleton at term. Sepsis, hemorrhage, and trauma are the principal complications. Fortunately maternal mortality is only slightly increased with multiple pregnancy.

Prognosis for fetuses

The perinatal mortality in multiple births is almost five times that of single term neonates. Moreover, the neonatal morbidity of twins is eight to ten times that of term singletons.

Gestational age is the best criterion for survival of a live-born neonate. Because gestational age may be in doubt in certain instances, a good guide is the observation that if the fetuses weigh more than 2500 gm each, they will have a good prognosis, perhaps better than a singleton of the same weight (who may be less mature).

Vertex presentation affords the best outlook for both twins. Spontaneous birth is better than required forceps delivery or version and extraction. The second twin is in greater jeopardy, since it usually is the smaller of the two and circulatory problems or trauma often complicate its birth.

• • •

Having twins or triplets can be a most rewarding experience. As the children develop, they experience a closeness unique for siblings. One twin, when asked how many brothers and sisters she had, answered, "three sisters and Pam (her twin)."

PREMATURE LABOR AND DELIVERY

Premature labor is that which occurs before the thirty-seventh week of gestation, resulting in the birth of an infant usually weighing less than 2500 gm (for details of care of premature infants, see pp. 554 to 563). Premature labor occurs in more than 10% of all pregnancies and is responsible for almost two thirds of infant deaths. Maternal, placental, and fetal causes may be identified, but in approximately two thirds of cases, no definite cause can be identified. Thirty to fifty percent of premature labors occur after premature rupture of the membranes. Iatrogenic prematurity, or delivery too early by induction or cesarean section, accounts for slightly less than 10% of preterm babies.

The importance of premature labor is that the infant is usually delivered too early for the growth and development necessary for uncomplicated adjustment to extrauterine life. Hence its prospects for survival or good health may be severely compromised.

Although certain problems may be identified, many so-called causes of premature labor may be coincidental. The following associations or causes are prominent in premature labor:

1. *Maternal problems.* Debilitating disorders, trauma, abdominal surgery, maternal injury, preeclampsia-eclampsia, uterine anomalies or tumors, cervical incompetence, and sepsis often are a prelude to premature labor.

2. *Placental disorders.* Gross placental abnormalities such as placental separation or extrachorial placenta are associated with premature labor.

3. *Fetal abnormalities.* Transplacental infections such as rubella, toxoplasmosis, or syphilis may be responsible for premature labor. Multiple pregnancy, hydramnios, and premature rupture of the membranes are also notable. Congenital adrenal hyperplasia is usually associated with premature labor.

4. *Iatrogenic causes.* Premature labor can result from elective delivery because of misjudgment of fetal maturity or miscalculation of the EDC.

The diagnosis of premature labor may be difficult to distinguish from painful Braxton Hicks contractions. Labor is progressive and associated with cervical dilatation, effacement, or both. It may be helpful to utilize external monitoring to record the frequency and intensity of contractions to be certain that labor is underway, as well as FHT monitoring.

Stopping premature labor

Exclusions to attempts to stop labor. Because premature labor is associated with an extremely high perinatal loss, one might think it best to try to quell uterine contraction in all women who threaten to deliver early. This is not reasonable, however, because many serious disorders cannot be diagnosed before labor. Moreover, early labor may spare the mother and infant. In other cases, the diagnosis of anomalies indicates that the mother should not have to carry the pregnancy to term.

It is apparent that labor cannot be stopped if the cervix is more than 3 to 4 cm dilated and more than 50% effaced and/or if the membranes have ruptured. In the final analysis, 20% of low birth weight fetuses are candidates for suppression of labor by drug therapy, assuming adequate maturity has been reached.

Permit labor to continue when the following exist:

1. Maternal disorders that jeopardize the pregnancy or make delivery the lesser risk (e.g., preeclampsia-eclampsia, abruptio placentae)
2. Fetal problems that become more threatening with time (e.g., severe Rh isoimmunization)
3. Other complications inimical to continuation of pregnancy (e.g., premature rupture of membranes, amnionitis)

Infants weighing more than 2500 gm and delivered after 37 weeks of pregnancy have the best prospects of survival. The mortality of newborns weighing 1500 to 2500 gm is approximately 10% if delivered earlier than 37 weeks' gestation and about 3% if delivered after 37 weeks. Hence the prognosis of low birth weight babies is more favorable if they weigh more than 1800 gm than if they weigh 1500 to 1800 gm. A mortality of less than 5% is likely if pregnancy has progressed to 35 weeks and the fetus weighs more than 2000 gm. With these guidelines, it is illogical to try to stop labor if the duration of pregnancy is 37 weeks or longer. The hazardous zone is 34 to 37 weeks, but the fetus should weigh more than 1800 gm.

The clinical appraisal of gestational age often is inaccurate, but amniotic fluid analysis (e.g., creatinine, bilirubin content), ultrasonography (e.g., biparietal diameter determination), or radiography (e.g., ossification centers) may enhance the estimate. Generally, it is prudent to suppress all labors that occur before 34 weeks' gestational age, assuming the exclusion of reasonable contraindications to the continuation of pregnancy.

In summary, attempts to arrest labor are justified only if the following conditions are present:

1. The fetus must be alive and weigh 1800 to 2500 gm.
2. No signs of fetal disease or distress must be present.
3. The membranes must be intact and the cervix less than 3 cm dilated or less than 50% effaced.
4. There must be no medical or obstetric disorder that is a contraindication to the continuation of pregnancy.

Pharmacologic control of labor. Hypnotics and sedatives are contraindicated. Narcotics may accelerate labor and often narcotize the neonate. Barbiturates are contraindicated because they suppress the respiratory center of the infant, and their effects cannot be reversed by drugs such as nalorphine (Nalline).

Effective tokolytic drugs include the following:

1. Ethyl alcohol: 100 ml 95% in 900 ml of 5% dextrose and water intravenously. The loading dose is 15 ml/kg body weight given in 2 hours. The maintenance dose is 1.5 ml/kg body weight given every hour.
2. Ritodrine (an improved analogue of isoxsuprine): 25 mg ritodrine diluted in 250 ml 5% glucose and water (100 μg/ml). The maintenance dose is 400 μg/min. Continue the drug therapy for longer than 2 hours after uterine contractions have ceased. The maximum dose is determined by maternal tachycardia.

Pharmacologic stimulation of fetal lung maturity. During process of arresting premature labor, betamethasone (Celestone), a glucocorticoid, may be used to hasten the production of alveolar surfactant in premature fetuses, thus increasing survival potential.

Conduct of irreversible or acceptable premature labor and delivery

The labor is conducted in accordance with the principles that apply to a low birth weight (easily compromised) fetus. If vaginal delivery is chosen, analgesia is limited. Utilize continuous fetal heart rate monitoring. Artificial rupture of membranes is delayed until the cervix is more than 6 cm dilated to achieve maximal cervical dilatation and effacement and to avoid prolapse of the cord.

Administer oxytocin continuously for augmentation of labor and with a low concentration of the drug in an intravenous solution. Pudendal block anesthesia is desirable along with a deep episiotomy. Outlet forceps are utilized for delivery unless easy spontaneous birth is likely. The neonate is permitted several breaths before clamping the cord; if resuscitation is required, the cord must be clamped and cut immediately. Oxygen is given by mask and warmth maintained.

Psychologic aspects of premature labor and delivery

Prematurity puts the infant and the family at risk. The parents face the threat of their infant's death. In the event that their infant may die, some parents pull away from any emotional attachment to this infant; anticipatory grieving is a protective mechanism. However, the danger inherent in grieving the loss prematurely lies in the infant's recovery and subsequent relationship to the parents:

1. The parents may be unable to reestablish a positive relationship and therefore have difficulty developing effective parenting patterns.
2. The parents may continue to view the child as being at risk, vulnerable to disease and dysfunction, and only on temporary loan to them.

3. The parents may become overprotective and over-indulgent or may place heavy demands or unrealistic expectations on the child's growth, development, and achievements.

Children of parents who grieved inappropriately after premature delivery and who have shown the behaviors just listed may demonstrate a variety of problems in psychosocial development such as the following:
- Difficulty with separation and dependency
- Sleep disturbances
- Failure to thrive
- School phobias
- Overconcern with bodily functions

Reactions to premature delivery. Grief reactions to the birth of a premature infant have been studied by Kaplan and Mason and others. The following four psychologic tasks must be faced and successfully resolved by the mother of a premature infant before effective relationships and parenting patterns can evolve:

1. *Anticipatory grief.* The mother withdraws from the normal process of bonding with her infant. She grieves in preparation for her infant's possible death, although she clings tenuously to the hope that the child will survive. This phase begins during labor and lasts until the infant expires or shows evidence of surviving.

2. *Confrontation and acknowledgment of her failure to deliver a normal full-term infant.* Grief and depression typify this phase, which persists until the infant is out of danger and is expected to survive.

3. *Resumption of the process of relating to the infant.* As the baby begins to improve—gains weight, feeds by nipple, and is weaned from the incubator—the mother should resume the process of developing the attachment or bonding to the infant that had been interrupted by his precarious condition at birth.

4. *Learning how this baby differs in his special needs and growth patterns.* The mother's fourth task is to learn, understand, and accept this infant's caretaking needs and growth and developmental expectations. In most instances, the special needs and developmental pattern differ only temporarily from that expected for normal full-term infants.

In the event that the infant survives, these psychologic tasks should be confronted and accomplished in the sequence given for the most successful outcomes for the mother and child.

If the infant dies during the neonatal period, the mother and her family are confronted with the mourning process.

Giving birth too early. The mother whose pregnancy terminates before term (1) has not had time to develop her fantasized mother role with this child, (2) may not have reached the phase of wanting to be rid of the pregnancy, and (3) may not have come to the point of anxiously anticipating the infant. Many women are not ready to give up the pregnant state when premature labor begins.

In the labor unit, the atmosphere surrounding the woman in premature labor is guarded, frequently tense. The focus is on the unborn:

1. Fetal status may be monitored electronically or frequently by fetoscope.

2. Decisions regarding analgesia and anesthesia are based on fetal tolerance.

3. Delivery is accomplished with episiotomy and forceps to minimize trauma to the infant.

4. The pediatrician is ready and all the equipment has been assembled if the delivery is to occur at this hospital. Occasionally the mother may be transferred to another hospital (which may be a distance from her home and family) with facilities for premature care.

5. A subdued air of silent anticipation prevails as the infant is born and its status evaluated.

The mother may or may not see the infant before highly skilled specialists surround him for resuscitative and other life-sustaining measures. If the mother sees the infant, she may see a small, glistening, limp, and often nonpink body, and she may hear his silence, gasping, or weak cry. The infant's appearance does not project the ego-enhancing image proffered by a robust, healthy newborn. The mother is often disregarded as attention focuses on the baby. If it is not possible to give explanations concomitantly with the infant's care, remember to do so later.

Mother-child relationship. As soon as possible, the mother should see and touch the infant so that she may begin to acknowledge the reality of the event, reaffirm the infant's true appearance and condition, and begin working through the psychologic tasks imposed by premature delivery.

A nurse or physician should be present when the mother (or father) visits the infant for the following reasons:

1. To help her "see" the infant rather than focus on the equipment

2. To provide the normal characteristics for an infant that age against which she can compare and contrast her infant instead of using norms for full-term infants for comparison

3. To encourage verbalization of feelings regarding the experience of pregnancy, labor, and delivery

4. To assess her perceptions of the infant to determine the appropriate time for her to become actively involved in his care

PLAN OF CARE: PREMATURE LABOR AND DELIVERY

PATIENT CARE OBJECTIVES

1. The mother retains a positive self-concept as a woman, mother, and sexual being.
2. The mother:
   a. Perceives the child as potentially normal (if this is medically substantiated).
   b. Provides the child with realistic care comfortably.
   c. Experiences pride and satisfaction in the care of the child.
3. The mother is able to organize her time and energies to meet the love, attention, and care needs of the other members of the family and herself as well.

NURSING INTERVENTIONS

Diagnostic	Therapeutic	Educational

Premature labor (≤37 weeks' gestation)

Diagnostic	Therapeutic	Educational

1. Assess patient's behavior:
  a. Angry or passive.
  b. Verbal or nonverbal.
  c. Crying, overtalkative, or quiet.
  d. Anxious.
2. Assess husband's (partner's) behavior:
  a. Supportive: positive response from patient. Verbal—coaching; nonverbal—stroking, looking.
  b. Nonsupportive: patient is distressed by his presence. Verbal—blaming, hostile to staff, and her; nonverbal—avoidance, distancing.
3. Check obstetric history:
  a. Length of this pregnancy; proximity to due date.
  b. Current symptoms: ruptured membranes, bleeding, degree of discomfort, in labor or not.
  c. Previous premature labors? Abortions?
	1. Focus on mother's feelings:
	  a. "All of this must leave you feeling confused and a little frightened."
	  b. "You are probably wondering how your baby will be."
	  c. "It's natural (OK) for you to ask for medication to stop the hurt. Let us see what we can do to help you with your discomfort."
	2. Keep her and husband informed of fetal and newborn status.
	3. Inform her of preparations for child (pediatrician is notified, etc.).
	4. Stay with patient; coach her; give verbal and nonverbal support with each contraction. *Avoid* "think of the baby . . ." type of statements.
		1. Patient is usually not tired of her pregnancy and not ready to let go of mother-fetus relationship.
		2. Woman may feel guilty or be made to feel guilty by husband, personnel, and others for egocentric behaviors during labor.
		3. In labor, women become self-centered. Reinforce normalcy of this to her (and to her family) during and after delivery.
		4. Concern for infant should not distract nurse from mother's need to be reassured that she did well in labor, etc.

After delivery of premature infant (≤37 weeks' gestation)

Tasks I and II

Diagnostic	Therapeutic	Educational

1. Assess mother's perception of situation:
  a. Realistic?
  b. Aware of problems or lack of problems?
  c. How she describes infant: "a plucked chicken," "a corpselike thing," "he," "she," "such a tiny baby."
2. Is mother able to focus on infant as well as on herself?
3. Assess mother's support system:
  a. Family members: who, present or not.
  b. Religious.
  c. Cultural.
4. Assess mother's behavior:
  a. Denial.
  b. Hopeful.
	1. Keep mother informed of infant's status; reassure regarding infant's viability, lack of deformities, defects, if true.
	2. Explain incubator, gadgetry, nursing procedures, and what mother can do if anything.
	3. Describe any defects, surgery, etc., and encourage her to vent feelings regarding same. This is done to reinforce what physician has told her. Repeat as often as necessary. Reassure her that it is OK for her to ask same questions over and over if she expresses feelings about this.
	
	Task I
	1. "It must be hard for you to let yourself love (get involved) with the
		1. For the mother with an obstetric history of difficulty conceiving or many abortions, this child may be closest evidence of success so far, and parents may feel gratified that they could carry an infant this far along.
		2. Working closely with mother (and her family) increases her sense of worth.
		3. Knowledge of situation and what to expect are ego strengthening. Even if knowledge is "bad news," mother has a chance to do worry work or grief work at that time to prepare herself for next event.

PLAN OF CARE: PREMATURE LABOR AND DELIVERY—cont'd

NURSING INTERVENTIONS—cont'd

Diagnostic	Therapeutic	Educational

After delivery of premature infant (≤37 weeks' gestation)—cont'd

Tasks I and II—cont'd

   c. Ready to become involved in infant's care.

Task I—cont'd

baby when you are not sure he will make it."

2. "Some women feel it would be better if the baby died if there may be something wrong with him." (This statement is made after she makes some reference to subject herself.)
3. "At times, the whole thing doesn't seem real."

Task II

1. Encourage her to verbalize feelings regarding this pregnancy, labor, and delivery and compare and contrast to previous experiences if any.
2. "Some women feel they may have caused an early labor themselves."

Task III

1. Assess mother's behaviors:
   a. Muscle tension or relaxation.
   b. Perspiration or not.
   c. Skin color changes.
   d. Eye contact with infant.
2. Assess mother's verbal responses:
   a. Perception of infant: "he," "she," or "it"; human or animal characteristics; potential viability or "corpselike."
   b. Appropriateness to infant or to her care of infant.

1. Assist mother to regard infant as he really is:
   a. Show her wet or soiled diapers.
   b. Inform her of amount he eats and how he eats.
   c. Point out his behaviors: frowns, yawns, stretching.
   d. Go over infant with her from head to toe.
2. Describe any improvements:
   a. Respiratory activity.
   b. Weight gain.
   c. Change from gavage to nipple feeding.
3. Support her interactions with infant:
   a. Stroking, fondling, holding, etc.
   b. Feeding, burping, changing diapers.
   c. Eliciting grasp reflex.
4. Help her vent feelings regarding infant's behavior while she is providing care (he may not wish to burp; he may regurgitate, etc.).
5. Assist her with identification of infant:
   a. Whose eyes? Chin? Nose?
   b. Size of feet—who does he take after?
   c. Who else had a birthmark? etc.

1. Parents must release fantasy baby and see this baby as individual with his own physical and behavioral characteristics. Psychologic tasks once accomplished enable mother to see and meet this infant's special needs.
2. Mother needs substantive data to reassure her that now it is safe to invest emotional energy in developing relationship with this infant.
3. Tactile, visual, and auditory stimuli are needed to assist mother in knowing her baby. These activities increase her self-confidence and self-esteem as she learns to care for infant.
4. Parents are acutely aware of how others regard infant. Nurse acts as role model by giving infant a gender, calling him by name, using positive statements regarding his behavior ("he drank a whole ounce of formula today" versus "he only drank half of his formula today"), handling him gently.
5. Parents can intellectualize that infant is as yet unaware of who is who (among his caretakers, including his parents), but they still feel rejected if infant does not look at them and pulls away from their touch and feel accepted if infant responds by rooting, grasping, burping, etc.

Continued.

PLAN OF CARE: PREMATURE LABOR AND DELIVERY—cont'd

NURSING INTERVENTIONS—cont'd

Diagnostic	Therapeutic	Educational

After delivery of premature infant (≤37 weeks' gestation)—cont'd

Task IV

Diagnostic	Therapeutic	Educational
1. As in Task III. 2. How often can mother come in to care for infant? How does mother (family) keep in touch? 3. Does mother have support of family members? Do others come in with her? 4. How much encouragement does mother need to take on tasks? 5. What are her comments as she interacts with infant?	1. Provide information and support as mother takes on care of infant. Allow her to pace herself. 2. Arrange for group meetings between mothers who share this experience; provide space, maybe even coffee, etc., and act as resource person as needed. 3. Arrange for home visit prior to infant's discharge and several afterward as circumstances allow. 4. Supply telephone numbers of those to call with questions. 5. Prepare mother for increase in anxiety as discharge date approaches. 6. Teach regarding expected growth and developmental patterns.	1. Mother's self-confidence may have been diminished by inability to carry to full-term and by seeing that infant required highly trained professionals and complex equipment previously. 2. Supporting mother's successes increase her confidence and help her build a positive concept of self as mother capable of caring for this infant.

REFERENCES

Barden, T. P., and others. 1972. Premature labor: its management and therapy. J. Reprod. Med. **9:**93.

Brenner, W. E., Bruce, R. D., and Hendricks, C. H. 1974. Characteristics and perils of breech presentation. Am. J. Obstet. Gynecol. **118:**700.

Bruce, S. J. 1962. Reactions of nurses and mothers to stillbirths. Nurs. Outlook **10:**88.

Burnell, G. 1974. Maternal reaction to the loss of multiple births. Arch. Gen. Psychiatry **30:**183.

Engel, G. L. 1964. Grief and grieving. Am. J. Nurs. **64:**9, Sept.

Hardgrove, C., and Warrick, L. H. 1974. How shall we tell the children? Am. J. Nurs. **74:**448.

Kaplan, D. M., and Mason, E. A. 1960. Maternal reactions to premature birth viewed as an acute emotional disorder. Am. J. Orthopsychiatry **30:**118, July.

McLenahan, I. G. 1962. Helping the mother who has no baby to take home. Am. J. Nurs. **62:**70, April.

Mercer, R. T. 1974. Response of mothers to the birth of an infant with a defect. In American Nurses' Association clinical sessions, 1974, San Francisco. New York, Appleton-Century-Crofts.

Rubin, R. 1963. Maternal touch. Nurs. Outlook **11:**828.

Saylor, D. E. 1975. Understanding presurgical anxiety. AORN J. **22:**624.

Waechter, E. H. 1970. The birth of an exceptional child. Nurs. Forum **9:**202.

Warrick, L. H. 1974. An aspect of perinatal nursing: support to the high-risk mother. In American Nurses' Association clinical sessions, 1974, San Francisco. New York, Appleton-Century-Crofts.

Zahourek, R., and Jensen, J. S. 1973. Grieving and the loss of the newborn. Am. J. Nurs. **73:**836.

Zuspan, F. P. 1972. Premature labor—its management and therapy: a symposium. J. Reprod. Med. **9:**93.

CHAPTER 26

Operative obstetrics

Many factors in modern maternity care continue to increase the margin of safety and comfort for both mother and infant. Improved methods for monitoring and assessing fetal-maternal well-being have contributed to more effective prevention and treatment of the medical and surgical complications of childbirth. Increased expertise in operative obstetrics has helped reduce the risk to mother and infant by *preventive* surgical procedures (episiotomy, forceps delivery, and cesarean section); and *therapeutic* surgical procedures (repair of lacerations to the birth canal and removal of the retained placenta).

Some procedures in operative obstetrics are complicated, whereas others are so frequently used as to make them adjuncts or aids to normal delivery. Episiotomy and forceps delivery comprise such a category. Cesarean section is used with increasing frequency because the problems that signal the need for nonvaginal delivery can be detected earlier and with greater accuracy. Surgical repair of birth injuries or surgical intervention in problems encountered with placental retention has markedly reduced maternal morbidity and mortality in the postnatal period.

The nurse must remember that the maternity patient whose management includes some type of surgical intervention will require postoperative as well as postdelivery care. This will, of course, include emotional as well as physiologic support.

EPISIOTOMY

An episiotomy is an incision made in the perineum to enlarge the vaginal outlet. It serves the following purposes:

1. Prevents tearing of the perineum. The clean and properly placed incision heals more promptly than does a ragged tear. Some conditions predisposing to perineal tearing and therefore indications for episiotomy are a large infant, rapid labors in which there is not sufficient time for stretching of the perineum to take place,

a narrow suprapubic arch with a constricted outlet, and malpresentations of the fetus (e.g., face).

2. May prevent prolonged and severe stretching of the muscles supporting the bladder or rectum, which may later lead to stress incontinence of urine or vaginal prolapse.

3. Reduces duration of the second stage, which may be important for maternal reasons (e.g., a hypertensive state) or fetal reasons (e.g., slowing heart rate below 100/min).

4. Enlarges the vagina in case manipulation is needed to deliver an infant, for example, in a breech presentation, or to apply forceps.

Types of episiotomy

The type of episiotomy is designated by the site and direction of the incision (Fig. 26-1).

Median episiotomy is the one most commonly employed. It is effective, easily repaired, and generally is the least painful. Occasionally there may be an extension through the rectal sphincter (third-degree laceration) or even into the anal canal (fourth-degree laceration). Fortunately primary healing and a good repair usually will be followed by good sphincter tone.

Mediolateral episiotomy frequently is employed in operative delivery when posterior extension is likely. Although a fourth-degree laceration may thus be avoided, a third-degree laceration may occur. Moreover, as compared with a median episiotomy, blood loss is greater and the repair more difficult and painful (Figs. 26-2 and 26-3).

FORCEPS DELIVERY

Two double-curved, spoonlike articulated blades comprise the obstetric forceps that is used to extract the fetal head, whether it be forecoming (vertex presentation) or aftercoming (breech presentation). This instrument, regarded by many as one of the greatest inventions of all time, was devised by Peter Chamberlen about

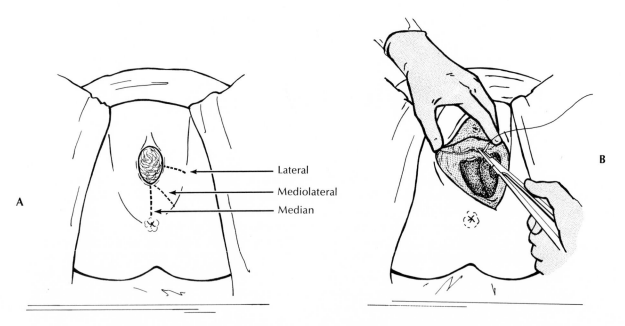

Lateral

Mediolateral

Median

Fig. 26-1. A, Types of episiotomy. **B,** Repair of left mediolateral episiotomy.

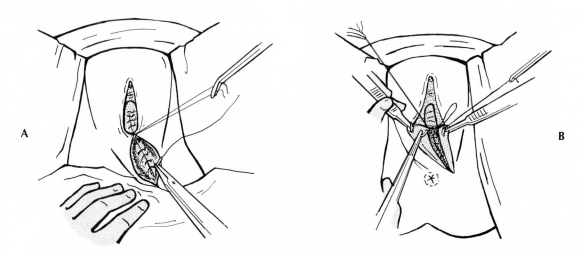

Fig. 26-2. A, Repair of levator muscle and its severed fascia. Attendant approximates cut edges of vaginal orifice using forceps to exert traction on suture. **B,** Repair of cut ends of bulbocavernosus muscle.

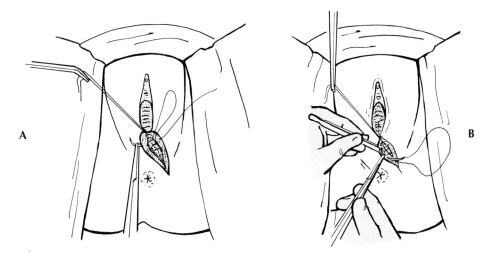

Fig. 26-3. A, Repair of muscle and fascial components of urogenital diaphragm. **B,** Closure of skin edges. Sutures are placed just under dermis so that no sutures are visible when skin edges are approximated.

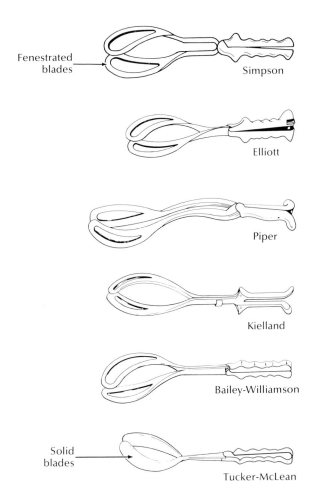

Fenestrated blades

Simpson

Elliott

Piper

Kielland

Bailey-Williamson

Solid blades

Tucker-McLean

Fig. 26-4. Types of forceps.

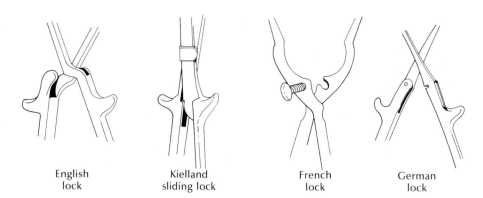

| English lock | Kielland sliding lock | French lock | German lock |

Fig. 26-5. Types of forceps locks. Note how blades cross (e.g., right blade crosses over to form left half of handle).

1625. Different *locks* (articulations) and varied curvature or length of the blades distinguish most of these forceps, which may have solid or fenestrated blades (Figs. 26-4 and 26-5). Some forceps are used for ordinary delivery (e.g., OA position); others are used for rotation of the vertex (e.g., LOP to OA position).

The commonly employed forceps has a cephalic curve shaped to that of the head and a pelvic curve that conforms to the pelvic axis. The blades are joined by a pin, screw, or groove arrangement.

Possible indications for forceps delivery are as follows:

- *Maternal*—to shorten the second stage in dystocia (difficult labor), when the mother's expulsive efforts are deficient (e.g., tired or after spinal anesthesia), or when the woman is endangered (e.g., cardiac decompensation)
- *Fetal*—to rescue a jeopardized fetus (e.g., premature labor or fetal distress close to delivery)

Forceps operations are subdivided into *required forceps delivery,* or when the procedure is imperative such as in status asthmaticus, and *elective forceps delivery,* or when the operation is assistive but not essential.

The incidence of forceps delivery depends on the proportion of simple to complicated cases treated at a particular hospital, whether light or heavy analgesia is popular, whether general or local infiltration anesthesia is favored, and the attitudes and skills of physicians or nurse-midwives in attendance.

There are literally hundreds of different obstetric forceps but only five major types that even the specialist may need to use:

1. An outlet forceps (e.g., Braun-Simpson forceps)
2. A rotational forceps without a pelvic curve for rotation of an OP to an OA position (e.g., Kielland's forceps)

3. A rotational forceps without a pelvic curve but a deep posterior and short-hinged anterior blade for rotation of OP to OA (e.g., Barton forceps)
4. An axis-traction forceps (e.g., Tarnier's forceps)
5. A forceps for the aftercoming head (e.g., Piper forceps)

Prerequisites for forceps operations

The following must apply for successful forceps delivery:

1. *Fully dilated cervix.* Severe lacerations and hemorrhage may ensue if a rim of cervix still remains.
2. *Head engaged.* The extraction of a mature fetus with a "high" (unengaged) head usually is disastrous.
3. *Vertex presentation or face presentation* (mentum anterior). Other presentations require wider than average bony pelvic diameters.
4. *Membranes ruptured* to ensure a firm grasp of the forceps on the fetal head.
5. *No cephalopelvic disproportion.* Assuming engagement, there must be no outlet contracture or gross sacral deformity.
6. *Empty bladder and bowel* to avoid visceral laceration and fistula formation.

Normally an episiotomy should be performed, particularly if a difficult midforceps delivery is likely or when a snug fit at the introitus is envisioned. To prevent undue blood loss, the episiotomy incision should be made at the time of perineal distention, well after locking and adjustment of the forceps.

Forceps designation relative to station of head

The station of the head determines the level of forceps application and, generally, the relative difficulty to be expected in forceps operations.

1. *High forceps.* The biparietal diameter of the vertex is above the ischial spines when the forceps are applied. When the head is unengaged or "floating," forceps delivery is difficult, hazardous, and never warranted. Most hospitals have policies against high-forceps application.

2. *Midforceps.* The vertex is at the ischial spines, almost to the ischial tuberosities on application of the forceps. The delivery often is difficult, depending on the size of the vertex, its position, and the pelvic architecture and diameters.

3. *Low forceps.* The vertex is deeply engaged and is on the pelvic floor, with the sagittal suture anteroposteriorly situated.

4. *Outlet forceps.* The vertex is distending the introitus with outlet forceps. This should be an "easy" forceps delivery. The blades are applied principally for control and guidance of the head (Figs. 26-6 to 26-13).

Before forceps are applied, an attendant checks, reports, and records FHT.

Forceps may be applied in two ways. First is the *cephalic application* in which each blade is applied carefully to the side of the head and adjusted correctly for the

Text continued on p. 400.

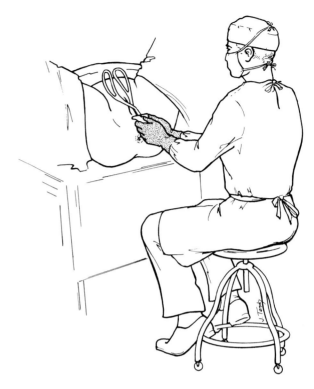

Fig. 26-6. Application of outlet forceps: OA. Physician checks forceps.

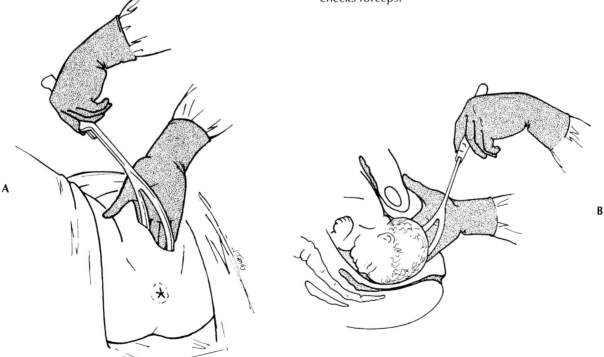

Fig. 26-7. Perineal view. **A,** Right hand determines blade placement and checks for cord. Left blade is then introduced into birth canal along palm of right hand. **B,** Internal view of maneuver.

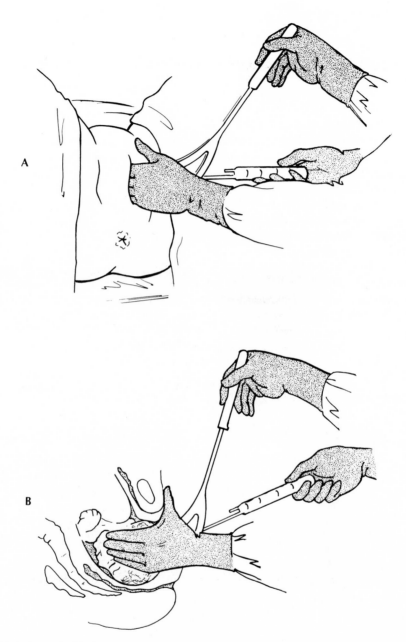

Fig. 26-8. A, Right blade is introduced with same precautions. Blade is brought down and locked with left blade. Blades should move and lock with ease or are removed and reapplied. **B,** Internal view of maneuver.

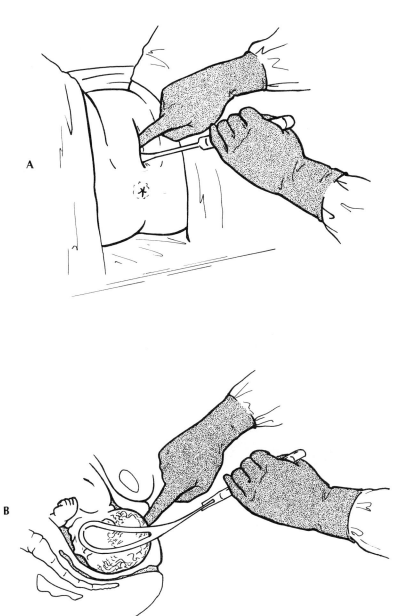

Fig. 26-9. A, Nurse checks FHT (to rule out cord compression) and physician checks application prior to exerting traction to advance head. **B,** Internal view of maneuver.

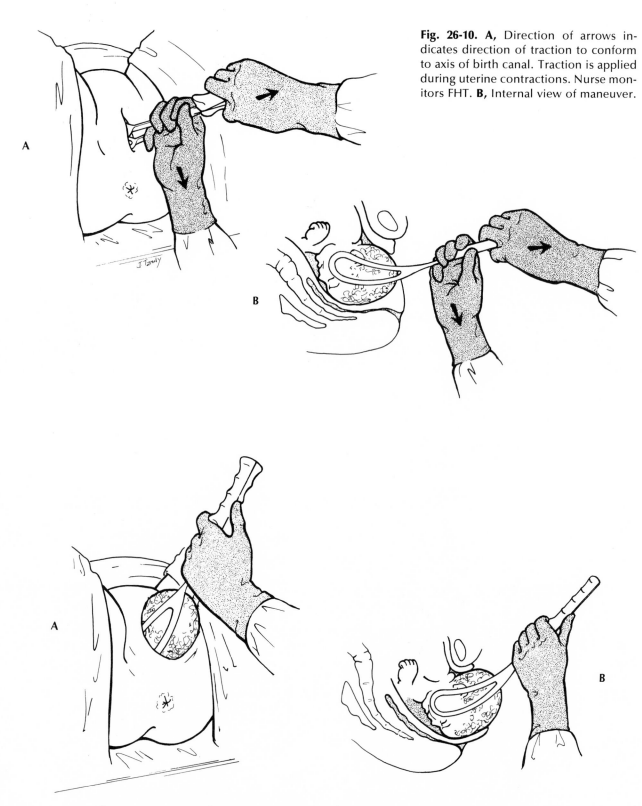

Fig. 26-10. **A,** Direction of arrows indicates direction of traction to conform to axis of birth canal. Traction is applied during uterine contractions. Nurse monitors FHT. **B,** Internal view of maneuver.

Fig. 26-11. **A,** Upward traction is exerted with extension of head; this conforms with axis of birth canal. **B,** Internal view of maneuver.

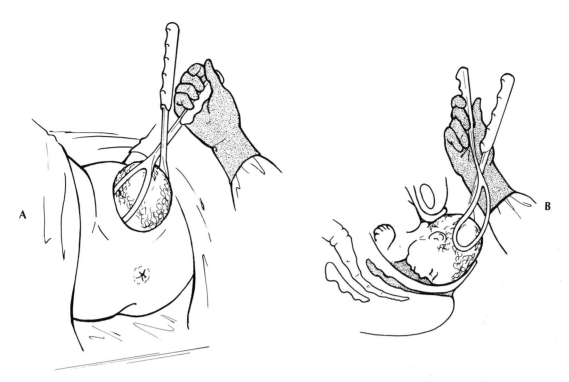

Fig. 26-12. A, Blades are unlocked; right blade is removed. **B,** Internal view of maneuver.

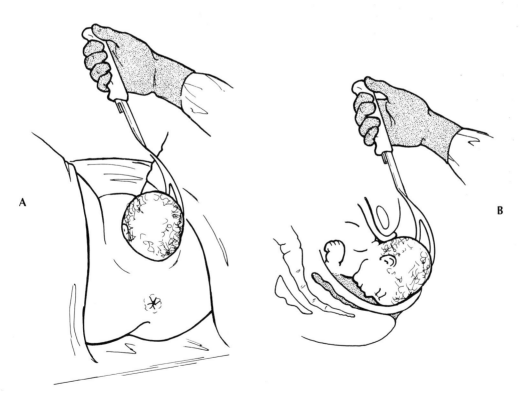

Fig. 26-13. A, Left blade is removed. Delivery is completed by applying pressure with drape-covered hand to perineum. **B,** Internal view of maneuver.

best fit. This is the proper method of forceps application and generally is not difficult unless the fetal head is arrested in the transverse position or markedly molded. The left blade is always applied first. The assistant hands the obstetrician the left blade first. The nurse can tell the mother that they fit like two tablespoons around an egg. The blades come over the baby's ears.

After forceps application and before traction is applied, the attendant rechecks the FHT. Compression of the cord between the fetal head and the forceps would cause a drop in FHT. The physician would then remove and reapply the forceps (Fig. 26-9).

The second method is the *pelvic application*. Each forceps blade is directed into the pelvis, one on the right and one on the left, without consideration of the position of the fetal head. Obviously misapplication often occurs because only when the vertex is directly OP or OA can the forceps be applied to the sides of the head. As a consequence, the fetus may be injured and maternal soft tissues lacerated. If the fetus is living, there is little excuse for pelvic application of forceps.

Axis-traction forceps

Axis-traction forceps were designed to aid in bringing the vertex down through the birth canal without undue pressure of the head of the fetus against the symphysis pubis. The rod connections from the heel of each Tarnier forceps blade to the traction bar favorably alter the direction of pull. All difficult midforceps or even low-forceps deliveries should be accomplished with axis-traction forceps.

A fetus in a mentum posterior position at term cannot be delivered as such through the birth canal. It may be possible to rotate the face anteriorly, however, but delivery by cesarean section is preferable.

Forceps application for aftercoming head

Although the usual forceps can be employed for the delivery of the aftercoming head in breech presentation, the shanks of the forceps frequently are too short. For this reason, Piper designed a forceps with a long, downward pelvic curve and elongated handles.

VACUUM EXTRACTION

Vacuum extraction is delivery of a fetus in vertex presentation with the use of a cup-suction device that is applied to the fetal scalp for traction. Indications for use of the vacuum extractor, or ventouse, are similar to those for simple forceps delivery. This rather expensive instrument, widely used in Europe, often speeds labor and delivery, obviating difficult forceps procedures or even cesarean section. The most popular device is the

Malstrom extractor, which permits controlled negative pressure of 0.7 to 0.8 kg beneath a metal cup available in various diameters.

The operator needs basic training in this method of delivery, and anesthesia is not required. The ventouse adds traction to the involuntary and voluntary efforts and is more physiologic than forceps extraction. It is easy to apply the ventouse to the occiput (away from a suture line or fontanel), and the device does not distort the head significantly. Although planned rotation cannot be effected with the ventouse because of lack of torque, natural rotation usually is encouraged. Because there is no increase in the volume of the presenting part, lacerations of the birth canal are uncommon.

The vacuum extractor cannot replace the obstetric forceps, however, because rotation (OP to OA) may be impossible without forceps and correction of asynclitism is not feasible. Moreover, for a difficult midpelvic arrest, axis traction is almost always required.

Extremely rapid delivery (for fetal or maternal distress) is impossible with a vacuum extractor. Face and breech presentations cannot be delivered with this instrument either.

Fetal scalp ecchymoses must be expected; even cephalhematomas occur with the ventouse. When there is prolonged application of the vacuum extractor (30 minutes), severe damage to the scalp or subgaleal hematomas may develop.

CESAREAN SECTION

Cesarean section is the delivery of a fetus through a uterine incision. Although the myth persists that Julius Caesar was delivered in this manner, the derivation of the term is more likely from the Latin word *caedo* meaning "to cut." Cesarean section generally is transabdominal, although vaginal cesarean section can be accomplished for delivery of a small fetus. The basic purpose of cesarean section is to preserve the life or health of the mother and/or her fetus. Cephalopelvic disproportion (CPD) is the most common indication for cesarean section. The need for this mode of delivery is highest in areas where contracted pelvis, tumors, and other such difficulties are more prevalent. Repeat cesarean sections, correctly or incorrectly justified on the basis of possible or probable rupture of the uterus, represent at least 30% of all cesarean sections in North America.

Maternal indications

In addition to fetopelvic disproportion, maternal indications for cesarean section include a questionably weak or defective uterine scar (after cesarean section, myomectomy, or unification operation), preeclampsia-eclampsia, placenta previa or premature separation of the normally implanted placenta, dystocia, pelvic tumors, maternal gonorrhea or herpes type 2 infections; serious maternal conditions that might be complicated by labor and delivery, such as recent fractures of the pelvis.

Fetal indications

Fetal distress (due to hypoxia or blood loss), insulin-dependent diabetes mellitus, prolapse of the cord in labor, hydrocephalus, and compound presentation are indications for cesarean section. When infertility, marriage late in life, and other factors place a ''high social premium'' on the baby, elective cesarean section may be warranted.

Types of cesarean section

There are five principal types of abdominal cesarean section (Fig. 26-14):

1. *Classical cesarean section.* This simplest of all cesarean section procedures is used when rapid delivery is necessary, in shoulder presentation, and in placenta previa when the placenta is implanted on the anterior wall. Classical cesarean section is useful when general anesthesia is unavailable, since this operation can be carried out under local infiltration anesthesia. A vertical incision is made through the visceral peritoneum and the contractile portion of the uterus above the bladder reflexion. Maternal bleeding may be considerable, especially if placenta previa is present, but no fetal blood loss usually occurs. The potential for rupture of the scar (1% to 2%) with a subsequent pregnancy and the frequent occurrence of small bowel adhesions to the anterior suture line have limited the use of this type of cesarean section.

2. *Low cervical or lower segment cesarean section.* This is possible by means of a transverse (preferred) or vertical incision through the lower uterine segment or after a transverse incision through the visceral peritoneum at the bladder reflexion and downward displacement of the bladder. A flap of peritoneum is used to cover the myometrial closure, and intraperitoneal drainage is minimized; adhesions are uncommon. Blood loss is rarely excessive, unless placenta previa is present. Good healing is the rule. Rupture of the scar with a later pregnancy occurs in about 0.5% of cases. This is the cesarean section most commonly employed.

3. *Peritoneal exclusion cesarean section.* This is useful when the intraperitoneal spill of infected fluid and blood should be avoided. The operation is merely a low cervical cesarean section with suture of the parietal peritoneum to the transversely incised visceral peritoneum prior to incision through the lower uterine segment. Drainage fluid has easy access to the surface, and the likelihood of peritonitis because of spill is greatly reduced. Although this procedure is not difficult and is theoretically valuable, avoidance of delay and intensive antibiotic therapy have reduced the need for this operation.

4. *Extraperitoneal cesarean section.* This may be the procedure of choice in neglected, grossly infected cases. The operation is technically difficult, the peritoneum often lacerated, and the bladder or ureter injured. The peritoneal exclusion operation and intensive, broad-spectrum antibiotic therapy probably will serve as well as the extraperitoneal cesarean section in most cases.

5. *Cesarean hysterectomy.* Total or subtotal hysterectomy may be elected, usually after a classic cesarean section. The indication may be uterine pathology such as large uterine myomata. Placenta previa accreta, antenatal bleeding, and palpable placental tissue at the internal os may be reasons for cesarean section. When the placenta will not separate at operation, the uterus must be removed. If severe amnionitis is present, it may be best to remove the uterus after delivery of the fetus from above.

The disadvantages of cesarean hysterectomy include considerable blood loss and injury to the bladder or ureters. Hence its acceptability as a mode of sterilization remains in question.

6. *Vaginal cesarean section.* Vaginal cesarean section, actually an extended anterior vaginal hysterotomy, may be appropriate to terminate an advanced pregnancy when the transabdominal approach is rejected, for example, in cases of fetal death and amnionitis at 34 weeks. Poor exposure, bleeding, bladder damage, and a limited area in which to work make this operation difficult and rarely feasible near term.

Postmortem cesarean section

Assuming a definitely viable fetus, a cesarean section within 5 to 10 minutes of the mother's death theoretically should result in a living fetus. Careful preparations for such a delivery are important, including permission for the operation. Actually few babies have survived postmortem cesarean section, principally because of hypoxia related to the maternal death and/or immaturity.

Prognosis after cesarean section

Maternal morbidity and mortality are related to the indication for cesarean section, type of operation, duration of rupture of the membranes and labor, and blood transfusion and antibiotic therapy given. In large hospitals in North America the maternal mortality with cesar-

SKIN INCISION   UTERINE INCISION

A

Vertical through skin
Vertical through uterus

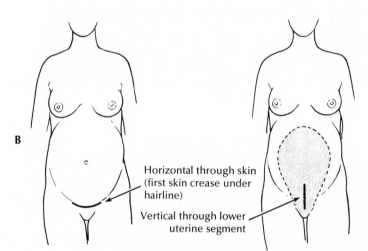

B

Horizontal through skin
(first skin crease under
hairline)

Vertical through lower
uterine segment

Fig. 26-14. Cesarean sections: skin and uterine incisions. **A,** Classical: skin and uterus—vertical incision. **B,** Low cervical: skin—horizontal; uterus—vertical. **C,** Low cervical: skin and uterus—horizontal.

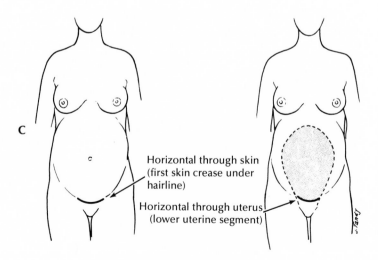

C

Horizontal through skin
(first skin crease under
hairline)

Horizontal through uterus
(lower uterine segment)

ean section is 0.1% to 0.2%. In communities where good maternity care is lacking, it may be five times this figure.

Perinatal mortality depends principally on fetal maturity, the problem for which the cesarean section was done, the anesthetic used, and the immediate postoperative support given. Actually it is the complications, for example, premature separation of the placenta, rather than the cesarean section that results in the perinatal death of at least 1% to 2% of children. In elective repeat cesarean section, however, a term perinatal mortality of 0.8% to 0.9% is achievable.

Delivery after cesarean section

If the original indication for the cesarean section is still present in a subsequent pregnancy near term, for example, a grossly contracted pelvis, repeat cesarean section is indicated. Moreover, women who sustained a classic cesarean section or any cesarean section marred by a septic course wherein questionable healing of the scar may rupture in labor, should be delivered by cesarean section.

When the original complication for which a cesarean section was initially done has not recurred (e.g., fetal distress due to cord compression at term during labor), one could permit a trial of labor under close observation with immediate cesarean section available in an emergency or elective low forceps at full dilatation. The alternative would be a repeat cesarean section because of concern for the strength of the uterine scar. Unless the patient is in a center with emergency surgical, anesthesia, and blood transfusion facilities available, a trial of labor and vaginal delivery are too great a risk for mother and fetus.

Surgical sterilization after two or more cesarean sections is difficult to justify on medical grounds, but the elective sterilization after even one cesarean section can be supported.

Management

Patients who must undergo cesarean section as the mode of delivery may be categorized in three groups. The first two are made up of women who have elective cesarean sections, and for them there is ample time for psychologic preparation. The psychic response of women in these groups may differ in that those scheduled for a repeat section may have disturbing memories of the conditions preceding the initial section, their experiences in the postoperative recovery period, and the added burden of care of an infant while recovering from a surgical operation as well as obstetrically. Those facing elective section for the first time share with other surgical patients

the same apprehensions concerning surgery coupled with the uncertainty of being able to cope with child care.

The third group are those women who face an emergency section as a result of a fetal or maternal response that suddenly necessitates changes in plans for vaginal delivery, postdelivery care, and care of self and infant at home. This may be an extremely traumatic experience. The patient approaches surgery usually tired and discouraged from a fruitless labor, worried and fretful about her own and the child's condition, and perhaps dehydrated and with low glycogen reserves. All preoperative procedures must be done quickly and competently. The time for explanation of procedures and of the operation is short, and since anxiety levels are high, much of what is said is forgotten or perhaps misconstrued. Postoperatively, time must be spent reviewing the events preceding the operation and the operation itself to assure these patients' understanding. Fatigue is often noticeable in these women, and they need much supportive care.

Most women usually feel some displeasure at not being able to have a normal vaginal delivery, and for a few, this can compound their problems of maintaining an adequate self-concept. Success in mothering activities and in the recovery process can do much to restore their self-esteem.

In addition to continuing careful monitoring of fetal and maternal well-being, the following preoperative preparation is carried out:

1. The abdomen is shaved beginning at the level of the xiphoid process and extending to the flank on both sides and down to the pubic area.

2. A retention catheter is inserted to ensure that the bladder remains empty during the operation. It is attached to a continuous drainage system. Since the urethra is 3 inches long (in nonpregnant women it is 1½ inches long), care must be taken to see that the catheter is properly placed and draining adequately.

3. Laboratory tests:
   a. Blood is sent for typing and cross matching. Two units of matched blood are kept in reserve for 48 hours after surgery.
   b. Urine is sent for routine analysis.

4. Maalox or other antacid is administered as ordered.

5. Intravenous infusion (e.g., 1000 ml Ringer's lactate solution in 5% dextrose in water) is started.

6. The patient is examined by the anesthesiologist, and the preoperative medication as ordered is administered.

7. Routine care is completed, including removal of dentures, contact lenses, rings, and fingernail polish and care of valuables.

8. The patient's chart is readied for use in surgery. Check if permission forms for care of the mother and infant are signed. Have the responsible adult accompanying the patient sign if the patient has received analgesia or anesthesia.

Figs. 26-15 to 26-20 depict the birth of an infant by cesarean section.

Once the surgery is completed, the mother is transferred to the recovery room for intensive care until her condition stabilizes. Then she is moved to the postnatal unit. Here the care is both postdelivery and postsurgical.

Care of mother after cesarean section. The following caretaking measures are necessary after cesarean section:

1. Prevention of hemorrhage:
   a. Check fundus gently but firmly. The uterus is sutured securely, so the procedure may cause discomfort but will not rupture the incised uterus. Oxytocin may be administered by intravenous infusion for 4 hours postoperatively.
   b. Check skin incision for signs of excessive bleeding.
   c. Check vital signs for evidence of shock.
2. Intake and output are recorded. Note if catheter is draining freely. Note and record character of drainage.

Fluids may be given orally when tolerated within 4 to 6 hours. The intravenous infusion (1000 ml/8 hours) is usually continued for 24 hours.

3. Postoperative pain and discomfort are controlled with the judicious use of medication, positioning the patient in bed, and splinting of incision while patient does deep breathing exercises. The pain arises from the stretching of the uterine musculature and supporting tissues, as well as from the incision site.

4. Coughing, deep breathing, paddling feet, and turning routines are instituted as for any postoperative patient. The patient may be allowed out of bed after 8 hours or after the anesthesia has completely worn off. The patient must be carefully watched for fainting episodes as a result of hypotension and use of sedative drugs.

5. The routine care for delivery patients is maintained, including sedation for afterpains or engorged breasts, breast care and perineal care for cleanliness, and temperature and blood pressure taken every 4 hours; showers may be taken by the second postoperative day if a spray dressing is used.

6. The mother must be shown her infant as soon as possible and given time to handle and examine the child. If the infant is in intensive care, she may be taken by wheelchair after the first day. The mother can participate in infant care as soon as she feels able. If feeding is

Text continued on p. 407.

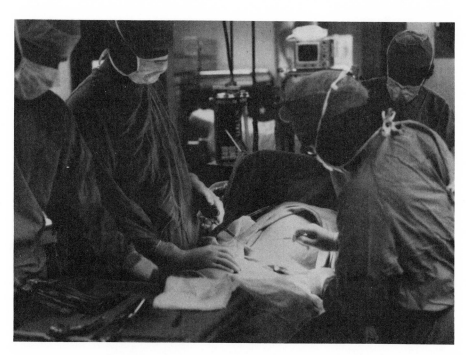

Fig. 26-15. Abdominal incision for cesarean section.

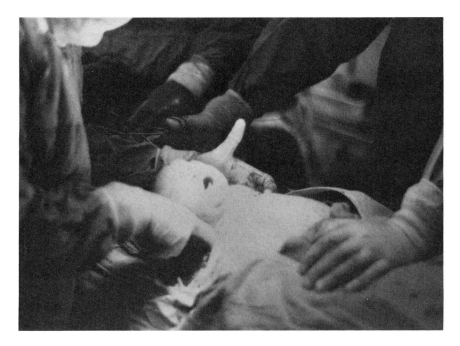

Fig. 26-16. Infant head guided through incision.

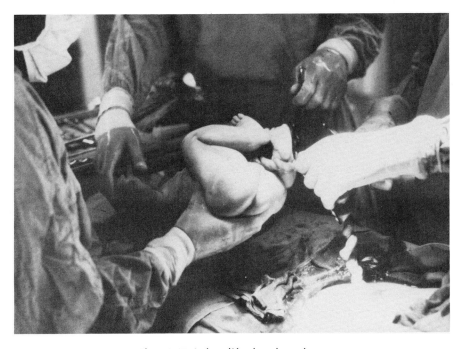

Fig. 26-17. Infant lifted and cord cut.

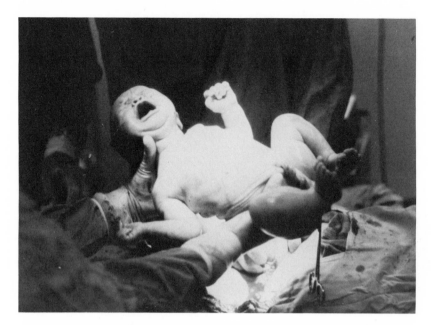

Fig. 26-18. Infant shown to mother.

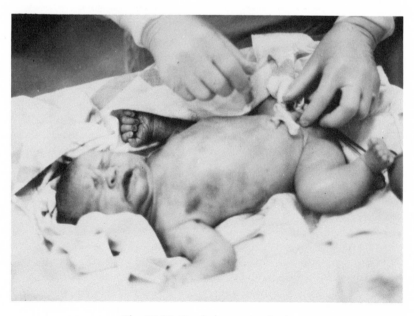

Fig. 26-19. Cord clamp attached.

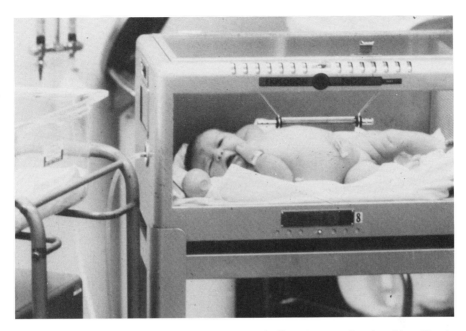

Fig. 26-20. Infant in warmed receiving crib. Note bulb syringe. Infant has identification band on wrist.

attempted, the infant can be supported on pillows to relieve pressure on the mother's abdomen. Some mothers find a side-lying position the most comfortable.

Those in rooming-in units usually are ready for these experiences by the third postoperative day.

Care of infant after cesarean section. These infants are considered to be at risk until there is evidence of physiologic stability after delivery. A warm crib and resuscitation equipment must be readied for surgery. A nurse or physician is delegated for the immediate care of the infant. These persons need to be expert in resuscitative techniques, as well as in observational skills for detecting abnormal infant responses. Depending on the physical state, the infant may be given to the mother to hold and examine before being transported to the transitional nursery. If compromised, the infant may be transported immediately to the infant intensive care unit.

REPAIR OF BIRTH CANAL INJURIES

Lacerations of the birth canal are second only to uterine atony as a major cause of postnatal hemorrhage. Therefore prevention, recognition, and prompt, effective treatment of birth canal lacerations are vitally important.

Continued bleeding despite efficient postnatal uterine contractions demands inspection or reinspection of the birth passage. Continuous bleeding from so-called minor sources may be just as dangerous as a sudden loss of a large amount of blood, although often it is ignored until shock develops. Birth canal lacerations may include injuries to the labia, perineum, vagina, and cervix.

Factors that influence the etiology and incidence of obstetric lacerations of the lower genital tract encompass operative delivery; aseptic or unattended spontaneous delivery; congenital abnormalities of the maternal soft parts; contracted pelvis; size, presentation, and position of the fetus; relative size of the presenting part and the birth canal; prior scarring from infection, injury, or surgery; the presence of vulvar, perineal, and vaginal varices; and abnormalities of uterine action, for example, precipitate delivery. Other associated problems may be abnormal tissue elasticity or friability, the presence of tumors, the general condition of the mother (e.g., exhaustion, dehydration), and the presence of complicating diseases. All these factors may exist alone or in combination.

The diagnosis of birth canal lacerations requires (1) an inherent awareness of their possible occurrence and (2) an immediate routine meticulous inspection of the entire lower birth canal after each delivery. Prerequisites for an adequate appraisal include aseptic technique (the patient who has "precipitated" must be prepared and draped), standard instruments for surgical repair, an assistant to provide exposure by retraction, and appropriate lighting.

Upward displacement of the cervix after its inspection by means of a "tailed" or "tagged" vaginal pack will greatly facilitate the inspection of the entire vaginal tract. Hence lacerations may be seen and repaired and hematomas identified and treated before they reach serious proportions. A vaginal pack also serves to elevate the uterus, enhancing its contractility and limiting blood loss during repair.

Proper anatomic reapproximation of all tissues is performed immediately after delivery for the following reasons:

1. To ensure hemostasis and to prevent hematomas
2. To eliminate open sources of puerperal infection
3. To correct problems (e.g., a poorly repaired old laceration of the rectal sphincter may be revised when increased vascularity and physiologic hypertrophy of pregnancy may favorably influence healing)

Blood replacement and the administration of appropriate antibiotic agents, when indicated, are important. A retention catheter may be required in specific cases.

Labial lacerations

Extreme vascularity in the labial and periclitoral areas often results in profuse bleeding. Immediate repair is required using fine catgut such as No. 4-0 on an atraumatic needle. Counterpressure with a gauze pad and a T binder may be required.

Lacerations of perineum

Lacerations of the perineum are the most common of all injuries in the lower genital tract. These are classified as follows:

- *First degree*—involves the mucosa and skin with some fibers of the superficial musculature
- *Second degree*—includes deeper structures of the perineum also
- *Third degree*—involves all the structures of the vaginal wall and the sphincter ani muscles are severed
- *Fourth degree*—involves all of aforementioned and the anal wall so that the anus is laid open

An episiotomy may extend to become either a third- or fourth-degree laceration.

Lacerations of vagina and vaginal hematomas

Prolonged pressure of the fetal head on the vaginal mucosa ultimately will interfere with the circulation and may produce ischemic or pressure necrosis. The state of the tissues therefore, together with the type of delivery, may result in deep vaginal lacerations and may predispose to vaginal hematomas.

Vaginal hematomas occur more frequently in association with forceps rotation of a fetus in an OP position; they are often found on the same side as the occiput, perhaps due to long continued pressure of the fetal head in one posterior quadrant of the vagina.

A vaginal hematoma should be diagnosed at the incipient or early stage. Most of them can usually be detected by routine inspection after delivery. Many vaginal hematomas occur beneath the mucosa opposite the ischial spines in the plane of the midpelvis. Therefore the physician will palpate the vaginal walls to detect a full, crepitant, or fluctuant area that may not have become visible yet. The large masses will be purple in color in contrast to the dark red of the remainder of the vaginal mucosa.

Many small hematomas undoubtedly go undetected and may even be self-limited. The underlying principle of treatment is the prevention of a large hematoma, however, because all hematomas have a small start. The sequelae include tissue devitalization, serious blood loss, shock, or infection.

During the postnatal period, if the patient complains of persistent perineal pain or feeling of fullness in the vagina, a careful inspection of the vulva is made. The patient assumes a side-lying position, the upper buttock is raised, and she is asked to bear down. A large purplish mass may be seen at the introitus.

She is then returned to the delivery unit where (after a suitable anesthetic has been administered) incision and evacuation of the hematoma is done, and deep sutures are placed for control of the bleeding area.

If the hematoma is larger than 5 cm in diameter, a catheter is placed in the bladder and a moderately tight vaginal pack inserted. A vaginal pack must be inserted carefully so as to avoid traumatizing the fibril tissues. To facilitate insertion of the pack, an antibiotic ointment may be spread on the pack or applied within the vagina. The catheter and pack may be removed in 6 to 8 hours. Antimicrobial agents for systemic action are not required routinely.

REMOVAL OF A RETAINED PLACENTA

The obstetrician must recognize the completion of the third stage of labor or complications may result. If the operator is hasty, for example, the placenta may not have an adequate opportunity to separate. If one waits too long, needless loss of blood may occur.

In the period after birth of the baby but before recovery of the placenta, some patients may have only slight bleeding, but others may have considerable blood loss. If no marked bleeding occurs and with proper management, the normally implanted placenta separates with the first or second strong uterine contraction after delivery of the infant, within 15 minutes in about 90% of patients.

Within 30 minutes after birth, an additional 5% of patients will have a separated placenta. If one waits 45 minutes after delivery, only another 1% to 2% of patients will achieve placental separation. Hence there is little to be gained by an extended wait-and-see attitude. If the placenta has not been recovered within 30 minutes of delivery, manual removal should be attempted.

If overly generous analgesia, such as morphine sulfate within 1 or 2 hours of delivery, or third-plane anesthesia with halothane or ether is given, prompt resumption of potent uterine contractions after the birth of the infant may be suppressed. Avoidance of sedation, administration of oxytocin intravenously or intramuscularly immediately after delivery, and elevation of the uterus without manual stimulation should aid separation of the placenta and reduce blood loss.

If excessive bleeding develops, manual separation and removal of the placenta is carried out immediately. No supplementary anesthesia will be needed for parturients who have had a block anesthetic for delivery. For other patients, administration of light nitrous oxide and oxygen inhalation anesthesia or intravenous thiopental (Pentothal) will suffice for intrauterine exploration, placental separation, and its recovery.

If delivery occurs early (fifth or sixth month) either spontaneously or by induced abortion, placental retention is the rule because of poor separation of the afterbirth. This may be due to an immature zone of separation, too weak uterine contractions, or a relatively large placenta.

Retained placenta may be the result of one of the following:

1. Partial separation of a normal placenta
2. Entrapment of the partially or completely separated placenta by an hour-glass constriction ring of the uterus or by mismanagement of the third stage of labor, for example, massage of the uterus (Credé) before separation of the placenta or ill-timed administration of ergot products
3. Abnormal adherence of the entire placenta or a portion of the placenta to the uterine wall

In all instances, postnatal hemorrhage or infection may be a critical complicating factor.

Some years ago, a popular procedure to shorten the third stage of labor was the administration of ergonovine or ergometrine, 1 ml intravenously, at the time of delivery of the fetal head or the anterior fetal shoulder. This promptly contracted the uterus, separated the placenta, and limited blood loss when given *precisely* at the correct time. If delayed or if some of the drug were injected outside the vein, the cervix would contract, and the placenta often was trapped so that general anesthesia was required to dilate the cervix for extraction of the placenta. Otherwise the physician might have to wait hours to recover the afterbirth.

Ergot products intravenously administered have a sudden marked pressor effect occasionally sufficient to cause an intracranial hemorrhage (e.g., rupture of a ''berry'' aneurysm). Because of the possible complications, ergot preparations should be given only *after* the recovery of the placenta, and they should always be given intramuscularly or orally, never intravenously.

Abnormal adherence of the placenta occurs for reasons unknown, but it is thought to be the result of zygote implantation in a zone of defective endometrium. Abnormal adherence of the placenta is diagnosed in only about 1 of every 12,000 deliveries. Approximately 90% of patients are multiparous, and many of these have also had abortions. The mother with an abnormally attached placenta is jeopardized mainly by postnatal hemorrhage leading to hypovolemic shock. Firm placental attachment is associated with increased maternal morbidity and mortality. Moreover, prematurity due to associated problems such as placenta previa accounts for increased perinatal loss.

Factors that predispose to abnormally firm placental attachment are (1) scarring of the uterus such as occurs after cesarean section, myomectomy, or vigorous curettage; (2) endometritis, associated with tuberculosis for example; (3) abnormal site of implantation such as the cervix, lower uterine segment, cornual region, or in one horn of a bicornuate uterus; or (4) malformation of the placenta, for example, extrachorial placenta.

Unusual placental adherence may be partial or complete, and the following degrees of attachment are recognized:

- *Placenta accreta (vera)*—slight penetration of the myometrium by placental trophoblast (rare)
- *Placenta increta*—deep penetration by the placenta (very rare)
- *Placenta percreta (destruans)*—perforation of the uterus by placenta (exceptional)

There are more cases of partial than complete placenta accreta.

In all types of abnormal adherence, placentation occurs in an area of deficient, sparse, or absent decidua. Thus the placenta develops on a surface partially or completely devoid of decidua (basalis). The uterine muscle is exposed, and invasion of the trophoblast and chorionic villi of the myometrium soon occurs. A dense fibrous area representing fusion of Nitabuch's layer and Rohr's stria develops, together with hyalinization of neighboring uterine muscle. There is no zone of separation; no cleavage plane can be developed between the placenta and the uterine wall. Attempts to remove the placenta in the usual manner are unsuccessful therefore, and laceration or perforation of the uterine wall may result.

In placenta percreta, complete penetration of the uterine wall by trophoblast often with intraperitoneal bleeding or rupture of the uterus may ensue.

At least 15% of abnormally adherent placenta (all types) are associated with placenta previa. Stated another way, about 3% of all placenta previas have a placenta accreta, increta, or percreta. Persistent bleeding in cases having a low-lying, abnormally adherent placenta is due to laceration of the dilated myometrial sinusoids by attempted manual removal of adjacent trophoblastic tissue, deficient thrombosis of vessels at the placental site, or poor contractility of the thinned, lower uterine segment musculature.

There are no sure signs of an abnormally adherent placenta during pregnancy. During late pregnancy, some patients with placenta increta or percreta may have considerable uterine pain, even suggestive of labor. Although these may be suspected by angiography, the diagnosis is almost invariably made intranatally.

Bleeding with complete or total placenta accreta does not occur unless separation of the placenta is attempted, but partial placenta accreta invariably is associated with excessive intranatal or postnatal bleeding. This is because vessels adjacent to the adherent placenta remain open, and free bleeding prevents clotting.

When manual removal of a placenta accreta is attempted, damage to placental tissue and decidua, both rich in thromboplastin, occurs. When this substance is released in quantity into the circulation, a consumption coagulopathy (disseminated intravascular coagulation) may develop.

At vaginal delivery the diagnosis of an abnormally adherent placenta generally is made when manual separation of a retained placenta is attempted. Placenta accreta or increta usually is diagnosed at cesarean section when a firmly applied placenta is discovered.

After vaginal delivery, if the placenta will not separate readily (even a portion), immediate abdominal hysterectomy may be indicated. Persistent attempts at placental removal rarely will be successful, and fatal hemorrhage may result.

If an abnormally adherent placenta is discovered at cesarean section, especially when surgery was indicated because of placenta previa, total hysterectomy may be the best treatment. If the patient is most desirous of a future pregnancy and is in good condition and if hemorrhage can be controlled, the risk of not removing the uterus may be justifiable. Small retained portions of the placenta may separate or be absorbed, but infection often is an added late complication. Reoperation may be necessary because of later hemorrhage. After a subsequent viable pregnancy, elective repeat cesarean section will be mandatory because another placenta accreta or increta is likely. Delivery should be followed immediately by total abdominal hysterectomy.

REFERENCES

Brenner, W. E., and others. 1974. Characteristics and perils of breech presentation. Am. J. Obstet. Gynecol. **118:**700.

Bright, M. V. 1974. Abdominal wound healing following cesarean section. J. R. Coll. Surg. Edinb. **19:**297.

Chalmers, J. A. 1975. The use of the vacuum extractor to accelerate the first and second stages of labor. Obstet. Gynecol. **2:**203.

Downing, J. W., and others. 1974. Lateral table tilt for cesarean section. Anesthesiology **29:**696.

Fox, H. 1972. Placenta accreta. Obstet. Gynecol. Survey **27:**475.

Hammond, H. 1972. Death from obstetric hemorrhage. Calif. Med. **117:**16.

Hibbard, L. T., and Schermann, W. R. 1973. Prophylactic external cephalic version in obstetric practice. Am. J. Obstet. Gynecol. **116:**511.

Kitchen, J. D., III, and others. 1975. Puerperal inversion of the uterus. Am. J. Obstet. Gynecol. **123:**51.

Malvern, J., and others. 1973. Ultrasonic scanning of the puerperal uterus following secondary postpartum hemorrhage. J. Obstet. Gynaecol. Br. Commonw. **80:**320.

Mingeot, R., and others. 1975. Breech delivery: a review of a consecutive series of 285 cases. Eur. J. Obstet. Gynecol. **5:**177.

Niswander, K. R., and Gordon, M. 1973. Safety of the low-forceps operation. Am. J. Obstet. Gynecol. **117:**619.

Ott, J. W. 1975. Vacuum extraction. Obstet. Gynecol. Survey **30:**643.

Phillips, R. D., and Freeman, M. 1974. Management of persistent occiput posterior position: review of 552 consecutive cases. Obstet. Gynecol. **43:**171.

Ranney, B. 1973. Gentle art of external version. Am. J. Obstet. Gynecol. **116:**239.

Rao, K. B. 1975. Maternal mortality in a teaching hospital in southern India. Obstet. Gynecol. **46:**397.

Rovinsky, J. J., and others. 1973. Management of breech presentation at term. Am. J. Obstet. Gynecol. **115:**497.

Serreyn, R., and others. 1973. Fetal hypoxia and breech delivery. Int. J. Gynaecol. Obstet. **11:**11.

UNIT EIGHT

Postdelivery period

CHAPTER 27

The puerperium

The puerperium or period of recovery from childbirth extends for 6 weeks after delivery. Repair of injury to the birth canal, involution of the uterus, and return of all systems to the prepregnant or nearly prepregnant state occurs during the puerperium. The process is both anabolic (lactation) and catabolic (involution of the uterus). Fatigue from the work of labor, sudden relief from discomfort, and a profound psychologic lift mark the period immediately succeeding the birth process.

PHYSIOLOGIC CHANGES
Vascular system

The pregnancy-induced hypervolemia (at least 40% increase near term) allows most women to tolerate a considerable blood loss at delivery. Many women lose 300 to 400 ml of blood at vaginal delivery and about twice this amount at cesarean section. This influences the blood volume and hematocrit changes during the puerperium.

After vaginal delivery, a declining blood volume usually is associated with a rise in hematocrit by the third to seventh day after delivery, suggesting that the loss of red blood cells is less than the reduction of vascular capacity (uterus and periphery) and that hemoconcentration results from the excretion of extracellular fluid.

After cesarean section, a more rapid decline in blood volume and hematocrit occurs, but there is a tendency for the hematocrit to stabilize or even decline slightly in the early puerperium.

By the third week after delivery, the blood volume usually is back to prenatal values. There is no red blood cell destruction during the puerperium, but any gain will disappear gradually in accordance with the life span of the red blood cell. In uncomplicated cases, the hematocrit will have returned to normal by the fourth or fifth postnatal week.

There is an extensive activation of blood clotting factors after delivery. This, together with immobility, trauma, or sepsis, encourages thromboembolization. Avoidance of tissue damage and infection, early ambulation, and limitation of estrogen therapy for suppression of lactation should reduce the risk of thromboembolic complications.

Genital tract

After delivery, the cervix is soft, appears bruised, and has some small lacerations. It remains easily distensible; two fingers may still be introduced easily by the tenth hour. By the eighteenth hour, it has shortened, has a firm consistency, and has regained its form. By the end of the first week, recovery is almost complete. The external os, however, does not regain its prepregnant appearance; it is no longer shaped like a circle but appears as a jagged slit (Fig. 14-2).

Estrogen deprivation is responsible for the thinness of the vaginal mucosa and the absence of rugae. The greatly distended, smooth-walled vagina gradually returns to its prenatal condition by about the third or fourth week. Most rugae may be permanently flattened, and the mucosa remains atrophic in the lactating woman at least until menstruation begins again. The torn hymen heals with the development of fibrosed nodules of mucosa called *carunculae hymenales*.

The uterus, which weighs about eleven times its prepregnant weight, rapidly involutes after delivery (Fig. 27-1). The uterus weighs approximately 1000 gm (2.2 pounds) immediately after delivery, 500 gm (1.1 pounds) a week after delivery, and 350 gm (11 to 12 ounces) 2 weeks after delivery. Estrogen-stimulated myometrial growth (hypertrophy and hyperplasia) is quickly reversed during the relative hypoestrogenism of the puerperium. Progesterone, which was responsible for much of the increased uterine weight and collagen formation during gestation, is not produced until the first ovulation weeks or even months in the future. It is not surprising, then, that progesterone cannot be detected after the first postnatal week.

Withdrawal of estrogen and progesterone is followed by the release of proteolytic enzymes and the migration of macrophages into the endometrium and myometrium. Uterine involution within 4 to 6 weeks occurs principally by a decrease in the size of individual myometrial cells.

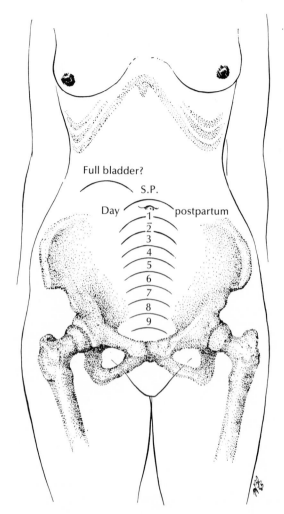

Full bladder?

S.P.

Day — postpartum
1
2
3
4
5
6
7
8
9

Fig. 27-1. Involution of uterus, showing various positions of fundus. *S.P.,* Level just after separation of placenta from uterine wall before its delivery. Immediately after delivery, fundus can be felt 2 cm below the umbilicus; within 12 hours, fundus returns to S.P. level, then begins its descent of about 1 cm/day. (From Ingalls, A. J., and Salerno, M. C. 1975. Maternal and child health nursing [ed. 3]. St. Louis, The C. V. Mosby Co.)

However, the augmentation of connective tissue and elastin in the myometrium and blood vessels and the increase in the total uterine cell number are permanent. Hence the uterine size usually is increased slightly after each pregnancy.

Uterine contractions persist after delivery of the placenta. In primiparas, the tone of the uterus is increased so that the fundus generally remains firm. Periodic relaxation and contraction are the rule for mul-

tiparas and may cause uncomfortable afterpains that persist for 2 or 3 days. Breast-feeding frequently intensifies these afterpains.

The placental site is partially obliterated by vascular constriction and thrombosis. Endometrial regeneration of the area follows promptly from stromal derivatives of the decidua basalis and mucosal elements from vestiges of glands in the placental site, leaving no scar on the endometrial lining. Endometrial regeneration is rapid and repair generally is complete by the fifth to sixth postnatal week.

Failure of the placental site to heal completely is called *subinvolution of the placental site*. Patients with this condition have persistent lochia and episodes of brisk, painless bleeding. Curettage usually is required.

Limitation of anesthesia, elevation of the uterus, and slight massage of the fundus usually will control excessive postnatal blood loss. Long-lasting oxytocics such as ergonovine or ergometrine are useful if uterine relaxation and active bleeding resumes. Oxytocin will not elevate the blood pressure, but ergot products may. Although ergot products are beneficial in the immediate treatment of uterine bleeding due to hypotonia, it is unlikely that these drugs are of value after the first 1 to 2 days.

Immediately after delivery, the nontender fundus should be about 2 cm *below* the umbilicus. On external palpation, the uterus feels firm and about the size of a grapefruit. Within 12 hours, with the "take-up" and improved tone of the uterine supports, the fundus should be approximately 1 cm *above* the umbilicus (Fig. 27-1), although a distended bladder may obscure the level. From then on, involution progresses rapidly. By the sixth postnatal day, the fundus normally will be one half the distance from the symphysis pubis to the umbilicus. The uterus should not be palpable abdominally after the ninth day after delivery.

Initially, postnatal vaginal discharge is bloody *(lochia rubra)* and lasts about 3 days. The flow pales, becoming pink or brown after several days *(lochia serosa)*. About 10 days after delivery, the drainage should be yellow to white *(lochia alba)* because of the presence of numerous leukocytes and cellular debris.

Persistence of lochia rubra early suggests retained placental fragments. Recurrence of bleeding after 3 to 4 weeks may be due to subinvolution of the placental site. Continued lochia serosa or lochia alba may indicate endometritis, particularly when fever, pain, or tenderness is associated. Lochia should smell like normal menstrual flow; an offensive odor usually indicates infection. Lochia clots, but normal menstrual flow does not.

Ovarian activity remains suspended for differing periods of time after delivery. For lactating women, amenorrhea or anovulatory periods may persist until the infant is weaned. If menstruation does begin, there is no need to discontinue nursing. However, it should be remembered that ovulation precedes menstruation, and a woman may therefore become pregnant while lactating. Approximately 90% of nonlactating primiparas and 30% of lactating primiparas begin menstruating within 3 months of delivery. Multiparas often start to menstruate earlier. The first menstrual period is much heavier than normal and anovulatory. Within 3 to 4 months, the amount of flow has returned to normal.

Urinary tract

Kidney function returns to normal, and ureteral dilatation gradually is reduced during the first month after delivery. Pelvic soreness due to the forces of labor, vaginal lacerations, or the episiotomy reduces or alters the voiding reflex. This, together with postnatal diuresis, may allow rapid filling of the bladder. If adequate voiding (less than 100 ml residual urine) does not occur after 24 hours, a retention catheter can be inserted for 48 hours, and a urinary antibiotic such as sulfisoxazole (Gantrisin) may be administered. The drug should be continued for at least 1 week whereupon a clean-catch urine specimen is obtained for culture and sensitivity to exclude persistence of bacteriuria.

Clean-catch or catheterized urine specimens after delivery often reveal hematuria due to bladder trauma. Later, hematuria may be a sign of urinary tract infection. Proteinuria may persist for at least a week in patients with preeclampsia-eclampsia. Acetonuria is common in diabetics and even uncomplicated patients after prolonged labor or dehydration. Lactosuria may be expected in lactating women. This cannot be detected by use of the Clinitest, since this test is specific for presence of glucose in the urine.

Normally a marked diuresis begins within 12 hours after delivery. This mechanism, whereby the excess tissue fluid accumulated during pregnancy is eliminated, is often referred to as the *reversal of the water metabolism of pregnancy*.

Gastrointestinal tract

The mother is usually hungry shortly after delivery and can tolerate a light diet.

A spontaneous bowel evacuation may be delayed several days after delivery. This can be explained by decreased muscle tone in the intestines; prelabor diarrhea or the predelivery enema, lack of food, dehydration, perineal tenderness due to the episiotomy, lacerations, or

hemorrhoids. For some women, regular bowel habits have to be reestablished after delivery. Attention to timing and dietary and fluid intake is essential.

Abdominal musculature

The muscles of the abdominal wall and pelvic floor and their fascia regain their tone during the puerperium and approximate their original length after the stresses of pregnancy are over. Lacerations or overstretching at the time of delivery may weaken the pelvic floor and predispose to genital hernias. Marked distension of the abdominal wall during gestation may result in diastasis of the recti muscles.

Vital signs

Temperature during the first 24 hours after delivery may elevate to 38° C (100.4° F) as a result of the dehydrating effects of labor. A diagnosis of puerperal sepsis is suggested, however, if a similar rise develops after the first 24 hours postdelivery and recurs or persists for 2 days. Other possibilities may be mastitis, urinary tract infections, or other systemic infections.

Bradycardia is a common finding for the first 6 to 8 days postdelivery. A pulse rate of between 50 to 70/min may be considered normal.

Blood pressure remains unchanged. A drop may indicate increased uterine bleeding. However, patients are prone to develop orthostatic hypotension before the cardiovascular system readjusts to the loss of intrapelvic pressure after delivery. An increased reading may indicate preeclampsia. Therefore patients who complain of headaches should be checked before administering any analgesia for relief of headache.

Endocrine status

During pregnancy, hormonal production changes considerably. The placenta, adrenals, thyroid, and anterior

Table 27-1. Hormonal reduction after delivery

Day 1	First week	Second to third weeks
HCG	Estrone	Estriol
Estrogen	Estradiol	
Aldosterone	Progesterone	
	Corticoids	
	17-Ketosteroids	
	11-Oxycorticosteroids	

pituitary act as major sources. Once delivery has occurred, there is a return to normal with reduction in some hormones (Table 27-1) and increases in the following:

1. Thyroid function: increased protein-bound iodine, butyl-extractible iodine, iodine uptake
2. Anterior pituitary gonadotropic hormones
3. Prolactin and oxytocin (in lactating women)

MANAGEMENT

The approach to care of women during the puerperium has changed from one modeled on the concept of "sick care" to one that is health oriented. It is now a collaborative effort on the part of all involved—mother, nurse, physician, and family—to prevent complications; to provide comfort, rest, and nourishment; to engage in teaching-learning activities related to self-care for the mother and the care of the newborn; and to foster the process of parent-child relationships. Although the care is concentrated in the first 3 to 5 days after delivery, health supervision should be continued for the 6-week period to ensure that adequate professional assistance is available during critical periods in child care and in readjustment to home and family.

Activity

Most patients can be ambulatory 6 to 8 hours after normal delivery, assuming local or light general anes-

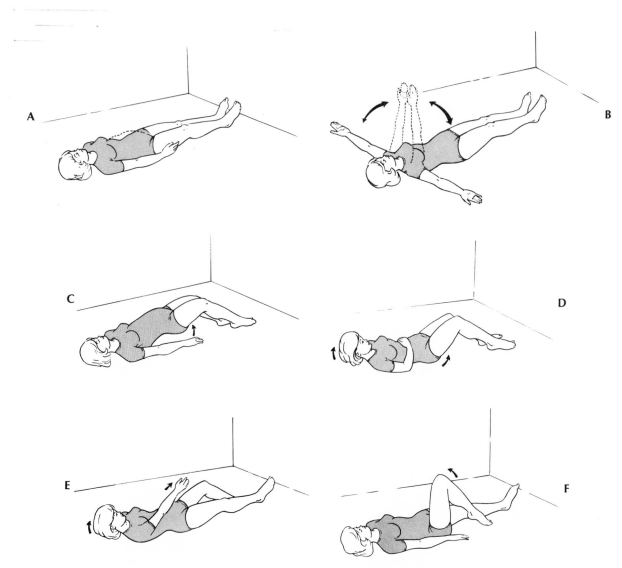

Fig. 27-2. A, First day; **B,** second day; **C,** third day; **D,** fourth day; **E,** fifth day; and **F,** sixth day.

thesia. To avoid headache, parturients who received intrathecal spinal anesthesia should remain flat in bed (one pillow) for a minimum of 8 hours before they are allowed to be up and around. This is not required for those who had epidural or caudal anesthesia.

The duration of hospitalization and the subsequent convalescence at home still are debated. Most uncomplicated patients who do not nurse may be dismissed from the hospital on the third postnatal day. Mothers who nurse probably should remain 1 or 2 days longer to ensure success of lactation. Patients with complications should be asymptomatic for at least 24 hours and capable of personal care after leaving the hospital.

Return visits and general instructions

Since biblical times, the puerperium has been considered to last for 6 weeks. Hence a return visit and examination have been scheduled traditionally 1½ months after delivery. This is illogical inasmuch as many problems such as leukorrhea may be identified and successfully treated earlier. Individualization is important therefore, but a more logical date for return to the physician or clinic would be 3 to 4 weeks postdelivery.

Advice and suggestions are welcomed particularly by primiparas. Recommendations must be suited to each patient's needs and circumstances. The following are reasonable for most patients:

1. Gradual increase in ambulation about the house is suggested. Stairs offer few problems. Avoidance of fatigue should be the rule. Light housekeeping can be resumed after the first week. Generally, the patient can drive her car about the tenth day. Moderate work can be accepted during the third week, but full activity should be delayed until after the postnatal visit and examination. Most women can resume all but the most physically tiring employment 4 to 5 weeks after childbirth. An increase in the amount of lochia rubra or its reappearance may indicate too much activity.

Patients should be told that they may have a "small period" or an episode of painless bleeding about 3 weeks after delivery (from the placental site). If bleeding becomes profuse or prolonged, however, the patient should call her physician for advice.

2. Postnatal exercises are helpful in trimming the figure and toning the musculature. If the patient is willing, calisthenics should be outlined; if she is not recep-

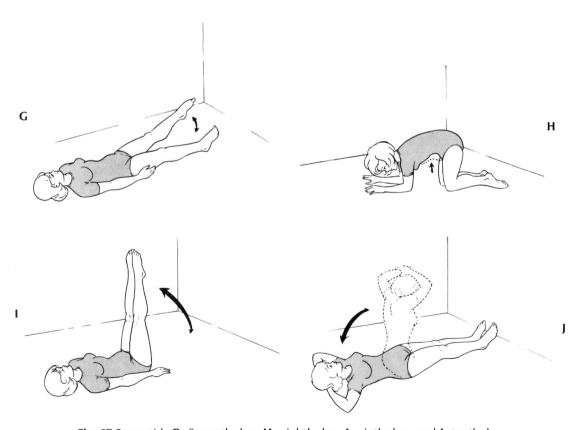

Fig. 27-2, cont'd. **G,** Seventh day; **H,** eighth day; **I,** ninth day; and **J,** tenth day.

tive, the value of household activities, that is, bending and stretching, is emphasized as beneficial exercise (Fig. 27-2).

3. The recommended food intake for lactating women is about 3000 calories, but approximately 2300 calories are suggested during the puerperium for those who are not nursing. Lactation requires slightly more food, including milk (e.g., more than 1 quart every day). Moreover, a daily vitamin-mineral supplement may be advisable for nursing mothers. If problems develop such as "caked breast" or fever or if the infant remains hungry despite the usual feedings and additional water, the physician should be contacted.

4. The couple can safely resume intercourse by the third to fourth week if bleeding has stopped and the episiotomy has healed. For the first 6 weeks to 6 months the vagina does not lubricate well because steroid depletion inhibits the vasocongestive response to sexual tension. A water-soluble gel or a contraceptive cream or jelly might therefore be recommended for lubrication. If there is some vaginal tenderness, the partner can be instructed to insert a few fingers into the vagina and rotate them around the vaginal os to help relax it and to identify possible areas of discomfort. A coital position in which the woman has control of the depth of penile penetration is also useful. The side-by-side or female-superior positions often are recommended.

Physiologic reactions to sexual stimulation for the first 3 postnatal months are marked by reduction in both rapidity and intensity of response. Vasocongestion of the labia majora and minora is delayed well into the plateau phase. The walls of the vagina are thin and pink, a condition similar to senile vaginitis. This is due to the hormonal starvation of the involutional period. Finally, the size of the orgasmic platform and strength of orgasmic contractions are reduced.

Some women have reported sexual stimulation to plateau and orgasmic levels when nursing their babies. It is interesting to note that although nursing mothers have a longer delay in ovarian steroid production, they are often interested in returning to sexual activity before nonnursing mothers. Nursing mothers also report higher levels of postnatal eroticism.

The woman should be instructed to follow the Kegal exercises to strengthen her pubococcygeal muscle. The pubococcygeal muscle is the major sphincter of the pelvis. It is associated not only with bowel and bladder function but also is associated with vaginal perception and response during intercourse.

5. Contraception should be discussed and a tentative program outlined before the patient leaves the hospital. If the mother is not nursing, she can resume oral contraceptives only under physician's directive. If she is nursing or wishes to use an IUD or diaphragm, temporary contraception such as the condom and/or foam should be provided, and the desired method can be instituted at the time of the postnatal examination.

PLAN OF CARE: PUERPERIUM—FIRST 2 WEEKS

PATIENT CARE OBJECTIVES

1. Involution of the uterus progresses normally.
   a. Size diminishes. Immediately after birth it is the size and consistency of a small grapefruit, the fundus located 2 cm below umbilicus. By the end of the second hour, as the uterine cavity fills with blood and clots, the fundus rises above the umbilicus. By the end of the twelfth hour, with intermittent massage and expelling of clots, the fundus is about 1 cm above the umbilicus. Thereafter the height of the fundus decreases 1 cm/day until the ninth day, when it is at the border of the upper level of the pubis. Throughout it remains in the midline or slightly to the right of midline.
   b. Uterine tone is maintained by contraction-retraction of uterine muscles. The uterus feels firm and contracts readily after massage, after expelling clots, or after emptying the bladder or rectum. By the second day it remains contracted. Contractions are noted when the infant suckles the breast.
   c. Lochia:
      (1) Color and consistency change. Lochia rubra contains blood, placental and decidual debris, and clots and is dark red in color. It persists from delivery through the third day. Lochia serosa is thin, serous, brownish in color, and lasts from the fourth to the tenth day. Lochia alba, a yellowish white discharge, contains an increased number of leukocytes, and lasts from the tenth day to as long as the sixth week.
      (2) Odor remains characteristically "fleshy," not foul.
      (3) Amount of discharge is moderate for the first 2 or 3 days, then scant. Some women may have none after 2 weeks; others persist until the sixth week.

PLAN OF CARE: PUERPERIUM—FIRST 2 WEEKS—cont'd

PATIENT CARE OBJECTIVES—cont'd

    d. Cervix regains its shape in a few days and the external os is contracted by the end of first week (introduction of a 1 cm probe difficult).

2. Vagina remains distensible; the introitus gapes when intra-abdominal pressure is increased by the bearing-down effort or coughing.

3. Abdominal wall is lax and weak in the midline where the recti muscles may be widely separated. The muscles feel like masses on either side of the abdomen and are not to be confused with the fundus of the uterus.

4. Pulse rate falls a short time after delivery (range 50 to 70/min), and bradycardia persists for 6 to 8 days.

5. Temperature is elevated to 38° C (100.4° F) in the first 24 hours after delivery. This is not unusual and if unaccompanied by other symptoms such as pain in calf of leg or foul odor of lochia, it is considered to be due to dehydration. If the temperature elevation persists for 48 hours, it is considered abnormal.

6. Blood pressure remains in accord with previous normal readings.

7. Body weight: There is an immediate weight loss of 10 to 12 pounds, then as excess tissue fluid is eliminated, a further loss of 4 to 5 pounds in the first 3 to 4 days. Further decrease occurs as the uterus involutes and plasma volume contracts.

8. Vascular system:

    a. Although a normal concentration of blood occurs as retained tissue fluids are released and the tendency to clot increases as a result of the absolute increase in the number of platelets, thrombi rarely develop.

    b. Hct reading by the third postnatal day is within a normal range (42% ± 3).

9. Breasts:

    a. For 2 to 3 days after delivery, the breasts secrete colostrum in increasing amounts.

    b. By the second day in multiparas and by the third in primiparas, the breasts become engorged, firm, tense, and tender. This is due to vascular stasis, and in 36 to 48 hours the pain disappears as the swelling spontaneously subsides.

    c. Soon after the onset of this engorgement, the true milk is formed, and the "let-down reflex" in response to the suckling of the baby or manual manipulation causes expression of milk.

10. Elimination:

    a. Most patients void spontaneously by the eighth hour postdelivery and thereafter frequent copious amounts for 48 hours as retained tissue fluids are released.

    b. Some patients defecate spontaneously by the third day. Others reestablish regular habits only with aid of laxatives or enemas.

11. Pain or discomfort: Many patients feel the stress and strain of labor and delivery for 1 to 2 days, and discomfort associated with an episiotomy, hemorrhoids, engorgement of the breasts, and other conditions may act to impede recovery for 3 to 5 days.

12. Emotional response: Patients exhibit typical dependent behaviors for 24 to 48 hours. These usually are superseded by a mixture of dependent-independent behaviors, which in turn give way to interdependent behaviors. Depressive reactions may begin by the end of the second postnatal day and persist for 1 to 3 days. Mother-child relationships may be positive immediately or show a "maternal lag," which does not interfere unduly with child-care activities (Chapter 29).

13. Skill in child-care activities increases with physical recovery and practice.

14. Records reflect care given and indicate areas of need for continued care.

NURSING INTERVENTIONS

Diagnostic	Therapeutic and educational

1. Receive report from nurse from labor unit: type of labor, time of delivery, progress, and care given during first to fourth hours postdelivery, plus any complicating conditions (e.g., postnatal hemorrhage, preeclampsia, depressive emotional state, etc.).	1. Admit to bed accommodation in postnatal unit and introduce to other patients sharing room.
	  a. Check for understanding of use of call bell; review routine of care: time of infant feeding, any visiting regulations, ordering diet preferences.
	  b. Describe and give rationale for procedures to be used in assessing recovery from childbirth and return of reproductive organs to prepregnant state (involution).
	  c. Provide comfort and cleanliness and advise patient to rest as much as possible for first 8 hours.

2. Review patient's record for information pertinent to plans for patient assuming care of self and child (patient profile).	2. Prevent hemorrhage. Explain necessity for frequent checking of uterus, its firmness and position relative to midline and umbilicus, intermittent, not constant, massage of fundus; expression of clots from uterine cavity; and

Continued.

PLAN OF CARE: PUERPERIUM—FIRST 2 WEEKS—cont'd

NURSING INTERVENTIONS—cont'd

Diagnostic   **Therapeutic and educational**

3. Establish routine for assessing physical recovery based on patient's condition. Minimal examinations:
   a. Fundus assessed for consistency and position in abdomen every 30 minutes for 4 hours; lochia assessed for amount, color, and odor every hour for 4 hours; episiotomy assessed for healing, signs of inflammation, hematomas every 8 hours for 3 days.
   b. Temperature, pulse, respirations taken every 4 hours.
   c. BP every 2 hours for 8 hours, every 8 hours for 3 days, and before administering analgesic if patient complains of headache.
   d. Check legs daily for signs of thrombosis (pain, warmth, and tenderness; swollen reddened vein that feels hard or solid to touch); may or may not be positive Homan's sign (dorsiflexure of foot causes calf muscles to compress tibial veins and produce pain if thrombosis is present).
   e. Breasts are checked daily.
   f. Voiding:
      (1) Bladder is checked for distention every 2 hours for 8 hours, then every 8 hours for 3 days.
      (2) Patient is requested to report if she is experiencing pain or burning on voiding, if she is voiding small amounts frequently, or if she is unable to void every 4 hours.
   g. Defecation: Patient is asked to report first bowel movement, and asked daily if regular habits have been established.
4. Determine patient's emotional status and extent of skill in self-care and infant care while carrying out other assessments and during teaching and counseling of patients.

emphasis on voiding and emptying bladder. Patient is asked to empty her bladder in preparation for examination of uterus and perineum. She lies in supine position with her knees flexed to relieve tension on abdomen. If episiotomy is not readily visible in this position, patient is turned to her side and buttocks raised to permit inspection of suture line. Good light source is essential for inspection of some episiotomies (e.g., in dark-skinned mothers).
3. Prevent infection.
   a. Personal hygiene:
      (1) Bed bath is given until patient's condition permits use of shower or tub, usually 24 hours after delivery. Patient must be instructed to use fresh washcloth and towel and to begin bath by washing nipples and breasts. Patient may require encouragement to wash perineum, including episiotomy incision, with mild soap and warm water at least once daily. Fear of "breaking the stitches" makes some patients reluctant to do this.
      (2) Routine cleansing of perineum after voiding or defecating is necessary. Soap and water and/or medicated wipe may be used. Patient is instructed to cleanse from pubis to anal area to prevent contamination of vagina and urethra with fecal material and to use sterile perineal pads. She is instructed to wash her hands before and after changing perineal pad. She is shown how to protect inner surface of pad from contamination and how to position pad from front to back. Soiled pads are wrapped and placed in separate covered containers. Mother is cautioned about placing infant on bedding (lower sheet) where she has been sitting to protect infant from infection. Spread can be drawn up over this area and used as base sheet for baby.
      (3) Vaginal discharge. Daily cleansing afforded by bath or shower in addition to careful cleansing after voiding and defecating is sufficient unless flow is profuse. Patients may require repeated instructions about frequent hand washing, technique of keeping sterile pad from being contaminated, expected amount and appearance of normal lochia and to report if a foul odor should occur. A foul odor is important symptom of uterine infection, and immediate therapy is indicated. Swab of vaginal contents may be ordered and sent to lab for culture (routine nose or throat swab sticks may be used for this procedure).
   b. Facilities and supplies: Bathroom and bed units must be kept scrupulously clean. Frequent changes of drawsheets and daily change of linen are recommended. Supervision of use of facilities to prevent cross infection among patients is necessary (e.g., common sitz bath must be scrubbed after each patient's use).
   c. Personnel must be conscientious about their hand-washing techniques to prevent cross infection. Use of face mask is required when carrying out perineal care in many institutions. Personnel with colds, coughs, or skin infections must not be in contact with these patients.
4. Prevent thrombosis:
   a. Patients with varicosities are encouraged to wear support hose.
   b. Exercise limbs if patient confined to bed longer than normal (8 hours) (e.g., patient with spinal anesthesia, cesarean section).
      (1) Alternate flexion and extension of feet.
      (2) Rotation of feet.
      (3) Alternate flexion and extension of legs.
      (4) Press back of knee to bed surface; relax.
      (5) Straight-leg raising.

PLAN OF CARE: PUERPERIUM—FIRST 2 WEEKS—cont'd

NURSING INTERVENTIONS—cont'd

Diagnostic	Therapeutic and educational

    c. Avoid use of estrogens to inhibit or suppress lactation.

    d. Encourage active walking about for true ambulation, not sitting immobile in chair. If thrombus is suspected, notify physician immediately; meanwhile, confine patient to bed with affected limb elevated on pillows.

5. Comfort measures:

    a. Episiotomy:

      (1) Dry heat from heat lamp positioned 20 inches from perineum may be used tid for 20-minute periods. At home, desk lamp makes effective heat lamp. In hospital, extendable over-bed lamp has proved successful. Patient may be instructed to lie with her head to foot of bed, perineal pad removed, lamp positioned, and patient draped for privacy and warmth. If portable heat lamp is shared by several patients, care must be taken to clean it between patients to prevent cross infection.

      (2) Moist heat (e.g., sitz bath) may be used by first postnatal day, twice a day or more often. Temperature of water is maintained at 38° to 43.2° C (100° F ± 10°). Call bell must be within reach in case patient feels faint. Mother will need assistance in sitting down in some sitz baths. Instruct mother to tighten her gluteal muscles until seated and then be sure to relax them; otherwise perineal area may remain dry (a shower taken prior to use of sitz bath helps to keep bath clean).

      (3) Anesthetic sprays, ointments, or medicated pads (Tucks) may be applied directly to sutured area.

      (4) Analgesics (e.g., Percodan, 1 or 2 tablets) may be offered for relief of pain. Some patients will require medication every 4 hours for first 2 postnatal days. Patient free of discomfort is able to concentrate her energies on her child and child care, so any needed medication should be administered 40 minutes prior to feeding period.

    b. Hemorrhoids:

      (1) Cold is effective in reducing hemorrhoidal swelling. Covered cold pack (rubber glove filled with small chips of ice works well) may be placed against hemorrhoids soon after delivery, left in position no longer than 20 minutes, and repeated every 4 hours. Cold witch hazel compresses are also effective.

      (2) Moist heat may also be used to reduce hemorrhoidal swelling. Patient may take sitz bath with water maintained at about 38° C (100° F) for 20-minute period. Careful observation of patient for feeling of faintness is necessary.

      (3) Instruct patient how to replace hemorrhoid gently in anorectal canal using lubricated finger cot or rubber glove. Once reduced, have patient maintain digital pressure for 1 to 2 minutes, or anal reflex will extrude hemorrhoid. This reduction process must be repeated after bowel movements or as necessary.

      (4) Judicious use of analgesics is indicated for first postnatal week. Patient can be reassured that unless rectal condition was present prior to pregnancy, it will correct itself once increased blood supply and pressure symptoms of pregnancy are diminished and regular bowel habits are reestablished.

    c. Breasts and nipples:

      (1) For mother who is breast-feeding, see Chapter 31.

      (2) For others who elect not to breast-feed, daily bath provides all cleaning necessary. Supportive tight brassiere may be worn until breasts attain their prepregnant size in about 6 weeks. If lactation-suppression medication has been administered, lactation rarely

Continued.

PLAN OF CARE: PUERPERIUM—FIRST 2 WEEKS—cont'd

NURSING INTERVENTIONS—cont'd

Diagnostic	Therapeutic and educational

occurs, and breasts may remain soft. If no medication is used, painful engorgement usually occurs about 48 to 72 hours after delivery. For treatment, see p. 487. It is also necessary to tell mother to avoid immersion of breasts in hot water when taking bath or shower and expressing milk present, measures designed to increase milk flow.

   d. Afterpains:

     (1) Massage uterus gently to expel clots.

     (2) Encourage early ambulation.

     (3) If severe enough during nursing to interfere with mother-infant responses, administer analgesics 40 minutes prior to nursing period.

     (4) Reassure mother these contractions are beneficial in that they empty uterus of clots, will occur with nursing infant in response to oxytocin release by pituitary, and will usually disappear in 48 hours.

6. Elimination:

   a. Voiding: Encourage mother to void at least every 3 or 4 hours during day. If bladder distention occurs and patient is unable to void, catheterization may be necessary. Postnatally, urethra may be difficult to visualize because of swelling about introitus; dry swab gently brushed downward from clitoris to vagina will cause urethra to gape and catheter can be inserted. Because this procedure causes patient considerable discomfort and possibility of causing bladder infection is high, every nursing measure to enhance mother's ability to void spontaneously should be used. Some of these are (1) turning tap on full because sound of running water can act as stimulus to voiding, (2) pouring warm water over vulva, and (3) having patient void while using sitz bath and follow with shower.

     Symptoms of bladder infection (pain and burning on voiding) or retention with overflow (small, frequent voidings) must be reported immediately to physician, since treatment with antibiotics and retention catheter may be indicated. Clean-catch specimen of urine should be obtained and sent to lab for culture and sensitivity studies.

   b. Defecating:

     (1) Laxative may be administered first, second, or third postnatal night (e.g., Senokot tablets or milk of magnesia, 30 ml). If patient is unable to have bowel movement by next morning, laxative suppository may be inserted, followed by hot drink. If this measure is unsuccessful, enema usually is necessary.

     (2) Reestablishment of regular bowel habits may be assisted by exercise, roughage in diet, and adequate fluid intake. Fear of discomfort because of episiotomy or from hemorrhoids may hinder woman from straining at stool; hence a stool softener such as Colace may be ordered and enema repeated every 2 days for the first week.

   c. Diaphoresis: Profuse diaphoresis, especially at night (night sweats), is not unusual for 2 or 3 days postnatally. Diaphoresis is mechanism to reduce retained fluids of pregnancy and usually is not symptom of infection. Comfort of bath and change of bed linen are required, however.

7. Rest and exercise:

   a. Bed rest for 8 hours after delivery is recommended for all patients. For those who have had spinal anesthetic, complete bed rest in a supine position is necessary for 24 hours. Bathroom privileges are curtailed and infant feeding by mother delayed until she can turn to her side or sit up. For those who have had anesthetics such as cervical and pudendal blocks, free movement is permitted unless analgesic has been administered. Once vital rest period is over, mother should be encouraged to

---

PLAN OF CARE: PUERPERIUM—FIRST 2 WEEKS—cont'd

NURSING INTERVENTIONS—cont'd

Diagnostic	Therapeutic and educational
	ambulate frequently. Early ambulation has proved successful in reducing incidence of thrombosis and in more rapid recovery of strength. Because orthostatic hypotension is frequent finding of first 24 hours, careful supervision for first use of bathroom or shower is necessary. Excitement and exhilaration experienced after birth of infant may make rest difficult and medication for sleep at night may be necessary. b Exercises may be started as soon as mother's condition permits, usually by first postnatal day. (Check obstetrician's directives.) 8. Nutrition (Chapter 13): Clear fluids may be offered immediately after delivery, then mother often elects either light or regular diet with between-meal and bedtime nourishment. Encourage use of protein, roughage, and ample fluid intake. 9. Infant care (Chapters 30 and 31): Mother's involvement will increase as her physical recovery and skill in caretaking activities permit.

PLAN OF CARE: PUERPERIUM—WEEKS 3 THROUGH 6

PATIENT CARE OBJECTIVES

1. Vaginal discharge, lochia, or menstruation may have returned to normal odor and appearance.
2. There are no urinary tract symptoms (e.g., frequency, urgency, dysuria, incontinence of urine).
3. Normal bowel function is reestablished without fecal incontinence.
4. Breasts do not reveal soreness or tenderness, and if not breast-feeding, no milk or only a small amount of milk may be expressed.
5. Hgb is 12 gm/100 ml or Hct is 37% ± 5.
6. Urinalysis reveals normal findings; proteinuria has disappeared. Lactose may be present if breast-feeding, but no pus cells are present. Culture reveals no organisms.
7. Vital signs, i.e., temperature, pulse, and respirations, are normal.
8. Blood pressure has returned to prepregnancy level.
9. Muscles of uterus reveal some degree of laxity, but tone is returning to prepregnancy level.
10. Weight has returned to prepregnant level.
11. Vulva and perineal area show no evidence of infection. The episiotomy scar usually is healed without undue contraction, and the introitus remains large enough to permit coitus without discomfort.
12. Pelvic floor has essentially regained its tone, permitting only a mild degree of uterine prolapse, cystocele, or rectocele.
13. Uterus is only slightly larger than in the prepregnant state and anteverted. If retroverted, it has developed free mobility.
14. Cervix is healed; the external os has assumed the typical transverse slit of the parous woman. Occasionally the glandular epithelium lining the cervical canal can be visualized as a bright red area surrounding the external os.
15. Pap smear reveals normal estrogen pattern.
16. Couple have begun practicing their chosen method of family planning.
17. Woman must be aware of the need for a medical reexamination in 6 months.
18. Record keeping is completed to date.

NURSING INTERVENTIONS

Diagnostic	Therapeutic and educational
1. Physical: a. Inquire concerning vaginal discharge, urinary problems, bowel	1. Welcome patient; inquire concerning general health of mother, child, and father if present. Have patient undress and put on examining gown. 2. Once BP and other details of examination have been obtained and re-

Continued.

PLAN OF CARE: PUERPERIUM—WEEKS 3 THROUGH 6—cont'd

NURSING INTERVENTIONS—cont'd

Diagnostic	Therapeutic and educational
action, condition of breasts, and what birth control methods if any are used. b. Take BP, temperature, and pulse, and weigh patient. c. Obtain blood for analysis and send to lab. d. Obtain clean-catch urine for analysis and culture and send to lab. e. Assist examiner with examination of breasts, abdomen, and pelvis and taking of cervical smear. 2. Psychologic: Assess for problems related to self, infant, or family.	corded, help patient position herself on table for examination of breasts, abdomen, and legs. Instruct her concerning self-examination of breasts. 3. Position her for pelvic examination; instruct patient about how to relax. Acquaint examiner with information obtained from patient and assist with examination. 4. Instruct patient as to use of desired birth control methods (Chapter 6). 5. Instruct patient as to reasons for 6-month reexamination. 6. Counsel regarding patient-centered problems (e.g., weaning infant) (Chapter 31).

REFERENCES

Edwards, M. 1973-1974. The crises of fourth trimester. Birth Fam. J. **1:**19, Winter.

Fein, R. A. 1976. The first weeks of fathering: the importance of choices and supports for new parents. Birth Fam. J. **3:**53, Summer.

Goldstein, P. J., Zalar, M. K., Grady, E. W., and Smith, R. W. 1973. Vocational education: a unique approach to adolescent pregnancy. J. Reprod. Med. **10:**77.

Hellman, L. M., and Pritchard, J. A. 1971. Williams obstetrics (ed. 14). New York, Appleton-Century-Crofts.

Ingalls, A. J., and Salerno, M. C. 1975. Maternal and child health nursing (ed. 3). St. Louis, The C. V. Mosby Co.

Klaus, M. H., and Kennell, J. H. 1976. Maternal-infant bonding: the impact of early separation or loss on family development. St. Louis, The C. V. Mosby Co.

LeMaster, E. E. 1965. Parenthood as crisis. In Parad, H. J. (ed.). Crisis interventions: selected readings. New York, Family Service Association of America.

Warrick, L. 1969. Femininity, sexuality and mothering. Nurs. Forum **8:**224.

Willson, J. R., Beecham, C. T., and Carrington, E. R. 1975. Obstetrics and gynecology (ed. 5). St. Louis, The C. V. Mosby Co.

Zalar, M. K. 1975. Human sexuality: a component of total patient care. Nurs. Dig. **3:**40, Nov.-Dec.

Zalar, M. K. 1976. Sexual counseling for pregnant couples. MCN Am. J. Mat. Child. Nurs. J. **1:**176, May-June.

CHAPTER 28

Complications of the puerperium

PUERPERAL INFECTION

Puerperal infection (puerperal sepsis) is any clinical infection of the genital canal that occurs within 28 days after abortion or delivery. Infections may result from bacteria commonly found within the vagina, an *endogenous infection,* or it may be due to the introduction of pathogens from outside the vagina, an *exogenous infection.* Lacerations of the vagina or cervix may open avenues for sepsis. Even more formidable, however, may be the large placental site. Here the denuded endometrium (decidua basalis) and residual blood after parturition make the uterus an ideal site for a wound infection. The virulence of infecting organisms, the patient's resistance, and the rapidity and specificity of therapy determine the efficacy of treatment. Puerperal sepsis occurs in about 6% of maternity patients in the United States, but fortunately body defenses generally limit the disease in most instances. Puerperal infection probably is the major cause of maternal morbidity and mortality throughout the world.

Pathogenesis

Only occasionally, perhaps after a traumatic delivery, does endogenous infection occur. Self-inoculation of bacteria from pyogenic skin lesions or unclean bedding, for example, may represent the means of contamination. Most puerperal infections, however, are exogenous, due to contamination by attendants who have respiratory or other infections or who inadvertently carry pathogens from another infected patient. Introduction of pathogens may be by respiratory droplet inoculation (poor masking), by hand or other contact (unsterile gloves or instruments, unwashed hands), or occasionally by dust or insect vectors.

The most common infecting organisms are the numerous streptococci. Fulminating epidemic puerperal sepsis classically is caused by the hemolytic streptococcus. The less virulent anaerobic streptococci may be responsible for other puerperal infections, however. *Staphylococcus aureus,* the gonococcus, the coliform bacteria and clostridia are less common but serious pathogenic organisms causative of puerperal infection.

Frequently, the infection is complicated by medical disorders such as anemia, malnutrition, or diabetes mellitus. Obstetric problems, including prolonged rupture of the membranes, a long exhausting labor, instrument delivery, hemorrhage, and retained products of conception, increase the likelihood and severity of puerperal sepsis.

Pathology

A variety of possible inflammatory sites are obvious. An episiotomy or laceration of the birth canal may be the primary focus, leading to parametritis, pelvic cellulitis, or thrombophlebitis. An endometritis, usually at the placental site, permits infection to begin. Localized infection may be followed by salpingitis, peritonitis, and pelvic abscess formation. (Tubal occlusion after salpingitis is a common cause of infertility.) Septicemia may develop, and secondary abcesses may arise in distant sites such as the lungs or liver. Pulmonary embolization or septic shock, often with disseminated intravascular coagulation, from any serious genital infection may prove fatal. Postnatal femoral thrombophlebitis (''milk leg'') may result in a swollen, painful leg.

Clinical findings

The symptomatology of puerperal infection may be mild or fulminating. Any fever, that is, a temperature of 38° C (100.4° F) or more on 2 successive days, not counting the first 24 hours after delivery, must be considered to be due to puerperal infection, in the absence of convincing proof of another cause, for example, tracheobronchitis or pyelonephritis.

General malaise, anorexia, chills, or fever may begin as early as the second postnatal day. Perineal discomfort or lower abdominal distress, nausea, and vomiting may soon develop. Foul or profuse lochia, hectic fever, tachycardia, ileus, pelvic pain, or tenderness characterize critical puerperal sepsis. Without improvement, bacteremic shock or death may ensue from sepsis.

General physical examination to identify nonpuerperal infection should be carried out. Careful abdominal evaluation is done to note uterine or adnexal pain. Examination of the perineum, episiotomy, or sutured lacerations and speculum visualization of the vagina and cervix, together with careful rectovaginal examination, are next in order.

Laboratory findings. Considerable leukocytosis, a shift to the left of the differential WBC and markedly increased RBC sedimentation rate are typical of puer-

peral infections. Anemia, often an accompaniment, is evidenced by reduced RBC, hemoglobin, and hematocrit values. Gram-stained smears of the lochia from within the cervix or uterus may suggest the type of infection; that is gram-negative cocci may be streptococci or staphylococci, and gram-positive, long bacilli may be clostridia. Intracervical or intrauterine bacterial cultures (aerobic and anaerobic) should reveal the offending pathogens within 36 to 48 hours.

X-ray findings. Rarely do x-ray films aid in the diagnosis of puerperal infection, but they may be invaluable in identifying nonpuerperal sepsis, for example, pneumonia.

Differential diagnosis

One must distinguish nongenital from genital sepsis. For example, mastitis, respiratory or urinary tract in-

---

PLAN OF CARE: PUERPERAL INFECTION

PATIENT CARE OBJECTIVES

1. Patient's response to treatment is positive.
   a. Culture reports are negative.
   b. Vital signs, temperature, pulse, respirations, blood pressure are within normal limits.
   c. Fluid-electrolyte balance is maintained.
   d. General health returns (e.g., energy, appetite, elimination).
2. Involution proceeds at a normal rate.
3. Effects of parent-child separation are resolved.
4. Records are complete and reflect the response of the patient to treatment.

NURSING INTERVENTIONS

Diagnostic	Therapeutic and educational
1. Send specimens—cervical, blood, urine—to lab for culture and sensitivity reactions and note results.	1. Institute (with physician) emergency measures required for treatment of septic shock and hemorrhage.
2. Check routinely for progress in involution (Chapter 27).	2. General measures:
3. Note and record vital signs every 4 hours or prn.	a. Isolate patient if highly communicable organisms are suspected (e.g., hemolytic streptococci, clostridia, C. diphtheria); obtain and send cervical, blood, and urine cultures and sensitivity reactions.
4. Note general reactions of patients to infection, i.e., malaise, perspiration, signs of shock.	b. Segregate patients with less fulminating puerperal sepsis (e.g., those due to E. coli or bacterioides).
5. Note intake and output and amount and character of urine.	c. Promote parent-child interactions:
6. Note parent's response to separation from infant.	(1) Every effort must be made to maintain contact between mother, father, and child. Frequent reports of infant's progress, bringing child to room entrance so mother can see him, and encouraging father to participate in infant's care and to bring reports to mother may ease pain and anxiety of separation.
	(2) Instruct as to general protective measures to use with child when contact is reestablished.
	3. Surgical measures: Dilatation and curettage (Chapter 6) should be effected for retained products of conception. Hysterectomy may be lifesaving for septic shock resulting from uterine rupture with infection. Colpotomy often is necessary for drainage of pelvic abscess. Septic embolization may require ligation or clipping of vena cava and ovarian veins.

fections, and enteritis must be considered in that order of probability.

Management

The most effective and cheapest treatment of puerperal infection is prevention, with measures such as antenatal nutrition to control anemia and intranatal control of hemorrhage. Good patient hygiene is essential. Strict adherence by all medical personnel to the best aseptic technique during the entire hospital or delivery period is mandatory. Coitus following rupture of the membranes is contraindicated. Dystocia or prolonged labor should be avoided, especially after leaking of amniotic fluid. Traumatic vaginal delivery must be avoided, blood loss replaced, and fluid-electrolyte balance maintained.

The virulence of the organisms, the resistance of the patient, and her likely response to treatment are the intangibles of *prognosis*. Prevention, supportive therapy, and prompt massive antibiotic administration have reduced the maternal mortality in the United States to less than 0.4%. Regrettably, in underdeveloped countries, the death rate may be more than ten to twenty times this figure.

SUBINVOLUTION OF UTERUS

Subinvolution of the uterus is the delayed return of the enlarged puerperal corpus to normal size and function. The causes of subinvolution include reduced circulation because of malposition and chronic passive congestion, myomata, retained products of conception, and infection.

Subinvolution may complicate the puerperium because of symptoms, for example, pelvic discomfort or backache. Or there may be signs of abnormality such as leukorrhea or bleeding from an enlarged, boggy, perhaps tender, uterus.

In the absence of frank bleeding, ergonovine (Ergotrate) 0.2 mg/4 hr for 2 or 3 days, antibiotic therapy, warm acetic douches, and manual replacement of a retroposed corpus and support by a suitable pessary may suffice. With hemorrhage, dilatation and curettage to remove retained secundines and to freshen the placental site for adequate healing generally are required together with oxytocics and antibiotics.

PROLAPSE OF UTERUS

Laceration or relaxation of the uterine supports may follow operative vaginal delivery or precipitate birth, particularly in primiparous patients. Uterocervical descensus generally is accompanied by cystocele, rectocele, or enterocele. Fortunately considerable ligamentous and other tissue take-up normally accompanies uterine involution. Pessary support may help but in severe cases, surgery may be required, for example, a Manchester-Fothergill procedure (shortening of the transverse cervical and uterosacral ligaments, usually with cystocele or rectocele repair) or hysterectomy. Operation is deferred for at least 6 months to permit maximum resolution to occur and to obtain the best surgical result.

MASTITIS

Mastitis, or breast infection, affects about 1% of puerperal patients, most of whom are primiparas who are nursing. Mastitis is almost always unilateral and develops well after the flow of milk has been established. The infecting organism generally is the hemolytic *S. aureus.* An infected nipple fissure usually is the initial lesion, but the ductal system is next involved. Inflammatory edema and engorgement of the breasts soon obstruct the flow of milk in a lobe, and regional, then generalized, mastitis follows. If prompt resolution of the septic process does not occur, a breast abscess is virtually inevitable.

Chills, fever, malaise, and local breast tenderness initiate the process. Eventual localization of sepsis and axillary adenopathy are delayed developments.

Intensive antibiotic therapy (e.g., cephalosporin and vancomycin, which are particularly useful drugs in staphylococcal infections), suppression of lactation, support of the breast, local heat (or cold), and analgesics are required. If an abscess develops, wide incision and drainage must be effected. Most patients respond to treatment, and an abscess can be prevented.

Almost all instances of acute mastitis can be avoided by proper nursing technique and the limitation of nursing time (Chapter 31).

POSTNATAL ANTERIOR PITUITARY NECROSIS

Postnatal anterior pituitary necrosis (Sheehan's syndrome, hypophyseal cachexia) follows hypovolemic shock in about 15% of survivors of severe postnatal hemorrhage. Infarction of much or all of the anterior hypophysis causes partial to total loss of thyroid, adrenocortical, and gonadal function. The degree of hormonal deficiency depends on the extent of gland destruction.

Patients with Sheehan's syndrome fail to lactate, and there is a decrease in breast size. Loss of axillary and pubic hair, genital atrophy, and amenorrhea are the rule. Such patients are apathetic and suffer easy fatigue.

Laboratory studies reveal a markedly reduced thyroid, adrenocortical, and ovarian function. Minimal treatment requires thyroid hormone, cortisone, and estrogen replacement.

The prognosis of Sheehan's syndrome depends on the degree of residual anterior pituitary function and the supplementary therapy required. Infertility, reduced resistance to infection, proneness to shock, and premature aging are problems of patients with pituitary cachexia.

PERSISTENT (ABNORMAL) LACTATION

Persistent postnatal lactation (postnatal galactorrhea, Chiari-Frommel syndrome) associated with amenorrhea and genital atrophy is a rare complication of pregnancy. The cause of this type of galactorrhea, often of profuse type, is unknown. Prolonged phenothiazine therapy or prolonged lactation may be responsible, but a tumor or degenerative lesion in the hypothalamus or pituitary should be sought. In the Chiari-Frommel syndrome, gonadotropin and estrogen urinary excretion is reduced or absent.

Treatment is disappointing. Clomiphene citrate may induce ovulation, pregnancy, or menstruation. A new drug, 2-bromergocryptine, will suppress abnormal lactation, and estrogen or oral contraceptive therapy may control galactorrhea, but the disorder will recur with termination of the medication.

PLACENTAL PATHOLOGY

So-called placental infarcts (red or white firm areas), extremely gross perivillous or intravascular fibrin deposition, may "choke" or inactivate many villi by reducing or eliminating the maternal circulation to the involved areas. Eventually ischemic necrosis of these villi develops because the placenta is dependent, just as the fetus, on the maternal blood supply.

Placentitis, or infection of the placenta, may be bacterial, viral, rickettsial, or protozoan. The most common agents are bacterial, which cause the greatest changes in the placenta. Chorioamnionitis, often secondary to premature rupture of the membranes, may be followed by placentitis, congenital pneumonia, omphalitis, or septicemia, often caused by enteric streptococci, colon aerogenes–type bacteria. Inflammatory leukocytes involve the membranes, which appear abnormally translucent and whitish. Perivascular white blood cell infiltration is notable in the chorion also and about the vessels of the cord. Even abscesses may form in the placenta. Placentitis often is followed by endometritis and parametritis—serious puerperal sepsis.

REFERENCES

Devereux, W. P. 1970. Acute puerperal mastitis: evaluation of its management. Am. J. Obstet. Gynecol. **108**:78.

Paydar, M., and Ostooarzadeh, M. 1974. Late postpartum hemorrhage. Int. J. Gynaecol. Obstet. **12**:141.

Sweet, R. L., and Ledger, W. J. 1973. Puerperal infectious morbidity: a two-year review. Am. J. Obstet. Gynecol. **117**: 1093.

CHAPTER 29

Parenthood

PARENTHOOD DEFINED

Biologic parenthood for both sexes begins with the union of ovum and sperm. During the antenatal (prebirth) period, the mother becomes the primary agent in providing an environment in which the fetus may develop and grow. This close symbiotic union of mother and child ends with birth, and others may assume partial or complete involvement in the infant's care. Whoever assumes the parental role, whether it be a biologic or surrogate parent, woman or man, enters into a crucial relationship with a child that will persist throughout the lifetime of each. Men and women, of course, may exist without a child, so in essence parenthood is optional. It may serve as a maturation factor in their lives and may or may not be biologically based. For the child, it is all important; his continued existence depends on the quantity and quality of care he receives.

The tasks, responsibilities, and attitudes that make up this care have been designated by Steele and Pollock (1968) as the "mothering function," a process in which an adult (a mature, capable, self-sufficient person) assumes the care of an infant (a helpless, dependent, immature person). They describe this process of mothering as one with two components: the first being practical or mechanical in nature and the other, emotional in nature. The first component includes child care activities such as "feeding, holding, clothing, and cleaning the infant, protecting it from harm, and providing motility for it." The second component includes attitudes of tenderness and awareness and concern for the child's needs and desires. This component of "motherliness" influences the environment of the child and has a profound effect on the manner in which the practical aspects are performed and on the emotional response of the child. Both components are essential to the infant's immediate well-being and future development.

Those components of the child's care that comprise the "practical" or "mechanical" aspects do not appear automatically as efficient caretaking behaviors at the birth of one's child. The human parent's ability in these respects has been altered by the effects of cultural and personal experiences. Many parents have to learn how to do these tasks, and this learning process can be a difficult one. If, however, the desire to learn is there and there are persons able and willing to support the parents' endeavors, the majority of parents become adept in care-taking activities.

The psychologic component in child care, *motherliness*, appears to stem from the parents' own earliest experiences with a loving, accepting mother-figure. In this sense the parents may be said to *inherit* the ability to show concern and tenderness and to pass on this ability to the next generation by repeating the kind of parent-child relationship they had experienced. Benedek (1950) describes a positive parent-child relationship as mutually rewarding and being fundamental to an individual's developing a feeling of confidence in the expectations that others will be willing to help and that he is worth helping. Erikson's concept (1959) of "basic trust" is similar, in that he postulates that such a psychologic entity forms the basis for the adult's eventual relationships with others and his ability to look to others for help. Those individuals whose dealings with others are characterized by a sense of trust tend to be social or outgoing in nature and able to seek and accept assistance from others. In contrast, those deficient in this sense tend to be alienated and isolated. They are more crisis prone because of their inability to make use of situational supports in times of stress.

Either parent may exhibit "motherliness"; it is now recognized to be a nongender-related ability. As Josselyn (1956) maintains, the ability to show gentleness, love, and understanding and to place another's welfare above one's own is not limited to women—it is a human characteristic.

PARENTAL BEHAVIORS

The quality of motherliness in the parent prompts nurturing as opposed to neglect and protection as opposed to abuse of the child. Cues indicating the presence or absence of this quality in maternal behavior appear early in the postnatal period as the mother reacts to her newborn child and begins the process of establishing a relationship. Its presence is manifested by behavior indicative of the parent's realistic perception and acceptance of the infant's needs, limited abilities, immature social responses, and helplessness (Steele and Pollock, 1968). According to Morris (1966), "Mother-infant unity can be said to be satisfactory when a mother can find pleasure in her infant and in the tasks for and with him; understand his emotional states and comfort him; read his cues for new experience and sense his fatigue points."

Those parents who are deficient in the quality of motherliness exhibit behavior that demonstrates their inability to respond appropriately to the needs of their infants. They expect responses from the infant far in excess of his ability to perform and interpret his inadequate responses as defiance or as negative judgment of parental capabilities. They obtain no pleasure from physical contact with their child, handle him roughly, let his head dangle without support, and do not cuddle him. The infant is seen as unattractive, and the tasks of bathing and changing the child are done with disgust or annoyance. There is a lack of discrimination in responding to the infant's signals relative to hunger, fatigue, need for soothing or stimulating speech, and need for comforting body or eye contact. These parents often show excessive concern over the health of their child and cannot distinguish between the expected minor illnesses of childhood and serious disabilities. It appears difficult for them to accept their child as healthy and happy (Morris, 1966).

Studies have shown that in the first contacts a mother has with her infant, an orderly and predictable pattern of behavior, or bonding, ensues regardless of whether the mother is young or old, a primipara or multipara, wed or unwed (Rubin, 1961; Klaus and others, 1970). The mother begins with a fingertip exploration of the infant's head and extremities; within a short time the open palm is used to caress the trunk, and eventually the infant is enfolded in the mother's arms. Interest in having eye contact was demonstrated again and again. Some mothers remarked that once their baby had looked at them, they felt much closer to him (Klaus and others, 1970). Others have also attested to this: "I was a mother and looked into his eyes so clear; fell into his eyes, and in love" (Lang, 1972). Once this initial contact is over, the new mother seems to relax and often sleep comes to both mother and child.

Other typical behaviors have been described as the *claiming process*. The mother enfolds the child physically in her arms, points out characteristics that the child shares with other family members, and indicates recognition of a relationship between them by commenting on the infant's responses to her as a parent as illustrated by the following: "Russ held him close and said, 'He's the image of his father,' but I found one part like me—his big toes are shaped like mine. Look, he's smiling; he likes his mother's jokes."

On the other hand, some mothers react negatively. The infant is claimed but in terms of the discomfort or pain he caused the mother, and the infant's normal responses are interpreted as being derogatory to the mother. The mother reacts to her child with dislike or indifference. The child is not held close or touched in such a way as to comfort him such as in the following example: "The nurse put the baby into Marie's arms. She promptly laid him across her knees and glanced up at the television. 'Stay still till I finish watching—you've been enough trouble already.'"

FACTORS INFLUENCING PARENTAL RESPONSES

Before introducing nursing measures designed to foster positive parent-child relationships, a number of factors need to be considered.

Physical condition of mother

Women who have experienced long and difficult labors often are too exhausted to respond other than in a perfunctory way to the newborn. They may be grateful for the infant being healthy and well and welcome the attention of others, but their primary need centers on recovery from a physical and emotional ordeal.

Physical condition of infant

Those infants born at risk either as a result of fetal or maternal disabilities usually are transferred to the intensive care nursery as quickly as possible. Concerns for their need for intensive medical and nursing care supersede concerns about providing close contact between the infant and the mother or father. Opportunities to view the infant in the intensive care nursery, to touch or hold him if this is at all possible, and provision for reports of the infant's progress must be part of the nursing plan (Fig. 33-4).

Parental expectations

Some parents are startled by the appearance of the infant—size, color, molding of the head, or bowed appearance of the legs. Many have never seen or had contact with a newborn infant and find themselves disturbed by their feelings. The physical characteristics normal in all newborns may be interpreted as physical or mental deficiencies by mothers and fathers. Many fathers have commented that they thought the odd shape of the child's head (molding) meant the child would be mentally retarded (Chapter 12).

Disappointment over the sex of the infant can take time to resolve. The mother or father may be able to give adequate physical mothering but find it difficult to be sincerely involved with the infant until these feelings have been resolved. As one mother remarked:

> I really wanted a boy. I know it is silly and irrational, but when they said "she's a lovely little girl" I was so disappointed and angry—yes angry—I could hardly look at her. Oh, I looked after her OK, her feedings and baths and things, but I couldn't feel excited. To tell the truth, I felt like a monster not liking my child. Then one day she was lying there and she turned her head and looked right at me. I felt a flooding of love for her come over me and we looked at each other a long time. It's OK now. I wouldn't change her for all the boys in the world.

Nursing care plans need to include time for explanations about the child's appearance and opportunities for parents to discuss the absence of feelings of motherliness freely without fear of censure or ridicule. Often just being able to express doubts and concerns comes as relief and makes it easier for parents to accept help with such feelings if necessary.

Social and economic conditions

Parents whose economic condition is made worse with the birth of each child and who are unable to utilize an acceptable method of family planning may be indifferent to the new baby. This indifference may be compounded by a health worry and a sense of helplessness.

Mothers who are alone, deserted by husband, family, and friends, or who are in an untenable economic state may view the birth of the child with dread. The difficulties in which they find themselves may overcome any desire for mothering the infant.

Nursing measures designed to help such patients are directed toward involving other community agencies, social and economic, as well as health agencies. Such problems often require long-term commitments from both the patient and community to effect satisfactory outcomes. The development of adequate situational supports may be instituted in the antenatal period.

Maternal age and maturity

Women having a child late in the childbearing years may find the care of the child exhausts their physical capabilities, and if economic and social conditions are also adverse, neglect of the child can result.

The youthfulness of some parents makes it difficult for them to assume the responsibilities that parenthood entails. They are involved in the crucial maturational task of moving from the dependence of childhood to the interdependency of the young adult. This task and the resultant preoccupation with their own needs for growth may blind them to the long-term needs of their child. Once the initial excitement of birth is over, the repetitive and time-consuming nature of infant care may erode their good intentions. There were approximately 207,000 babies born to young women under 18 years of age in 1970, and this number has been increasing at the rate of approximately 3000 a year (U.S. Department of Health, Education, and Welfare, 1975). Their needs and the needs of their babies represent one of the largest health problems in maternity care (Gershenson, 1973; Osofsky, 1976; Wright, 1976). The physical problems encountered by this vulnerable group are discussed in Chapter 15. Meeting their psychologic and maturational needs is also a cause for national concern. Efforts are being made to determine the young mother's feelings toward her infant, the quality of the interaction between mother and infant, her knowledge of and attitude toward infant caretaking activities, and her understanding of her infant's growth and developmental needs. In addition, it is vital to determine the kind of support those close to these young mothers are able or prepared to give and the kinds of community aid that can supplement this. The chart on p. 433, developed by Poole (1976), gives sample interview questions that the nurse may use to obtain this information, which then serves as the data base for care.

Since many of these young women have not completed their basic education, programs for continuing education are being developed across the nation. These attempt to combine learning self-care (including contraceptional care), prenatal preparation for labor and delivery, and child care activities with the traditional classroom subjects. Some school districts provide separate schooling, whereas others stress maintenance of the young parent in her original environment among existing friends (Howard, 1968; Hartman, 1970; Smith, 1971). Counselors and teachers hope to provide these young people with alternate methods of coping with life relationships and the need for closeness to and acceptance by another person that are appropriate for their age levels and resources.

However, those who work with young parents stress the need to recognize the maturational differences within the age groups. The following descriptions of three 17-year-olds illustrate the differing attitudes, acceptance of the pregnancy, readiness for parenthood, and amount and kind of outside support available.

1. Sharon, 17 years old with an attractive outgoing personality, was married 3 months before the birth of her baby. She was enthusiastic about attending parent craft classes, and her husband, Bob, came to those relating to support in labor. She stated that he was to finish high school in June, 2 months before the baby was born, and she expected him to go to work immediately in a local gas station. Their parents were going to help them for 6 months by paying the rent on a small three-room apartment, but they were expected to provide for other necessities. Bob made a cradle for the baby, and she made most of the baby clothes. They were going to use old furniture, but the baby had a new crib. Both families were excited about the baby and nonjudgmental in their attitudes toward Sharon and her husband.

Sharon had a normal pregnancy and delivery. She was pleased and happy with her baby and found caring for the child rewarding. Bob did well in his job and accepted his new responsibilities. When they began to feel too confined to home and child care, the young couple decided that Sharon would supplement the family income by caring for neighbors' children rather than Bob's getting a second nighttime job, since they needed the time to be together. The additional money would be spent on recreation for themselves.

2. Mary Lou, 17 years old, was a small, fragile-looking young woman. Mary Lou was the youngest of four sisters, all of whom were married and away from home. She had numerous relatives—aunts, uncles, and cousins—in the vicinity. Both her mother and father worked.

Mary Lou never divulged the name of the father of her child. She had no intention of giving the baby up for adoption. She intended to stay home and care for it herself. She refused to attend group classes but was eager and willing for the nurse to teach her individually. When she was taken on a tour of the hospital facilities, she clung to the nurse and needed much reassurance and mothering. The birth was normal, and she had a baby boy. This was an occasion for great family rejoicing, since there had not been a boy for three generations and her sisters had girls. Mary Lou came to the hospital with a suitcase of pretty clothes for herself and lovely baby clothes. The extended family accompanied her to the hospital and were there to greet the new baby. On the first visit to the home, the nurse was extremely aware of the overwhelming presence of the family, particularly Mary Lou's father. Mary Lou was feeding the baby his bottle in a correct but perfunctory manner. Subsequent visits found her increasingly trying to isolate herself. The nurse encouraged Mary Lou to seek additional counseling because she was concerned with Mary Lou's lack of affective response. Mary Lou refused, and within a week ran away from home, leaving the baby boy behind.

3. Betty, 17 years old, was an overweight young woman. She refused to wear maternity clothes and bought herself an overlarge dress in a dark brown material with small red flowers. She took no other interest in her appearance. She talked repeatedly about how the father of the child had taken advantage of her, that she was a good girl, and "that he was bad." The baby was to be put up for adoption. She refused to discuss her relationships with her parents, who lived in another city.

Betty had a long, difficult labor. At one time she struck the nurse caring for her and screamed for the nurse "to get this monster out of me." She refused to see the baby or to talk about the child. She appeared to deny the whole experience. When the time came for her to return to her home, the nurse accompanied her to the bus. She boarded the bus, an overweight girl in an unattractive dark brown dress. The bus pulled away, the nurse waved, but Betty did not look back.

It is obvious that to each of these teenagers, pregnancy had a different meaning; their perceptions of themselves varied as did their needs. A stereotyped approach to the young is no more successful than a stereotyped approach to the older pregnant woman.

If the baby is placed for adoption after birth, the event may be accepted by young parents with varying emotional responses. For some, as with Betty, it may be another episode in a "bad" experience. With others, the birth of the child and the arrangement for his care are undertaken with little or no apparent understanding of a child's needs as indicated by the following:

The baby, whom the couple will call _____, is under county care at the _____ and will probably be given to foster parents—although the couple would like to see their daughter live with in-laws.

The couple are now staying with friends in a small apartment above a garage in _____, but talked happily about the rush of events that brought them a daughter last Saturday night.

"We're happy to have a baby even though the doctors at the hospital told us it wasn't a very good idea," said the young mother.

"I was so happy that I bought her $50 worth of new clothes," said her husband, tugging at his wife's burgundy double knit slacks.

_____, the mother, smiled, puffed on her cigarette, and said she could hardly recall much of her moments during childbirth.

"I remember the patients helping me walk. I remember there were some nurses and technicians and a doctor at the end. And I remember a baby too. That was nice," she said.*

---

*From San Francisco Chronicle, Nov. 17, 1976, p. 24.

SAMPLE INTERVIEW QUESTIONS*

Often girls your age when they become mothers find their lives to be very different from what they had planned for themselves. They sometimes must drop out of school and it may be very hard for them to find a job that they like. Plans they once had for themselves may just seem like unreachable dreams. Let's talk about how you feel regarding these things.

1. Are you going to school now?
    What do you feel about that?
        If necessary: Are you glad that you are?
            or   Do you wish that you were?
2. Do you have any kind of job right now?
    What do you feel about it?
        If necessary: Do you like your job?
                        Does it seem adequate to meet your needs?
                        Do you wish you were working?
3. What would you most like to be doing with your life right now if you could do anything that you wished?
4. What would you most like to do in the future if you had the choice of doing anything that you wanted to do?
    Is this a possible goal for you?
    What do you feel about that?

Young mothers often find their lives totally filled with school, job, and caring for their babies. Often they do not have time to do the things they like to do such as visit with their friends, make new friends or be with their husband or boyfriends. Sometimes their own mothers seem to use the baby as a means of controlling what their daughters do and do not do. This can sometimes be very frustrating.

5. Do you seem to be able to find time to be by yourself?
    What do you feel about that?
    What do you usually do when you have free time for yourself?
    What would you most like to do during this time?
6. Do you find time to be with your friends?
    Are you able to see them as often as you would like to?
    What do you feel about that?
    Have you made any new friends since you had the baby?
    If unmarried—Have you been able to be with your boyfriend or meet and date new guys since you had the baby?
    What do you feel about that?
7. Do you feel as if your mother puts a lot of pressure on you to do the things that she thinks you should do?
    What do you feel about that?

Husbands or boyfriends sometimes get involved with the baby and sometimes they do not. Young mothers often feel isolated and alone and resent the fact that the father is not helping much with the baby. Sometimes mothers feel that they do not get along with their husbands or boyfriends as well as they did before the baby came.

8. Does your baby's father seem to enjoy the baby?
    What type of things does he do with him (her)?
        Change diapers?
        Bathe?
        Feed?
        Play?
        Other?
    Do you get enough help from him?
        What do you feel about that?
    Do you seem to be closer, less close or about the same to him as you were before the baby was born?
        What do you feel about that?

It is important what some people think about us but with other people we do not really care what they think. I'm going to give you a list of people and I want you to tell me whether or not they would agree with the way you take care of your baby and how you feel about whether they agree or not.

9. mother   social worker
   father   nurse
   baby's father   doctor
   baby's father's parents church members
   teacher   minister or priest
   employer   neighbors
   friends   relatives
   nutritionist

Some things about caring for the baby are fun but others may be very irritating to a mother. I'm going to ask you about different things you do in caring for your baby and about what your baby does. Tell me what you feel about them.

10. First, feeding your baby?
    What do you feel about this?
    How much time does it usually take?
    Does it seem to take a lot out of you?
11. Now let's consider changing your baby's diapers.
    What do you feel about that?
12. How about bathing your baby?
13. How about playing with your baby?
    What do you feel about that?
    Do you find time to play with your baby often?
    Do you feel that it is important for you to play with him (her)?
14. Does your baby try to annoy you sometimes?
    What does he do that really annoys you?
        What do you feel about that?
    What do you usually do about it?
    Do you ever find that you need to punish your baby?
    What types of things does he do that he needs to be punished for?
    How do you usually punish him (her) when he (she) needs it?

*From Poole, C. J. 1976. Adolescent mothers: can they be helped. Pediatr. Nurs. **2**:10, March-April.

On the other hand, giving a baby up for adoption may be attended by all the symptoms of grief one would expect at the death of a newborn:

She is only 15 but she loves the baby. Her parents won't take it so she has to give her up. It was heartbreaking. On the day she went home she came into the nursery to hold her baby for one last time.

The grief of the young parent at her loss has to be balanced with the need of her infant for continued care and nurturing.

Medical and nursing personnel need to assess the long-term capabilities of parents through their contacts during the antenatal and natal periods not only to help them cope with the present but also to plan into the future.

Interference with personal aspirations

The resentment some women feel toward parenthood (that it interferes or curtails their plans for personal freedom or advancement in a career) may not have been resolved during the antenatal period. If not, the anger and/or disappointment spill over into the caretaking activities and may result in indifference and neglect or, conversely, to oversolicitousness and the setting of impossibly high standards for their behavior or the child's performance (Shainess, 1970).

Nursing intervention needs to include opportunities for parents to vent their feelings freely to an objective listener to discuss measures to permit personal growth of the parent, for example, by means of part-time employment, volunteer work, and agencies that provide baby-sitting care or mother-substitutes during parent vacations, as well as to learn care of the child.

Early and sustained contact and the bonding process

Research with mammals other than humans indicates that early contact between mother and offspring is important in developing future relationships. Although there is little scientific evidence to support or deny the importance of early first contacts between the human

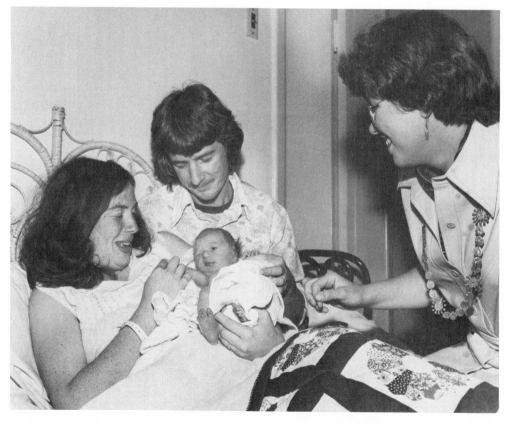

Fig. 29-1. Family after birth in Alternative Birth Center at Mount Zion Hospital and Medical Center in San Francisco. One of their physicians is visiting family. (Courtesy Mount Zion Hospital and Medical Center, San Francisco, Calif.)

mother and her child, recent research in this regard is suggestive of a similar need. Klaus and co-workers (1972) found that the addition of 16 extra hours of mothering contact with the infant during the first 3 days had positive effects on maternal behavior that persisted for the 30 days included in their study.

Traditional in many hospital settings, the practice of separating mother and child immediately after birth and limiting the time the mother and family spend with the newborn in the first few days would seem to contravene the natural responses of mother to child and increase anxiety. This is illustrated in the following excerpt from *A Proper Marriage* by Doris Lessing:

It [the door] opened, and the pink nurse entered with five babies balanced all over her arms. They were yelling, with hungry open mouths. The babies were plopped neatly one after another onto the beds, and gathered in by the waiting mothers. The pink nurse, empty-armed, arrived at Martha's bed, and inquired, ''Well, how are you?''

''Where's my baby?'' asked Martha anxiously.

''She's having a nice rest,'' said the nurse, already on her way out.

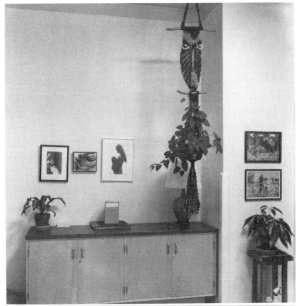

A

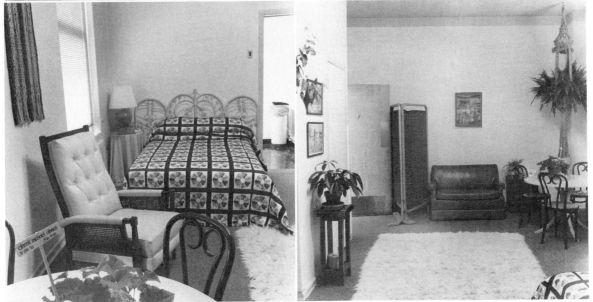

B

C

Fig. 29-2. Homelike atmosphere is created for uncomplicated labor and birth in Alternative Birth Center at Mount Zion Hospital and Medical Center in San Francisco. Hospital delivery suite, intensive care nursery, and staff are in immediate facility to meet any emergency situation. (Courtesy Mount Zion Hospital and Medical Center, San Francisco, Calif.)

"But I haven't seen her yet," said Martha, weak tears behind her lids.

"You don't want to disturb her, do you?" said the nurse disprovingly.

The door shut. The woman, whose long full breast sloped already into the baby's mouth, looked up and said, "You'd better do as they want, dear. It saves trouble. They've got their own ideas."

Martha, cheated and empty, lay and watched the other women suckle their babies. It was intolerable that after nine months of close companionship with the creature, now announced as a girl, she might not even make its acquaintance. There was something impossible in the idea that yesterday the child had been folded in her flesh and it now lay rooms away, washed and clothed, in a cradle with its name on it. It made her uneasy; she wanted to see—she even felt irrationally that the child might have died at birth and they were lying to her.*

The recent upsurge in demand by parents for home as opposed to hospital delivery is attributable in some measure to the parents' desire to share the birth process and for immediate and continuous contact with their child. The development in hospitals of family-centered maternity care units also reflects this demand (Figs. 29-1 and 29-2). One widely used method is the provision of facilities for the mother and her baby to room-in. The infant is transferred to the area from the transitional nursery after evidencing satisfactory postnatal adjustment. The father is encouraged to visit as often and as long as he wishes and to participate in the care of the infant. Some hospitals are experimenting with "birth rooms." The mother is accompanied by the father during the delivery of the infant, and all three may remain together until discharged. Medical and nursing personnel are available for any care necessary for the mother and child. Other hospitals arrange for the discharge of mother and infant anywhere from 2 to 24 hours after delivery if the condition of the mother and that of the child warrant it. Follow-up care with nursing personnel from a public health agency is part of this plan.

PROCESS OF ASSUMING PARENTAL ROLE

Emotional adjustment in the postnatal period relates predominantly to recovery from the labor of birth and to adaptation to the parental role. The *reality phase* of this adaptive process now occurs, and the mother's ability to advance through the developmental stages of dependent behavior, a mixture of independent and dependent

behavior and finally interdependent behavior, marks the success of attaining a new role in life. This developmental sequence is similar to any other; mastery at one stage permits a moving on and a mastery of the next.

Nursing care during this period is based on an assessment of the mother's perceptual acuity and the amount of physical and psychic energy she possesses. From these assessments, plans of care may be developed to enhance physical recovery, participation in the care of herself and her baby, and return to family commitments. These plans include the strengthening of the family's coping mechanisms, enlisting adequate situational supports and role-modeling interaction with the newborn (Fig. 29-3). This period is a crucial one with crisis potential for the family (Gordon and Gordon, 1960; Larsen and others, 1966; Donner, 1972).

Stage I: Dependent behavior

During the 1- to 2-day period after delivery, the mother's dependency needs predominate, and to the extent that these needs are met by others, the mother is able to divert her psychic energy to her child rather than to herself. She needs "mothering" in order to "mother." Rubin (1961) has aptly described these few days as the "taking-in phase"—a time when nurturing and protective care is required by the new mother.

These mature and apparently healthy women appear to suspend involvement in everyday responsibilities and rely on others to respond to their needs for comfort, rest, nourishment, and closeness to their families and newborn.

Physical discomfort, arising as it may from an episiotomy, sore nipples, hemorrhoids, aftercontractions, and occasionally a sprained coccygeal joint, can interfere with the mother's need for rest and relaxation. The judicious use of comfort measures and medication depends on the nurse. Many women hesitate to ask for medication, believing that any pain they experience is normal and to be accepted; few have a knowledge of the use of heat or cold to relieve local pain.

This is a time of great excitement, and most parents are extremely talkative. They need to verbalize all the happenings of pregnancy and their experience of birth to bring it into focus, analyze it, and accept it so that it can be put aside mentally, permitting them to move on to another phase. Some are able to use the staff or other patients as "audience"; others cannot, and for them, the opportunity to be with family or friends is imperative.

Anxiety and preoccupation with her new role often narrow a mother's perceptual field so that information must be repeated. She may require reminders to rest or,

---

*From Lessing, D. 1970. A proper marriage. New York, Simon & Schuster, Inc., p. 147.

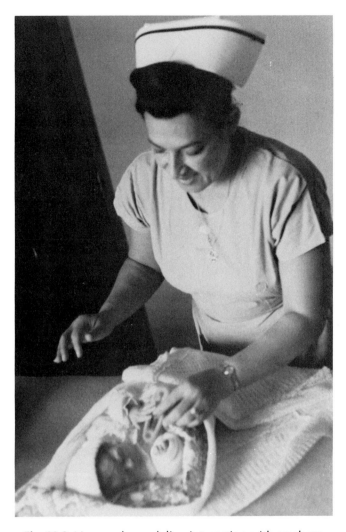

Fig. 29-3. Nurse role-modeling interaction with newborn.

conversely, to ambulate enough to promote recovery. Ward routines do not necessarily loom large in the new mother's order of priorities; showers are taken when the physicians are due for examinations, and telephone conversations preclude "being ready" for the baby. Regulations seem cumbersome, and mothers and their families find it difficult at times to accept such rules when they interfere with their needs to share reactions about their child.

Stage II: Dependent-independent behavior

If the mother has received adequate nurturing in the first few days, by the third day her desire for independent action reasserts itself, and she responds enthusiastically

to opportunities to learn and practice the care of the baby or, if an accomplished mother, to carry out or direct this care.

Professional care during this period often is somewhat limited. The concept of the "naturalness of being a mother" deemphasizes the new parent's needs and problems. Regardless of the desire for a baby and the amount of antenatal preparation undertaken, the reality of parenthood has to be experienced to be understood fully on a personal level. One young mother expressed it as follows:

But then in my second week, as my strength began to return, my energies began to focus on the overwhelming task of motherhood that stood before me. And I realized then that I faced that task alone. Not that my husband wouldn't stand by me, not that my friends would not share experiences with me, but I stood alone with the realization that only I could be the child's mother.*

In this period of 4 to 5 weeks, the adjustments made to reality and the mastery of the tasks of parenthood are crucial for the subsequent functioning of the family as a unit. It has been found that those mothers who experience the most difficulty in adjusting are primiparas, women with careers, women who feel deeply the isolation of themselves with their babies and resent the endless coping with home responsibilities as well as those associated with child care, women who miss the lack of outside stimulation, particularly if accustomed to a busy work environment, and those who lack friendships or other people with whom to share delights and concerns. Unless some intervention is instituted, these everyday types of problems accumulate until a crisis situation develops.

Nursing must be aimed at increasing the mother's mastery of the "art of motherhood," thereby increasing or sustaining her self-esteem. These interventions may be grouped under those pertaining to perception, coping mechanisms, and situational supports.

Perception. One of the main concepts to be stressed repeatedly is that parenthood is a learned role. As any other learned role, it takes time to master, improves with experience, and evolves gradually and continually as the needs of the adults and child change.

Teaching should stem from the mother's prior knowledge and competency. For some, a simple review of points forgotten is all that is needed; others require detailed information, demonstrations done slowly and carefully to permit imitation, and supportive supervision. The need for repetitious teaching is to be expected if the mother's anxiety level distorts her ability to learn. As the mother's condition permits, she assumes more and more responsibility for her own hygienic care and the reporting of abnormalities in her progress. Therefore she will require careful explanation of what care is necessary and what symptoms would be considered abnormal (for patients experiencing their first delivery, all symptoms are new and strange) and reportable.

Care of the newborn may be limited to feeding during the first few days. When the mother's strength returns, she may wish to bathe and change the infant also. Demonstrations of these techniques and supervision of her efforts are incorporated into the nursing care. Recognition of her successes and praise increase the mother's feeling of security in her ability to function.

Because of the sheltered environment provided after delivery, women may misjudge the actual amount of physical and psychic energy they possess. They may expect to resume tasks too soon and then feel discouraged when they are not able to do so. In addition, the baby's behavior does not always meet expectations. Sore nipples, worry about adequate milk supply, or even lack of sensations anticipated with breast-feeding can lead to a mother's disappointment. Some babies cry more than expected or do not seem satisfied with their feedings. Many babies have fussy periods that do not respond to any ministrations:

But my husband, too, was disconcerted at first, for the intense, unending plaintive cries of our firstborn reached to the very depths of our hearts. And, we both had really believed that, somehow, a baby born naturally at home and never separated from its mother would not be so fretful. However, it becomes apparent that all babies cry.*

Occasionally fatigue accumulates during the last month of pregnancy when sleep is interrupted by shortness of breath, urinary frequency, leg cramps, or inability to lie in a comfortable position. After delivery this fatigue is accentuated by the round-the-clock demands of the new baby.

Sibling rivalry may require parental time and attention to handle successfully. Even if the children have participated in planning for the new baby, they may be unable to accept the reality of diminished parental attention; their behavior may reflect their feelings of frustration (Fig. 29-4).

Forewarning about the possibility of such happenings even in the best regulated homes permits the parents to judge themselves less harshly and to be better prepared to seek assistance, change routine, or accept the happening as a passing phase.

A young mother described such an experience to a student nurse on a postnatal visit to the home:

When you cautioned me that last day in the hospital about not getting involved with my clients too soon, I just didn't believe you. I felt so well and on top of things. But when we got home, everything seemed to fall to pieces. My episiotomy hurt dreadfully, the baby never slept at night. I just had to phone and cancel out. If you hadn't said that, I would have figured I was a failure and I don't know what I would have done. Now everything is coming around.

Depressive states are not uncommon during this stage. Feelings of extreme vulnerability may arise from a number of factors. Psychologically the mother may be over-

---

*From Lang, R. 1972. Birth book. Ben Lomond, Calif., Genesis Press.

*From Lang, R. 1972. Birth book. Ben Lomond, Calif., Genesis Press.

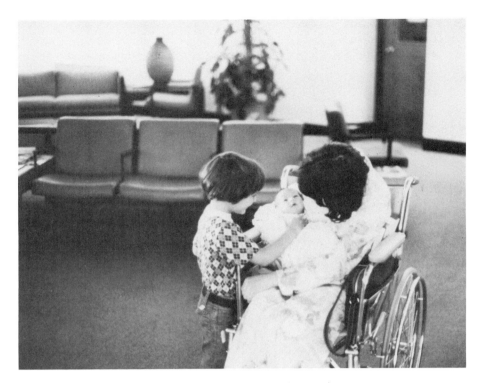

Fig. 29-4. Meeting new sister in hospital setting.

whelmed by the actuality of parental responsibilities or feel deprived of the pregnancy state, with its concomitant supportive care of family members and friends. Others regret the loss of the mother-fetal relationship and mourn its passing. Still others experience a ''let down feeling'' once labor and the ordeal of birth is complete. They had girded themselves for an elemental experience, a walk ''through the shadows,'' and now it was safely over.

Once immediate tasks and adjustments have been undertaken and brought under control, a plateau is reached. At this time the lifelong effects of their new responsibilities come into focus, and some parents experience a feeling of ''being trapped'' and of wondering ''what it is all about.''

Such reactions are not necessarily expressed verbally, but the depressive state is signified by typical behaviors—withdrawal, loss of interest in surroundings, and crying.

Physiologically it has been suggested that a lowered level of circulating glucocorticoids or a condition of subclinical hypothyroidism may exist during the puerperium. This could explain some minor degrees of depression.

Whatever the cause, the depressive reaction should not be dismissed lightly. Its prevalence and its name of ''the baby blues'' have deprived many women of the support they need. Recognition of the state, helping the woman to verbalize her feelings, conveying warmth in touch and tone of voice, and setting up tasks she can accomplish easily and successfully are interventions that can help to counteract these feelings.

Situational supports. Because this culture has emphasized the instinctual components of motherhood, many parents are hesitant in seeking help from nurses, physicians, family, and friends. Gordon and Gordon (1960) found that long-term support by nurses or physicians was a positive factor in the ultimate adjustment of the family. Parents need to be encouraged to communicate openly with each other regarding their stresses. Relatives or friends assisting with housework and baby-sitting older children and eventually the new baby are specific ways others can help. Being able to share experiences verbally with others who are interested and experienced also tends to reassure the new mother.

A mother, in discussing visits by the family to see the new baby, commented:

I want the family to come. You people praise him so and think he is the most wonderful baby. All my friends have their own babies and are too busy trying to get compliments for them to give us any. All babies need aunties and grandmothers!

Being given information about the availability of health facilities and how to get in touch with the nurse or physician relieves new parents of feeling total responsibility for the health of the new baby. A physician reported one aspect of his plan for new mothers as follows:

I make sure they have my phone number and ask them to call me day or night if they are worried. Since I've done this, the frantic calls have decreased to almost nothing. Knowing they can call seems to take the "steam" out of their concern. I feel it has worked both ways, for their benefit and mine.

Visits by nurses to the home may be spaced to take into account potential stress times such as 2 to 3 days after the return home, between the third and fourth week, and in the sixth week. One woman, cared for throughout pregnancy and the postnatal period by a nursing student, had anticipated a "kind of nervous breakdown." It did not materialize and in the final visit with the student, she said, "You've been the best nerve medicine I've ever had."

The supportive care given at such times includes the entire family. Parents are as concerned with the ups and downs of other family members as they are of mother and child. It may consist of listening to accounts of successes and failures, individual's feelings about the new baby, and comments about expectations of others in their new roles. One prime requisite is to set up a climate for the safe expression of doubts and anger, as well as happiness. The family will test the nurse's intent and knowledge, and she must recognize and accept this. The following dialogue is an example of this:

Patient: "I phoned the hospital and they said just what you said about the sitz bath."
Nurse: "Well, I'll give myself a star."
(Both laughed.)
Nurse: "Did it help any?"

Coping mechanisms. In addition to new parents learning the techniques for care of themselves and their babies, other suggestions have proved helpful to parents in coping with readjusting their lives (Gordon and Gordon, 1960). A list of these could be given to new parents, but discussion of their specific ways of handling these suggestions is also necessary.

1. Set priorities for tasks. Many tasks can be left for a later period or done by others. Be adamant about not taking on extra tasks for family, friends, or community.

2. Do not become overconcerned with "appearances"—tidiness in the home is not as important as time spent with the family. Taking up the role of "super housekeeper" can be postponed until other adjustments are made.

3. Get plenty of rest and sleep; rearrange schedules to fit this. Naps may not be possible if there are other children in the family, so early-to-bed is recommended. Do not attempt to nurse another relative at this point; such responsibilities should be undertaken by other family members.

4. Try not to schedule a move to a new location soon after giving birth.

5. Arrange for some time away from the baby; enlist help of friends, family, or others for baby-sitting. Relaxation for both husband and wife is necessary.

6. Learn what health facilities are available and how to get in touch with the physician or nurse.

7. Get out of the house at least once a day. Access to a car and being able to drive are assets, and taking the baby out for a walk or even going shopping make for breaks in routine.

8. Be open in your communication with others. Share incidents of delight or of worry with others; give open indications of your needs for support and for sharing experiences.

It is to be hoped that toward the end of stage II the tasks and adjustments of daily routine will begin to follow a pattern. The new baby begins to take an established position in the family, and many of the feeding problems, whether related to breast- or bottle-feeding, have been largely resolved. The mother's physical energy and strength return, and by the fifth week the infant has had a postnatal checkup by the physician and the mother has had hers or has made arrangements for one.

The time for moving on to the next stage of adjustment has come.

Stage III: Interdependent behavior

In this stage of adjustment, interdependent behavior reasserts itself, and the family moves forward in time as a system with interreacting members.

The relationship of husband and wife, although forever altered by the introduction of a child, resumes many of its former characteristics. A primary need is to establish a life-style that includes the children but is in some respects exclusive of them. Emphasis must be placed on husband and wife sharing interests and activities that are adult in scope. This time is often one of stress for the parental pair. Career patterns of men in their twenties and thirties show intensive activity centering around advancement in their profession or job. This often necessitates long hours away from the home or moving from one locality to another. Meanwhile, the woman is engrossed in home activities directed toward care of the young children. Interests and needs diverge, and a gradual estrangement may occur that is glossed over for the time being by the "business" of each. A special effort must be undertaken to strengthen the adult-to-adult relationship as a basis for the family unit.

Most couples begin intercourse by the third or fourth week after the child is born and some begin earlier, as soon as this can be accomplished without discomfort for the wife. This increases the man-woman aspect of the family, and the adult pair shares a closeness denied to the other family members. Many new fathers speak of the alienation experienced when they observe the intimate mother-child relationship, and some are frank in expressing feelings of jealousy toward the interloper. The resumption of marital relationships seems to bring the parents' relationship back into focus.

As soon as intercourse is resumed, the possibility of pregnancy arises, since in some women, ovulation and impregnation may occur as early as the sixth or seventh postnatal week. This phenomenon is delayed in women who are breast-feeding, but this delay is scarcely a phase of infertility, and pregnancy can occur. Planning for such an eventuality is necessary before intercourse begins.

Baby-sitting, if at all possible, must be planned and a regular schedule developed. This includes time off for the mother during the day so that she can get away from the home and its responsibilities. In some localities, church or other agencies have developed programs attuned to the needs of mothers. Women come to the center, the young child is cared for, and the mothers take part in activities with other mothers. This serves to help them establish relationships with others who are also involved in the care of young children. A mutual sharing of successes and failures in this regard helps the new mother maintain a feeling of equilibrium.

Most women are physically able to return to work by the end of the sixth week. If this is done, it will occasion certain adjustments for child care. Ideally a substitute parent would be one who could come to the home and provide love as well as care to the child. Some parents are fortunate enough to have grandparents or other relatives to fill such a role. Others must take the child to another person's home or a day-care center early in the morning and pick the child up at night. Such care as is provided by day-care centers is needed by some children whose mothers must work to help support them or who are the sole support of the child in some single-parent families. For those who require this type of service, assistance in locating such help can be obtained from the local health department. There are unfortunately not enough quality placements for all children requiring this care.

Ideally parents make plans for care prior to the birth of the baby; however, if this is not done, medical personnel should be cognizant of the sources of assistance on a local level, and they must make sure that parents are aware of them also. This may serve to alert parents to the many health services available to them in the community (e.g., well-baby centers and immunization clinics).

Relationships with siblings take on more permanence as the new baby assumes his position in the sibling hierarchy. Many parents show much ingenuity in introducing the baby to brothers and sisters. Jealous reactions are to be expected once the initial excitement of "having a new baby" is over, since the baby absorbs the time and attention of the significant persons in the other children's lives. The new parent can learn many innovative techniques by listening to other parents describe their efforts to ease the older siblings' acceptance of the new child.

Regression to an infantile level of behavior is frequently seen in the other children. Some will revert to bed-wetting, whining, or refusal to feed themselves. Much patience is required of parents to weather this phase. Plans must be undertaken to divert aggressive behavior directed toward the baby to other safer outlets. A special time may be set aside for additional attention to older children when the baby is sleeping. For example, fathers can spend more time with older siblings, and be attentive to the baby when the older children are in bed at night.

Both girls and boys seem to enjoy helping in the care of the baby or a substitute baby (doll). Many parents relate difficulties with siblings when they are devoting attention to feeding the infant, either by breast or bottle. The other children seem to sense the closeness of the mother and child in this act and resent it. To counter these reactions some mothers have let the older children drink from a bottle or breast too. The tediousness and effort needed to obtain milk or fruit juice by this method often rapidly discourages them. One mother reported that her young son routinely "breast-fed" his doll while she breast-fed the new baby. They had conversations at this time, and she believed that by sharing this experience he seemed to take pride in his adult behavior of drinking from a cup.

Another difficulty arises when well-meaning relatives or friends concentrate on the new baby to the exclusion of the older children. Thoughtful adults often bring gifts to and shower attention on the older children as well as the baby.

To expect a young child to accept automatically and love a rival for parents' affection is assuming a too-mature response. Sibling love grows as does other love, by being with another person and sharing experiences.

PLAN OF CARE: PARENT-CHILD RELATIONSHIPS—INITIATING THE RELATIONSHIP

PATIENT CARE OBJECTIVES

1. Parents are reassured of the normalcy of infant characteristics:
   a. Appearance (e.g., molding of head, milia, lanugo, forceps marks).
   b. Behavior (e.g., sleeping, waking, crying).
   c. Responses (e.g., eating, regurgitating, defecating, voiding, gaining weight).
2. Parents are aware of the criteria they will use in assessing the success or failure of the care they give their child:
   a. Infant responses: The mother may feel successful if her infant snuggles against her, looks at her, stops crying when she holds him, or burps when feeding. The mother may feel unsuccessful if the child persists in crying, is unable to breast-feed, "frowns" at her, or will not wake up.
   b. Maternal competence in caretaking activities: The mother may feel inadequate to the extent to which she feels incompetent in handling or holding the child.
   c. Opinions of significant others: Mothers may expect that others will be supportive and accepting of their beginning attempts or critical and intolerant of their less-than-perfect efforts. These expectations can prompt them to seek assistance or to avoid it.
3. Infant's identity is established:
   a. Through the claiming process. Parents look for similarities or differences of their infant compared to other family members as to size, weight, sex, appearance, behavior, and responses.
   b. By checking the identifying wristband.

NURSING INTERVENTIONS

Diagnostic	Therapeutic	Educational
1. Maternal behaviors are assessed for cues as to needs for learning and teaching, for support to reduce tension levels, and for counseling with reference to presence or absence of motherliness. a. Mother gradually increases physical contact in that she (1) begins with fingertip touching of head and extremities, changes to whole hand to caress and hold, and finally enfolds infant in her arms; (2) scrutinizes infant's body carefully, notes variations in what she deems normal, and looks for reassurance; (3) seeks eye contact and wants baby to wake up if sleeping; and (4) goes through claiming process. b. She reacts in her own personal manner to emotional excitement (e.g., crys, laughs, talks, remains silent). c. She shows level of competence in handling and holding child consonant with previous experience and level of anxiety. d. She responds to infant going to sleep, stopping crying, etc., with lessening of tension and increasing relaxation. 2. Maternal behaviors are correlated with mother's level of physical and psychic energy, anxiety level, freedom from discomfort, and ability.	1. Contacts between mother and infant are (a) timed to make use of infant's normal patterns of sleeping and waking at birth, at about 4 to 6 hours, and every 2 to 5 hours thereafter, and (b) long enough (at least 1 hour) to permit mother to hold, examine, and enjoy her child. 2. Mother is given report on infant's examination (physical) and progress to date. 3. Nursing personnel are available to give infant care as indicated to reassure mother regarding normalcy of her infant and to assist with maternal caretaking activities.	1. Normal characteristics of newborn are reviewed. 2. Infant care activities are demonstrated and practice supervised: a. Hospital routines when infant goes from nursery area to mother's bedside, such as identification of infant, emergency care of infant if gagging or choking episode occurs (p. 476), protective measures used to minimize possibilities of cross infection. b. Infant feeding techniques (Chapter 31). 3. Maternal criteria for success in mothering skills, i.e., infant responses and competence in caretaking activities, and opinions of significant others are discussed; examples used of behavior noted; and praise given for success.

PLAN OF CARE: PARENT-CHILD RELATIONSHIPS—CONSOLIDATING THE RELATIONSHIP

PATIENT CARE OBJECTIVES

1. Parents develop a satisfactory level of competence in the routine caretaking activities of bathing, feeding, holding, and clothing the infant.
2. Parents establish realistic criteria for use in evaluating their efforts in mothering relative to the following:
   a. Infant responses: acceptance of a mixture of success and failure in the control they can exert in such infant behaviors as crying, fussing, eating, sleeping and waking, growing, and gaining weight.
   b. Parental competence in caretaking activities:
      (1) Self-esteem grows as skill in caretaking activities increases.
      (2) Recognition develops of what care is essential for the well-being of the infant as opposed to the prior expectations of the mother.
      (3) A flexible schedule for infant care is accepted.
   c. Opinion of significant others: Assistance from others is accepted or rejected as knowledge and skill grow. Parents have awareness of vulnerability to praise or criticism of own mothers, spouse, and close relatives.
3. Infant's identity expands with parental awareness of his particular rhythms of sleeping, waking, hunger, and satiety and his cues for expressing his need for sleep, food, soothing, socializing, relief from pain or discomfort.

NURSING INTERVENTIONS

Diagnostic	Therapeutic	Educational

1. Maternal (paternal) behaviors assessed during feeding periods when mother or father is giving general care to infant. These parent-child contacts provide additional opportunities to assess mother's attitude toward herself and her new responsibility, and father's commitment to child care. Indications of motherliness, that quality which enriches and makes human the care activities, become more apparent.
  a. Do they seem to enjoy handling and touching baby and stroking and patting him, or do they minimize any body contact? Touch gentle or rough? Personal or impersonal?
  b. It is difficult to assess modes of address used by parents to their infants, but tone of voice may be indicative of meaning behind terms used.
  c. Do they seek and maintain eye contact? Do they stare fixedly into baby's eyes.
  d. Is mother able to overcome natural reluctance to handle excrements of infant?
  e. Do they have rigid plans for baby routines and expectations of infant fitting into these plans?
2. Maternal behaviors are correlated with mother's physical and psychic condition. Fatigue, discomfort, anxiety about assuming full responsibility for the child, and adverse social and/or economic factors
	1. When in hospital, mother is given daily report on infant's progress and behaviors (e.g., eating, sleeping, voiding, defecating).
	2. Infant is examined in mother's presence, and findings are reviewed with mother. Written instructions as to feeding, medications, etc., are provided.
	3. Mother and father are encouraged to participate in infant care, and whenever possible techniques developed by mother are used.
	4. Discuss problems experienced (e.g., infant crying, sleeping), and assistance with solutions is given.
	5. Discuss successes and failures in caretaking activities, and help with accumulating successful coping mechanisms and discarding unsuccessful ones.
	  a. Mother conserves her energy by having rest period when infant sleeps, by not becoming involved in "perfect housekeeper" image, by encouraging infant to sleep through at night by waking for feeding at 10 or 11 PM; by enlisting help of others, relatives or friends, to help with household chores; and accepting baby-sitting offers.
	  b. She takes time to study her baby (e.g., what different types of crying mean, when he likes being awake—morning, afternoon, or evening).
	  c. She is open-minded about expectations of her role and oth-
		1. This represents a period of intensive learning and mastering of following practical aspects of child care:
		  a. Demonstrate and supervise practice of bathing, changing, and holding infant, and continued assistance with feeding.
		  b. Discuss normal rhythms of child and mother's awareness of how child communicates his needs.
		  c. Discuss normal responses of parents to complex role of parent.

Continued.

PLAN OF CARE: PARENT-CHILD RELATIONSHIPS—CONSOLIDATING
THE RELATIONSHIP—cont'd

NURSING INTERVENTIONS—cont'd

Diagnostic	Therapeutic	Educational

need to be taken into account because they can affect manner and interest displayed to child and can cloud true relationship.
3. Paternal behaviors are correlated with father's shared cultural and personal concepts of fathering role and previous experience with infants.
4. Both parental patterns are checked against data collected earlier to establish evidence of consistent pattern of reaction to child and parental role.
	ers' roles (e.g., father's) and infant's abilities.
	6. Discuss mother's and/or father's reactions to parenthood role; offer opportunity for safe revelation of their feelings.
	7. For some parents whose behavior indicates consistent rejection of infancy of child and his dependency needs, above interventions apply; however, additional care is needed as follows:
	  a. Repeated contacts with parents are planned and carried out.
	  b. Other supportive personnel such as social worker can be enlisted to help.	

PLAN OF CARE: PARENT-CHILD RELATIONSHIPS—GROWTH IN PARENTAL ROLE

PATIENT CARE OBJECTIVES

1. Parents become knowledgeable about abnormal responses of the infant and those responses for which professional consultation is required and develop knowledge of the normal growth and development of the infant.
2. Criteria for success in parenting are flexible with reference to the following:
   a. Infant responses: Infant's dependency needs are recognized and accepted as a beginning level of development. Parents are aware of parental actions being an important factor in the behavior exhibited by the infant. Adaptation of the mother and infant's normal rhythms and responses begins as a process of mutual behavior modification.
   b. Parental competence in caretaking activities: Parents recognize that the skills required will change with growth and development of the child and that it is reasonable to seek guidance and support as new needs arise.
   c. Opinion of significant others: Parents recognize that this dependency will continue, but in its negative sense, it can be countered with mastery of parental tasks and a growing self-esteem as a parent.
3. Infant's identity continues to expand as he becomes part of a family group with siblings, birth order, etc.

NURSING INTERVENTIONS

Diagnostic	Therapeutic	Educational
1. Parental behaviors are assessed during hospital stay, during postnatal visits to home and at visit to pediatrician's office or well-baby clinic for fourth-week checkup of infant. How is child held by mother? Is her hand grasp and touch gentle? Does she look at child's face or at examiner? Does she participate in restraining and comfort-	1. Examine infant and review findings with parents. 2. Provide opportunity for mother (family) to discuss problems: parents' reactions to child, child's needs and demands, feeling of depression or helplessness and how such feelings affect care mother can give her child. 3. Recognize success of parental ef-	1. Discuss signs and symptoms of illness and measures instituted to effect cure or obtain medical assistance. 2. Discuss the infant's developmental needs: a. Accommodation to physical growth (e.g., introduction of solid foods into the diet) or weaning.

PLAN OF CARE: PARENT-CHILD RELATIONSHIPS—GROWTH IN PARENTAL ROLE—cont'd

NURSING INTERVENTIONS—cont'd

Diagnostic	Therapeutic	Educational
ing child? Is she overly concerned about child's health? Is child isolated except for necessary caretaking activities? 2. Physical examination shows healthy developing child or evidence of neglect or abuse. 3. Information regarding physical responses of child such as appetite, bowel movements, voiding, or rashes is elicited. 4. Concern with responsibilities: How does mother manage child's crying? Household chores? Isolation from community? Keeping up her career? Repetitive nature of care? Inability to get unbroken rest? 5. Coping mechanisms being used: Does mother get away from home responsibilities occasionally? Do other family members help? Is there someone she can talk to? Can she express her feelings about new responsibilities freely? Does she only allow expressions of idealized mothering feelings?	forts in mothering their child and help with areas of concern. 4. Institute future nursing interventions: a. Plan for next routine visit. b. Help family obtain further assistance if needed to develop more adequate coping mechanisms; use of public health agency personnel or social workers. Some communities have established round-the-clock telephone centers where parents can obtain help for emotionally based problems with their child. These are in addition to emergency medical services. c. Refer child to other agencies for correction of defects noted. d. Discuss facilities for child care outside the home by other than immediate family.	b. Use of longer wakeful periods to increase social stimulation of infant and interactions with siblings and other family members. c. Adaptation to infant's persisting dependency and his inability to conform socially or show social awareness of other's needs. 3. Discuss balancing infant's needs with those of other family members (e.g., jealousy of siblings, husband's or wife's feelings of alienation), parents' need to modify infant's behavior to meet their expectation (e.g., toilet training, sleeping patterns, stopping crying when admonished), and infant's ability to conform.

REFERENCES

Adams, M. 1963. Early concerns of primigravida mothers regarding infant care activities. Nurs. Res. **12**:72.

Ainsworth, M. D. 1970. The development of infant-mother attachment. In Caldwell, B. M., and Reccurti, H. N. (eds.). Review of child development research (vol. 3). New York, Russell Sage Foundation.

Baldwin, W. H. 1976. Adolescent pregnancy and childbearing—growing concerns for Americans. Population Bull. **31** (2).

Barbero, G., Morris, M., and Redford, M. 1963. Malidentification of mother, baby, father relationships expressed in infant failure to thrive. In The neglected battered child syndrome. New York, Child Welfare League of America.

Barneel, C. R., and others. 1970. Neonatal separation: the maternal side of interactional deprivation. Pediatrics **54**:197.

Benedek, T. 1950. Adaptation to reality in early infancy. Psychoanal. Q. **7**:200.

Benedek, T. 1970. Motherhood and nurturing. In Anthony, E. J., and Benedek, T. (eds.). Parenthood: its psychology and psychopathology. Little, Brown & Co.

Bernal, J. 1972. Crying during the first ten days of life and maternal responses. Dev. Med. Child Neurol. **14**:362.

Broussard, E. R., and Hartner, M. S. 1970. Maternal perception of the neonate as related to development. Child Psychiatry Human Dev. **1**:16, Fall.

Burstein, I., and others. 1974. Anxiety, pregnancy, labor and the neonate. Am. J. Obstet. Gynecol. **118**:195.

Dareid, M., and Appell, G. 1969. Mother-child relations. In Howells, J. A. (ed.). Modern perspectives in international child psychiatry. Edinburgh, Oliver & Boyd.

Davis, L., and Grace, H. 1971. Anticipatory counseling of unwed pregnant adolescents. Nurs. Clin. North Am. **6**: 581.

Donner, G. J. 1972. Parenthood as a crisis. Perspect. Psychiatr. Care **10**:84, April-June.

Erikson, E. H. 1959. Identity and the life cycle: selected papapers. In Psychological issues (vol. 1). New York, International Press.

Fry, B., and Barham, B. 1975. Reaching out to pregnant adolescents. Am. J. Nurs. **75**:1502.

Gershenson, C. 1973. Child development, infant day care and adolescent parents: a national overview. Presented at Improving Care for Infants of School Age Parents, an Invitational Workshop, Summer.

Gordon, R., and Gordon, K. 1960. Social factors in prevention of postpartum emotional problems. Obstet. Gynecol. **15**: 453.

Hartman, E. 1970. Involvement of a maternity and infant care project in a pregnant school girl program in Minneapolis, Minnesota. J. Sch. Health **40**:224, May.

Helfer, R. E., and Kempe, C. H. 1965. The battered child. Chicago, The University of Chicago Press.

Howard, M. 1968. Comprehensive service programs for school-age pregnant girls. Children 13:193, Sept.-Oct.

Josselyn, I. M. 1956. Cultural forces: motherliness and fatherliness. Am. J. Orthopsychiatry 26:264.

Kaufman, I. 1973. Psychiatric implications of physical abuse of children. In Protecting the battered child. Denver, Children's Division, American Humane Association.

Kennell, J., and others. Maternal behavior one year after early and extended postpartum contact. Dev. Med. Child Neurol. 16:172.

Klaus, M. H., and Kennell, J. H. 1970. Mothers separated from their newborn infants. Pediatr. Clin. North Am. 17: 1015.

Klaus, M. H., and Kennell, J. H. 1976. Maternal-infant bonding. St. Louis, The C. V. Mosby Co.

Klaus, M. H., and others. 1970. Human maternal behavior at the first contact with her young. Pediatrics 46:187.

Klaus, M. H., and others. 1972. Maternal attachment: importance of the first post-partum days. N. Engl. J. Med. 286: 460.

Klaus, M. H., and others. 1975. Does human maternal behavior after delivery show a characteristic pattern? In Parent-child interaction, Ciba Foundation Symposium No. 33 (new series). Amsterdam, Associated Scientific Publishers.

Klaus, M. H., and others. 1975. Evidence for a sensitive period in the human mother. In Parent-child interaction, Ciba Foundation Symposium No. 33 (new series). Amsterdam, Associated Scientific Publishers.

Klein, L. 1974. Early teenage pregnancy, contraception and repeat pregnancy. Am. J. Obstet. Gynecol. 120:249.

Lang, R. 1972. Birth book. Ben Lomond, Calif., Genesis Press.

Larson, V., and others. 1966. Difference between new mothers: psychiatric admissions vs. normals. Presented at the Washington State Medical Association's Annual Meeting, Sept., 1966, Spokane, Wash.

LeMasters, E. E. 1965. Parenthood as a crisis. In Parad, H. J. (ed.). Crisis interventions: selected readings. New York, Family Service Association of America.

Lessing, D. 1970. A proper marriage. New York, Simon & Schuster, Inc.

Luffer, A. D., and others. 1972. Effects of mother-infant separation on maternal attachment behavior. Child Dev. 43:1203.

Mercer, R. 1976. Becoming a mother at sixteen. MCN Am. J. Mat. Child Nurs. 1:44, Jan.-Feb.

Morris, M. 1965. Maternal claiming-identification process: their meaning for mother-infant mental health. Am. J. Orthopsychiatry 35:302.

Morris, M. 1966. Psychological miscarriage: an end to mother love. Transaction, p. 11, Jan.-Feb.

Morris, M. G., and Gould, R. W. 1963. Role reversal: a concept in dealing with the neglected/battered child syndrome. In The neglected battered child syndrome. New York, Child Welfare League of America.

National Institute of Child Health and Human Development, U.S. Department of Health, Education, and Welfare. 1971. Optimal health care for mothers and children: a national priority. Washington, D.C., U.S. Government Printing Office.

Nelson, S. 1973. School age parents. Child. Today 2:31, March-April.

Noren, C. H. 1974. Family. MS, November, p. 12.

Osofsky, H. J. 1976. The pregnant teenager: a medical, educational and social analysis. Springfield, Ill., Charles C Thomas, Publisher.

Parke, R. D. 1972. Mother-father-newborn interaction: effects of maternal medication, labor and sex of infant. In Proceedings of the Eightieth Annual Convention of the American Psychological Association, Honolulu, Hawaii.

Poole, C. 1976. Adolescent mothers: can they be helped. Pediatr. Nurs. 2:7, March-April.

Ringler, N. M., and others. 1975. Mother-to-child speech at two years—effects of early postnatal contact. J. Pediatr. 86:143.

Robertson, J. 1962. Mothering as an influence on early development. Psychoanal. Study Child. 17:245.

Rubin, R. 1961. Maternal behavior. Nurs. Outlook 9:682.

San Francisco Chronicle. Nov. 17, 1976, p. 24.

Shainess, N. 1970. Abortion is no man's business. Psychology Today, p. 18, March.

Smith, E., and others. 1971. A team approach. Children 18: 209, Nov.-Dec.

Steele, B., and Pollock, C. 1968. A psychiatric study of parents who abuse infants and small children. In Helfer, R. E., and Kempe, C. (eds.). The battered child. Chicago, The University of Chicago Press.

U.S. Department of Health, Education, and Welfare. 1975. Vital statistics of the United States, 1970: natality (vol. 1). Washington, D.C., U.S. Government Printing Office.

Williams, T. M. 1974. Childbearing practices of young mothers: what we know, how it matters, why so little. Am. J. Orthopsychiatry 44:70.

Wright, M. K. 1976. Comprehensive services of adolescent unwed mothers. Children 13:170, Sept.-Oct.

UNIT NINE

Normal newborn

CHAPTER 30

Management of normal newborn: general care

MANAGEMENT

Although most infants make the necessary physiologic adjustment to extrauterine existence without undue difficulty, their continued life depends on the care received from others (see Appendix B). The extent and nature of that care will be determined by the infant's physiologic ability to (1) establish and maintain respirations; (2) complete the cardiovascular adjustment initiated at birth; (3) ingest, retain, and digest nutrients; and (4) eliminate waste by voiding and defecating. In addition, care is dictated by the infant's need for (1) close observation and monitoring of physiologic responses to permit early detection of distress and institution of corrective medical or nursing interventions; (2) protection from infection and trauma; (3) provision of warmth, nutrition (Chapter 31), and body hygiene; and (4) mothering.

In the hospital, the newborn's environment consists of the personnel who assume responsibility for his care, the facilities provided for his care, and his parents, who may or may not participate in his care. These three components are linked by policies, administrative, medical, and nursing, which reflect the standards of care the agency undertakes to provide for the newborn.

Increased interest on the part of medical groups in the study of the fetus and care of the neonate during the perinatal period has led to the development of ''perinatology'' as a branch of health care. This specialty manages the normal and abnormal infant and the varying environmental influences that increase or detract from the probability of optimal development. Nursing personnel may vary in degree and kind of preparation, but all need to demonstrate ability in detecting abnormal responses in infant or parent and in instituting necessary diagnostic and supportive nursing measures.

A system designed for the delivery of health care services to the neonate is illustrated in Fig. 30-1. The infant is transferred from the delivery unit to the observational area (transitional nursery). Its location, types of equipment, supplies, and skills of assigned personnel reflect the infant's need for intensive care during the critical transitional period. Once stabilized, the infant can be admitted to a mother-infant unit. These units may be *rooming-in units,* wherein the infant shares accommodations with the mother and full participation of parents in the infant's care is encouraged. These units provide excellent learning areas for new mothers and serve to foster early and sustained parent-child relationships. In areas where rooming-in units are not feasible, or the mother either prefers less direct involvement in infant care or is not physically able to participate, the infant may be lodged in a normal newborn nursery. The implementation of family-centered care is possible under these circumstances through instituting longer mother-child contacts at feeding times and providing demonstrations and lectures relating to infant care. In some areas, early discharge to the home is being introduced. This requires careful preparation of parents, a healthy infant, and regular follow-up services if the infant is not to be placed in jeopardy.

For the infant designated as ''high risk,'' transfer to an intensive care unit is indicated (Chapters 32 and 34).

Construction, maintenance, and operation of nurseries in accredited hospitals is directed by national professional organizations such as the American Academy of Pediatrics and local or state governing bodies. Prescribed standards include areas such as the following:

1. *Environmental factors:* provision of adequate lighting, elimination of potential fire hazards, safety of electrical appliances, adequate ventilation, controlled temperature (warm and free of drafts) and humidity (lower than 50%)
2. *Measures to control infection:* adequate floor space to permit positioning bassinets at least 24 inches apart, hand-washing facilities, techniques for safe formula preparation and storage, and cleaning and sterilizing of equipment and supplies (Fig. 30-2)

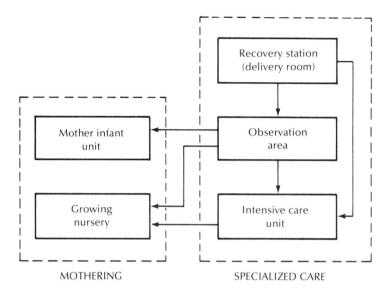

Fig. 30-1. Method for division of care of newborn. This system allows special consideration of infants during their early hours in observation nursery, intensive care nursery when necessary, and a "mothering" nursery for full development of maternal-infant relationship so important in first days of life. In small maternity areas, observation area may also serve as combined nursery for growing infants and those who require specialized care. (From Babson, S. G., Benson, R. C., Pernoll, M. L., and Benda, G. I. 1975. Management of high-risk pregnancy and intensive care of the newborn [ed. 3]. St. Louis, The C. V. Mosby Co.; modified from Silverman, W. H. 1970. Clin. Obstet. Gynecol. **13:**87.)

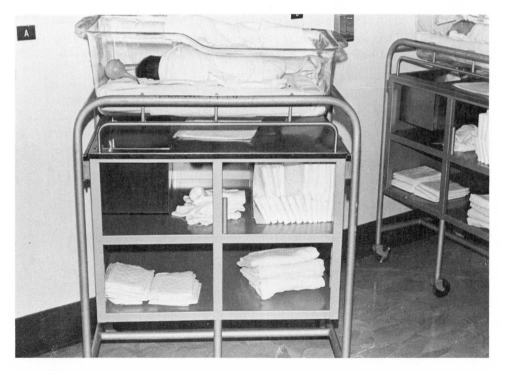

Fig. 30-2. Individual nursery bassinet. Each infant has own supply of clothes, and bulb syringe is kept readily available. Cribs are plastic to permit easier visualization of infant.

In addition, hospital personnel develop their own policies and procedures directed toward protection of the neonates under their care. For example:

1. Nursery personnel are restricted to those directly involved in the care of mothers and/or infants. This restriction minimizes the number of persons to whom each infant is exposed, thereby reducing the introduction of pathologic organisms. In this respect, those children born at home are at an advantage because those who come in contact usually are family members. In hospitals this home environment is somewhat duplicated when the infant and mother ''room together'' and the mother and father are active in the care, thereby reducing the number of nursing personnel involved. In many hospitals, nurseries are constructed with anterooms, where physicians carry out examinations and procedures such as circumcisions, or where parents may come to feed or hold their infants who must remain in the hospital for care.

2. Personnel assigned to the nursery wear special uniforms or cover gowns and before beginning the care of infants carry out a hand-washing technique.

3. Any persons coming from an ''outside'' area are expected to gown and wash their hands prior to contact with either infants or equipment. Such persons include nurses, physicians, parents, department supervisors, electricians, or housekeepers.

4. Individuals with infectious conditions are excluded from contact with neonates, including those with upper respiratory tract infections, gastrointestinal tract infections, and infectious skin conditions. Most agencies have now coupled this day-to-day screening of personnel with yearly health examinations.

More detailed information concerning standards of care for newborn nurseries may be obtained from the following sources:

The American Academy of Pediatrics, 1801 Hinman Ave., Evanston, Ill. 60202
  Standards and Recommendations for Hospital Care of the Newborn, 1971
  Standards of Child Health Care, Council on Pediatric Practice (ed. 2), 1972
American College of Obstetricians and Gynecologists, 1 East Wacker Drive, Chicago, Ill. 60601
  Standards for Obstetric-Gynecological Hospital Service, 1969
American Hospital Association, 840 North Lake Dr., Chicago, Ill. 60611
  Infection Control in the Hospital, 1970

PHYSICAL ASSESSMENT*

During the neonatal period, the antenatal and postnatal characteristics of the infant emerge, and only grad-

---

*Students are advised to review Chapter 8 for the neonate's physiologic states.

ually do the former disappear as the infant continues to grow and mature in the extrauterine environment. The first physical assessment of the infant is done at birth using the Apgar scoring technique and a physical assessment (p. 327). A second more thorough physical examination is done on each newborn within 24 hours after delivery. The goal is to provide a complete record of the newborn that will act as a data base for subsequent assessments and care. Having the parents present during the examination permits prompt discussion of parental concerns and actively involves the parents in health care of their child right from birth. At the same time, parental interactions with the child can be observed and early diagnosis of problems in parent-child relationships facilitated.

The area used for the examination should be well lighted, warm, and free of drafts. The child is undressed as needed and placed on a firm flat surface. The infant may need to be picked up and cuddled at times for reassurance. The examination can be carried out in a systematic manner, beginning with a general evaluation of such characteristics as appearance, maturity, nutritional status, activity, and state of well-being, and then specific observations can be made (Table 30-1).

Posture

The presentation and position of the fetus determines the posture of the newborn and certain of his characteristics. For example, if the fetus presents as a vertex, the newborn readily assumes the fetal position. The arms and legs are held in moderate flexion, and the fists are clinched. Newborn infants resist having their extremities extended for examination or measurement and will cry when this is attempted. Usually the crying will cease when the infant is allowed to assume the curled-up, fetal position. A frank breech presentation, on the other hand, appears more straight and stiff, so that the infant will assume his intrauterine position in repose for a few days at least. In addition, antenatal pressure of a hand or arm against the face may result in some facial asymmetry, but this is temporary in most instances (Fig. 30-3).

Skin

The term infant has an erythematous skin (beefy red) for a few hours after birth, after which it fades to its normal color. It often appears blotchy, especially over the extremities, and slightly cyanotic. This bluish discoloration *acrocyanosis,* is caused by vasomotor instability, capillary stasis, and high hemoglobin; it is normal, transient in occurrence, and persists over the first 7 to 10 days, especially with exposure to cold. The amount of *vernix caseosa,* a whitish greasy material, varies, but the

Table 30-1. Checklist of significant observations in newborns*

DATE					
TIME					

ACTIVITY	✔	ACTIVE				
	+	Activity decreased				
	+	Tires easily				
	+	Lethargic				
	+	Floppy				
	+	Irritable				
	+	Pacifier required				
	+	Frantic				
	+	Swaddled				
	+	Tremors				
	+	Twitching				
	+	Rigid				
	+	Opisthotonos				
	+	Moro poor or absent				
APPEARANCE	✔	COLOR STABLE				
	+	Pallor				
	+	Plethora				
	+	Mottled				
	+	Harlequin syndrome				
	+	Jaundice				
	+	Dusky				
	+	Cyanosis: Generalized				
	+	Circumoral				
	+	Circumocular				
	+	Extremities				
	+	Tearing				
	+	Eye discharge				

DATE					
TIME					

RESPIRATIONS	✔	CRY GOOD				
	+	Cry high-pitched				
	+	Cry weak				
	+	Sneezes				
	+	Stuffy nose				
	+	Yawning				
	+	Hoarseness				
	+	Stridor				
	✔	RESPIRATIONS REGULAR				
	+	Shallow				
	+	Labored				
	+	Deep				
	+	Irregular				
	+	Seesaw				
	+	Periodic breathing				
	+	Rest periods: <10 seconds				
	+	10 to 30 seconds				
	+	Apnea >30 seconds				
	+	Alae nasi dilated				
	+	Cough				
	+	Grunting				
	+	Retraction				

DIRECTIONS: This record is completed by the nurse indicating presence of findings (✔), severity (+, ++, +++), timing (ac, pc), etc. This checklist is used instead of routine nursing notes. Capitalized items indicate normal findings. Each column signifies a period of observations. Significant additional data are recorded in the Progress Notes. A 24-hour summary of nursing observations is given to the physician at morning rounds. These observations and the physician's findings provide the necessary data base on which a decision is made concerning illness.

*From Kempe, C. H., Silver, H. K., and O'Brien, D. (eds.). 1976. Current pediatric diagnosis and treatment (ed. 4). Los Altos, Calif., Lange Medical Publications; modified from Lubchenco, L. O. 1961. Pediatr. Clin. North Am. **8:**471.

Table 30-1. Checklist of significant observations in newborns—cont'd

DATE						DATE					
TIME						TIME					
	✔ HUNGRY						✔ SKIN NORMAL				
	✔ DEMANDING					+	Dry and peeling				
	✔ SUCKS WELL					+	Irritated				
	+ Sucks poorly					+	Petechiae (area)				
	✔ GAVAGED WELL					+	Ecchymosis (area)				
FEEDINGS (GASTROINTESTINAL)	✔ Gavaged well/slowly					+	Bleeding (area)				
	+ Gavaged poorly					+	Dehydrated				
	+ Gavage resisted					+	Edema				
	+ Mucus on tube					+	Pustular rash				
	+ Mucus, other					+	Erythema toxicum				
	+ Drooled					+	Other rash (specify)				
	+ Gagged					+	Abscess (area)				
	+ Regurgitated					+	Sclerema				
	+ Abdomen distended					+	Umbilical redness				
	cm Abdomen, circumference					+	Umbilical oozing				
	+ Hiccup										
	+ Sore buttocks										

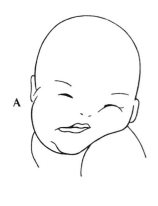

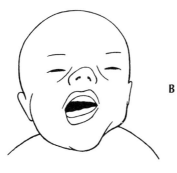

A

B

Fig. 30-3. A, Facial asymmetry. Asymmetric appearance is caused by displacement of mandible and presence of more or less pronounced fossa, or excavation, in neck, representing former position of shoulder. Some malocclusion is apparent. Confirmatory evidence may be provided by observing position of comfort that newborn often assumes. **B,** Lopsided appearance disappears spontaneously in few weeks or months, depending on its severity. (Courtesy Mead Johnson Laboratories, Evansville, Ind.)

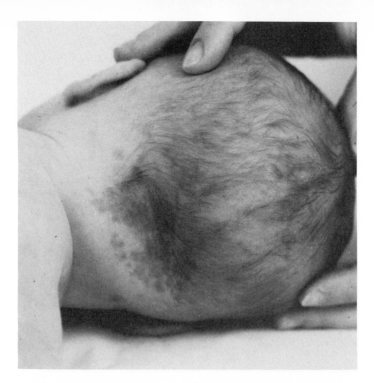

Fig. 30-4. Stork bite (telangiectatic nevi). Pale pink or mauve spots seen frequently on eyelids, glabella, and occiptal areas of newborn infants are considered by some to be type of nevus flammeus, or true vascular nevus. Certainly they behave differently from nevus flammeus in other skin areas. They are lighter in color, blanch on pressure, and almost invariably fade promptly and disappear completely before end of first year. They are rare in older infants and so common among light-complexioned newborns as to be almost routine finding. (Courtesy Mead Johnson Laboratories, Evansville, Ind.)

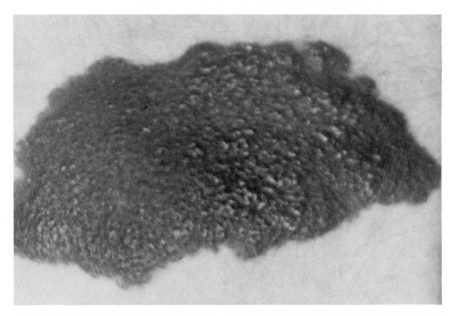

Fig. 30-5. Nevus vasculosus, or strawberry mark, is second most common type of capillary hemangioma and consists of dilated, newly formed capillaries occupying entire dermal and subdermal layers, with associated connective tissue hypertrophy. Typical lesion is raised, sharply demarcated, bright or dark red, and rough-surfaced swelling that resembles an outside slice of ripe strawberry. Lesions are usually single but may be multiple, and 75% occur in the head region. (Courtesy Mead Johnson Laboratories, Evansville, Ind.)

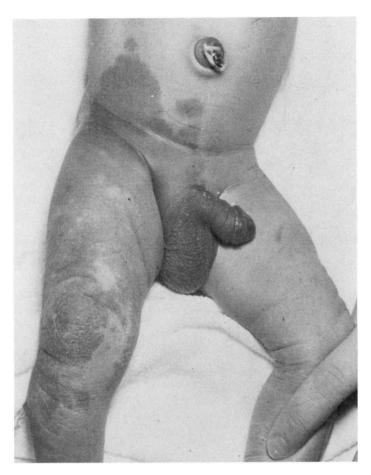

Fig. 30-6. Port wine stain, or nevus flameus, is usually observed at birth and is composed of plexus of newly formed capillaries in papillary layer of corium. It is red to purple in color; variable in size, shape, and location; and not elevated. True port wine stains do not blanch on pressure and do not disappear spontaneously. (Courtesy Mead Johnson Laboratories, Evansville, Ind.)

infant at term or beyond the second week postterm usually has minimal vernix and slight peeling of the skin, particularly over the palms of the hands and soles of the feet. The healthy term newborn is plump and the skin may feel slightly tight, suggesting fluid retention. Fine *lanugo hair* may be noted over the face, shoulders, and back. Distended sebaceous glands, or *milia*, are often seen over the face, particularly on the cheeks or the nose, and disappear as the infant matures. Actual edema of the face and *ecchymosis* (bruising) may be noted as a result of face presentation or forceps delivery. *Mongolian spots,* bluish black area of pigmentation over the back and buttocks, are seen more frequently in the dark-skinned races. They fade gradually over a period of months or years. *Telangiectatic nevi,* known as "stork bites," are pink in color and easily blanched (Fig. 30-4). They appear on the upper eyelids, nose, upper lip, lower occiput bone, and nape of the neck. They have no clinical significance and fade between the first and second years. Other birthmarks include nevus vasculosus (strawberry mark) (Fig. 30-5) and nevus flammeus (port wine stain) (Fig. 30-6). An evanescent rash, *erythema toxicum* (also called *erythema neonatorum,* or "flea-bite" dermatitis), with lesions in different stages, erythematous macules or papules or small vesicles, may appear suddenly anywhere on the body. The cause is unknown and although the appearance is alarming, it has no clinical significance and requires no treatment. Since the skin is fragile and easily debrided, it presents an inadequate barrier to infection.

Head

The newborn's head is large in comparison with his body, about one fourth of the body length, with the face smaller than the cranium (in the adult, the head is one eighth of the body length). Considerable molding of the head in vertex presentations is usual. Some overriding of the cranial bones may be noted. In babies born by cesarean section or breech birth, the head is usually very round and symmetrical if no labor was experienced. At birth the head circumference is ±35 cm (13 to 14 inches). Once molding has disappeared (around 2 weeks), a more accurate measurement can be made. By 6 weeks, an increase of 3 cm is normal. The head circumference is normally greater than the chest circumference (±33 cm, 12 to 13 inches) at birth, and they are about equal by 1 year of age. Measure the head at the greatest diameter (occipitofrontal) over the ears and center of forehead. Measure the chest at the nipple line.

A *caput succedaneum*, or soft scalp swelling, is an edematous area that extends across suture lines and is found over the most dependent part of the head in vertex presentations at birth. It results from pressure during the birth process. A *cephalhematoma* is formed by bleeding into the subperiosteal space on the surface of a skull bone and is circumscribed by the borders of the particular skull bone. It is not visible at birth and increases in size until the bleeding stops over the first 2 days. It requires no treatment and gradually is reabsorbed (Fig. 32-4).

Both fontanels are easily felt. The anterior fontanel closes at about the eighteenth month, whereas the posterior fontanel is usually closed between the eighth and twelfth week of life.

The eyes may show slight subconjunctival hemorrhages. The iris will be slate blue in white infants but brownish in black, brown, or yellow infants. Tears may be produced by the baby when he cries. The ability to follow a light with the eyes is notable. The infant will look toward a light and may focus briefly on the examiner's face. By the end of 4 weeks, the infant focuses his eyes on an object put in line of vision. The pupils are moderately constricted for about 3 days after delivery.

The infant is checked for nasal obstruction because nasal breathing is the natural type during the neonatal period, and nasal obstructions cause restlessness, crying, and cyanosis as the infant experiences difficulty in swallowing and breathing simultaneously.

The mouth can be visualized when the infant is crying and the chin gently depressed. In the normally hydrated infant the mucous membrane appears moist and pink. Pallor cyanosis of the mucus normally is not noted. Some drooling of mucus is common in the first few hours after birth; excessive drooling occurs with esophageal atresia. The palate is visualized to rule out clefts. Retention cysts, small whitish areas, are commonly found on the gum margins and at the juncture of the hard and soft palate. The cheeks appear to be full because of well-developed sucking pads. These, like the labial tubercles (sucking calluses) on the upper lip, disappear when the sucking period is over.

The ears are well-formed in most instances, but gross malformations or low-set ears may be indicative of other abnormalities, particularly of the genitourinary tract. The pinna, in term or near-term infants, shows noticeable but variable stiffness. Minor anomalies are common and occur as preauricular fistulas and tubercles.

The infant can *hear* at bith. Response to sound (ringing a bell) is evidenced by a slight startle reflex or a flickering of the eyelids. The fact that infants have no "social response" to the sound of others crying does not mean they cannot hear. As early as the first week of life, the infant may respond with grimacing and body movements to the sound of a human voice. Infants with significant hearing loss can be fitted with hearing aids even at 1 month.

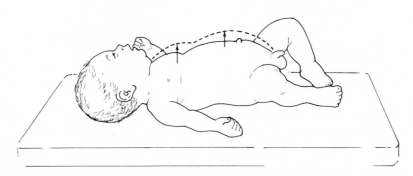

Fig. 30-7. Normal respiration. Chest and abdomen rise with inspiration. (Courtesy Mead Johnson Laboratories, Evansville, Ind.)

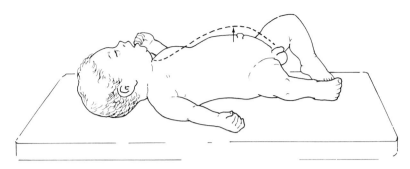

Fig. 30-8. Seesaw respiration. Chest wall retracts as abdomen rises with inspiration. (Courtesy Mead Johnson Laboratories, Evansville, Ind.)

The neck is characteristically short and squat. Creases may be visualized by supporting the infant's shoulders and raising them about 2 inches. In a short time the head will drop back to the table surface, exposing the creases.

Chest

A small amount of breast tissue (7 to 10 mm) is palpable in infants of both sexes. Breast engorgement, which subsides within 2 weeks, is a response to the presence of circulating maternal hormones. It requires no treatment and recedes naturally.

Respirations are abdominal; the breaths may be irregular and shallow, and the respiratory rate is about 30 to 60 breaths/min. Breath sounds are mainly bronchial or tracheobronchial. Occasionally, rales are noted and rhonchi are not unusual. Compare normal respiratory movement (Fig. 30-7) with abnormal movement (Fig. 30-8).

The maximal impulse of the heart should be felt just lateral to the midclavicular line in the third or fourth interspace (lower left sternal border). The pulse rate averages about 110 to 130/min and may be slightly irregular because of sinus arrhythmia. Systolic blood pressure is 60 to 100. Inconstant murmurs may be heard.

The clavicles are palpated to reveal fractures. Tenderness, crepitus at the fracture site, and limited movement of the arm are reported and treated (p. 518).

Abdomen

Generally, one can palpate the liver, the kidneys, and occasionally the spleen. A relaxed umbilical ring may be noted, especially in black babies, but true herniation is rare. The umbilical cord begins to dry soon after birth, detaches from the underlying skin by the fourth to fifth day, and falls off by the tenth to fifteenth day.

Genitals

In female infants the labia are relatively large and approximated. Slight mucoid discharge often may exude

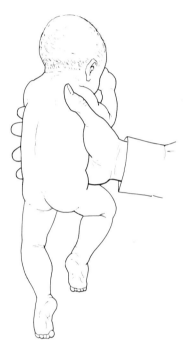

Fig. 30-9. Examining back. Infant's back should be slightly flexed, freely movable, and free of defects. Infant should kick both legs.

from the vaginal introitus. Occasionally blood-tinged vaginal discharge is seen. This persists over the first 2 weeks as a response to maternal hormones still present in the infant's circulation. Nearly all female infants have a fleshy pink tag protruding from the base of the vaginal opening. This is the *hymenal tag*, which gradually atrophies and usually disappears by the end of the fourth week.

In male infants the scrotum is pendulous with rugae completely covering the sac. Usually the testes can be felt in the scrotum. An adherent prepuce must be expected, and complete retraction of the foreskin can take up to 6 months. Wide variations in size of scrotum and penis are to be expected. The urethral meatus should be near the tip of the penis and easily visualized.

Anus

A patent anal canal and meconium should be apparent on insertion and removal of a gloved little finger, soft rubber catheter, or thermometer. Transient obstruction can result until the passage of a firm meconium plug.

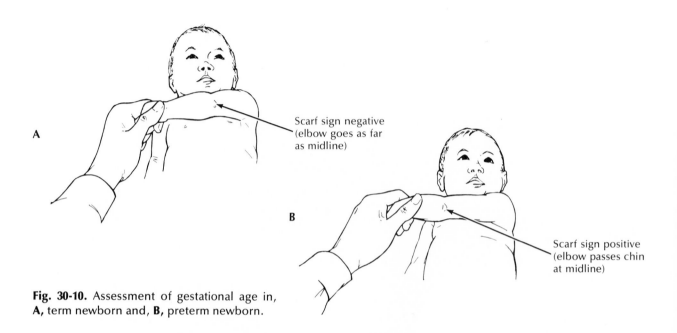

A

Scarf sign negative (elbow goes as far as midline)

B

Scarf sign positive (elbow passes chin at midline)

Fig. 30-10. Assessment of gestational age in, **A,** term newborn and, **B,** preterm newborn.

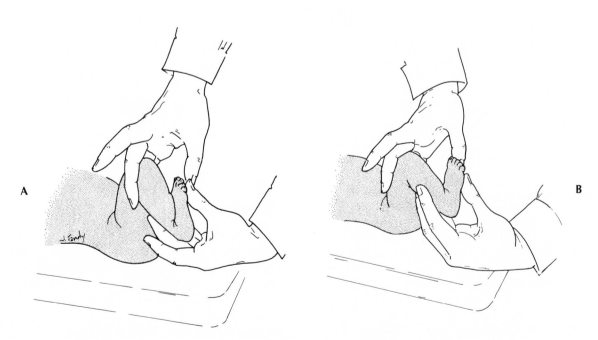

A

B

Fig. 30-11. Ankle dorsiflexion. **A,** 0-degree angle in term newborn. **B,** 90% or 20-degree angle in preterm newborn. (See Figs. 34-3 and 34-4, A and B.)

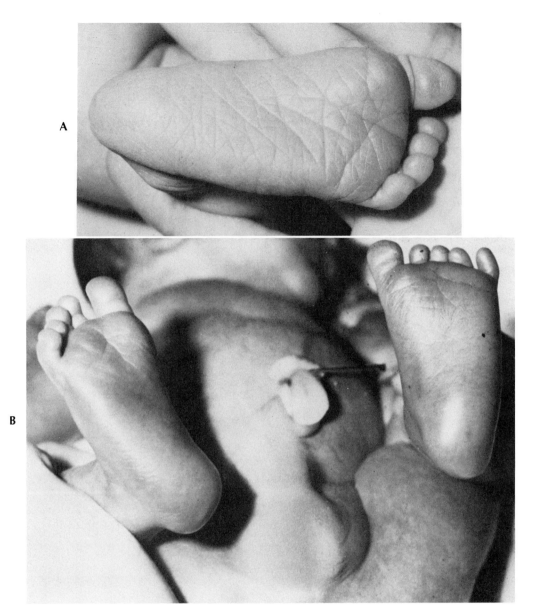

Fig. 30-12. A, Normal sole creases of full-term newborn. **B,** Sole of foot of premature infant. (See Fig. 34-4, *A.*)

Trunk and extremities

The back is examined for curvature (Fig. 30-9) and spinal defects and the base of the spine checked for dimples, tuft of hair, or an open sinus. This may be indicative of an occult spina bifida.

The arms and legs should be symmetric in shape and function. The difference in arm and ankle movements between term and premature infants is demonstrated in Figs. 30-10 and 30-11. These serve as two criteria for the estimate of gestational age (Chapter 34). The hands and feet are examined for webbing and extra or missing digits, and feet are examined for clubfoot and sole creases (Fig. 30-12). The hands are examined for palmar creases (Chapter 7). The hips are checked for dislocation by placing the hand so that the thumb is on the inner aspect of the infant's thigh and the fingers extend from the knee to the tip of the femur. The hips are pressed downward and abducted 90 degrees. The index finger palpates the movement of the joint, and a click may be felt if a dislocation is present (Ortalani's sign). The creases at the buttocks should be in the same line and the legs equal in length (Fig. 35-12).

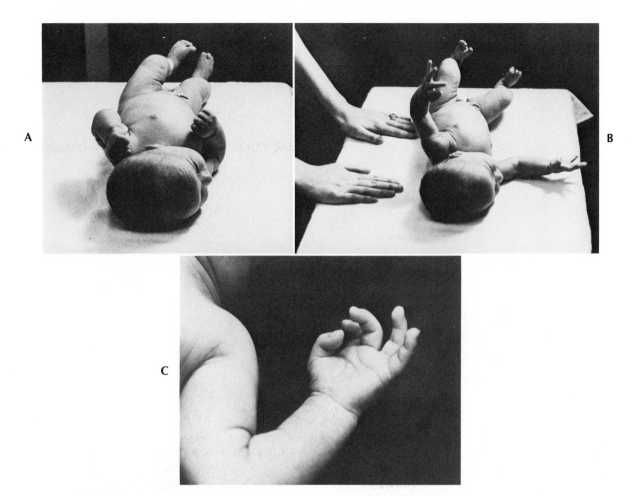

Fig. 30-13. A, Position of rest. **B,** Moro reflex consists predominately of abduction and extension of arms. **C,** Interesting subtlety of Moro response in newborn infants is C position of fingers: digits extend, except index finger and thumb, which are often semiflexed, forming shape of C. (Courtesy Mead Johnson Laboratories, Evansville, Ind.)

Activity

Neurologic reflexes. The neurologic examination screens CNS immaturity or damage. Severe impairment of reflexes can affect the infant's ability to exist in the extrauterine environment. Certain reflexes act to protect the infant such as blinking, sneezing, gagging, and withdrawal. Others are essential for the feeding process such as rooting, sucking, and swallowing. Others can be utilized in behavioral control processes at a later date, for example, the gastrocolic reflex can be used in toilet training. Still others act to promote social interactions; the infant grasping the mother's finger or hair usually elicits a warm response of the mother, a sense of the infant belonging to the parent. The startle reflex (Moro) may act to increase a new mother's anxiety as she interprets the startle as a negative response to her handling of the child.

The presence of other reflexes necessitates protective measures; for example, if the newborn is placed in the prone position, the crawling reflex is stimulated, which means that the neonate can "crawl" to the side or top of the crib. Therefore crib sides need to be covered to prevent the infant from pushing his head through the crib bars.

The neurologic examination can be tiring for the infant so it may be carried out in stages. All the reflexes described in the following discussion should be present.

Moro (startle) reflex (Fig. 30-13). The Moro reflex may be elicited in a number of ways: (1) hold the infant in both hands and lower both hands rapidly an inch so that a sensation of falling is experienced; (2) hold the infant's hands, lift his body and neck but not his head off the examining table, and quickly let go; or (3) lift the

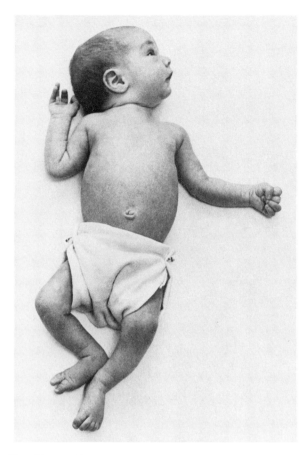

Fig. 30-14. Classic pose in spontaneous tonic neck reflex finds infant on his back with head turned to one side and arm and leg on same side extended. If baby's head is passively rotated in opposite direction, reversal of position of extremities may occur. (Courtesy Mead Johnson Laboratories, Evansville, Ind.)

head of the crib and inch and let it drop. Note the arms, the hands, and the cry. The arms abduct at the shoulders and extend at the elbow, and then the arms are abducted. The fingers spread or extend, forming the letter "C." The response should be immediate, bilateral, and symmetric. A vigorous cry follows the startle response.

Tonic neck reflex (fencing position) (Fig. 30-14). This is a spontaneous postural reflex in which the infant in the supine position turns the head to one side, extends that arm and leg, and flexes the arm and leg on the opposite side. It may not be seen during the first few days of life. Once present it persists until about the third month.

Grasping reflex (Fig. 30-15, *A*). If the palm of the hand is stimulated by touch, the fingers will close. The grasp should be strong enough by term so that the infant may be lifted from the table by holding onto the ex-

aminer's finger. Touching the sole of the foot elicits the same response. Note the difference in the grasp reflex in the premature and term neonate (Fig. 30-15, *B* and *C*).

Sucking reflex. This can be assessed by placing a clean finger in the infant's mouth and noting the vigor of the sucking and the amount of suction produced. (Mothers can test this reaction before beginning nursing. It helps waken the baby, and the strength of the response encourages them to begin with limited sucking time on each breast.)

Rooting reflex (Fig. 30-16). This reflex is well developed in the fetus, so its absence in the term infant is a cause for concern. It can be elicited by touching either corner of the mouth or the middle of the upper or lower lip. The infant opens his mouth and turns his head toward the stimulus. The reflex tends to disappear after sufficient food has been taken.

Swallowing and gagging. It is essential that these reflexes are present if the infant is to be fed by breast or bottle.

Sneezing. The infant will sneeze to clear the air passage. ("Blowing the nose" is a learned behavior.) Mothers unaware of this may think the baby has a cold.

Babinski (plantar) reflex. Stroking of the lateral plantar surface (not the ball of the foot) will cause the toes to flare open.

Deep tendon reflexes. The examiner can use a finger rather than a percussion hammer to elicit the patellar or knee jerk reflex. The infant must be relaxed, and even then a nonselective overall reaction can occur.

Cremasteric reflex. The testes retract when the skin is stroked on the front inner side of the thigh or if the infant is chilled.

Incurvature of trunk. If the infant is held in a prone position, stroking parallel to the spine causes the pelvis to turn to the stimulated side.

Righting reaction. If a term infant is held upright with his feet touching a surface, he will straighten first his legs, then his trunk, then his head.

Automatic walking (Fig. 30-17). If an infant is held upright over a firm surface and inclined forward, as the sole of one foot touches the surface, he will right himself with that leg and then flex the other. As the other foot touches the table, the reverse occurs. Term infants walk on the soles of their feet, and premature infants, on their toes.

Crawling in prone position. If the term infant is placed in the prone position, he will tuck his legs up under the abdomen and turn his head to one side. Note the difference in position of the premature and term infant as shown in Fig. 30-18. Thrusts with the legs will cause him to "creep" up to the top of the crib.

Hand-to-mouth movement. This random placing of the

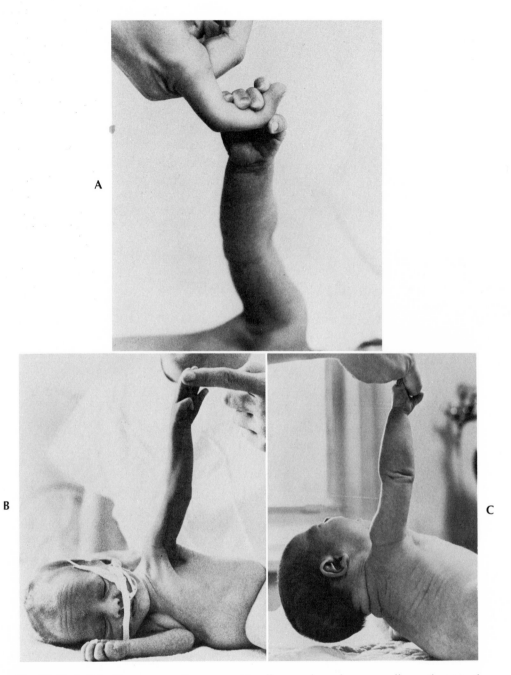

Fig. 30-15. A, Primitive grasp reflex present in all normal newborn usually weakens and disappears after 3 months. When palm is stimulated by finger, infant will grasp it. Full-term infant reinforces his grip as finger is drawn upward. Dorsum of hand should not be touched, since this excites opposite reflex, and hand opens. **B,** Grasp reflex, present in premature infant is distinct from that noted in term intant. Grip can be obtained and arm drawn upward, but when traction is applied, grip opens and there is much less muscle tension. **C,** Once grasp is obtained in term infant, grip is reinforced when his arm is drawn upward. There is progressive tensing of muscles until baby hangs momentarily. (**B** and **C** courtesy Mead Johnson Laboratories, Evansville, Ind.)

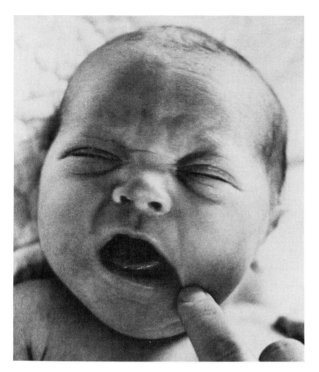

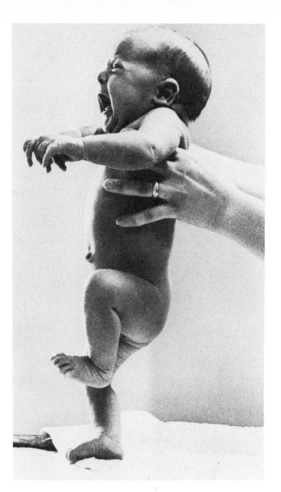

Fig. 30-16. Rooting reflex is apparent when corner of newborn infant's mouth is touched. Bottom lip lowers on same side; tongue moves toward stimulus. (Courtesy Mead Johnson Laboratories, Evansville, Ind.)

Fig. 30-17. Walking reflex is phase of neuromuscular maturity from which infant normally graduates after 3 or 4 weeks. If infant is held so that sole of his foot touches table, reciprocal flexion and extension of leg occur, simulating walking. (Courtesy Mead Johnson Laboratories, Evansville, Ind.)

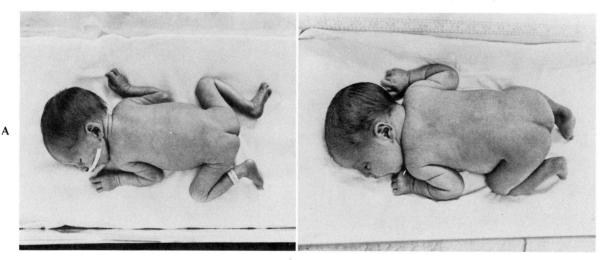

A

B

Fig. 30-18. A, In prone position, premature infant lies with pelvis flat and legs splayed out sideways like frog. **B,** Normal full-term infant lies with his limbs flexed, pelvis raised, and knees usually drawn under abdomen. (See Fig. 34-4, *A.*) (Courtesy Mead Johnson Laboratories, Evansville, Ind.)

hand to the mouth and sucking of fingers has been seen in utero. It is well developed at birth and is intensified with hunger.

Gastrocolic reflex. Distention of the stomach muscles causes a corresponding relaxation and contraction of muscles of the colon. As a result, infants often have bowel movements during or just after a feeding. This reflex has been noted but not tested.

Behavioral patterns. Brazelton (1973) and others* have brought the behavioral states of the neonate into prominence. It is their contention that the behavioral responses of infants are more indicative of their cortical control and responsiveness and eventual management of the infant environment than is the Apgar rating or the traditional reflex assessment (the reflexes may be found intact in anencephalic infants). They emphasize the importance of the infant-parent interaction. The infant through his responses acts to either consolidate relationships or alienate the persons in his immediate environment. By his actions he may encourage or discourage attachment and caretaking activities. The development of parent-child love does not occur without feedback; either the absence of feedback because of separation (p. 562) or incorrectly interpreted feedback can act to impair the growth of parental love.

One of the first tasks parents have to accomplish is to become aware of the unique behavioral responses of their child. This coupled with stimulation of the infant physically (holding, cuddling) and socially (talking to, smiling at) is necessary for the eventual growth and development of the child.

Feeding patterns. Variations among infants in interest in food, symptoms of hunger, and amount ingested at any one time are noticeable from birth. If put to breast, some infants nurse immediately, whereas others require a learning period of up to 48 hours before nursing can be said to be effective. The number of ounces taken at any one bottle-feeding depends, of course, on the size of the infant, but other factors also seem to play a part.

The mother reported her 6-day-old infant (5 pounds 13 ounces) had taken 3 ounces at 11 PM, 1½ ounces at 3 AM, 1 ounce at 6 PM, and now at the 10 AM feeding, "was sleepy and seemed to want only 1½ oz." The nurse suggested she keep track of the total amount taken over 24 hours. The mother interrupted to say, "I know what is wrong—yesterday all the relatives visited and held him. I think he's tired out." The nurse agreed that this could be so.

The next day the mother reported he was eating very well

*Students are encouraged to become proficient in the use of the Neonatal Behavioral Assessment Scale by Dr. T. B. Brazelton. See also "Newborn Assessment Tool" by Dr. Ann Clark in *Childbearing: A Nursing Perspective.*

and commented "I'm glad my instincts were right—it was just too busy a day for him."

Mothers need positive feedback to develop a feeling of confidence in their own ability. Often just listening and praising is the most effective intervention. Feeding is an emotionally charged area of infant care. Culturally, the size and growth of an infant is equated with excellence and evidence of mothering ability. The infant who is a fussy eater can serve to raise parental anxiety levels very high. The anxious parent appears to compound the problem, and a vicious cycle can develop. If relatives or friends can take over a feeding period or two, this seems to break the cycle so that the mother can view the feeding session in a more relaxed manner, not as a condemnation of her care.

Social patterns. Social patterns refer to the following infant behavior patterns:

1. *Crying.* Most mothers can describe the difference in their infants' cries as they experience hunger, pain, desire for attention, or fussiness.

I can tell when she's hungry. It starts in a plaintive way and then becomes more and more demanding. When she is hurt, she lets out a startled yell as though she couldn't believe it was happening to her. Sometimes when she is put down to sleep, she starts a kind of talking cry, jerky and demanding, and then it gets louder and if nothing happens, fades away in little spurts. The fussy cry is the hardest to take—nothing seems to work—such a complaining sound, it goes on and on.

A report such as this means that this mother and baby are communicating effectively.

2. *Smiling and vocalizing.* Even by the end of the first week of life, smiling is evident in a surprising number of infants. They seem to watch their parents faces carefully and respond to others talking to them; with body movements, including fleeting smiles, they seem to be reaching out to accept others. Some begin a type of cooing while feeding, even at 2 weeks.

Sleeping and waking behavior (Fig. 30-19). Desmond and associates (1966) noted that infants pass through phases of psychologic instability in the first 6 to 8 hours after birth, which they termed the *transitional period* between intrauterine and extrauterine existence. The first phase lasts up to 30 minutes after birth and is called the *first period of reactivity.* The *second period of reactivity* occurs at about the fourth to eighth hour. This sequence occurs in all neonates, regardless of gestational age or type of delivery, vaginal or cesarean section. There will be variations, however, in the length of time the periods last, depending on amount and kind of stress experienced by the fetus. Following are the clinical findings in the first period:

1. Infant is awake, alert, and active; his eyes are

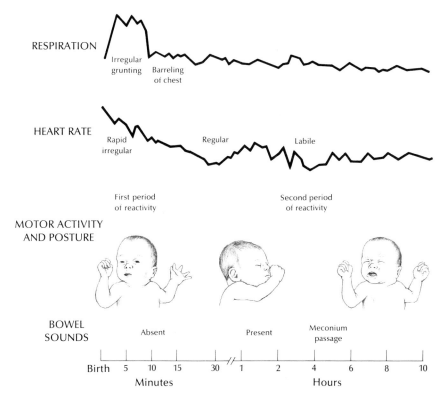

Fig. 30-19. Some physiologic changes occurring in neonate in his adjustment to extrauterine life. (From Pierog, S., and Ferrara, A. 1976. Medical care of the sick newborn [ed. 2]. St. Louis, The C. V. Mosby Co.; modified from Desmond, M. M.,
Rudolph, A. J., and Phitaksphraiwan, P. 1966. Pediatr. Clin. North Am. **13:**651.)

open, he looks around, and he may appear hungry, with
good sucking reflex.

2. Respirations are rapid and irregular; there may be
some grunting and barreling of chest.

3. Heart rate is rapid (tachycardia) with some irregularity.

4. Body temperature falls.

Then the infant's activity gradually diminishes, his
alertness fades, and sleep comes. Air enters the gastrointestinal tract and by about the end of the first hour
bowel sounds can be heard.

In the second period the infant again wakens and is
alert. There is usually a gagging episode with regurgitation of mucus and debris from the birth canal. The meconium stool is usually passed, and the infant again appears hungry and ready to suck.

Once these periods are completed, the infant stabilizes
with waking periods every 3 to 4 hours. For the first few
weeks these seem dictated by hunger, but soon thereafter
a need for socializing appears to function as well. In all,
the neonate sleeps about 17 hours a day, with the periods
of wakefulness gradually increasing. By the fourth week

of life some infants are staying awake from one feeding
session to the next.

Elimination patterns. The infant develops an elimination pattern by the second week of life. It appears to be
associated with the frequency (gastrocolic reflex) and
amount of feedings. The stools of breast-fed and bottle-
fed babies differ (pp. 499 and 507). The stress in this culture for daily bowel movements (regularity) makes most
mothers see this process as an indication of health and
therefore a judgment concerning the quality of the care
they have given. Addition of solid food changes the characteristics of the stool, and mothers need to be aware of
the change.

Urination increases from about three to four times in
the first few days to five to six times later in the first
week; voiding six to ten times a day is a good indicator
of adequate fluid intake (hydration) thereafter.

Weight (United States and Canada)

At 40 weeks, the normal infant's weight may range
between 5½ to 9½ pounds (2500 to 4300 gm); however, most weigh 7 to 7½ pounds (3200 to 3400 gm),

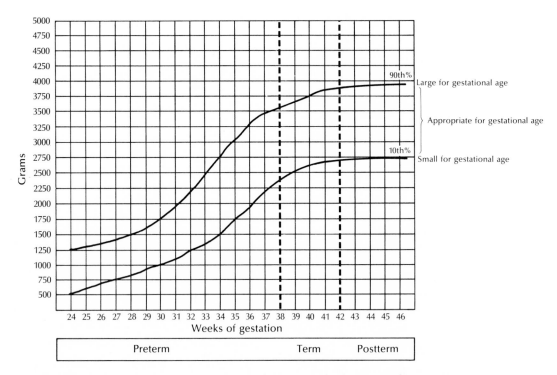

Fig. 30-20. Intrauterine growth status as determined by birth weight at various gestational ages.

the males slightly heavier than females. See Fig. 30-20 for variations in weights according to gestational age.

Length (United States and Canada)

The newborn will be approximately 51 cm in crown-heel length and 33.5 cm in crown-rump length. By 6 weeks length increases about 10%.

Laboratory data

Blood findings in the normal infant are as follows:

RBC: 4.1 to 7.5 million/mm³ (average 5.9 million).
Hgb: 14 to 24 gm (average 19 gm), of which one half to three fourths are fetal hemoglobin
WBC: 8000 to 38,000/mm³ (average 17,000)
  PMNs: 60%
  Lymphocytes: 20%
  Monocytes: 10%
  Immature white cells: 10%
Platelets: 350,000 mm³
Nucleated red cells: <500/mm³
Reticulocytes: 3%
Sedimentation rate: markedly accelerated
Hct: 54% ± 10 mm
MCV: 85 to 125 μ^3
MCHC: 36%
MCH: 35 to 40 $\mu\mu$g
Prothrombin, plasma thromboplastin component (factor IX),

proconvertin (factor VII), and Stuart factor (factor X): low
Proaccelerin (factor V): normal or slightly elevated

Urine findings in the normal infant are as follows:

Total protein: 6.1 mg/100 ml
Cholesterol: 50 to 100 mg/100 ml
PKU: negative finding (Chapter 7)

About 30 to 60 ml of urine with low specific gravity are normally voided the first day. Protein and acetone are often present. Occasionally casts, red cells, and white cells may be present. Uric acid crystals (a normal finding) are often the cause of pink urine. (See Appendix H.)

CHILD CARE ACTIVITIES

Included in the general care of infants are activities related to assessing the infant's condition, maintenance of respirations and temperature, hygiene, clothing and holding the infant, and care of the circumcision if performed. Much of the mother's knowledge concerning this care will stem directly from previous experience with infants, folkways indigenous to her ethnic or social group, and teaching of professionals during parentcraft classes. For the new parent with little skill in child care, these areas may occasion much anxiety. Support from the nursing staff in the mother's beginning efforts can be an important factor in her seeking and accepting help in the future.

Maintaining respirations and adequate oxygen supply

The first consideration is maintaining an open airway. The infant may be turned to the side and supported in this position with a rolled blanket at the back to facilitate drainage. If there is excessive mucus present, elevate the foot of the crib and aspirate the oral pharynx with a catheter and DeLee mucous trap. Administer oxygen by mask if the neonate shows excessive mottling or has cyanosis of the face. All mothers need instruction in the care of an infant having a gagging or choking episode: the infant is turned onto his stomach (prone) with the head lowered to permit drainage of mucus or milk. A bulb syringe may be used to aspirate the mouth and nose. Once the episode is resolved, the infant needs cuddling and reassuring.

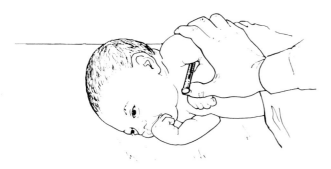

Fig. 30-21. Taking axillary temperature.

Determining infant's temperature

The temperature may be taken either by axilla or rectum every hour until stabilized (Figs. 30-21 and 30-22). For details regarding procedures see Chapter 37. The former is preferred because there is less danger of injuring the infant, but it takes at least 10 minutes to obtain a true reading. Initial temperatures as low as 36° C (96.8° F) are not uncommon. By the twelfth hour the temperatue should stabilize at 36.5° C (97.6° F). By the fourth week it is maintained at 36.5° to 37.3° C (97.6° to 99° F). Although it is not an exact method, the mother can determine if the baby is too warm or too cold by placing her hand on his abdomen. If it feels moderately warm to the touch, the infant may be considered to be comfortable.

Determining heart rate and rhythm

The apical beat is assessed for a full minute to assess rate and rhythm. The sounds should be clearly audible, 120 to 160 beats/min, and once the transition period is over, regular in rhythm. Functional murmurs are common for the first 48 hours.

Assessing growth

The infant is weighed daily while in the hospital and results recorded (Fig. 30-23). A total weight loss of more than 10% in the first 3 to 4 days indicates the need for clinical reappraisal. The head and chest circumference and body length are measured at birth and again in the fourth-week follow-up visit and compared with established norms.

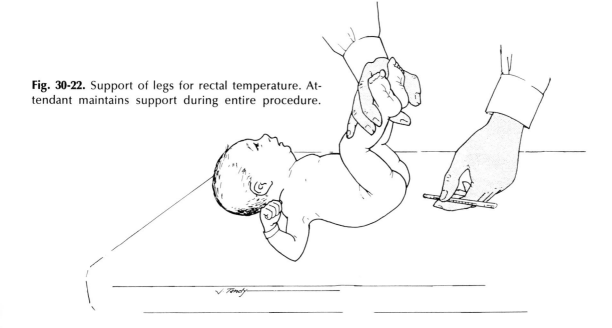

Fig. 30-22. Support of legs for rectal temperature. Attendant maintains support during entire procedure.

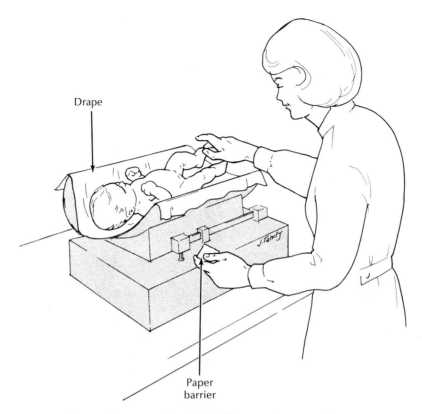

Drape

Paper barrier

Fig. 30-23. Weighing infant. Note hand is held over infant as safety measure. Scale is covered to provide warmth and protection against cross infection. Scale is adjusted to zero reading after cover is in place. Note nurse uses paper barrier as another precaution against cross infection.

Bathing the infant

Bathing serves a number of purposes. It provides opportunities for (1) a complete cleansing of the infant, (2) observing the infant's condition, (3) promoting comfort, and (4) parent-child-family socializing. The initial bath is postponed until the infant's temperature stabilizes at 36.5° C. Heat loss in the infant is disproportionate to the adult because of the relatively large skin surface to body mass. This loss is counteracted to some degree by the presence of "brown fat," unique to neonates, which has greater thermogenic activity than ordinary fat. The shivering mechanism of heat production is rarely operative in the neonate. The neonate increases heat production mostly by increasing metabolic activity. Heat loss occurs in four ways:

1. *Convection:* the flow of heat from the body surface to cooler ambient air
2. *Radiation:* the loss of heat from the body surface to cooler solid surfaces not in direct contact
3. *Evaporation:* the loss of heat that occurs when a liquid is converted to a vapor
4. *Conduction:* the loss of heat from the body surface to cooler surfaces in direct contact

Loss of heat in these ways must be controlled during the bath period to conserve the infant's energy. The ambient temperature of the room should be 22.2° C (72° F) and the bathing area free of drafts. Bathing quickly, exposing only a portion of the body at a time, and thorough drying are therefore part of the bathing technique. After the initial bath, a daily bath may be given at any time convenient to the parents but not immediately following a feeding period, since the increased handling may cause regurgitation of the feeding. In some hospitals the infant is given an initial bath, and then cleansing the genitals as necessary is deemed sufficient for the first 3 to 4 days.

CLEANSING THE INFANT

The fragility of the infant's *skin* lessens its effectiveness as a barrier to infectious agents as well as to the absorption of chemical substances applied to the skin. Gentle cleansing of skin surfaces and use of a mild soap without perfume or coloring are recommended.

If amnionitis complicated the intranatal period or if skin infections have occurred recently in the nursery, the newborn may be bathed with dilute pHisoHex (less than 3%), followed by thorough rinsing of the skin. This detergent is a potential neurotoxin, particularly for infants who weigh less than 2000 gm, and its use has been restricted in many areas.

If stool or other debris has caked and dried on the skin, soak to remove it. Do not attempt to rub it off because debridement may result. *Creases* under the chin and arms and in the groin need daily cleansing. Vernix may be left on for 48 hours; if it persists beyond that time, it may be washed off. The crease under the chin may be exposed by elevating the infant's shoulders 2 inches and letting the head drop back. The *scalp* is washed daily with water and a mild soap. The scalp must be rinsed well. Scalp desquamation, called *cradle cap,* can often be prevented by removing any scales with a fine-toothed comb or brush after washing. If the condition persists, the physician may order an ointment to massage into the skin.

Cleanse the *eyes* from the inner canthus outward, using a clean washcloth. A discharge may be noted for the first 2 to 3 days, resulting from the reaction of the conjunctiva to the silver nitrate used as a prophylactic measure against gonorrheal infection. Once the eyes have recovered from this irritation, any discharge should be considered abnormal and reported to the physician.

Avoid contamination of one eye with the discharge from the other by using a separate cotton swab and water source for each eye.

Cleanse the *ears* and *nose* with twists made of moistened cotton.

The *fingernails* and *toenails* can be cut more readily with manicure scissors when the infant is asleep. Hold the skin back from the nail and cut straight across. The nails are kept short; otherwise they can be snagged by clothing, and the infant can scratch himself during normal random hand and leg movements. Wash and dry between the fingers and toes daily.

The *genitals* of both male and female infants need daily cleansing at least. For uncircumcised males, the foreskin is retracted gently. If adhesions are present, complete retraction may take 1 to 2 weeks and in some instances up to 6 months. Do not use force. Cleanse glans with soap and water to remove smegma and always replace the foreskin.

For the female, daily cleansing of the genitals may be done by separating the labia and washing from the pubic area to the anus.

CIRCUMCISION

Circumcision (Figs. 30-24 to 30-26) is a minor surgical operation in which the congenitally adherent prepuce of the penis is separated from the glans and a part of the prepuce is excised to permit retraction of the foreskin or to completely expose the glans for better male hygiene. This operation, long a rite in many early cultures and a ritual in the Jewish religion, is recommended by many physicians, principally because the procedure improves the individual's cleanliness and comfort. Moreover, the incidence of cancer of the penis is much lower in circumcised men, and the frequency of cervical cancer may be lower in the wives of men who have been circumcised. Others claim that the operation is unnecessary because continued retraction of the foreskin from birth

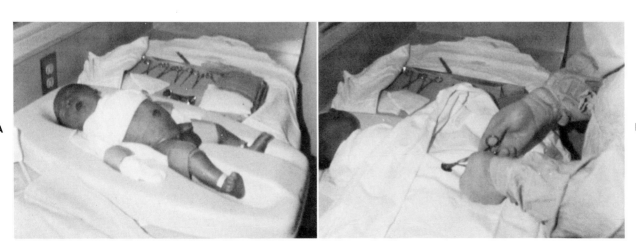

A

B

Fig. 30-24. A, Proper positioning of infant in Circumstraint. **B,** Physician performing circumcision.

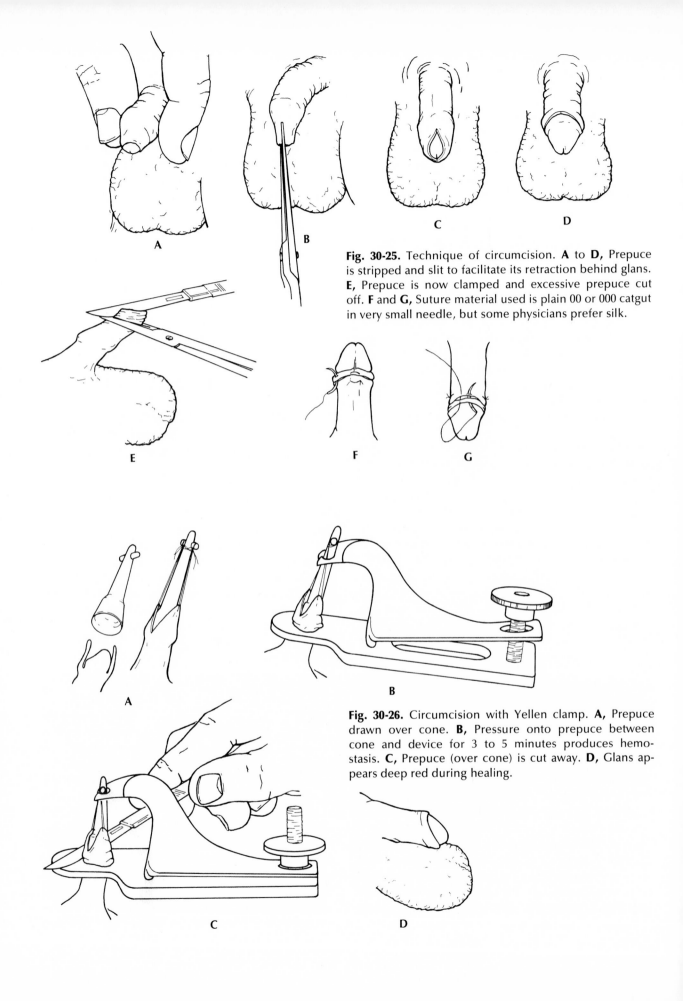

Fig. 30-25. Technique of circumcision. **A** to **D,** Prepuce is stripped and slit to facilitate its retraction behind glans. **E,** Prepuce is now clamped and excessive prepuce cut off. **F** and **G,** Suture material used is plain 00 or 000 catgut in very small needle, but some physicians prefer silk.

Fig. 30-26. Circumcision with Yellen clamp. **A,** Prepuce drawn over cone. **B,** Pressure onto prepuce between cone and device for 3 to 5 minutes produces hemostasis. **C,** Prepuce (over cone) is cut away. **D,** Glans appears deep red during healing.

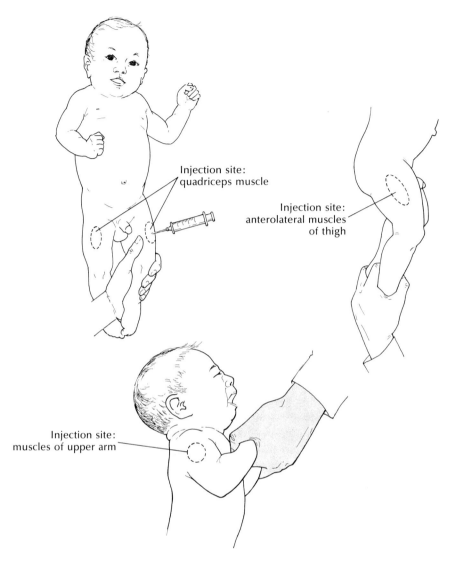

Injection site:
quadriceps muscle

Injection site:
anterolateral muscles
of thigh

Injection site:
muscles of upper arm

Fig. 30-27. Injection sites for infant. (Courtesy Ross Laboratories, Columbus, Ohio.)

should facilitate cleansing of the glans, and removal of the foreskin may dull sexual satisfaction.

The operation is performed in the hospital prior to the baby being discharged with the mother. Vitamin K (Aquamephyton) is administered intramuscularly (Fig. 30-27) to minimize the effect of the normal drop in the clotting factors after birth. Since these factors return to prebirth levels by the end of the first week, performing a circumcision then would have a firmer physiologic basis (Jewish ritual performed on the eighth day). The procedure is no longer done immediately after birth because the amount of cold stress has proved detrimental to the infant.

For this procedure, the infant is positioned on a plastic restraint form so that his movements are restricted. The penis is cleansed with soap and water. The infant is draped to provide warmth and a sterile area. The sterile equipment is readied for use (Fig. 30-24).

Numerous instruments have been devised for circumcision (Fig. 30-28). The Yellen clamp, for instance, may make this an almost bloodless operation (Fig. 30-26). Once the operation is completed, a small petrolatum gauze dressing may be applied for the first day to prevent adherence of the diaper. The infant is then comforted, dressed, and returned to his crib. These infants are usually "fussy" for about 2 to 3 hours and may refuse a

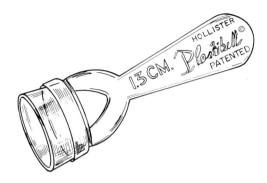

Fig. 30-28. Plastibell is device used by some hospitals for circumcision. Plastic bell remains in place over glans until healing occurs when bell falls off. (From Lerch, C. 1974. Maternity nursing [ed. 2]. St. Louis, The C. V. Mosby Co.)

feeding. Complications include undesirable primary or secondary bleeding, infection, or distortion of the penis by scar tissue.

The penis must be checked hourly for bleeding for 12 hours. By the second day, a yellowish white exudate may cover the glans as part of the healing process. This is not clinically significant because it is not an infective process. The penis may be washed gently and patted dry. No attempt is made to remove the exudate, which persists for 2 to 3 days. The incised area at the base of the glans remains tender for 2 to 3 days, so the diaper must be pinned loosely.

OBSERVATIONS

Color of the skin. Development of *jaundice* before 48 hours may be indicative of a blood dyscrasia and requires immediate medical investigation (p. 592). Jaundice may be expected to occur between 48 and 72 hours as a consequence of the normal physiologic breakdown of fetal red blood cells and relative immaturity of the liver. Rarely does the circulating bilirubin derived from this source reach levels that result in the infant developing kernicterus (pp. 593 and 598). Infants who are SGA, have received an extra infusion of blood from the placenta, or have an inadequate fluid intake may be particularly susceptible.

Cyanosis of hands and feet (acrocyanosis, or "mitten and bootie" cyanosis) is not pathologic and is replaced by normal skin coloring by days 7 to 10. Circumoral pallor and cyanosis may be noticeable during crying or feeding. Report this finding to the physician. It may be indicative of cardiopulmonary pathology, generalized infection, or hypoglycemia. Report to the physician if

the infant appears pale (anemia) or ruddy (polycythemia).

Evidence of adequate hydration. Lack of skin turgor is not a symptom of dehydration until the prebirth accumulation of fluid is lost by the third to fourth day. Subsequent to that, dehydration may be assessed by examining the skin of the abdomen or inner thighs. Depression of the fontanel and softness of the eyeball are the most reliable indicators of dehydration.

Evidence of increased intracranial pressure. Bulging of the fontanel when the infant is at rest may indicate increased intracranial pressure and is reported to the physician.

Bulging of the fontanel also occurs normally when the infant cries or strains at stool because intracranial pressure is increased at these times.

Bruises or other evidence of trauma. A *bruise on the cheek* can result from forceps pressure. Note whether forceps were applied during delivery. Two small puncture wounds on the scalp may be from the electrode attached to the scalp for fetal monitoring during labor or the site where a specimen of blood was taken from the scalp. *Bruises of the scalp* and petechiae on the face are sometimes found on infants who have sustained great and prolonged pressure during passage through the birth canal or when the umbilical cord had been tightly wound around their necks before birth.

Petechiae on the trunk and lower extremities are abnormal and are reported.

Bruising and swelling of the genitals and buttocks are common findings in those infants born in breech presentation. All these may be expected to subside by the end of the first week.

Rashes. A rash over the genitals and buttocks may appear by the second day of life. Meconium is not irritating to the skin because of its composition, but the transitional and later stool of bottle-fed infants and urine of all infants are irritating although the latter is sterile. Cleansing with water is indicated with each diaper change. Diaper rash can vary from mild to severe. The mild form resembles chafing, with reddened, nonraised areas, and exposure to air and frequent changing of diapers usually will clear the condition. A more severe type called *ammoniacal diaper rash* is characterized by bright red papules that erupt and keep forming craterlike ulcers. This requires exposure to heat as well as air, forcing fluid to dilute the urine, and immediate change of diaper after voiding or defecating. The most severe type occurs when the area becomes infected, indurated, and tender. Medical advice should be sought and a specifically ordered medication applied. A rash on the face may result from the infant scratching himself or excoriation caused by rubbing his face against the sheets, particularly if regurgitated stomach contents are not washed off.

Mouth. The inside of the mouth can be inspected when the infant is crying. If white curdy deposits are noted, give the infant some water to drink and see whether the white plaques are washed away. If they are not, do not attempt to remove them; notify the physician, since the infant may have developed thrush (candidiasis) (p. 607). Sucking calluses may eventually form on the lips. These are not injurious and need no treatment. Note the shape of the infant's mouth when crying. If it drags to one side, it may indicate facial paralysis and should be reported to the physician. The infant's tongue appears large in comparison with his mouth. Its growth is forward from the base, the frenulum. Tongue-tie (the inability to lift the tip of the tongue because of a too short frenulum) is a rare condition.

CLOTHING THE INFANT

A shirt and diaper are sufficient clothing for the young infant indoors. A bonnet to protect the scalp and minimize heat loss and to shade the eyes can be added when taking the infant outside in summer. Wrapping the infant snugly in a blanket serves to maintain body temperature and to give a feeling of security. Overdressing in warm temperatures can cause discomfort and prickly heat; underdressing in cold temperatures can also cause discomfort. Cheeks, fingers, and toes can readily become frostbitten.

When dressing the child, avoid pulling shirts roughly over the face and catching fingers in shirt sleeves. Form a mask with the fingers over the baby's face as the shirt is pulled on or off. Diapering the infant may be done prior to and after feeding (Fig. 30-29). It is not necessary to wake the infant for changing, since the above routine means about twelve changes a day. To increase absorbency the bulk of the diaper can be brought to the front area for males and to the back for females. This will help absorb urine so that the skin surface is protected. The diaper between the infant's legs should not be bulky, since it can cause outward displacement of the hips. A soaker pad can be placed under the infant as a protection for the wrapping blanket. The continued use of rubber or plastic pants may lead to diaper rash.

Care of the infant's clothes and bedding is directed toward minimizing cross infection and removing residues from soap, feces, or urine that may irritate the infant's skin. In the hospital, it is washed separately from other linen and is autoclaved. At home, it should be washed separately, with a mild detergent or soap and hot water. A double rinse usually removes traces of the cleansing agent or acid residue from the urine or stool. If possible, dry the clothing and bedding in the sun to neutralize residues.

Bedding requires frequent changing. The plastic-coated firm mattress must be washed daily and the crib or bassinet damp dusted. A pillowcase makes an efficient bottom sheet for a bassinet.

The infant's toilet articles may be kept separate and convenient for use in a box or basket.

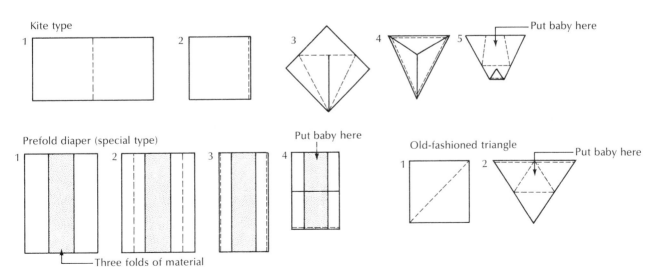

Fig. 30-29. Diapering infant. Dotted lines indicate folds. For kite type, start with large, regular diaper if single thickness is thin.

POSITIONING AND HOLDING THE INFANT

Positioning the infant in the crib on his side permits drainage of mucus from the mouth and applies no pressure to the cord or to the sensitive circumcised penis. Anatomically, the infant's shape—barrel chest, flat spine, and Moro reflex—makes rolling over a simple procedure. A rolled blanket against the spine will prevent his rolling to the prone position and adds a feeling of security. Care must be taken to prevent him from rolling from flat unguarded surfaces. He must never be left alone on the bath table. If the attendant has to leave, either the infant should be taken along or put back into the crib. If left on the parent's bed, he should be "walled in" with pillows to prevent his rolling off. Changing the position from side to side may be done after the feeding period to assist in developing even contours of the head as well as easing pressure on other parts of the body.

An infant must be held securely with support for the head, since the infant is unable to maintain erect head posture for more than a few moments; if the head jerks, a whiplash injury can result. Figs. 30-30 to 30-32 illustrate various positions for holding an infant with adequate support. Too much stimulation or roughhousing should be avoided after feeding and before a sleep period. After feeding, positioning the infant on his right side or prone promotes gastric emptying.

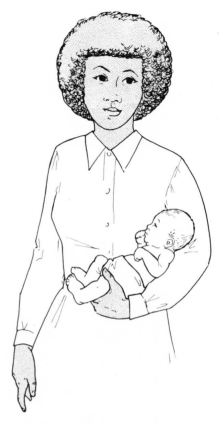

Fig. 30-31. Cradle hold.

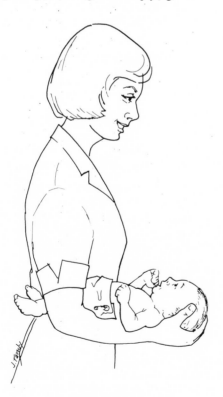

Fig. 30-30. Football hold

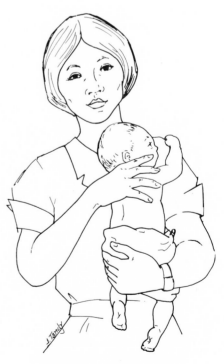

Fig. 30-32. Upright position.

PLAN OF CARE: NORMAL NEWBORN—GENERAL CARE—FIRST DAY OF LIFE

PATIENT CARE OBJECTIVES

Physiologic adjustment to extrauterine existence

1. Respirations: Airway is open and respirations stabilized at forty to sixty breaths/min with short periods of apnea. Breathing is quiet (no grunting or wheezing). The chest and abdomen rise and fall in synchronized motion, and there is no sternal retraction. The infant breathes through the nose; the nares do not flare on inspiration. Color is consistent with basic skin tone. Cyanosis may be present in hands and feet.
2. Temperature: Body temperature is stabilized by the twelfth hour and maintained between 36.5° and 37.2° C (97.6° to 98.9° F).
3. Heart rate and regularity in rhythm is stabilized between 120 and 160 by the twelfth hour; it may drop to 100 in deep sleep but returns immediately with activity. The heart rate increases with stress or activity. Heart murmurs are normal for 48 hours.
4. Acceptance and swallowing of nutrients and fluids by the twelfth hour. Amount of regurgitation of mucus and/or nutrients and fluids is within normal limits by the twenty-fourth hour.
5a. There is adequate healing of cord, that is, no oozing of blood and no evidence of inflammation.
  b. There is adequate healing of circumcised penis if a circumcision was performed, that is, no excessive bleeding and no evidence of inflammation.
6. Defecation: Meconium stool may be passed at birth or any time thereafter until the twenty-fourth hour.
7. Urination: Some infants void at birth; most void between the twelfth and twenty-fourth hours after birth.
8. Appearance and activity (reflexes and behavior patterns) are within normal limits.

Caretaking activities

1. A plan of care is instituted that
   (a) requires skilled personnel and adequate facilities to ensure continuous assessment, protection against infection or trauma, and care in case of emergency
   (b) reflects consideration of the needs of a particular infant with a unique history, constitution, and membership in a particular family group
   (c) includes complete medical and nursing records
2. Assessment of the infant by twenty-fourth hour by professional personnel reveals satisfactory adjustment of the infant and his physical status.
3. Nutrition: Initial feeding of infant is done by the sixth hour. Mother begins feeding process (Chapter 31).
4. Hygiene: Initial bath is given once the infant's temperature is stabilized and routine of hygienic care is established.

Parenthood

1. Initial and subsequent contacts between parents and infant promotes close parent-child-family ties (Chapter 29).

NURSING INTERVENTIONS

Diagnostic	Therapeutic	Educational

1. Respirations:
a. Check respiratory effort every 15 minutes for 4 hours, then every hour until stable. Record findings every hour.
  (1) Count respirations by observing chest wall. Note if sternum retracts or nares flare and chin lags on inspiration (Fig. 33-7).
  (2) Note if infant is normal nose breather (i.e., sleeps with mouth closed, does not have to interrupt feedings to breathe).
  (3) Note abnormal sounds—grunting, wheezing—during inspiration or expiration.
  (4) Note efficiency of gagging, sneezing, swallowing reflexes related to maintaining clear airway.
	1. Placement:
	a. Infant is transferred from labor unit to transitional nursery. Infant's identification is checked. Nursery personnel are alerted to data of immediate significance to care, such as following:
	  (1) Gestational history (e.g., age of mother, any social problems, EDC, and any physical problems).
	  (2) Labor and birth experience (e.g., labor lengthy and difficult, maternal medications and/or anesthesia, cord around neck, type of delivery, Apgar score).
	  (3) Care at birth (e.g., prophylaxis to eyes completed).
	  (4) General condition and activity (e.g., alert, respirations
		1. Mother's responses are noted while she examines and holds infant, and assessment of mother's knowledge of and skill in infant care is made.
		2. Demonstration and supervised practice of care that is required if infant chokes or regurgitates at feeding time; demonstration given while nurse is present at first feeding.
		3. Information is given as to infant's progress (sleeping, waking, crying, feeding, urination, defecating, weight) and normalcy of infant's characteristics, including cord, genitals, and appearance of stool.

Continued.

PLAN OF CARE: NORMAL NEWBORN—GENERAL CARE—FIRST DAY OF LIFE—cont'd

NURSING INTERVENTIONS—cont'd

Diagnostic	Therapeutic	Educational

Diagnostic

b. Be alert for bouts of rapid and irregular respirations, gagging, and regurgitation of mucus, etc., during "reactivity" periods.
  (1) Following birth.
  (2) After 4 to 6 hours of life.
c. Color: Color over head and trunk and mucous membrane is indicative of adequate oxygenation. Feet and hands remain cyanotic for 48 hours.
2. Temperature: Take and record temperature on admission to unit, then every hour until stabilized. After that, take temperature every 4 hours for remainder of first 24 hours by one of following methods:
  a. Rectal temperature (at least once to establish patency of anus).
  b. Axillary temperature.
  c. Skin temperature by sensor.
3. Cardiovascular system: Heart rate checked every 4 hours. Note regularity and presence of heart murmurs.
4. Cord and circumcised penis:
  a. Check every 30 minutes for 4 hours for excessive bleeding.
  b. Healing process: By 24 hours cord appears dry (becomes black and stiff like twig) with no bleeding or signs of inflammation (odor, discharge, reddened skin at base), and clamp or cord tie may be removed. Incised area of penis should appear clean with no odor or discharge.
5. Defecation:
  a. Note evidence of passage of meconium (vernix stained yellow, report of meconium-stained amniotic fluid, or passage of meconium at birth) prior to admission to nursery.
  b. Record passage of meconium; may be anticipated by 4 to 6 hours or at beginning of waking periods and after feedings (gastrocolic reflex). Patency of lower gastrointestinal tract can then be assumed.
  c. If there is delay in passage of meconium (24 hours or more), check for patency of anus, abdominal distention, bowel sounds; assess amount of fluid

Therapeutic

normal, has voided, number of vessels in cord).
b. Infant is placed in area where constant surveillance, external heat sources, and emergency care are available. Ambient temperature of nursery unit should be maintained at 22° C (70° to 72° F). Crib and area for bathing, changing, and examining should be away from windows and drafts.
c. Infant transferred to normal newborn nursery when respirations are stable, behavior and temperature are normal, and acceptance and swallowing of water are satisfactory (usually 6 to 10 hours).
d. Infant may be transferred to rooming-in unit or home when regurgitation episodes are controlled and passage of meconium stools and urine are noted and recorded (usually by 24 hours).
2. Respirations:
  a. Carry out procedures for clearing airway of mucus as needed.
    (1) Position infant on side to facilitate drainage from mouth.
    (2) Hold infant in prone position with head slightly lowered and aspirate mouth and nose using bulb syringe.
    (3) Clear airway of mucus using DeLee trap or nasal suction apparatus.
    (4) If mucous regurgitation is excessive, empty stomach using DeLee trap.
    (5) After bout of gagging, etc., comfort infant.
  b. If abnormal symptoms occur, further intervention is indicated (pp. 531 to 536).
3. Temperature:
  a. Stabilization.
    (1) Wipe infant free of blood and excessive vernix, dress in shirt and diaper, wrap snugly in blanket, position on side in bassinet, cover with light blanket, and then place under heat lamp until

---

PLAN OF CARE: NORMAL NEWBORN—GENERAL CARE—FIRST DAY OF LIFE—cont'd

NURSING INTERVENTIONS—cont'd

Diagnostic	Therapeutic	Educational

intake, and notify physician of findings. Some healthy infants do not defecate for 48 hours (Kempe and others, 1976).

6. Urination:
   a. Note evidence of voiding before admission to nursery (report of voiding at birth or diaper wet).
   b. Record voiding when noted (some infants void as part of delivery process; most void by 12 hours; rarely, some may not void for 2 to 3 days, depending on amount of fluid in bladder at birth and fluid intake (Kempe and others, 1976).
   c. After 24 hours, if infant has not voided, check bladder for distention and note if infant is restless or appears in pain as pressure is applied to bladder; assess fluid intake, and notify physician of findings. Physician may aspirate bladder to ascertain if urine is present. Position infant as for circumcision. Suprapubic area is exposed and cleansed. Physician will require sterile gloves, syringe (30 ml), and long needle.
   d. Note presence of (1) urates, which appear as pink (copper dust) staining on diaper that dissolves and disappears when diaper is placed in water and are not significant, and (2) blood, which does not disappear when diaper is soaked in water. Blood may result from pseudomenstruation in female, bleeding from circumcision, or too forceful retraction of foreskin in male. If not from these sources, report to physician.

7. Physical assessment (p. 451):
   a. By physician or nursing practitioner before twenty-fourth hour of life.
   b. By nursery personnel during caretaking activities.

8. Nutrition (Chapter 31).

9. Parenthood (Chapter 29).

temperature is stabilized. Check body temperature every hour to prevent hyperthermia.

   (2) Or infant may be placed thoroughly dried under radiant heat panel without clothing until temperature has stabilized. Check body temperature every hour to prevent hyperthermia. Then bathe and, if temperature drops, place under heat panel until temperature is stabilized.

   b. Minimize loss of heat by doing examinations under heat panel and postpone initial bath until temperature reaches 36.5° C (98° F).

4. Cardiovascular system: Avoid stress through provision of warmth, fluids, nutrients, and comforting as needed, and protect from infection and trauma.

5. Cord and circumcised penis: Cutting cord and circumcising infant are surgical procedures and necessitate institution of routine measures related to postsurgical care.

   a. Administer prescribed dosage of Vitamin K_1 preparation intramuscularly (Aquamephyton) (Fig. 30-27).

   b. Control of excessive bleeding: Apply gentle pressure using folded 4 × 4 gauze as pad to site of bleeding.
      (1) From cord: Check clamp or tie and double clamp if necessary.
      (2) From penis: If bleeding is not controlled, vessel may need to be ligated. Notify physician and prepare equipment (circumcision tray and suture). Maintain pressure intermittently until physician arrives.

   c. Prevention of infection:
      (1) Cord: Cleanse around cord with prescribed preparation (e.g., alcohol); put on diaper so that umbilicus is exposed to air. Notify physician of odor or discharge, and if

Continued.

PLAN OF CARE: NORMAL NEWBORN—GENERAL CARE—FIRST DAY OF LIFE—cont'd

NURSING INTERVENTIONS—cont'd

Diagnostic	Therapeutic	Educational
	skin area around cord becomes inflamed.	

     (2) Circumcised penis: Wash penis gently with water to remove urine or feces. Glans may appear red and sore, and within 24 hours yellowish exudate forms. This is normal healing, not an infective process. If the Plastibell apparatus (Fig. 30-28) is used, the plastic bell covering the circumcised penis prevents hemorrhage, infection, and trauma. When the incision has healed, the plastic bell falls off.

  d. Alleviation of discomfort:

     (1) Cord contains no nerve endings for pain, so incision is painless. However, bulk of clamp or dryness of cord may act as irritant if pressure is present. Avoid pressure with diaper (or belly band if mother insists on its use), and position infant on side to sleep.

     (2) Circumcision incision (at base of glans) may be painful; apply diaper loosely and position infant on side to sleep.

6. Hygiene:

  a. Initial sponge bath given when temperature stabilizes.

  b. Soiled diapers are changed before and after feedings; infant is not wakened from sleep to change diaper. First stool, meconium, is nonirritating to skin. However, it adheres to skin as it dries, and efforts to remove it may irritate skin surface. Soak off with sufficient water; do not rub.

7. Weighing: Infant is weighed (in hospital) once a day at routine time. Mother is kept aware of changes in weight.

8. Initial feeding (Chapter 31).

9. Close observation of infant is necessary at all times, particularly when giving care. Findings are recorded promptly, and significant deviations are reported immediately, so additional care can be instituted.

PLAN OF CARE: NORMAL NEWBORN—DAYS 2 TO 14

PATIENT CARE OBJECTIVES
Physiologic responses
1. Respirations are stabilized within normal limits (30 to 60/min). Mother is aware of normal variations in breathing rhythm and rate. Mother is able to keep the infant's airway clear by positioning the infant in bassinet or crib on side to facilitate drainage; or if choking occurs, by turning the infant onto his abdomen with his head down and removing mucus with bulb syringe.
2. Temperature: Body temperature is maintained within normal limits. Mother becomes adept at using a thermometer and is aware of the influence of heat, cold, and dehydration on infant's temperature.
3. a. Healing of cord continues; cord drops off between 4 and 15 days after birth. There is no evidence of inflammation.
   b. Healing of the circumcised penis continues. Yellowish exudate forms over glans; the incised site remains tender for 2 to 3 days.
4. Defecation: Number of stools varies on the basis of type of feeding, breast or bottle. Stools go through a transitional process from meconium, to greenish yellow curdy stool, to a yellow, more formed stool if bottle-feeding, or remain golden yellow and loose if breast-feeding.
5. Urination: The infant voids six to ten times in 24 hours; urine is pale and straw colored.
6. Birth weight regained by end of second week.
7. Appearance and behavior.
   a. Molding of the head lessens and head assumes more rounded contours by the second or third day.
   b. Icterus neonatorum begins 48 hours or later after birth (in ±50%), reaches a peak on the fourth or fifth day, and then subsides.
   c. Melanin in skin responds to light, and color tone changes from ruddy tones at birth to black, yellow, brown, or pink, depending on amount of melanin present.
   d. Rashes are of transitory nature; skin may appear dry and peel, especially in skin folds.
   e. Activity: Infant sleeps about 17 hours a day. Muscle tone is good; infant wakens for feedings and is alert and responsive. Cry is lusty, sustained, and demanding in tone. Smiles; moves arms and legs in response to human voice.

Caretaking activities
1. Sources of readily available emergency care are known to parents.
2. Protection is continued against infection and trauma.
3. Nutrition: The intake of nutrients and fluids is adequate for growth and hydration (Chapter 31).
4. Hygiene.
   a. Hygienic care and examination of the infant is practiced as a daily routine. Mother is aware of normal characteristics and responses of infant.
   b. Mother practices safe techniques for bathing and changing infant, including care of scalp, eyes, nose, mouth, cord, nails, body creases, buttocks, and genitals.
   c. Mother is knowledgeable about dressing the infant and care of infant's clothing.
   d. Mother is aware of measures used to control discomforts; diaper rash, prickly heat rash, etc.
5. Regular evaluation of the degree to which the desired outcomes have been attained and the tasks still to be accomplished is carried out.

Parenthood
1. Parents become increasingly:
   a. Aware of infant's behavior as "cues" for type of care needed (food, fluids, easing of discomfort, reassurance, cuddling, exercise, changing, social contacts).
   b. Adept at caretaking activities.
   c. Knowledgeable as to "normal" versus "abnormal" responses of infant and where and how to seek assistance for infant problems and parenthood concerns.

NURSING INTERVENTIONS

Diagnostic	Therapeutic	Educational
1. Respiration: Observe respirations and record every 8 hours while in hospital.	1. Respirations: Maintain open airway.	1. Discuss normal growth and development of infant and his changing needs for exercise and social contacts.
2. Temperature: a. Take and record temperature every 8 hours while in hospital.	2. Temperature: a. Dress infant in clothing suitable to maintain warmth in varying ambient temperatures.	2. Demonstrate and supervise practice in bathing and cleaning, chang-

Continued.

PLAN OF CARE: NORMAL NEWBORN—DAYS 2 TO 14—cont'd

NURSING INTERVENTIONS—cont'd

Diagnostic	Therapeutic	Educational

Diagnostic

b. Take temperature if fever is suspected, but as temperature is not reliable indicator of infection, since infant may be septic with reduced temperature, check other signs and symtoms.

3. Serum PKU test is done 48 hours after ingestion of protein (milk or breast milk). (See Chapter 7 and p. 632.)

4. Tests for bilirubin levels are done if jaundice is severe (usually third day) and repeated as needed.

5. While infant is in hospital, note and record changes in stool color and consistency and pattern infant establishes (e.g., four times every day or every 2 days) for defecation.

6. Note and record color and concentration of urine and number of voidings while infant is in hospital.

7. Note changes in skin (color and rashes).

8. Note healing of circumcised penis and cord. When cord drops off, small beads of blood may appear for 1 to 2 days when infant cries or strains at stool. The navel may be protuberant.

9. Weigh daily while in hospital; weigh at end of second week.

Therapeutic

b. If temperature is elevated, rule out inanition (dehydration) fever or overheating, give up to 4 ounces sterile water, remove some of infant's coverings. Recheck temperature in 1 hour. If elevated temperature persists, institute further interventions (p. 530).

3. Bathing:
   a. Give daily sponge bath, including scalp. Use mild nonperfumed soap but not on face or body if skin is dry. Baby lotion may be used but avoid powder and oil.
   b. Tub bath may be substituted for sponge bath when cord drops off.
   c. Select area to bathe infant that is warm and free of drafts, with surface large enough so that infant will not roll off.
   d. Preparation for bathing should be completed before infant is brought to area, with clothing organized and available.
   e. Form habit of keeping instruments, pins, scissors, etc., closed and well out of reach of infant.
   f. Nails may be cut using manicure or special infant nail scissors when infant is soundly asleep.
   g. Genitals:
      (1) Change diapers when soiled but do not rouse infant from sleep to change him.
      (2) Rashes over buttocks may appear by second or third day. Wash area and dry, expose buttocks to air, and use heat lamp if severe. Position light source (25 watts) at least 24 inches above infant; secure infant so he cannot move and come into direct contact with light source.
      (3) Retract foreskin of uncircumcised infant; cleanse glans and replace foreskin.

Educational

ing diapers, using thermometer, and holding infant.

3. Discuss pertinent information relating to following:
   a. Temperature:
      (1) Review causes of elevation in body temperature such as exercise, stress with resultant vasoconstriction and minimal sweating response to pyrogens (germs), and fact that infant is a homoiotherm (body temperature same as environment).
      (2) Review symptoms to be reported such as high or low temperatures with accompanying symptoms of fussiness, stuffy nose, lethargy, irritability, poor feeding, and crying.
      (3) Review use of interventions for reducing body temperature such as cool tub bath, dressing infant appropriately in relation to ambient temperature, protection from long exposure to sunlight, and warm wraps in cold weather.

4. Respirations:
   a. Review normal variations in rate and rhythm.
   b. Review reflexes, such as sneezing to clear air passage.
   c. Review need for protection of infant from individuals with upper respiratory tract infections (efficient mask can be made from toilet paper if mother has cold).
   d. Review symptoms of common cold: nasal congestion, coughing, sneezing, difficulty in swallowing (sore throat), minimal fever. Advise on measures to help infant: for example, feed more frequently to avoid overtiring child, hold in upright position to feed, offer extra sterile water; in sleeping, raise mattress 30 degrees (do not use pillow) to raise chest and head; avoid drafts; do not overdress; use only medications prescribed by physician (do not use nose

PLAN OF CARE: NORMAL NEWBORN—DAYS 2 TO 14—cont'd

NURSING INTERVENTIONS—cont'd

Diagnostic	Therapeutic	Educational

		drops, since aspiration may result in lung involvement); cover upper lip with light film of petrolatum to minimize excoriation.
		5. Elimination:
		  a. Review changes to be expected in color of stool and number of bowel evacuations plus odor for breast- or bottle-fed infants.
		  b. Review color of normal urine and number of voidings to expect each day.
		6. Inform parents whom to contact if assistance is needed, what community agencies are available, what symptoms require medical attention (e.g., fever persists beyond 24 hours, infant rubs ear, infant coughs up purulent material, vomiting, refusal of feedings, diarrhea, lethargy), and what to report (e.g., specific symptoms and how long they have persisted, temperature reading, what corrective measures have been undertaken and with what effect).

PLAN OF CARE: NORMAL NEWBORN—DAYS 15 TO 28

PATIENT CARE OBJECTIVES

Physiologic responses

1. Respirations are stabilized within normal limits, and lungs sound normal. The family is aware of signs and symptoms of respiratory distress, whom to call, and what to communicate. The family practices protective measures to minimize respiratory tract infections.
2. Temperature: Maintenance of body temperature within normal limits, i.e., 36.5° to 37.3° C (97.6° to 99° F). Family is aware of signs and symptoms of fever, what measures to institute to reduce fever, and whom to contact for assistance.
3. Umbilicus may protrude slightly; parents are aware of cause and effect. No treatment is necessary; however, culturally motivated care is accepted and supervised.
4. Defecation: The infant establishes own pattern, varying from three to four times a day to once or twice a week. Stools are yellow-brown in color and of soft consistency.
5. Urination: Voiding six to ten times a day continues; urine is pale, straw-colored.
6. Appearance and behavior. Assessment of the infant reveals following:
   a. Normal growth and weight for age and body structure.
   b. Vision and hearing normal.
   c. Skin soft, no evidence of bruising, no excoriation of buttocks or creases.
   d. Muscle tone good.
   e. No evidence of malformation of or injury to bones and joints.
   f. Infant alert and responsive (smiles, some cooing, follows people and objects with his eyes, and is desirous of social contacts.
   g. Sleep pattern is established (awake between one or two feedings; fussy period may be consistent).

Continued.

PLAN OF CARE: NORMAL NEWBORN—DAYS 15 TO 28—cont'd

PATIENT CARE OBJECTIVES—cont'd

Caretaking activities

1. Plan for periodic assessment of the infant is established, with either a private physical or well-baby clinic.
2. Protection against infection or trauma continues.
3. Parents are knowledgeable as to community sources of assistance for the infant and/or for themselves.
4. Routine observation of infant's growth and developmental needs is established as a component of family's daily care of infant.
5. Nutrition: Child appears healthy and is satisfied with nutritional intake (Chapter 31).
6. Hygiene: Child appears clean, and the skin is in good condition; routine of care has been established and use made of these caretaking activities as modes for expression of parent-child relationships; opportunities of increasing socialization with other family members; and verbal, tactile, and visual stimulation of the infant.

Parenthood

1. Child is accepted as individual with persisting infantile dependency needs and as an integral part of a family unit.

NURSING INTERVENTIONS

Diagnostic	**Therapeutic and educational**
1. Weigh (Appendix H).	1. Welcome parents and infant.
2. Measure height and head circumference (Appendix H).	2. Explain routine to be followed (e.g., physical assessment, discussion of changes to be expected, and assistance with problems).
3. Assess all body systems using techniques of observation, inspection, palpation, auscultation, and percussion.	3. Have parent undress and dress infant and help with examination (provides opportunity to assess parental approach to infant).
4. Assess motor development; neurologic status (reflexes), including hearing (turns head to source of sound) and sight (follows moving object, raises head and looks about room); and nutritional status.	4. Review plan of well-baby supervision (e.g., at 2 to 4 weeks of age, then every 2 months until 6 to 7 months of age, then every 3 months until 18 months, at 2 years, 3 years, preschool, and every 2 years thereafter*).
5. Laboratory tests (hemoglobin or hematocrit, urinalysis, intradermal tuberculin test) are usually left until infant is 10 to 12 months of age.	5. Give information about changes in growth and development to be expected over next 2 months.
6. Assess general condition of infant: alert, skin soft and clear, no rashes or evidences of trauma.	6. Give information about disease processes and what to report to physician or health nurse.
7. Assess parents' relationship with child and knowledge of normal growth and development and symptoms of disease.	7. Review immunizations and schedule (Appendix I).
	8. Assist parents in coping with problems. (General statement such as "Tell me how you and the baby spend your day" is preferable to "Are you having any problems?" which can be answered by flat "no", or to "Are you bathing the baby every day?" which can place mother on defensive.)

*Committee on Standards of Health Care, American Academy of Pediatrics. 1972. Standards of child health care (ed. 2). Evanston, Ill., The Academy.

REFERENCES

Adams, M. 1963. Early concerns of primigravida mothers regarding infant care activities. Nurs. Res. **12:**128, Spring.

American Academy of Pediatrics. 1974. Report of the Committee on Infectious Diseases (ed. 17). Evanston, Ill., The Academy.

Babson, S. G., Benson, R. C., Pernoll, M. L., and Benda, G. I. 1975. Management of high-risk pregnancy and intensive care of the neonate (ed. 3). St. Louis, The C. V. Mosby Co.

Bernal, J. 1972. Crying during the first 10 days of life and maternal responses. Dev. Med. Child Neurol. **14:**362.

Bowlby, J. 1960. Attachment and loss (vol. 1). New York, Basic Books.

Brazelton, T. B. 1973. Neonatal Behavioral Assessment Scale. National Spastics Society Monograph (No. 50). London, William Heinemann, Ltd.

Brazelton, T. B. 1974. Does the neonate shape his environment? Birth Defects **10:**131.

Chinn, P. L., and Leitch, C. J. 1974. Child care maintenance: a guide to clinical assessment. St. Louis, The C. V. Mosby Co.

Clark, A., and Affonso, D. 1976. Childbearing: a nursing perspective. Philadelphia, F. A. Davis Co.

Clark, L. 1974. Care of the well child: introducing mother and baby. Am. J. Nurs. **74:**1483.

Craig, M. 1970. Normal neonatal behavior patterns the first week of extrauterine life. Child Fam. **9:**303.

Desmond, M. M., and others. 1966. The transitional care nursery. Pediatr. Clin. North Am. **13:**651.

Eoff, M., and others. 1974. Temperature measurements in infants, Nurs. Res. **23:**457.

Farmby, D. 1967. Maternal recognition of infant's cry. Dev. Med. Child Neurol. **9:**293.

Foss, B. M. (ed.). 1963. Determinants of human behavior. New York, John Wiley & Sons.

Fouts, G. Elimination of an infant's crying through response prevention. Percept. Mot. Skills **38:**225.

Frantz, R. L. 1966. Pattern discrimination and selective attention as determinants of perceptual development from birth. In Kidd, A. J., and Rivaire, J. L. (eds.). Perceptual development in children. New York, International Universities Press.

Gordon, T., and Foss, B. M. 1966. The role of stimulation in the delay of onset of crying in the newborn infant. Q. J. Exp. Psychol. **18:**79.

Greenberg, M. M. N. 1974. Engrossment: the newborn impact upon the father. Am. J. Orthopsychiatry **44:**520.

Haire, D., and others. 1972. Implementing family centered maternity care with a central nursery. Heelock, N.J., Childbirth Education Association of New Jersey.

Honig, A. 1970. The role of the nurse in stimulating early learning. J. Nurs. Educ. **9:**11.

Horoniety, E., and others. 1971. Newborn and four week retest on a normative population using the Brazelton newborn assessment procedure. Paper presented at the Annual Meeting of the Society for Research in Child Development, Minneapolis.

Kempe, C. H., and Helfer, R. E. 1972. Helping the battered child and his family. Philadelphia, J. B. Lippincott Co.

Kempe, C. H., Silver, H. K., and O'Brien, D. (eds.). 1976. Current pediatric diagnosis and treatment. Los Altos, Calif., Lange Medical Publications

Mingeot, R., and Herbert, M. 1973. The functional status of the newborn infant. A study of 5,370 consecutive infants. Am. J. Obstet. Gynecol. **115:**1138.

Pierog, S. H., and Ferrara, A. 1976. Medical care of the sick newborn (ed. 2). St. Louis, The C. V. Mosby Co.

Porter, C. 1973. Maladaptive mothering patterns: nursing interventions. In American Nurses' Association. Clinical sessions, 1972. New York, Appleton-Century-Crofts.

Rheingold, H. L. 1968. Infancy. In Sills, D. L. (ed.). International encyclopedia of the social sciences. New York, Macmillan, Inc.

Slumek, M. 1971. Screening infants for hearing loss, Nurs. Outlook **19:**115.

Vaughan, V. C., and McKay, R. J. (eds.). 1975. Nelson textbook of pediatrics (ed. 10). Philadelphia, W. B. Saunders Co.

Waechter, E., and Blake, F. 1976. Nursing care of children. Philadelphia, J. B. Lippincott Co.

Whitner, W., and Thompson, M. 1970. The influence of bathing on the infant's body temperature. Nurs. Res. **19:**30.

Wolff, P. H. 1969. Observations on newborn infants. Psychosom. Med. **21:**110.

Wolff, P. H. 1969. The natural history of crying and other vocalizations in early infancy. In Foss, B. M. (ed.). Determinants of infant behavior (vol. 4). New York, Barnes & Noble.

Yu, V. 1975. Body position and gastric emptying. Arch Dis. Child. **50:**500.

CHAPTER 31

Infant nutrition

FEEDING THE INFANT

Feeding periods are important to the infant and young child because, in addition to food, they derive significant emotional and psychologic benefits. Hence eating and drinking episodes can be sources of great satisfaction for both mother and child. These experiences and the treatment received from those who care for him constitute the infant's introduction to everyday life.

There is much variation in the nutritional needs and desires of infants. Moreover, considerable variation may be noted in any one infant without apparent reason. Therefore individualization and simplicity have come to be two important precepts in infant feeding in most cases; neither strict adherence to a feeding schedule nor slavish feeding each time the infant cries is advisable. Most mothers will develop a reasonably flexible schedule based on need, desire, demand, and availability.

Infant feedings are best initiated when the infant is awake, alert, and responsive. All infants progress through two wakeful episodes during the transitional period, the first occurring just at birth and the second 4 to 8 hours later. Thereafter they wake every 2 to 5 hours, and their behavior typically signifies hunger. The crying can be momentarily quieted by holding them upright or rocking them, but eventually crying begins again and has an angry sound. Infants will suck on a fist or finger, and rooting and swallowing reflexes can be elicited. For the first 24 hours, gagging and vomiting of mucus are common occurrences at the beginning of the wakeful periods. Once the infant has completed the transitional period, with the stomach emptied of the accumulation of mucus and the bowel of meconium, he often appears hungrier and accepts and retains feedings more readily.

Regardless of the method of feeding, both staff and parents must be aware of the infant's natural rhythm of sleeping and waking and hunger and satiety. Utilization of this knowledge assists in developing a more effective feeding routine for both infant and mother.

BREAST-FEEDING*

There are both advantages and disadvantages to breast-feeding an infant. The decision of the parents should be respected, and the provision of help and support for whatever method is chosen is the nurse's responsibility. The nurse's bias may be difficult to conceal as the following report indicates:

Mrs. S planned throughout her pregnancy to bottle-feed her baby. The topic of breast-feeding was discussed by the nurse, but Mrs. S remained decided about the method to be used. When the nurse visited her after the baby was born, the mother remarked, "You will be glad to hear I'm breast-feeding."

The nurse asked, "You feel I would be glad?"

Mrs. S replied, "Yes, every time we talked about bottle-feeding your voice got tight and remote so I knew you didn't approve."

With regard to its advantages, breast-feeding is a more convenient method and for most women provides great emotional satisfaction. Nursing speeds uterine involution by stimulating fundal contraction. It is not less expensive than bottle-feeding, however, when one considers the high-protein diet the mother requires. The composition of breast milk is ideal for most infants' needs, and it is superior to formula (even with vitamin supplements). The protein of human milk is more easily digested by human babies than that of cows or other milk-producing animals. Breast milk is aseptic and delivered at the proper temperature without the mother expending effort. Breast milk contains certain antibacterial and antiviral substances that add to the transplacental immunity and may increase resistance to certain infections.

Although immature, weak, or ill infants or ones with cleft palates may not be able to suck, they do benefit from breast milk. Many women express their milk and

---

*Information about breast-feeding may be obtained from the LaLeche League Information, Inc., 9616 Minneapolis Ave., Franklin Park, Ill. 60131; and the Nursing Mothers' Council, 2817 Carlson Circle, Palo Alto, Calif. 94306.

bring it to the intensive care unit for their child. When the infant has recovered, breast-feeding can be instituted. This "giving" of breast milk has made many mothers feel that they are participating actively in the care of their child. Holding and cuddling the baby while breast-feeding also aid in the bonding process.

The disadvantages relate more to the restrictive nature of breast-feeding than to any pathology that can occur (e.g., mastitis). Mothers who must return to work often do not wish to wean and leave the baby at the same time.

Many other factors can enter into the decision to breast-feed or to continue breast-feeding. Some women and men are repelled by the idea of breast-feeding, and such feelings may not be easily overcome. Some women will breast-feed a second child but not a first child, and the following comment explains why: "For the first baby, everything was just too strange and I was too tense. Now I'm more relaxed and sure of myself and I would like to try it."

Therefore nurses must bring up the topic antenatally even if the multiparous patient has not breast-fed previously. Other family members can also affect the choice, especially the new mother's mother. As one mother explained:

I tried to breast-feed Kathy, but my mother kept saying how thin she was and how I probably didn't have enough milk so I gave up. For Karen I no longer needed my mother's advice so I had no trouble at all. I surprised her (the mother).

By skillful antenatal interviewing, such blocks to breast-feeding can be brought out and explored.

If a mother is unsuccessful in her attempt to breast-feed, support for her decision to change is necessary.

Every effort should be forthcoming to help her cope with any sense of failure in her child-caring ability. The feeling of failure can act to impair her relationship with her child.

Lactation process

Numerous hormones are required for lactation. About the time of puberty, increased ovarian estrogen production causes proliferation of the mammary ducts. With the occurrence of ovulation during adolescence, progestogens from the corpus luteum then induce development of the breast lobules and alveoli (Fig. 31-1).

Considerable enlargement of the breasts occurs during gestation in response to the large amounts of estrogen and progestogen, produced principally by the placenta. Small amounts of premilk secretion, colostrum, collect in the milk ducts, and this may even be expressed as early as the sixth or seventh month of gestation. This slightly yellowish, viscid fluid slowly increases until term. However, 2 or 3 days after delivery a surge of actual milk may be expected in the nursing mother. Even after a late abortion or preterm delivery, some milk is produced, indicating that evacuation of the uterus in advanced pregnancy triggers lactation.

The exact mechanism of lactation still is debated, but prolactin secretion rises rapidly after delivery, probably in response to a sharp drop in circulating estrogen and progestogen. An increase in the glucocorticoid production associated with the stresses of labor and delivery may also be a factor in the onset of lactation. Although the interrelationships are not completely understood, the numerous anterior pituitary hormones (e.g., ACTH and TSH), the gonadotropins (FSH and LH), prolactin (lactogenic hormone), and perhaps somatotropin

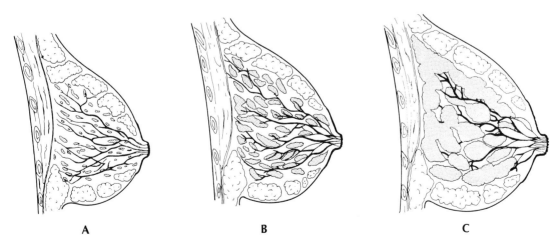

Fig. 31-1. Mammary glands. **A,** Nonpregnant. **B,** During pregnancy. **C,** During lactation. (Courtesy Ross Laboratories, Columbus, Ohio.)

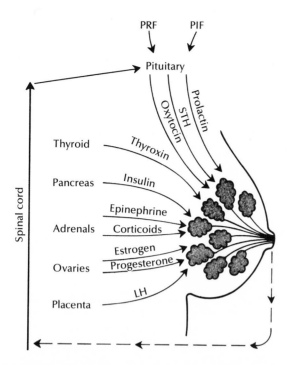

Fig. 31-2. Multiple hormonal influences on human lactation. (From Bergersen, B. S. 1976. Pharmacology in nursing [ed. 13]. St. Louis, The C. V. Mosby Co; modified from Catz, C. S., and Giacoia, G. P. 1972. Pediatr. Clin. North Am. **19:**151.)

(growth hormone) are required for the production of milk, which accumulates in the lacteal ducts (Fig. 31-2). Suckling during the puerperium causes the release of oxytocin, a hormone developed in the hypothalamus but stored in the posterior pituitary. Tactile stimuli from the breasts, carried by afferent tracts in the spinal cord to the brain, trigger its release. Oxytocin contracts the myoepithelial cells that line the walls of the milk ducts, and this causes ejection (milk ''let-down'') of the fluid through the nipple during the process of nursing.

Elevated prolactin levels inhibit the production of FSH and LH. Hence ovarian function, particularly ovulation, is delayed. If lactation is suppressed or terminated, ovarian follicular development resumes, and menstruation normally occurs soon thereafter. This is demonstrated by the occurrence of a period 6 or 7 weeks after delivery in mothers who do not nurse. Actually many of these new mothers ovulate within the first 2 months after parturition. For this reason, early contraception may be important.

Prelactation phase. Colostrum, or premilk fluid, is a yellowish breast secretion generally present during the last trimester of pregnancy and produced in increasing amounts for several days after delivery. It is of a higher specific gravity than milk and contains more protein, vitamin A, and minerals than milk. In contrast, colostrum has a lower carbohydrate and fat content. Although colostrum contains antibodies, it is doubtful that they are absorbed from the intestine and therefore do little to augment the immunity of the infant. Colostrum is a natural and ideal starter food and has a slight desirable laxative effect that aids in the evacuation of meconium.

Although colostrum may have been produced for weeks before delivery, the mother is told that true milk will not be produced (''come in'') until 2 to 4 days after childbirth. Prelactation expression or nursing may increase the milk supply later. The initial engorgement usually is less if the neonate nurses soon after delivery, and in addition, this may allow mother and infant more opportunity to become accustomed to each other and encourage the bonding process.

The infant feeds at both breasts but not more often than every 2 or 3 hours, and for the first day, nursing is limited to 3 or 4 minutes on each side. If the mother elects to sleep through the first 2 or 3 nights after delivery (prior to milk production), the infant may be satisfied by periodic oral glucose feedings.

Lactation phase. Milk may be expected to appear 48 to 96 hours after delivery. Initially considerable engorgement due to circulatory turgescense, not milk retention, may be noted. After 8 to 12 hours, softening of the breasts and free flow of milk can be expected.

Breast milk is an ideal food for the neonate. Once lactation is established, the milk contains protein (casein and lactalbumin), 1.25%; carbohydrate, 7.5%; fat, 3.5% to 4%; mineral salts, 0.2%; and an energy value of 20 calories to the ounce. The first milk produced by the breast is low in fat, and in comparison, the last milk is high in fat. Therefore any analysis of breast milk should contain the whole nursing sample. The milk has a bluish white appearance because the fat is white, not yellow as it is in cow's milk. It contains vitamins, if the mother's intake of vitamins is sufficient, and calcium derived from maternal stores (bones). So as not to deplete her own body stores of nutrients, the mother must ingest not only adequate amounts of protein, minerals, and vitamins but also sufficient calories to make up for the energy value of 350 to 700 calories in the milk secreted every day (500 ml to 1000 ml). Recommended daily allowances (Food and Nutrition Board, 1974) are as follows:

Calories	3000
Protein	100 gm
Calcium	1200 mg
Vitamin A	6000 IU
Thiamin	1.5 mg

Ascorbic acid (vitamin C)	80 mg
Riboflavin	2 mg
Niacin	19 mg
Vitamin D	400 IU

If the mother does not like milk (a quart a day is recommended), protein, fluids, and calcium must be supplied in other forms. The daily diet should include eggs; one or more servings of meat, fish, or poultry; and abundant fruits and vegetables. If the child seems colicky, the mother can experiment with adjusting her diet by eating sweets in moderation and foregoing gaseous vegetables such as cauliflower.

Breast milk production on the second day after the milk comes in will be about 120 ml. On the third day 180 ml is likely, and by the fourth day the mother may be producing a total of 240 ml of milk. For a practical estimate of milk production during the first postnatal week, multiply the number of days after the milk comes in by 60. This will equal the approximate number of milliliters of milk secreted in that 24-hour period.

If no complications develop, sustained milk production is achieved after the first 10 to 14 days. Frequently, 120 to 180 ml of milk per feeding is produced by most lactating women after the second week.

The infant is encouraged to nurse at each hungry period, that is, about every 3 or 4 hours, day and night.

It is best to increase gradually the sucking time at each breast to protect the nipples from laceration, fissure formation, and infection. After free flow is established, milk actually runs out, and an overabundance is usual. If the infant needs more food for some reason, more frequent nursing, for example, every 2 or 3 hours for about 2 to 3 days will increase the supply.

Inadequate early lactation may be due to failure to empty the breasts (e.g., small or compromised infants, poor nursing procedure, inadequate nutritional intake). Emotional problems, such as an aversion to breast-feeding, or medical disorders, such as severe sepsis or Sheehan's syndrome, can also cause inadequate lactation.

Suppression of lactation. If the mother does not wish to suckle her infant or if this is medically contraindicated, lactation can be prevented by mechanical means or by the administration of estrogens and/or androgens.

If mechanical suppression is chosen, nursing, expression of milk, or pumping of the breast must be discontinued. A tight compression ''uplift'' binder is applied for about 72 hours, after which a snug brassiere is advised. The breasts will become distended, firm, and tender, but after 48 to 72 hours, lactation and discomfort will cease. Ice packs and analgesics may be used if necessary. Fluid restriction or laxatives are not helpful. Involution will be complete in about a month.

Hormonal suppression of lactation may be accomplished by giving ethinyl estradiol (TACE), 1.3 mg (twenty-six tablets of 0.05 mg each) or its equivalent in the following sequence:

1. Four tablets (0.2 mg) twice a day on postnatal day 1
2. Three tablets (0.15 mg) twice a day on postnatal day 2
3. Two tablets (0.1 mg) twice a day on postnatal day 3
4. One tablet (0.05 mg) twice a day on postnatal days 4 through 7

Depoestrogen such as estradiol valerate (Delestrogen), 3 mg of a solution containing 10 mg/ml intramuscularly, immediately after delivery is effective in suppression of lactation.

Depoestrogen and androgen are effective also, for example, testosterone enanthate, 90 mg/ml, and estradiol valerate, 4 mg/ml, 3 ml injected promptly after delivery.

Estrogens have been implicated in the occurrence of thromboembolization postdelivery particularly after cesarean section or a complicated vaginal delivery. In such patients, mechanical suppression of lactation probably should be elected.

Secretion of drugs in breast milk. The ingestion of certain drugs by the mother results in their secretion in breast milk, and as a result the infant is exposed to them. Drugs that are secreted in large amounts include barbiturates, bromides, salicylates, iodides, thiouracils, ergot, and cascara. Toxicity for the infant is likely only when the mother's intake of such drugs is excessive. Drugs that are secreted in small, nontoxic amounts after the average dose of maternal administration include the opiates, alcohol, nicotine, atropine, caffeine, sulfa drugs, penicillin, and phenolphthalein. A complete list of drugs secreted in breast milk is given in Table 31-1.

Techniques of nursing

If put to breast at birth, some infants will begin to suck immediately; others only nuzzle the breast or nipple. The close body and eye contact this encourages affords both mother and infant much pleasure and reassurance, and the abrupt severance of the mother-fetal unit is modified by gradualness. The infant must be kept dry and warm during this process to minimize heat loss and the consequent use of vital energy to replace it. Since the important element at this time is the early establishment of the mother-child relationship, not the infant's need for nourishment, holding and examining the infant will serve the same purpose.

Infants awaken from their first sleep about 4 to 6 hours

Text continued on p. 496.

Table 31-1. Drugs excreted in human milk and possible significance for nursing infants*

Drug	Excreted	Quantity excreted	Significance
Antihistamine drugs			
Diphenhydramine (Benadryl)	Yes		Not significant in therapeutic doses to affect child
Trimeprazine tartrate (Temaril)	Yes		Not significant in therapeutic doses to affect child
Tripelennamine (Pyribenzamine)	Yes		Only bovine studies reported to date; apparently not enough is excreted to be significant in therapeutic doses
Anti-infective agents			
Amantadine (Symmetrel)	Possible		Not to be administered; personal correspondence with manufacturer suggests it will be found in maternal milk; may cause vomiting, urinary retention, skin rash
Ampicillin (Polycillin, Amcill, Omnipen, Penbritin, Principen, others)	Yes	0.07 μg/ml	Not significant in therapeutic doses to affect child
Carbenicillin disodium (Pyopen, Geopen)	Yes	0.265 μg/ml 1 hour after administration of 1 Gm	Not significant in therapeutic doses to affect child
Cephalexin (Keflex)	No		
Cephalothin (Keflin)	No		
Chloramphenicol (Chloromycetin)	Yes	Half blood level 2.5 mg/100 ml	Infants have underdeveloped enzyme system, immature liver and renal function, may not have glycuronide system adequately developed to conjugate chloramphenicol; caution advised
Chloroquine (Aralen)	No	After daily dose of 0.6 Gm no traces could be found in milk of 105 subjects	Not significant in therapeutic doses to affect child
Demeclocycline (Declomycin)	Yes	0.2 to 0.3 mg/500 ml	Not significant in therapeutic doses to affect child
Erythromycin (Ilosone, E-mycin, Erythrocin)	Yes	0.05 to 0.1 mg/100 ml 3.6 to 6.2 μg/ml	Higher concentrations have been reported in milk than in plasma
Isoniazid (Nydrazid)	Yes	0.6 to 1.2 mg/100 ml same concentration in milk as in maternal serum	Infant should be monitored for possible signs of isoniazid toxicity
Kanamycin (Kantrex)	Yes	1 Gm given intramuscularly gave a concentration of 18.4 μg/ml	Infant should be monitored for possible signs of kanamycin toxicity
Lincomycin (Lincocin)	Yes	0.5 to 2.4 μg/ml	Not significant in therapeutic doses to affect child
Mandelic acid	Yes	0.3 Gm/24 hr following maternal dose of 12 Gm/day	Not significant in therapeutic doses to affect child
Methacycline (Rondomycin)	Yes		Same precautions as with tetracyclines
Methenamine (Hexamine)	Yes		Not significant in therapeutic doses to affect child
Metronidazole (Flagyl)	Yes	Level comparable to serum	Apparently not significant in therapeutic doses; caution should be exercised due to its high milk concentrations

*From O'Brien, T. E. 1974. Excretion of drugs in human milk. Am. J. Hosp. Pharm. **31**:844; copyright © 1974, American Society of Hospital Pharmacists, Inc. All rights reserved.

Table 31-1. Drugs excreted in human milk and possible significance for nursing infants—cont'd

Drug	Excreted	Quantity excreted	Significance
Anti-infective agents—cont'd			
Nitrofurantoin (Furadantin)	Yes		Not significant in therapeutic doses to affect child
Nalidixic acid (NegGram)	Yes	3.9 μg/ℓ	Not significant in therapeutic doses; however one case of hemolytic anemia in an infant was attributed to nalidixic acid
Novobiocin (Albamycin, Cardelmycin)	Yes	0.36 to 0.54 mg/100 ml	This antibiotic has been used to treat infections among infants with no untoward effects reported
Oxacillin (Prostaphlin)	No		
Paraamino salicylic acid	No		
Penethamate (Leocillin)	No	24 to 74 μg/100 ml	Animal study suggests it be avoided
Penicillin G potassium	Yes	Up to 6 units/100 ml	Controversy exists among clinicians: some feel that risk of sensitivity symptoms must be looked for, others feel small amount is insignificant; parent should be told to inform physician that infant has been exposed to penicillin
Penicillin, benzathine (Bicillin)	Yes	10 to 12 units/100 ml	Clinical need should supersede possible allergic responses
Pyrimethamine (Daraprim)	Yes		Detected in human milk but no conclusions drawn; apparently not significant in therapeutic doses
Quinine sulfate	Yes	0 to 0.1 mg/100 ml after maternal dose of 300-600 mg	Not significant in therapeutic doses to affect child
Sodium fusidate	Yes	0.02 μg/ml	Not significant in therapeutic doses to affect child
Streptomycin	Yes	Present for long periods in slight amounts given as dihydrostreptomycin	Risk should outweigh benefit of nursing; to be avoided
Sulfanilamide	Yes	After maternal dose of 2 to 4 Gm daily 9 mg/100 ml in milk	Not significant in therapeutic doses; may cause rash
Sulfapyridine	Yes	3 to 13 mg/100 ml after maternal dose of 3 Gm daily	To be avoided; has caused skin rash
Sulfathiazole	Yes	0.5 mg/100 ml after dose of 3 Gm/day	Not significant in therapeutic doses to affect child
Sulfisoxazole (Gantrisin)	Yes	Concentration similar to plasma level	To be avoided during first 2 postpartum weeks; may cause kernicterus
Tetracycline HCl (Achromycin, Steclin, Sumycin, others)	Yes	0.5 to 2.6 μg/ml after maternal dose of 500 mg qid	Not enough to treat an infection in an infant; however, it has been hypothesized that there may be sufficient amount to cause discoloration of teeth in infant; antibiotic, however, may be largely bound to milk calcium
Antineoplastics			
Cyclophosphamide (Cytoxan)	Yes		To be avoided, as are other antineoplastic drugs; nursing should be discontinued
Automatic drugs			
Atropine sulfate (ingredient in many products, both pre-	Yes	Less than 0.1 mg/100 ml	Should not be administered for two main reasons: (1) it inhibits lactation, and (2) it may cause atropine intoxication in infant

Continued.

Table 31-1. Drugs excreted in human milk and possible significance for nursing infants—cont'd

Drug	Excreted	Quantity excreted	Significance
Automatic drugs—cont'd			
scription and non-prescription)			
Carisoprodol (Soma, Rela)	Yes	May be present in breast milk at concentrations four times maternal plasma	Not to be administered, based upon manufacturer's recommendation; infant may be exposed to series of adverse reactions ranging from CNS depression to gastrointestinal upset
Ergot (Cafergot)	Yes		Avoid where possible; may cause symptoms in infants ranging from vomiting and diarrhea to weak pulse and unstable blood pressure
Hyoscine	Yes	Trace amounts	Not significant in therapeutic doses to affect child
Mepenzolate bromide (Cantil)	No		
Methocarbamol (Robaxin)	Yes	Small amounts	Not significant in therapeutic doses to affect child
Propantheline bromide (Pro-Banthine)	No		
Scopolamine	Yes		Not significant in therapeutic doses to affect child
Blood formation and coagulation			
Dicumarol	Yes		Therapeutic doses can be administered without deleterious effect on infant; infant should be monitored with mother
Ethyl biscoumacetate (Tromexan)	Yes	0 to 0.17 mg/100 ml; no correlation with dosage	Not significant in therapeutic doses; infant should be monitored with mother
Iron	Yes		Not significant in therapeutic doses to affect child
Ferrous sulfate			
Iron-dextran (Feosol, Imferon)			
Phenindione (Hedulin, Dindevan)	Yes		To be avoided; may produce prothrombin deficiency in infant; one case of massive hematoma reported in infant receiving drug in maternal milk
Warfarin sodium (Coumadin)	Yes		Infant should be monitored with mother; benefit should outweigh possible risk
Cardiovascular drugs			
Dextrothyroxine (Choloxin)	Yes		Not significant in therapeutic doses to affect child
Guanethidine (Ismelin)	Yes		Not significant in therapeutic doses to affect child
Methyclothiazide, deserpidine (Enduronyl)	Yes		Same precautions as with reserpine and thiazide diuretics
Methyldopa (Aldomet)	Yes		Studies performed on bovines; nothing reported in humans
Propranolol (Inderal)	No		
Reserpine (Serpasil, others)	Yes		May produce galactorrhea

Table 31-1. Drugs excreted in human milk and possible significance for nursing infants—cont'd

Drug	Excreted	Quantity excreted	Significance
Central nervous system drugs			
Alcohol	Yes	Small amounts	It appears that moderate amounts of alcohol have little, if any, effect on nursing infant
Amitriptyline (Elavil)	No		
Aspirin	Yes	Moderate amounts	It could cause bleeding tendency by interfering with function of infant's platelets or by decreasing amount of prothrombin in blood. Risk is minimal if mother takes aspirin just after nursing and if infant has adequate store of vitamin K
Barbiturates	Yes		It appears that in therapeutic doses barbiturates have little or no effect on infant; one case was reported where high doses had a hypnotic effect on one infant; it is best to avoid administering, since barbiturates serve as inducing agents for hepatic drug metabolizing enzymes
Barbital (Veronal)	Yes	4 to 5 mg of diethylbarbituric acid/500 ml of milk detected after a single dose of 500 mg	Significant quantities, avoid administration; produced marked sedation in infant
Bromides (Bromo-Seltzer; many non-prescription sleeping aids)	Yes	0 to 6.6 mg/100 ml	Not to be administered based upon manufacturer's recommendation; may cause drowsiness
Caffeine	Yes	1% of that ingested	Not significant in usual amounts to affect child
Chloroform	Yes		One study performed in 1908 reported that nursing infant slept for 8 hours; not significant in therapeutic doses
Chloral hydrate (Noctec, Somnos)	Yes	0 to 1.5 mg/100 ml	Not significant in therapeutic doses
Chlorazepate (Tranxene)	Yes		Not to be administered based upon manufacturer's recommendation; may cause drowsiness
Chlordiazepoxide (Librium)	Yes		Not significant in therapeutic doses to affect child
Chlorpromazine (Thorazine)	Yes	4.15 mg/ml after daily dose of 200 mg in dogs	Not significant; may cause galactorrhea
Codeine	Yes		Not significant in therapeutic doses to affect child
Cycloheptenyl ethyl barbituric acid (Medomin)	Yes		Not significant in therapeutic doses to affect child
Desipramine (Norpramin)	No		
Dextroamphetamine (Dexedrine)	No		
Diacetylmorphine (Heroin)	Yes		Not enough to prevent withdrawal in addicted infants
Diazepam (Valium)	Yes	51 ng/ml after 4 days of diazepam; 28 ng/ml of N-dimethyldiazepam	Recent studies recommend that this drug be avoided during nursing; infant reported as lethargic and experienced weight loss; may cause hyperbilirubinemia
Diphenhydramine (Benadryl)	Yes		Not significant in therapeutic doses to affect child

Continued.

Table 31-1. Drugs excreted in human milk and possible significance for nursing infants—cont'd

Drug	Excreted	Quantity excreted	Significance
Central nervous system drugs—cont'd			
Flutenamic acid (Arlef)	Yes		Excreted in small amounts; no recommendations
Hydroxyphenbuta-zone (Tandearil)	Yes	0 in 53 of 55 mothers	Conflicting reports; both conclude that it would have no significant effect in therapeutic doses
Imipramine (Tofranil)	No		
Indomethacin (Indocin)	Yes		Not significant in therapeutic doses to affect child
Lithium carbonate (Eskalith, Lithane, Lithonate)	Yes	Same in child's serum as in mother's milk, 0.3 mEq	Infant should be monitored for possible signs of lithium toxicity
Mefenamic acid (Ponstel)	Yes		Not significant in therapeutic doses to affect child
Meperidine (Demerol)	Yes		Not significant in therapeutic doses to affect child
Meprobamate (Mil-town, Equanil)	Yes	Present in milk two to four times maternal plasma level	Infant should be monitored for possible signs of meprobamate toxication if therapy is to be continued
Mesoridazine besylate (Serentil)	Yes		Not significant in therapeutic doses to affect child
Morphine	Yes	Small amounts	Not significant in therapeutic doses to affect child
Pentazocine (Talwin)	No		
Phenobarbital (Lumi-nal, others)	Yes		To be avoided where possible; serves as inducing agent for hepatic drug metabolizing enzymes
Phenylbutazone (Butazolidin)	No	0.63 mg/100 ml 1½ hours after mother injected (IM) with 750 mg	No side effects noted among group studied, but because of possible lethal reactions infant should be closely monitored
Phenytoin (Dilantin)	Yes		Not significant in therapeutic doses although one case of methemoglobinemia was associated with phenytoin
Piperacetazine (Quide)	Yes		Manufacturer suggests it may have great potential for excretion in milk
Primidone (Mysoline)	Yes		To be avoided, may cause undue somnolence and drowsiness
Prochlorperazine (Compazine)	Yes	0.4 to 1.5 mg/100 ml in dogs after daily dose of 200 mg	Not significant in therapeutic doses to affect child
Propoxyphene HCl (Darvon)	Yes	0.4% of dose to mother found in stomach of nursing rat	Not significant in therapeutic doses to affect child
Salicylates	Yes	1.0 to 3.0 mg/100 ml of sodium salicylate detected 4 hours after maternal dose of 4 Gm	Not significant in therapeutic doses; high doses (5 Gm/day) have been reported to cause rash in infant
Thiopental sodium (Pentothal)	Yes		Not significant in therapeutic doses to affect child
Thioridazine (Mellaril)	Yes		Not significant in therapeutic doses to affect child
Tranylcypromine (Parnate)	Yes		Not significant in therapeutic doses to affect child
Trifluoperazine (Stelazine)	Yes	0.4 to 1.5 mg/100 ml in dogs after daily dose of 200 mg	Not significant in therapeutic doses to affect child

Table 31-1. Drugs excreted in human milk and possible significance for nursing infants—cont'd

Drug	Excreted	Quantity excreted	Significance
Diagnostic agents			
Carotene (natural product found in carrots)	Yes		One incident reported where infant turned yellow; mother ate 2 to 3 lb. of carrots per week; not significant in average quantities
Iopanoic acid (Telepaque)	Yes		Not significant in therapeutic doses to affect child
Electrolytic, caloric, and water balance			
Cyclopenthiazide (Navidrix)	No		
Cyclamate (Sucaryl)	Yes		Not significant in therapeutic doses to affect child
Furosemide (Lasix)	No		
Hydrochlorothiazide (Hydrodiuril, Esidrix, others)	Yes		To be avoided, based on manufacturer's recommendation; no specific adverse effects reported in infants to date
Spironolactone (Aldactone)	No		
Thiazides	Yes		To be avoided based on manufacturer's recommendation; no specific adverse reactions reported in infants to date
Expectorants and cough preparations			
Potassium iodide	Yes	3 mg/100 ml	To be avoided, may affect infant's thyroid
Gastrointestinal drugs			
Aloe	Yes		Controversial, one author claims it may give rise to catharsis in some infants; others feel its presence is insignificant
Anthraquinone (Dorbane, Dorbantyl, Danthron, Peri-Colace, Doxidan, Dialose-Plus)	Yes		One animal study found it present in milk and in "significant" amounts; another human study did not detect it; third human study detected it and felt it best not to administer it to nursing mothers, as it may cause catharsis in infant
Cascara	Yes		Avoid where possible; reported to have increased gastric motility in infant
Emodin (found in cascara sagrada)	Yes		Avoid where possible; reported to have increased gastric motility in infant
Phenolphthalein (found in many nonprescription laxative products)	Yes		Not significant in therapeutic doses to affect child
Rhubarb	Yes		Not significant in therapeutic doses to affect child
Senna	Yes		Not significant in therapeutic doses; high doses may cause diarrhea in nursing infant
Hormones and synthetic substitutes			
Carbimazole (Neo-Mercazole)	Yes		Not to be administered; antithyroid may cause goiter in nursing infant
Chlormadione (Estalor-21)	Yes		Possible effects must be weighed against risk of pregnancy; see contraceptives (oral)

Continued.

Table 31-1. Drugs excreted in human milk and possible significance for nursing infants—cont'd

Drug	Excreted	Quantity excreted	Significance
Hormones and synthetic substitutes—cont'd			
Chlorotrianisene (TACE)	Yes		Avoid where possible estrogenic substances may be in breast secretions
Contraceptives (oral)	Yes		Possible effects must be weighed against risk of pregnancy; may inhibit lactation if administered during first postnatal weeks; possible gynecomastia in male infant
Corticotropin	Yes		Destroyed during passage through gastrointestinal tract; its presence in milk is unimportant
Cortisone	Yes		No human study; among animals a 50% lower weight than control, retarded sexual development, exophthalmos
Dihydrotachysterol (Hytakerol)	Yes		May cause hypercalcemia
Estrogen (oral contraceptives)	Yes	0.17 μg/100 mg	Possible effects must be weighed against risk of pregnancy; see contraceptives (oral)
Ethisterone (Pranone)	Yes		To be avoided; may cause significant skeletal advancement
Fluoxymesterone (Halotestin, Ora-testryl, Ultandren)			Used to suppress lactation
Iodides (nonradioactive)	Yes	After a dose of 0.6 Gm (as potassium salt) 68 mg was recovered	To be avoided, chronic use may affect infant's thyroid gland
Liothyronine sodium (Cytomel)	No		
Lyndiol	Yes		To be avoided; caused diminution in milk protein and milk fat
Lynestrenol (oral contraceptive under investigation)	Yes		Possible effects must be weighed against risk of pregnancy; see contraceptives (oral)
Medroxyprogesterone acetate (Provera)	No		
Mestranol (estrogenic compound found in several oral contraceptives)	Yes		Possible effects must be weighed against risk of pregnancy; see contraceptives (oral)
Norethisterone ethanate (progesterone contraceptives)	Yes		Possible effects must be weighed against risk of pregnancy; see contraceptives (oral)
Norethynodrel (Enovid)	Yes	1.1% of dose	Possible effects must be weighed against risk of pregnancy; see contraceptives (oral)
Norethindrone (Norlutin)	Yes		Possible effects must be weighed against risk of pregnancy; see contraceptives (oral)
Phenformin HCl (DBI)	Yes		Not significant; does not exert hypoglycemic effect on normal subject
Pregnane-3 (α), 20 (β)-diol	Yes		Although it may cause unconjugated hyperbilirubinemia in breast-fed infants, it was regarded as not being significant enough to stop nursing
Thiouracil	Yes	Higher in milk than in blood 9 to 12 mg/100 ml	To be avoided; may cause goiter in nursing infant or agranulocytosis
Thyroid	Yes		Not significant in therapeutic doses to affect child
Tolbutamide (Orinase)	Yes		Not significant in therapeutic doses to affect child

Table 31-1. Drugs excreted in human milk and possible significance for nursing infants—cont'd

Drug	Excreted	Quantity excreted	Significance
Radioactive agents			
Gallium 67 (gallium citrate)	Yes		Avoid where possible, radionuclides are generally contraindicated during nursing; or nursing should be temporarily stopped
Iodine, radioactive (^{131}I)	Yes	Total in 48 hours of milk; 1.3 μCi after maternal dose of 29.5 μCi	To be avoided; affects infant's thyroid gland
Sodium, radioactive, as sodium chloride	Yes	0.5 to 1.3% of dose per liter of milk	Not significant in therapeutic dose, although it is best to avoid radionuclides if possible
Serums, toxoids, and vaccines			
Diphtheria antibodies	Yes	Less then 0.30% of dose administered	Of no value in conferring passive immunity to infant
Skin and mucous membrane preparations			
DDT	Yes	5 mg/100 ml	Concentration is higher in human milk than in bovine milk; DDT poisoning
Vitamins			
Calciferol (vitamin D)	Yes		Caution advised; may cause hypercalcemia
Cyanocobalamin (vitamin B$_{12}$)	Yes	0.1 to 0.4 μg/ℓ	Not significant in therapeutic doses to affect child
Folic acid	Yes	0.7 μg/ℓ	Not significant in therapeutic doses to affect child
Phytonadione (vitamin K$_1$, Aquamephyton)	Yes		Not significant in therapeutic doses to affect child
Thiamin (vitamin B$_1$) deficiency	Yes	10 to 13 μg/ℓ	Lack of this B vitamin in nursing mother (beriberi) causes excretion of toxic substance, methylglyoxal, which has caused infant death
Miscellaneous agents			
Allergens (eggs, wheat flax seed, peanuts, cottonseed, etc.)	Yes		May cause allergic response in sensitive child
Colchicine	Yes		1929 study indicated that this drug may pass into milk; no adverse effect reported
Fluorides (found in many toothpastes)	Yes		Not significant in quantities ingested; excess could affect tooth enamel
Hexachlorobenzene[1,23]	No		Avoid use as insecticide; has caused infant mortality
Mercury	Yes		Environmental contaminant; signs of mercury intoxication and CNS effects
Nicotine	Yes	0.4 to 0.5 mg/ℓ ; 11 to 20 cigarettes/day	In moderation, no effect; not more than 20 cigarettes/day
Ribonucleic acid (RNA)	Yes		Particles from human milk contain a reverse transcriptase and high molecular weight RNA that serves as template; these particles have two features diagnostic of known RNA tumor viruses

after birth and again are alert and hungry. Gagging episodes and vomiting of mucus are almost invariably present during the early portion of the wakeful time, and the staff needs to be alert to provide the care necessary in maintaining an unobstructed airway (p. 467). To assess the infant's ability to ingest and retain nutrients, a bottle-feeding of up to 4 ounces of sterile water is given. Sterile water is used so that if the infant aspirates, it will be absorbed by the lung tissue with no damaging effect. Reflexes (sucking, swallowing, gagging) required for feeding must be present. Infants should exhibit tolerance for the stress of sucking. If they appear tired by the process, a softer nipple or a nipple with larger holes may resolve the difficulty. If evidence of stress persists, respirations increase, and circumoral pallor develops, notify the physician, since these symptoms may be indicative of cardiovascular problems (p. 583). This initial feeding also permits detection of structural anomalies that require immediate medical attention. If an infant has a tracheoesophageal fistula, the infant swallows, then gagging, choking episodes occur with regurgitation of bubbly mucus, and the infant appears cyanotic and in distress. If the esophagus ends in a blind pouch, the infant will swallow a small amount satisfactorily and then regurgitate the entire amount unchanged by gastric contents. A stomach tube may be passed to determine if the esophagus is patent (p. 513).

In addition to the previous assessment measures, the nurse must note excessive abdominal distention, the amount of water taken, and the coordination of the feeding reflexes. These then are recorded.

If infants respond normally, they may then be put to the breast; however, the feeding of the sterile water often appeases their hunger. If so, it is better perhaps for the mother to use this time for holding, cuddling, and examining her infant, waiting until the next wakeful period to begin breast-feeding. In some areas, the bottle-feeding of sterile water is being omitted to permit as early a beginning of breast-feeding as possible. The infant who appears to have difficulty at the breast will then be reassessed, using the bottle technique.

In the beginning, many breast-fed babies nurse every 2 to 3 hours during the day and once or twice at night. It is advocated by some that the night feedings not be omitted during the period before the milk comes in. Regular emptying of the breasts of colostrum appears to bring the milk in earlier and minimizes the discomfort from engorgement. Appetite spurts are normal in children and occur at fairly regular intervals. In the young infant, the mother will notice that the baby seems hungrier and dissatisfied with the amount of milk received at about 4 to 8 days after birth, 5 to 6 weeks of age, and

again about the third month. Increasing the frequency of breast-feedings for a few days increases the amount of milk produced, the infant's hunger is appeased, and he reverts to longer intervals between feedings.

The mother should wash her hands before breast-feeding to help protect her baby from infection. She may assume any position that she finds comfortable, allows the breast to fall forward without tension, and leaves one hand free to guide the nipple into the child's mouth. The infant is held so that his cheek touches the breast; the pressure against the outer angle of the lip elicits the rooting reflex, and the infant turns toward the nipple. The odor or taste of the colostrum or milk seems to rouse the infant's interest, and he usually turns in the direction of its source.

To initiate nursing, the nipple and surrounding areolar tissue are guided into the infant's mouth and over the tongue by placing a finger on either side of the nipple and compressing the areolar area (Figs. 31-3 and 31-4). The mother often can sense whether the infant has drawn enough areolar tissue into the mouth along with the nipple. If not, the nurse may check the infant's position

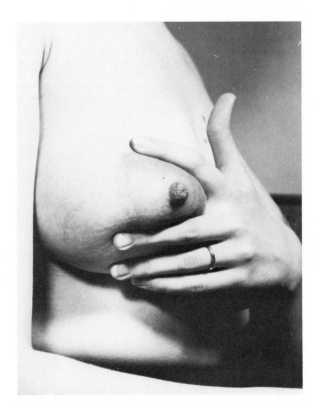

Fig. 31-3. Pointing nipple. (Courtesy Ross Laboratories, Columbus, Ohio.)

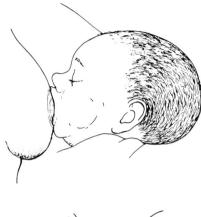

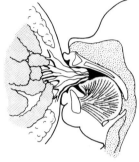

Fig. 31-4. Proper position of infant's mouth on breast. (Courtesy Ross Laboratories, Columbus, Ohio.)

and note whether the areolar area is being drawn into the mouth as sucking proceeds. If the infant is positioned and sucking properly, the facial muscles contract and pull the ear lobes forward. Loud sucking noises usually indicate that the child is grasping just the nipple. Because lengthy sucking on the nipple may cause erosion, soreness, and eventually cracking, the infant must be removed and the procedure begun again. The mother is cautioned not to pull the infant away from the breast but to release the suction by gently depressing the infant's chin or inserting a clean finger into the baby's mouth (Fig. 31-5).

Gradually increasing the length of time the baby is at the breast permits the nipple to develop tolerance to the vigorous sucking. The mother may start with 3 minutes on each breast the first day, and increase the time by 2 minutes a day until the infant is sucking 7 minutes on the first breast and up to 7 minutes on the other at each feeding. If the baby's sucking needs seem unsatisfied, it is better to increase the frequency of feedings rather than to allow longer sucking at any one time.

Once the baby is properly positioned, the mother can make a "dimple" in the tissue near his nose so he can breathe freely (Fig. 31-6). Burping the infant is suggested prior to feeding if the baby has been crying and after the feeding at each breast. During this procedure the infant is held upright and the back gently rubbed (Fig. 31-7).

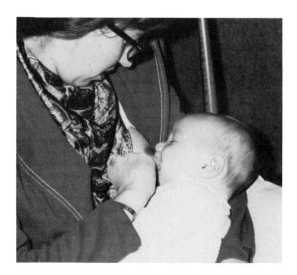

Fig. 31-5. Inserting clean finger into baby's mouth releases suction so he may be removed from breast. (From Duell, D. 1970. Technique of breast-feeding [unpublished master's thesis] San Jose, Calif., San Jose State University.)

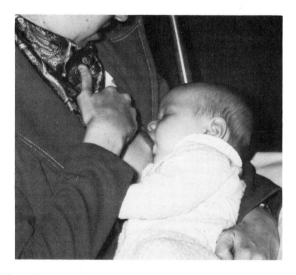

Fig. 31-6. Making sure infant has room to breathe properly. (From Duell, D. 1970. Technique of breast-feeding [unpublished master's thesis]. San Jose, Calif., San Jose State University.)

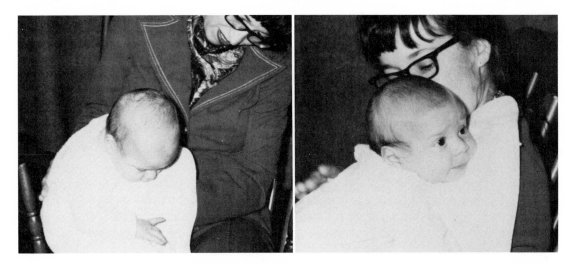

Fig. 31-7. Burping infant. (From Duell, D. 1970. Technique of breast-feeding [unpublished master's thesis]. San Jose, Calif., San Jose State University.)

Common difficulties and concerns in breast-feeding

Initial. Following are common problems and suggestions for dealing with them:

1. The mother's nipple may appear retracted, and the infant may not be able to grasp it. Have the mother roll the nipple gently between her fingers until it is erect and suggest she do this prior to subsequent feedings.

2. The baby's mouth may not open wide enough to grasp the nipple. Have the mother depress the infant's lower jaw with one finger as she guides the nipple into the mouth.

3. The infant may grasp the nipple and areolar tissue correctly, but he will not suck. Have the mother stimulate sucking motions by pressing upward under the baby's chin. Expression of colostrum results, and the infant is stimulated by the taste to begin sucking.

4. The infant may make frantic rooting, mouthing motions but he will not grasp the nipple and eventually begins to cry and stiffens his body in apparent frustration. Have the mother interrupt the feeding, comfort the infant, and take time to relax herself, and then she may begin again.

5. The infant may suck for a few minutes and then fall asleep. Have the mother interrupt the feeding and take time to waken the infant. Stimulation may include loosening the wraps, holding him upright, talking to him, or gently rubbing his back or the soles of his feet. A sleepy infant will not nurse satisfactorily. If it is impossible to wake the baby, it is better to postpone the feeding.

6. By the third or fourth postnatal day, the breasts may become so full and distended with milk that the nipples appear retracted, and the infant may be unable to nurse. The lag between the production of milk and the efficiency of the ejection reflexes often results in engorgement of the breasts for up to 48 hours after the milk comes in. The mother often complains that the breast is tender and that the tenderness extends into the axilla. The breasts usually feel firm, tense, and warm as a result of the increased blood supply, and the skin may appear shiny and taut. The unyielding areolas make it difficult for the infant to grasp the nipple. Hence nursing can be uncomfortable to the mother and frustrating for both mother and infant. Expression of milk manually or by using a breast pump generally will start the flow of milk and relieve the engorgement. In some instances, moist warmth (e.g., shower, cloths) will also start the flow. A mild analgesic may also be ordered for use prior to nursing. The mother should be encouraged to wear her supportive nursing brassiere most of the time. Careful attention to the general comfort of the mother during the nursing period is important. Selection of a comfortable position, use of pillows for support, and the presence of an attentive, unhurried nurse do much to help the mother weather these few days.

7. The infant may start by sucking vigorously and, as the milk flows freely, develop a long, slow, rhythmic sucking. This may then change to a short, rapid sucking, with frequent rest periods. This behavior indicates a slowing of the flow of milk. Alternate massage of the breasts starts the milk flowing freely again, and the infant should revert to the slow, rhythmic sucking. As

soon as this begins, the massage is discontinued so that the infant will not be overwhelmed and choked by the milk flowing too rapidly.

Later. Once the technique of breast-feeding has been mastered, the mother's concerns tend to center on the quantity and quality of the milk produced. The following information* can be given in response to her queries.

1. Milk production and supply.
   a. The amount of milk produced can be considered satisfactory if the infant has six to ten voidings of pale, straw-colored urine in 24 hours.
   b. The more frequently the infant suckles the greater the milk production.
   c. Both breasts should be used and emptied at each feeding. Eventually by the end of the fourth week, the child can suckle 10 to 15 minutes on the first breast and up to 20 minutes on the second without injury to the nipple tissue.
   d. Once the milk supply has been established, the mother may express the milk and freeze it for a bottle-feeding later if she wishes to be away at the scheduled feeding time. If she should be absent longer than 6 to 8 hours, the milk may be expressed from both breasts, since the milk supply will lessen if the breasts are not emptied regularly.
   e. Bottle-feedings of extra water should be limited to warm weather. Increasing the frequency of feedings during the day may be all that is required to control thirst.
   f. The breast-feeding mother requires extra fluids. These can be taken routinely before each feeding. Glasses of water, fruit juices, tea, or milk can be alternated.
   g. Because tension tends to lessen milk production, the mother's family should respect her need for adequate rest. The first few days after the mother comes home with the new baby are often filled with excitement and anxiety about mothering activities. Entertaining company or undertaking extended family commitments may have to be curtailed.
   h. When introducing solids, the infant is nursed prior to feeding the solid food. Otherwise disinterest in and reduction of suckling reduce the necessary stimulation to the milk supply.

*Modified from "Instructions for Nursing Your Baby," by Doris Haire. Reprints of the pamphlet may be obtained from ICEA Supplies Center, 208 Duty Bldg., Bellevue, Wash. 98004.

2. Quality of the milk.
   a. Normal breast milk has a thin, watery consistency and bluish white color. Although it does not look "rich," it has the right composition of nutrients for the child (Table 31-2).
   b. The stools of breast-fed babies are very loose. Some infants have a bowel movement at each feeding, whereas others may go up to 5 days without one. Babies who are fed only breast milk do not become constipated, although they may strain considerably in passing the stool. The stool is not irritating to the skin.
   c. If menstruation occurs, the mother can continue to breast-feed. Although some babies may act fussy, the quality and quantity of the milk are not affected.
   d. No infant has been found to be allergic to breast milk itself, but a baby can react to certain foods that the mother eats. Avoidance of these foods is all that is necessary to curtail the reaction. The mother determines which foods to avoid primarily by means of trial and error.

Nursing twins

Nursing twins takes planning and patience. If the mother elects to room-in, the added care of two infants may prove too taxing to her strength, although many mothers have stated that the early adjustment made going home easier. It is suggested that these mothers remain longer in the hospital unless there is help at home. It is important to establish a feeding schedule as soon as possible. The mother may use a modified demand schedule, that is, feeding the first baby who wakes up and then awakening the second baby, or she may waken both and feed simultaneously. A record of the feeding times, which breast was used by which baby, and which side was used first is essential during the early weeks. If one twin nurses more readily than the other, an effort should be made to have that twin nurse on alternate breasts so as to equalize stimulation. If feeding simultaneously, the mother should experiment with positions; for example, each baby may be supported on pillows and in the football hold, or one may be held in the football hold and the other in the cradle hold. Obviously the mother with twins will need extra assistance from her family, extra nourishment, and extra rest if she is to have sufficient energy not only to care for and nurse each baby but also to provide the mothering each needs.

Care of breasts

Daily washing of the breasts with water is sufficient for cleanliness. In addition, for the first 2 to 3 weeks the nipple and areolar tissue is washed and dried after each feeding, since the remaining colostrum or milk can contribute to the development of sore nipples. A lubricant such as liquid petrolatum may then be massaged gently into the nipple area, and if feasible, the breasts can be exposed to the air for 20 to 30 minutes. The lubricant used should not contain alcohol, since the drying effects of the alcohol tend to encourage cracking of the tissue. Some infants object to either the taste or smell of ointments and will refuse to nurse until the breast has been washed.

The nursing brassiere needs to be well fitted, with broad shoulder straps and the flaps over the breasts large enough to release the breasts without discomfort. Milk leaking from the breasts, particularly just prior to the next feeding (ejection reflex), can be uncomfortable and embarrassing, but lining the brassiere cup with plastic material is not recommended, since moisture tends to soften the nipple and predispose to erosion. It is better to pad the brassiere with folded squares of soft cotton, a perineal pad cut in two, or commercially designed pads. A tingling sensation in the nipple area precedes leaking of the milk. Pressure with the heel of both hands over the nipple areas will often prevent the milk forming, and the leaking from the breast is forestalled.

Regardless of careful antenatal preparation of the breasts and nipples and attention and care postnatally, by the end of the first week some women will have developed sore nipples. When examined, the nipples will be found to be eroded, with fissures or cracks. Occasionally "blood blisters" form around the nipple, and when they break, blood seeps into the infant's mouth. This blood is not detrimental to the infant; the discomfort to the mother is the concern. The mother will need encouragement and support if she is to persist and successfully breast-feed her infant. Until the eroded and cracked nipples heal, the mother is instructed to try the following measures in addition to those prescribed in the general care:

1. Use a heat lamp to dry the nipples after the feeding (40-watt bulb in a desk lamp, positioned 18 inches from breast).

2. Limit sucking time to 5 minutes on each breast, the time it takes to empty the breasts of milk.

3. Use a pacifier if the infant's sucking needs have not been met.

4. Use a nipple shield.

5. Discontinue nursing for 48 hours. During this time the milk is expressed manually or with a breast pump, collected in a sterilized glass, and given to the baby by bottle. Precautions for maintaining the milk in a safe condition must be followed. Bottles and nipples must be sterilized by immersing them in water and boiling for 10 minutes; any milk not immediately consumed must be refrigerated or frozen.

The nursing mother may note an increase in lochial flow once nursing begins. At times afterpains are intensified to such a degree that the mother becomes uncomfortable, and her tension interferes with nursing the infant. A medication for pain such as Percodan may be offered 30 minutes prior to the nursing period, and the mother may be reassured that this discomfort is transitory and will be gone in 2 days. For some women, the rhythmic contractions of the uterus occurring while nursing are akin to those experienced during orgasm. These unexpected sexual sensations within the context of child care may be disturbing, and women may need to be reassured as to the normalcy of these feelings.

BOTTLE-FEEDING

The initial feeding and care of the infant to be bottle-fed parallels that of the breast-fed baby. About 4 to 6 hours after birth the infant is fed up to 4 ounces of sterile water to assess the normalcy of reflexes and the absence

Table 31-2. Composition of milk and milk formulas*

Percentage of calories from	Human milk	Cow's milk	Diluted cow's milk + 10% carbohydrate	Evaporated milk 13 ounces Water 19 ounces Carbohydrate 1½ ounces
Protein	8%	20%	10%	15%
Fat	50%	50%	25%	39%
Carbohydrate	42%	30%	65%	46%

*From Kempe, C. H., Silver, H. K., O'Brien, D. (eds.). 1976. Current pediatric diagnosis and treatment (ed. 4). Los Altos, Calif., Lange Medical Publications.

of structural anomalies. Thereafter the baby wakens every 2 to 5 hours for feeding. Within a few weeks, the pattern generally stabilizes, with feedings usually every 3 or 4 hours (but by feeding the child at 10 or 11 PM, even if it means waking him, the mother can often get 5 to 6 hours of uninterrupted sleep). The night feeding usually persists until about the sixth week. The bottle-fed infant will experience the same appetite spurts as does the breast-fed baby, that is, at 4 to 8 days after birth, at 5 to 6 weeks, and at about the third month. During this time, more frequent feedings are in order.

As long as his fluid and calorie requirements are met, the baby is permitted to regulate the volume and frequency of feeding within the range of not more than every 2 hours and not less than every 5 to 6 hours.

Composition of formulas

The chemical composition of cow's milk differs from that of breast milk. Protein concentration is more than

twice (3.4%). The quality of the protein also differs in that cow's milk has a higher content of casein (2.8% as opposed to 0.4%) and lactalbumin (0.4% as opposed to 0.8%) than human milk. The casein coagulates and forms large curds when mixed with gastric juices, whereas the lactalbumin remains in solution. As a result the higher concentration of casein in cow's milk slows digestion, gastric emptying time, and later, absorption. Therefore formula preparation includes a process to partially digest casein before it is ingested. This may be done by boiling and diluting the milk; by adding an acid, alkali, or proteolytic enzyme; or by evaporation and drying.

Since infants have a wide range of digestive tolerance, exact duplication of breast milk by a formula preparation is not necessary. The energy value per ounce is the same (20 calories/ounce), and the differences in protein and carbohydrate content balance each other in the yield of calories (Table 31-2).

A comparison of the electrolyte content of infant foods is shown in Table 31-3.

The addition of water to a formula reduces the amount of protein and fat in a given quantity as the addition of glucose increases the relative amount of carbohydrate. In this way the formula approximates the composition of human milk. A full-strength milk formula (20 calories/ounce) contains 13 ounces of evaporated milk, 19 ounces of water and 1 or 2 tablespoons of Karo syrup.

There is a wide range of commercially prepared formulas to choose from that both meet the infant's normal and special nutritional requirements (Table 31-4).

Table 31-3. Electrolyte content of infant foods (mEq/ℓ)

Food	Na$^+$	K$^+$	Ca^{++}	PO$^+$	Cl$^-$
Human milk	7	14	17	9	12
Cow's milk	25	36	61	53	34
Typical commercial modified formula	17	23	42	37	19

Table 31-4. Normal and special infant formulas*

	Manufacturer	Carbohydrate source	Fat source	Indications for use	Comments (nutritional adequacy)
Milk and milk-based formulas					
Cow's milk Evaporated milk	Several brands	Lactose, sucrose	Butterfat	Feeding of full-term and premature infants with no special nutritional requirements	Supplemented with iron and vitamins C and D if not fortified
Commercial infant formulas					
SMA	Wyeth	Lactose	Safflower oil	Feeding of full-term and premature infants with no special nutritional requirements	Supplemented with iron, 12 mg/ℓ

*From Kempe, C. H., Silver, H. K., and O'Brien, D. (eds.). 1976. Current pediatric diagnosis and treatment (ed. 4). Los Altos, Calif., Lange Medical Publications.

Continued.

Table 31-4. Normal and special infant formulas—cont'd

	Manu-facturer	Carbohydrate source	Fat source	Indications for use	Comments (nutritional adequacy)
Commercial infant formulas—cont'd					

Enfamil
  Ready to use
  Concentrated liquid
  Powder
	Mead Johnson	Lactose	Coconut, corn, oleo, soy, lecithin	Feeding of full-term and premature infants with no special nutritional requirements	Available fortified with 12 mg iron/ℓ

Similac
  Ready to feed
  Concentrated liquid
  Powder
	Ross	Lactose	Coconut, corn, soy	Feeding of full-term and premature infants with no special nutritional requirements	Available fortified with 12 mg iron/ℓ

Products for milk protein-sensitive infants ("milk allergy")					
Neo-Mull-Soy liquid	Syntex	Sucrose	Soy		Soy protein isolate
Prosobee	Mead Johnson	Corn sugar,* sucrose	Soy		Soy protein isolate Zero band antigen
Isomil	Ross	Corn sugar,* sucrose, cornstarch	Corn, coconut, soy		Soy protein isolate
Meat base	Gerber	Modified tapioca starch	Sesame, beef lipids		
Elemental diets for tube feeding and products for oral supplements					
Vivonex	Eaton	Glucose, glucose oligosaccharides	Safflower oil	Used as a general dietary supplement or as a sole nutritional source in malabsorption	Synthetic amino acid base Also high in nitrogen
Flexical	Mead Johnson	Sucrose, dextrin	20% medium chain triglycerides, 80% soy	Fat malabsorption	
Ensure	Ross	Sucrose, corn syrup solids	Corn oil	Lactose intolerance	Soy protein plus calcium caseinate
Hycal	Beecham	Glucose			A flavored product for calorie supplementation only
Polycose	Ross	Glucose polymers			A powdered calorie supplement
Low-sodium formulas					
Lonalac powder	Mead Johnson	Lactose	Coconut	Management of children with congestive cardiac failure	For long-term management, additional sodium must be given Supplement with vitamins C and D and iron Na = 1 mEq/ℓ

*Composed of glucose, maltose, and dextrins.

Table 31-4. Normal and special infant formulas—cont'd

	Manu-facturer	Carbohydrate source	Fat source	Indications for use	Comments (nutritional adequacy)
Low-sodium formulas—cont'd					
Partially demineralized whey formulas					
SMA S-26 Concentrated liquid or powder	Wyeth	Lactose	Safflower oil	Use where a low-salt diet is indicated	Relatively low solute load Na = 7 mEq/ℓ
Similac PM 60/40 Powder	Ross	Lactose	Coconut, corn	Use where a low-salt diet is indicated	Relatively low solute load Na = 7 mEq/ℓ
Products for infants with malabsorption syndromes					
Vivonex	Eaton	Glucose, glucose oligosaccharides	Safflower oil	Elemental diet in chronic secretory diarrheas	Synthetic amino acid base
Portagen	Mead Johnson	Corn sugar,* sucrose	Medium chain triglycerides (coconut source) and safflower	Management of chyluria, intestinal lymphangiectasia, various forms of steatorrhea, biliary atresia	Fat in medium chain triglycerides and safflower oil
Alacta (available internationally but not in USA)	Mead Johnson	Lactose	Butterfat	Infants with poor fat tolerance or poor fat absorption	Supplement with vitamins A, D, and C and iron. To increase calories supplement with carbohydrates Renal solute load is high if powder only is used to increase calories to 67 Cal/100 ml
Nutramigen	Mead Johnson	Sucrose, tapioca	Corn	Feeding of infants and children intolerant to food proteins Use in galactosemic patients	Enzymatic hydrolysate of casein
Pregestimil	Mead Johnson	Glucose, tapioca	Medium chain triglycerides (coconut and corn source)	Malabsorption syndromes, especially after diarrhea and in malnutrition	Contains added iron and vitamins Protein is enzymatically hydrolyzed milk protein
Cho-Free	Syntex	None	Soybean oil	Infants intolerant to carbohydrate	Carbohydrate-free soy oil and protein Add carbohydrates to increase calories
For infants with phenylketonuria					
Lofenalac	Mead Johnson	Corn sugar,* sucrose	Corn	Infants and children with phenylketonuria	
Albumaid XP	Ross (Milner)			Older children with phenylketonuria	Very low phenylalanine content permits increased supplementation with normal foods

Nutritional needs of infant

Since the infant's nutritional needs are related to his weight and activity, the formula strength and amount need to be increased as the child grows. At birth the infant's stomach will dilate to contain 10 to 20 ml. By the end of the first week, stomach capacity has increased to 30 to 90 ml; by 2 to 3 weeks, 75 to 100 ml; and by the end of neonatal period, 90 to 150 ml.

Table 31-5 is useful in predicting the composition and schedule of feeding of infants.

Conformity to established height and weight percentiles and a history of a well-balanced adequate diet are usually sufficient to assess if the child's nutritional status is normal.

Most companies that supply baby foods prepare illustrated booklets with detailed instructions in the steps in preparation of formula. If such booklets are used (free on request), the nurse reviews their contents with the mother before discharge. The physician prescribes the exact ingredients and number of feedings per day of formula based on the infant's weight and growth needs and provides written as well as verbal instructions. These will suffice until the mother brings the baby for the fourth-week checkup, at which time the strength of the formula and number of ounces per feeding are increased.

Preparation of formula*

1. Equipment needed:
   a. A regular bottle sterilizer, available at a baby-care store, or a large kettle with a lid.
   b. A wire rack (one should come with a commercial sterilizer), or a clean towel. This item is used to separate bottles from the sterilizer or kettle bottom.
   c. A can opener.
   d. Tablespoon, slotted spoon, or eggbeater.
   e. Seven nursing bottles, together with nipples, caps, and collars.
   f. Bottle and nipple brushes.
   g. Tongs for sterile handling of bottles.
   h. A can of the selected baby formula.
2. Washing and rinsing bottles and nipples:
   a. Scrub bottles, nipples, collars, and caps with the bottle brush, detergent, and hot water.
   b. Squeeze the water through nipple holes during washing and rinsing.
   c. Rinse bottles and nipples with hot, running water.

*Modified from the booklet "Preparing Similac Infant Formula for Your Baby," published by Ross Laboratories, Columbus, Ohio.

Table 31-5. Composition and schedule of milk feedings for infants up to 1 year of age*

Age (months)	0	1	2	3	4	5	6	7	8	9	10	11	12
Calories per day†	130 to 100/kg (60 to 45/pound)						110 to 100/kg (50 to 45/pound)				100 to 90/kg (45 to 40/pound)		
Fluid per day (ml)	130 to 200/kg (2 to 3 ounces/pound)				130 to 165/kg (2 to 2½ ounces/pound)					130/kg (2 ounces/pound)			
Number of feedings per day‡	6 or 7			4 or 5				3 or 4				3	
Ounces per feeding	2½ to 4	3½ to 5	4 to 6	5 to 7	6 to 8	7 to 9							
Milk Evaporated Whole	65 ml/kg (1 ounce/pound) up to a total of 13 ounces (1 can) daily 130 ml/kg (2 ounces/pound) up to a total of 28 to 32 ounces daily												
Sugar per day	1 to 1½ ounces					§	None						

*From Kempe, C. H., Silver, H. K., and O'Brien, D. (eds.). 1976. Current pediatric diagnosis and treatment (ed. 4). Los Altos, Calif., Lange Medical Publications; modified from Silver, H. K., Kempe, C. H., and Bruyn, H. 1975. Handbook of pediatrics (ed. 11). Los Altos, Calif., Lange Medical Publications.
†The larger amount should be used for the younger infant.
‡Will vary somewhat with individual babies.
§Decrease sugar by ½ ounce every 2 weeks.

3. Techniques for sterilizing formula preparations or drinking water (when the infant is old enough, a clean technique of preparation may be used):
   a. Terminal heating method: Bottles are filled with the prescribed amount of formula and nipples, caps, and collars are put on loosely. The filled bottles are placed on a wire rack or towel in a sterilizer or deep kettle. Water to 3 inches is added to the sterilizer. When the water in the sterilizer starts to boil, cover and let boil for 25 minutes. Remove the sterilizer from heat and leave covered until the sterilizer has cooled to touch. When the bottles are cool enough to handle, remove them from the sterilizer, tighten caps, and store in refrigerator.
   b. Aseptic method:
      (1) Place the bottle, nipples, collars, caps, mixing spoon, can opener, measuring pitcher, and tongs on a rack or towel in a sterilizer or deep kettle. Cover with water, and place over heat. Add the prescribed amount of water needed to make formula in a clean pan. Place over heat. When the water in both the sterilizer and pan come to a boil, cover and boil 5 minutes.
      (2) Wash top of a can of milk with soap and water and dry. Shake the can well. Make two puncture holes in the top with sterile can opener and mix prescribed amount of milk and boiled water.
      (3) Pour the correct number of ounces of formula into each nursing bottle. Put nipples, collars, and caps on bottles. Store in the refrigerator until needed.

Bottle-feeding the infant

For the first few feedings, until the baby becomes familiar with the process, the baby can be held slightly away from the mother's body while the nipple is being put into his mouth and he begins to suck. When the baby is held close to the mother, the rooting reflex is elicited, and the mother may find it more difficult to introduce the nipple.

The bottle-fed baby ingests more air while sucking than does the breast-fed baby; therefore it is important to hold the bottle at such an angle that the milk covers

---

PLAN OF CARE: NUTRITION OF NORMAL NEWBORN—FIRST DAY OF LIFE

PATIENT CARE OBJECTIVES

1. Reflexes (rooting, sucking, swallowing, gagging, regurgitating) are present and sufficiently developed to permit infant feeding by breast or bottle.
2. Periods of wakefulness when infant is alert and hungry are utilized to facilitate initiation of the feeding process and to promote a satisfying mother-child interaction.
3. Mother begins feeding her infant by breast or bottle.
4. Infant accepts, swallows, and retains feedings.
5. Regurgitation or vomiting episodes are controlled, and the mother is able to care for the infant so that an open airway is maintained.

NURSING INTERVENTIONS

Diagnostic	Therapeutic	Educational
1. Assess reflexes, sucking, swallowing, gagging to determine whether infant is able to be breast- or bottle-fed. 2. Assess infant readiness for feeding (rooting reflex readily elicited, alert, and responsive). 3. Assess mother's level of knowledge about feeding her infant and skills she possesses. 4. Note condition of nipples if mother is to breast-feed.	1. Utilize wakeful periods for feeding infant. 2. Initiate feeding of infant by mother (breast or bottle) as soon as possible. 3. Assist mother with feeding technique she has chosen.	1. Instruct as to nutritional needs of infant during first few days of life. 2. Instruct as to feeding abilities of infants (e.g., their sucking needs, how to burp them, that learning nursing process may require practice; that there are variations in appetite). 3. Demonstrate and supervise care needed if infant gags, chokes, or spits up during feeding process. 4. Instruct mother who is breast-feeding in care of her breasts to prevent erosion of nipples, to augment supply of milk, and to prevent infection of breast or infant.

PLAN OF CARE: NUTRITION OF NORMAL NEWBORN—DAYS 2 TO 14

PATIENT CARE OBJECTIVES

1. Infant nutritional state is satisfactory. Evidence includes following: weight gain, skin turgor adequate, skin soft, fontanels not depressed, active and alert when awake, good muscle tone, sleeps contentedly 2 to 5 hours between feedings, crying from stress of hunger appeased by feeding, has soft stools, voids pale straw-colored urine six to ten times a day.
2. Mother is adept at techniques relative to breast- or bottle-feeding.
   a. Breast-feeding: (1) initiating and terminating the feeding session, (2) enhancing the supply of milk, (3) protecting her nipples from erosion and fissures, (4) adjusting the number of feedings to meet the infant's need for increased food intake, and (5) utilizing alternative methods of feeding the infant to free her to take part in other activities.
   b. Bottle-feeding: (1) preparation of formula, (2) initiating and terminating feedings, (3) adjusting the schedule and formula to meet the infant's need for increased food intake, and (4) adopting practices that ensure infant-mother contact.
3. Mother is aware of infant's nutritional needs for growth; that is, she supplements the diet with solid foods, vitamins, and minerals and knows when and how to introduce them.
4. Mother is aware of the symptoms indicative of gastrointestinal disturbances, which are as follows: fontanels depressed, skin dry, eyes lack luster, diarrhea with green curdy stools, fever, refusal of feedings and fluids, lethargy, irritability, and a diminished number of voidings of urine. Mother is aware of the need to obtain medical care promptly to arrest lethal processes of dehydration and acid-base imbalance, as well as the procedure for obtaining assistance.

NURSING INTERVENTIONS

Diagnostic	Therapeutic	Educational
1. Examine general condition of infant as part of routine care.	1. Establish relaxed environment in which mother undertakes feeding process (free from pain, comfortable position, assistance from interested patient and knowledgeable nurse, and privacy).	1. Continue instruction as to nutritional needs of infant.
2. Obtain reports from mother (family) concerning satisfaction of infant (e.g., whether infant sleeps soundly and is hungry every 2 to 5 hours and his crying is appeased by nourishment).	2. Continue assistance with technique of breast- or bottle-feeding.	2. Assist mother (family) in recognizing cues infant uses and pattern of hunger and satiety each infant develops.
3. Observe mother when she is engaged in feeding infant to determine skills and areas in which further assistance is needed.	3. For breast-feeding mother, provide adequate diet ($\uparrow$ protein $\uparrow$ fluids) and daily routine for care of breasts.	3. Instruct family as to symptoms indicative of gastrointestinal disturbances.
4. Observe infant during and after feeding process to note ability to suck, swallow, and retain feedings.	4. Assist mother in dealing with concerns as to her ability to provide adequate nourishment for her child.	4. Discuss techniques relative to weaning, introduction of other nutrients to diet.
5. Check mother's knowledge of care of breasts if she is breast-feeding.		

---

the neck of the bottle. The baby may be burped prior to beginning the feeding, especially if he has been crying, after about an ounce of formula has been taken, and at the end of the feeding. To do this, the mother holds the infant in an upright position and gently massages his back (Fig. 31-7).

Once the baby begins sucking properly, the mother can hold him close so he may relax against her warmth. Every infant needs physical contact with the mother. The feeding period offers one of the most natural ways for infant and adult to share, to give, and to experience nurturing.

It is a dangerous practice to "prop the bottle" when feeding an infant. The nipple can lodge against the back of the throat and block the air passage or if the infant regurgitates, the fluid may be aspirated, causing death or a lung infection. There is a higher incidence of otitis media in infants who are propped and suck in the horizontal position. The eustachian tube orifice opens during swallowing, and mucus from the nose can drain into the duct and occlude it (Kempe and others, 1974). The infant should never be left alone when feeding until he is old enough to hold the bottle and to remove it from his mouth by himself.

PLAN OF CARE: NOURISHMENT OF NORMAL INFANT—DAYS 15 TO 28

PATIENT CARE OBJECTIVES

1. Infant's nutritional status remains satisfactory; growth, weight gain, and pattern of weight gain are within normal limits.
2. Mother is adept at adjusting feeding process to meet infant's nutritional needs for growth, infant's need for socializing, and mother's need for widening scope of other activities.
3. Mother is aware of nutritional needs that may arise over next 2 months.
4. Mother is aware of techniques of weaning the infant from breast or bottle.
5. Mother is able to discuss current problems related to feeding her infant, explore methods of solution, and recognize and use measures instituted successfully in the past.
6. Mother-infant relationship is positive as evidenced by her behavior toward the infant and the type of feeding and interactive processes instituted.
7. Mother is knowledgeable about signs and symptoms of gastrointestinal disturbances and what procedures to follow to obtain medical help.

NURSING INTERVENTIONS

Diagnostic	Therapeutic and educational
1. Examination of infant by medical or nursing personnel reveals satisfactory nutritional status. 2. Assess mother's (family's) knowledge of future nutritional needs of infant, process of weaning from breast or bottle, symptoms of digestive problems requiring medical assistance. 3. Assess mother-child relationship.	1. Counsel about problems related to feeding infant by breast or bottle. 2. Discuss process of weaning, introduction of solids, etc., infant's diet. 3. Provide information as to nutritional needs over next few months, and review symptoms of gastrointestinal conditions requiring prompt medical attention.

Common concerns

The following are common concerns of mothers who are bottle-feeding their infants, with suggestions for dealing with the problems:

1. The infant tires quickly and goes to sleep. The mother may try a softer nipple and/or enlarge the holes in the nipple. This may be done by heating a needle stuck into a cork as a handle and inserting the hot needle into the nipple holes. New nipples may be softened by boiling 5 minutes before using.

2. The infant takes "forever" to feed. This is not uncommon, particularly in smaller babies. Slow, patient feeding, keeping the infant awake, and encouraging him to suck by massaging upward under his chin may be necessary. Regardless of the time involved, the infant needs to consume approximately the total number of calories per day prescribed as normal for his weight.

3. The infant gulps down the formula, chokes, and regurgitates. The mother checks to see if holes in the nipple are too large. If the bottle is held upside down, the milk should come out in drops, not in a stream. Help the infant learn to drink more slowly by stopping the feeding after each ounce, burping, cuddling, and then resuming the feeding.

4. The temperature of the warmed formula (place the bottle in a pan of hot water) can be checked by letting a few drops fall on the inside of the wrist. If it feels comfortably warm to the mother, it is the correct temperature. (Commercially prepared formula stored at room temperature does not need warming.)

5. Once a bottle of formula has been used for a feeding, the remaining formula should not be kept for the next infant feeding. It may be stored in the refrigerator and used as coffee or cereal cream by the adults in the family.

6. The stools of bottle-fed babies are soft but formed. They are light yellow in color and have a characteristic foul odor. The composition of the stool is irritating to the infant's skin; therefore the buttocks need frequent cleaning. By the end of the second week the number of stools has decreased from about five to one to two stools a day.

REFERENCES

Adams, M. 1963. Early concerns of primigravida mothers regarding infant care activities. Nurs. Res. **12:**72, Spring.

Countryman, B. 1971. Hospital care of the breast-fed newborn. Am. J. Nurs. **71:**2365.

Countryman, B. 1973. Editorial. Obstet. Gynecol. News **8:**6, March 15.

Food and Nutrition Board. 1974. Recommended dietary allowances (ed. 8). Washington, D.C., National Academy of Sciences–National Research Council.

Haire, D. 1970. Instructions for nursing your baby. Bellevue, Wash., ICEA Supplies Center.

Haire, D. 1970. How the breast functions. Bellevue, Wash., ICEA Supplies Center.

Hemingway, L. 1973. Breast feeding and the family doctor. 2. Lactation problems. Aust. Fam. Phys. **2:**90.

Iffig, M. C. 1968. Nursing care and success in breast feeding. Nurs. Clin. North Am. **111:**347.

Kempe, C. H., Silver, H. K., and O'Brien, D. (eds.). 1976. Current pediatric diagnosis and treatment. Los Altos, Calif., Lange Medical Publications.

Schwartz, D. J., and others. 1973. A clinical study of lactation suppression. Obstet. Gynecol. **42:**599.

Vaughan, V. C., and McKay, R. J. (eds.). 1975. Nelson textbook of pediatrics (ed. 10). Philadelphia, W. B. Saunders Co.

Zuckerman, H., and Carmel, S. 1973. The suppression of lactation by clomiphene. J. Obstet. Gynaecol. Br. Commonw. **80:**822.

UNIT TEN

High-risk newborn

CHAPTER 32

Identification of infant at risk

Each year 250,000 infants are born with significant structural and functional intrauterine growth deviations (IUGD). The seriousness of this community health problem is reflected in the more than 6 million hospital days and $200 billion a year allocated to the care and treatment of these neonates. Prevention and detection procedures are being improved continuously; methods of promoting the availability of these services to populations at risk challenge the community health delivery systems. An interdisciplinary team approach is imperative to provide holistic care: surgery, rehabilitation, and education of the child and social, psychologic, and financial assistance to the parents. Parental disappointment and disillusion and the nurse's own negative feelings toward (or stigmatization of) the infant's disorder add to the complexity of nursing care.

IUGD comprise those disorders present at birth or detectable during the nursery period. Major, life-threatening malformations include such conditions as meningocele, omphalocele, cyanotic cardiovascular anomaly, hydrocephalus, esophageal atresia, and tracheoesophageal fistula. Fortunately many IUGD are minor abnormalities such as clubfoot and polydactyly that do not pose a serious deterrant to the realization of a normal potential and life expectancy.

Most infants move from intrauterine to extrauterine life with little difficulty. For some, however, birth is complicated by many factors, and survival is jeopardized. These high-risk infants' survival and well-being depend on advanced and often aggressive medical management and a suitably controlled environment.

The responsibility of the obstetric team for the reduction of perinatal mobidity and mortality cannot be minimized. Two thirds of all deaths in the first year occur in the first 28 days, and most of these are recorded in the first 24 hours of life. More individuals die in the first day of life than at any other time. One in every ten infants born in the United States sustains some lifelong impairment because of sequelae related to high-risk problems.

Saving the life of the neonate is not sufficient if serious, perhaps permanent injury is sustained. Prompt recognition and immediate appropriate intervention will improve the quality of life. Intact survival is the goal.

Not every institution is equipped for intensive care of the newborn. Each hospital must have a trained staff and emergency equipment to care for any fetus or infant at risk until transfer to a suitable intensive care unit can be effected.

Some of the most common problems that may be anticipated on any maternity service will be described. Terminology is stressed to facilitate observation, recording, and reporting of the symptoms of pathologic states. Procedures, their purposes, and rationale will be reviewed in detail (Chapter 37). Nursing procedures and nursing actions related to medical care have been included. In most hospitals, nurses are responsible for ordering and maintaining equipment, assisting the physician, and monitoring and recording the infant's responses.

When studying and utilizing this content, the student is asked to keep an open mind. New data are constantly being identified. Some of the appropriate procedures and treatments of the recent past are considered ineffective and even hazardous today. To support the goal of intact survival, therapy must be continuously reviewed and improved in light of advancing progress.

Nurses who plan to work in a neonatal intensive care unit are referred to the references at the end of this chapter.

OVERALL GOALS OF MEDICAL-NURSING CARE OF HIGH-RISK INFANT

1. Anticipate and diagnose premonitory or early disease.

2. Minimize the effects of the disorder to avoid disability of the child.

3. Treat disease promptly and appropriately when possible.

4. Facilitate a positive parent-child relationship.

See Appendix L.

HIGH-RISK FACTORS

A detailed listing of maternal, familial, fetal, and newborn criteria to aid in the identification of the neonate who may be at risk is found in Chapter 15.

Not all problems of the infant can be anticipated or diagnosed during the first 24 hours of life; some may not be apparent until the infant is in the general nursery or until after discharge from the hospital. To ensure early recognition of problems, the nurse must remain alert to the symptoms that signal deviations from normal growth and development and provide anticipatory guidance to parents to assist them in alerting the physician promptly if the need arises.

TRANSITION OR OBSERVATION NURSERY
General considerations

Transition from intrauterine to extrauterine life is a critical period of adaptation for every neonate. The first 24 hours after birth is a recovery period for all infants; each must be watched as carefully as any postoperative patient.

Prematurity and obvious external disorders are easily discernible in the delivery room. These infants are sent immediately to premature or intensive care facilities. A self-contained, portable unit may be used to transport the neonate safely (Fig. 32-1). However, many newborn problems are not obvious at birth. Careful observation of the neonate during the transitional period may lead to the early detection and treatment of the less obvious congenital anomalies. The skilled nurse, in collaboration with the medical staff, is in a position to identify and report possible problems for early diagnosis and appropriate treatment.

Nursery setup

Whether large or small, the hospital offering any maternity service must have a designated area for the careful monitoring of the newly born normal infant. Necessary equipment includes heat sources, such as overhead radiant heaters with thermistor probes, Servo-Control incubators, and resuscitative equipment. Neonates should be grouped to facilitate closer observation by the nursing staff. All personnel in contact with the infant are trained to observe the earliest percepti-

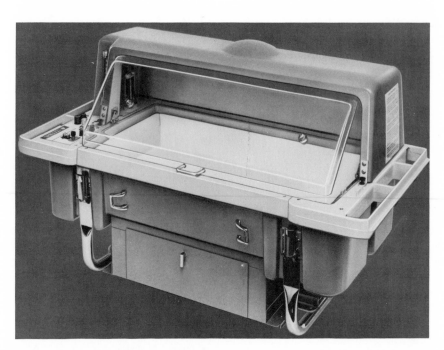

Fig. 32-1. Transport incubator. Compartments contain medications and equipment to administer oxygen and to suction. Unit ensures thermoneutral environment. (Courtesy Air-Shields, Inc., Hatboro, Pa.)

ble changes or signs before life-threatening situations arise.

CONDITIONS NOT READILY APPARENT AT BIRTH

While in the transition or observation nursery, the neonate is observed for any deviations from the norm:

- Hidden congenital anomalies
- Effects of birth trauma or birth anoxia
- Anemia and polycythemia
- Neonatal shock
- Hypoglycemia
- Sepsis

Hidden congenital anomalies

Amount of amniotic fluid. An excessive amount of amniotic fluid, polyhydramnios, is frequently associated with congenital anomalies in the neonate. The infant should be examined closely at the earliest possible time. In the presence of polyhydramnios, any of the following may be suspected:

1. Cephalocaudal malformations
   a. Hydrocephaly
   b. Microcephaly
   c. Anencephaly
   d. Spina bifida
2. Orogastrointestinal malformations
   a. Cleft palate
   b. Esophageal atresia with or without a tracheal fistula
   c. Pyloric stenosis
   d. Volvulus
   e. Imperforate anus
3. Miscellaneous conditions
   a. Down's syndrome
   b. Congenital heart disease
   c. Deformed extremities
   d. Infants of diabetic or prediabetic mothers
4. Prematurity

Oliogohydramnios may be accompanied by agenesis of the ears. In the presence of oligohydramnios, observe for genitourinary tract anomalies, particularly renal agenesis.

Gastrointestinal tract. Screening for gastrointestinal tract malformations is performed on a routine basis for all infants. Obstructions occur in about 1 in 3000 newborns. With proper training the evaluative procedures may be carried out by personnel with various levels of preparation (Table 32-1).

Respiratory tract. Screening for congenital anomalies of the respiratory tract is necessary even for the infant who is apparently normal at birth (Table 32-2).

Table 32-1. Evaluation: gastrointestinal tract

Perinatal criteria	Probable problem
Amount of amniotic fluid	See above
Abdomen	
Scaphoid contour	Diaphragmatic hernia
Distended contour	Tumor, ascites, air (from tracheoesophageal fistula, meconium ileus)
Umbilical vessels (one artery)	Urinary anomaly; chromosome abnormalities (16-19 trisomy)
Advancement of feeding tube prior to first feeding (Fig. 32-2)	Inability to pass tube into stomach suggests esophageal atresia
Stomach contents: color; amount	Fluid more than 25 ml or yellow in color suggests duodenal or ileal atresia
Insertion of rectal thermometer or gloved small finger into rectum (Fig. 32-3)	Inability to pass thermometer suggests imperforate anus, rectal atresia, anal stenosis
Absence of meconium	Probable obstruction; with abdominal distention, probable meconium ileus
Feeding behavior	
Changes in respirations or color	Esophageal or tracheoesophageal anomaly; congenital heart anomalies
Regurgitation of unchanged feeding	Esophageal atresia
Bile-stained or fecal vomiting	Intestinal obstruction

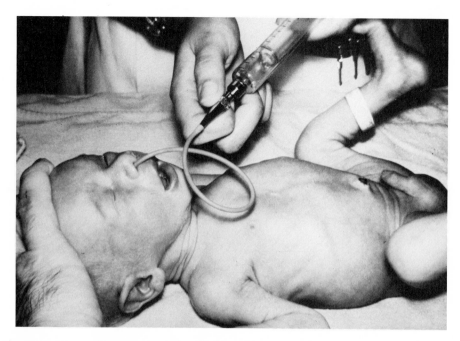

Fig. 32-2. Diagnostic nasogastric intubation. (Courtesy John R. Campbell, M.D., University of Oregon Health Sciences Center, Portland, Ore.)

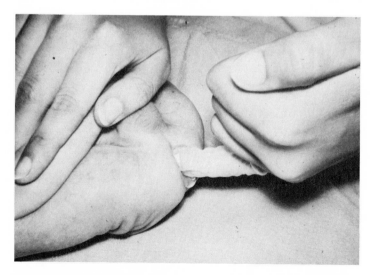

Fig. 32-3. Technique of rectal examination in newborn. (Courtesy John R. Campbell, M.D., University of Oregon. Health Sciences Center, Portland, Ore.)

Respiratory distress (Chapter 33) at birth or shortly thereafter may be due to anomalous development. Congenital laryngeal web and bilateral choanal atresia are readily apparent at birth. Both require emergency surgery (Chapter 35).

Some simple procedures may add substantive data when the neonate exhibits respiratory distress after transfer to the nursery.

Urogenital tract. Careful notation of perinatal events and observations aids in the identification and confirmation of existing congenital anomalies (Table 32-3). To facilitate initiation of a positive parent-child relationship, the sex identity of the neonate must be established as quickly as possible.

Cardiovascular system. Severe congenital cardiovascular disorders often are evident immediately after birth (Table 32-4). These infants usually are transferred directly to special nurseries or pediatric units. Some problems, such as a small patent ductus arteriosus or a minimal coarctation of the descending aorta, become apparent only as the infant is exposed to stresses such as growth demands of later infancy and early childhood, or infection. In about 75% of cases, the cardiovascular anomalies are unexpected.

Neurologic system. Neurologic symptoms may reflect hidden congenital anomalies as well as numerous other conditions. Many neonatal responses are nonspecific. Each symptom must be evaluated carefully

---

Table 32-2. Evaluation: respiratory tract

Perinatal criteria	Probable problem
Polyhydramnios	Orogastrointestinal malformation
Abdomen	
Scaphoid	Diaphragmatic hernia with hypoplastic lung
Distended	Tracheoesophageal fistula
Cyanosis, snoring respirations when at rest; cyanosis is relieved as infant cries	Partial obstruction of posterior nares or unilateral choanal atresia
Stridor	Diaphragmatic hernia
	Vascular rings compressing trachea

Table 32-3. Evaluation: urogenital tract

Perinatal criteria	Probable problem
Voiding	
Absence of, with or without bladder distention	Lack of voiding suggests agenesis of all or part of urinary tract; rectal or vaginal fistulas
With distressed crying	Stenosis of urinary meatus
Oligohydramnios with or without low placement of ears	Urinary tract abnormality
Anatomic appearance	
Meatal placement	Hypospadias or epispadias in male
Adequacy of size of opening	Stenosis is possible in male or female
Phimosis in male	May affect ability to void; may be cause of infant colic
Ambiguous genitals	Chromosomal studies are necessary; parental concern about not knowing sex of child
Absence of testes in scrotum in term neonate; make sure baby is not cold; testes will retract in cold (cremasteric reflex)	Rule out genitourinary tract anomaly
Low-set ears	Probable renal agenesis

Table 32-4. Evaluation: cardiovascular system

Perinatal criteria	Probable problem
Prematurity: 37 weeks or less and 2500 gm or less	Increased incidence of anomalous cardiovascular system development
Obstetric history	
Thalidomide ingestion	Cardiomyopathy
Rubella; coxsackievirus, type B	Incidence is 50% if infected in first trimester
High altitude	Patent ductus arteriosus (PDA)
Diabetes	Variable problems
Major chromosomal disorders	
Down's syndrome	Incidence 40% of cardiovascular problems
Turner's syndrome	Incidence 44% of cardiovascular problems
Neonate's spontaneous activity and response to stimuli absent or reduced (e.g., flaccid, apathetic)	Myocarditis; left heart hypoplasia
Breathing patterns	
Tachypnea at rest	
Full-term infant, 45/min or more	
Low birth weight infant, 60/min or more	
Increased depth of respiration	Cyanotic heart disease
Flaring of alae nasi	Heart disease with pulmonary overcirculation
Apneic spells	Left heart hypoplasia with hypoglycemia
Arterial pulses; blood pressure	
Radial, posterior tibial, dorsalis pedis, and femoral pulses not readily palpable	Variety of stenoses, coarctation
Discrepancy of blood pressure in extremities	Aortic coarctation
Pitting edema on backs of hands and dorsa of feet	Heart failure
Physical signs	Heart failure
Tachypnea at rest with no respiratory distress	
Tachycardia at rest (180/min or more)	
Feeding difficulties, such as poor suck and fatigability	
Peripheral edema	
Sweating at room temperature	
Gallop rhythm	

before appropriate therapy may be instituted (Table 32-5).

One of the therapeutic contributions the nurse can make is to identify the neonate who is "just not right," even when there is a negative antenatal history or unreported laboratory or other data. This feeling that something may be wrong is the beginning of the statement of a hypothesis. The nurse thus alerted can mobilize and initiate further diagnostic procedures to institute corrective or palliative therapy.

Effects of birth trauma or birth anoxia

All newborns, but particularly those exposed to dystotic labor or delivery or both, are observed closely for associated birth injuries. The nurse's critical contributions to the welfare of the newborn are early observation, accurate recording, and prompt reporting of signs in-

dicative of deviations from normal. Of equal importance is the nurse's support of the parents of the infant with birth injury (pp. 99 to 101). Some of the most common neonatal birth injuries and the accepted therapies are presented on the following pages.

Cephalhematoma. Cephalhematoma is a collection of blood between the skullbone and its periosteum. Cephalhematoma is due to pressure during a delivery. This bleeding may occur with spontaneous delivery (from pressure against the maternal bony pelvis) or easy forceps delivery, as well as difficult forceps rotation and extraction. This soft, fluctuating, irreducible fullness does not pulsate or bulge when the infant cries. A cephalhematoma never crosses a cranial suture line (Fig. 32-4). It appears several hours after birth or the day after delivery or becomes apparent following absorption of a caput succedaneum. It is usually largest on the

Table 32-5. Evaluation: neurologic system

Perinatal criteria	Possible problem
Obstetric history 　Preterm neonate 　Drug addiction 　History of congenital malformations in family or in 　　other children Neonate's symptomatology 　Need for resuscitation at birth 　Gestational age and weight 　Muscle tone: hypotonia; hypertonia 　Reflexes: absent; difficult to elicit; hyperreflexia 　Response to stimuli: poor; absent; exaggerated 　Cry: high-pitched; weak; abnormal sounding 　Excitability: jitteriness; seizure activity 　Activity: hyperactive; lethargic 　Feeding behavior: poor 　Low-set ears	This listing not matched to specific perinatal criteria; 　range of possible problems includes following: 　Malformations 　　Hydrocephalus 　　Microcephaly 　Kernicterus 　Chromosomal aberration; probable mental retar- 　　dation 　　Down's syndrome 　　Cri du chat syndrome 　Infection: sepsis 　Hypoglycemia 　Drug dependency 　Increased intracranial pressure 　　Hydrocephalus 　　Hemorrhage 　　Neoplasm 　　Infection: sepsis

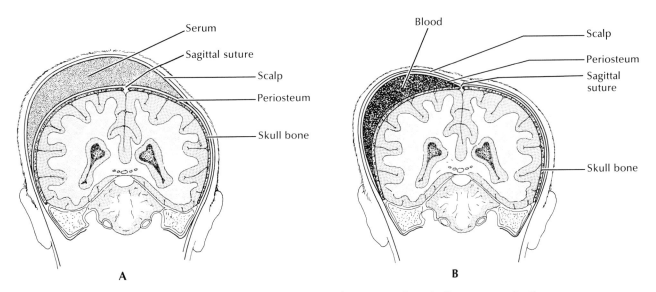

Fig. 32-4. Differences between caput succedaneum and cephalhematoma. **A,** Caput succedaneum: edema of scalp noted at birth and crosses suture lines. **B,** Cephalhematoma: bleeding between periosteum and skullbone, appears within first 2 days, and does not cross suture lines.

second or third day when the bleeding stops. The fullness of cephalhematoma spontaneously resolves in 3 to 6 weeks. It is not aspirated, or infection may develop.

Nursing care is directed primarily to supporting the parents. The physician's explanations may need to be reaffirmed, that is, the bleeding is not into the brain and

no treatment is warranted. The parents may need to talk about their reactions to having a child with a misshapen head, albeit a temporary disfigurement.

Hyperbilirubinemia may occur as the hematoma resolves. Jaundice may not appear until the neonate is home. Therefore the parents are instructed to observe the newborn for jaundice and may be asked to bring the infant in to be rechecked prior to the usual 4-week schedule.

Intracranial hemorrhage. Birth trauma and hypoxia are the most common causes of intracranial hemorrhage, and premature infants are especially prone to this condition. Subarachnoid hemorrhage (bleeding into the cerebrospinal fluid) or dural bleeding (cerebrospinal fluid clear) may develop.

The hemorrhage may occur anywhere within the cranial vault. Tears in the tentorial membrane result in bleeding into the cerebellum, pons, or medulla oblongata; the prognosis is grave. Regulatory centers for respiratory control and muscle movement and coordination are located within these structures.

The symptoms of intracranial hemorrhage are generally noted immediately after birth but may not be seen until several hours or days later. Abnormal respiration with cyanosis, reduced responsiveness, irritability, opisthotonos, high-pitched shrill cry, tense fontanel, twitching, or convulsions may be noted. Twitching of the lower jaw with salivation often is a sign of convulsions. A positive Moro reflex, present at birth but which disappears later, or a negative Moro reflex from birth may be recorded. Actual paralysis is a later development of intracranial hemorrhage.

The cerebrospinal fluid pressure may be elevated with intracranial hemorrhage. Normal infants may have occasional red blood cells in the cerebrospinal fluid, but bloody fluid suggests gross subarachnoid hemorrhage or a traumatic tap.

Treatment consists of elevation of the head several inches higher than the hips, warmth, oxygen to relieve cyanosis, vitamins K and C to assist in controlling hemorrhage, and intravenous fluids or other suitable method of meeting the neonate's food and fluid needs. Subdural hemorrhage requires repeated evacuation, especially if the head size is increasing and the fontanel is bulging. Prophylactic antibiotic therapy has many advocates, but few authorities recommend repeat spinal taps to reduce pressure. Therapy for hyperbilirubinemia may be required. Recovery depends on the extent and location of the hemorrhage and the degree of CNS damage, as well as other complications such as atelectasis. Minimal handling to promote rest guides nursing care.

The newborn's prognosis is grave, and death may ensue at any time. Survivors may develop cerebral palsy, mental retardation, or both. Therefore avoid reassuring statements. Couch statements in terms such as, "He is responding to therapy at this time"; "Her vital signs are stable this morning." Adequate explanation and active listening are important functions in the supportive care of parents.

Fracture of clavicle. The clavicle is the bone most often fractured during delivery. Generally the break is in the middle third of the bone. Dystocia, particularly shoulder impaction, may be the predisposing problem. Limitation of motion of the arm, crepitus of the bone, and absent Moro reflex on the affected side are diagnostic. Treatment requires immobilization of the shoulder and arm. Immobilization is usually by a "figure-of-eight" bandage to hold the shoulders in good alignment. The prognosis is good.

The humerus and femur are other bones that may be fractured during difficult deliveries. Fractures in newborns heal rapidly as a rule. Immobilization is accomplished with slings, splints, swaddling, and other devices. The parents need support in handling these infants because they are often fearful of hurting them. Parents are encouraged to practice handling, changing, and feeding the affected newborns so that their confidence and knowledge are assured and bonding is facilitated. A plan for follow-up therapy is developed with the parents so that the times and arrangements for checkups for therapy are workable and acceptable to them, as well as to those providing the therapy.

Brachial palsy. Paralysis of the arm may be high (Erb-Duchenne) because of damage to the spinal nerve C5-6 or lower (Klumpke) from injury to C7 and T1. These nerves course down the neck through the shoulder toward the arm. Injury may occur with excessive stretching of the neck during delivery. Although it is more frequently seen with breech delivery, occasionally vertex delivery may result in this injury. Erb-Duchenne paralysis is the most common (Fig. 32-5).

A flaccid arm with the elbow extended and the hand rotated inward, a negative Moro reflex on the affected side, sensory loss over the lateral aspect of the arm, and an intact grasp reflex are typical of upper arm brachial palsy.

Treatment consists of intermittent immobilization, proper positioning, and exercise to maintain the range of motion of joints. Gentle manipulation and range of motion exercises are delayed until about the tenth day to prevent additional injury to the brachial plexus.

Immobilization may be accomplished with a brace or splint or by pinning the infant's sleeve to the mattress. Position for 2 to 3 hours at a time in the following manner: abduct arm 90 degrees, externally rotate the shoulder; flex the elbow 90 degrees; supinate the wrist with palm directed slightly toward the face (Fig. 32-6). The arm should be free periodically for good skin care. About the tenth day, gentle massage and range of motion exercises are begun to prevent contractures.

With lower arm paralysis, the wrist and hand are flaccid, the grasp reflex is absent, deep tendon reflexes

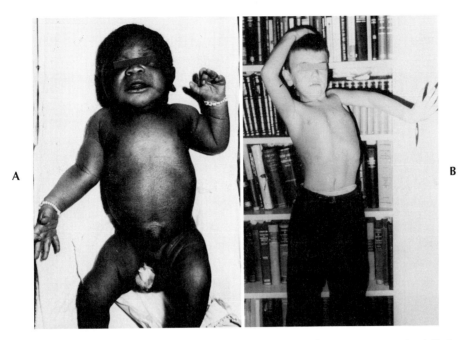

Fig. 32-5. A, Erb-Duchenne palsy in newborn infant. Right upper extremity failed to participate in Moro response. Recovery was complete. **B,** Residual of Erb-Duchenne paralysis. Left arm was short; it could not be raised above level shown. (From Shirkey, H. C. [ed.]. 1975. Pediatric therapy [ed. 5]. St. Louis, The C. V. Mosby Co.)

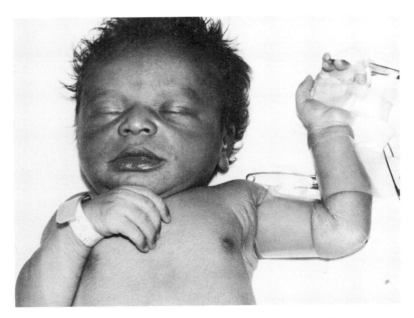

Fig. 32-6. Recommended corrective positioning for treatment of Erb-Duchenne. Note abduction and external rotation at shoulder, flexion at elbow, supination of forearm, and slight dorsiflexion at wrist. (From Behrman, R. E. [ed.]. 1973. Neonatology: diseases of the fetus and infant. St. Louis, The C. V. Mosby Co.)

are present, and dependent edema and cyanosis may be apparent (in the affected hand). Treatment consists of placing the hand in a neutral position, padding the fist, and gently exercising the wrist and fingers.

Parents are taught to position and immobilize the arm and/or wrist and to gently massage and manipulate the muscles to prevent contractures while the arm is healing. If edema or hemorrhage are responsible for the paralysis, the prognosis is good, and recovery may be expected in a few weeks. If laceration of the nerves has occurred and healing does not result in return of function within a few months (3 to 6 months or 2 years at the most), surgery may be indicated; little or no function will develop, however.

Phrenic nerve injury (diaphragmatic paralysis). Lateral hyperextension of the neck during difficult breech delivery may result in injury to spinal roots C3-5. Cyanosis and irregular thoracic respirations with no abdominal movement on inspiration are characteristic of paralysis of the diaphragm. Paralysis is usually one-sided (hemidiaphragmatic). Diagnosis is confirmed by x-ray visualization of the elevated diaphragm and consequent displacement of the thoracic organs.

Treatment is nonspecific: position the neonate on the involved side, administer oxygen as needed, and provide food and fluids by the route best suited for the infant (intravenously, gavage, nipple). Most infants recover spontaneously within 6 weeks to a year. Untreated, many infants succumb to pneumonia in the atelectatic lung during the first 3 months. Surgery to tighten and thereby lower the diaphragm may be necessary for the infant with severe respiratory distress. Infants generally do well after surgery, even if the phrenic nerve is permanently damaged.

This condition frequently accompanies brachial plexus injury.

Facial palsy (Fig. 32-7). Facial palsy is generally due to misapplication of forceps and pressure by one blade against the facial nerve during delivery. The face on the affected side is flattened and unresponsive to the grimace of crying or stimulation, and the eye may remain open. Moreover, the forehead will not wrinkle. Often the condition is transitory, resolving within hours or days of birth. Permanent paralysis is rare.

Treatment involves careful, patient feeding, prevention of damage to the cornea of the open eye, and supportive care of the parents. Frequently, the infant looks grotesque, especially when crying. Feeding may be prolonged with the formula flowing out of the neonate's mouth around the nipple on the affected side. The mother may need understanding and sympathetic encouragement while learning how to feed and care for the infant and to hold and cuddle the infant.

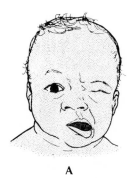
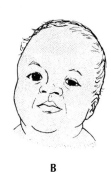

A   **B**

Fig. 32-7. A, Paralysis of left side of face 15 minutes after forceps delivery. **B,** Same infant 24 hours later. Recovery was complete in another 24 hours.

Hematologic status: anemia and polycythemia

Anemia. Neonatal anemia may be difficult to recognize by clinical evaluation alone. Anemia may be due to hypovolemia. The causes of hypovolemia include the following:

1. Placenta previa or abruptio placentae
2. Bleeding from the umbilical cord, for example, caused by holding the infant higher than the placenta prior to the cessation of pulsation in the cord
3. Iatrogenic factors, for example, incision of placenta during a cesarean section

Polycythemia. Polycythemia is not fully understood. The most likely cause is iatrogenic, such as "milking" the cord prior to clamping and cutting the cord or holding the neonate below the level of the placenta prior to cessation of pulsation in the cord. Other possible causes are infection and cardiovascular anomaly. Polycythemia increases blood viscosity, thereby diminishing perfusion of tissues and adding to the cardiac workload. Intravascular coagulation may occur.

Neonatal shock

Signs of hypovolemic shock are similar to those of asphyxia. The infant who has suffered an acute hemorrhage generally has the following symptoms at birth:

- Pallor with cyanosis
- Tachycardia
- Tachypnea
- Gasping breaths
- Retractions
- Feeble or absent pulses
- Weak cry
- Absent or diminished spontaneous movements
- Hypotonia

Immediate transfusion is lifesaving. Proper treatment is predicated on correct diagnosis. Clinical differentiation often may be accomplished by assessing the three criteria shown below.

	Hypovolemic shock	**Asphyxia**
Heart rate	160/min (unless hypoxic)	Bradycardia
Cyanosis	Unrelieved by oxygen	Relieved by oxygen
Respiratory rate	Rapid	Slow

Sepsis

The high-risk infant is more susceptible than the normal term infant to infection for the following reasons:

1. Paucity of energy reserves
2. Exposure to many tests and treatments (e.g., injections, suctioning, resuscitative measures), which may compromise his resistance further
3. Coexisting energy-consuming conditions such as respiratory distress or sepsis

Hypoglycemia

Definition. Blood sugar is 45% or less in term infants and 20% or less in premature infants.

Symptoms. The following symptoms evidence CNS disturbance:

1. Feeding difficulty, hunger
2. Apnea
3. Irregular respiratory effort
4. Cyanosis
5. Weak, high-pitched cry
6. Jitteriness, twitching, eye-rolling, convulsions
7. Lethargy

Infants at risk. Those infants who are more vulnerable to hypoglycemia include the following:

1. Low birth weight infants
2. Dysmature infants
3. Infants of diabetic or prediabetic mothers
4. Infants of preeclamptic-eclamptic mothers
5. Polycythemic infants
6. Cold infants

Prevention. Do Dextrostix test on admission to nursery and initiate early infant feeding. Term infants may be fed at 6 to 12 hours of age or earlier, as necessary. Small neonates or those born of diabetic mothers may need to be fed at 1 hour of age.

PLAN OF CARE: HEMATOLOGIC STATUS—ANEMIA AND POLYCYTHEMIA

PATIENT CARE OBJECTIVES

1. There is adequate perfusion and ventilation of tissues.
2. There are no episodes of hypoglycemia.

NURSING INTERVENTIONS

Diagnostic	Therapeutic and educational
Anemia	
1. Heel stick before 1 hour of age. Infant is anemic if (a) Hct is below 40% or (b) Hct is between 40% and 50%. Watch this baby closely, so as to note drop below 40%. 2. Skin color is pale.	1. Do transfusion with fresh,* whole, adult blood, 10 to 20 ml/kg or exchange transfusion with 100 to 200 ml blood. See procedure on exchange transfusion (p. 626). 2. Observe. 3. Put neonate on constant cardiac/respiratory monitor, or monitor manually continuously. Assemble equipment for intubation, blood transfusion, and umbilical catheterization.
Polycythemia	
1. Venous (central) Hct is 60% or more; in severe polycythemia, Hct is 70% or more. 2. Hypoglycemia. 3. Plethora (deep red skin color) at rest or duskiness (cyanosis) when crying. 4. Episodes of apnea or respiratory distress. 5. Poor feeding. 6. Jaundice or hyperbilirubinemia.	1. Partial exchange transfusion with fresh, frozen plasma may be done. 2. Phlebotomy with electrolyte and fluid replacement may be done, but phlebotomy alone is unacceptable. 3. Hypoglycemia with polycythemia is intractable (e.g., does not respond to therapy). 4. Feed by gavage if necessary. 5. Observe for apnea (use monitor); stimulate infant to breathe as necessary. 6. Assist parents in coping with situation.

*Enzyme, 2,3-diphosphoglycerate (2,3-DPG), which facilitates release of oxygen from red blood cells into tissues, is present in fresh blood. 2,3-DPG is not present in infant blood or adult blood over 24 hours old.

PLAN OF CARE: NEONATAL SHOCK

PATIENT CARE OBJECTIVE

1. Neonate survives hypovolemic shock with no adverse sequelae.

NURSING INTERVENTIONS

Diagnostic	Therapeutic

1. Observe for symptoms (p. 520).
2. Assess infant's response to administration of O_2.
3. Observe infant's response to umbilical catheterization and transfusion (pp. 626 and 627).
	1. Record observations accurately and thoroughly. If assessing infant at home, transfer to hospital immediately.
	2. Assist physician.
	  a. Resuscitation: Provide warmth, suction, O_2; accurately monitor and record neonate's responses.
	  b. Transfusion:
	    (1) Order blood typing and cross matching immediately.
	    (2) Obtain transfusion setup.
	    (3) Assist with transfusion (p. 626).
	    (4) Maintain accurate record of transfusion and neonate's response.
	3. Support parents: keep them informed, promote eye contact with and attachment to infant, and encourage expression of feelings and questions.

PLAN OF CARE: SEPSIS

PATIENT CARE OBJECTIVES

1. Sepsis is prevented if possible.
2. Sepsis is recognized and treated early with minimal or no adverse sequelae:
   a. Appropriate weight gain is maintained.
   b. Absence of fluid-electrolyte imbalance.
   c. Absence of untoward reactions to medications.
   d. No neurologic or other sequelae.

NURSING INTERVENTIONS

Diagnostic	Therapeutic and educational*

1. Assess perinatal history:
  a. Maternal signs and symptoms of infection, venereal or other.
  b. Amniocentesis.
  c. Premature rupture of membranes.
  d. Character (odor, color) of amniotic fluid.
  e. Prolonged labor.
  f. Operative delivery, such as forceps rotation and extraction or cesarean section.
  g. Resuscitative measures employed after delivery.
  h. "Born out of asepsis" (BOA).
  i. Internal fetal monitoring during labor.
2. Assess neonate's signs.
  a. Feeding:
    (1) Poor suck.†
    (2) Anorexia.
    (3) Regurgitation of feedings.
    (4) Diarrhea.
	1. Personnel health practices: No personnel should work with infants if they have any infection (e.g., sore throat, "cold sore" [herpes simplex 2 causes serious illness in neonates], gastrointestinal upset).
	2. Be alert to possible complications associated with perinatal events.
	3. Take cultures of infant's skin: groin and axillas, any suspicious lesions, or site of electrode attachment to fetal scalp. Send oropharyngeal aspirate to laboratory.
	4. Isolate any infant who is suspect.
	5. Provide incubator care: heat, O_2 as needed, isolation. In incubator, infant can be exposed for better visualization.
	6. Assist respirations: Position on side, change position at least every hour, suction as needed, administer O_2 to relieve cyanosis, pass nasogastric tube to relieve abdominal distention, gently stimulate when apneic.
	7. Assist with and record treatments; record infant's re-

*Also see pp. 602 to 607 for discussion of neonatal infections.
†Cardinal symptom of sepsis.

PLAN OF CARE: SEPSIS—cont'd

NURSING INTERVENTIONS—cont'd

Diagnostic	Therapeutic and educational

b. Lack of weight gain, weight loss, dehydration.

c. Neurologic:

    (1) Lethargy, especially if it develops after 24 hours of age.†

    (2) Irritability.

    (3) Hyperreflexia or hyporeflexia.

    (4) Tremors, convulsive activity.

d. Color:

    (1) Jaundice.†

    (2) Pallor.

    (3) Cyanosis.

    (4) Hemorrhage into skin—petechiae.

e. Temperature: may show drop >1° to 2° F or an increase of >1° F.

f. Respirations:

    (1) Bradypnea.

    (2) Apneic episodes.

g. Shock: cool, clammy skin.

3. Assess infant's reactions to treatment.

4. Vital signs: Use assessment checkoff list every hour until signs are stable (Table 30-1 and Appendix K).

sponse and modify treatment as necessary.

a. Parenteral fluids; monitor degree of hydration.

b. Intake and output.

c. Weigh every 8, 12, or 24 hours, as ordered.

d. Medications.

e. Blood gases, bilirubin level, and pH.

f. Lumbar punctures, blood cultures, Bili-Lite, other procedures

8. Observe for and give supportive care during convulsive activity.

9. Keep parents informed.

PLAN OF CARE: HYPOGLYCEMIA

PATIENT CARE OBJECTIVES

1. There are no hypoglycemic episodes.
2. There is no brain damage.

NURSING INTERVENTIONS

Diagnostic	Therapeutic

1. Heel stick: Dextrostix, Clinistix.

a. Frequency of test is determined by condition of neonate:

    (1) For normal term infant, test is done at 45 minutes, 2 hours, and 6 hours of age.

    (2) For the infant at risk, test is done at following intervals:

30 minutes of age	9 hours of age
1½ hours of age	12 hours of age
2½ hours of age	24 hours of age
4 hours of age	Once daily for 8 days
6 hours of age	

b. Blood sugar is ≤45% in term infant and ≤20% in premature infant. Order blood sugar test by lab immediately.

2. Symptoms of hypoglycemia.

1. Feed 10% glucose orally. This procedure may be done by nurse.

2. Administer 15% to 20% glucose in water intravenously (done by physician).

REFERENCES

Behrman, R. E. (ed.). 1973. Neonatology: diseases of the fetus and infant. St. Louis, The C. V. Mosby Co.

Shirkey, H. C. (ed.). 1975. Pediatric therapy. ed. 5. St. Louis, The C. V. Mosby Co.

Van Leeuwen, G. 1973. The nurse in prevention and intervention in the neonatal period. Nurs. Clin. North Am. **8:** 509.

CHAPTER 33

Therapeutic approach to infant at risk

Neonatal intensive care challenges the health team's modes of curative, protective, and nurturant approaches and techniques. The high-risk infant is subject to the same problems that the normal newborn faces, which may be compounded by those related to development and maturity. Health care must support the high-risk newborn's basic functioning while compensating for his inadequacies and weaknesses (Fig. 33-1). "Normal" values and parameters vary with the infant's level of maturity and his developmental problems. Assessment and therefore supportive care are complicated further by the infant's inability to speak and his nonspecific, generalized responses to dysfunctional problems. Assessment rests heavily on historical data provided by the mother and obstetric team and on current levels of knowledge related to gestational age, dysfunctions, and disorders of the neonate. In addition to the emotional aspects of development, the physiologic maintenance of warmth, respiration, and nutrition are discussed in this chapter.

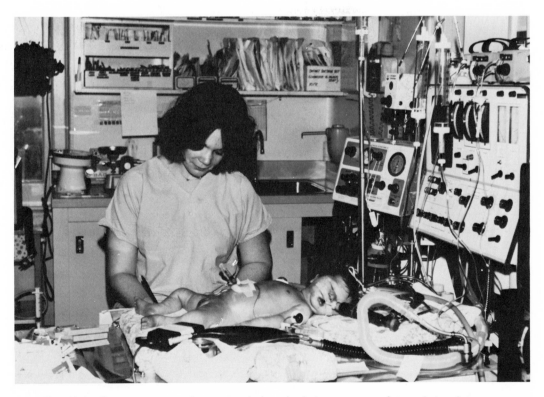

Fig. 33-1. One-to-one nursing around the clock is essence of true intensive care. (Courtesy Mount Zion Hospital and Medical Center, San Francisco, Calif.)

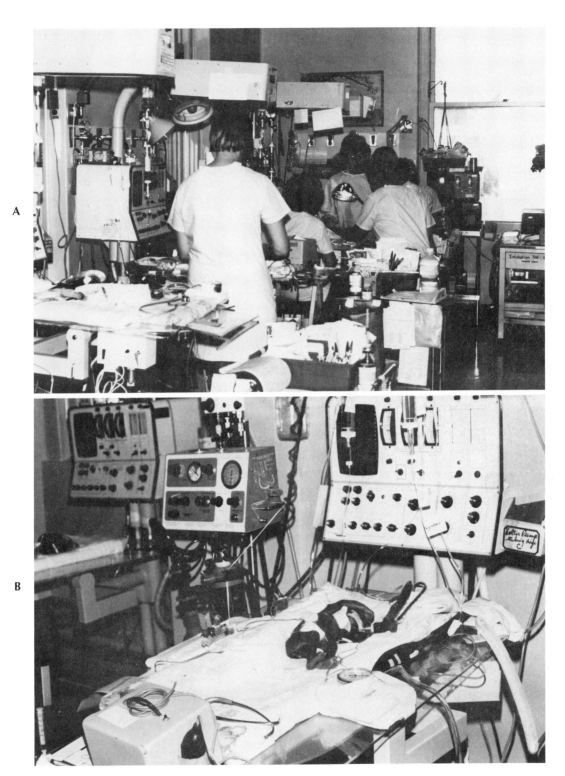

Fig. 33-2. A, Intensive care requires close cooperation of physicians and nurses working in maze of equipment. **B,** 1000 gm infant receiving intensive care. (Courtesy Mount Zion Hospital and Medical Center, San Francisco, Calif.)

EMOTIONAL ASPECTS OF CARE
Neonate's emotional needs

Premature and sick infants have at least the same emotional developmental needs as those of the normal term infant. It may be difficult for the infant at risk to meet his developmental needs. The sick infant who needs intravenous therapy, nasogastric feedings, heel sticks, oxygen by plastic hood, or continuous positive airway pressure cannot be cuddled, fondled, or played with as can the term infant. Instead he must experience many painful stimuli, including numerous intrusive procedures such as electronic leads taped to and removed from his chest wall, blurred views through the plastic walls of the incubator, and a cacophony of sounds inside his closed-in world (e.g., motors, hiss of oxygen).

Without adequate attention to his emotional and developmental needs, the premature and sick infant exposed to these life-supportive measures and separated from a constant mothering and comforting person, may begin to show signs of great anxiety and tension, including the following:

- Failure to thrive (slow or absent recovery, growth, weight gain)
- Looking away from or to the side of the people who are caring for him
- Absent, weak, or infrequent crying (as if to say, "What's the use?")

Supportive care

The infant's sense of trust develops when he learns the feel, sound, and smell of the same mothering person who comforts him and who removes uncomfortable stimuli (e.g., hunger, wet or soiled clothing). He even learns to anticipate these happenings. He soon learns that his cries bring this mothering person. These conditions cannot be duplicated in the nursery, but some modifications often can be made in the nursing care plan. In the technologic environment of a premature or sick baby nursery (Figs. 33-2 and 33-3), nursing's focus must be on people, not on equipment. The possibilities are limited only by the parameters of human creativity. Following are some suggestions:

1. Assign one nurse per shift to be the identifiable person caring for the infant.

2. Schedule time from treatments to stroke the infant's skin. The parent(s) may touch the infant through portholes.

3. Insert mobiles and decals that can be changed frequently inside the incubator.

4. Respond to his efforts to cry by reassuring him and

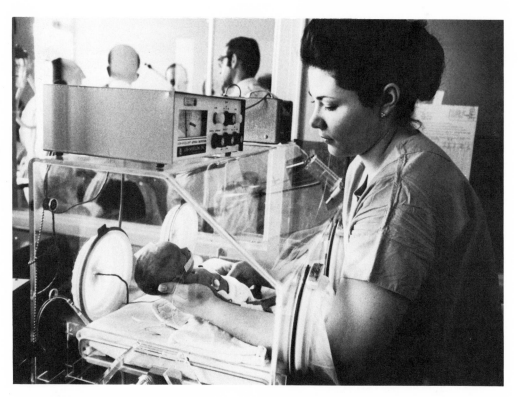

Fig. 33-3. Isolette infant incubator. (Courtesy Air-Shields, Inc., Hatboro, Pa.)

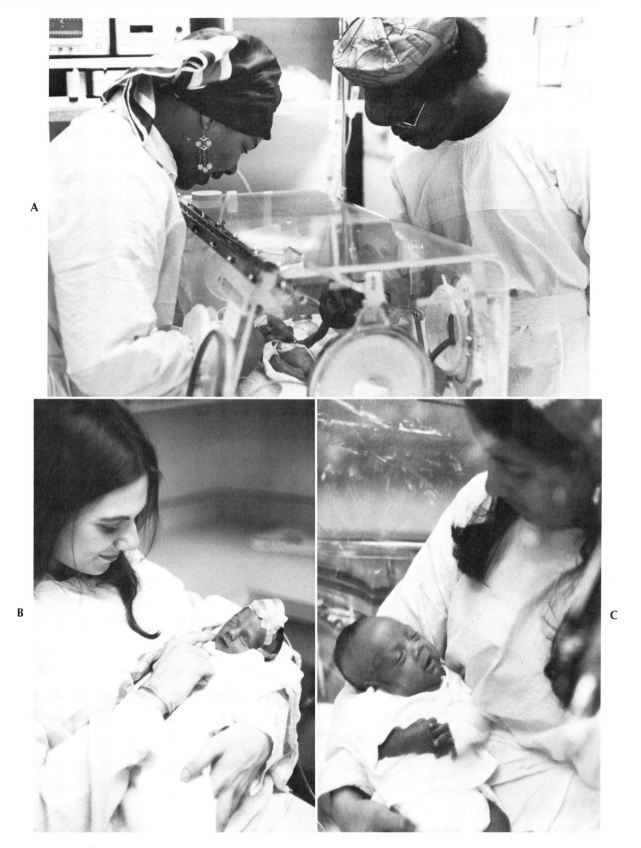

Fig. 33-4. Parents are actively encouraged to visit, touch, and, when possible, hold their premature babies. There is no restriction on visiting hours. **A,** Note father with one hand in incubator holding infant's hand. **B,** Note mother's tentative fingertip exploration of infant. **C,** Infant's response to mother aids in mother-infant bonding. Note infant's shaved head where intravenous fluids had been given. (Courtesy Children's Hospital of San Francisco, Newborn Intensive Care Unit; photo by Patricia Ryan, R.N.)

offering a pacifier while stroking and talking to the infant.

5. When the infant can tolerate being out of the incubator, even for short periods of time, remove him, cuddle and rock him, and sing to him, especially during his feedings—even when feeding by gavage or gastrostomy. Or take him out and hold him while helping him raise bubbles of air from his stomach. If the mother (or father) is able to visit frequently, she and the infant benefit immeasurably from this activity (Fig. 33-4).

6. If the infant must have feedings by gavage or gastrostomy, offer a pacifier during the feeding process (in the absence of respiratory distress). He will get sucking satisfaction and begin to associate this pleasant, self-gratifying, and self-initiated activity with the comforting feeling of a filling stomach.

7. Talk, sing, and hum to him whenever possible. Avoid loud talking and excessive discordant noise around the newborns. Some nurseries permit the placement of windup musical box toys in the incubator or crib.

8. Hold the newborn so that he can see your face. Focus your eyes on his as you talk or sing to him.

9. Even if the infant is undergoing phototherapy, some time out from under the lamp is possible. Remove his blindfold so that he can see your face or the parent's face during periodic, short, comforting sessions.

PHYSICAL ASPECTS OF CARE
Warmth and thermogenesis

General considerations. Effective neonatal care is predicated on the maintenance of an optimal thermal environment. In homoiothermic individuals, the narrow limits of normal body temperature are maintained by producing heat in response to its dissipation. Hypothermia due to excessive heat loss is a prevalent and dangerous problem in neonates. Although the newborn infant's ability to produce heat often approaches the capacity of the adult, his tendency toward rapid heat loss in a suboptimal thermal environment is increased and often hazardous to his well-being.

The neonate rarely can generate heat through shivering. Thermogenesis is accomplished primarily by increased metabolic activity in the brain, heart, and liver. An additional source of heat, unique to the newborn, is *brown fat*. Thermogenic activity of brown fat is greater than ordinary fat, and brown fat has a richer vascular and nerve supply. Heat produced by intense lipid metabolic activity can warm the neonate. Reserves of brown fat, usually present for several weeks after birth, are rapidly depleted with cold stress. The less mature the infant, the less reserve he has of this essential fat at birth.

Cold stress. Cold stress imposes metabolic and physiologic problems on all infants, regardless of gestational age and condition. Oxygen consumption and energy in the cold-stressed infant are diverted from maintaining normal brain cell and cardiac function and growth to thermogenesis for survival.

If the infant cannot maintain an adequate oxygen tension, vasoconstriction follows and jeopardizes pulmonary perfusion. As a consequence, certain blood gases exceed normal limits ($Po_2\downarrow$, $Pco_2\uparrow$), and the blood pH drops. These changes aggravate existing respiratory distress syndrome (RDS), or hyaline membrane disease (HMD). Moreover, decreased pulmonary perfusion and oxygen tension may maintain or reopen the right-to-left vascular shunt of fetal circulation.

The basal metabolic rate will be increased with cold stress, and if protracted, anaerobic glycolysis occurs, resulting in increased production of acids. Metabolic acidosis and respiratory acidosis develop. Excessive fatty acids combine with bilirubin, thus increasing the risk of kernicterus even at serum bilirubin levels of 10 mg/100 ml or less.

Temperature regulation. Anatomic and physiologic differences between the neonate, child, and adult are notable:

1. The neonate's thermal insulation is less. The blood vessels are closer to the surface of the skin. Changes in environmental temperature alter that of blood, thereby influencing temperature-regulating centers in the hypothalamus.

2. The neonate has a larger body surface to body weight (mass) ratio.

3. Vasomotor control is less well developed in the neonate.

4. Heat is produced primarily by nonshivering thermogenesis.

5. Although present, the neonate's sweat glands have little homoiothermic function until the fourth week or later of extrauterine life.

The normal term infant, in response to lower environmental temperature, may try to increase his body temperature by crying, by increasing his respiratory rate, or by increased motor activity. His usual flexed position also is a safeguard against heat loss. Crying increases his work load, and the cost of energy (calories) may be expensive.

The premature infant is less capable of controlling temperature than the normal infant at term because of the following:

1. Relatively larger surface area per body weight
2. Paucity of subcutaneous tissues (including brown fat) and muscle mass

3. Limited sweat and shiver response
4. Limited glycogen stores
5. Nonflexed posture
6. Inactivity

The infant in respiratory distress (poor oxygenation) or suffering from intrauterine malnutrition (diminished glycogen stores) is severely compromised with the additional stress of chilling. An increased metabolic rate potentiates any existing respiratory acidosis.

In the presence of oxygen deprivation (arterial P_{O_2} 40 mm Hg or less), the infant's metabolic response to chilling is depressed or eliminated.

Dissipation of body heat. Body heat is dissipated through evaporation, radiation, convection, and conduction. (See discussions on normal newborn bathing on p. 468, technique for regulation of warmth and humidity in infant's environment on p. 615, and techniques for maintaining thermoneutral environment on pp. 616 to 618.)

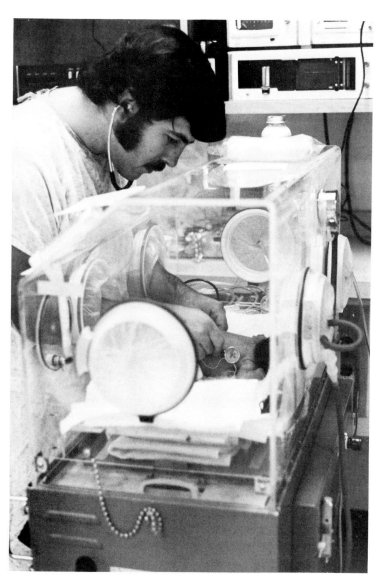

Fig. 33-5. Examination of sick preterm infant. The baby can be examined within the incubator without cooling or altering ambient oxygen. (Courtesy Children's Hospital of San Francisco, Newborn Intensive Care Unit; photo by Patricia Ryan, R.N.)

PLAN OF CARE: TEMPERATURE SUPPORT AND REGULATION

PATIENT CARE OBJECTIVES
1. Skin temperature is maintained at 36.1° ± 0.5° C (97° ± 1° F).
2. No apneic spells of ≥15 seconds occur.
3. Adequate weight is gained.
4. Sequelae of cold stress do not develop, i.e., sclerema, oxygen deprivation to tissues, metabolic acidosis, hypoglycemia, abnormal blood gases, and dysfunction of CNS.

NURSING INTERVENTIONS

Diagnostic	Therapeutic

---

1. Know anatomy and physiology of infant, principles of heat loss, conditions of environment that affect heat loss and its conservation.

1. Nursing care should be planned and implemented to prevent or minimize cold stress.
   a. Quickly dry newly born infant in warm, absorbent blanket, taking particular care to dry and cover head (one fourth of body length). (If infant is of good weight and in good condition, he may be given to mother to hold). Prevent cold air from blowing over face. Receptors in facial skin are exquisitely sensitive to cold.
   b. Place wrapped infant in warm incubator, Krieslman, or other heated carrier. Infant may be placed unwrapped under radiant heat shield.
   c. All procedures and observations on unwrapped infant are done in incubator, under radiant heat, on warm surfaces, etc. (Fig. 33-5).
   d. All surfaces and materials touching infant are warm.
   e. Bath is given taking precaution to prevent cold stress.
   f. Caretakers' hands should be warm when handling neonate.
   g. O_2 or air administered to infant is warmed.
   h. Warm oral feedings.

2. Determine infant's temperature by monitoring following (pp. 616 to 618):
   a. Overhead radiant heat shield with thermistor probe to skin.
   b. Servo-Control incubator.
      (1) Thermistor probe taped to skin.
      (2) Thermometer on incubator wall.
   c. Anal (core) temperature.
   d. Axillary temperature.
   e. Coolness or warmth to touch of infant's body and extremities.

2. Maintain equipment in excellent operative condition. Know procedures and rationale for procedures.
   a. Maintain abdominal skin temperature at 35.1° ± 0.5° C (97° ± 1° F), axillary temperature at 36.5° C (97.8° F).
      (1) Report any rise in temperature over 37.3° C (99° F) or a drop of 0.6° to 1° C (1° to 2° F).
   b. Equipment is plugged in and operative. Thermostat is set on control panel. Probe is in contact with skin. Portholes and lid are closed. Incubator is placed away from windows, air conditioning units, etc.
   c. Know procedures: anal temperature; axillary.
   d. Place bassinet away from drafts, sources of heat, or cold. Take temperatures by thermometer periodically to check accuracy of equipment.

3. High or low core temperature:
   a. Recheck temperature after completing therapeutic interventions.
   b. Observe for other signs, symptoms (color, behavior).
   c. Evaluate environment and procedures on infant for excessive sensory stimulation (tactile, auditory, bright lights).
   d. If no change, notify physician of findings.

3. Alter environment to return infant to desired body temperature.
   a. Check and readjust thermostat setting as necessary. Is equipment plugged into electrical outlet?
   b. Check and reapply probe as necessary. Wet or detached probe may lead to hyperthermia.
   c. Are portholes closed? Open? Is sleeve off track (on incubators with plastic sleeve covers)?
   d. Increase or decrease amount of clothing and blankets as necessary.
   e. Lighting: If gooseneck lamp is directly over infant, it may increase his temperature.
   f. Check placement of incubators, cribs, etc.
   g. Use different thermometer.
   h. Decrease excessive sensory stimuli wherever possible.

4. Subnormal or erratic core temperature.

4. Check for signs of infections. Record and report following immediately:
   a. Poor feeding.
   b. Vomiting.
   c. Diarrhea.
   d. Lethargy.
   e. Pallor.

PLAN OF CARE: TEMPERATURE SUPPORT AND REGULATION—cont'd

NURSING INTERVENTIONS—cont'd

Diagnostic	Therapeutic

5. Possible physiologic signs of cold stress:
  a. In stronger, more mature infant: increased physical activity, crying.
  b. Increased respiratory rate.
  c. Color change:
    (1) Deepening acrocyanosis.
    (2) Appearance of generalized cyanosis.
    (3) Mottling of skin (cutis marmorata).
  d. In male with descended testes, activated cremasteric reflex. Cremasteric reflex: on exposure to cold, testes are pulled back up into inguinal canal.
	5. Alter environment to warm infant.
	  a. If not already in incubator or under radiant heat source, place infant there now (pp. 616 to 618).
	  b. Monitor until desired temperature is achieved, then wean slowly from heat source as infant's condition warrants.

Respiratory function

GENERAL CONSIDERATIONS

Normal respiratory function is dependent on the following factors:

1. Adequacy of the oxygen available
2. Patency of the respiratory tract
3. Capacity of alveoli to expand and remain open
4. Functional capability of the cardiovascular system
   a. Heart
   b. Maintenance of blood pH
   c. Maturity and integrity of capillary network in the lungs to promote gaseous exchange and in the brain to support the function of the respiratory center
   d. Hematocrit and hemoglobin
5. Functional capability of brain tissue, nerves, nerve pathways, and reflex responses.
6. Maturity of diaphragm and intercostal and abdominal musculature to initiate and maintain adequate ventilation

Several significant differences exist between the respiratory tract of the infant and that of the adult:

1. Infants are obligate nose breathers.
2. The infant's tongue is relatively large (macroglossia), whereas the glottis and trachea are small.
3. All lumens of the infant are narrower and more easily collapsed.
4. Respiratory tract secretions of the infant are more abundant than the adult's.
5. The mucous membranes of the infant are more delicate and therefore more susceptible to trauma. The ciliated columnar epithelium just below the vocal cords is especially prone to edema.

6. The alveoli of the infant are more sensitive to changes in pressures.

7. The capillary network of the infant is less well developed. Capillaries are more friable with less well-developed vasoconstrictive and dilatative ability.

8. The infant's bony rib cage and respiratory muscles are not as well developed.

NURSING NEONATE WITH RESPIRATORY DISTRESS

Any neonate with respiratory difficulty is in jeopardy. The infant's response to prompt, appropriate treatment bears a direct relationship to the cause, his maturity, and other medical problems.

Breathing is a new experience for the infant. In priority of care, it ranks second only to massive hemorrhage. Because of its high priority and its challenging nursing aspects, considerable space in the delivery room is devoted to the initiation and maintenance of respirations.

The alert nurse often is the pivotal point between functional and dysfunctional survival for the infant in respiratory distress. Nursing care of the premature baby in respiratory distress is discussed on pp. 555 and 556. The plan of care for respiratory functioning in general is on p. 536. Procedures, nursing actions, and rationale are covered in Chapter 37. The outline for supportive care

SUPPORTIVE CARE FOR RESPIRATORY FUNCTIONING

Diagnostic criteria

Clinical significance

A. Antenatal history
  1. Obesity, diabetes, maternal bleeding, anemia
  2. Heroin addiction, poor nutrition, prolonged rupture of fetal membranes, fetal asphyxia from maternal hypertension, mother receiving steroid therapy

  1. Predisposition to idiopathic RDS
  2. Less likely to develop RDS

B. Intranatal events
  1. Prolonged rupture of fetal membranes
  2. Meconium-stained amniotic fluid with fetal distress (increased fetal activity, fetal heart deceleration)
  3. Elective cesarean section before labor starts
  4. Intravenous administration to mother of 5% dextrose in water only (no electrolytes)

  1. Possible pulmonary infection
  2. Possible meconium aspiration with chemical pneumonitis (especially starting from 6 hours of age)
  3. Possible RDS (secondary to premature delivery)
  4. Fetal hyponatremia—neonate flaccid, cyanotic

C. Neonatal status
  1. Amount of resuscitation performed

     a. Low Apgar score noted at 1, 5, and 15 minutes.
     b. Did neonate need medication to counteract anesthesia or analgesia?
     c. Was endotracheal intubation necessary?

     d. Was gastric suctioning performed?
  2. Gestational age and weight
     a. Under 37 weeks appropriate or large for date
     b. Postmature (meconium-stained)

  3. Miscellaneous
     a. Multiple gestation

     b. Breech presentation

     c. Congenital anomalies
        (1) Funnel chest
        (2) Diaphragmatic hernia
        (3) Choanal atresia
        (4) Cleft palate
        (5) Tracheoesophageal atresia

  1. Possibility of respiratory distress following birth asphyxia and resuscitative procedures
     a. Possible respiratory depression
     b. Same as a

     c. Possible edema of mucosa; possible aspiration pneumonia
     d. Same as c
  2.
     a. Periodic breathing; possible RDS
     b. Spontaneous pneumothorax; pneumomediastinum; aspiration syndrome

  3.
     a. Second child may be depressed; aspiration syndrome

     b. Aspiration syndrome; direct trauma to phrenic nerve, spinal cord, and/or cranial tissue
     c. Respiratory distress
        (1) and (2) Mild to severe respiratory distress

        (3) Cyanosis when quiet, but relieved when crying
        (4) and (5) Aspiration pneumonia; airway obstruction

Care of compromised neonate in delivery room

Procedures for immediate ventilatory assistance (pp. 367 to 372 and Chapter 37):
  1. Suctioning
  2. Mask oxygen
  3. Physical stimulation
  4. Ventilatory resuscitation procedures
     a. Mouth-to-mouth
     b. Bag and mask with adaptor for oxygen input
     c. Endotracheal intubation
  5. Cardiac massage
  6. Heated environment for infant resuscitation and other procedures
     a. Overhead radiant heat shield
     b. Krieselman or comparable resuscitator
     c. Sunlamps

Transportation

Transportation of the sick newborn to a regional neonatal intensive care center should be effected immediately if such care is not available at the institution of birth (pp. 512 and 554).

SUPPORTIVE CARE FOR RESPIRATORY FUNCTIONING—cont'd

Nursery care

Procedures for continuing ventilatory assistance (Chapters 25 and 37):

1. Observe for signs and symptoms of respiratory distress.
2. Maintain a neutral thermal environment.
   a. Overhead radiant heat shield.
   b. Servo-Control incubator.
3. Administer and monitor oxygen (oximeter; heel sticks for blood gases).
4. Assist ventilation.
   a. Bag and mask.
   b. Endotracheal intubation with continuous positive air pressure or other.
   c. Respirator.
5. Maintain acid-base balance.

Table 33-1. Commonly occurring complications in infants with respiratory distress

Condition	Symptom (problem)	Medical and nursing management	Rationale

Tension pneumothorax	Sudden dyspnea
	Cyanosis or pallor
	Bulging of chest wall on affected side
	Heart sounds displaced toward unaffected side
		T: 100% oxygen by plastic hood or mask (*no* positive pressure)
		T: Notify physician*
		D: Prepare to assist with following:
		  1. Needle aspiration of pleural cavity (thoracentesis tray, chest tube, suction)†
		  2. Radiographs
			Assist resolution of air in pleural space and prevent further accumulation
			
			Reduce pneumothorax
			
			Visualize effect of treatment and degree of involvement

Pneumomediastinum	Symptoms usually mild With massive accumulation of air around heart and compression of vena cava: tachypnea, cyanosis; distant or barely audible heart sounds, which are pathognomonic; crepitus of neck	T: Administer 100% oxygen by plastic hood or mask (no positive pressure) T: Notify physician* D: Assist with x-ray examination	Treatment of choice to resolve air in mediastinum (needle aspiration is ineffective) Visualize and monitor progress of condition

Cardiac failure	Tachypnea (50 to 100 breaths/min at rest)
	Tachycardia (140 to 180 beats/min at rest) and pulse irregularities
	Poor feeding; fatigue
	Pulmonary rales or ronchi
	Palpable liver, spleen
	Increasing edema
		T: Maintain warmth (skin temperature, 36° C)
		T: Maintain O$_2$ between 30% to 35% (ambient)
		T: Raise head and shoulders (raise mattress 10 to 20 degrees)
		D: Put on cardiac monitor
		T: Physician's orders:
		  Digitalization—discontinue if heart rate under 100
		  Fluids-electrolytes
		  Diuretics
		D: X-rays and ECG
			Decrease oxygen need, spare energy, avoid acidosis.
			Prevent hypoxia
			Detect abnormalities (obtain cardiograph)
			Facilitate respiratory effort and relieve diaphragm and pool fluids in lower body
			Support body systems

T = Therapeutic interventions; D = diagnostic interventions; educational intervention: parents are kept informed of progress and details of infant's condition and treatment to extent of their understanding.
*One nurse does this while another assists distressed infant.
†Pleur-evac underwater seal drainage of pleural cavity may be used.

on pp. 532 and 533 is presented to emphasize ventilatory problems and their treatment. The nurse's alertness and informed observations place her in a preventive as well as therapeutic role. For example, if a child is born at night with a history of premature rupture of membranes 36 hours or more before delivery, the nurse should obtain cultures from his axillas, groin, and buccal mucosa even if he is momentarily asymptomatic. Should symptoms appear after the infant has been bathed, the cultures have already been obtained, and the number of hours before results are available will have been shortened.

In other circumstances, for example, a postmature neonate born bathed in meconium, the nurse orders a thoracentesis tray and other equipment to have immediately available should symptoms of tension pneumothorax appear (Table 33-1).

Although respiratory complications occur occasionally in normal newborns, the neonatal nurse must be constantly alert for the conditions listed in Table 33-1 in the high-risk infant, especially one with a history of resuscitation.

General appearance of infant with respiratory distress. The infant in distress at birth is immediately identifiable. Some infants who at birth appear pink, vigorous, with good muscle tone, and with respiratory rates and rhythms within normal range, become distressed soon thereafter. Respiratory difficulty may appear suddenly with cyanosis and retractions such as occur after aspiration or tension pneumothorax. More commonly, respiratory difficulty follows a progressive sequential pattern:

1. The respiratory rate initially may increase in rate without a change in rhythm.

2. The apical pulse increases in rate.

3. Retractions, depending on the cause, begin as subcostal and xiphoid, then progress upward to intercostal, suprasternal, and clavicular retractions (Fig. 33-6).

4. The color changes from pink to circumoral pallor, to circumoral cyanosis, and then to generalized cyanosis; acrocyanosis deepens.

5. Respiratory effort and deepening distress are indicated by the following (Fig. 33-7):
   a. Flaring of nares
   b. Chin tug
   c. Expiratory grunt
   d. Abdominal seesaw breathing patterns (Fig. 30-8)
   e. Increase in number of apneic episodes

6. The temperature may begin to drop as energy is diverted from thermogenesis to respiratory effort. Avoid rapid warming of neonate because this may evoke apneic episodes.

7. Impending cardiac failure is evidenced by palpable liver and spleen and developing edema.

Positioning. The neonate's respiratory efforts must be supported by careful positioning. After aspiration of excessive mucus, the head of the mattress is elevated 10 degrees. The infant's neck may be slightly extended by a small folded towel placed under the shoulders. He can be prevented from slipping down by a rolled towel placed under his thighs. When on his back, his arms will be at his side, flexed and slightly abducted. Diapers if used must be pinned loosely. (For more detail, see p. 611.)

When positioning the infant, the nurse notes the following:

1. Avoid hyperextending the neck because this may interfere with respirations and swallowing of secretions.

2. Avoid the prone position. The weight of the body increases respiratory efforts.

Suctioning. An open airway usually decreases the neonate's labored breathing by improving ventilation. See discussion of suctioning procedures (p. 610).

Oxygen needs and administration. Oxygen therapy may be lifesaving, but its administration must be care-

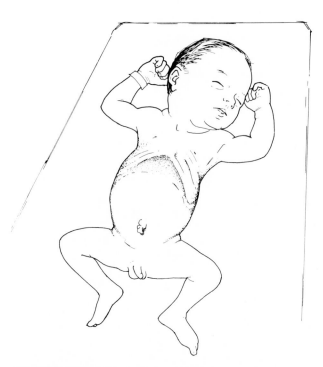

Fig. 33-6. Retraction: substernal, subcostal, and intercostal retractions are evident. (Courtesy Ross Laboratories, Columbus, Ohio.)

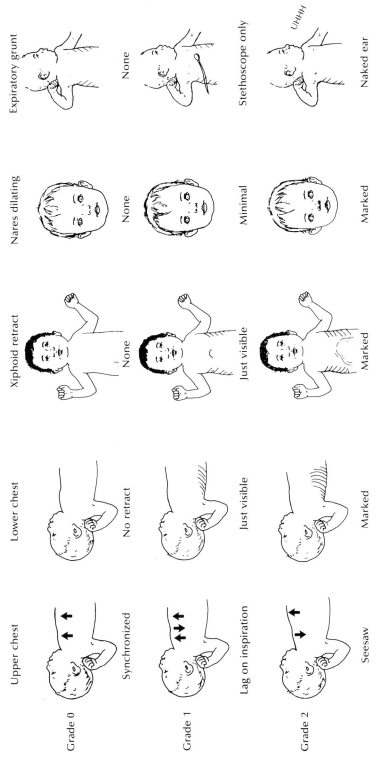

Fig. 33-7. Observation of retractions. Silverman-Anderson index of respiratory distress is determined by grading each of five arbitrary criteria: *grade 0* indicates no difficulty; *grade 1*, moderate difficulty; and *grade 2*, maximum respiratory difficulty. Retraction score is sum of these values; total score of 0 indicates no dyspnea, whereas total score of 10 denotes maximal respiratory distress. (Modified from Silverman, W., and Anderson, D. 1956. Pediatrics **17**:1.)

PLAN OF CARE: RESPIRATORY FUNCTIONING

PATIENT CARE OBJECTIVES

1. Respirations are maintained:
   a. Right-to-left circulatory shunts do not recur.
   b. Bronchopulmonary dysplasia and retrolental fibroplasia do not develop.
   c. Metabolism meets needs of repair, maintenance, and growth.
   d. Respiratory needs of all tissues are met:
      (1) Blood gases and acid-base balance are maintained within normal limits.
      (2) Vasoconstriction does not occur.
   e. Congenital dysfunctions or anomalies are recognized early and appropriate treatment initiated.
2. Parents are able to cope constructively with the situation and to relate to the infant as a person.

NURSING INTERVENTIONS

Diagnostic	Therapeutic

1. Note respiratory rate, rhythm, and depth:
  a. Tachypnea: rate >15 respirations/min over baseline at birth or >60 breaths/min.
  b. Bradypnea: rate <30 respirations/min is grave sign.
  c. Apneic episodes: failure to breathe ≥15 seconds.
  d. Shallow, rapid respirations.
  e. Deep, slow respirations.
2. Evaluate retractions:
  a. Location: unilateral or bilateral, subcostal or substernal, intercostal, supraclavicular or suprasternal.
  b. Degree of in-drawing (see Fig. 33-7).
3. Observe for following:
  a. Flaring of alae nasi on inspiration.
  b. Chin tug (or lag).
  c. Seesaw respirations.
  d. Inspiratory stridor.
  e. Expiratory grunt (heard by ear or with a stethoscope) or sigh.
  f. Nasal and/or oropharyngeal discharge.
  g. Scaphoid abdomen and/or overinflated chest.
4. Evaluate skin color:
  a. Plethora.
  b. Pallor.
  c. Cyanosis: generalized, circumoral, aggravated when asleep or when active and crying.
  d. Mottled skin (cutis marmorata) in absence of chilling or inactivity.
5. Monitor O_2 concentration:
  a. Oximeter.
  b. Order lab work for arterial blood gases and pH.
6. Evaluate for other signs of progressing anoxia:
  a. Muscle tone: from generalized flexion to flaccidity.
  b. Froglike posture.
  c. Lax, open mouth.
  d. Heart rate: <100 beats/min; >160/mm (for more than 1 minute); irregular.
  e. Hypothermia.
  f. Progressive weakness, exhaustion.
	For techniques involved, see Chapter 37.
	1. Ensure patency of respiratory tract:
	  a. Suction prn.
	  b. Position.
	  c. Feeding technique.
	  d. Check for choanal atresia or tracheoesophageal anomalies, etc.
	2. Support infant's capacity to produce surfactant:
	  a. Monitor pressure of O_2 or air entering respiratory tree (high pressures decrease surfactant production).
	  b. Avoid high concentrations of O_2 for prolonged periods, since this impairs capacity of alveolar walls to secrete surfactant.
	3. Decrease infant's need for O_2.
	  a. Maintain skin temperature.
	  b. Warm and humidify O_2/air.
	  c. Plan for periods of rest.
	  d. Feed warmed formula by gavage as necessary.
	4. Assist infant's respiratory efforts:
	  a. Continuous positive airway pressure; continuous end expiratory pressure.
	  b. Position infant so that chest expansion is not compromised.
	  c. Feeding technique: Avoid abdominal distention.
	5. Prepare infant for lab work:
	  a. Warm foot for heel stick, or do heel stick.
	  b. Irrigate umbilical artery with heparinized solution per physician's orders.
	6. O_2 therapy: Concentration and rate of flow governed by lab work (blood gases, pH).
	7. Remind infant to breathe by following measures:
	  a. Gentle stimulation.
	  b. Resuscitate if gentle stimulation is ineffective:
	    (1) Mouth-to-mouth.
	    (2) Mask.
	    (3) Laryngoscopy.

fully monitored as with any drug. Indiscriminate use of oxygen may be hazardous and result in retrolental fibroplasia and bronchopulmonary dysplasia. See the discussion on oxygen therapy (p. 612), the plan of care on the opposite page, and the discussions on retrolental fibroplasia and pulmonary dysplasia (p. 561).

Warmth. A neutral thermal environment is essential for metabolic homeostasis. Cold stress is detrimental to the well-being of any infant but especially the infant at risk. For a discussion of thermogenesis and the prevention of cold stress, see p. 528.

Feeding. Feeding the infant in respiratory distress is as much of a challenge to the nurse as it is for the infant. The extra work of breathing taxes his energy reserves and demands greater caloric input. Breast- and bottle-feeding may be possible for the neonate in mild distress. A softer nipple with an adequate opening is used (e.g., when inverted, fluid should drip at 1 drop/sec). The airway must be cleared prior to and during feeding as necessary. Moreover, the infant is bubbled prior to feedings.

If the infant is feeding at the breast, the nurse remains at the bedside with a bulb syringe at hand. This provides reassurance for the mother and avoids a buildup of tension, which might be transferred from mother to infant. Should the infant gag or choke, the nurse can show the mother how to manage such a situation.

The infant should be able to complete a feeding in 30 minutes without signs of fatigue. His need for sucking satisfaction may be great, but his energies are needed for recovery and growth at this time.

Depending on the infant's energy and degree of distress, he may benefit from feeding from the bottle or breast for 5 to 10 minutes, with the remainder of the feeding accomplished by gavage. The neonate in severe distress may require gavage feeding exclusively. Parenteral feeding may be required for the neonate who cannot tolerate either oral or gavage feedings.

The following is noted:

1. Milk tends to stimulate mucus production, thereby increasing the danger of aspiration. Substitution of clear fluids may be necessary.

2. Abdominal distension (Fig. 33-8) compromises respiratory effort. Avoid overfeeding, bubble frequently, and avoid rapid feeding.

3. An overdistended stomach and fatigue also predispose to aspiration and compromised respirations. Feed smaller quantities more frequently, or select an alternative method of feeding, for example, gavage, intravenous alimentation, or parenteral fluids exclusively or in combination with gavage or nipple.

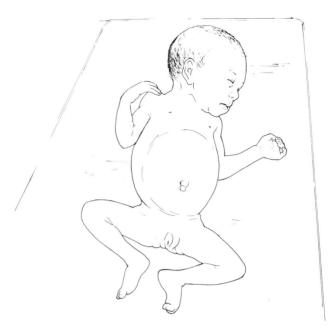

Fig. 33-8. Sudden abdominal distention. (Courtesy Ross Laboratories, Columbus, Ohio.)

The infant's sucking needs can be met even if feeding by gavage is necessary for an extended period of time. Enlarge the opening of a "premie" nipple so that it will fit snugly around a feeding tube. Measure and mark the appropriate distance on the tube. Thread the orogastric feeding tube to the mark and proceed with gavage feeding (pp. 618 and 619).

Feeding and elimination
GENERAL CONSIDERATIONS

Small neonates comprise the largest number of high-risk infants. Of these, about one third are of low birth weight for gestational age, whereas about two thirds are preterm.

The feeding and nutrition of the high-risk infant warrant careful consideration. The extent to which nutritional needs are met is directly related to the infant's immediate and long-range well-being. For example, if the full-term, low birth weight (SGA) (dysmature) infant with low glycogen stores is not fed promptly, the resultant symptomatic or asymptomatic hypoglycemia may seriously damage his carbohydrate-dependent brain cells.

The preterm infant often suffers several physiologic handicaps whose severity increase as gestational age decreases (Table 33-2).

Table 33-2. Immaturity and resultant problems

Developmental immaturity	Physiologic handicap
CNS	Sucking reflex may be absent, poorly developed, or uncoordinated with swallowing reflex; aspiration is constant danger Poor gag reflex
Gastrointestinal tract	Small gastric capacity Variable food transit times through gastrointestinal tract, affecting digestion and absorption Poor tolerance for fats (especially saturated); fat lost in stool decreases calories available to neonate and is accompanied by loss of minerals and fat-soluble vitamins. Lax abdominal musculature, ↓ HCl, weak cardiac sphincter
Metabolism (enzyme systems)	Inefficient handling of metabolic breakdown products (e.g., blood tyrosine levels from metabolism of protein rise, capable of causing positive PKU test even if baby does not have PKU)
Urinary system	Impaired water conservation Reduced selectivity in reabsorption of electrolytes
Limited glucose stores	Increases danger of hypoglycemia, hyperbilirubinemia, and protein catabolism and their sequelae, e.g., brain damage

Table 33-3. Caloric requirements (appropriate weight for gestation—preterm infants)*

Item	Calories/kg/24 hr	
Resting	40 to 50	(depending on age)
Activity	10 to 15	
Cold stress	5 to 10	(depending on environmental temperature)
Specific dynamic action	8 to 8	
Fecal loss	2† to 12	
Growth	25 to 25	
Total	90 120	

*From Babson, S. G., Benson, R. C., Pernoll, M. I., and Benda, G. I. 1975. Management of high-risk pregnancy and intensive care of the neonate (ed. 3). St. Louis, The C. V. Mosby Co., p. 108.
†On parenteral feedings.

Oral feeding and infant's reactivity periods. In the first 24 hours of life, the neonate experiences reactivity periods when excessive mucous secretion and regurgitation may occur. The second reactivity period appears about 4 to 12 hours after birth. In timing the initial feeding, the nurse should be aware that food at this time may be taken poorly or even aspirated.

NUTRITIONAL REQUISITES

Caloric, nutrient, and fluid requirements of the infant at risk (Tables 33-3 to 33-5) are greater for many reasons, some of which follow:

1. Limited stores—preterm or dysmature (malnourished) neonate.
2. Depleted stores—neonate who is stressed by one or a combination of the following factors:
   a. Birth asphyxia.
   b. Increased respirations or respiratory effort.
   c. Insensitive fluid loss by evaporation when under radiant heat or during phototherapy.
   d. Hypothermic environment.
3. Immature systems:
   a. Gastrointestinal tract—losses through vomiting, diarrhea, dysfunctional absorption.
   b. Kidneys—losses caused by inability to concentrate urine and maintain an adequate rate of urea excretion and an inadequate response to antidiuretic hormone (ADH).

Early feeding. Early feeding, within 6 to 8 hours of birth of term neonates (earlier in preterm infants), either orally or parenterally, is necessary for the following reasons:

- To prevent dehydration
- To spare the available stores of glycogen
- To maintain blood glucose levels
- To lessen initial weight loss
- To keep serum bilirubin levels within normal limits
- To curtail protein catabolism that would result in metabolic acidosis, hyperkalemia, or elevated BUN
- To conserve energy for growth
- To stimulate sucking response

Table 33-4. Daily vitamin requirements (National Research Council)*

A	1500	IU
Thiamine	0.2	mg
Riboflavin	0.4	mg
Pyridoxine	0.2	mg
B_{12}	1.0	μg
C	35	mg
D	400	IU
E	5	IU
Niacin	6.0	mg
Panthenol	—	
Folic acid	0.05	mg
K	1.0	mg†

*From Babson, S. G., Benson, R. C., Pernoll, M. I., and Benda, G. I. 1975. Management of high-risk pregnancy and intensive care of the neonate (ed. 3). St. Louis, The C. V. Mosby Co., p. 110.
†By injection on first day of life (p. 471); added to diet by third day.

Table 33-5. Range in daily feeding requirements of low birth weight infants per kilogram of body weight*

Nutrient requirements		First week of life	Active growth period
Water (ml)		80-200	130-200
Calories		50-100	110-150†
Protein	⎫	1-2	3-4
Glucose	⎬ (gm)	7-12	12-15
Fat	⎭	3-4	5-8
Sodium	⎫	1-2	2-3
Potassium	⎪	1-2	2-4
Chloride	⎬ (mEq)	1-2	2-3
Calcium	⎪	1-2	3-5
Phosphorus	⎪	1-2	2-4
Magnesium	⎭	—	0.5-1.0
Iron (mg)		—	1.5-2.0

*From Babson, S. G., Benson, R. C., Pernoll, M. L., and Benda, G. I. 1975. Management of high-risk pregnancy and intensive care of the neonate (ed. 3). St. Louis, The C. V. Mosby Co., p. 109.
†Calorie requirements of over 120/kg apply to infants with perinatal undergrowth.

4. Growth demands: The preterm neonate's growth rate approximates that of fetal growth rate, that is, growth rate during the last trimester is two or more times that of an infant after delivery at term.

WEIGHT AND FLUID LOSS

Up to 85% of the preterm neonate's body weight consists of water, most of which occupies the extracellular fluid compartment. Even with early fluid and nutritional intake, the preterm infant's weight and fluid losses seem exaggerated. Factors predisposing to weight and fluid losses include the following:

1. Inadequate fluid intake (e.g., from delayed administration or insufficient volume).
2. Evaporative losses (4 ml/kg/hr or more) through thin skin with poor capillary control (e.g., from an overheated incubator, radiant heater, phototherapy). The total body surface (skin and lining of the respiratory tract) is large in comparison to body mass.
3. Insensitive fluid loss (15 ml/kg/24 hr or more) through lungs (e.g., from increased respiratory rates or low-humidity environment).
4. Greater fluid demands to meet increased cellular metabolic processes (e.g., from stress, repair, or growth).
5. Fluid loss through immature kidney functioning.

6. Fluid loss through the gastrointestinal tract (e.g., from meconium or loose stools of dysfunctional origin, or from overfeeding, phototherapy, or sepsis).

The limits of acceptable weight loss are as follows: During the neonate's first 3 days of extrauterine life, the preterm infant can lose 12% or less of birth weight. For the term infant, a 10% or less weight loss is acceptable for neonates of normal weight for gestational age; 15% or less weight loss is acceptable for infants weighing 4500 gm (9 pounds 14 ounces) or more. For dysmature SGA infants, a loss of 5% or less of birth weight is acceptable.

After the first 3 days, a preterm neonate's loss or gain per each 24 hours should not exceed 2% of the previous day's weight.

The following examples illustrate how to calculate weight loss and gain, suggesting causes and nursing actions for each case.

Example 1

Day 4   1750 gm
Day 5   1730 gm
         20 gm loss

$$\frac{20}{1750} = \frac{x\%}{100\%}$$

$$1750x = 2000$$

$$1750 \overline{)\,2000.0\,}^{\;1.1\%}$$

$$x = 1.1\% \text{ weight loss}$$

Probable causes: Stool passage
　　　　　　　　Inadequate fluid: amount and type
　　Action: Record and report
　　　　　　Observe infant
　　　　　　Do Dextrostix

Example 2

Day 4	1750 gm
Day 5	1790 gm
	40 gm gain

$$\frac{40}{1750} = \frac{x\%}{100\%}$$

$$1750x = 4000$$

$$1750 \overline{)4000.0} \quad 2.3$$

$$x = 2.3\% \text{ gain}$$

Probable causes: Overfeeding
　　　　　　　　Fluid retention
　　Action: Record and report
　　　　　　Observe neonate for other symptoms
　　　　　　Collect urine in bag: check amount, specific gravity
　　　　　　Do Dextrostix

Example 3

Day 4	1750 gm
Day 5	1715 gm
	35 gm loss

$$\frac{35}{1750} = \frac{x\%}{100\%}$$

$$1750x = 3500$$

$$1750 \overline{)3500.0} \quad 2.0$$

$$x = 2\% \text{ weight loss}$$

Table 33-6. Laboratory monitoring of parenteral fluids*

Weight	Once or twice daily
Length	Weekly
Head circumference	Weekly
Electrolytes	Daily until stabilized; then 3 times weekly
BUN	Twice weekly
Blood glucose	(see p. 523)
Calcium	Daily times 3; if satisfactory, weekly
Base deficit	Daily times 3; if satisfactory, weekly
Hematocrit	Weekly
SGOT	Weekly
Albumin or total protein	Weekly
Bilirubin	As indicated

*From Babson, S. G., Benson, R. C., Pernoll, M. L., and Benda, G. I. 1975. Management of high-risk pregnancy and intensive care of the neonate (ed. 3). St. Louis, The C. V. Mosby Co., p. 117.

Probable causes: Excessive stooling, voiding
　　　　　　　　Excessive evaporative losses
　　　　　　　　Inadequate amount and type of fluid
　　　　　　　　Malabsorption problem
　　Action: Record and report
　　　　　　Check incubator and infant for temperature; check incubator for humidity
　　　　　　Observe neonate for other symptoms
　　　　　　Collect urine in bag: check urine for amount and specific gravity; Clinistix
　　　　　　Do Dextrostix

FORMULA AND FEEDING SCHEDULES

The formula and feeding schedule of the infant at risk are based on the following criteria:

1. Infant's birth weight and pattern of weight gain or loss
2. Estimated gestational age
3. Physical condition: pharyngeal coordination (sucking, swallowing reflexes are present and coordinated), fatigability, malformations, amount of urine excreted per hour
4. Laboratory values: nitrogen balance, electrolyte imbalance, glucose level, serum bilirubin, and other results

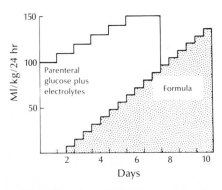

Fig. 33-9. Example of combined parenteral and oral feeding in milliliters per kilogram per day for newborn infant weighing less than 1500 gm at birth who is unable to suck. Increases of 2 ml/kg/24 hr of oral feeding from an initial intake of 2 to 3 ml achieve an intake of approximately 100 ml/kg/24 hr by 7 days of age. Many infants will not tolerate this volume of intake without abdominal distention, regurgitation, and risk of aspiration; continuation of parenteral fluids is advisable for these infants. (From Babson, S. G., Benson, R. C., Pernoll, M. L., and Benda, G. I. 1975. Management of high-risk pregnancy and intensive care of the neonate [ed. 3.]. St. Louis, The C. V. Mosby Co.; modified from Babson, S. G. 1971. J. Pediatr. **79:**694.)

The following variants influence the feeding of the infant at risk:

1. Fluid volume given
2. Caloric requirements
3. Mode of feeding
4. Formula: predigested, breast milk, calories per ounce

Parenteral fluids or intravenous alimentation. The very small neonate or those unable to suck because of developmental or respiratory problems (especially those on assisted ventilation) are sustained by parenteral infusions (Chapter 37). The electrolytes and nutrients per milliliter as well as milliliters per kilogram of body weight per hour are carefully calculated by the physician. The nurse monitors the functioning of infusion equipment (tubing, infusion pump), assures asepsis, secures and protects the needle (catheter) at insertion site, and assesses and records the neonate's responses (Table 33-6).

Weaning from parenteral therapy. As the neonate's condition improves, he may be offered fluids by nipple. As the amount of oral feedings are increased and tolerated, the amount of infused milliliters per 24 hours is decreased (Fig. 33-9).

Oral preparations. Many infants at risk are capable of nippling formula soon after birth. The nurse assists in assessing the neonate's tolerance for this mode of feeding by noting the following:

- Pharyngeal coordination (suck and swallow reflexes present and synchronized)
- Presence and degree of respiratory distress or apneic episodes if any
- Presence of bowel sounds and absence of abdominal distention
- Gastric residual of 2 ml or less prior to feeding

Various milk formulas are available. These formulas vary in calories, protein, and mineral content per ounce (Table 33-7). Formulas are fed by nipple, gavage, or both. Each neonate must be evaluated for his ability to handle solute and fluid load.

Oral feedings begin with sterile water. After three successful feedings, a formula preparation is offered. Feedings are advanced by increasing the amount of fluid *or* the number of calories per ounce (per 30 ml) at any one feeding, and the neonate's tolerance is observed. Infants under approximately 1800 gm (4 pounds) have feedings advanced more slowly. Too rapid advancement may lead to the following:

1. Vomiting, diarrhea, abdominal distention
2. Apneic episodes
3. Residual feeding of 2 ml or more at the time of the next feeding
4. Retention of fluid with cardiopulmonary embarrassment or marked diuresis with loss of Na^+ leading to hyponatremia
5. Regurgitation—aspiration pneumonia

Table 33-7. Contents of various milks/100 ml*

	Human	Cow	Enfamil With Iron	Similac With Iron	Similac 24 With Iron	PM 60/40	SMA	SMA 27
Protein (gm)	1.3	3.3	1.5	1.8	2.2	1.6	1.5	2.0
Fat (gm)	3.5	3.7	3.7	3.6	4.3	3.5	3.5	4.9
CHO (gm)	7.0	4.8	7.0	7.0	8.4	7.5	7.0	9.7
Na^+ (mEq)	0.65	2.5	1.1	1.3	1.6	0.65	0.65	0.9
K^+ (mEq)	1.4	3.5	1.9	2.6	2.6	1.5	1.4	1.9
Ca^{++} (mEq)	1.7	6.0	3.2	3.5	4.0	1.7	2.2	3.0
PO_4 (mEq)	1.0	6.2	2.9	2.9	3.5	1.2	2.1	2.8
Cl^- (mEq)	1.0	2.7	1.1	1.8	1.9	1.3	1.0	1.4
Calories	67.0	67.0	67.0	67.0	80.0	67.0	67.0	90.0
Iron (mg)	—	—	1.25	1.2	1.2	0.2	1.25	1.69
Renal solute load (mOsm)	8.25	21.9	10.1	12.9	14.9	9.9	9.1	12.2

*From Babson, S. G., Benson, R. C., Pernoll, M. L., and Benda, G. I. 1975. Management of high-risk pregnancy and intensive care of the neonate (ed. 3). St. Louis, The C. V. Mosby Co., p. 109.

PLAN OF CARE: NUTRITION OF HIGH-RISK INFANT

PATIENT CARE OBJECTIVES

1. Hypoglycemic reactions are avoided.
2. Acceptable fluid-electrolyte balance is maintained.
3. Feeding is accomplished with the following results:
   a. Minimal respiratory distress; no aspiration or aspiration pneumonia.
   b. Minimal expenditure of energy.
   c. No abdominal distention.
   d. No trauma to tissues of the gastrointestinal tract.
   e. No diarrhea.
4. Sucking satisfaction is maximized.
5. Nutrition is sufficient to accomplish the following:
   a. Meet resting metabolic requirements.
   b. Provide sufficient energy for physical activity.
   c. Counter losses through gastrointestinal and urinary tracts.
   d. Supply constituents for growth. The infant establishes a steady pattern of weight gain appropriate for him.
6. Parent-child relationship is fostered in the following ways:
   a. Involvement in the feeding process in light of the infant's physical capabilities and desired degree of involvement.
   b. Infant begins to associate feeding and eating with pleasure as he develops a sense of trust.
   c. At discharge, the parents are comfortable with the feeding method needed by the infant whether that method is breast, bottle, gavage, or by gastrostomy.

NURSING INTERVENTIONS

Diagnostic	Therapeutic	Educational

Diagnosis is based on persistent symptoms, condition of infant over period of time (is he developing signs of shock, sepsis, jaundice, dehydration, lethargy, increased paroxysmal crying?). Many normal infants, under normal conditions, exhibit one or more symptoms or episodes.	Appropriate fluid or formula preparations are essential to meet infant's nutritional requirements. Nurse's observations contribute to physician's decisions regarding type of fluids and formula and their mode of administration.
	
	Infants with metabolic disorders or malabsorption syndromes benefit from early diet management to prevent or modify accumulation of toxic metabolites and to ensure nutrients necessary for repair, maintenance, and growth.
		Encourage parent participation.
		1. As soon as infant's condition permits, nurse involves parents in feeding process (if they wish). They may:
		  a. Observe infant being fed by bottle, gavage, and/or other technique.
		  b. Participate in feeding the infant.
		2. Nurse initiates discussions of infant's nutritional needs and how these are met.
		3. Nurse counsels parents concerning their fears and questions on feeding small or handicapped infant.
		4. Nurse acts as role model in providing physical and psychosocial care of infant so that parents and infant may thrive.

1. Antenatal history:
  a. Maternal history of metabolic disorders (e.g., diabetes).
  b. Presence of polyhydramnios, oligohydramnios.
  c. Therapy for preeclampsia-eclampsia (magnesium sulfate, diuretics).
	1. Antenatal history:
	  a. Screen all infants for hypoglycemia. If necessary, feed early.
	  b. Observe infants carefully for congenital dysfunction and anomalies: metabolic disorders; malabsorptive syndromes; tracheoesophageal fistula; esophageal atresia; anal atresia; renal anomaly. Record and report for prompt diagnosis and appropriate therapy.
	  c. Treat electrolyte imbalance (e.g., hypermagnesemia) as early as possible.	

2. Fetal status:
  a. Preterm.
  b. SGA.
	2. Fetal status:
	  a. Screen all infants for hypoglycemia, and feed as necessary.	

PLAN OF CARE: NUTRITION OF HIGH-RISK INFANT—cont'd

NURSING INTERVENTIONS—cont'd

Diagnostic	Therapeutic	Educational
c. LGA. d. Postterm.	b. Assess readiness and ability to feed: energy level, maturity, suck and swallow reflexes and their synchronization, and amount of and ability to handle mucus. Choose appropriate feeding method.	
3. Observe infant for following: a. Irritability, continual hunger (e.g., possible narcotic withdrawal syndrome). b. Convulsive states (e.g., hypoglycemia, abnormal blood chemistries, intracranial hemorrhage. To recognize convulsive states in the neonate, see pp. 518, 557, and 569. c. Paroxysmal bouts of crying? Are crying episodes accompanied by apparent peristaltic waves? d. Gastrointestinal anomalies (p. 513.	3. Based on observations: a. Screen for hypoglycemia, and feed as necessary. b. If the child is drug-dependent: give frequent, small feedings, swaddle, hold often (for other treatment, see pp. 601 and 602). c. If child convulses, maintain airway during convulsion, give oxygen for cyanosis, note character of convulsion, call physician, do Dextrostix for hypoglycemia.	
4. Laboratory values (Appendix H): a. Blood serum levels for glucose, calcium, magnesium, etc. b. Urinalysis: infections, reducing substances. c. Hemoglobin, hematocrit: Check for anemia.	4. Laboratory values: a. Amount of calcium, magnesium, and other minerals will modify feeding and other medicinal regimen (e.g., calcium gluconate is given for hypermagnesemia). b. Tests for reducing substances in urine (e.g., glucose, galactose, phenylketonuria, alkaptonuria, etc.) may reveal metabolic disorders that would alter feeding and medical regimen. c. To prevent or treat iron-deficiency anemia, elemental iron may be ordered by 2 months of age. Multivitamin mixtures including vitamin E and pyridoxine may be begun by the third day of life. d. Assist with blood transfusion as necessary (pp. 626 and 627). e. Give ascorbic acid *between* feedings per order.	
5. Weight is plotted on growth grid: a. Admission. b. Daily: What is weight loss? What is rate of weight gain?	5. Weight: a. Accuracy is imperative as basis for prescription of dietary regimen. b. Deviations from normal in weight losses or gains guide future diagnostic evaluations	

Continued.

PLAN OF CARE: NUTRITION OF HIGH-RISK INFANT—cont'd

NURSING INTERVENTIONS—cont'd

Diagnostic	Therapeutic	Educational
	to determine cause and treatment.	

6. Elimination patterns:
  a. Frequency of urination.
  b. Amount, frequency, and character of stool:
    (1) Obstipation and/or constipation.
    (2) Diarrhea.
    (3) Loss of fats (steatorrhea).
	6. Elimination behavior is observed to determine patency and functioning of gastrointestinal and urinary tracts and provides basis for diagnosis and treatment (medical).	

7. Oral feedings:
  a. Type of formula; calories/ounce.
  b. Volume.
  c. Behavior during feeding:
    (1) Attempts at sucking.
    (2) Abdominal distention.
    (3) Vomiting, regurgitation.
    (4) Cyanosis.
    (5) Amount of mucus.
  d. Time necessary to feed.
	7. Observe oral feedings for ongoing evaluation and readjustment of nursing care regarding type of nipple to use ("premie," regular, breast), type of feeding (continue with oral, combine oral and gavage, gavage only), amount, frequency, when to involve mother or father in actual feeding.	

8. Gavage feedings:
  a. Observe as for oral feedings.
  b. Size of feeding tube; nasogastric or orogastric route.
	8. Observe gavage feedings for ongoing evaluation and readjustment of nursing care regarding continuation of gavage feedings, attempting oral feedings, providing simultaneous sucking satisfaction as soon as possible (before tenth day of life gavage through nipple if nothing else) (p. 537), type and amount of formula, frequency of feedings, when to teach mother how to do gavage feedings if child will go home with this need.	

9. Abdominal distention:
  a. Note time, degree, effect on respiratory effort.
  b. Assist with x-ray examination.
	9. Abdominal distention:
	  a. Identify for early treatment.
	  b. Avoid overfeeding.
	  c. Burp or "bubble" infant as necessary; readjust positioning during feeding.
	  d. Prepare for and assist with x-ray examination (avoid heat loss during).	

10. Vomiting and/or regurgitation:
  a. Note color, amount, time in relation to feeding, character (e.g., forceful? spill over?)
  b. Pass nasogastric tube for diagnosis as necessary.
	10. Vomiting and/or regurgitation:
	  a. Early recognition of condition for correction: high or low gastrointestinal obstructions, anomalous bile ducts.
	  b. Avoid overfeeding—evaluate by checking amount of residual prior to subsequent feeding; refeed residual and subtract	

PLAN OF CARE: NUTRITION OF HIGH-RISK INFANT—cont'd

NURSING INTERVENTIONS—cont'd

Diagnostic*	Therapeutic*	Educational
	this amount from this feeding; decrease amount of feeding; feed more frequently. c. Prepare for gastrointestinal studies. d. Pass nasogastric or orogastric tube per physician's order.	
11. Diarrhea: a. Note color, amount, frequency, type of expulsion. b. Obtain stool for pH, culture. c. Do rectal swabs for culture. d. Initiate isolation technique until return of culture.	11. Diarrhea: Early recognition of condition is necessary for correction to prevent fluid-electrolyte imbalance and to direct medical management, to treat any existing sepsis, to correct a surgical problem (Hirschsprung's disease).	
12. Check for symptoms of dehydration. Note following: a. Skin turgor over abdomen and inner thighs. b. Presence of sunken fontanel. c. Softness of eyeball; sunken eyeball. d. Presence of dry mucous membranes. e. Amount and frequency of urination. f. Collect specimen of urine for specific gravity and visual evaluation, for urinalysis, for culture. 　(1) Collect in urine bag. 　(2) Catheterize or arrange for suprapubic puncture.	12. Dehydration: a. Early recognition to prevent fluid-electrolyte imbalance and to direct medical management. b. Prepare for blood work, intravenous therapy. c. Carefully monitor all intake and output; monitor progression of symptoms or their regression.	
13. Obstipation and/or constipation: a. Note absence of meconium or small amounts of meconium (or small, hard balls). b. Do sweat test. c. Check for imperforate anus (p. 513).	13. Obstipation and/or constipation: a. Early recognition of congenital dysfunction or anomaly (cystic fibrosis, imperforate anus, gastrointestinal obstruction or of bile production and bile duct system). b. Give infant enema per order.	
14. Observe for jaundice: a. Time of occurrence. b. Degree of coloration. c. Other signs and symptoms (e.g., signs of sepsis). d. Is infant breast-feeding?	14. Jaundice: a. Early recognition of blood incompatibility, sepsis, or other problems so that effective therapy can be instituted to prevent feeding problems, kernicterus, anemia, etc. b. Phototherapy. c. Exchange transfusion.	
15. Parenteral fluids.	15. Parenteral therapy.	
16. Alimentation.	16. Intravenous alimentation.	

*For techniques involved, see Chapter 37.

REFERENCES

Babson, S. G., Benson, R. C., Pernoll, M. L., and Benda, G. I. 1975. Management of high-risk pregnancy and intensive care of the neonate (ed. 3). St. Louis, The C. V. Mosby Co.

Behrman, R. E. (ed.). 1973. Neonatology: diseases of the fetus and infant. St. Louis, The C. V. Mosby Co.

Clark, A. L., and Affonso, D. 1976. Childbearing: a nursing perspective. Philadelphia, F. A. Davis Co.

Gillon, J. E. 1973. Behavior of newborns with cardiac distress. Am. J. Nurs. **73:**254.

Klaus, M. H., and Fanaroff, A. A. 1973. Care of the high risk neonate. Philadelphia, W. B. Saunders Co.

Korones, S. B. 1976. High-risk newborn infants—the basis for intensive nursing care (ed. 2). St. Louis, The C. V. Mosby Co.

Van Leeuwen, G. 1973. The nurse in prevention and intervention in the neonatal period. Nurs. Clin. North Am. **8:**509.

CHAPTER 34

Problems related to gestational age and birth weight

GENERAL CONSIDERATIONS

Preterm or *premature* refers to the neonate born at 37 weeks' gestation or earlier, regardless of birth weight. *Term* refers to the neonate born between 38 and 42 weeks' gestation. *Postterm* or *postmature* refers to the neonate whose gestational age exceeds 42 weeks.

The weight of the embryo or fetus has a normal range for each gestational week (Fig. 34-1). If at any week the weight of the embryo or fetus is 2 or more standard deviations above the norm, it is said to be *large for gestational age* (LGA), or *large for dates;* if its weight is 2 or more standard deviations below the norm, it is termed *small for gestational age* (SGA), or *small for dates.*

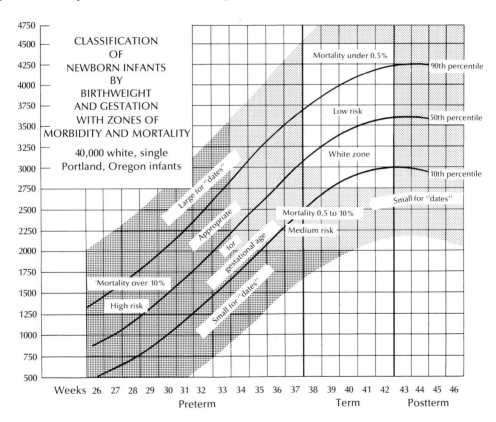

Fig. 34-1. Zones of mortality and morbidity in relation to both weight and gestation. (From Babson, S. G., Benson, R. C., Pernoll, M. L., and Benda, G. I. 1975. Management of high-risk pregnancy and intensive care of the neonate [ed. 3]. St. Louis, The C. V. Mosby Co.)

LGA neonates may be preterm, term, or postterm. Common causes for LGA neonates include gestational or true maternal diabetes or heredity. SGA neonates may also be preterm, term, or postterm. Frequently, SGA neonates are born of hypertensive mothers or mothers with preeclampsia-eclampsia and occur in multiple gestation and discordant twin pregnancies. High altitude, rubella, or other intrauterine infection and malnutrition may predispose to the birth of SGA neonates.

Terminology is yet to be standardized. The SGA infant may also be called *dysmature* or *pseudopremature*. *Fetal malnutrition, intrauterine growth retardation,* and *chronic fetal distress* refer to some of the processes that may result in the birth of neonates who are SGA.

PRETERM INFANTS

By definition, the preterm or premature infant is one born prior to the thirty-seventh week of gestation. Estimation of gestational age based on the last normal menstrual cycle is unreliable. Other parameters for determining gestational age and maturity are now

available. These are presented later in this chapter.

The optimal environment for fetal growth and development is within the uterus of a healthy, well-nourished woman for 38 to 42 weeks. The extrauterine environment of the preterm neonate must approximate a healthy intrauterine environment for the normal sequence of growth and development to continue. Morbidity and mortality among true premature infants occur at a rate three to four times that of older infants of comparable weight (Fig. 34-2).

The actual or potential problems of the preterm infant of 2000 gm differ from those of the term or postterm infant of equal weight. The premature infant is at a distinct disadvantage when he faces the transition from intrauterine to extrauterine life. The degree of disadvantage depends primarily on his level of maturity. Physiologic disorders and anomalous malformations affect his response to treatment as well. In general, the closer he is to the normal term infant in gestational age and weight the easier his adjustment to the external environment.

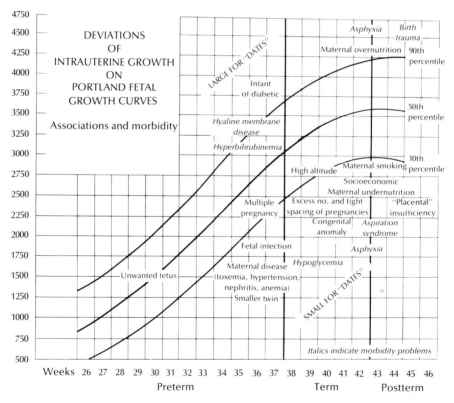

Fig. 34-2. Important associations and morbidity factors of accelerated or reduced fetal growth above 90th percentile and below 10th percentile for gestational age using Portland curves. Fetal growth data obtained from 40,000 single, white, middle-class infants born near sea level. (From Babson, S. G., Benson, R. C., Pernoll, M. L., and Benda, G. I. 1975. Management of high-risk pregnancy and intensive care of the neonate [ed. 3]. St. Louis, The C. V. Mosby Co.)

Admission to nursery

Admission of a premature newborn to the nursery usually is an emergency situation. A rapid initial evaluation is needed to ascertain the need for lifesaving treatment. Resuscitative measures should be instituted in the delivery room. The neonate's need for warmth and oxygen must be ensured during his transfer from the delivery room to the nursery.

The premature infant's external environmental support consists of the following:

1. Incubator control for body temperature
2. Air or oxygen administration, depending on the infant's color and respirations
3. Electronic monitors* as needed for the observation of respiratory and cardiac functions

Metabolic support consists of measures such as the following:

1. Parenteral therapy to assist in supporting normal blood gas and acid-base homeostasis
2. Parenteral fluids to facilitate antibiotic therapy if sepsis is a concern
3. Blood specimen analyses to monitor blood gases, pH, hypoglycemia, and sepsis

During these emergency treatments and procedures, the nurse must begin to chart signs and symptoms that may reveal the infant's condition and his response to therapy.

Pertinent observations

Vital signs. Initial emergency measures completed, nursing observations and maintenance activities advance to primary importance. The nurse must note, record, and evaluate vital signs frequently. Values obtained during the first 24 hours will serve as a data base.

Temperature. The temperature may be labile and should be monitored frequently. (See the plan of care on p. 530 and procedures on p. 616.) Check every hour until it is stable between 36.1° ± 0.5° C (97° ± 1° F).

Apical pulse. The apical pulse is counted for a full minute. Normally the pulse tends to be weak, rapid, and irregular but readily audible. The normal range is 120 to 160/min.

Respirations. Respirations are counted for a full minute and recorded if they were counted with the infant awake or resting. Rates associated with low morbidity and mortality are as follows:

1. Respirations 40/min from birth without significant fluctuations

2. Respirations 60/min after the first hour of birth, followed by no significant increase or decrease (e.g., ±15 respirations/min)

Periodic breathing is a phenomenon of prematurity. Periods of periodic breathing must not exceed 10 seconds.

Apneic episodes must be monitored electronically. Stimulate the infant to breathe, as necessary, if apneic episodes occur and last for 15 seconds or more.

Blood pressure. The blood pressure is rarely monitored. It may be obtained by biometric instrumentation or approximated by the flush method (p. 630).

Other observations. Other observations are noted at specified intervals. The institution usually has a printed form for recording the findings. Information regarding the following is important:

1. Intravenous therapy: which fluid is infusing, rate of flow, cumulative amounts each hour, medications added (when, how much, what kind, etc.)
2. Elimination: voiding, stools (number, color, character)
3. Weight: daily
4. Skin
   a. Color
      (1) Cyanosis: location, degree, when it appears, does oxygen relieve it and how much oxygen was needed to relieve or eliminate the cyanosis?
      (2) Jaundice
      (3) Plethora
      (4) Pallor
   b. Petechiae, ecchymoses, oozing at the umbilicus or from injection sites, other signs
   c. Turgor
   d. Edema: generalized, eyelids, extremities
   e. Broken, irritated skin; rashes: kind, location
   f. Dry, peeling
5. Degree of hydration
   a. Skin turgor: over abdomen, on inner thigh (not reliable if infant is edematous)
   b. Eyeballs: sunken, soft, normal
   c. Fontanel: sunken, full, flush with cranial bones
6. CNS
   a. Feeding poor
   b. Cry weak, whining, high-pitched
   c. Fontanel bulging
   d. Reflexes (for evaluation of reflexes, see pp. 460 to 464)
   e. Muscle tone
   f. Irritability, hyperactivity, or lethargy

---

*All nurses must be cognizant of electrical and other hazards whenever electronic and inhalation equipment is used. Precautions must be observed constantly (Chapter 38).

g. Opisthotonos

h. Convulsions, twitching of one or more parts of body, increased chewing movements

7. Gastrointestinal tract (for procedures, see Chapter 37)

a. Gavage feeding: any residual, which nostril was used if by nasogastric route, amount, response to feeding

b. Oral feeding: type of nipple needed, amount of time used (to avoid fatigue, no oral feeding should exceed 20 minutes), response to feeding

c. Reflexes: gag, cough, swallow, suck; pharyngeal coordination

d. Formula: kind, amount

e. Time of feeding

f. Regurgitation: type, amount, color, odor, time in relation to feeding

g. Vomiting: type, amount, color, time in relation to feeding, force of, odor

h. Abdominal distention

i. Stools: number, amount, color, condition of buttocks

8. Hypoglycemia: may be asymptomatic but can be approximated or anticipated under the following conditions

a. 50% of all premature infants within 24 hours of birth

b. After abrupt discontinuation of parenteral therapy or hyperalimentation

c. In presence of respiratory distress or sepsis, which are energy-consuming conditions

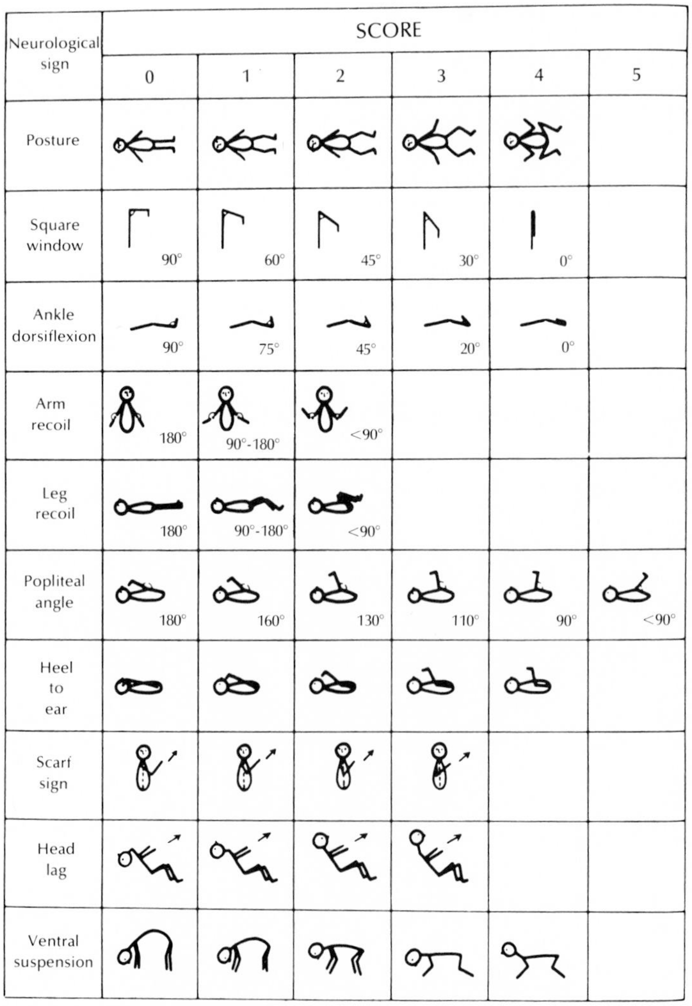

Fig. 34-3. Scoring system of neurologic signs for assessment of gestational age. (From Dubowitz, L. M. S., Dubowitz, V., and Goldberg, C. 1970. J. Pediatr. **77:**1.)

PATIENT'S NAME

⌂ **Examination First Hours**

CLINICAL ESTIMATION
OF GESTATIONAL AGE
An Approximation Based on Published Data*

PHYSICAL FINDINGS		WEEKS GESTATION
VERNIX		APPEARS — COVERS BODY, THICK LAYER — ON BACK, SCALP, IN CREASES — SCANT, IN CREASES — NO VERNIX
BREAST TISSUE AND AREOLA		AREOLA & NIPPLE BARELY VISIBLE NO PALPABLE BREAST TISSUE — AREOLA RAISED — 1-2 MM NODULE — 3-5 MM — 5-6 MM — 7-10 MM — ?12 MM
EAR	FORM	FLAT, SHAPELESS — BEGINNING INCURVING SUPERIOR — INCURVING UPPER 2/3 PINNAE — WELL-DEFINED INCURVING TO LOBE
	CARTILAGE	PINNA SOFT, STAYS FOLDED — CARTILAGE SCANT RETURNS SLOWLY FROM FOLDING — THIN CARTILAGE SPRINGS BACK FROM FOLDING — PINNA FIRM, REMAINS ERECT FROM HEAD
SOLE CREASES		SMOOTH SOLES ̄ CREASES — 1-2 ANTERIOR CREASES — 2-3 ANTERIOR 2/3 CREASES — CREASES ANTERIOR 2/3 SOLE — CREASES INVOLVING HEEL — DEEPER CREASES OVER ENTIRE SOLE
SKIN	THICKNESS & APPEARANCE	THIN, TRANSLUCENT SKIN, PLETHORIC, VENULES OVER ABDOMEN EDEMA — SMOOTH THICKER NO EDEMA — PINK — SOME DESQUAMATION PALE PINK — THICK, PALE, DESQUAMATION OVER ENTIRE BODY
		AP. PEAR — FEW VESSELS
NAIL PLATES		AP. PEARS — NAILS TO FINGER TIPS — NAILS EXTEND WELL BEYOND FINGER TIPS
HAIR		APPEARS ON HEAD — EYE BROWS & LASHES — FINE, WOOLLY, BUNCHES OUT FROM HEAD — SILKY, SINGLE STRANDS LAYS FLAT — RECEDING HAIRLINE OR LOSS OF BABY HAIR SHORT, FINE UNDERNEATH
LANUGO		APPEARS — COVERS ENTIRE BODY — VANISHES FROM FACE — PRESENT ON SHOULDERS — NO LANUGO
GENITALIA	TESTES	TESTES PALPABLE IN INGUINAL CANAL — IN UPPER SCROTUM — IN LOWER SCROTUM
	SCROTUM	FEW RUGAE — RUGAE, ANTERIOR PORTION — RUGAE COVER — PENDULOUS
	LABIA & CLITORIS	PROMINENT CLITORIS LABIA MAJORA SMALL WIDELY SEPARATED — LABIA MAJORA LARGER NEARLY COVERED CLITORIS — LABIA MINORA & CLITORIS COVERED
SKULL FIRMNESS		BONES ARE SOFT — SOFT TO 1" FROM ANTERIOR FONTANELLE — SPONGY AT EDGES OF FONTANELLE CENTER FIRM — BONES HARD SUTURES EASILY DISPLACED — BONES HARD, CANNOT BE DISPLACED
POSTURE	RESTING	HYPOTONIC — HYPOTONIC LATERAL DECUBITUS — BEGINNING FLEXION THIGH — STRONGER HIP FLEXION — FROG-LIKE — FLEXION ALL LIMBS — HYPERTONIC — VERY HYPERTONIC
RECOIL – LEG		NO RECOIL — PARTIAL RECOIL — PROMPT RECOIL
	ARM	NO RECOIL — BEGIN FLEXION NO RECOIL — PROMPT RECOIL MAY BE INHIBITED — PROMPT RECOIL AFTER 30" INHIBITION

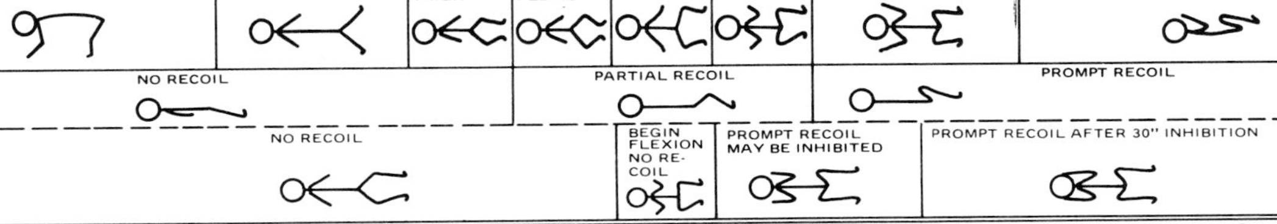

20 21 22 23 24 25 26 27 28 29 30 31 32 33 34 35 36 37 38 39 40 41 42 43 44 45 46 47 48

A

Fig. 34-4. Clinical estimation of gestational age. **A,** Preliminary examination. **B,** Neurologic examination. **C,** Score sheet. (From Brazie, J. V., and Lubchenco. L. O. 1974. In Kempe, C. H., Silver, H. K., and O'Brien, D. [eds.]. Current pediatric diagnosis and treatment [ed. 3]. Los Altos, Calif., Lange Medical Publications.)

Confirmatory Neurologic Examination to be Done After 24 Hours

MeadJohnson LABORATORIES

WEEKS GESTATION: 20 21 22 23 24 25 26 27 28 29 30 31 32 33 34 35 36 37 38 39 40 41 42 43 44 45 46 47 48

PHYSICAL FINDINGS

TONE

Finding	Progression across gestation
HEEL TO EAR	NO RESISTANCE → SOME RESISTANCE → IMPOSSIBLE
SCARF SIGN	NO RESISTANCE → ELBOW PASSES MIDLINE → ELBOW AT MIDLINE → ELBOW DOES NOT REACH MIDLINE
NECK FLEXORS (HEAD LAG)	ABSENT → HEAD IN PLANE OF BODY → HOLDS HEAD
NECK EXTENSORS	HEAD BEGINS TO RIGHT ITSELF FROM FLEXED POSITION → GOOD RIGHTING CANNOT HOLD IT → HOLDS HEAD FEW SECONDS → KEEPS HEAD IN LINE c̄ TRUNK >40" → TURNS HEAD FROM SIDE TO SIDE
BODY EXTENSORS	STRAIGHTENING OF LEGS → STRAIGHTENING OF TRUNK → STRAIGHTENING OF HEAD & TRUNK TOGETHER
VERTICAL POSITIONS	WHEN HELD UNDER ARMS, BODY SLIPS THROUGH HANDS → ARMS HOLD BABY LEGS EXTENDED → LEGS FLEXED GOOD SUPPORT c̄ ARMS → HEAD ABOVE BACK
HORIZONTAL POSITIONS	HYPOTONIC ARMS & LEGS STRAIGHT → ARMS AND LEGS FLEXED → HEAD & BACK EVEN FLEXED EXTREMITIES

FLEXION ANGLES

Finding	Progression across gestation
POPLITEAL	NO RESISTANCE → 150° → 110° → 100° → 90° → 80° (A PRE-TERM WHO HAS REACHED 40 WEEKS STILL HAS A 40° ANGLE)
ANKLE	45° → 60° → 45° → 20° → 0°
WRIST (SQUARE WINDOW)	90° → 60° → 45° → 30° → 0°

REFLEXES

Finding	Progression across gestation
SUCKING	WEAK NOT SYNCHRONIZED c̄ SWALLOWING → STRONGER SYNCHRONIZED → PERFECT
ROOTING	LONG LATENCY PERIOD SLOW, IMPERFECT → HAND TO MOUTH → BRISK, COMPLETE, DURABLE → PERFECT HAND TO MOUTH
GRASP	FINGER GRASP IS GOOD STRENGTH IS POOR → STRONGER → CAN LIFT BABY OFF BED INVOLVES ARMS → COMPLETE → HANDS OPEN
MORO	BARELY APPARENT → WEAK NOT ELICITED EVERY TIME → STRONGER → COMPLETE c̄ ARM EXTENSION OPEN FINGERS, CRY → ARM ADDUCTION ADDED → ?BEGINS TO LOSE MORO
CROSSED EXTENSION	FLEXION & EXTENSION IN A RANDOM, PURPOSELESS PATTERN → EXTENSION BUT NO ADDUCTION → STILL INCOMPLETE → EXTENSION ADDUCTION FANNING OF TOES → COMPLETE.
AUTOMATIC WALK	MINIMAL → BEGINS TIPTOEING GOOD SUPPORT ON SOLE → FAST TIPTOEING → HEEL-TOE PROGRESSION WHOLE SOLE OF FOOT → A PRE-TERM WHO HAS REACHED 40 WEEKS WALKS ON TOES → ?BEGINS TO LOSE AUTOMATIC WALK
PUPILLARY REFLEX	ABSENT → APPEARS → PRESENT
GLABELLAR TAP	ABSENT → APPEARS → PRESENT
TONIC NECK REFLEX	ABSENT → APPEARS
NECK-RIGHTING	ABSENT → PRESENT AFTER 37 WEEKS

B

Fig. 34-4, cont'd. For legend see p. 551.

EXAM FOR GESTATIONAL AGE

Clinical	<36	37-38	39+
Sole creases			
Breast nodule			
Scalp hair			
Earlobe			
Testes and scrotum			

Neurologic	28	29	30	31	32	33	34	35	36	37	38	39	40	41
Pupillary reaction to light														
Traction reflex														
Glabellar tap														
Neck righting														
Head to light														

Posture and passive tone
Posture
Heel to ear
Popliteal angle
Dorsiflexion foot
Scarf sign
Forearm flexion

Active tone
Lower extremity
Trunk
Neck-sitting
Neck-lying

Reflexes
Sucking
Rooting
Grasp
Moro
Crossed extension
Walking

C

LMP_____
EDC_____
Weeks gestation_____

Weight_____
Length_____
Head circumference_____

Date of exam_____

Grams_____%
Centimeters_____%
Centimeters_____%

Gestational age by exam
Clinical_____weeks
Neurological_____weeks

Date of birth_____

Signature_____ M.D.

Fig. 34-4, cont'd. For legend see p. 551.

Transfer from community (hospital or home) to regional neonatal care center

Hospitals that are not staffed or equipped to care for high-risk infants arrange for their immediate transfer to specialized centers. During transport to a center, the following are necessary to meet the infant's needs:

1. Prewarmed blankets, prewarmed incubator, or improvise: surround the infant with hot-water bottles at a distance of 5 to 10 cm from his body
2. Portable oxygen and suction apparatuses
3. Bulb syringe or DeLee mucous trap catheter
4. Intravenous setup with a battery-powered infusion pump
5. Medications as ordered by physician
6. Appropriate attendant(s)

Examination for gestational age

The physician usually conducts the initial examination to determine the probable gestational age. The nurse's correct knowledge of the indicators for gestational age and maturity and the methods of evaluation of these will increase her therapeutic potential at the cribside of all newborns, preterm or otherwise. See Figs. 34-3 and 34-4 for the clinical estimation of gestational age.

Nursing the premature infant

Prematurity implies some immaturity of physiologic functioning and a paucity of reserves. Physiologic problems of immature body systems govern the plan of care of these infants. Nursing actions are based on knowledge of the physiologic problems imposed on the preterm infant and on his need to conserve energy for repair, maintenance, and growth. The physiologic problems, nursing actions, and possible complications follow.

PLAN OF CARE: PRETERM INFANT

PATIENT CARE OBJECTIVES
1. Respirations are initiated and maintained.
2. Body temperature is maintained.
3. The infant is adequately nourished.
4. CNS trauma is prevented or minimized.
5. Infection is prevented.
6. Renal function is supported.
7. Hematologic problems are prevented or minimized.
8. Musculoskeletal problems are prevented or minimized.
9. Retinal damage is prevented or minimized.
10. A positive parent-child relationship and socialization are begun.

PHYSIOLOGIC PROBLEMS
1. Initiation and maintenance of respirations:
   a. Paucity of functional alveoli.
   b. Smaller lumen and greater collapsibility or obstruction of respiratory passages.
   c. Weakness of respiratory musculature.
   d. Insufficient calcification of bony thorax.
   e. Absent or weak gag, cough reflex.
   f. Immature and friable capillaries in brain and lungs.
   g. Infants less than 28 weeks gestational age have few functional alveoli and are usually nonviable. Infants at 29 to 30 weeks are marginal for this function.
2. Maintenance of body temperature: The smaller the infant the more difficult it is for him to maintain a normal body temperature.
   a. Large surface area in relation to body weight (mass).
   b. Absent or poor reflex control of skin capillaries (no shiver response).
   c. Small, inadequate muscle mass activity.
   d. Paucity of insulating subcutaneous fat.
   e. Immature temperature regulating center in brain plus friable capillaries in brain.
3. Maintenance of adequate nutrition.
   a. Mechanical feeding problems:
      (1) Absent or weak sucking and swallow reflexes; unsynchronized.
      (2) Absent or weak gag and cough reflexes.
      (3) Small stomach capacity.

PLAN OF CARE: PRETERM INFANT—cont'd

PHYSIOLOGIC PROBLEMS—cont'd

(4) Immature cardiac sphincter.

(5) Lax abdominal musculature.

b. Absorption and assimilation problems:

(1) Paucity of stored nutrients: vitamins A and C; calcium, phosphorus, iron; glycogen; fat; protein. Loss of fat and fat-soluble vitamins in stool.

(2) Immature absorption, decreased amount of HCl.

(3) Impaired metabolism (enzyme systems) or enzyme pathology.

4. CNS trauma:

a. Birth trauma: damage to immature structures.

b. Fragile capillaries and impaired coagulation process; prolonged prothrombin time.

c. Recurrent anoxic episodes.

d. Tendency to hypoglycemia.

5. Poor resistance to infection:

a. Paucity of stored nutrients from mother.

b. Paucity of stored immunoglobulins from mother.

c. Impaired ability to synthesize nucleoproteins (antibodies).

d. Thin skin and fragile capillaries near surface.

e. Impaired ability to muster white blood cells.

6. Maintenance of renal function:

a. Impaired renal clearance of metabolites, drugs.

b. Inability to maintain acid-base and electrolyte homeostasis.

c. Impaired ability to concentrate urine.

7. Minimization of hematologic problems:

a. Increased capillary friability and permeability.

b. Low plasma prothrombin levels (increased tendency to bleed).

c. Relatively slowed erythropoietic activity in bone marrow.

d. Relatively increased rate of hemolysis.

e. Loss of blood to lab specimens.

8. Immature musculoskeletal system:

a. Weak, underdeveloped muscles.

b. Immature skeletal system (bones, joints).

c. Paucity of subcutaneous fat and its cushioning effect.

9. Retinal immaturity, coupled with respiratory immaturity and distress, low birth weight, and other unidentified factors.

NURSING INTERVENTIONS

Diagnostic	Therapeutic*
Respiratory function	
1. Check respiration rate, depth, regularity:	1. Maintain warmth to decrease O_2 consumption and sequelae of cold stress.
a. Periodic breathing.	2. Suction as needed.
b. Apnea.	3. Administer warmed and humidified compressed air and O_2 at levels to relieve cyanosis and dyspnea.
c. Seesaw respirations.	
d. Expiratory grunt.	a. Analyze O_2 concentration every 1 to 4 hours.
e. Chin tug.	b. Blood gases and electrolytes: order, assist with, record time, procedure, amount of blood drawn, infant's response.
f. Retractions.	
g. Flaring of alae nasi.	
2. Cry: feeble, whining, high-pitched.	4. Position infant to assist ventilatory effort (p. 534).
3. Check heart rate.	5. Feeding technique appropriate for this infant (pp. 542 to 545).
4. Cyanosis:	
a. When it occurs.	6. Keep on respiratory monitor until infant weighs 4

*Educational interventions are not included per se in this plan. The nursing-medical team (1) explains to the parents equipment and procedures, the appearance and positioning of the infant, and the infant's responses; (2) provides support during the grieving process; (3) facilitates parent-child bonding by encouraging parents to visit and touch and to voice feelings and concerns; and (4) assists parents to prepare family for receiving infant. For further discussion refer to Chapters 7, 29, and 33.

Continued.

PLAN OF CARE: PRETERM INFANT—cont'd

NURSING INTERVENTIONS—cont'd

Diagnostic	Therapeutic

Respiratory function—cont'd

    b. Where (circumoral, generalized).
    c. Relieved by O_2 or not; amount O_2 needed.
    d. Accompanied by pallor.
5. Check reflexes: presence and condition of gag, swallow, cough.
6. Prebirth history:
    a. Was mother treated with betamethasone?
    b. Preeclampsia? (Sedatives, magnesium sulfate, diuretics?)
    c. Maternal temperature.
    d. Maternal infection.
    e. Premature rupture of membranes: length of time prior to delivery, color, odor, culture, amount of fluid.

pounds or condition stabilizes; check rate every 1 to 2 hours and when necessary.

Temperature regulation

1. Check for variations in body temperature by following:
    a. Thermister probe to skin.
    b. Axillary temperature.
    c. Rectal method (not recommended).
2. Temperature of extremities should feel warm to touch.
3. Check for dehydration:
    a. Soft, sunken eyeball.
    b. Depressed fontanel.
    c. Poor skin turgor over abdomen, inner thigh.
4. Observe for apneic pauses.
    a. Number.
    b. Duration.
    c. Whether accompanied by cyanosis or not.
    d. Does infant pick up same respiratory rate after apneic episode or is rate increased? Decreased?

1. Maintain temperature:
    a. Skin: 36.7° C (98° F).
    b. Axillary: 36.5° C (97.8° F).
    c. Incubator: usually 33.5° to 35° C (92° to 95° F).
2. Keep incubator away from windows, air conditioners.
3. Ensure warmth during all procedures:
    a. Ambient warm air, draft-free.
    b. Warmed blankets and equipment.
    c. Blood transfusion warmed by passing tube through warm bath.
    d. Nurse's hands are warm.
    e. Incubator lid and portholes are closed.
    f. Warm air or O_2 to infant.
4. Conserve infant's energy whenever possible. Handle as little and as gently as possible.

Nutrition

Feeding

1. Check reflex maturity:
    a. Suck and swallow.
    b. Gag and cough.
2. Assess energy level.
    a. Length of time needed to eat.
    b. Degree of fatigability.
3. Observe for following:
    a. Diarrhea.
    b. Dehydration.
    c. Vomiting or regurgitation.
    d. Gastric residual.
    e. Color, amount, character of stools.
4. Plot daily weight on growth grid.
5. Measure for growth every week:
    a. Head circumference.
    b. Body length.

1. Institute appropriate method for this infant:
    a. Oral.
    b. Gavage.
    c. Do not use nipple if respirations ≥60/min.
2. Feed early:
    a. To prevent depletion of reserves.
    b. To support biochemical homeostasis.
3. Start feedings with sterile water, then proceed to glucose, then to formula if feeding by oral route.
4. Timing of feedings:
    a. Infant under 1250 gm (2 pounds 12 ounces), every 2 hours.
    b. Infant between 1500 and 1800 gm (3½ to 4 pounds), every 3 hours.
    c. Infants in good condition and with active peristalsis, start first feeding between 6 and 12 hours after birth.
    d. Infant with respiratory distress, give parenteral fluids.

PLAN OF CARE: PRETERM INFANT—cont'd

NURSING INTERVENTIONS—cont'd

Diagnostic	Therapeutic
Absorption and assimilation	

1. Observe for following:
  a. Steatorrhea.
  b. Activity level: active or lethargic?
  c. Color: pallor?
  d. Symptoms of hypoglycemia.
2. Test for hypoglycemia with Dextrostix (≤20 mg/100 ml blood for preterm infant). May be otherwise asymptomatic.
3. Assess for edema.
	1. As above.
	2. Administer and record vitamins and minerals per physician order (vitamins A, C, D, E; iron).
	3. Adjust formula, feeding method, etc., to infant's responses and changing needs.

CNS	

1. Observe for symptoms of increased intracranial pressure.
2. Observe for convulsions:
  a. Twitching.
  b. Increased chewing movements.
  c. Eye rolling.
3. Observe for behavior changes.
	1. Maintain adequate oxygenation to relieve cyanosis.
	2. Maintain open airway.
	3. Prevent or promptly identify and relieve hypoglycemia, hypocalcemia.

Infection	

1. Note following:
  a. Feeding behavior.
  b. Skin: irritations, rashes, jaundice.
  c. Drainage from eyes, umbilicus; nasal congestion.
  d. Frequency of stools.
  e. Body temperature (unreliable).
  f. Behavior change: "just not right," lethargic, listless.
  g. Respiratory rate increase or decrease (persistent) for 24 hours.
2. Check antenatal record: exposure to infections, fever, genital herpes. Rupture of membranes: time and duration, odor, color.
	1. Meticulous hand-washing is imperative; check personnel's health.
	2. Use aseptic technique for anything puncturing skin and for umbilical catheterization.
	3. Prevent skin breakdown:
	  a. Under monitor leads, tapes, restraints.
	  b. Over bony prominences. Use flotation pad or sheepskin.
	4. Gentle insertion of orogastric or nasogastric tubes.
	5. Supervise parents' hand-washing, gowning when visiting.
	6. Monitor administration of medications.
	7. Restrict visitors, repairmen, equipment change, etc.

Renal function	

1. Note following:
  a. Urinary output:
    (1) Diaper saturation; number of diapers/day.
    (2) Collect and measure; check specific gravity.
  b. Edema.
  c. Tachypnea.
  d. Vomiting.
  e. Abdominal distension.
	1. Assist kidney function by decreasing demands on that system:
	  a. Provide formula with right concentration of solute.
	  b. Support respirations, normal body temperature, nutrition, fluid balance.
	  c. Prevent infection.

Hematologic problems	

1. Note following:
  a. Skin manifestations: ecchymoses, petechiae, jaundice, pallor.
  b. Increased bleeding or oozing around cord, injection sites, etc.
  c. Symptoms of cerebral irritation (or increased intracranial pressure from hemorrhage).
	1. Handle infant gently and as little as possible.
	2. Give intramuscular injection of vitamin K (one dose) if not being given antibiotics that hamper its synthesis in gastrointestinal tract. If being given these antibiotics, more doses will be needed.
	3. Treat to reduce hyperbilirubinemia with phototherapy or assist with exchange transfusions.
	4. Monitor withdrawal of blood for lab examinations and evaluations. Assist with blood replacement as necessary.

Continued.

PLAN OF CARE: PRETERM INFANT—cont'd

NURSING INTERVENTIONS—cont'd

Diagnostic	Therapeutic
Immature musculoskeletal system	
1. Molding of cranial bones is noted.	1. Position infant:
2. Also note following:	a. Change position frequently.
a. Unnatural rotation or extension of joints.	b. Place in correct body alignment. Watch position of feet; position laterally to aid in walking later.
b. Asymmetric contours of body.	2. If diapers are used (infant under 1500 gm should not be diapered), cut to size; pin or tape with posterior flap overlapping anterior flap.
c. Muscle tone, muscle mass.	
d. Pressure areas over bony prominences.	3. Pad areas over bony prominences (sheepskin, bubble pads, other).
Retinal immaturity	
1. Monitor following:	1. Supervise collection of blood for study: method, time, amount.
a. Blood gas values.	
b. O_2 concentration of inspired air.	2. Monitor amount and duration of O_2 therapy to keep P_aO_2 between 50 and 70 mm Hg or better.
2. Note and record respiratory distress and amount and duration of O_2 therapy required to relieve distress.	

POSSIBLE COMPLICATIONS

1. Respiratory problems: atelectasis, apnea, anoxia, asphyxia, pneumothorax, altered blood gases and pH, retrolental fibroplasia, bronchopulmonary dysplasia, RDS (HMD).
2. Inadequate temperature maintenance:
   a. Cold stress with oxygen deprivation, respiratory acidosis, metabolic acidosis, depletion of glycogen stores (hypoglycemia), sclerema.
   b. Hyperthermia with apneic episodes.
   c. Dehydration.
3. Nutrition:
   a. Feeding problems: aspiration, aspiration pneumonia, abdominal distention, diarrhea, dehydration, electrolyte imbalance, inadequate weight gain, hypoglycemia with neurologic sequelae.
   b. Absorption and assimilation problems: edema, anemia, rickets, scurvy, incomplete metabolism of phenylalanine and tyrosine, electrolyte imbalance.
4. CNS trauma: mental retardation, cerebral palsy, neuromuscular impairment, psychosocial impairment, perceptual problems.
5. Infection: septicemia, sepsis, shock, hypoglycemia.
6. Renal problems:
   a. Acidosis.
   b. Edema.
   c. Azotemia.
   d. Vomiting and aspiration and abdominal distention compromise adequate ventilation.
   e. Electrolyte imbalance.
   f. Dehydration.
7. Hematologic problems:
   a. Hyperbilirubinemia, kernicterus, anemia, intracranial hemorrhage.
   b. Too many or inappropriately placed heel sticks for bloods may cause heel cord shortening and problems in walking later on (p. 615).
8. Immature musculoskeletal system:
   a. Hip dislocation: hyperextension and external rotation.
   b. Misshapen skull.
9. Retinal immaturity:
   a. Retrolental fibroplasia, with severity ranging from impaired vision to retinal detachment and total blindness.

Nutritional requirements

The nutritional requirements for low birth weight infants are given in Table 33-5.

Nutritional supplementation of the following vitamins and minerals frequently is warranted for both the premature and SGA infant:

1. Vitamin A is lost if the neonate has steatorrhea.
2. Vitamin C is required to metabolize phenylalanine and tyrosine.
3. Vitamin D and calcium are in great demand to promote bone and tissue growth and to replace losses through steatorrhea.
4. Vitamin E and pyridoxine are essential in the prevention of anemia and edema and may be added to the infant's formula by the third day of life.
5. Vitamin K_1 (not an analog that may predispose to hyperbilirubinemia), 0.5 to 1 mg intramuscularly, is given soon after birth. Depending on gestational age, the neonate may have difficulty in synthesizing vitamin K_1. If the infant is receiving antibiotic therapy (which destroys intestinal flora), has diarrhea, is lacking the ability to absorb nutrients, or is receiving parenteral fluids, additional doses of vitamin K_1 may be indicated.
6. Elemental iron is added to the infant's formula by 2 months of age.

Diseases of prematurity

Respiratory distress syndrome (RDS), also known as *hyaline membrane disease* (HMD), retrolental fibroplasia, and bronchopulmonary dysplasia are seen almost exclusively in preterm neonates. RDS claims a significant number of lives, whereas the impaired vision or blindness resulting from retrolental fibroplasia places a serious burden on the survivors and their families.

The cause, clinical course, supportive measures, and prognosis of these diseases are discussed here in some detail. The rationale is to provide the nurse with a substantial theory base to accomplish the following:

- Recognize predisposing obstetric factors and refer pregnant women at risk to appropriate facilities. This is especially critical for the many nurses in outlying districts who bear considerable responsibility in providing maternity and newborn services.
- Assure knowledgeable assessment of the infant's status initially and during therapy
- Implement and modify prescribed therapies judiciously
- Facilitate parental support and education

RDS

Incidence. RDS is a leading cause of morbidity and mortality among preterm infants, affecting about 20,000 per year in North America. Generally, the smaller the preterm infant the higher the mortality rate. Occasionally a full-term neonate is affected.

Pathophysiology. The central lesion is atelectasis. The *membrane* is composed in part of fibrin derived from the pulmonary circulation and is not the result of aspirated fluid or an irritant. Accompanying problems such as hypoxia, metabolic and respiratory acidosis, and pulmonary hypoperfusion with right-to-left shunting are secondary to atelectasis.

Cause. The development of a hyaline membrane within the proximal bronchial tree of neonates dying of respiratory distress within a few hours after birth still is a cryptic disorder. The role of surfactant in preventing alveolar collapse at the end of expiration has been established. A deficiency in surfactant production may be the basis for RDS.

Surfactant (or surface factor) designates a group of surface-active phospholipids. Of this group, lecithin may be the crucial phospholipid responsible for alveolar stability. This biochemical compound is present on the surface of the alveolar cells, creating the minimal surface tension necessary to keep these spaces open on expiration. Lungs must remain partially expanded at all times. This process is analogous to powdering rubber gloves so that they do not stick together.

A deficiency in this surfactant forces the infant to work to reexpand the lungs with each inspiration. The result is fatigue, depletion of energy reserves, hypoxia and hypercapnia, progressive atelectasis, and diminishing lung compliance (or increasing ''stiffness''). Factors that impair the production of surfactant are hypoxia, acidosis, and reduced pulmonary blood circulation. Thus a vicious cycle is established. The normal newborn expends more calories and consumes more oxygen to breathe than does the adult. For the infant in respiratory distress this expenditure may be as much as six times that of the normal term newborn.

Lecithin production. Enzyme systems necessary for the production of lecithin are normally activated between the thirty-second and thirty-sixth week of gestation. From the thirty-fourth to thirty-sixth week of intrauterine life, the fetus resides in a high cortisol milieu, and there is reason to conclude that it is the high glucocorticoid levels that are normally responsible for accelerating surfactant synthesis and lung maturation. These biochemical pathways seem to be prodded into earlier maturation and secretion of lecithin in conditions such as the following:

1. Partial premature separation of placenta (abruptio placentae)

2. Prolonged rupture of fetal membranes, intrauterine infection, or both
3. Maternal hypertension regardless of origin (preeclampsia, other hypertensive states)
4. Maternal heroin addition

These stressors force earlier lung maturation and frequently preclude the development of RDS.

In the late 1960s a synthetic steroidlike hormone (betamethasone) that stimulates fetal lung maturity if given to the pregnant woman 2 to 3 days before the anticipated premature birth was identified. This is only effective at select times, between 28 and 32 weeks' gestation. Betamethasone, given for a brief period, neither affects the growth or development of other vital fetal organs nor does the drug disturb the mother. The incidence of RDS in treated neonates is greatly reduced. Therefore the cost of caring for these infants is reduced from several thousands of dollars to a few dollars.

If this promising prophylactic treatment proves successful and without adverse side effects, clinic and labor nurses need to be well informed to provide parental support while competently assisting in the procedures involved.

Other conditions such as maternal diabetes and erythroblastosis fetalis seem to have the opposite effect by delaying lung maturity and the production of pulmonary lecithin. It is as yet unclear if maternal diabetes delays lung maturity or if the incidence appears greater because infants of diabetic mothers tend to be delivered electively before term.

Onset. RDS may be apparent in the infant at birth. This neonate has a low Apgar score and frequently requires resuscitation and ventilatory assistance. Other symptoms generally appear within the first 6 hours. Initially expiratory grunting and nasal flaring are evident. As the disease progresses, tachypnea (60 respirations/ min or more), retractions, and even cyanosis in room air may be noted. Hypotension and shock may be evident. Apneic pauses replace the expiratory grunting. An arterial Po_2 of 40 mm Hg or less in room air is a constant finding. Symptoms often peak in 48 to 72 hours.

Diagnosis. X-ray films usually reveal a generalized granular or reticular alteration in both lungs and diminished lung volume. Patchy atelectasis may be present also but distinguishable from RDS. Bronchial air shadows may highlight the films. A reduced blood pH value but increased serum nonprotein nitrogen, potassium, and phosphorous values are typical of RDS. Arterial blood gases show decreased arterial Po_2 and often a combined metabolic and respiratory acidosis. Scattered visceral and peripheral hemorrhages may develop in critical cases.

Treatment. Therapy of the infant with RDS is primarily supportive. Specific and general supportive methods are discussed.

Specific supportive methods. Until the neonate can produce lecithin, oxygenation and ventilation are as follows:

1. The neonate with mild involvement may be supported by increased oxygenation of inspired air. A common practice is to administer the oxygen (60% or less) by means of a hood.
2. Continuous positive airway pressure (CPAP) may be administered by means of an intratracheal tube, face mask, nasal prongs, or hood (p. 614).
3. Continuous negative airway pressure (CNAP) is a respirator that works in the same manner as CPAP but exerts negative pressure on the neonate's body while its head is exposed. The neonate may breathe room air or an air-oxygen mix by means of a mask or prongs.
4. Continuous end expiratory pressure (CEEP) may be administered (p. 614).
5. Mechanical respiratory aids may be needed to maintain ventilation in the event that other methods do not relieve respiratory distress such as hypoxia, apnea, or respiratory failure.

In addition, intratracheal intubation is accompanied by risks of infection, blockage with secretions, and inflammation of the mucosa.

The following caution is observed: Injudicious use of oxygen and mechanical devices to deliver oxygen or air under high pressures must be avoided because these may be detrimental. (See opposite page for detailed description of oxygen toxicity.) Often they may result in any one or a combination of the following:

- Destruction or diminution of the lung cells' capacity to produce lecithin
- Pneumothorax or pneumomediastinum
- Bronchopulmonary dysplasia
- Retrolental fibroplasia

Regarding the treatment for acidosis, energetic treatment with sodium bicarbonate tromethamine (THAM) is being questioned. Its possible relationship to increased incidence of intracranial hemorrhage and persistent patent ductus arteriosus is under study. Infusions of blood and albumin are being used to correct acidemia instead of sodium bicarbonate. Favorable results have been reported. (It had previously been noted that the infants who subsequently developed RDS had low cord proteins, whether preterm or term. If cord proteins were high, any respiratory distress noted was because of problems other than RDS.)

Adjustment of fluid-electrolyte imbalance is also important in RDS.

General supportive methods. The following measures are important in the treatment of the infant with RDS:

1. A thermoneutral environment is provided so that the infant's body temperature is maintained between 36.5° to 37° C (97.8° to 98.6° F).

2. Gentle handling of the neonate is necessary. This infant is disturbed as little as possible.

3. Caloric intake is sufficient to prevent catabolism (40 calories/kg/24 hr or more).

4. Replace blood if excessive amount is lost, usually as a result of samples taken for laboratory analysis.

5. Control serum bilirubin levels by phototherapy, exchange transfusion, or both. Low serum albumin levels, hypoxia, and acidosis interfere with the binding of bilirubin and therefore subject these infants to kernicterus at low serum bilirubin levels (10 mg/100 ml or less).

6. Digitalize as needed.

7. Prophylactic antibiotic therapy is controversial but is indicated if umbilical catheterization is performed.

Prognosis. Formerly if the infant survived the first 48 to 72 hours, his clinical condition improved slowly until recovery at about 10 to 12 days. However, newer methods and equipment may sustain the infant longer, and recovery or death may ensue several weeks after birth.

Antenatal diagnosis of lung maturity is relatively accurate (p. 192). The technique for analyzing amniotic fluid for the L/S ratio provides data from which to determine the best possible time for cesarean delivery if this is contemplated, to determine if treatment with betamethasone or its equivalent is indicated, or to decide whether to transfer the mother to a regional neonatal care center for delivery. Thus the infant's immediate needs are anticipated, and precious time is not lost in obtaining adequate medical and nursing care.

PREMATURITY AND OXYGEN TOXICITY

Retrolental fibroplasia and bronchopulmonary dysplasia are diseases of prematurity secondary to oxygen therapy. Both conditions are relatively "new" disorders, recognized since the advent of methods of administering high concentrations of oxygen beginning in the 1940s. Although oxygen therapy may be lifesaving and occasionally must be given in high concentrations for extended periods of time, it is also potentially hazardous and must be administered judiciously (p. 612).

Retrolental fibroplasia. The retinal changes in retrolental fibroplasia were first described in 1942. The occurrence of this condition has been found to be related to the following factors:

- Incomplete retinal differentiation and completion of vascularization

- High arterial oxygen tension levels
- Prolonged duration of oxygen therapy

P_aO_2 between 45 and 70 mm Hg (arterialized heel stick levels between 35 and 45 mm Hg) may be within safe limits. The most crucial period for toxic levels to occur is during the recovery phase from RDS and other respiratory distress. The exact level of arterial oxygen tension needed to prevent RDS is unknown.

Oxygen tensions that are too high for the level of retinal maturity initially result in vasoconstriction. Subsequently, after oxygen therapy is discontinued, neovascularization in the retina and vitreous occurs with capillary hemorrhages, fibrotic resolution, and possible retinal detachment. Cicatricial tissue formation and consequent visual impairment may be mild or severe. The entire disease process in severe cases may take as long as 5 months to evolve. Examination by an ophthalmologist before discharge and a schedule for repeat examinations thereafter are recommended to direct anticipatory guidance of parents.

Bronchopulmonary dysplasia. Bronchopulmonary dysplasia (BPD) is a possible sequela to treatment with positive pressure ventilation (rarely found in neonates supported by negative pressure apparatuses) and high levels of inspired oxygen (60% or more). Changes in the lung fields resemble those of Mikity-Wilson syndrome. The coarse cystic changes result in focal areas of emphysema. Respiratory distress, tachypnea, and increased effort appears. It is difficult to wean the infant from the positive-pressure ventilator. This finding may be the first indication of the disease process. Cor pulmonale and cardiac failure may occur.

Prognosis. The first sign that the infant is recovering is a decreasing dependence on oxygen therapy. Recovery may take several months. The mortality rate is between 30% and 50%.

NEONATAL NECROTIZING ENTEROCOLITIS

Necrotizing enterocolitis (NEC) is an inflammatory disease of the gastrointestinal mucosa, frequently complicated by perforation. This often fatal disease appears in about 5% of neonates in intensive care nurseries. Although its etiology is unknown, several possibilities are suspect:

1. Immaturity (approximately 25% of preterm infants weighing 1300 gm or less develop this disease)
2. Hypoxemia
3. High solute feedings
4. Excessive amounts of feeding
5. Septicemia

In addition, NEC does not develop in infants fed with breast milk.

Signs of developing NEC are nonspecific as is characteristic of many neonatal disease processes. The infant's color is poor. Apneic periods increase in number. Abdominal distention may be noted. Frequently, gastric residuals are 2 ml or more prior to feedings. Stool may be positive for occult blood (positive guaiac). Diagnosis is confirmed by x-ray examination.

Treatment is supportive. Oral or tube feedings are discontinued to rest the gastrointestinal tract. Parenteral therapy (often by alimentation) is begun. Antibiotic therapy may be instituted. Surgery is performed when necessary. Therapy may be prolonged, since recovery may be delayed by adhesions, complications of bowel resection (malabsorption), and intolerance for oral feedings.

Prognosis for preterm infants

Baseline examination. An examination is performed to provide baseline data. From these data, handicapping conditions may be identified early and appropriate treatment begun. In addition, the infant's progress may be plotted and tentative prognosis proferred. Suggested evaluative tests include growth grids adjusted to gestational age, the Denver Developmental Screening Test, and a neurologic examination.

Favorable outcome criteria. Although it is impossible to predict with complete accuracy the growth and developmental potential of each premature neonate, some findings support an anticipated favorable outcome. The growth and development landmarks are corrected for gestational age.

The age of a preterm neonate is corrected by adding the gestational age and the postnatal age. For example, if an infant was born at 32 weeks' gestation a month ago, today she is 36 weeks of age according to her gestational life (age since her mother's LMP). Six months after her birthdate, the child's corrected age is 4 months. Her responses are evaluated against the norm expected of a 4-month-old infant.

Favorable findings that support the prediction of a growth and developmental pattern within the norm include the following:

1. At discharge from the hospital, which usually occurs between 37 and 40 weeks after the LMP, the infant is assessed for the following characteristics:

    a. When prone, the infant can raise his head. He is able to hold his head parallel with his body when tested for the traction response. (When pulled up by the hands, the infant's head lags, but then his head and chest will be in line as the infant reaches the upright position. This alignment will be held momentarily before the head falls forward.)

    b. When the infant is hungry, he cries with vigor.

    c. The growth grid shows appropriate weight gain and pattern of weight gain.

    d. The neurologic examination reveals appropriate responses for age. The retina appears normal.

2. At 39 to 40 weeks since the LMP, the infant is able to focus on the examiner or parent's face and is able to follow it with his eyes.

3. At the corrected ages of 6 and 12 months, the infant is assessed again for age-appropriate responses.

The infant is suspect if he displays any of the following behaviors:

- Was and continues to be a poor feeder
- Is irritable
- Displays sensory, perceptual, intellectual, or motor deviations as he matures
- Displays or develops hypertonia or hypotonia.

These behaviors must be interpreted with caution and the infant reevaluated by an interdisciplinary team at frequent intervals. Parents will need continued support and attention should these signs appear. Minor behavioral deviations should be diagnosed also so that the parents can be assisted in their understanding and acceptance of the child. Deviations such as clumsiness, varying degrees of incoordination, slowness in reading and writing, and other similar problems may be distressing to the parents and other family members.

Child abuse and neglect. The incidence of physical and emotional abuse is three times greater toward the infant who by virtue of prematurity or illness was separated from his mother for a period of time after his birth. Physical abuse includes varying degrees of poor nutrition and poor hygiene; emotional abuse ranges from subtle to outright dislike of the child; preferential treatment for siblings, nagging, extremely high expectations of the child, and various other types of overt or covert negative responses by one or both parents.

Factors surrounding the birth such as parental pain and anxiety, heavy financial burden for his care, unresolved anticipatory grief and threat to self-esteem, unwanted pregnancy, and many others may predispose parents to subconsciously or overtly reject the child. The goal of the helping professionals is to reduce the incidence of child abuse and neglect.

A carefully devised medical-nursing care plan may help to reduce this threat to the infant born at risk. Parents who have negative feelings about the pregnancy, and/or the infant at risk need support. Their feelings can be acknowledged as valid, including the burden they are experiencing financially and emotionally and their understandable feelings toward the infant. Parents are prepared for the procedures and gadgetry of the intensive care unit. Soon after delivery, the parents, especially the mother, should have the opportunity to meet the infant in the *en face* position, to touch him, and to see his favorable characteristics. As soon as possible, depending primarily on the mother's physical condition, the mother is allowed to visit the nursery at will and assist with the infant's care. When she is not able to be physically present, the staff devises appropriate methods to keep the family in almost constant touch with the neonate (p. 100). Some hospitals have instituted a parents' club for parents of infants in intensive care nurseries. These clubs encourage those who are experiencing the same anxiety and grief to share their feelings. An "older" member often takes over a "new" member and provides additional support.* Incorporating these actions into the infant's care plan is to acknowledge and support nature's design in engaging and maintaining a bond between the mother and infant that ensures for the infant the continued care he needs for physical and emotional survival at an optimal level.

---

*For further information write to Ms. Terry Gardner, c/o Margaret Jensen, San Jose State University, San Jose, Calif. 95126.

SGA (DYSMATURE) INFANTS
General considerations

Infants whose birth weight, for reasons other than heredity, falls below the tenth percentile expected at term are considered at high risk (mortality greater than 10%). Fetal growth retardation is attributable to the following possible causes:

- Deficient supply of nutrients (intrauterine malnutrition)
- Intrauterine infections
- Congenital malformations
- Heredity

Intrauterine growth retardation related to malnutrition will be discussed here. Two types of growth retardation are identified by the examination of cellular characteristics:

1. Hypoplasia or deficient number of cells, although each cell has a normal amount of cytoplasm
2. Diminished cell size resulting from a reduced amount of cytoplasm, although the total number of cells is unaffected

Malnutrition early in embryonic development results

PLAN OF CARE: SGA INFANT

PATIENT CARE OBJECTIVES
1. Adequate ventilation is initiated and maintained.
2. Adequate nutritional state is achieved and maintained.
3. Body temperature is maintained.
4. CNS trauma is prevented or minimized.
5. Infection is prevented.
6. Musculoskeletal problems are prevented or minimized.
7. Positive parent-child relationship and socialization are begun.

PHYSIOLOGIC PROBLEMS*
1. Initiation and maintenance of respirations:
   a. Chronic intrauterine hypoxia, perinatal asphyxia.
   b. Aspiration syndrome: ball-valve obstruction.
2. Maintenance of adequate nutrition: chronic intrauterine malnutrition with paucity of stored fat and glycogen.
3. Maintenance of body temperature:
   a. Depleted subcutaneous fat and glycogen reserves.
   b. Diminished muscle mass.
   c. Large body surface compared to body weight.
4. CNS trauma:
   a. Tendency to hypoglycemia.
   b. Chronic intrauterine hypoxia, perinatal asphyxia.
5. Poor resistance to infection:
   a. Growth retardation may be due totally or in part to exposure to intrauterine infection.
   b. Paucity of fat and glycogen stores.
6. Musculoskeletal system:
   a. Inadequate bone growth: wide cranial sutures.
   b. Diminished muscle mass, especially over buttocks, cheeks.
   c. Paucity of subcutaneous fat and its cushioning effect.

---

*Related to intrauterine nutritional growth retardation.

Continued.

PLAN OF CARE: SGA INFANT—cont'd

NURSING INTERVENTIONS

Diagnostic	Therapeutic*
Respiratory function	
1. Same as for preterm infant.	1. Same as for preterm infant.
2. Alert, wide-eyed appearance.	2. Suction as needed: endotracheal intubation with tracheobronchial suction.
Nutrition	
1. Same as for preterm infant.	1. Same as for preterm infant with exception of timing of feedings.
2. Hunger: cries, fusses for feeding; large capacity for feedings.	2. Initiate feeding at 2 to 4 hours of age.
3. Weigh every day.	3. Safeguard energy reserves:
4. Check intake and output.	a. Facilitate respiratory efforts.
	b. Maintain body warmth.
	c. If on parenteral fluids, monitor carefully; wean slowly.
Temperature regulation	
1. Same as for preterm infant.	1. Same as for preterm infant.
CNS trauma	
1. Signs and symptoms of hypoglycemia.	1. Maintain adequate oxygenation.
2. Muscle tone.	2. Identify promptly or prevent hypoglycemia.
3. Irritability and reactivity.	
4. Reflex responses: difficult to elicit, absent, asymmetric.	
Infection	
1. Same as for preterm infant.	1. Same as for preterm infant.
Musculoskeletal system	
1. Pressure areas over bony prominences.	1. Same as for preterm infant.
2. Body contour and alignment; symmetry.	

POSSIBLE COMPLICATIONS

1. Respiratory functions: altered blood gases and pH, asphyxia, aspiration pneumonia, atelectasis, pneumomediastinum, pneumothorax.
2. Nutrition:
   a. Same as for preterm infant.
   b. Hypoglycemia with neurologic sequelae.
3. Inadequate temperature maintenance: same as for preterm infant.
4. CNS trauma: same as for preterm infant.
5. Infection: same as for preterm infant.
6. Musculoskeletal system:
   a. Skin breakdown, infection.
   b. Misshapen skull.

*For educational interventions, see plan of care on p. 555.

in hypoplasia; later in fetal life, it results in reduced cell size. For a more detailed discussion of intrauterine growth retardation refer to the references at the end of this chapter.

Physical characteristics

Several physical findings are characteristic of the growth-retarded neonate:

1. Reduced subcutaneous fat
2. Loose and dry skin
3. Diminished muscle mass especially over buttocks and cheeks
4. Sunken abdomen (scaphoid) as opposed to being normally well-rounded
5. Thin, yellowish, dry, and dull umbilical cord (normal cord is gray, glistening, round, and moist)
6. Sparse scalp hair
7. Wide skull sutures (inadequate bone growth)

Neonatal morbidity

An increased susceptibility to neonatal illness is obvious in these SGA infants. The following problems are the most commonly diagnosed and are mentioned here to alert the neonatal nurse.

Perinatal asphyxia. Frequently, SGA infants have been exposed to chronic hypoxia for varying periods of time prior to labor and delivery. Labor is stressful to even a normal fetus and is more serious for one suffering from growth retardation. The chronically hypoxic infant is severely compromised by even a normal labor and has difficulty compensating after birth. The alert, wide-eyed appearance of the neonate is attributed to prolonged prenatal hypoxia. Appropriate management and resuscitation are essential for the depressed infant.

A maternal history of heavy cigarette smoking, preeclampsia-eclampsia, low socioeconomic status, multiple gestation, gestational infections such as rubella and syphilis, advanced diabetes mellitus, and cardiac problems is associated with small infants predisposed to perinatal asphyxia. When a women with this background arrives in labor, the nursery staff must be alerted to possible perinatal asphyxia.

Aspiration syndrome. Two fetal responses to intrauterine hypoxia are the passage of meconium through a relaxed anal sphincter and reflex gasping. Gasping draws amniotic fluid and any particulate matter contained deep into the bronchial tree. At birth, more aspiration may occur, and symptoms of respiratory distress often appear.

Hypoglycemia. Hypoglycemia is frequently encountered in SGA neonates, term or preterm. The incidence may be as high as 40%. Hypoglycemia in low birth weight infants is considered to be a glucose level of 20 mg/100 ml of blood or less. This disorder may occur anytime from birth until about the fourth day of life. If it is untreated, neurologic sequelae can be anticipated. One monitors blood glucose levels by laboratory biochemical study and Dextrostix.

Heat loss. Diminution of subcutaneous fat and a large body surface compared to body weight subject the SGA neonate to problems of thermoregulation. Cold stress jeopardizes recovery from asphyxia. The paucity of fat and glycogen reserves increases such an infant's vulnerability to cold and other stress.

Prognosis. Neonatal mortality rates are higher for the SGA term infant when compared to the infant of appropriate growth for gestational age (AGA) of the same age. Korones (1976) states, "Generally the immediate prognosis for survival and the long-term outlook for normal function seem to be better in small-for-dates infants than in those who are premature and normally grown, yet neither of these groups fares as well as the normal-sized term infant."

POSTTERM INFANTS

Postterm, or *postmaturity,* refers to gestation prolonged beyond 42 *completed* weeks from the first day of the last menstrual cycle. Postmaturity implies progressive placental insufficiency and a dysmature or SGA neonate or an oversized neonate.

Weights of postmature infants usually fall within the normal range for gestational age. However, the infant may be SGA because of deteriorating metabolic exchange in the aging placenta. Fetal malnutrition and hypoxia result in the wasted appearance of this dysmature infant.

General appearance

The wasted postterm infant has the following physical characteristics:

1. Dry, cracked skin (desquamating), parchmentlike
2. Nails of hard consistency extending beyond the fingertips
3. Profuse scalp hair
4. Subcutaneous fat layers depleted, leaving skin loose and giving an "old man" appearance
5. Long and thin body contour
6. Absent vernix
7. Often meconium stain (golden yellow to green) of skin, nails, and cord
8. May have an alert, wide-eyed appearance symptomatic of chronic intrauterine hypoxia

The majority of postterm infants are oversized but otherwise normal, with an advanced development and bone age.

PLAN OF CARE: POSTTERM INFANT

PATIENT CARE OBJECTIVES

Antenatal

1. Maternal emotional stress with prolonged gestation and tests to evaluate fetoplacental status are minimized.
2. Safe maternal-fetal outcome of evaluative tests such as OCT and amniocentesis is obtained.
3. Parents understand the situation.

Intranatal

1. Physically safe outcome for mother and fetus:
   a. Hypoxia is eliminated or minimized.
   b. Fetus suffers no birth trauma such as fractures, palsies, or intracranial hemorrhage.
   c. Dystotic labor, maternal infection, and bleeding are absent.
2. Parental fears are identified and minimized.

Early neonatal period

1. Asphyxia and/or birth trauma are averted or minimized.
2. There are no hypoglycemic episodes.
3. A positive parent-child relationship is initiated.

PHYSIOLOGIC PROBLEMS

1. Initiation and maintenance of respirations:
   a. Intrauterine hypoxia, perinatal asphyxia.
   b. Aspiration syndrome: ball-valve obstruction.
2. Maintenance of body temperature:
   a. Depleted subcutaneous fat and glycogen reserves.
   b. Large body surface to body weight.
3. Maintenance of adequate nutrition:
   a. Depleted fat and glycogen stores.
   b. Tendency to hypoglycemia.
4. CNS trauma:
   a. Oversized infant may cause cephalopelvic disproportion with possible birth trauma.
   b. Intrauterine hypoxia, perinatal asphyxia.
   c. Tendency to hypoglycemia
5. Resistance to infection:
   a. Diminished energy stores.
   b. Skin dry, cracked, loose; vernix absent.
   c. May have been exposed to infection during amniocentesis or application of internal fetal electrodes.

NURSING INTERVENTIONS

Diagnostic	Therapeutic and educational
Antenatal	
1. Assess mother's feelings and understanding of situation. 2. Note results of evaluative tests for fetoplacental status. 3. Assess family's need for supportive services: homemaker, transportation, financial assistance; assess stress from relatives and friends. 4. Recalculate EDC.	1. Initiate discussion and allow time for expression of feelings and fears. Prepare mother for friends and relatives asking, "Are you still here?" 2. Reinforce, repeat, simplify, or clarify physician's explanations of procedures, findings, proposed management. 3. Alert appropriate resources such as social worker, public health nurse.
Intranatal	

1. During labor or precesarean section:
   a. Monitor labor: contractions, dilatation, effacement, station, rupture of membranes, degree of molding.
   b. Monitor fetal status: fetal heart rate, fetal activity level, character of amniotic fluid.
 2. Assess parental response to situation and medical management.
	1. Explain all procedures; call mother and her family by name; stay with mother.
	 2. Cautious induction with fetal monitoring is necessary. Physician must be present during induction. If physician leaves unit, discontinue induction.
	 3. Maximize oxygenation of fetus:
	   a. Assist women to stay in high Fowler's position or

PLAN OF CARE: POSTTERM INFANT—cont'd

NURSING INTERVENTIONS—cont'd

Diagnostic	Therapeutic and educational
Intranatal—cont'd	in side-lying position; start and maintain IV fluid; prevent high-activity contraction patterns (decrease Pitocin induction; position her on side). b. Administer O_2 as necessary for fetal heart rate deceleration. 4. Prepare mother and family for cesarean section. 5. Prepare for resuscitation of neonate.
Early neonatal period 1. Assess newborn status: Apgar, meconium staining, retractions, need for resuscitative measures; evaluate for gestational age; check for hypoglycemia. 2. Assess parental responses to infant and to mode of delivery. 3. Assess for parental fears regarding infant and his condition. 4. Observe infant for signs and symptoms of birth trauma.	1. Assist physician in immediate care of newborn. 2. Observe infant for signs and symptoms of birth trauma: fractures, intracranial hemorrhage, hypoglycemia, palsies; report and record. 3. Cover hands with mitts to prevent scratching self with long nails. 4. Initiate discussion and allow time for mother (and father) to express feelings about condition of neonate, mode of delivery. Explain and repeat physician's explanation of situation and infant's condition and treatment.

POSSIBLE COMPLICATIONS

1. Respiratory function: altered blood gases and pH, asphyxia, aspiration pneumonia, atelectasis, pneumomediastinum, pneumothorax.
2. Inadequate temperature maintenance: same as for preterm infant.
3. Nutrition:
   a. Same as for preterm infant.
   b. Hypoglycemia with neurologic sequelae.
4. CNS trauma: same as for preterm infant.
5. Infection: same as for preterm infant.

Possible hazards

Hazards to the neonate include the following:

1. The neonate may be exposed to the hazards of the OCT (possible hypoxia), and amniocentesis (possible infection, bleeding, direct trauma to infant).

2. All postterm neonates (AGA or SGA) may tolerate the stress of labor poorly. Late fetal heart rate deceleration patterns with a slow return to the baseline rate, meconium-stained amniotic fluid, oligohydramnios, and a fetal scalp blood pH of 7.2 or less are indices of fetal jeopardy. Delivery by cesarean section is a frequent necessity.

3. The oversized neonate may be exposed to excessive trauma such as fractures and intracranial hemorrhage and to asphyxia during a dystotic labor.

The mother also is exposed to possible hazards:

1. She often undergoes tests to evaluate placental sufficiency and fetal status (e.g., OCT, amniocentesis),

and if indicated, labor is induced or cesarean section is performed.

2. Dystocia may accompany fetopelvic disproportion.

Prognosis

The mortality rate for neonates whose gestational age is 42 weeks or more is two to three times greater than that for the term infant. Of infants who succumb, 75% to 85% of deaths occur during labor.

LGA INFANTS

The large or oversized infant traditionally has been one who weighs 4000 gm or more at birth (8 pounds 13 ounces). About 10% of neonates are of this weight, and about 2% weigh 4500 gm or more (9 pounds 15 ounces). Moreover, most of these newborns have other proportionately larger measurements. Many are deliv-

---

PLAN OF CARE: LGA INFANTS

PATIENT CARE OBJECTIVES
1. Infant experiences no birth trauma.
2. Birth trauma is corrected or its effects minimized.

NURSING INTERVENTIONS

Diagnostic	Therapeutic	Educational
1. Assess infant for hypoglycemia: a. Blood glucose level. b. Symptoms.	1. Treat hypoglycemia.	1. Reinforce, simplify, or clarify physician's explanations of procedures, findings, and medical-surgical management.
2. Assess for gestational age.	2. Evaluate for and institute appropriate nursing care based on gestational age.	2. Initiate discussion and allow time for mother (and father) to express feelings about condition of infant, mode of delivery, prognosis, etc.
3. After delivery by cesarean section: a. Assess for pallor: usually due to iatrogenic bleeding. b. If in labor prior to surgery, assess for anoxia, depressed skull fracture, possible palsies; later for cephalhematoma. c. If fetal distress had been noted, observe for aspiration.	3. After cesarean section, record and report observations. Assist physician with treatments: a. Possible transfusion. b. Preoperative and postoperative care for reduction of depressed skull fracture; reemphasize to parents physician's explanation of cause and management of of cephalhematoma, palsies. c. Administer O$_2$; position infant; medications as necessary.	3. Encourage parent to visit, touch, and assist in care of infant when appropriate. Be available to assist parents at cribside. Help parents keep in touch with infant until his discharge.

4. After delivery by vaginal route:
 a. If fetal distress had been noted, observe for aspiration.
 b. Neurologic problems:
 (1) Brachial palsy: Erb-Duchenne type. Symptoms on affected side:
   (a) Arm: abducted and internally rotated.
   (b) Wrist: flexed.
   (c) Palm: limp, grasp reflex present.
   (d) Moro reflex: absent.
 (2) Paralysis of phrenic nerve:
   (a) Color: cyanotic.
   (b) Breath sounds: diminished.
   (c) Respirations: labored, rapid.
   (d) Abdomen: no rise with inspiration.
   (e) Cry: weak or hoarse.
 (3) Facial palsy (symptoms on affected side):
   (a) Facial contour and movement: asymmetric.
   (b) Cheek: flattened.
   (c) Eye: open.
	4. After vaginal delivery:
	 a. Facilitate respirations.
	
	 b. Neurologic problems:
	 (1) Brachial palsy: No definitive treatment is given. Self-limited usually. Position neonate in good body alignment to aid healing; prevent further injury; prevent deformity (p. 518).
	
	 (2) Phrenic nerve paralysis: Position infant with head of mattress up. Place in optimal position to facilitate respiratory effort (p. 520).
	
	 (3) Facial palsy: If eye stays open, keep moist; close eye and apply patch to protect it from corneal abrasions. Support infant in upright position during feeding. Take	

PLAN OF CARE: LGA INFANTS—cont'd

NURSING INTERVENTIONS—cont'd

Diagnostic	Therapeutic	Educational

Diagnostic

(d) Poor suck, drooling of formula on affected side.

(4) Brain injury from anoxia and/or direct trauma:
  (a) Convulsions*: clonic, tonic, localized; apneic spells. Symptoms include altered respiratory pattern, altered level of consciousness, abnormal eye movements, abnormal chewing movements.
  (b) Bulging fontanel; wide sutures.
  (c) Muscle tone: hypotonic; hypertonic.
  (d) Reflexes: hyperreflexic, difficult to elicit; absent; asymmetry of response.

c. Orthopedic problems:
  (1) After vertex delivery: fractured clavicle. Symptoms on affected side:
    (a) Arm: decreased or absent movement; pain response on passive movement.
    (b) Deformity of clavicle over fracture site is sometimes seen and felt: distal part of clavicle is movable on palpation.
  (2) After breech delivery: fractured femur. Symptoms on affected side:
    (a) Movement: absent; asymmetric Moro response; pain response on passive movement.
    (b) Deformity of femur is sometimes seen and felt.

5. Soft tissue trauma:
  a. Abrasions from bony pelvis or forceps.

Therapeutic

extra time to feed. Do not force, since this may cause aspiration (p. 520).

(4) Brain injury: Order and assist with lab workup for differential diagnosis to rule out other causes for convulsions:
  (a) EEG, subdural tap, skull films.
  (b) Workup for sepsis: blood culture, urinalysis, lumbar puncture; chest x-ray film.
  (c) Workup for metabolic problems.
  (d) Workup for structural defects.
  (e) O_2 to relieve cyanosis.
(5) Position to facilitate respirations. Suction as necessary.
(6) Nutrition: nipple with caution, IV.
(7) IV therapy: Administer medications, anticoagulants, antibiotics.
(8) Minimize stimuli: auditory, visual, tactile.

c. Orthopedic: Maintain good body alignment to prevent further injury and to prevent deformity. Prevent pressure areas on skin.
  (1) Fractured clavicle (p. 518): figure-of-eight bandage over infant's shoulders across back to immobilize clavicle to facilitate healing, prevent deformity.
  (2) Fractured femur: Both legs are placed in traction-suspension (Bryant's traction) with or without a spica cast for 3 to 4 weeks until adequate callus is formed.

5. Soft tissue trauma:
  a. Prevent infection through broken skin.

*For other causes of convulsions, see pp. 523 and 543.

Continued.

PLAN OF CARE: LGA INFANTS—cont'd

NURSING INTERVENTIONS—cont'd

Diagnostic	Therapeutic	Educational

b. Ecchymoses from bony pelvis or forceps.
c. Petechiae over traumatized area only from bony pelvis or forceps.
d. After first or second day, cephalhematoma.
e. Subconjunctival hemorrhage from rupture of scleral capillaries.
6. Miscellaneous:
  a. Long fingernails.
  b. Macerated, dry, peeling skin.
	b. Observe for hyperbilirubinemia as hemorrhagic areas are resolved.
	c. Continue to observe and record changes in petechiae (e.g., progressive resolution vs increase in number and distribution)
	6. Miscellaneous:
	  a. Cover hands with mitts to prevent self-inflicted scratches.
	  b. Dry, dead skin in bedding will not injure child. Small amounts of lotion may be used; avoid unnecessary bathing.	

---

ered well after the EDC. Better maternal health and nutrition probably are responsible for this greater growth during recent generations.

Maternal pelvic diameters have not kept pace with these changes; hence fetopelvic disproportion often occurs, particularly in obese women, women who gain 35 pounds or more during gestation, or diabetic mothers who are prone to large babies. Birth trauma, especially associated with breech or shoulder dystocia, is a serious hazard for the oversized neonate. Asphyxia and/or CNS injury may also occur.

A biparietal diameter greater than 10 cm found by fetometry (ultrasound or x-ray examination) or a uterine fundal measurement (McDonald) greater than 42 cm in the absence of polyhydramnios, and only average or smaller interior pelvic diameters are frequent findings. One should reevaluate all pregnancies of longer than 42 weeks' gestation. All large fetuses are monitored during a trial of labor and preparation made for a cesarean section if fetal distress or poor progress ensues.

The prognosis for the mother may entail lacerations to the birth canal if operative vaginal delivery is permitted. Cesarean section usually is indicated, particularly with borderline cephalopelvic disproportion or in breech presentation, even in multiparas who previously have delivered oversized fetuses. LGA neonates may be preterm, term, or postterm; children of diabetic (or prediabetic) mothers; and dysmature.

Each of these categories has special concerns, which are discussed elsewhere in this chapter. Regardless of coexisting potential problems, the oversized infant is at risk by virtue of his size alone.

Any one or a combination of injuries discussed in the plan of care for LGA infants may occur in normal or small-sized infants. Factors other than the large size of the infant that predispose to birth trauma include the following:

- Premature labor and delivery
- Length of labor
- Size and shape of maternal pelvis
- Fetal presentation, attitude, and lie

SUMMARY

Infants whose gestational age and birth weights exceed the defined parameters of normal are considered to be at risk. The survival and well-being of the infant are dependent on the collaborative efforts of the medical and paramedical team. The nurse's skills in observation and recording often form the foundation for early diagnosis and appropriate treatment of medical and surgical conditions. Furthermore, the nurse's role in facilitating the development of a positive parent-child relationship cannot be overemphasized.

As discussed earlier, preparation of parents begins long before the infant is discharged from the hospital. Preparation of the older children also needs to be undertaken prior to the infant coming home. The very young child can easily "forget" the existence of a brother or sister in the hospital. If possible, visits to see the new baby should be encouraged. For the older child the idea of an imperfect baby can be clarified by seeing him and having a chance to discuss fears and misconceptions. One 8-year-old was given the job of "explaining" all about his premature sister to the visiting grandparents. He discussed the care of the baby and use of supportive equipment surprisingly well.

If, however, death is the outcome of this episode, the older children will be affected as well as the parents. A small child who cannot understand verbal explanations needs demonstrations of love and affection to provide reassurance and security. He may be unable to express frightening thoughts that he may be experiencing. Occasionally the small child may resort to misbehavior to draw attention or cling excessively to his parents.

Older children need verbal explanation as well as assistance in voicing feelings and thoughts. Discussion about the fetal/newborn death as well as death in general should be an open subject in the family. The cause of the death should be openly presented so that the child may cope with any existing feelings of guilt.

Avoid references such as "the baby went away (or to sleep)" or "God took him." These euphemisms are usually meant to help the child but more often can be threatening. Regardless of the way parents handle the reaction to the death, some children may manifest their inner disturbance by nightmares, bed-wetting, school problems, or other ways.

REFERENCES

Aladjem, S., and Brown, A. K. (eds.). 1974. Clinical perinatology. St. Louis, The C. V. Mosby Co.

Babson, S. G., Benson, R. C., Pernoll, M. L., and Benda, G. I. 1975. Management of high-risk pregnancy and intensive care of the neonate (ed. 3). St. Louis, The C. V. Mosby Co.

Bliss, V. J. 1976. Nursing care for infants with neonatal necrotizing enterocolitis. MCN Am. J. Mat. Child Nurs. **1**:37, Jan.-Feb.

Christensen, A. 1977. Coping with the crisis of premature birth—one couple's story. MCN Am. J. Mat. Child Nurs. **2**:24, Jan.-Feb.

Clausen, J., and others. 1976. Maternity nursing today. McGraw-Hill Book Co.

Gluck, L., and others. 1974. Interpretation and significance of the lecithin/sphingomyelin ratio in amniotic fluid. Am. J. Obstet. Gynecol. **120**:142.

Goldstein, A. S., and others. 1974. A comparison of the lecithin/sphingomyelin ratio and shake test for estimating fetal pulmonary maturity. Am. J. Obstet. Gynecol. **118**:1132.

Hardgrove, C., and Warrick, L. H. 1974. How shall we tell the children. Am. J. Nurs. **74**:448.

Horney, K. 1977. Caring perceptively for the relinquishing mother. MCN Am. J. Mat. Child Nurs. **2**:29, Jan.-Feb.

Kastenbaum, R. 1959. Time and death in adolescence. In Feifel, H. (ed.). The meaning of death. New York, McGraw-Hill Book Co.

Korones, S. 1976. High-risk newborn infants—the basis for intensive nursing care (ed. 2). St. Louis, The C. V. Mosby Co.

Kowalski, K., and Obborn, M. 1977. Helping mothers of stillborn infants to grieve. MCN Am. J. Mat. Child Nurs. **2**:29, Jan.-Feb.

Low, J. A., and Galbraith, R. S. 1974. Pregnancy characteristics of intrauterine growth retardation. Obstet. Gynecol. **44**:122.

Masson, G. M. 1973. Plasma estriol in retarded intrauterine fetal growth. J. Obstet. Gynaecol. Br. Commonw. **80**:423.

Nagy, M. H. 1959. The child's view of death. In Feifel, H. (ed.). The meaning of death. New York, McGraw-Hill Book Co.

Pierog, S. H., and Ferrara, A. 1976. Medical care of the sick newborn (ed. 2). St. Louis, The C. V. Mosby Co.

Shephard, B., Buhi, W., and Spellacy, W. 1974. Critical analysis of the amniotic fluid shake test. Obstet. Gynecol. **43**:558.

Tucker, S., and others. 1975. Patient care standards, St. Louis, The C. V. Mosby Co.

Young, R. 1977. Chronic sorrow: parents' response to the birth of a child with a defect. MCN Am. J. Mat. Child. Nurs. **2**:38, Jan.-Feb.

CHAPTER 35

Congenital anomalies

Many congenital anomalies require surgical intervention soon after birth. Careful assessment alerts the medical-nursing team to the infant's need for surgical therapy.

GENERAL PREOPERATIVE AND POSTOPERATIVE CARE

The neonate withstands the stress of surgery surprisingly well, provided it is done as soon after birth as feasible and the facilities available for care are adequately equipped and staffed. The medical-nursing team must be specially trained to anticipate and meet the neonate's physiologic needs. The surgical team consists of the radiologist, surgeon, anesthesiologist, and nurse. Diagnostic studies are kept to a minimum, and consideration of the neonate's immaturity is kept in mind. For example, air is used rather than standard radiopaque materials for diagnostic x-ray examinations because of the danger of regurgitation and aspiration, and microtechniques are utilized for the necessary blood chemistry studies (e.g., preoperative hemoglobin levels) to minimize blood loss.

The infant is transported to the operating room in an Isolette incubator and is accompanied by an intensive care nursery nurse. Preanesthesia preparation includes administration of preoperative medications, usually minute amounts of atropine or scopolamine, insertion of an endotracheal tube, and gastric emptying.

During the operation, blood loss is constantly monitored, and blood is replaced milliliter by milliliter because the neonate's remarkable ability to maintain blood circulation through vasoconstriction means vital signs remain unaltered until sudden and complete collapse occurs as the compensatory system is overtaxed. Temperature is maintained by positioning the infant on a thermal mattress and draping suitably.

Once the operation is completed, the infant is returned to the intensive care nursery. The first hour postoperation is a crucial one, and constant surveillance of recovery from the anesthesia is imperative. Body temperature is maintained between 36.1° to 36.7° C (97° to

98° F). An open airway is maintained by means of positioning of the head, suctioning, and use of high humidity. (If the respiratory rate increases, suctioning is indicated.) Oxygen dosage is prescribed on the basis of arterial blood gas values (e.g., Po_2). Fluid-electrolyte balance is monitored, and intravenous replacement is given as ordered. Postural drainage and percussion are

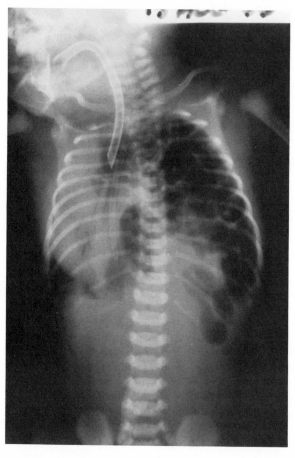

Fig. 35-1. Diaphragmatic hernia. (Courtesy John R. Campbell, M.D., University of Oregon Health Sciences Center, Portland, Ore.)

572

ordered as necessary. The infant is turned from side to side to equalize pressure areas. An indwelling gastric catheter attached to intermittent suction removes gastric secretions to prevent their possible aspiration because the cough reflex is inadequate.

MOST COMMON SURGICAL EMERGENCIES

The following five congenital anomalies account for more than 90% of surgical emergencies of the neonate:

1. Diaphragmatic hernia
2. Tracheoesophageal anomalies
3. Omphalocele
4. Intestinal obstruction
5. Imperforate anus

Diaphragmatic hernia

Diaphragmatic hernia (Fig. 35-1) is the most urgent of the neonatal emergencies. Incomplete embryonic development of the diaphragm allows herniation of abdominal viscera into the thoracic cavity. The defect and herniation may be minimal and easily reparable or so extensive that the viscera present in the thoracic cavity during embryonic life precluded the normal develop-ment of pulmonary tissue. Most cases involve a postero-lateral defect, usually on the left. The extent of the defect, the severity, and timing of the symptomatology determine the seriousness of the problem.

Prompt surgical repair is imperative after correction of acidosis, insertion of a nasogastric tube and aspira-tion, and oxygen therapy.

The prognosis depends largely on the degree of pulmo-nary development and the success of diaphragmatic closure. Prognosis in severe cases is guarded.

Tracheoesophageal anomalies

Esophageal atresia is an urgent congenital anomaly. Various types are recognized, depending on the presence or absence of an associated tracheoesophageal fistula, the site of the fistula, and the point and degree of esoph-ageal obstruction (Figs. 35-2 and 35-3). The most com-mon variety is associated with moderate polyhydram-nios.

Immediate surgical correction of the anomaly is man-datory. The prognosis is dependent on the degree of maturity of the neonate and the presence of a fistula or pneumonia. Cardiac and other gastrointestinal anomalies commonly are associated with esophageal atresia.

PLAN OF CARE: DIAPHRAGMATIC HERNIA

PATIENT CARE OBJECTIVES
1. Respiratory distress and its sequelae are minimal. Neonate is adequately ventilated.
2. Neonate is adequately nourished.

NURSING INTERVENTIONS

Diagnostic	Therapeutic and educational

1. Minimal diaphragmatic herniation: asymptomatic or mild respiratory distress.
2. Extensive diaphragmatic herniation:
  a. Constant respiratory distress from birth that be-comes increasingly severe as bowels fill with air.
    (1) Large or asymmetric chest contour.
    (2) Dullness to percussion on affected side.
    (3) Bowel sounds are heard in thoracic cavity.
    (4) Breath sounds are diminished.
  b. Scaphoid (flat) or plate-shaped abdomen.
  c. X-ray films confirm presence of intestines in thorax, as well as mediastinal displacement.
	1. Report findings to physician immediately.
	2. Place infant in semi-Fowler's position (infant seat may be used).
	3. Give O_2 as necessary to relieve cyanosis. NOTE: If it is necessary to employ pulmonary ventilation, endo-tracheal tube must be passed to avoid distention of stomach. Avoid positive ventilation pressure >30 mm Hg, or alveolar rupture, pneumothorax, and death may result.
	4. Summary of preoperative and postoperative care:
	  a. Neonate: hydration, freedom from infection, ventila-tion.
	  b. Parents:
	    (1) Reinforce, clarify physician's discussion of ana-tomic and physiologic defect, surgery, and prognosis.
	    (2) Assist parents in coping with situation: grieving; arrange and facilitate parental involvement in touching and holding infant and making deci-sions.

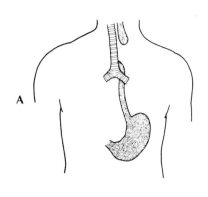
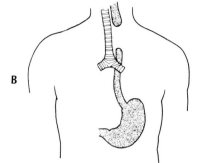
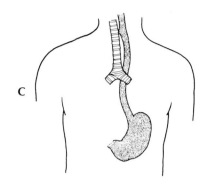
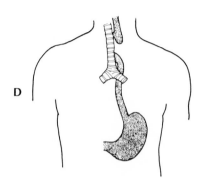
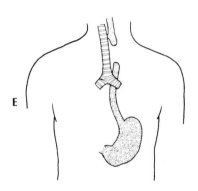

Fig. 35-2. Congenital atresia of esophagus and tracheoesophageal fistula. **A,** About 87%. Upper segment of esophagus ends in blind pouch; lower segment connects with trachea by small fistulous tract. **B,** About 8%. Upper and lower segments of esophagus end in blind sac. **C,** About 4%. Esophagus is continuous but connects by fistulous tract to trachea; known as *H-type.* **D,** Less than 1%. Both segments of esophagus connect by fistulous tracts to trachea. Infant may drown with first feeding. **E,** Less than 1%. Upper segment of esophagus ends in atresia and connects to trachea by fistulous tract. Infant may drown with first feeding.

Fig. 35-3. Esophageal atresia with catheter coiled in pouch. (Courtesy John R. Campbell, M.D., University of Oregon Health Sciences Center, Portland, Ore.)

PLAN OF CARE: TRACHEOESOPHAGEAL ANOMALIES

PATIENT CARE OBJECTIVES
1. Respiratory distress is absent or minimized.
2. Nutrition is adequate.
3. Infant remains in good physical condition to withstand the stress of surgery.
4. A positive parent-child relationship is initiated and maintained.

NURSING INTERVENTIONS

Diagnostic	Therapeutic and educational

1. Atresia of esophagus: Esophagus terminates in blind pouch.
  a. Observe for distinctive symptoms:
    (1) Excessive oral secretions with drooling.
    (2) Progressive respiratory distress as unswallowed secretions spill over into trachea.
    (3) Feeding intolerance:
      (a) Choking, coughing, and cyanosis follows even small amount of fluid taken by mouth.
      (b) Regurgitation of unaltered formula (unmixed with stomach secretions or bile) soon after first feeding is initiated.
  b. Inability to pass catheter into stomach (and aspirate mucus) indicates tentative diagnosis of esophageal atresia.
2. Atresia of esophagus with fistulous tract between esophagus distal to atresia and trachea.
  a. Observe for distinctive symptoms:
    (1) Symptoms as described above.
    (2) Abdominal distention that begins to develop soon after birth.
3. H-type fistula: If fistulous tract is small, this malformation may not be diagnosed in very young infant. It may be diagnosed soon after birth. Examiner may become suspicious if infant experiences recurring aspiration pneumonia. Radiologic examination confirms presence of H-type fistulous anomaly.
	1. In presence of excessive oral secretions and respiratory distress, *do not feed* infant orally before consulting physician.
	2. First feeding of all infants is done by skilled nurse. (If mother wishes to breast-feed immediately, infant should be examined prior to nursing at breast, even though there frequently is little if any colostrum taken at this time.)
	  a. Feed sterile water. Discontinue feeding in presence of feeding intolerance and respiratory distress.
	  b. Position neonate with head down to facilitate drainage of secretions *except* in presence of abdominal distention, intracranial hemorrhage, or prematurity.
	3. In presence of abdominal distention, place neonate in semi-Fowler's position and raise head ≥30 degrees (infant seat may be used). This position facilitates respiratory efforts and discourages reflux (spillage) of stomach secretions into respiratory tree with resultant chemical bronchitis and pneumonitis.
	4. On physician order or per standing orders, insert suction tube into blind pouch. Connect to low, intermittent suction.
	5. Assist parents in coping with situation:
	  a. Reinforce and clarify physician's description of anatomy and physiology of malformation, surgical repair, preoperative and postoperative care, and prognosis.
	  b. Help parents cope with having given birth to imperfect child (p. 99).
	  c. Facilitate and arrange for parent-child touch and eye contact.

Omphalocele

Omphalocele is a herniation noted at birth in which part of the intestine protrudes through a defect in the abdominal wall at the umbilicus (Fig. 35-4). Failure of migration of the midgut in embryonic development probably is responsible for omphalocele. The protruding bowel is covered only by a thin, transparent membrane composed of amnion.

Prompt closure of defects of less than 5 cm in diameter usually is successful. Larger defects may require closure in stages. The general prognosis is related to associated anomalies.

Nursing management. There is usually only a short span of time between the neonate's birth and surgical intervention. In addition to the usual preoperative orders, preparation of the infant for surgery includes protecting the defect from infection, rupture, and drying. The physician prescribes that the omphalocele be protected by one of the following:

1. Sterile towels or sponges kept moist with sterile saline solution that has been warmed to body temperature.
2. Protective sterile petrolatum dressings and a firm plastic or metal covering.

Planning for the provision of support to the parents is an essential aspect of nursing care (p. 99).

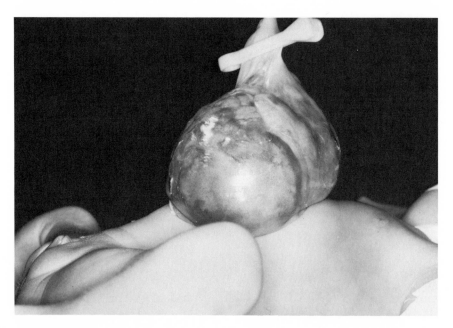

Fig. 35-4. Omphalocele containing liver. (Courtesy John R. Campbell, M.D., University of Oregon Health Sciences Center, Portland, Ore.)

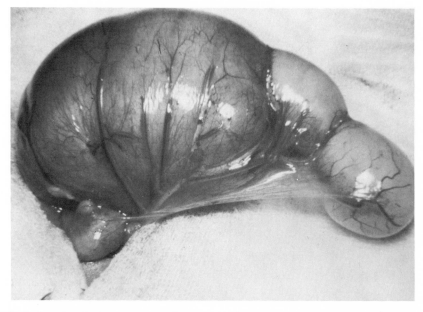

Fig. 35-5. Atresia of jejunum. Note distention of intestine just proximal to obstruction. Obstruction is removed, and two segments of bowel are anastomosed to establish continuity. (Courtesy John R. Campbell, M.D., University of Oregon Health Sciences Center, Portland, Ore.)

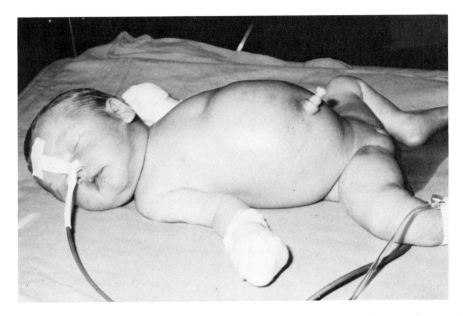

Fig. 35-6. Meconium ileus with midgut volvulus. Meconium ileus is frequently associated with cystic fibrosis. Normal meconium stool is not passed, and abdomen distends progressively. Treatment is directed at removal of mechanical obstruction and at prevention of complications of cystic fibrosis. (Courtesy John R. Campbell, M.D., University of Oregon Health Sciences Center, Portland, Ore.)

PLAN OF CARE: INTESTINAL OBSTRUCTION

PATIENT CARE OBJECTIVES
1. Fluid-electrolyte balance is good.
2. Nutritional status is good.
3. Respiratory problems are avoided or minimized.
4. Positive parent-child relationship is initiated and maintained.

NURSING INTERVENTIONS

Diagnostic	Therapeutic and educational

1. Pass small orogastric catheter to aspirate stomach contents. Report immediately:
  a. Fluid ≥25 ml.
  b. Bile-stained fluid.
2. Abdominal distention: progressive.
3. Bile-stained or fecal vomitus.
4. Absence of meconium or passage of light-colored, inspissated stool.
	1. Stop oral feedings. Monitor IV therapy (pp. 620 to 622).
	2. Prevent aspiration. Suction gastric contents per physician order. Indwelling catheter to low, intermittent suction may be ordered.
	3. Position infant in semi-Fowler's to facilitate respiration.
	4. Follow preoperative orders. Neonate may be transferred to another facility or pediatric unit postsurgery.
	5. Support parents (p. 99).

Intestinal obstruction

Congenital jejunal or ileal obstruction is suspected when distention and bile-stained or fecal vomiting occurs in a newborn in the first 24 to 48 hours of life (Fig. 35-5). Although this condition is uncommon, premature infants and those with other anomalies may be affected.

X-ray films of the abdomen usually show a dilated small bowel without gas in the colon. A barium enema may be helpful in determining the cause of the obstruction. Hirschsprung's disease, ileus secondary to sepsis, meconium ileus, and volvulus must be considered in the differential diagnosis (Fig. 35-6). Prompt surgery usually provides a good result.

Imperforate anus

Imperforate anus is a congenital disorder that is more common in males than in females (Fig. 35-7). About 85% of affected females will have developed a small fistula (Fig. 35-8), but this is rare in males (Fig. 35-9). The obstruction may be of the low type (anal membrane) or the high type (anal or rectal atresia).

Since continence for a life time may be dependent on the proper corrective surgery, a pediatric surgeon is consulted at once. Surgery may be as simple as an incision of an anal membrane, but with anorectal agenesis, a prompt colostomy will be necessary.

Survival is expected. Continence, on the other hand, is dependent on several factors, including sacral anomalies and proper surgery.

PLAN OF CARE: IMPERFORATE ANUS

PATIENT CARE OBJECTIVES
1. Fluid-electrolyte balance is good.
2. Nutritional status is good.
3. Respiratory problems are avoided or minimized.
4. Positive parent-child relationship is initiated and maintained.

NURSING INTERVENTIONS

Diagnostic

1. Anatomic appearance: Abnormal placement or configuration may overlay internal atypical development:
   a. Placement of anus.
   b. Number of anal openings.
   c. Check for normal "wink" response of normal sphincter muscle.
   d. Insert well-lubricated probe (thermometer, tubing, small finger) gently.
2. Physiologic function:
   a. Observe for passage of meconium or other discharge.
   b. Seek other signs of gastrointestinal obstruction (e.g., abdominal distention).

Therapeutic and educational

1. Careful observation, notation, and reporting of anatomic signs and physiologic functions hasten diagnosis and initiation of appropriate treatment.
2. Initial insertion of probe (thermometer) into anal canal is done with *extra* caution until patency is established.
3. Nurture parents (p. 99).

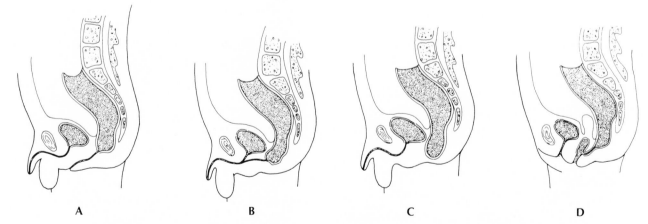

| A | B | C | D |

Fig. 35-7. Types of imperforate anus. Anal sphincter muscle may be present and intact. **A,** High lesion opening onto perineum through narrow fistulous tract. **B,** High lesion ending in fistulous tract to urinary tract. **C,** Low lesion in bowel passes through puborectal muscle. **D,** High lesion ending in fistulous tract to vagina.

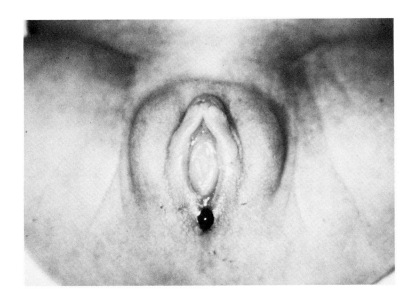

Fig. 35-8. Imperforate anus: fourchette fistula. Note meconium draining through fistula. (Courtesy John R. Campbell, M.D., University of Oregon Health Sciences Center, Portland, Ore.)

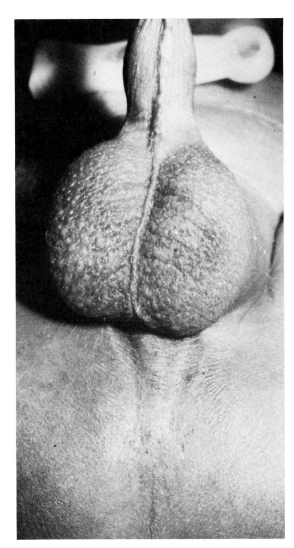

Fig. 35-9. Imperforate anus with rectopectal penile fistula. (Courtesy John R. Campbell, M.D., University of Oregon Health Sciences Center, Portland, Ore.)

PLAN OF CARE: MENINGOMYELOCELE

PATIENT CARE OBJECTIVES

1. Defect is repaired, or neurologic and musculoskeletal problems are minimized.
2. Infection of cerebrospinal fluid is avoided.
3. A positive parent-child relationship is initiated, or parents are supported in decision making regarding the placement of their child.

NURSING INTERVENTIONS

Diagnostic	Therapeutic and educational

1. Symptoms depend on location and extent of defect:
  a. No apparent neurologic involvement distal to defect.
  b. Neurologic involvement:
    (1) Paralysis.
    (2) Flaccidity and spasticity of muscles below defect.
    (3) Sphincter control: check character and number of voidings and stools; observe for leakage.
  c. Injury to defect:
    (1) Rupture or leakage of cerebrospinal fluid.
    (2) Infection.
    (3) Irritation of area.
2. Assess for associated problems that may occur:
  a. Symptoms of developing hydrocephalus:
    (1) Head circumference, every day.
    (2) Status of anterior fontanel, every day.
  b. Clubfoot (p. 587).
	1. Write detailed record of observations. Note and report any changes.
	2. Position with care:
	  a. Position prone or side-lying with rolled towels to prevent pressure or injury to defect, thereby providing portal of entry for infectious agents.
	  b. Change position every hour to prevent pressure areas.
	  c. If physician permits infant to be held, exercise caution to avoid injury to defect.
	3. Skin care: Skin around defect is cleansed and dried carefully to prevent breakdown, thus establishing portal of entry for infectious agents. Apply physician-ordered dressings, ointments, etc.
	4. Nurture parent (p. 99).
	5. Meet infant's touching and cuddling needs.

COMMON MALFORMATIONS (INTRAUTERINE GROWTH DEVIATIONS)
Meningomyelocele

Meningomyelocele, a neural tube defect, is a herniation of the meninges containing cerebrospinal fluid and CNS tissue through a defect in the vertebral column or skull. The defect often occurs in the lower back. The accompanying spinal malformation is *spina bifida*. The meningomyelocele extrudes out through the opening of the spinal column, caused by a congenital absence of one or more vertebral arches. Occasionally a familial history (5% recurrence rate) of this anomaly is identified, but most cases are of unknown (?infectious) origin. A *meningocele* is also a herniation of the meninges and contains cerebrospinal fluid but does not contain CNS tissue (brain, cord, or nerve roots).

Antenatal diagnosis of neural tube defects (meningomyelocele, meningocele, anencephaly) is now possible. Three methods are available:

1. The levels of α-fetoprotein in the maternal serum and amniotic fluid increases in the presence of neural tube defects. Serum assays may be utilized for screening; and amniotic fluid determinations are needed for definitive diagnosis.
2. Ultrasound.
3. Amniography.

The couple may be advised of the existence of the defect and assisted in arriving at their own decision regarding the affected pregnancy.

Surgical repair often can be done in the neonatal period. If other anomalies are present such as hydrocephalus, delayed correction may be elected. Permanent impairment of neuromuscular function below the level of the defect depends on the amount of CNS tissue involved. In severe cases, voluntary and involuntary function is absent. The prognosis is guarded. Only about 60% of cases are operable, and many of these children die or achieve only partial function.

The parents will need considerable support and instruction regarding the infant's care. In some instances, parents may require assistance in placing the child in a special care facility.

Hydrocephalus

Hydrocephalus is encountered in approximately 1 fetus in 2000 (about 12% of all malformations). It is a condition characterized by an abnormal accumulation of fluid in the cranial vault, accompanied by enlargement of the head, prominence of the forehead, atrophy of the brain, weakness, and convulsions. Several types are known: *external hydrocephalus,* which implies an abnormal accumulation of fluid between the brain and the

---

PLAN OF CARE: HYDROCEPHALUS

PATIENT CARE OBJECTIVES
1. Neurologic sequelae are minimized.
2. Coexisting defects are corrected, or appropriate treatment is initiated.
3. A positive parent-child relationship is initiated when possible or applicable.

NURSING INTERVENTIONS

Diagnostic	Therapeutic and educational

1. Changes in head size every day:
  a. Width of sutures.
  b. Size and tension of anterior fontanel.
  c. Head circumference.
2. Facial appearance:
  a. Flat, broad bridge of nose.
  b. Bulging forehead.
  c. "Setting-sun" effect as eyes are displaced downward by pressure from accumulating fluid.
3. Neurologic signs:
  a. High pitched, shrill cry.
  b. Irritability or restlessness.
  c. Poor feeding or changes in feeding pattern from good to poor.
  d. Behavior changes.
	1. Carefully note and report observations and changes.
	2. Provide skin care to prevent infection:
	  a. Prevent pressure areas. Use lamb's wool, sheepskin, flotation mattress, frequent position changes.
	  b. Keep clean and dry.
	3. Support head carefully when holding or turning infant.
	4. Feeding:
	  a. Choose method, amount, and frequency of feeding to accommodate infant's tolerance and energy level.
	  b. Be alert for vomiting and possible aspiration.
	5. Meet infant's touching and cuddling needs.
	6. Nurture parent: provide support and information regarding defect and treatment.

---

dura mater; and *internal hydrocephalus* in which the excessive accumulation of cerebrospinal fluid is in the ventricular system of the brain. Spina bifida occurs in approximately one third of neonates born with hydrocephalus.

The fetus with hydrocephalus frequently assumes the breech presentation in utero. Severe dystocia due to cephalopelvic disproportion is encountered; delivery by cesarean section is usual. In cases in which a vaginal delivery is attempted, puncture of the fetal head and drainage of the excess fluid may be necessary before the head can be delivered. Fetal mortality rate after this procedure is approximately 3 deaths out of every 4 deliveries.

Regardless of the route of delivery, the experience is emotionally traumatic for the parents.

Surgery is usually performed soon after birth. If surgical shunting is not accomplished, increasing intracranial pressure will eventuate in irreversible neurologic damage. A period of observation is necessary, however, to determine the type of operation required. Meanwhile, nursing care is individualized.

Anencephaly and microcephaly

Anencephaly and microcephaly are congenital fetal deformities in which the head is considerably smaller than normal. About 70% of anencephalics are female.

In this anomaly, there is complete or partial absence of the brain and of the overlying skull. Because the pituitary gland is absent or vestigial, the adrenal cortex is diminutive (for lack of ACTH stimulation). This condition is frequently accompanied by polyhydramnios. The cause of anencephaly is unknown, but multiple environmental factors have been postulated. A 3% recurrence rate in familial histories has been noted.

In microcephaly the head generally is well formed but small. X-ray exposure of the woman has been followed by microcephaly in that child. Rubella, cytomegalic inclusion disease, and perhaps other infectious processes are the causes in some cases.

Anencephaly is incompatible with life; warmth and fluid are provided until the neonate's death, which is usually before the end of the first 24 hours after birth. Microcephaly patients require specific nursing care and medical observation to appraise the extent of psychomotor retardation that almost always accompanies this abnormality. The nurse's supportive role with parents is considerable.

Choanal atresia

Choanal atresia, or stenosis, is the complete or partial blockage of the posterior nares by membrane, cartilage, or bone (Fig. 35-10).

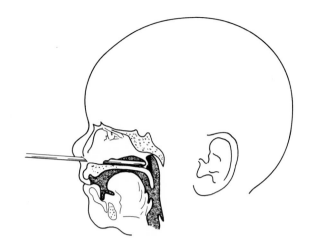

Fig. 35-10. Choanal atresia. Posterior nares are obstructed by membrane or bone either bilaterally or unilaterally. (Courtesy Ross Laboratories, Columbus, Ohio.)

PLAN OF CARE: CHOANAL ATRESIA

PATIENT CARE OBJECTIVES
1. Adequate ventilation is initiated and maintained.
2. Adequate nutrition is maintained.
3. Surgery is curative.

NURSING INTERVENTIONS

Diagnostic	Therapeutic and educational

1. Infant becomes cyanotic at rest. An obligate nose breather at birth, neonate does not learn to open mouth to breathe for 2 to 3 weeks. With crying, neonate's color improves.
2. Inspiratory efforts may be accompanied by sucking in of closed lips with thoracic retractions.
3. Nasal discharge.
4. Snorting respirations, often observed in presence of choanal stenosis or unilateral atresia, with increased respiratory effort.
5. Feeding difficulties. Neonate may be unable to breathe and eat at same time.
6. Diagnosis:
  a. Inability to pass small feeding tube through one or both nares.
  b. Presence of above symptoms
	1. Short-term measures:
	  a. Tape or tie in place small plastic airway to keep infant's mouth open preventing airway from becoming clogged or dislodged and from causing irritation or infection of esophagus.
	  b. Feed by nasogastric or orogastric tube until infant learns to breathe and eat at same time (p. 618).
	  c. Support parents.
	2. Long-term measures:
	  a. Surgical repair of membranous or cartilaginous obstruction may be easily accomplished. Repair of bony obstruction may be more difficult and may be deferred until infant is older.
	  b. Assist parents in coping with situation of having infant with defect; assist parents to help prepare infant for surgery (adequate nutrition, absence of infection).

Cleft lip or palate

Cleft lip and/or palate is a common congenital midline fissure or opening in the lip or palate; one or both deformities may occur. The incidence is approximately 1 in 700 white neonates and 1 in 2000 black neonates. Polygenetic factors are causative in some cases but fetal viral infection, maternal corticosteroid therapy, radiation, dietary influence, and hypoxia have been associated factors. The combination of cleft lip and palate effects more males than females.

Treatment requires special feeding techniques, for example, the use of uniquely designed nipples (p. 624).

Cleft lip repair may be done soon after delivery if the neonate is free of infection, in good condition, and weighs 2500 gm (5 pounds and 9 ounces). Cleft lip repair is best done when the infant weighs 4500 gm (10 pounds) or more, however, since there is more tissue to work with. Advantages of earlier labial repair include facilitating a positive parent-child relationship and permitting the infant to learn to use and strengthen musculature around the mouth. Infants with palatolabial fissures often look grotesque and repulsive to the parents. After repair and with collaborative health team support, the mother frequently is able to assume responsibility for the newborn's care until palatal repair is feasible between 16 to 24 months of age (20 pounds weight or more). The plastic surgeon, pediatrician, orthodontist, hospital and community nurses, speech therapists, and social workers comprise the collaborative health team that has made possible the effective treatment available today. Until repair of the palate is performed, a prosthesis is fitted to aid the infant's feeding and speech development and to reduce respiratory tract infections.

The grief reaction to having a child with this defect and the nursing care involved is discussed in Chapter 7. Parents also benefit from seeing before and after pictures of other babies born with this defect. Coupled with other verbal and nonverbal supportive care, this visual reassurance is effective. Parents can be referred to other parents (or organizations of parents such as the Cleft Palate Club) for continuing mutual support.

Cardiovascular disorders

Cardiovascular defects occur in 3 of every 1000 births; congenital heart disease is implicated in approximately 50% of deaths from malformations during the first year of life (Fig. 35-11). Etiology is still unclear, although a familial tendency is evident in many cases. Coexisting congenital defects are frequent in neonates with cardiovascular anomalies. Maternal disease during pregnancy has been implicated. Symptoms characteristically are first evident after the umbilical cord is severed.

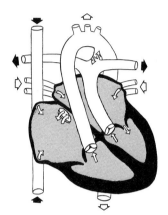

Complete transposition of great vessels

The anomaly is an embryologic defect caused by a straight division of the bulbar trunk without normal spiraling. As a result, the aorta originates from the right ventricle, and the pulmonary artery from the left ventricle. An abnormal communication between the two circulations must be present to sustain life.

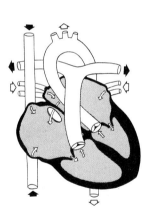

Atrial septal defects

An atrial septal defect is an abnormal opening between the right and left atria. Basically, three types of abnormalities result from incorrect development of the atrial septum. An incompetent foramen ovale is the most common defect. The high ostium secundum defect results from abnormal development of the septum secundum. Improper development of the septum primum produces a basal opening known as an ostium primum defect, frequently involving the atrioventricular valves. In general, left to right shunting of blood occurs in all atrial septal defects.

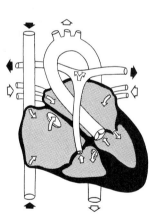

Tricuspid atresia

Tricuspid valvular atresia is characterized by a small right ventricle, large left ventricle, and usually a diminished pulmonary circulation. Blood from the right atrium passes through an atrial septal defect into the left atrium, mixes with oxygenated blood returning from the lungs, flows into the left ventricle, and is propelled into the systemic circulation. The lungs may receive blood through one of three routes: (1) a small ventricular septal defect, (2) patent ductus arteriosus, (3) bronchial vessels.

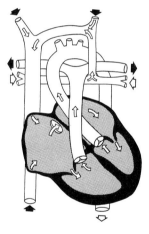

Anomalous venous return

Oxygenated blood returning from the lungs is carried abnormally to the right heart by one or more pulmonary veins emptying directly, or indirectly, through venous channels into the right atrium. Partial anomalous return of the pulmonary veins to the right atrium functions the same as an atrial septal defect. In complete anomalous return of the pulmonary veins, an interatrial communication is necessary for survival.

Continued.

Fig. 35-11. Congenital heart abnormalities. (Courtesy Ross Laboratories, Columbus, Ohio.)

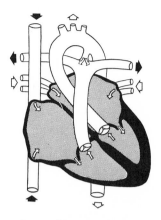

Patent ductus arteriosus

The patent ductus arteriosus is a vascular connection that, during fetal life, short circuits the pulmonary vascular bed and directs blood from the pulmonary artery to the aorta. Functional closure of the ductus normally occurs soon after birth. If the ductus remains patent after birth, the direction of blood flow in the ductus is reversed by the higher pressure in the aorta.

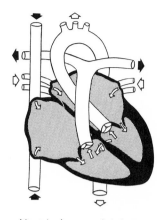

Ventricular septal defects

A ventricular septal defect is an abnormal opening between the right and left ventricle. Ventricular septal defects vary in size and may occur in either the membranous or muscular portion of the ventricular septum. Due to higher pressure in the left ventricle, a shunting of blood from the left to right ventricle occurs during systole. If pulmonary vascular resistance produces pulmonary hypertension, the shunt of blood is then reversed from the right to the left ventricle, with cyanosis resulting.

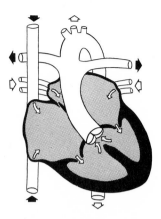

Truncus arteriosus

Truncus arteriosus is a retention of the embryologic bulbar trunk. It results from the failure of normal septation and division of this trunk into an aorta and pulmonary artery. This single arterial trunk overrides the ventricles and receives blood from them through a ventricular septal defect. The entire pulmonary and systemic circulation is supplied from this common arterial trunk.

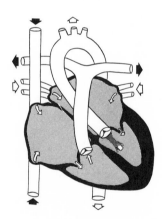

Subaortic stenosis

In many instances, the stenosis is valvular with thickening and fusion of the cusps. Subaortic stenosis is caused by a fibrous ring below the aortic valve in the outflow tract of the left ventricle. At times, both valvular and subaortic stenosis exist in combination. The obstruction presents an increased work load for the normal output of the left ventricular blood and results in left ventricular enlargement.

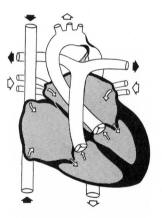

Coarctation of the aorta

Coarctation of the aorta is characterized by a narrowed aortic lumen. It exists as a preductal or postductal obstruction, depending on the position of the obstruction in relation to the ductus arteriosus. Coarctations exist with great variation in anatomic features. The lesion produces an obstruction to the flow of blood through the aorta causing an increased left ventricular pressure and work load.

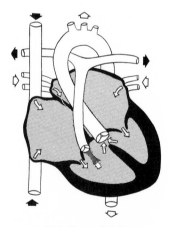

Tetralogy of Fallot

Tetralogy of Fallot is characterized by the combination of four defects: (1) pulmonary stenosis, (2) ventricular septal defect, (3) overriding aorta, (4) hypertrophy of right ventricle. It is the most common defect causing cyanosis in patients surviving beyond two years of age. The severity of symptoms depends on the degree of pulmonary stenosis, the size of the ventricular septal defect, and the degree to which the aorta overrides the septal defect.

Fig. 35-11, cont'd. For legend see p. 583.

PLAN OF CARE: CARDIOVASCULAR DISORDERS

PATIENT CARE OBJECTIVES
1. Adequate oxygenation of tissues is maintained.
2. The infant is protected from additional stresses such as infection, inadequate nutrition, and cold stress.
3. Corrective or palliative surgery is performed.
4. Parents have an understanding and beginning acceptance of the problem and its treatment and any necessary continuing care after discharge.
5. Parents are able to initiate and maintain a positive parent-child relationship.

NURSING INTERVENTIONS

Diagnostic

1. Check mother's previous and present obstetric histories; check maternal and paternal medical histories.
2. Cry: weak and muffled, loud and breathless.
3. Color:
   a. Cyanotic: usually generalized; increases in supine position; often unrelieved by oxygen*; usually deepens with crying; gray, dusky; mild, moderate, severe.
   b. Acyanotic: pale, with or without mottling with exertion.
4. Activity level:
   a. Restless.
   b. Lethargic.
   c. Unresponsive except to pain.
   d. Lack of movement of arms and legs when crying (severe distress).
   e. Arms become flaccid when eating.
5. Posturing:
   a. Hypotonic; flaccid even when sleeping.
   b. Hyperextension of neck.
   c. Opisthotonos.
   d. Dyspnea when supine.
   e. Favors knee-chest position.
6. Persistent bradycardia ≤120/min or persistent tachycardia ≥160/min.
7. Respirations: Count when neonate is sleeping to identify problem early.
   a. Tachypnea ≥60/min.
   b. Retractions with nasal flaring or tachypnea.
   c. Dyspnea with diaphoresis† or grunting.
   d. Gasping followed in 2 or 3 minutes by respiratory arrest if untreated promptly.
   e. Chronic cough (not often seen).
   f. Grunting with exertion such as crying or feeding by nipple.
8. Feeding behavior:
   a. Anorexic.
   b. Poor suck: from lack of energy or when unable to close mouth around nipple due to dyspnea.
   c. Difficulty coordinating suck, swallow, breathing; pulls away from nipple to take breath.
   d. Slow, with pauses to rest.
   e. Unable to feed by nipple.

Therapeutic and educational

1. General care: Support respiratory effort and decrease work of heart.
   a. Administer O_2 as necessary to relieve cyanosis.
   b. Suction.
   c. Provide warmth.
   d. Position for optimal respiratory effort:
      (1) Knee-chest, prone, side-lying.
      (2) Hold upright over nurse's shoulder
      (3) See respiratory distress, p. 531.
   e. Omit oral feedings until physician arrives. If oral feedings are ordered, offer small amounts more frequently to avoid overdistending stomach and compromising respirations and to avoid fatigue.
   f. If oral feedings are discontinued, prepare for gavage feeding or parenteral therapy.
2. Record and report all findings to provide current data base for continuing therapy:
   a. Degree and extent of cyanosis: nail beds, mucosa, scrotum.
   b. General body color: pale, grayish, cyanotic.
   c. Muscle tone when active and when at rest.
   d. Effect of O_2 on cyanosis; how much was needed to relieve symptoms; changes with change in activity level.
   e. Heart rate. Heart sounds: loudness, location.
   f. Respirations.
   g. Fatigability.
3. Painful procedures (e.g., venipuncture, increase distress) especially in cyanotic baby. Minimize distress:
   a. Place infant in prone position.
   b. Administer O_2 by mask during procedure.
   c. Keep infant warm.
   d. Request technician to stop before infant begins to gasp.
4. Prevent stress: infection, hypoglycemia.
5. Medicate per physician order and observe infant response:
   a. Digitalis preparation: When preparing digitalis dose, second nurse should double-check amount drawn into syringe. Take apical beat; if heart rate is below 100/min, report to physician before administering drug.
   b. Diuretic.
6. Support parents.

---

*Suspect hematologic problem as well (e.g., methemoglobinemia).
†Diaphoresis: uncommon response in normal newborn.

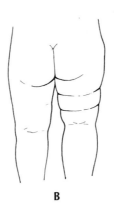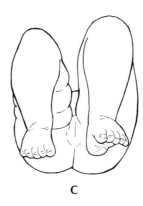

A B C

Fig. 35-12. Congenital dysplasia of hip. **A,** Normal gluteal and popliteal skin creases. **B,** Abnormal skin creases and asymmetry of skin folds. **C,** Apparent shortening of femur. Femur head is displaced. (Courtesy Ross Laboratories, Columbus, Ohio.)

PLAN OF CARE: CONGENITAL HIP DYSPLASIA

PATIENT CARE OBJECTIVES

1. Parents understand and accept the condition and are committed to the immediate and long-term treatment necessary to effect correction.
2. The infant's condition is corrected without residual deformity or impaired function.

NURSING INTERVENTIONS

Diagnostic

1. Note type of delivery. Breech presentation, especially in female neonates, may affect incidence.
2. Signs on affected side:
   a. Asymmetry of gluteal dorsal surface of thigh and inguinal folds. Folds appear higher than those on unaffected side.
   b. Leg appears shorter, since head of femur often overrides the acetabulum.
   c. Limited abduction of affected leg (e.g., <60%).
   d. Click sound heard during passive abduction of hip.
   e. Femoral pulse is not felt over head of femur when hip is flexed and leg is abducted.
3. Check for adequate circulation in legs when appliance is in place:
   a. Color.
   b. Warmth.
   c. Pedal pulses.
   d. Pressure areas.

Therapeutic and educational

1. Nurse may discover signs initially. Record and report findings to physician or clinic.
2. Institute physician-ordered therapy: Treatment involves pressing femoral head into acetabulum to form adequate socket before ossification is complete.
   a. Thick diapers used to abduct and externally rotate leg and flex hip; pin anterior flaps of diapers under posterior flaps.
   b. Frejka pillow: apply diapers and plastic pants, then apply pillow. Later this appliance will be followed by spica cast in most instances.
3. Parents:
   a. Reinforce, repeat, and simplify physician's explanations to parents of this condition and its treatment.
   b. Support mother and father as they learn how to apply corrective appliance and to hold, feed, and play with infant wearing appliance.
   c. Reinforce need for long-term treatment; involve them in planning to increase their commitment and motivation.
   d. Help them verbalize feelings regarding ability to meet treatment demands.
   e. Refer to social services or other appropriate community resource.
4. Some cultures (American Indian) swaddle infants to board during first year of life. This may cause permanent damage that could cause deformity and impair function even if corrective treatment is instituted immediately after first year of life.

Musculoskeletal problems

The two most common musculoskeletal deviations seen in the neonatal period are congenital dysplasia of the hip and congenital clubfoot. Both conditions are easily recognized. Early detection and definitive treatment are mandatory for successful correction; delay makes repair more difficult and prognosis less favorable.

Congenital hip dysplasia (congenital dislocation of the hip). This often hereditary disorder occurs more commonly in females (Fig. 35-12). The pelvis is more appropriate for this to happen because of its architecture. The acetabulum is abnormally shallow so that the head of the femur becomes dislocated upward and backward to lie on the dorsal aspect of the ilium where a false acetabulum may be formed. A stretched joint capsule results, and ossification of the femoral head is delayed.

Before dislocation occurs, reduced movement, splinting of the affected hip, limited abduction, and asymmetry of the hip may be noted. After dislocation, all these signs will be present, together with the external rotation and shortening of the leg. A clicking sound may be noted on gentle forced abduction of the leg, and a bulge of the femoral head is felt. X-ray films will reveal a deformity in congenital dysplasia of the hip.

Treatment generally involves closed reduction and a cast to maintain abduction, extension, and internal rotation, usually with the infant in a "frog-leg" position.

Talipes equinovarus. Talipes, or clubfoot, is a congenital fixed postural deformity in which the foot is twisted out of shape or position. The heel is turned inward from the midline of the leg, the foot is plantar flexed, and the achilles tendon is shortened.

Before the infant is 2 months old, often during his nursery stay, successive plaster casts are applied first to correct the heel inversion and adduction of the forefoot and later the equinus deformity. Special shoes with lower leg braces will be necessary when the child learns to walk, and surgery may even be required in childhood if correction is incomplete. The prognosis depends on the extent of the deformity and the response to progressive orthopedic treatment.

Phocomelia. Phocomelia, or "seal-like limbs," is a developmental anomaly, typified by absence of the arms and/or legs or stunting of the extremities. In the early

---

PLAN OF CARE: TALIPES EQUINOVARUS

PATIENT CARE OBJECTIVES

1. Parents understand and accept the condition and are committed to the immediate and long-term treatment necessary to effect correction.
2. The infant's condition is corrected without residual deformity or impaired function.

NURSING INTERVENTIONS

Diagnostic	Therapeutic and educational

1. Sex of infant: Incidence in male is twice that in female.
2. Symptoms on affected side(s): equinovarus.
  a. Entire foot is inverted (e.g., soles face midline).
  b. Heel of foot is drawn upward, with plantar flexion.
  c. Forefoot is adducted, with soft tissue contractures.
  d. Deep crease transverses sole of foot.
  e. Crying aggravates deformity. (If this were positional defect, foot would regain its normal position as infant cries.)
3. Observe for other associated defects: spina bifida, meningomyelocele.
	1. Equinovarus type of clubfoot comprises 95% of affected infants.
	2. Record and report observations to physician.
	3. Institute physician's orders:
	  a. Transfer to pediatric unit.
	  b. Order corrective appliance.
	4. Support parents:
	  a. Reemphasize, repeat, and simplify physician's explanation of cause, condition, proposed long-term treatment.
	  b. Support mother as she learns to give passive exercise and massage to foot or as she learns to care for corrective appliance (casts, etc.).
	  c. Reinforce infant's need for long-term treatment.
	  d. Encourage exploration and venting of feelings.
	  e. Avoid comments such as, "It could have been something worse."
	  f. Refer to social worker or other community resources.

1960s the drug thalidomide was implicated as the causative agent for the limb deformities of many thousands of infants, especially in Germany. As a result the United States Food and Drug Administration tightened its regulations governing drug approval. Painfully apparent was evidence that drugs ingested during pregnancy may have tragic implications for fetal development. Thalidomide (and perhaps imipramine, or Tofranil) is a cause of this condition; sporadic cases of congenital amputation or stunting are of unknown etiology.

The child born with these deformities requires special care as follows:

1. Rehabilitative problems are often complex. The prostheses require frequent refitting as the child grows. The child requires careful guidance and training in achieving the optimal level of functioning possible. Approximately fifteen child amputee centers are located throughout the United States.

2. Psychosocial developmental problems are significant. The kinesthetic satisfaction derived from kicking the legs and waving the arms is not possible. The hand-to-mouth movement behavior pattern, necessary for self-gratification and exploration of one's environment, is missing. The child learns about his environment by pushing the trunk up by the arms; a pillow prop under the infant's chest will compensate for this somewhat. The child's concerns about body image and obvious differences from others will require attention in later years. Any child reflects the attitudes and sentiments of those around him; if that child senses positive attitudes toward him and his defect, he will incorporate these into a positive self-concept.

3. Supportive care of the parents must begin at the birth of the child and continue for years. After the initial grief reaction, the parents need information regarding the rehabilitative and psychosocial components of their child's care.

Polydactyly. Extra digits on the hands or feet occur occasionally (Fig. 35-13). In some instances it is hereditary. If there is little or no bone involvement, the extra digit is tied with silk suture soon after birth. The finger falls off within a few days, leaving a small scar. When there is bone involvement, surgical repair is indicated.

Genitourinary tract anomalies

Abnormally low-set ears may indicate other, often genitourinary, anomalies (e.g., renal agenesis) (Fig. 35-14).

Exstrophy of the bladder (Fig. 35-15). In this congenital anomaly of unknown etiology, a separation of the symphysis pubis and anterior abdominal wall structures results in exterioration of the bladder trigone and surrounding mucosa. The exposed mucosa is deep red, has numerous folds and is sensitive to touch. A direct passage of urine to the outside occurs. Associated

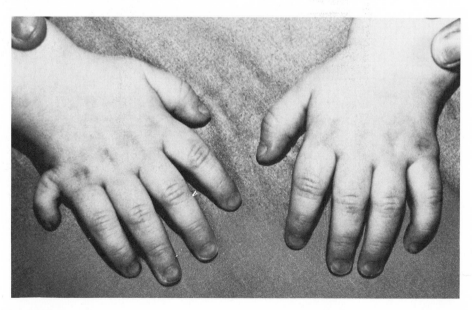

Fig. 35-13. Polydactyly: supernumerary digit of right hand. Most common congenital anomaly of upper extremity and is occasionally seen in conjunction with other congenital malformations. (Courtesy Mead Johnson Laboratories, Evansville, Ind.)

anomalies should be sought, such as undescended testes, inguinal hernia, absence of the vagina, or bowel defects. Surgical correction, often elimination of the bladder and construction of an ileal conduit, is rarely justified in the neonatal period. A prosthesis for collection of the urine and protection of the bladder may be employed.

Nursing management in the presence of exstrophy of the bladder involves the following:

1. Prevent urinary tract infection.
2. Prevent ulceration of adjacent skin from the constant seepage of urine.
3. Meet the infant's touching and cuddling needs.
4. Support parents.
5. Teach parents to care for the defect if surgery is scheduled when the infant is several weeks or months of age.

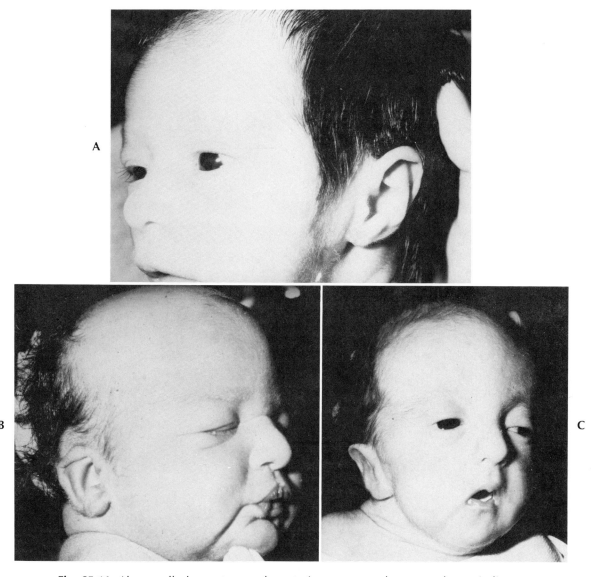

Fig. 35-14. Abnormally low-set ears characterize many syndromes and may indicate abnormality of internal organs, especially bilateral renal agenesis (Potter's syndrome). **A,** In normal infant, insertion of ear to scalp falls on extension of line drawn across inner and outer canthus of eye. **B,** If ear is twisted or rotated, it may give false impression of being low set. **C,** True low-set ear. (Courtesy Mead Johnson Laboratories, Evansville, Ind.)

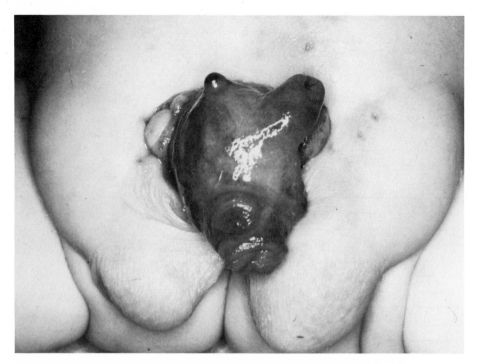

Fig. 35-15. Exstrophy of bladder. (Courtesy Edward S. Tank, M.D., Division of Urology, University of Oregon Health Sciences Center, Portland, Ore.)

Hypospadias and epispadias. Hypospadias is a developmental anomaly of the urethral meatus. In the male, the meatus opens in the midline of the under-surface of the penis or on the perineum. In the female, the meatus opens into the vagina. This condition tends to be hereditary.

Epispadias, also occurring in both sexes but predominating in males, is a congenital absence of the upper urethral wall. In the female it is often associated with exstrophy of the bladder. In the male, the meatal opening is located anywhere along the dorsum of the penis.

Most instances of hypospadias are minor and require no corrective surgery. Pronounced defects require extensive urethroplasty. If needed, surgery is completed before the boy enters school so that he can urinate from a standing position like other boys. The more serious defects often coexist with other multiple anomalies.

Nursing management of the physical care of the infant with hypospadias is the same as that for the normal infant. Supportive care of parents of a child with a disorder is discussed in Chapter 7. Should urethroplasty be required, no circumcision is done, since the foreskin is used in the surgical procedure. In these cases, the parents are taught how to care for the urethral meatus and foreskin to prevent infection and promote cleanliness.

Sexual ambiguity. Sexual ambiguity in the neonate often is discovered by the nurse who has more time and perhaps a better opportunity to examine the infant than the obstetrician who may be concerned with maternal complications (Fig. 35-16).

Erroneous or abnormal sexual differentiation may be a genetic aberration (e.g., congenital adrenal hypoplasia) or be due to maternal problems (e.g., steroid sex hormone therapy for threatened abortion). It is imperative to establish the genetic sex and the sex of rearing as soon as possible not only to save embarrassment for reporting the birth of a (genetic) male who in fact is a female or the opposite, but to permit the surgical correction of anomalies before an individual or social pattern is set.

Prompt consultation with a surgeon who is experienced in the area of intersex should be arranged without delay. Meanwhile parents need supportive care as they await the decision.

Teratoma

Teratoma, a solid or semisolid neoplasm, is composed of the three embryonal tissue types (ectoderm, mesoderm, entoderm). A teratoma in the newborn may occur in the skull, mediastinum, or abdomen, but a solid or semisolid tumor in the sacral area also may prove to be a teratoma. It is protected by sterile dressings prior to surgical removal. Many teratomas diagnosed in the new-

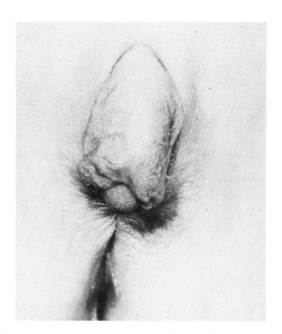

Fig. 35-16. Ambiguous external genitals. (Courtesy Edward S. Tank, M.D., Division of Urology, University of Oregon Health Sciences Center, Portland, Ore.)

born are malignant. If the lesion cannot be entirely removed by surgery, x-ray therapy and chemotherapy are used. Long-term survival rate for infants with sacrococcygeal teratoma is 85% after surgical removal in the neonatal period but only 50% if surgery is delayed until the infant is more than 1 month old. Rectal and anal function can always be preserved.

SUMMARY

The nursing care to meet the physical needs of the neonate born with an anomaly requiring immediate surgical intervention presents a challenge. The neonate's physiologic functioning must be supported, infection prevented, and a protective environment provided (pediatric unit, neonatal intensive care nursery).

In addition, the nurse and other members of the interdisciplinary team must consider the psychosocial needs of the parents. The child may survive the surgical insult well. However, the way that parents feel about the child and the emotional (and financial) disruption imposed by the anomaly and its treatment influence the quality of the parent-child relationship. The relationship affects the child's self-concept and ability to achieve his potential during his lifetime.

REFERENCES

Babson, S. G., Benson, R. C., Pernoll, M. L., and Benda, G. I. 1975. Management of high-risk pregnancy and intensive care of the neonate (ed. 3). St. Louis, The C. V. Mosby Co.

Behrman, R. E. (ed.). 1973. Neonatology: diseases of the fetus and infant. St. Louis, The C. V. Mosby Co.

Clark, A. L., and Affonso, D. 1976. Childbearing: a nursing perspective. Philadelphia, F. A. Davis Co.

Clausen, J., and others. 1976. Maternity nursing today. New York, McGraw-Hill Book Co.

Nelson, W. E. (ed.). 1969. Textbook of pediatrics (ed. 9). Philadelphia, W. B. Saunders Co.

Reeder, S. P., and others. 1976. Maternity nursing (ed. 13). Philadelphia, J. B. Lippincott Co.

Shirkey, H. C. (ed.). 1975. Pediatric therapy (ed. 5). St. Louis, The C. V. Mosby Co.

Tucker, S., and others. 1975. Patient care standards. St. Louis, The C. V. Mosby Co.

CHAPTER 36

Neonatal disorders of maternal origin

JAUNDICE AND THE NEONATE

The pigment bilirubin is one breakdown product of hemoglobin. Total serum bilirubin is the sum of conjugated (direct or water-soluble) and unconjugated (indirect or free) bilirubin.

Unconjugated or free bilirubin can leave the vascular system and be deposited in body tissues (e.g., the skin and sclera). The resultant yellow coloring is termed *jaundice*. To be removed (or cleared) from the body, bilirubin must be conjugated into the water-soluble or direct form. Direct bilirubin is excreted by the liver into the bile and then into the gut for excretion in the feces.

Conjugation is a function of a mature liver, available serum albumin-binding sites, and the rate of hemolysis. The full-term neonate's liver is usually sufficiently mature and the production of glucuronyl transferase adequate enough to prevent pathologic levels of bilirubin (12 mg/100 ml or more). In the absence of asphyxia neonatorum, cold stress, hypoglycemia, and maternal ingestion of drugs such as sulfa and aspirin (salicylates), adequate serum albumin-binding sites should be available. The number and kind of vascular cell elements necessary to the fetus, but superfluous in the neonate, are broken down in the early neonatal period. About 50% of full-term and 80% of preterm neonates will demonstrate physiologic jaundice *after* 24 hours of life.

Physiologic jaundice

Physiologic jaundice is considered a normal occurrence in the neonatal period. Bilirubin is produced by normal hemolysis of excess intravascular cell elements (red blood cells). Fetal red blood cells have a shorter life span than adult red blood cells; therefore the end products of their destruction accumulate more rapidly. In the term infant, the levels for serum bilirubin (total) increase as follows: up to 24 hours, 2 to 6 mg/100 ml; up to 48 hours, 6 to 7 mg/100 ml; and up to 3 to 5 days, 4 to 12 mg/100 ml. In the premature infant, the levels

are as follows: up to 24 hours, 1 to 6 mg/100 ml; up to 48 hours, 6 to 8 mg/100 ml; and up to 3 to 5 days, 10 to 15 mg/100 ml. Jaundice appears when the level reaches about 7 mg/100 ml (usually second to third day). Hence jaundice is not apparent until the second or third day and does not exceed 12 mg/100 ml.

Bilirubin concentration in the premature infant peaks between the sixth and eighth day and usually does not exceed 15 mg/100 ml.

Several nursery practices may influence the appearance and degree of jaundice. For example, early feeding tends to keep the serum bilirubin level low; chilling the neonate encourages higher levels. Early feeding stimulates intestinal activity and the passage of meconium and stool. Removal of intestinal contents prevents the reabsorption (and recycling) of bilirubin from the gut, a residual mechanism left over from fetal life. Chilling the neonate results in acidosis, a condition that decreases the amount of available serum albumin-binding sites.

Pathologic jaundice

Elevated serum levels, especially of unconjugated indirect bilirubin, pose a grave danger to the neonate, especially the premature infant. Physiologic jaundice may become pathologic and require a diagnostic workup and plan of care if any of the following conditions pertain:

- Appearance of jaundice during the first 24 hours
- Jaundice lasting longer than 7 days for the full-term and 10 days for the preterm neonate
- Serum bilirubin levels increasing more than 5 mg/100 ml/24 hr
- Serum bilirubin levels greater than 12 mg/100 ml for a full-term neonate or greater than 15 mg/100 ml for a preterm neonate
- Direct bilirubin greater than 1.5 mg/100 ml

The nurse can observe the appearance and persistence

of jaundice and the neonate's behavior and alert the physician. Laboratory studies for serum bilirubin are not routine. The nurse and physician must be alert to conditions favoring hyperbilirubinemia.

Hyperbilirubinemia

Serum bilirubin levels above accepted norms constitute hyperbilirubinemia. Several conditions are associated with this condition including the following:

1. Maturity of liver (e.g., premature versus term neonate)
2. Rate of hemolysis: Rh or ABO incompatibility, enclosed hemorrhage (cephalhematoma), abnormal red blood cells (spherocytosis), maternal infection, injections of vitamin K analog to mother during labor or to neonate
3. Interference with conjugation and/or competition for albumin-binding sites: metabolic factors (cold stress, asphyxia, hypoglycemia); breast milk inhibitor of glucuronyl transferase; drugs (novobiocin, long-acting sulfas, aspirin, tranquilizers); lower serum albumin levels (common in premature neonates)
4. Interference with excretion of conjugated bilirubin: obstruction or atresia of biliary duct or lower gastrointestinal tract; hepatitis

Prevention of hyperbilirubinemia is the most desirable approach. Early recognition and management of maternal infection and judicious drug therapy may be possible. Give proper blood transfusions. An active program directed toward prevention of premature delivery that includes adequate nutrition, family planning (maternal age at conception, spacing of pregnancies), and acceptable antenatal care available to everyone is long overdue.

Screening measures are useful both in the prevention and management of hyperbilirubinemia:

1. Familial and mother's obstetric histories are taken and reviewed. (Note all abortions and term pregnancies.)
2. Blood typing and Rh determination of infant is done at birth and compared to mother's, and RhoGAM is given to mother if appropriate (p. 599).
3. Coomb's test and Hemantigen screen are performed when necessary.
4. A careful record of maternal infection is kept, including the time of occurrence during pregnancy, results of cultures, and therapy.
5. Amniocentesis is performed in selected cases (pp. 597 and 598).

The objective of management of hyperbilirubinemia is to keep the serum bilirubin below toxic levels (pp. 625 to 627). There are three available interventions directed toward controlling this condition:

1. Phototherapy is a photochemical method that alters the nature of bilirubin in two ways. First, it renders bilirubin less toxic and presumably suitable for hepatic excretion, and second, it photo-oxidizes and removes bilirubin directly by way of the skin.
2. Exchange transfusion removes serum bilirubin and maternal hemolytic antibodies and corrects anemia.
3. Enzyme induction is stimulated to enhance liver function. Certain drugs (phenobarbital, alcohol, morphine) have been considered to facilitate hepatic function. The effectiveness and appropriateness of these methods are still questionable and controversial (p. 627).

In cases in which low serum albumin levels exist, intravenous infusions of albumin may be administered to aid in conjugation.

Kernicterus

Unconjugated bilirubin can leak through vascular walls and enter the susceptible neurons in the basal ganglia of the CNS. The presence of bilirubin in these cells interferes with cell metabolism, and cellular death ensues (p. 598). Cerebral palsy, epilepsy, and mental retardation are expected in survivors.

Breast milk jaundice

Jaundice from ingestion of breast milk occurs in a small proportion of full-term infants. Unconjugated bilirubin levels rise beyond physiologic limits usually by the seventh day. The levels subside by the fifth day after breast-feeding is discontinued. (Breast-feeding is only discontinued if bilirubin levels rise above accepted norms.) Despite high serum bilirubin levels (equal to 20 mg/100 ml), kernicterus has not been reported.

An enzyme present in the milk of some women inhibits the enzyme (glucuronyl transferase) necessary for conjugation of bilirubin. Treatment consists of substituting formula for breast milk.

HEMOLYTIC DISEASE OF THE NEWBORN (ERYTHROBLASTOSIS, Rh OR ABO INCOMPATIBILITY)

Hemolytic disease of the newborn, or erythroblastosis fetalis, is a disorder of the blood and blood-forming organs of the fetus and neonate characterized by hemolytic anemia and compensatory erythropoiesis. Blood group differences between the mother and father result in the formation of maternal isohemoglutinins. A transfer of these red blood cell–destroying antibodies from the mother to her fetus causes erythroblastosis. Once the mother is sensitized, increasingly serious disease tends to develop in subsequent children of the opposite blood group. Hemolytic disease of the newborn occurred in 0.5% to 1% of all mature pregnancies in North America before prophylactic $Rh_o(D)$ human immune globulin (RhoGAM) became available in the mid-1960s. Many children died or were seriously affected. Since immunization against this antigen began, however, the incidence of severe erythroblastosis has been drastically reduced.

Pathogenesis and pathology

During antibody studies in the 1940s, it was observed that the injection of red blood cells of rhesus monkeys into rabbits caused the production of an antiserum that agglutinated the red blood cells of these monkeys and of most humans as well. Consequently, red blood cells that could be agglutinated by this specific antiserum possessed the rhesus (Rh) antigen and were called *Rh positive*, whereas those red blood cells that could not be agglutinated were called *Rh negative*. Subsequently, it was revealed that the Rh factor is not a single antigen but a complex blood system with a number of variants.

Six common Rh (rhesus) antigens are identified as follows: C, D, E, c, d, e. Antibody formation results from the presence of one or more of these (and other less common) antigens. Because two chromosomes are present in every cell, one derived from each parent, the genetic constitution of an individual with reference to these antigens might be, for example, DD, dd, or Dd.

Different combinations allow eight Rh genotypes, each with a single Rh chromosome (e.g., CDE, cde, cDE, etc.). Actually, thirty-six different combinations (genotypes) are possible. The order of antigenetic potency of these antigens is D, C, E, c, e, and d.

Soon after the Rh factor was reported, it was found that erythroblastosis, hydrops fetalis, and icterus gravis —variations of hemolytic disease of the newborn—were caused by the hemolysis of fetal red blood cells due to maternal antibodies. Later studies showed that slightly more than 90% of cases of clinically evident hemolytic disease of the newborn followed sensitization of isoimmunization of an Rh-negative woman by the Rh factor in the red blood cells of her fetus. Moreover, not only can inheritance of the Rh factor from an Rh-positive father cause the maternal isoimmunization, but transfusion or intramuscular injection of Rh-positive blood may also be responsible.

Between 10% and 15% of marriages of white persons will involve Rh-incompatible partners. About 5% of

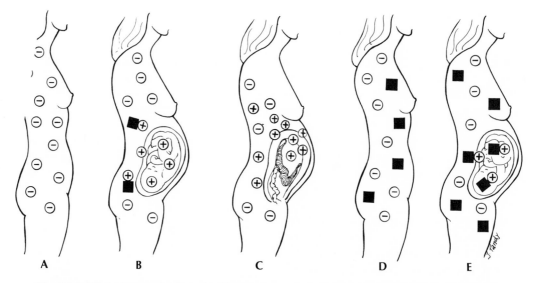

Fig. 36-1. Rh isoimmunization. **A,** Rh-negative woman before pregnancy. **B,** Pregnancy with Rh-positive fetus. Some Rh-positive blood passes into mother's blood. **C,** During separation of placenta, a massive inoculation of mother by Rh-positive red blood cells occurs. **D,** After delivery, mother becomes sensitized to Rh-positive blood and develops anti–Rh-positive antibodies shown as darkened squares. She now has increased titer or positive Coombs' test. **E,** During subsequent pregnancy with Rh-positive fetus, maternal anti–Rh-positive antibodies enter fetal circulation, attach to Rh-positive red blood cells, and subject them to hemolysis.

black parents will be Rh incompatible, but only rarely an Oriental couple will be similarly affected.

Not all Rh-positive men are homozygous for the Rh factor, or will all children of Rh-positive men married to Rh-negative women be Rh positive. About 50% of the progeny of Rh-positive men who are heterozygous will be Rh positive; the remainder will be Rh negative. Actually, approximately 65% of newborns of Rh-incompatible marriages are Rh positive.

The risk of maternal sensitization is less than expected. In the first pregnancy, only 0.1% of mothers will be sensitized. In the second and third pregnancies, 11% will be affected, and 15% in the fourth or subsequent Rh-positive pregnancies will be affected. About 5% of Rh-incompatible matings produce affected infants.

Hemolytic disease of the newborn develops according to the following sequence (Fig. 36-1):

1. Isoimmunization of an Rh-negative woman (by the administration of Rh-positive blood or Rh-positive fetal red blood cells) stimulates the production of anti-Rh antibodies.

2. Transplacental passage of the woman's anti-Rh antibodies to her fetus causes hemolysis of its red blood cells, together with other abnormal processes in utero and in neonatal life.

Sensitization of an Rh-negative woman must preceed intrauterine transfer of antibodies and fetal damage. Therefore the first child rarely is affected unless the mother has been sensitized by the administration of improperly typed (Rh-positive) blood.

ABO incompatibility between the mother and her fetus may occur more frequently than Rh incompatibility. Most cases of ABO incompatibility are mild, often not recognized clinically, and rarely require treatment.

Other less common red blood cell antigens also capable of transplacental isoimmunization include Kell, Duffy, and Kidd. Fortunately, serious fetal damage from these factors is unlikely, because there is no specific preventive measure as yet available to any but $Rh_o(D)$ sensitization.

The placenta of the seriously affected fetus is larger than normal. Increased villous size, persistence of Langhans' cells, and foci of erythropoiesis are apparent. Frequently, the amniotic fluid is yellowish, that is, pigment-stained (from the decomposition of bilirubin).

Severe Rh incompatibility results in marked fetal hemolytic anemia with erythroid hyperplasia of bone marrow and extramedullary hematopoiesis. The placenta clears the released blood pigments fairly well, however, so that only in extreme cases is the fetus icteric (yellow or jaundiced) (e.g., icterus gravis). The marked anemia leads to cardiac decompensation, cardiomegaly, hepatomegaly, and splenomegaly. Edema, ascites, and hydrothorax develop. Anemia is responsible for pulmonary and other hemorrhage. Intrauterine or early neonatal death may occur.

Once delivery has occurred, the erythroblastotic newborn becomes icteric because it cannot excrete the considerable residue of red blood cell hemolysis. Yellowish pigmentation of cerebral basal nuclei often develops (kernicterus) when the serum bilirubin is greater than 20 mg/100 ml, and serious CNS abnormalities may develop and persist as spasticity, for example, if the infant survives.

Clinical findings

Maternal. The diagnosis of hemolytic disease of the newborn in women sensitized to the $Rh_o(D)$ or other blood factors is likely when a Hemantigen test or its equivalent (cell pool containing all the common antigens) done on maternal serum at about midpregnancy is positive. If the test is negative initially, it should be repeated at 32 to 36 weeks. If the maternal serum antibody titer is greater than 1:16, amniocentesis is done after the twenty-sixth week.

The amount of pigment from the decomposition of bilirubin can be measured when in solution. Therefore a spectrophotometric examination of amniotic fluid obtained by amniocentesis is helpful in diagnosing the extent of hemolytic activity in the fetus of an Rh-sensitized woman.

Three zones (A, B, and C) of optical density (ΔOD) of the amniotic fluid have been identified (Lilley, 1961) as being indicative of the severity of hemolytic disease of the newborn, which is an aid in the obstetric-pediatric management. The interpretation of the results of amniocentesis are as follows:

1. When increased ΔOD at 450 nm persists within the A zone, a normal or only slightly anemic fetus is likely. Under these circumstances, the pregnancy is allowed to continue to delivery at term. The prognosis for the newborn is good, although replacement transfusion may be required.

2. Significantly increased ΔOD at 450 nm within the B zone is indicative of a moderately anemic fetus or one that may be hydropic or even stillborn at term. Once definite viability is established, delivery should be accomplished, even by cesarean section, if uncomplicated, induced vaginal delivery does not ensue. Exchange transfusions will be required for such a premature neonate. A fair prognosis is likely under the best of circumstances.

3. When C zone ΔOD readings are evaluated, it is certain that the fetus is severely affected (Fig. 36-2). If

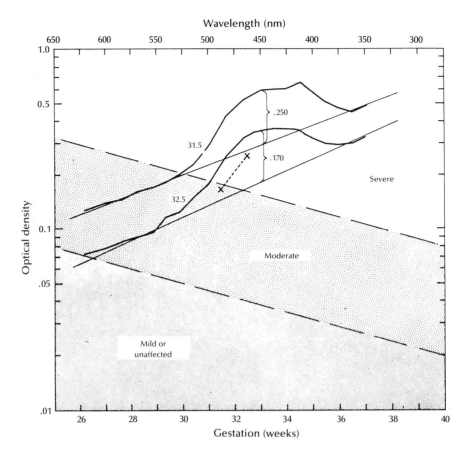

Fig. 36-2. Transabdominal amniocentesis: spectrophotometric analysis of amniotic fluid surrounding erythroblastotic fetus. Amniocentesis was performed at 31½ and 32½ weeks. Spectral absorption curve was obtained by plotting optical densities at various wavelengths on two-cycle semilogarithmic graph paper. Tangential line joining lowest portions of this curve approximates unstained amniotic fluid and is baseline for calculations. Difference between involved and uninvolved curves is measured at 450 nm. (Maximum absorption by bilirubin or bilirubin-like products occurs at 450 nm.) This difference is plotted at appropriate number of weeks of gestation (see dotted line). Case illustrated shows rapid progression from moderate to severe disease. Under such conditions, fetal death is often imminent. Prompt delivery usually must be accomplished if gestational age will permit; otherwise, intrauterine fetal transfusion may be considered. (From Babson, S. G., Benson, R. C., Pernoll, M. L., and Benda, G. I. 1975. Management of high-risk pregnancy and intensive care of the neonate [ed 3]. St. Louis, The C. V. Mosby Co.)

the fetus is between 26 and 32 weeks gestational age, an intrauterine transfusion should be considered every 1 to 2 weeks until viability has been reached, whereupon prompt delivery, generally by cesarean section, will be necessary to save the child. Exchange transfusions will be required. Treatment of the mother and neonate at a maternity center is usually arranged because special pediatric and laboratory care will be essential.

Fetal. The diagnosis of hemolytic disease of the newborn involves the following:

1. Placental enlargement (e.g., alteration of the average fetal to placental weight at term of 1:6 to 1:2 or 3:4)
2. Fetal edema (hydrops fetalis), pleural and pericardial effusions, and ascites, which indicate cardiac failure (many of these infants are stillborn)
3. Neonatal pallor with jaundice generally appearing during the first 24 to 36 hours
4. Hemolytic anemia of a progressive type
5. Hepatosplenomegaly
6. CNS signs if kernicterus develops

7. Fetal bleeding tendencies occasionally
8. Yellow-stained vernix

Laboratory findings

Laboratory findings include the following:
1. Neonate Rh positive; mother Rh negative
2. Maternal anti-Rh titer increased
3. Occasionally a sensitized Rh-positive infant that is typed as Rh negative because of so-called blocking antibodies
4. Positive direct Coombs' test (antihuman globulin)
5. Increased erythropoiesis; many nucleated red blood cells in peripheral blood
6. Anemia often present at birth or developing in the early neonatal period; other evidence of erythroblastosis may occur in the absence of obvious anemia, however
7. Indirect and occasionally direct serum bilirubin increase in cord blood
8. Anti-Rh agglutinins usually present in infant serum; hypoglycemia may be asymptomatic
9. Reduced globulin-binding capacity
10. Increased spectrophotometric ΔOD of the amniotic fluid at 450 nm (amniocentesis)

Management

Maternal. Rh (and ABO) typing should be done early in pregnancy. The antibody titer for Rh and ABO antigens should be obtained in all Rh-negative patients, in those women with a history of having received blood products, or when a history of possible blood factor complications in a previous pregnancy is revealed.

Amniocentesis should be accomplished in Rh-sensitized women. Subsequent management will depend on the severity of the sensitization as described previously.

Fetal. Intrauterine exchange and replacement transfusions require fresh type O, Rh-negative blood. Exchange transfusions may be necessary in the presence of the following factors:
- Severe hemolytic disease of the newborn in a previous child
- Anti-Rh titer of the mother greater than 1:16
- Clinical hemolytic disease of the newborn at birth or within the first 24 hours
- Cord serum bilirubin level greater than 3.5 mg/100 ml
- Positive direct Coombs' test
- Serum bilirubin level greater than 15 mg/100 ml during the first 24 hours or greater than 20 mg/100 ml within the first week

Repeat exchange transfusions may be required if the serum bilirubin level exceeds 20 mg/100 ml after a previous exchange transfusion.

Separate measures for the neonate include the following:
1. Digitalize infant if signs of cardiac decompensation develop. (Restrict intravenous calcium to avoid bradycardia or arrhythmia.)
2. Obtain daily hemoglobin values until a stable state has been reached. After this, hemoglobin determinations every 2 weeks for 2 months is good practice.
3. Breast-feeding may be allowed if the neonate can nurse.

Prophylaxis. Rh immunoglobulin is a preventive measure against Rh isoimmunization. It is not a treatment for patients who are already sensitized. Therefore it is recommended only for nonsensitized Rh-negative women at risk of developing Rh isoimmunization.

The United States Public Health Service recommendations are as follows:
1. Rh immunoglobulin (RhIG) is given only to a woman postdelivery or postabortion who is $Rh_o(D)$ negative and D^u (allelomorph variant) negative and whose fetus is $Rh_o(D)$ positive or D^u positive. It is *never* given to an infant or father.
2. RhIG is not useful in a patient who has Rh antibodies.
3. RhIG should be given intramuscularly, not into fatty tissue or intravenously.

Prevention of isoimmunization of an Rh-negative woman to the Rh factor in her fetus is now possible in over 95% of cases by RhIG administered within 72 hours of evacuation of the uterus (by abortion or more advanced pregnancy).

Prognosis

In the United States, Rh hemolytic disease of the newborn occurs once in approximately 150 to 200 full-term deliveries. At least 200,000 children are affected by Rh isoimmunization each year, of which 5000 are stillborn. If severe hemolytic disease of the newborn is untreated, about 10% of infants will develop kernicterus. Approximately 70% of newborns with kernicterus die in the neonatal period. The survivors usually have serious neurologic sequelae, including cerebral palsy, mental retardation, and serious sensory deficiencies. With intrauterine (fetal) transfusions, about 40% of these can be saved despite maternal and fetal hazards of the procedure. Amniocentesis studies, early delivery of affected fetuses, and exchange as well as replacement transfusions save many more.

Complete recovery may be expected in most infants who do not develop kernicterus. If hyperbilirubinemia is treated promptly and effectively, most infants recover without residua or sequelae.

PLAN OF CARE: JAUNDICE

PATIENT CARE OBJECTIVES
1. Hyperbilirubinemia and its sequel kernicterus are absent.
2. There is minimal or no sequelae from hyperbilirubinemia and its treatment.

NURSING INTERVENTIONS

Diagnostic	Therapeutic	Educational

1. Infant behavior:
  a. Changes in feeding and sleeping patterns.
  b. Color and consistency of stools; dark, concentrated urine.
  c. Pallor.
  d. Neurologic signs (appear 2 to 10 days after birth) of kernicterus:
    (1) Depression: coma, lethargy, depressed or absent Moro reflex, flaccidity, diminished or absent sucking or rooting reflexes.
    (2) Excitation: muscular irritability or rigidity, twitching, convulsions, hyperreflexia, high-pitched cry.
    (3) Bulging anterior fontanel.
2. Identification of predisposing factors for jaundice from antenatal and perinatal history:
  a. Vitamin K injection, novobiocin.
  b. Maternal ingestion of sulfisoxazole (Gantrisin).
  c. Maternal-fetal rubella and other infections.
  d. Maternal diabetes.
  e. Maternal and fetal blood types and Rh factors; results of Coombs' test; fetal spherocytosis.
  f. Anomalies such as atresia of bile duct.
  g. Gestational age (Chapter 34)
  h. Cephalhematoma.
  i. Breast-feeding (p. 595).
3. Identification of jaundice:
  a. Order lab work in suspected cases: serum bilirubin, CO_2-combining power. (Serum bilirubin increases and CO_2-combining power decreases as rate of red blood cell destruction increases.)
  b. Note time of onset: hours in first day of life, after 24 hours the day of appearance of jaundice. Degree of jaundice: Jaundice is first apparent when serum bilirubin reaches 5 to 7 mg/100 ml blood.
	1. Record and report immediately for prompt diagnosis and treatment.
	2. Maintain phototherapy (pp. 625 and 626).
	3. Assist with exchange transfusion (pp. 626 and 627).
	4. Prevent respiratory and metabolic acidosis and cold stress, since these impede albumin binding of pigment and thus increase susceptibility to kernicterus at lower serum bilirubin levels.
	5. Give RhoGAM IM. RhoGAM must be typed and cross matched with mother's blood. Prior to injecting medication, check mother's name and hospital number and fill out forms that accompany package. Follow pharmacy's directions. Observe mother for adverse reactions.
		1. Keep parents informed; support parents:
		  a. Explain physiologic and pathologic jaundice; explain need for adequate fluid intake (e.g., offer water between breast- and bottle-feedings).
		  b. Reinforce physician's explanations regarding disease, its treatment, infant's condition, and possible prognosis.
		  c. Especially if mother is discharged with infant soon after delivery, teach her how to identify jaundice and when to call physician.
		  d. Involve parents with infant's care when possible.

PLAN OF CARE: JAUNDICE—cont'd

NURSING INTERVENTIONS—cont'd

Diagnostic	Therapeutic	Educational

c. Tests for jaundice: Jaundice is best viewed in daylight. (Artificial light, color of nursery walls may distort color.)
   (1) Blanch area over bony area (forehead) with thumb. Skin will look yellow before area is perfused again.
   (2) Check conjunctival sacs and buccal mucosa in darker skinned infants.

MATERNAL CONDITIONS AFFECTING THE INFANT
Infants of diabetic mothers

Hypoglycemia in infants of diabetic mothers (IDM) is due primarily to a temporary state of hyperinsulinism in response to the high glucose load imposed by the mother. The neonate's larger glycogen stores thus are rapidly depleted. The higher the level of glucose in cord blood the more immediate the danger of hypoglycemia.

Augmented fat tissue and glycogen stores as well as organ enlargement, for example, cardiomegaly, hepatosplenomegaly, and splanchnomegaly (accompanied by an enlarged umbilical cord), result in macrosomia evident in IDM. The brain is the only organ that is not enlarged. Frequently, the neonate is plethoric and chubby, with a cushingoid facies. Although most IDM are LGA, those born of mothers with vascular complications are SGA and suffer the following associated problems (Fig. 36-3):

1. RDS (HMD) is now attributed to the IDM born prematurely and is not a consequence of the maternal disease process.
2. Hyperbilirubinemia:
   a. Hyperbilirubinemia may be directly related to gestational age rather than to maternal diabetes. Fifty percent of neonates of 32 to 34 weeks' gestation develop hyperbilirubinemia; 15% of infants born at 37 weeks' gestation manifest this condition.
   b. Many neonates are plethoric with polycythemia. This increases the potential bilirubin load that the neonate must clear. The excessive red blood cells are produced in extramedullary foci (liver and spleen), in addition to the usual sites in bone marrow. Therefore both liver function and bilirubin clearance may be adversely affected.
   c. In the early neonatal period, IDM experience a relative dehydration resulting from diuresis to clear the excess glucose.
3. Blood hyperviscosity: polycythemia increases blood viscosity and thereby impairs circulation. Renal vein thrombosis, a rare condition that is seen primarily in IDM, frequently is fatal.
4. Hypocalcemia occurs in 30% of IDM and infants of mothers with gestational diabetes (IGDM). This condition is related to the associated high incidence of preterm delivery and perinatal asphyxia.
5. Birth trauma and perinatal asphyxia occurs in 20% of IGDM and 35% of IDM. Examples include the following:
   a. Cephalhematoma.
   b. Paralysis of the facial nerve.
   c. Fracture of the clavicle.
   d. Brachial plexus palsy, usually Erb-Duchenne (upper arm palsy).
   e. Phrenic nerve palsy, usually diaphragmatic hemiparalysis.
6. Congenital anomalies occur in about 6% of IDM. The incidence is greatest among the SGA neonates. The most frequently occurring anomalies include the following:
   a. CNS—anencephaly, encephalocele, meningomyelocele, hydrocephalus.

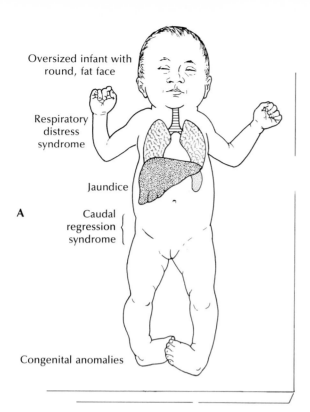

Oversized infant with round, fat face

Respiratory distress syndrome

Jaundice

A

Caudal regression syndrome

Congenital anomalies

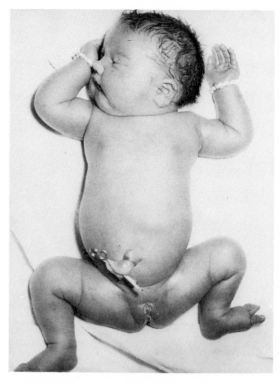

B

Fig. 36-3. A, Factors contributing to neonatal jeopardy of infant of diabetic mother (IDM). **B,** Infant of diabetic mother. (**B** from Shirkey, H. C. [ed.]. 1975. Pediatric therapy [ed. 5]. St. Louis, The C. V. Mosby Co.)

PLAN OF CARE: INFANT OF DIABETIC MOTHER

PATIENT CARE OBJECTIVES

1. A liveborn infant is delivered.
2. Infant is delivered as near to term as possible.
3. Hypoglycemia must be prevented or minimized.
4. Congenital anomalies or disorders are identified promptly and appropriate treatment instituted.
5. Infant suffers no birth trauma such as from cephalopelvic disproportion secondary to macrosomia.

NURSING INTERVENTIONS

Diagnostic

1. Evaluate for respiratory distress; ventilatory adequacy.
2. Observe for signs of following:
   a. Hypoglycemia.
   b. Birth trauma.
   c. Respiratory maturity.
   d. Gestational age.
   e. Congenital anomalies or disorders (incidence is 6% compared to 2% in all deliveries).
   f. Jaundice.
   g. Meconium aspiration (if amniotic fluid was stained or if skin, nails, or cord are stained).
   h. Hypermagnesemia; electrolyte imbalance.
3. Note results of evaluative tests of maternal-fetal status:
   a. OCT.
   b. Amniocentesis.
   c. Other.
4. Birth weight and pattern of weight gain (tendency for fetus to be LGA).
5. Note if mother had been treated for preeclampsia-eclampsia (magnesium sulfate, diuretics), which would further compromise neonate.

Therapeutic and educational

1. Resuscitate as necessary.
2. Treat as if infant is premature, regardless of weight, until gestational age and respiratory maturity is established.
   a. Place in incubator that has been set between 32° and 36° C (90° and 97° F) (depending on infant's maturity, size).
   b. Attach thermistor probe or take axillary temperature every 15 minutes until stabilized and then hourly. Temperature should stabilize at 36° C (97° F).
   c. Check respiratory rate every 15 minutes for 6 hours; place neonate on respiratory monitor if irregular.
   d. Have O_2 and resuscitative equipment available.
3. Feed as necessary (glucose, calcium). Monitor parenteral fluid therapy.
4. Promptly report and record any signs of anomalies, dysfunction, or disorder.
5. Keep parents informed. Nurse is available to parents for their questions, discussion of feelings, etc.
6. Infant's condition is not reflection of infant diabetes, but that of maternal condition.
7. Minimize auditory, visual, and tactile stimuli to promote neonate's rest.

b. Caudal regression syndrome—sacral agenesis with weakness and/or deformities of the lower extremities, malformation and fixation of the hip joints, and shortening or deformity of the femurs.
c. Tracheoesophageal fistula.
d. Congenital heart malformations.

Narcotic drug dependence

Drug abuse implicates many preparations, including alcohol. However, the morphine derivatives or synthetic opioids are the most serious for the newborn whose mother is an addict. The perinatal mortality of these neonates is six to eight times higher than that of a proper control group. Abortion, premature birth, stillbirth, and neonatal complications are the major reasons.

The nurse is frequently the first to observe the symptoms of drug dependence in the neonate. Typical signs, which are due to withdrawal rather than narcosis, appear soon after birth or after several hours, depending on the length of maternal addiction, the amount of drug taken, and time of injection prior to birth. The newborn may be depressed initially.

The onset of withdrawal signs in the neonate generally begins within 24 hours after birth. The neonate may be jittery and hyperactive. Frequently, the cry is shrill and persistent. The infant may yawn or sneeze frequently. The tendon reflexes are increased but the Moro reflex decreased. If untreated, the infant may develop fever, vomiting, diarrhea, dehydration, apnea, and convulsions and die.

Therapeutic programs that have been effective include the following:

1. Phenobarbital, 6 mg/kg/24 hr intramuscularly or 2 mg orally four times a day for 3 to 4 days, then reducing the dose by one third every 2 days but continuing to treat for about 2 weeks
2. Compound tincture of opium (paregoric) 2 to 4 drops/kg orally every 4 to 6 hours initially to as much as 20 to 30 drops/kg orally every 4 to 6 hours, depending on the symptomatology

Methadone should not be given to the newborn, even

PLAN OF CARE: NARCOTIC DRUG–DEPENDENT NEONATE

PATIENT CARE OBJECTIVES
1. Neonate is successfully weaned from the drug with no sequelae (e.g., aspiration, trauma to skin and other tissues, brain damage).
2. Neonate is placed in appropriate home.

NURSING INTERVENTIONS

Diagnostic	Therapeutic and educational
1. Check antenatal record: type of drug, extent of addiction of mother if known.	1. Provide warmth. Swaddle (bundle infant up snugly) and prop in side-lying position.
2. Note neonate's signs:	2. Place on cardiac and respiratory monitor or perform following:

a. Activity: tremors, irritability, hypertonicity, twitching, convulsions, difficulty sleeping. First indication may be reddened abrasions on nose and knees of infant from friction of movement on linen.	a. Check pulse and respirations every 15 to 30 minutes until stable.
	  b. Administer O_2 as necessary.
	  c. Stimulate gently if apnea occurs.

	3. Minimize visual, auditory, and tactile stimuli:
b. Cry: high-pitched, shrill; note duration of crying.	a. If neonate convulses, give O_2, suction, resuscitate as necessary.
c. Gastrointestinal tract function: frantic sucking of fists, regurgitation, vomiting, poor feeding, diarrhea. Assess for dehydration.	4. Suction as necessary and before and after feedings. 5. Offer small, frequent feedings. Swaddle and hold infant close to body during feedings. 6. Monitor parenteral therapy, if instituted. 7. Give medications in diminishing doses as ordered: IM, oral, or IV. Any of following may be ordered: paregoric, phenobarbital, chlorpromazine hydrochloride (Thorazine), diazepam (Valium) (do not use if neonate is jaundiced) (see above).

d. Respiratory function: respiratory distress, yawning, sneezing,	8. Place infant in side-lying position.
	9. Protect from injury:
	  a. Pad crib sides.
	  b. Cover hands with mitts.

Continued.

PLAN OF CARE: NARCOTIC DRUG–DEPENDENT NEONATE—cont'd

NURSING INTERVENTIONS—cont'd

Diagnostic	Therapeutic and educational
excessive mucus, cyanosis, apneic episodes.	c. Place sheepskin pad under neonate.
e. Diaphoresis.	10. Offer pacifier, as necessary.
f. Pyrexia.	11. Skin care:
3. Appraise mother:	a. Keep clean and dry, especially neck folds, groin, buttocks.
a. Assess her desire to keep or relinquish infant.	b. If skin is excoriated: apply zinc oxide ointment, karaya powder; expose to air and/or heat lamp.
b. Assess manner: angry? accusatory?	12. Care of mother:
4. Evaluate symptoms to differentiate between drug dependence and other conditions: tracheoesophageal fistula, CNS disorder, sepsis, hypoglycemia, electrolyte imbalance.	a. Keep mother informed. Involve her with decision making when possible.
	b. Involve mother with infant care if she is willing. Promote mother-child attachment.
	c. Avoid angry, argumentative encounters with mother. Respond with patience and sympathy.
	d. Support mother's positive maternal responses and feelings, even if she is relinquishing her infant.
	e. Involve infant's father if possible.
	f. Refer to social worker.

---

if the mother is on methadone maintenance, because of possible addiction.

With treatment, the prognosis for the neonate is good; without treatment, at least one third of infants of narcotic addicts will die.

Drug dependence in the neonate is physiologic, not psychologic, so that there is no predisposition to dependence later in life. However, the psychosocial environment in which the infant is raised may predispose to addiction.

Contradictory reports on observations of methadone-dependent neonates indicate that withdrawal symptoms may occur more frequently and be more prolonged than in heroin-dependent neonates, as well as that most infants are asymptomatic and normal by 10 days of age. Crib death has been linked to methadone-dependence. Further study of the short-term and long-term effects of methadone on the neonate and young child is needed.

Sepsis

Sepsis of the newborn may begin in the antenatal or postnatal period. Fulminating or persistent sepsis generally is apparent at birth; other infections may be obscure and become manifest later. Many organisms are capable of causing sepsis of the newborn, but most of these are enteric bacteria associated with maternal amnionitis. Infections of the neonate generally are blood-borne. Infectious organisms may enter the blood through the skin, mucous membrane, or umbilicus or from an infected viscus such as the lung.

Clinical findings may include lethargy, restlessness, or poor weight gain. Fever may be recorded; there may be leukocytosis; C-reactive protein may or may not be elevated. Vomiting, diarrhea, or CNS signs such as convulsions, may be apparent. Examination usually reveals the presence of jaundice, hepatomegaly, or splenomegaly—notable after well-established sepsis. Hemorrhage may be an associated sign in sepsis.

Cultures from the blood, nasopharynx, cerebrospinal fluid, and umbilicus should be obtained, together with sensitivity to antibiotics of the organisms identified.

If sepsis is suspected, the infant should be isolated, and a broad-spectrum antibiotic such as ampicillin may be given. Otherwise, symptomatic therapy should be prescribed and, if cultures are positive in 24 to 48 hours, specific antibiotics given in suitable doses. Delay in diagnosis may alter the prognosis, especially if infection becomes localized. Most term neonates recover.

Congenital syphilis. There is transplacental transfer of the causative organism *Treponema pallidum* after the sixteenth week of gestation (Fig. 36-4).

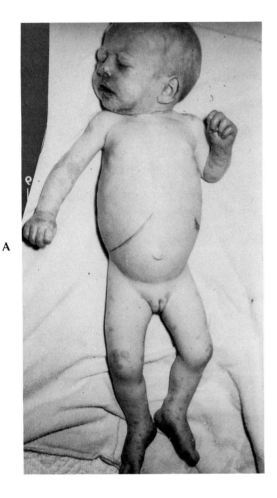

A

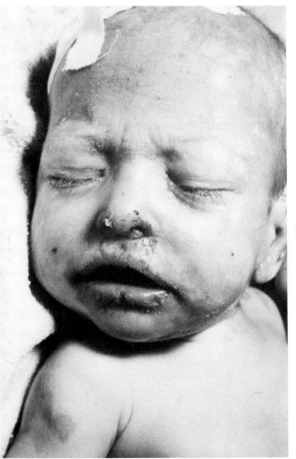

B

Fig. 36-4. Early congenital syphilis apparent at birth, which corresponds to secondary syphilis in the adult. (Late congenital syphilis, corresponding to tertiary syphilis, becomes apparent after 2 years of age.) **A,** Cutaneous lesions of congenital syphilis. Lines drawn on body indicate hepatosplenomegaly. No destruction of bridge of nose (common finding in congenital syphilis) is noted on this infant. **B,** Rhinitis (snuffles) resulting in rhagades and excoriation of upper lip. Red-colored rash is around mouth and on chin. (From Shirkey, H. C. [ed.]. 1975. Pediatric therapy [ed. 5]. St. Louis, The C. V. Mosby Co.)

PLAN OF CARE: CONGENITAL SYPHILIS

PATIENT CARE OBJECTIVES
1. Effects of congenital syphilis are minimized.
2. Parents receive education regarding cause, transmission, therapy, prevention, and early detection.
3. Parents learn the necessary follow-up care for the infant.
4. Personnel do not contract the disease.

NURSING INTERVENTIONS

Diagnostic	Therapeutic and educational

1. Assess maternal history:
  a. History of stillbirths, recurrent abortions (spontaneous).
  b. Note large, boggy placenta.
2. Check and assess neonate's signs:
  a. Elevated cord serum IgM; positive serology.
  b. Vesicular or bullous cutaneous or mucous membrane lesions, especially over palms and soles.
  c. Rash:
    (1) Copper-colored rash over face, palms, soles.
    (2) Red-colored rash around mouth, anus.
  d. Hepatosplenomegaly.
  e. Pseudoparalysis or painful extremities.
  f. Bone lesions.
  g. Edema: over joints, generalized.
  h. Anemia, pallor.
  i. Jaundice.
  j. Rhinitis (snuffles); rhagades and excoriated upper lip.
  k. Pyrexia.
  l. Irritability.
  m. SGA and failure to thrive.
	1. Use isolation technique, handwashing, gloves. After adequate treatment (48 hours), infant should not be contagious.
	2. Medicate: Penicillin is still drug of choice.
	  a. Treatment of woman during second and third trimesters (before seventh month of gestation) cures fetal infection.
	  b. Even with adequate treatment, child's blood tests for treponemal antibody may remain positive for years.
	3. Provide general care:
	  a. Take axillary temperature every 3 or 4 hours.
	  b. Record intake and output.
	  c. Feed per infant tolerance: nipple, "premie" nipple, gavage.
	  d. Swaddle for comfort.
	  e. Assist with specimen collections.
	  f. Cover neonate's hands with mitts to prevent self-inflicted scratches.
	4. Inform parents that bone lesions are reversible with adequate therapy.
	5. Support parents:
	  a. Avoid blaming parents for infant's condition.
	  b. Educate parents regarding transmission, treatment, prevention.
	  c. Assist parents with communication with pediatricians.
	  d. Involve parents with care if possible. Facilitate early and frequent parent-child contact. Acknowledge positive parent involvement (e.g., interest, cooperation, care of infant).

Herpesvirus hominis **type 2 infection.** Neonatal infection is relatively rare, occurring in an estimated 1 in 3500 to 1 in 30,000 live births. Neonatal infection with herpesvirus type 2 (genital herpes) is often fatal (Fig. 36-5). The neonate may acquire the virus by any of four modes of transmission:

- Transplacental infection
- Ascending infection by way of the birth canal
- Direct contamination during passage through an infected birth canal
- Direct transmission from infected personnel

Fetal infection may be prevented if the following conditions are obtained:

1. Active cases of genital tract herpetic lesions are diagnosed prior to labor and the mother is delivered by cesarean section.
2. Amniotic membranes remain intact.

Genital herpes should be ruled out prior to artificial rupture of membranes or application of fetal scalp electrodes.

Fetal infection is almost certain if the mother has viremia, which occasions transplacental viral transfer, or in the presence of genital herpes, if the amniotic membranes have been ruptured for more than 4 hours.

The nurse should note that this disease is highly contagious. Although herpesvirus type 2 is responsible for herpetic infections primarily occurring "below the waist," the nurse's ungloved hands may pick up the virus through breaks in the skin when infected lesions are touched.

Prognosis. Prognosis is grave in severe infections. Ocular or neurologic damage is significant sequela in survivors.

PLAN OF CARE: HERPESVIRUS TYPE 2 INFECTION

PATIENT CARE OBJECTIVES
1. Fetal-neonatal infection is prevented or its effects minimized.
2. Parents receive education regarding cause, transmission, and early detection.

NURSING INTERVENTIONS

Diagnostic	Therapeutic	Educational

1. Review antenatal record. Note following maternal signs and symptoms prior to or during pregnancy:
  a. Vaginal discharge or notable vaginal pain on examination and dyspareunia.
  b. Burning on urination and/or urinary retention.
  c. Perianal discomfort.
  d. Presence of lesions that may appear as vesicles surrounded by erythematous zones or raised areas with necrotic centers.
2. Note if genital herpes was diagnosed prior to delivery, which should be by cesarean section.
3. Note time elapsed between rupture of membranes and birth of infant.
4. Observe infant for signs and symptoms:
  a. Fever.
  b. Coryza.
  c. Tachycardia.
  d. Hemorrhage, often evidenced by hemoptysis, bloody stools.
5. Note if diagnosis is confirmed by viral studies.
	1. Deliver by cesarean section. Nurse prepares patient for surgery.
	2. Prevent contact between infected individuals and neonates.
	3. Institute strict isolation technique in caring for infected mothers and infants.
	4. Implement physician's orders of supportive care, since no specific curative treatment is available at present.
		1. Support parents throughout neonate's illness, treatment, or death.
		2. Educate parents regarding transmission and prevention of disease. If nurse feels unprepared or hesitant to provide necessary sexual counseling, parents should be referred. Avoid critical attitude toward parents.
		3. Oral herpes frequently becomes genital herpes.

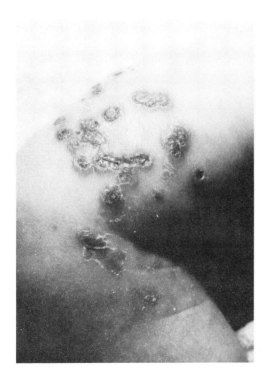

Fig. 36-5. Neonatal herpesvirus infection. (From Behrman, R. E. [ed.]. 1973. Neonatology: diseases of the fetus and infant. St. Louis, The C. V. Mosby Co.)

PLAN OF CARE: GONORRHEA

PATIENT CARE OBJECTIVES
1. Fetal infection is prevented.
2. Spread of the infection to other infants and personnel is avoided.
3. Normal vision (sight) is maintained.

NURSING INTERVENTIONS

Diagnostic	Therapeutic	Educational

1. Observe infant for symptoms:
  a. Unstable temperature.
  b. Hypotonia.
  c. Poor feeding behavior.
2. Endocervical (maternal) cultures for *N. gonorrhoeae*.
	1. Instill $AgNO_3$ into conjunctival sacs.
	2. Obtain orogastric aspirate from infant for culture and sensitivity. Medicate per order.
	3. Isolate infant and institute isolation techniques.
	4. Place in incubator with Servo-Control mechanism to maintain thermoneutral environment.
	5. Feed by method most appropriate (e.g., IV, tube feeding).
		1. Keep parents informed. Involve parents in care of infant whenever possible.
		2. Help parents understand cause, prevention, and treatment of this disease.

Gonorrhea. Gonorrheal infection, other than ophthalmia neonatorum, is an infrequent but significant cause of neonatal morbidity. Maternal gonorrheal infection may be responsible for any of the following:

• Premature rupture of membranes
• Amnionitis
• Premature labor
• Low birth weight neonate (SGA)

Endocervical cultures for *Neisseria gonorrhoeae* should be obtained routinely during pregnancy and appropriate treatment instituted when necessary to prevent fetal-neonatal infection.

Prognosis. The neonate with a mild infection often recovers completely with appropriate treatment. Occasionally infants succumb in the early neonatal period to overwhelming infection, pneumonia, or RDS secondary to prematurity.

Rubella. The congenital rubella syndrome frequently results in spontaneous abortion, congenital cataract, microcephaly, nerve deafness, or cardiac anomalies when infection occurs between 5 and 10 weeks of pregnancy. Rubella acquired later in gestation may lead to intrauterine growth retardation or premature delivery.

Numerous infants whose mothers had rubella during gestation are born alive with active viral infection (Fig. 36-6). This so-called extended rubella syndrome is typified by one or more of the following disorders: encephalitis, ocular abnormalities, pneumonitis, cardiac maldevelopment, hepatosplenomegaly and jaundice, and

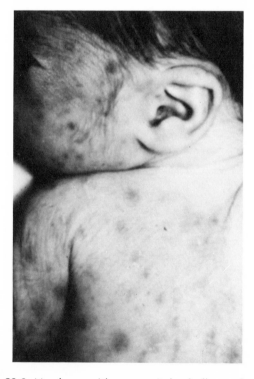

Fig. 36-6. Newborn with congenital rubella syndrome, showing multiple purpuric lesions over face, trunk, and upper arm. (From Behrman, R. E. [ed.]. 1973. Neonatology: diseases of the fetus and infant. St. Louis, The C. V. Mosby Co.)

thrombocytopenia or purpura. A tendency for infants born with rubella syndrome to develop leukemia during childhood has been noted (p. 97).

Although many of these babies die in early infancy, others survive longer with active rubella. Because the rubella virus has been cultured in babies for 1 to 1½ years after delivery, these infants are a serious source of infection to susceptible individuals, particularly potentially or actually pregnant women. Extended pediatric isolation is mandatory until the noncontagious stage of rubella has been reached.

Oral thrush. Oral thrush, or mycotic stomatitis, is caused by *Candida albicans*. This infection results from direct contact with a contaminated maternal birth canal, hands (mother or other's), feeding equipment or breast, and bedding. The appearance of white plaques on the oral mucosa, gums, and tongue is characteristic. The white patches are easily differentiated from milk curds; the patches cannot be removed and tend to bleed when touched. In most cases the infant does not seem to be discomforted by the infection; a few newborns seem to have some difficulty swallowing.

Infants who are sick, debilitated, or receiving antibiotic therapy are more susceptible. Those with conditions such as cleft lip and/or palate, neoplasms, and hyperparathyroidism seem to be more vulnerable to mycotic infection.

The objectives of management are to eradicate the causative organism, control exposure to *C. albicans,* and improve the infant's resistance. Interventions include the following:

1. Maintain scrupulous cleanliness to prevent reinfection (nursing personnel, parents, others).
    a. Use good handwashing technique.
    b. Provide clean surfaces for neonates (newborn is never placed directly on sheets on which the mother has been sitting)
    c. Clean and store feeding equipment well.
2. Support the compromised neonate's physiologic function (Chapter 33).
3. Administer chemotherapy:
    a. Apply aqueous solution of gentian violet (1%

to 2%) with swab to oral mucosa, gums, tongue. (Guard against permanent stain on skin, clothes, equipment.)
    b. Instill nystatin (Mycostatin) into mouth with a medicine dropper. Give infant sterile water to wash out milk prior to giving nystatin. Nystatin may also be swabbed over mucosa, gums, or tongue.

To give medication or vitamins by medicine dropper, position the infant's head to the side or support the infant in a semi-Fowler position. Insert the dropper into the oral cavity so that the tip rests against the cheek, alongside the tongue. Wait until the infant begins to suck on the dropper, and then squeeze the rubber end slowly until the dropper is empty.

Neonatal conditions in which the mother is implicated for hereditary reasons (diabetes, Rh-negative or O blood type) or because of infection are ego-threatening for the mother. She and the family need considerable support as the neonate's condition is assessed and diagnosed and the appropriate treatment instituted.

REFERENCES

Aladjem, S. (ed.). 1975. Risks in the practice of modern obstetrics (ed. 2). St. Louis, The C. V. Mosby Co.

Behrman, R. E. (ed.). 1973. Neonatology: diseases of the fetus and infant. St. Louis, The C. V. Mosby Co.

Clark, A. L., and Affonso, D. 1976. Childbearing: a nursing perspective. Philadelphia, F. A. Davis Co.

Clausen, J., and others. 1976. Maternity nursing today. New York, McGraw-Hill Book Co.

Finnegan, L. P., and Macnew, B. A. 1974. Nursing care of the addicted infant. Am. J. Nurs. **74:**685.

Goplerud, C. P., and others. 1973. The first Rh-isoimmunized pregnancy. Am. J. Obstet. Gynecol. **115:**632.

Lilly, A. W. 1961. Liquor amnii analysis in the management of pregnancy complicated by rhesus sensitization. Am. J. Obstet. Gynecol. **82:**1359.

Massi, G. B., and others. 1974. Low dosage anti-immunoglobulin in the prevention of rhesus isoimmunization. J. Obstet. Gynaecol. Br. Commonw. **81:**87.

Neeson, J. D. 1975. Herpesvirus genitalis: a nursing perspective. Nurs. Clin. North Am. **10:**599.

Reeder, S. R., and others. 1976. Maternity nursing (ed. 13). Philadelphia, J. B. Lippincott Co.

CHAPTER 37

Techniques for the nursing care of high-risk neonates

Knowledge of physiologic processes is basic to the learning and implementation of procedures. Memorization of the steps in any procedure without thorough knowledge of the supportive rationales and the physiologic processes that have gone awry accounts for many of the blunders and complications in the management of high-risk infants. The nurse's quality of performance improves proportionately with her level of understanding of rationale.

The procedures discussed in this chapter require manipulation of the newborn infant. He must be positioned to prevent damage to delicate tissues and to achieve the goal of the procedure. Internal manipulation includes the passage of tubes, activation of uncomfortable reflexes (gagging), penetration of needles and the displacement of tissue by the injected fluid, compression of tissues (tourniquets), and jarring alarms of the monitors. Many of his tactile proprioceptions are discomforting.

Normal psychosocial development of infants requires pleasant sounds, relief from bright lights, sucking, gentle, comforting stroking, and the touch of warm, pliant human skin. Whenever possible, these ingredients are incorporated into the nursing care plan. The rewards are significant for the infant and gratifying for the nurse. The infant responds to comforting measures, looks at and later recognizes his attendants (including his mother), and gains weight more readily.

VENTILATORY RESUSCITATION
Physical stimulation

Physical stimulation should be brief and gentle. Acceptable methods include the following:

1. Clear the infant's mouth of mucus, then stimulate sensitive receptors at the entrance of the nares with a bulb syringe or suction catheter. A gasp is the usual response.

2. Give a brisk slap to the bottom of feet.

3. Gently rub the infant's back.

4. Later if the infant is in an incubator, tie a strip of gauze loosely about a leg or arm and thread the strip out a porthole for easy access. If infant "forgets" to breathe (the apnea monitor alarm sounds), a gentle tug on the gauze usually suffices to "remind" infant.

If this method is insufficient, institute the most appropriate of the following resuscitative procedures: mouth-to-mouth resuscitation, face bag and mask resuscitation, or laryngoscopy-endotracheal intubation.

The following archaic forms of tactile stimulation are hazardous to the infant because capillaries in vital organs may be ruptured, excessive heat may be lost, shock may ensue, and time for effective resuscitation may be lost. In the past, these techniques were practiced immediately after delivery of depressed infants and are mentioned here only to condemn:

- Alternate hot and cold tubbing
- Forceful dilatation of the anal sphincter with the operator's little finger
- Rocking the infant from head-up to head-down position
- Jackknifing the infant's body
- Spanking
- Compressing the chest

Mouth-to-mouth resuscitation

The emergency procedure of mouth-to-mouth resuscitation requires no equipment and can be initiated at a moment's notice. All personnel should be trained in this technique:

Technique	Rationale
1. Clear airway of any mucus or debris.	1. Prevents impelling debris down airway.
2. Position infant. Place small rolled towel under	2. Opens airway by straightening trachea and per-

Technique—cont'd

    shoulders to extend neck slightly to "sniffing" posture.
3. Insert plastic airway if available.

4. Place your mouth over infant's nose and mouth to create a seal.
5. Repeat the word *ho* as you gently puff volume of air *in your cheeks* into infant. *Do not* force air.*
6. Repeat puffs at rate of 30/min.
7. Infant's chest should rise slightly with each puff; keep fingers on chest wall to sense air entry.
8. Allow chest to fall by passive recoil.
9. If available, place tubing of O_2 in your mouth as you inhale quickly between puffs.

Rationale—cont'd

    mitting back of tongue to fall away from posterior pharynx.
3. Provides unobstructed airway (especially from tongue if infant is flaccid).
4. Permits insufflation under pressure.

5. Prevents injury to lung tissue (e.g., pneumothorax, pneumomediastinum).
6. Approximates normal respiratory rhythm.
7. Determines if air is reaching alveolar level.

8. Allows removal of insufflated air.
9. Increases O_2 content in insufflated air.

If chest wall does not rise and infant's vital responses do not improve in 30 seconds, consider airway obstruction. Infant may need laryngoscopy-endotracheal intubation aspiration.

Bag and mask resuscitation

Emergency equipment is in constant readiness. It must be checked at the beginning of each shift, restocked immediately after each use, and includes the following:
1. Masks of assorted sizes, small enough to fit only over mouth and nose
2. Adequate oxygen supply with pressure-regulating gauges
3. Plastic airways (sizes 00, 0, 1)
4. Infant laryngoscope with premature blade and spare batteries
5. Endotracheal tubes with obturators and adapter for bag insufflation
6. Bulb syringe
7. DeLee mucous trap with two-hole catheter
8. French two-hole suction catheters
9. Mechanical aspiration equipment
10. Resuscitation surface, such as Krieselman crib or other type with radiant heat source (e.g., over-head radiant shield, spotlights of 150 watts such as Sylvania or GE)
11. Miscellaneous: sterile water for suction tubing, gloves, towel roll, infusion sets with intravenous fluids
12. Medications (e.g., naloxone, nalorphine, caffeine)

The bag and mask resuscitation procedure is as follows (Fig. 25-6):

Technique

1. Clear airway of any mucus or debris.
2. Position infant. Place small rolled towel under shoulder to extend neck slightly to "sniffing" posture.
3. Introduce plastic airway between tongue and palate.
4. Fit mask over nose and mouth to create seal. Do not allow mask to extend over eyes.
5. Insufflate at 15 to 20 mm H_2O pressure (initial pressure may be as high as 40 mm H_2O. As soon as chest rises, drop down to 15 to 20 mm H_2O pressure) for 1 to 2 seconds at 50 times/min; chest wall should rise.
6. Rest 1 to 2 seconds for expiration.
7. O_2 is administered at 100%. Humidified O_2 is preferred.

8. Keep fingers halfway between umbilicus and rib cage.
9. Observe infant's response:
   a. Spontaneous respiratory effort.
   b. Color improvement.
   c. Increased muscle tone.
   d. Increased and/or stabilized heart rate.

Rationale

1. Prevents forcing debris down airway.
2. Opens airway by straightening trachea and permitting back of tongue to fall away from posterior pharynx.
3. Ensures an open airway.

4. Permits insufflation under pressure. Avoids injury to eyes.

5. Prevents overexpansion of alveoli and rupture.

6. Expiration is passive resulting from elastic recoil of chest wall.
7. O_2 is powerful stimulant for respiratory effort but is drying to mucosa and thickens mucus.
8. Prevents abdominal distention, which compromises respiratory effort.
9. If infant response is not prompt, other therapy is needed: report immediately.

Endotracheal intubation

Generally, mask oxygen and bag ventilation of a mild to moderately depressed infant are sufficient for resuscitation. However, in profound depression or if meconium has been aspirated, immediate endotracheal intubation usually is necessary to clear the airway prior to oxygenation (Fig. 25-3). To prevent cold stress, this

---

*It is recommended that all personnel do the following: Using positive-pressure manometer (if none is available in nursery or delivery room, check with anesthesia department), test pressure exerted by "puffing" into machine. Practice until pressure does not exceed 25 mm/H_2O and feel of this becomes automatic.

procedure must be performed in a warm environment (e.g., overhead radiant heater). All resuscitative procedures are performed on a firm surface, preferably warmed and covered with preheated absorbent blanketing (Fig. 25-1). The profoundly depressed infant may require external cardiac massage if the heart rate does not respond within 20 seconds of intubation and adequate ventilation, together with the measures employed for the moderately depressed neonate (Fig. 25-2).

RELIEF OF RESPIRATORY DISTRESS
Suctioning newborn

For the normal or distressed infant, the nurse's knowledge and skill in suctioning may be critical in assisting him to establish and/or maintain adequate respirations.

The equipment includes the following:
1. Bulb syringe (intact and fairly firm)
2. DeLee mucous-trap catheter (available in reusable glass or disposable plastic), with a two-holed tip
3. Catheters (external suction source and container of sterile water are needed also)
   a. French, rubber (moderately firm): sizes 10, 12, and 14; whistle-tip; two-hole tip
   b. French, plastic disposable: sizes 8, 10, and 12; finger control; two-hole tip

The bulb syringe, catheters, and all tubing are sterile and wrapped.

During all procedures, the infant's heat loss must be avoided or minimized by drying and wrapping the infant and placing him in a warmed Krieselman or comparable crib or under overhead radiant heat or another source of heat. In addition a humidified oxygen source and equipment for the administration of oxygen must be readily available.

Upper airway aspiration: mouth and nose. A clear airway is fundamental to establishing adequate ventilation. Generally, the normal full-term infant born vaginally has little difficulty in clearing his air passages. Most secretions are drained by gravity, propelled to the oropharynx by the cough reflex to be drained or swallowed. Swallow and cough reflexes in premature infants may be absent or not well developed, however.

To assist gravity drainage, the nurse supports the wrapped infant on the arm or on the hip (in the football hold), positioning his head downward. *Do not* hold him by his ankles in the head-down position because this raises cerebral venous pressure, which may result in hemorrhage, increases the risk of accidentally dropping the infant, and hyperextends and stretches the spine.

Mucus from the mouth and nose is easily removed with a bulb syringe. The technique and rationale for suctioning with a bulb syringe are as follows:

Technique	Rationale
1. Suction mouth first.	1. Sensitive receptors around nares respond to stimuli by initiating gasp. Any mucus present could be pulled into lower airway.
2. Compress the bulb *prior* to insertion, creating suction.	2. Prevents blowing secretions deeper into mouth and nose.
3. Insert syringe into space between cheek and gums, and release compression gradually (to suck out mucus).	3. Prevents tissue trauma and removes secretions.
4. Remove from mouth. Compress syringe to empty it and to create new vacuum to repeat procedure.	
5. Repeat steps 2 and 3 as needed in mouth, then in nose. Stop suctioning when cry is clear (infant does not sound mucousy or bubbly).	

Midairway (nasopharynx, oropharynx) and stomach aspiration. Catheters are necessary for deeper suctioning. Position the infant for resuscitation as follows:

1. Place the infant on his back.

2. Place a folded towel under the shoulders to *slightly* extend the neck to a "sniffing" posture to (a) separate tongue from pharyngeal wall and (b) prevent obstruction from newborn's normally low palate and macroglossia.

Several precautions must be taken when suctioning with catheters:

Precaution	Rationale
1. Keep deep suctioning to minimum.	1. Hazards: a. Direct trauma to mucosa with edema formation and/or bleeding or increased secretions. b. Stimulation of vagal reflex: bradycardia, cardiac arrhythmias, laryngospasm, and apnea, especially if this type of suctioning is done within first few minutes of infant's birth.
2. Limit suctioning to 10 seconds or less.	2. Prolonged suctioning stimulates laryngospasm and reduces air (O_2) content in airway.
3. Suction is *off* as tube is put into position.	3. Prevents direct tissue trauma.
4. Avoid forcing catheter.	4. Hazard: direct tissue trau-

Precaution—cont'd	Rationale—cont'd
	ma and/or perforation in presence of congenital anomalies such as choanal, esophageal, or intestinal atresia.
5. Apply suction only as tube is being withdrawn.	5. Prevents direct tissue trauma.
6. Rotate catheter when suctioning.	6. Prevents tissue trauma consequent to tissue being drawn into eye of catheter.
7. Observe infant's response. Withdraw tube to suction posterior nasopharynx.	7. Gagging indicates entrance into esophagus; coughing indicates entrance into trachea.

Suctioning with DeLee mucous-trap catheter. Catheter suction is supplied by the operator: no extra equipment is necessary; excess negative pressure is not attained. The mucous trap can be detached and the enclosed specimen sent to the laboratory for examination and culture as necessary.

Aspirate the mouth and throat first, then the nose to prevent inhalation of pharyngeal contents.

Discontinue suctioning when (1) the cry is clear, and (2) air entry into lungs is heard by stethoscope.

Use of nasopharyngeal catheter with mechanical suction apparatus. Negative pressure on portable and wall gauges should be adjusted to avoid excessive suction. The technique and rationale for using a nasopharyngeal catheter with suction apparatus are as follows:

Technique	Rationale
1. Lubricate catheter in sterile water.*	1. Facilitates passage of tube and prevents infection.
2. Insert catheter:	2. Decreases risk of laryngeal spasm and reflex apnea.
a. Orally along base of tongue.	
b. Nasally, horizontally into nares, then raising it to advance it beyond bend at back of nares.	
3. With catheter in place, place thumb over finger control to create suction. Rotate tubing between fingers while withdrawing catheter.	3. Prevents direct trauma by drawing mucosa into eye of catheter.
4. Limit each suctioning to ≤10 seconds.	4. Prevents laryngospasm and oxygen depletion.
5. If infant is active, an attendant may be needed to stabilize infant's head. Or if there is time, "mummy" infant prior to this procedure (p. 628).	5. Prevents trauma and effects suctioning. Both hands are needed to manipulate catheter and finger control of suction pressure.

*A 4-ounce bottle of sterile water for feeding is convenient, already comes in a sterile container, and decreases risk of contamination possible with large stock bottles.

Suctioning gastric contents. The DeLee mucous trap or French catheters may be used also to suction stomach contents. This procedure is not recommended for all infants. Occasionally suctioning of stomach contents may be useful for the infant with excessive mucus to prevent regurgitation and possible aspiration. Respirations should be well established before this is done, since the catheter may cause apnea or laryngeal spasm.

If secretions of airway mucus are green in color, gastric suctioning is recommended. Green color (or excessive mucus) may be indicative of intestinal obstruction.

With premature rupture of membranes, fluid may be sent to the laboratory for examination. The presence of polymorphonuclear leukocytes indicates an intrauterine inflammatory process and potential neonatal infection.

The technique and rationale for this procedure are as follows:

Technique	Rationale
1. Position infant as for nasopharyngeal suctioning.	1. Extends and straightens esophagus.
2. Insert catheter through mouth or nose, advancing it slowly (as for nasopharyngeal suctioning).	2. Prevents tissue trauma.
3. Stop advancement momentarily, pull back on tubing, and redirect tip if infant gags.	3. Avoids curling of catheter in nasopharynx, entry into trachea, vagal stimulation, and regurgitation of stomach contents.
4. Advance tubing, and wait for swallow. Advance tubing as infant swallows.	4. Assures entry into stomach. Stimulates esophageal peristalsis and opens cardiac sphincter.
5. Suction for ≤5 seconds.	5. Empties stomach contents.
6. Withdraw tube while rotating it between fingers, and suction for remaining ≤5 seconds.	6. Drains esophagus.
7. Record amount of fluid obtained.	7. Amounts exceeding 15 to 25 ml are suspicious of high intestinal obstruction.

Additional comments. "Milking" the trachea is ineffectual. This procedure may injure cartilage and will often delay effective suctioning.

In addition, if the infant is premature or is suspected of having intracranial hemorrhage, his head is kept level with his body to prevent increasing intracranial pressure and possible bleeding as a result of gravity.

Positioning newborn

Positioning the infant in respiratory distress must be carefully individualized in the nursing care plan. The infant's particular needs are considered: the amount of secretions; the maturity of gag, swallow, and cough reflexes; and the maturity of neuromuscular and skeletal systems. Following are the technique and rationale for positioning the infant:

Technique	Rationale
1. Elevate head of mattress.	1. Gravity keeps weight of abdominal contents off diaphragm.
2. Flex and abduct infant's arms and place at his sides.	2. Weight of arms is kept off chest. Facilitates greater thoracic expansion.
3. Avoid use of diapers, or or pin diapers on loosely.	3. Assists infant's efforts to utilize abdominal muscles for respirations.
4. Extend neck slightly to "sniffing" position by placing folded towel or diaper under shoulders (Fig. 25-3).	4. Lessens tracheal obstruction by extending trachea. Prevents hyperextension obstruction from low palate or macroglossia. Overextension may make it difficult if not impossible for infant to swallow secretions.
5. Check towel placement frequently.	5. Obstruction may occur from flexion or overextension of neck (towel under head).
6. Turn from side to side every 1 to 2 hours.	6. Facilitates drainage of pulmonary secretions, and prevents skin breakdown.
7. *Do not* place infant in prone position.	7. Respiratory effort is impaired by full weight of infant on chest and abdomen.

Oxygen therapy

The administration of oxygen must be as carefully monitored as any drug. Oxygen overdosage results in tissue damage. The histologic change noted in pulmonary tissue is a thickening of the alveolar walls, epithelial lining, and basement membranes (Wilson-Mikity syndrome, BPD). In the retina, oxygen overdosage causes vasoconstriction and, later, ischemia. About 2 months after the cessation of oxygen therapy, these retinal vessels dilate, leading to edema, scarring, and detachment. Eyesight may be slightly to severely impaired, or total blindness (retrolental fibroplasia) may ensue.

Oxygen may be vital to an infant at birth to counteract acidosis, promote pulmonary blood flow and closure of the ductus arteriosus, and maintain capillary integrity.

Hypoxemia. An infant is presumed to be hypoxemic if he presents symptoms such as the following: (1) bradycardia—heart rate of less than 100/min, (2) hypothermia—temperature of less than 35.5° C (95.9° F), (3) prolonged periods of apnea—apneic episodes of greater than 15 seconds, or (4) anemia.

Clinical measurements may be insufficient to determine oxygen need, since some noncyanotic infants are hypoxemic. Laboratory assessments are essential for accurate evaluation of blood gases and acid-base status.

Regulating oxygen dosage. Oxygen dosage should be sufficient to relieve cyanosis. If the infant has a cyanotic episode, the nurse may administer 100% oxygen by mask or bag for short periods. If the condition persists, the physician may order an increase in oxygen dosage above 40% (e.g., if Po_2 is 40 mm Hg, oxygen dosage may be increased to 50%). The infant's response is recorded every 30 minutes. With improvement in color and response, oxygen dosage is lowered to 40% or less. Laboratory values are used to determine dosage:

1. Blood pH between 7.35 and 7.44
2. Arterial Po_2 between 40 and 90 mm Hg (For the very premature infant, 90 mm Hg may be too high and may expose him to sequelae of oxygen overdosage. Although the precise figure is unknown, an arterial Po_2 of 65 mm Hg should be safer.)
3. Arterial hemoglobin saturation between 85% and 90% (based on fetal maturity)

In addition, ambient oxygen is tested on an oximeter and recorded.*

Methods of oxygen administration

Incubator. The maintenance of a high and constant level of oxygen in an incubator is almost impossible because (1) the mechanism cannot achieve concentrations beyond 60% to 70% ambient oxygen, and (2) opening of the incubator's portholes or lid rapidly dissipates oxygen into the room.

Plastic hood. The hood is suitable for administering 40% to 50% oxygen at fairly constant levels, warmed to 31° to 34° C, and humidified. In addition, it is useful within incubators. Portholes or lid can be opened without affecting oxygen levels within the hood (Fig. 37-1).

Another advantage is that the plastic hood is practical outside of the incubator when the infant is being treated. An overhead radiant heater maintains a thermoneutral environment for the infant at this time.

Bag and mask: manual ventilatory assistance. This technique is appropriate for intermittent and assisted ventilation over protracted periods of days to maintain blood gas and acid-base levels within normal limits. The procedure is usually ordered for 10 minutes every 30 minutes to 1 hour and utilized when ventilating by intubation or other means.

The infant's mouth and nose are tightly covered with

---

*Some neonatologists believe that if cyanosis is present, the concentration of insufflated oxygen can be increased beyond 40% until cyanosis is relieved without development of untoward sequelae (lung and retinal damage). Careful monitoring of this procedure is essential.

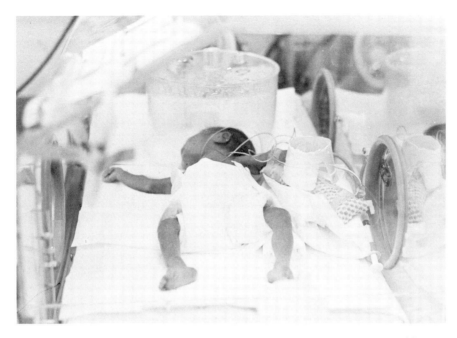

Fig. 37-1. Premature infant in incubator with oxyhood. Note cut disposable cup to protect infusion site. Syringe near porthole contains heparinized saline for irrigation of umbilical vein.

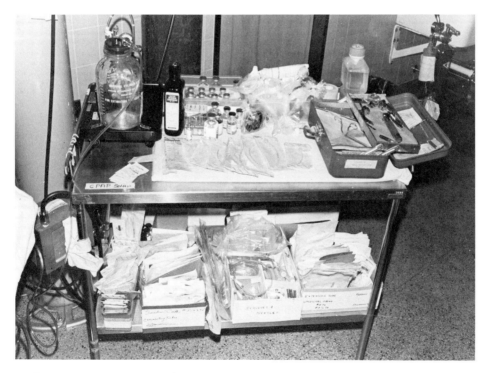

Fig. 37-2. CPAP setup cart for care of high-risk neonate with respiratory distress.

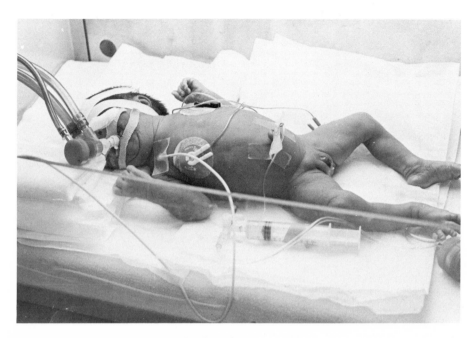

Fig. 37-3. High-risk neonate (under heat lamp not shown). Note CPAP, eye patches (under phototherapy), thermistor probe (near right shoulder), probe (left) for heartbeat, probe (right) for respirations, umbilical catheter from three-way stopcock, and syringe filled with heparinized saline. Note enlarged labia.

the mask. Pressure, trauma, and extending the mask over the eyes are to be avoided.*

Most bag and mask devices can deliver variable percentages of oxygen, but some cannot go above 40%.

Gastric distention is avoided by passing an orogastric or nasogastric tube prior to the procedure. Abdominal distention compromises respiratory effort by applying pressure against the diaphragm.

Continuous positive airway pressure (CPAP). This technique is appropriate for use with nasal prongs, a nasotracheal tube, and a face mask and bag (Figs. 37-2 and 37-3). The purposes of this technique include the following:

1. Employs same principle as the expiratory grunt (the expiratory grunt is a physiologic adaptation to trap air within the lungs, keeping alveoli open to prevent atelectasis on expiration)
2. Increases functional residual capacity
3. Improves oxygenation
4. Decreases pulmonary shunting

Continuous end expiratory pressure (CEEP). With this procedure, positive pressure is exerted during expiration. Its function is similar to CPAP.

The disadvantage of CEEP is that it changes intrathoracic pressure from negative to positive, thereby decreasing cardiac output.

Monitoring oxygen therapy

Oxygen analyzer. The oxygen analyzer is used as follows:

Technique	Rationale
1. Calibrate O_2 analyzer with room air prior to each reading. With tubing open to room air, compress bulb three times to fill analyzer; depress button. Analyzer should read O_2 in room air at 20%; adjust dial as necessary.*	1. Reduces error in reading O_2 concentration in incubator or plastic hood.
2. Place tubing close to infant's nose, compress bulb between three and six times to fill analyzer, and depress button; read and *record* findings.	2. Determines percentage of ambient O_2 available to infant.
3. Adjust O_2 flow based on findings.	3. Maintains percentage of O_2 ordered.
4. Check analyzer with 100% O_2 at least once each day.	4. Double-checks equipment accuracy.

*In some hospitals, eye patches (like those used for phototherapy) are applied prior to this procedure.

*Newer oximeters automatically adjust and calibrate to room air.

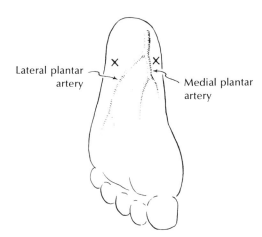

Lateral plantar artery

Medial plantar artery

Fig. 37-4. Puncture sites (x) on sole of infant's foot for heel stick for capillary blood. (From Babson, S. G., and Benson, R. C. 1971. Management of high-risk pregnancy and intensive care of the neonate [ed. 2]. St. Louis, The C. V. Mosby Co.)

Heel stick. A common laboratory procedure is the heel stick (Fig. 37-4). The test is done to obtain blood for the determination of pH and arterial P_{O_2}. The nurse's role is as follows:

Technique	Rationale
1. Request procedure to be done at same time as O_2 analyzer determination.	1. Correlates administration of O_2 with its effectiveness, blood pH, $P_{a_{O_2}}$.
2. Warm foot (heel) of infant by applying moist warm pack for at least 5 minutes to dilate capillaries and arterioles.	2. Capillary blood gives inaccurate reading. Arterialized capillary blood is needed.
3. Complete determinations at once.	3. Delay and storage of specimen at room temperature result in drop in pH and rise in P_{CO_2} (in red blood cells, glycolysis continues, resulting in rise in lactic acid).
4. Protect specimen from room air.	4. pH rises, P_{CO_2} falls; P_{O_2} falls as O_2 from specimen equilibrates to ambient O_2 tension.
5. Store specimen in ice bath if delay is necessary. Determinations must be done before 2 hours, however.	5. Affords accuracy in readings of pH and blood gases.

In some institutions, the nurse is responsible for inserting the heel stick, which involves the following procedure*:

*Residual scars and corn formation may be sequelae if this procedure is not done in the proper area of the heel.

1. Cleanse heel by rubbing with 70% alcohol.
2. Dry with sterile cotton pledget or gauze square.
3. Using Bard-Parker No. 11 or Redi-Lance blade, puncture heel deep enough to get free flow of blood.
4. Discard first drop.
5. Quickly collect blood into appropriate capillary tubes.

The test for PKU is also done on blood obtained by heel stick.

Regulation of warmth and humidity in infant's environment. A thermoneutral environment is mandatory to spare the infant's energy sources by reducing the need to increase metabolic activity, which increases his need for more oxygen. Ambient humidity prevents drying of airway membranes, with direct trauma to the tissues, and facilitates the transfer of oxygen molecules across pulmonary capillary walls.

Maintenance of a thermoneutral environment involves the following:

Technique	Rationale
1. Maintain humidity between 40% and 60% if no plastic head hood is available, so that no visible misting occurs on incubator walls.	1. Permits better visualization of infant. Prevents infant from becoming wet from "rain." Controls development of organisms in humidity equipment.
2. Warm (31° to 34° C) and humidify the oxygen-air mixture within plastic head hoods.	2. Prevents heat loss and cold stress. Liquefies secretions. Assists movement of O_2 across capillary walls.
3. Minimize opening of incubator lid and portholes, especially if no plastic head hood is used.	3. Avoids loss of heat, humidity, and O_2.

High humidity is best provided by ultrasonic nebulization (smaller droplet size) and is reserved for the following situations:

- High concentration oxygen therapy because oxygen is drying to mucous membranes
- Meconium aspiration syndrome if there is evidence of respiratory distress
- Presence of excessive or thickened mucus
- Tracheostomy or intubation for prolonged periods of time

Monitoring and recording of infant responses. The following are assessed and recorded:

1. Respiratory rate, rhythm, and effort. If apnea monitor is used, set at 15 to 20 seconds.
2. Heart rate. If cardiac monitor is used, set lower level at 80 to 100 beats/min.
3. Skin color.
4. Activity level and muscle tone.
5. Feeding behavior.

Weaning from oxygen therapy. The techniques and rationale for weaning the infant from oxygen therapy are as follows:

Technique	Rationale
1. Weaning process is gradual.	1. The longer infant has received O_2 therapy the greater the hazards of sudden cyanosis and respiratory collapse.
2. Examples of rates of weaning (one of following): a. Decrease by 1 ℓ/min every 2 hours. b. Decrease by 10% every 30 to 60 minutes (or 2 to 4 hours) as child improves.	2. Too rapid weaning with hypoxia can reopen right-to-left shunts: foramen ovale, ductus arteriosus.
3. Monitor lab values simultaneously: blood pH, P_aO_2, P_aCO_2, arterial hemoglobin concentration.	3. Provides data for modifying rate of weaning process.
4. Observe infant closely for following: a. Pulse. b. Respiratory effort. c. Skin color. If these symptoms occur, increase oxygen and proceed with slower weaning schedule.	4. Adverse reactions to weaning: a. Pulse elevation. b. Respiratory distress. c. Cyanosis.

MAINTAINING THERMONEUTRAL ENVIRONMENT
Techniques for assessing body temperature

Axillary temperature with clinical thermometer. The technique for taking the axillary temperature is the same for all infants. It is important to coordinate the procedure with the maintenance of incubator temperature.

When an incubator cannot supply the heat necessary to maintain the desired skin temperature of the infant, direct a 150-watt bulb (Sylvania or comparable lamp) over the infant through the top of the incubator from a distance of about 1 meter (3 feet).

The technique for taking the axillary temperature is as follows:

1. Clinical thermometer capable of registering 29° C (84° F) is employed.

2. Check thermometer for intactness.

3. Shake mercury down in thermometer.

4. Hold thermometer firmly in axilla for 10 minutes.

5. Desired temperature to stabilize at 36.1° ± 0.5° C (97° ± 1° F):

    a. Take axillary temperature and readjust incu-

bator temperature control occasionally until it stabilizes at proper level.

    b. Monitor axillary and incubator temperatures.

6. Recheck temperature and monitor until properly maintained after procedures which necessitate the opening of portholes and/or lid. Record incubator temperature in Fahrenheit to distinguish it from baby's.

Rectal temperatures. Rectal temperatures are discouraged. The thermometer (1) irritates the rectal mucosa and exposes the infant to tissue trauma—even to perforation of rectal mucosa, (2) stimulates bowel movements, and (3) misleads the nurse regarding the infant's progress. A normal core temperature reading may exist in an infant exposed to cold stress. A significant drop in temperature occurs only after the body's metabolic efforts to provide heat can no longer keep up with the heat loss.

Heat support: controlling the environment

Overhead radiant heat shield. The heater thermostat should register between 36.1° ± 0.5° C (97° ± 1° F). It must be kept plugged into electrical outlet at all times. The heat shield is used as follows:

Technique	Rationale
1. Dry newly born infant with warm absorbent blanket and place him under radiant heat shield.	1. Reduces heat loss by evaporation, conduction, convection, and radiation.
2. Adjust bassinet in head-down position (about 10 degrees).	2. Allows for gravity drainage of mucus in respiratory tract.*
3. Remove gross soiling (meconium, blood).	3. Facilitates observation of skin coloring and any changes.
4. Check the thermostat setting for accuracy.	4. Avoids overheating or underheating.
5. Apply thermistor probe (metal side next to infant) with paper tape or nonirritating plastic tape (e.g., Hy-tape) to anterior abdominal wall between navel and xiphoid process; avoid placement over bony rib cage.	5. Improves accurate reading of skin temperature. Sensors in skin respond more quickly to change.
6. Check frequently to ensure that probe retains skin contact.	6. Avoids overheating or underheating.
7. Observe infant for color change; crying, restlessness; increased respiratory rate.	7. Determines if abnormal behavior is due to cold stress or other factors (debility, sepsis).

*If the infant is suspected of having intracranial hemorrhage, keep his head on the same level as his body or slightly elevated if mucus is not excessive.

Technique—cont'd	**Rationale**—cont'd
8. Note previous symptoms, then check axillary temperature with thermometer; recheck probe, thermostat setting, and heater contact.	8. Rules out equipment malfunction.
9. Record findings.	9. Effects communication with other caretakers.

Servo-Control incubator. Servo-Control incubators or equivalents utilize the same principle as the thermostat in maintaining an even temperature in an oven or a room (Fig. 37-5). The infant's skin temperature, as opposed to the circulating air, provides the point of control.

The skin is a very sensitive indicator of the infant's thermal state. Receptors note even minor changes resulting from peripheral vasoconstriction, dilatation, or increased metabolism long before a change in deep (core) body temperature develops. Measurements of skin temperature provide a more reliable indicator of the energy exchange between the infant and his environment therefore.

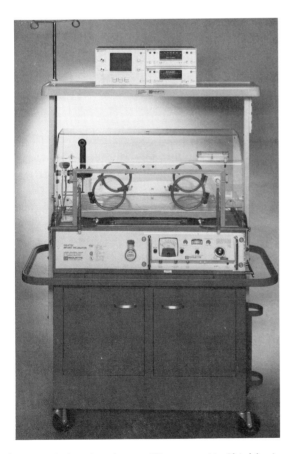

Fig. 37-5. Infant incubator. (Courtesy Air-Shields, Inc., Hatboro, Pa.)

For automatic control of temperature using Servo-Control incubators, the following measures are necessary:

1. Set the incubator control panel at the physician-ordered predetermined level, usually between 36° and 37° C (96.8° and 98.6° F).

2. Tape a thermistor probe (automatic sensor) from the control panel to the infant's skin, preferably over the anterior abdomen.

3. Check the sensor periodically for its continued firm application to skin; check and record the core temperature (axillary, rectal) with a clinical thermometer; record incubator temperature readings.

4. Record the core and incubator temperatures every 2 to 4 hours after the infant's temperature is stabilized.

5. Record the infant's general appearance and behavior.

Servo-Control incubators are also designed to regulate relative humidity. A low humidity (30% or less) for a prolonged period such as 2 weeks or more is detrimental. This continued low humidity is associated with fluctuations in temperature balance, poor weight gain, episodes of diarrhea, and increased mortality among premature infants. A relative humidity between 40% to 50% is recommended.

For infection control, care of humidifying equipment includes the following:

- Establishment of humidity at approximately 50%
- Change of the water reservoirs and vaporizers each day
- Decontamination of the incubator and humidifying equipment on a regular schedule and, when necessary, between infants.

Warming hypothermic infant. Rapid warming or cooling may occasion apneic spells and acidosis in an infant. Therefore the warming process is increased slowly over a period of hours or days.

The nurse places the infant in a Servo-Control incubator and proceeds as follows:

1. Set incubator temperature on control panel at 1.2° C (2° F) above skin temperature even if lower than normal.

2. Tape thermistor probe to skin of anterior abdominal wall.

3. When skin temperature reaches predetermined, set incubator temperature, repeat process until abdominal skin temperature of 36.1° ± 0.5° C (97° ± 1° F) is achieved.

Weaning infant from Servo-Control incubator. The weaning process is accomplished slowly over a period of hours or days as follows:

1. Dress infant in diaper and shirt.

2. Lower incubator temperature; record temperatures of infant and incubator.

3. Assess baby's response.

4. Repeat steps 2 and 3 until incubator temperature equals room temperature, and infant's axillary temperature is 36.1° to 36.6° C (97° to 97.8° F).

5. Wrap infant in blanket, open incubator portholes, and assess infant response.

6. Remove baby to open crib if axillary temperature is adequate.

FEEDING HIGH-RISK NEONATE
Oral feedings: initial feeding

Several factors must be considered when one prepares to give the initial feeding to any infant as follows:

Factor	Rationale
1. Neonate's age in hours or infant's age in days.	1. During reactivity periods, excessive mucus with gagging may occur. Feeding increases the danger of aspiration. In general, reactivity times occur at birth and at 4 to 6 hours of age.
2. Condition at birth.	2. Infants with Apgar scores of 6 or less (depressed) or the infant with low birth weight (2500 gm or less) may display a delayed reactivity. This may occur after 12 to 18 hours of age.
3. Possibility of congenital anomalies of gastrointestinal and/or respiratory tract. Incidence of congenital anomalies is higher in preterm infants.	3. With choanal atresia, neonate may be unable to breathe and feed simultaneously. With esophageal atresia, infant often will regurgitate and may aspirate. With tracheoesophageal fistula, feeding may enter trachea directly. With lower gastrointestinal tract obstruction (stenosis, atresia), regurgitation, or vomiting, abdominal distention may compromise respirations.
4. Gastric capacity.	4. Limited stomach capacity dictates smaller feedings (p. 504). To provide adequate nutrition, feedings are scheduled more frequently. For suggested initial amounts, see p. 541.
5. CNS maturity.	5. Sucking and swallowing reflexes may not be well developed and synchronized (even in a term baby, the suck and swal-

Factor—cont'd	Rationale—cont'd
	low reflex may not be well coordinated during first few hours).
6. Energy level.	6. Premature infant or infant with respiratory distress may not have sufficient energy to divert to the process of feeding. Use "premie" nipple, or utilize gavage feedings (see below).
7. Type of feeding: plain sterile water.	7. Until infant's ability to feed is assessed, danger of aspiration exists. Plain sterile water is least irritating to respiratory tree: a. Formula may cause aspiration pneumonia. b. Glucose water may cause inflammatory response in respiratory tree similar to aspirated formula.

Gavage feeding

Feeding by gavage is the method of choice for the infant who is (1) compromised by respiratory distress, (2) immature and/or has a weak suck or uncoordinated sucking-swallowing behavior, or (3) easily fatigued even when using a "premie" nipple.

Necessary equipment for either the nasal or oral route includes the following:

1. Sterile feeding tube: rubber or plastic, rounded tip, sizes 5 to 10, infant lengths
2. Syringe for feeding clearly calibrated
3. Stethoscope and sterile medication syringe without needle
4. Sterile water for lubrication
5. Feeding formula
6. Medications

Tests for correct placement of feeding tube. Fortunately the infant's anatomy makes it difficult to enter his trachea. One or more of the following tests are done to determine correct stomach placement:

1. Using sterile syringe, inject 0.5 ml of air through catheter into stomach. Simultaneously, listen for sound of air bubbling or "growling" in stomach with stethoscope over epigastric region.

2. Aspirate small amount of stomach contents. Fill tube with stomach contents, and pinch off tube; add syringe containing feeding. This avoids allowing air into stomach with feeding.

3. Less reliable test is as follows:
   a. After inserting tube, place other end into small container of sterile water.

b. If some bubbles appear initially and subsequently stop, tip is probably in stomach.

c. If bubbles appear synchronized with respirations, tip is probably in trachea. This would be accompanied by coughing, gagging, apnea, cyanotic episode, or other signs of respiratory distress. Remove quickly and allow infant to rest few minutes before reinserting tube.

Oral insertion: intermittent or indwelling catheter

Technique	Rationale
1. Position infant: head of mattress up one notch, folded towel under shoulders to slightly extend neck.	1. Opens oropharynx. Extends and straightens esophagus.
2. Select size 8 French feeding tube.	2. Is adequate size for feeding. Less apt to fold over or curl up.
3. Measure distance between bridge of nose and lower end of xiphoid process. Mark distance with 2 inch thin strip of paper tape. Fold tape over tube, leaving two long ends with which to secure tube when it is in place.	3. Determines length necessary to reach into stomach without folding back on itself. Facilitates anchoring tubing, if it is to be indwelling. Paper tape is usually less irritating to skin.
4. Lubricate tube in sterile water.	4. Prevents trauma and infection.
5. Pass tube along base of tongue, advancing it into esophagus as infant swallows.	5. Offers less risk of vagal stimulation or of accidental entry into trachea. Stimulates esophageal peristalsis and opens cardiac sphincter.
6. Test placement of tube.	6. Avoids introduction of formula, vitamins, and medicines into trachea or esophagus.
7. Aspirate and measure any residual in stomach. If ≤ 1 ml, subtract same amount from this feeding. If >1 ml, physician may wish to have this feeding skipped.	7. Avoids overfeeding. Excessive fluid in stomach suggests intestinal obstruction.
8. Slowly pour warmed formula into syringe barrel and allow it to flow by gravity into stomach; hold reservoir 15 to 20 cm (6 to 8 inches) above infant's head. If gravity flow is too rapid, lower syringe, or insert plunger into syringe, and inject *slowly*. Feeding time	8. Rapid entry of formula into stomach causes rapid rebound response with regurgitation, thus increasing danger of aspiration or abdominal distention, which compromises respiratory effort.

Technique—cont'd	Rationale—cont'd
should approximate that of nipple feedings (20 minutes or about 1 ml/min).	
9. Do not allow level of formula to go below neck of syringe.	9. Prevents entry of air into stomach to minimize risks of regurgitation and distention.
10. Observe infant's response.	10. Prevents respiratory distress. Assist gastrointestinal functioning.
11. Follow formula with specified amount of sterile water.	11. Gets all formula into stomach and clears tubing of formula.
12. Pinch tubing (or clamp it off) and withdraw it rapidly.	12. Prevents entry of air into stomach. Creates vacuum to hold fluid in tubing to prevent dripping it into trachea on withdrawal.
13. Burp or bubble infant. With left hand, support infant's head and shoulders. Raise to a sitting position and lean infant onto right hand. Right hand supports infant's chest with palm and jaw with thumb and forefinger. Gently rub his back with left hand.	13. Increases comfort. Prevents regurgitation.
14. Position on right side with small rolled drape or towel.	14. Facilitates stomach emptying.
15. Record following: a. Amount of residual. b. Type and amount of feeding, medicine. c. Time of feeding. d. Infant response: fatigue, peaceful sleep, abdominal distention, respiratory distress, type and amount of vomiting or regurgitation; heart and respiratory rate.	15. Provides basis for evaluation and readjustment of feeding regimen. Facilitates communication among personnel.

Nasal route: intermittent or indwelling catheter
(Fig. 37-6)

Technique	Rationale
1. Position as for oral route.	1. Opens oropharynx. Extends and straightens esophagus.
2. Select size 3½ to 5 French feeding tube:	2. Is adequate size for feeding and small enough to allow breathing space around it, since neonates are obligate nose breathers.

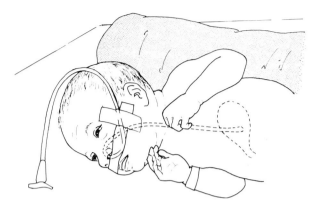

Fig. 37-6. Indwelling gavage tube: nasal route. Infant is propped on his right side to facilitate emptying of stomach. Note rolled towel for support.

Technique—cont'd

  a. If indwelling, change every 2 to 3 days (48 to 72 hours) or more frequently, if otitis is present, alternating sides of nares.

  b. Observe infant for respiratory distress.

  c. May be preferred route for indwelling tube for continuous drip feeding.

3. Measure distance from bridge of nose to xiphoid process (just beyond tip of sternum). Mark spot with 2-inch thin strip of paper tape, and overlap tube, leaving ends free.
4. Lubricate with sterile water.
5. Insert tube, holding it horizontally until it reaches back of nares, then lift tubing slightly and continue to advance. Allow infant to swallow tube down while it is being advanced.
6 to 15. Same as for oral route.

Rationale—cont'd

  a. Prevents infection, irritation; excess mucus, ulceration, bleeding.

  b. If distress due to tube, remove it. Use oral route.

  c. Very small preterm often tolerates feeding better by continuous drip; stomach is not overloaded.

3. Provides adequate length to reach stomach without curling. Facilitates anchoring of tubing. Decreases risk of skin irritation from tape.

4. Prevents tissue trauma.

5. Accommodates to bend in back of nares and minimizes direct tissue damage. Stimulates peristalsis and opens cardiac sphincter.

6 to 15. Same as for oral route.

Additional comments. Burp the infant gently after feedings. Turn his head or position him on right side after feeding and burping. In addition, postpone postural drainage and percussion for a minimum of 1 hour after feeding.

Avoid feeding the infant within an hour prior to a laboratory test for blood glucose.

A premature or sick infant will indicate readiness to feed from the nipple instead of by tube by (1) hand-to-mouth gestures and (2) mouthing the feeding tube.

Monitoring parenteral fluid administration

For parenteral fluid administration, one needs equipment to start and/or maintain intravenous therapy by way of a peripheral vein, venous cutdown, or umbilical catheter.

In addition, the following are needed to prevent accidental overhydration:
1. 250 ml bottles of infusate
2. Administration sets with inclosed reservoirs and minidropper
3. Infusion pump with automatic alarm to signal an empty fluid chamber
4. Application of medicine cup (paper) or other appliance to protect insertion site

The technique and rationale of parenteral fluid administration follow (Fig. 37-7):

Technique

1. Prepare equipment.

2. Restrain infant.

3. Provide pacifier to infant if appropriate.

4. Continue care of IV. Regulate rate of flow:
  a. Infusion pump: check setting; double-check by counting drops/min every hour, and note amount infused every 4 hours.
  b. Reposition extremity or infant's head.

  c. *Do not* make up deficiency or excess by changing rate of flow without consulting with physician.

5. Check infusion site every hour:

Rationale

1. Avoids searching for missing articles after procedure is begun.

2. For infant safety and increased ease of starting parenteral fluids.

3. Provides comfort for the infant who can handle a pacifier.

4. For adequate infusion:

  a. Assures a more accurate and constant flow rate. Double-checks for equipment malfunction.

  b. Assures proper body alignment and prevents breakdown of skin. Protects infusion site.

  c. Fluid may overload infant's system. If infant has received more than prescribed amount for period, he must be assessed for overhydration and cardiac decompensation.

5. Prevents trauma to tissues. Assures adequate

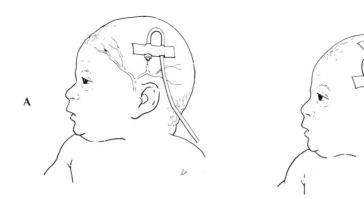

Fig. 37-7. A, Venipuncture of scalp vein. **B,** With paper cup to protect venipuncture site.

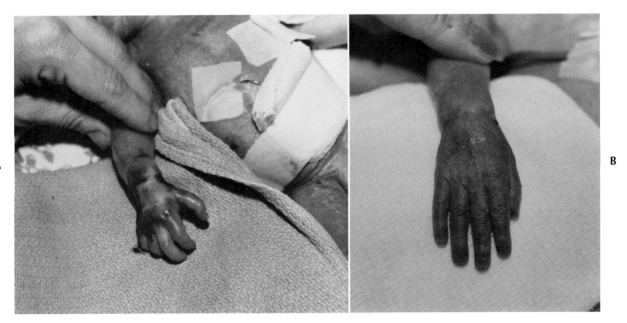

Fig. 37-8. A, Intravenous infiltration in small infant can cause severe ischemia. **B,** Fortunately, preterm infant has remarkable regeneration abilities (same hand 1 week later). (Courtesy Mount Zion Hospital and Medical Center, San Francisco, Calif.)

Technique—cont'd	**Rationale**—cont'd	**Technique**—cont'd	**Rationale**—cont'd
	hydration. Possible complications:	face for symmetry of contour and movement.	into surrounding tissues and possible tissue breakdown.
a. Tissue infiltration (swelling).	a. Infection.	6. Evaluate infant's hydration every hour:	6. Determines adequate rate of flow.
b. Tissue trauma: color, temperature.	b. Thrombophlebitis.	a. Urine output: collect or weigh diapers.	a. Assesses amount of urine excreted.
c. If needle is in extremity, compare and contrast with other extremity.	c. Tissue and vein trauma (Fig. 37-8).	b. Specific gravity of urine. See pp. 631 and 632 for use of urine collectors.	b. Assists in assessing appropriate solute/fluid infant needs and/or his kidney function.
d. If needle is in scalp vein, check head and	d. Needle out of vein with injection of fluid		

Technique—cont'd

c. Weight: may be weighed every 8, 12, or 24 hours.

d. Urine: Check for glucose every 8 to 24 hours.
e. Stools: number, character.

f. Other: tissue turgor; fever; bulging or sunken fontanels; soft, sunken eyeballs; behavior changes.
7. Record:
a. Type of fluid being used.
b. Amount of fluid absorbed every hour and amount scheduled to have been absorbed.
c. Amount of fluid in bottle or fluid chamber.
d. Flow rate.

e. Infant's condition.

8. Change IV tubing and bottle every 24 hours.
9. Irrigate IV:

a. Three-way stopcock may be used to connect tubing to needle.

b. Without three-way stopcock, clamp IV tubing and disconnect at junction with needle. Keep tubing end sterile. Attach syringe containing 1 to 3 ml of normal saline or heparinized saline to needle.
c. *Slowly* inject fluid into vein. Disconnect syringe and reconnect to IV tubing. Unclamp IV tubing and regulate flow of infusate.
10. After IV is discontinued:

Rationale—cont'd

c. Weight gain or loss >100 gm (4 ounces) in 24 hours indicates need to alter rate of flow.
d. Assesses adequacy of glucose intake and/or kidney function.
e. Assists in assessing adequacy of fluid and/or solute/fluid ratio.
f. Assesses state of hydration.

7. Provides complete data:
a. Evaluates treatment.

b. Meets infant's changing needs.

c. Identifies possible cause of any existing or new problem.
d. Provides baseline for continuation at present rate or change in rate.
e. Indicates infant's response to this regimen and readiness for progression.
8. Decreases possibility of infection.
9. Maintains patency of system:
a. Facilitates flushing needle while decreasing chance of contamination and loss of blood during procedure.
b. Clears out small occluding clots; prevents formation of clots.

c. Prevents trauma to vein or dislodging the needle.

10. Ensures adequate nutrition and hydration:

Technique—cont'd

a. Observe infant for hypoglycemia for 24 hours.

b. Observe infant for adequacy of nutrition and hydration.

c. Continue to assess infant for thrombophlebitis at previous insertion site and sloughing.

Hyperalimentation

Hyperalimentation is designed to provide complete nutrition by the intravenous route for extended periods of time. The prefix *hyper* is somewhat misleading: more or larger feedings are not given, but the route of feedings is exclusively by vein.

The infusion solution consists of protein hydrolysate, glucose, electrolytes, minerals, and vitamins. The infusion is continuous at a prescribed rate through an indwelling catheter threaded into the vena cava (Figs. 37-9 to 37-11).

Hyperalimentation is the method of choice for the infant who (1) requires several surgeries for repair of gastrointestinal anomalies or obstruction, (2) suffers from chronic diarrhea, or (3) has malabsorption syndrome.

Equipment necessary for hyperalimentation includes the following:
1. Instruments for starting intravenous infusion or a cutdown
2. Silastic catheter of appropriate size
3. Millipore intravenous filter
4. Constant infusion pump (Holter or other)
5. Hyperalimentation solution (infusate)
6. Pacifier and mobiles
7. Restraints as necessary

The procedure may be done in the operating room. Nursing action is the same as that for the care of an infant receiving intravenous fluid therapy, except for the following notable additions:
1. Avoid using the catheter for purposes other than infusate (e.g., not used for blood or medications).
2. Avoid making up excess or deficit by altering the drip rate without consulting the physician.

The hyperalimentation procedure is as follows:

Technique

1. Order prescribed mixture from pharmacy, or mix under aseptic conditions.

Rationale—cont'd

a. Hypoglycemia often is seen after discontinuation of parenteral therapy.
b. Assesses infant's ability to take and utilize nutrients and fluids by mouth or gavage.
c. Begins definitive treatment and prevents tissue damage.

Rationale

1. Assures accuracy of amounts. Prevents microbial contamination.

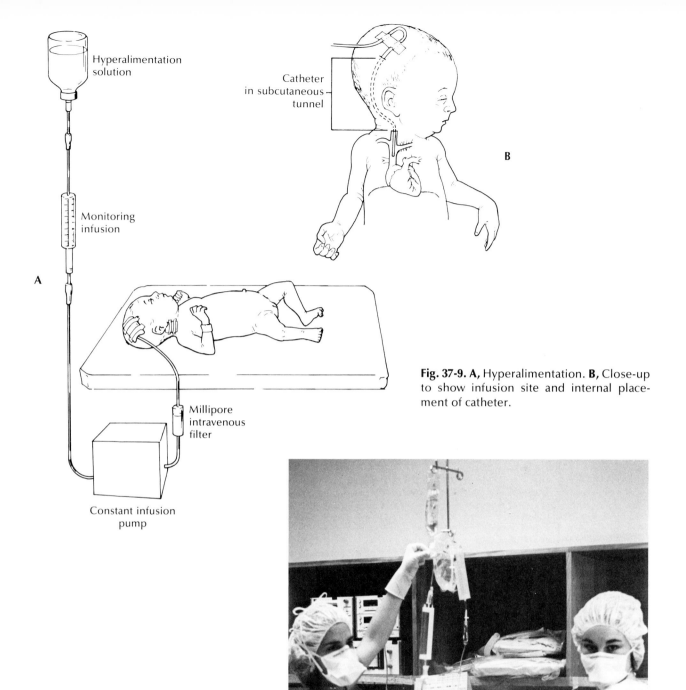

Hyperalimentation
solution

Monitoring
infusion

A

Catheter
in subcutaneous
tunnel

B

Millipore
intravenous
filter

Constant infusion
pump

Fig. 37-9. A, Hyperalimentation. **B,** Close-up to show infusion site and internal placement of catheter.

Fig. 37-10. Preparation of intravenous alimentation by nurses. Solution is carefully calculated for glucose, protein, electrolytes, and volume by physician, made up by pharmacy under linear air in sterile hood, and administered through Volutrol filter and tubing by nurse under sterile conditions. Solution is changed every 24 hours. (Courtesy Children's Hospital of San Francisco, Newborn Intensive Care Unit; photo by Patricia Ryan, R.N.)

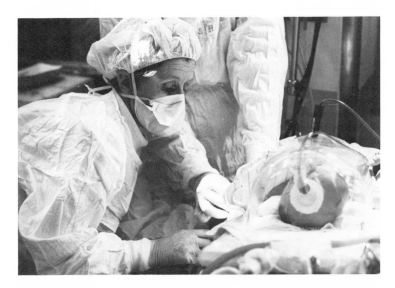

Fig. 37-11. Placement of percutaneous Silastic feeding catheter (1/25,000 inch) in arm vein of infant with diaphragmatic hernia and inability to feed by mouth. Catheter is threaded through vein into right atrium. There is no scar, and infection is extremely uncommon with percutaneous route. (Courtesy Children's Hospital of San Francisco, Newborn Intensive Care Unit; photo by Patricia Ryan, R.N.)

Technique—cont'd

2. Check on rate of flow:
   a. Check pump setting.
   b. Check amount given from calibrated, enclosed reservoir every 2 to 4 hours.
3. Change bottle, tubing, and Millipore filter every 1 to 2 days. Culture filter after use.
4. Change dressing around catheter.

5. Monitor infant's weight daily at same times on same scales.
6. Provide pacifier and mobiles.

7. Observe infant for complications associated with hyperalimentation:
   a. Catheter and its insertion: local skin infection, septicemia, blood vessel thrombosis, obstruction or dislodgment of catheter, cardiac symptoms such as arrhythmia.
   b. Infusate—type and amount: glucosuria, dehydration, acidosis, amino acid imbalance.

Rationale—cont'd

2. Avoids overfeeding or underfeeding. Checks equipment for malfunction.

3. Decreases risk of microbial contamination.

4. Prevents infection and for observation of area of needle insertion.
5. Provides index of response to this form of therapy.
6. Provides sucking satisfaction and some visual stimulation.
7. Facilitates prompt identification and treatment of problems:
   a. Sepsis accounts for 50% of complications.

   b. Metabolic complications.

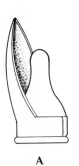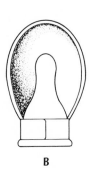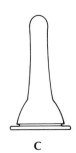

A   **B**   **C**

Fig. 37-12. Cleft-palate nipples. **A,** Side view and, **B,** front view of rubber flange that covers defect during feeding. Flange can be cut to fit. **C,** Lamb's nipple. Nipple carries formula beyond defect.

Feeding newborn with cleft lip and palate

The following feeding devices are suggested for the newborn whose defect precludes his ability to create a vacuum and to suck (Fig. 37-12):

1. Lamb's nipple
2. Duckey nipple, with flange to fit over defect
3. Brecht feeder
4. Rubber-tipped Asepto syringe

A thickened formula may be ordered as a means of utilizing gravity flow to prevent aspiration. The formula is thickened with a dried rice cereal. A larger hole is made in the standard nipple.

During feeding, observe for the following signs:
- Aspiration—choking and cyanosis
- Swallowed air—abdominal distention

The technique and rationale for feeding an infant with cleft lip and palate are as follows:

Technique	Rationale
1. Check infant for clear airway.	1. Minimizes possibility of aspiration.
2. Hold infant in upright position.	2. Minimizes possibility of aspiration and return of fluid through nose. Aids swallowing.
3. Interact with infant as if he were a normal infant: talk to him, etc.	3. Is important for his psychosocial development. If mother sees nurse doing this, it may facilitate her acceptance of child.
4. Burp or bubble infant frequently.	4. More air is swallowed when there is unnatural passage between nose and mouth. Increases infant's comfort. Minimizes regurgitation and aspiration.

When feeding the infant with a rubber-tipped Asepto syringe, place the rubber tip on top of and to the side of the infant's tongue. Offer feeding slowly to allow the infant time to swallow. (NOTE: If the child has only a cleft lip, he may be able to feed well with a regular or "premie" nipple.)

THERAPY FOR HYPERBILIRUBINEMIA

The goal of therapy is to assist the neonate in reducing serum levels of unconjugated bilirubin. To be excreted by the liver, bilirubin must be conjugated (in water-soluble form). In the premature infant especially, body systems are functioning but immature. The conjugation system is overwhelmed, the serum levels of unconjugated bilirubin rise, and the risk of kernicterus increases.

There are two principle methods available to reduce serum bilirubin levels: phototherapy and exchange blood transfusion. In addition, phenobarbital therapy may be used.

Exchange transfusion is the treatment of choice in the presence of an hemolytic process (isoimmunization) to remove the antibodies responsible for hemolysis and to correct anemia.

Phototherapy

Light therapy is helpful because blue light, between 400 and 500 nm in the spectral band, photo-oxidizes bilirubin down to colorless and apparently nontoxic compounds. This decomposition occurs in the skin. A commercial fluorescent white tube of 200 to 400 footcandles

may be used; care must be taken that the light is not used beyond 200 hours because then the output in the 400 to 500 nm range decreases. (Vita-Lite bulbs may remain effective for a year.)

For the hyperbilirubinemic infant, the procedure is as follows:

Technique	Rationale
1. Unclothe infant:	1. Exposes as much skin areas as possible to light.
a. Protect infant's eyes with eye patches (Fig. 37-13).	a. Prevents possible injury to conjunctiva and/or retina.*
(1) Be sure eyes are closed.	(1) Prevents corneal abrasions.
(2) Check eyes for drainage each shift.	(2) Prevents or allows prompt treatment of purulent conjunctivitis, should it occur.
b. Cover head with stockinette.	b. This precaution is controversial and may differ from hospital to hospital.
c. For diapering, paper face mask may be used.	c. This "string bikini" is scanty enough to allow skin exposure, yet sufficient to protect bedding.
2. Monitor skin temperature. If infant is in incubator,	2. Prevents hyperthermia or hypothermia.

---

*There are no known sequelae from exposure of the eyes to the Bili-Lite as yet. Exposure to light may alter biorhythms, however.

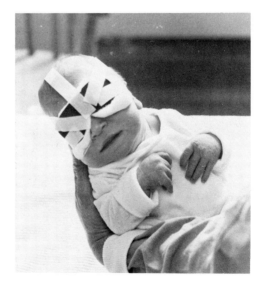

Fig. 37-13. Olympic Bili-Mask. (Courtesy Olympic Medical Corp., Seattle, Wash.)

Technique—cont'd | **Rationale**—cont'd

temperature dial on control panel may need to be turned to maintain proper temperature.

3. Periodically and especially with parents' visits discontinue phototherapy for few minutes and remove eye patches. Unwrap eyes and hold for feeding.

3. Necessary for normal psychosocial contact. Infant may visualize his contacts. Parent has opportunity to look into baby's eyes—a necessary activity to develop attachment to infant.

4. Observe infant's behavior:
   a. Record and report eating and sleeping patterns.
   b. Loose greenish stools, green urine.
   c. Priapism.

4. Effect of phototherapy on biologic rhythms is uncertain. Data base is needed to evaluate common side effects that need appropriate treatment.

5. Replace fluid losses; protect skin from excoriation.

5. Prevents dehydration. Prevents infection of broken-down skin areas.

Exchange transfusion

The purposes of exchange transfusion are as follows:
- To reduce serum bilirubin levels
- To correct the anemia
- To remove antibodies (or other causative agents) responsible for hemolysis

The nurse is alert to the fact that a significant risk (mortality rate of 50%) exists with this procedure.

An exchange transfusion is accomplished by alternately removing a small amount of the infant's blood and replacing it with a like amount of donor blood. Depending on the infant's size, maturity, and condition, amounts of 5 to 20 ml are slowly exchanged at a time. The total amount of blood exchanged approximates 170 ml/kg of body weight (80 ml/pound) or between 75% and 85% of the infant's total blood volume.

This procedure is done under conditions that prevent cold stress to the infant, as with other procedures. The following equipment is necessary:

1. Disposable exchange transfusion set
2. Fresh donor's blood (under 3 days old and heparinized), 2 units on hand in case of error or contamination
3. Monitoring equipment
4. Transfusion record
5. Water bath (38° C, or 100° F) to warm the blood
6. Medications: calcium gluconate in 5 ml syringe with No. 24 needle; 50% glucose solution in 10 ml syringe with No. 24 needle; sodium bicarbonate or tromethamine (THAM) in 10 ml syringe with No. 24 needle
7. Sterile gowns, drapes, gloves, caps, and masks
8. Cleansing solution with sterile cotton pledgets or gauze sponges

9. Adequate lighting
10. Heat source to keep the infant warm

The exchange transfusion procedure is as follows:

Technique | **Rationale**

1. Prepare and adjust heat lamps or overhead radiant heat shield; have warmed blankets available for infant.

1. Prevents cold stress.

2. Infant is kept NPO for 3 to 4 hours, or aspirate stomach contents by gastric tube.

2. Prevents aspiration.

3. Assemble resuscitative equipment: O_2 source, masks, breathing bag, airways, laryngoscope (extra batteries), endotracheal tube with obturator, suction, medication (see equipment).

3. Is readily available if needed for immediate supportive therapy.

4. Position infant on back and restrain. Take and record vital signs.

4. Facilitates treatment. Prevents dislodging catheter and tissue trauma. Provides baseline to evaluate change.

5. Assemble electronic monitoring equipment or stethoscope. Attach electrodes, or keep stethoscope over apex of heart. Monitor and record results continuously during procedure.

5. Hazards of procedure include apnea, bradycardia (≤ 100/min), cardiac arrhythmia or arrest.

6. Physician *and* nurse check donor blood: type, Rh, age.

6. Minimizes chance of error.

7. Run tubing from bottle (bag) through warm water bath to infant.

7. Avoids cold stress, ventricular fibrillation, vasospasm, or decrease in blood viscosity.

8. Before starting transfusion assist physician as necessary:
   a. Cleanse site of cutdown (jugular or femoral arteries) or umbilical stump (umbilical vein).
   b. Drape.
   c. Put on gown and gloves.

8. Prevents microbial contamination.

9. During transfusion:
   a. Physician measures CVP prior to initiating transfusion.
   b. Nurse notes and records time exchange is begun.
   c. For *each* successive

9a. Change from 10 to 12 cm pressure is indication to stop and reassess infant's status.
   b. Maintains accurate record.
   c. Maintains accurate

Technique—cont'd

withdrawal of infant's blood *and* injection of donor's blood, nurse records time, amounts in and out, cumulative amounts in and out.
  d. After 100 ml have been exchanged, physician gives calcium gluconate; nurse monitors heart and respiratory rates and records.
  e. Nurse records pertinent comments.
  f. Nurse records medications: time, type, amount, infant response.
10. After transfusion (catheter may be removed or left in place with dressing):
  a. Nurse finishes charting.
  b. Nurse continues to observe and record infant's behavior closely for 24 to 48 hours:
    (1) Vital signs: heart rate, respirations, temperatures, pedal pulses.
    (2) Lethargy, jitteriness, convulsions.
    (3) Dark urine.
    (4) Edema.

Rationale—cont'd

continuous record to assist with ongoing procedure and provides index of infant response.

  d. Possibility of cardiac irritability is minimized.

  e. Maintains accurate record.
  f. Maintains accurate record.

10. Infant is observed to prevent hemorrhage from site and to detect and treat promptly any complications of blood transfusion such as heart failure, hypocalcemia, hypoglycemia and acidosis,* sepsis, shock, thrombus formation.

Phenobarbital therapy

Phenobarbital may promote hepatic clearance of bilirubin (p. 593). The drug is given to the mother before delivery and to the newborn for several days after birth.

The advantages of phenobarbital therapy include the following: Neonates of women treated with phenobarbital during pregnancy have lower levels of serum bilirubin. The number of transfusions needed for their premature infants is decreased. Disadvantages are that neonates of epileptic mothers on long-term phenobarbital therapy have shown an increased tendency to bleed (vitamin K factors are suppressed), excretion of barbiturates is variable in neonates, and several days (4 to 5) of treatment are necessary before serum bilirubin levels are significantly reduced. In addition, some neonates, especially those that are premature, do not respond at all when jaundice is already present.

MISCELLANEOUS TECHNIQUES
Umbilical catheterization

The purposes of umbilical catheterization are as follows:

- To obtain blood samples
- For parenteral fluid therapy
- For exchange transfusion

The dangers of this procedure include the development of emboli, thrombi, and sepsis.

A heat source is necessary to prevent cold stress: (e.g., acidosis, apnea). Emergency drugs and oxygen, suction, and resuscitation equipment should be available if needed. It is also necessary to check to see that all electrical equipment is grounded to prevent electric shock or burn to infant.

The technique and rationale are as follows:

Technique

Physician

1. Prepare area; drape neonate.
2. Insert catheter into artery; location of catheter confirmed by x-ray film.

3. Apply antibiotic ointment and/or bandage over area.

Nurse

1. Monitors vital signs every 10 to 15 minutes until stable, after procedure.
2. If bleeding from site occurs, apply direct pressure.
3. Observe color and warmth of legs and peripheral pulses.
4. Maintain patency of line per order (e.g., heparinized solution).
5. Record. Keep physician informed.

Rationale

1. Sterile procedure.

2. Placement must be accurate. If in vein, may cause thrombosis and liver damage. Arterial lines may be left in place ≤2 weeks.

3. Prevents infection: redness, edema, drainage, elevated temperature.

1. Assesses neonatal tolerance of procedure.

2. Prevents blood loss.

3. Catheter may have entered femoral artery, or thrombus may have formed.
4. Prevents clogging and emboli.

5. Is legal record and facilitates communication among staff. Provides baseline to evaluate change.

Restraining neonate

The purposes of restraining an infant include the following:

- Protects the infant from injury
- Facilitates examinations and limits discomfort during tests, procedures, and specimen collections

---

*Red blood cells continue anaerobic glycolysis with production of acid metabolites after removal from donor.

When restraining an infant, there are special considerations one must keep in mind:

1. Check the infant frequently.

2. Apply restraints, and check them frequently to prevent skin irritation and circulatory impairment.

3. Maintain proper body alignment.

4. Apply restraints without use of knots or pins if possible. If knots are necessary, they are the kind that can be released quickly. Pins are used with care to prevent puncture wounds and pressure areas—and to prevent the infant's swallowing one of them.

5. If the infant is in an incubator, secure the infant to the mattress to protect the extremities, especially when the lid is raised or the mattress moved.

Restraining techniques include the following.

Mummy. This technique is used for the stronger, more vigorous newborn. It is used for examinations, treatments, or specimen collections that involve the head and neck.

Equipment includes a blanket and one or two large safety pins (Fig. 37-14).

The procedure is as follows:

1. Spread blanket on flat surface; crib should suffice.

2. Fold over one corner (12 o'clock).

3. Lay newborn on blanket so that neck is at fold.

4. Fold 9 o'clock corner over right shoulder; tuck that corner securely under infant's left side.

5. Bring 6 o'clock corner up over feet and tuck it either under infant's left side or, if long enough, fold over blanket crossing it under infant's chin.

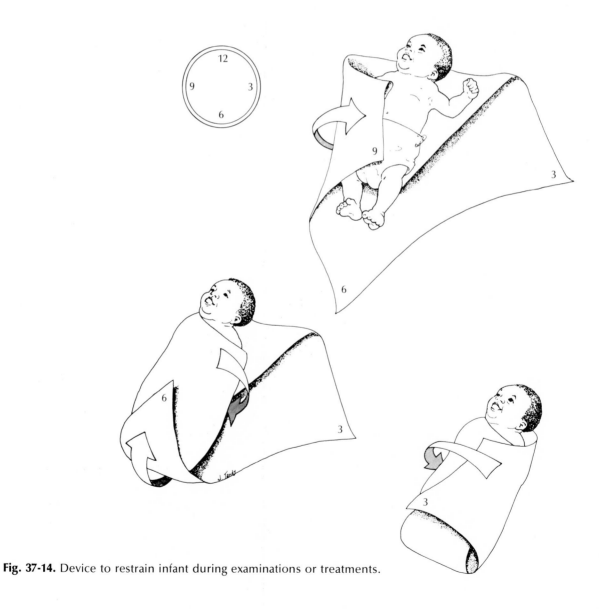

Fig. 37-14. Device to restrain infant during examinations or treatments.

6. Swing 3 o'clock corner snugly over infant and fold under his right side. Pin this corner into place.

Extremity restraints. This technique is used to control movements of the infant's arm(s) or leg(s).

Equipment includes gauze strips or wide strips of soft material and cotton wadding; pins are optional.

The procedure depends on which one of the many kinds available is used. Examples are as follows:

1. *Pad extremity with cotton wadding.* Fold one end of gauze strip over the extremity and pin. Pin other end to mattress.

2. *Clove-hitch restraint.* Arrange strip of long, 2-inch wide material as shown in Fig. 37-15. Loop device over extremity, which has been padded with cotton; pin loose ends to mattress. Clove-hitch does not tighten even if infant's movements tug on restraint.

Towel support. Although this is not a true restraint, it serves to control the infant's position and movement. It may be rolled and placed at his back or sides or folded and placed under his neck or upper back.

1. It provides comfort and security by stabilizing his position.

2. It maintains positioning to assist respiratory effort and gastrointestinal functions and prevent skin breakdown.

3. It prevents the infant from rolling against the incubator wall where he may lose heat by convection.

4. It prevents the infant from falling out of the incubator when the lid is lifted.

Restraint without appliance. The nurse may restrain the infant with the use of hands and body. Fig. 37-16 illustrates restraining the infant in position for lumbar puncture.

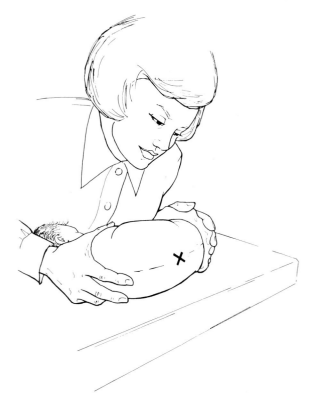

Fig. 37-16. Position for lumbar puncture.

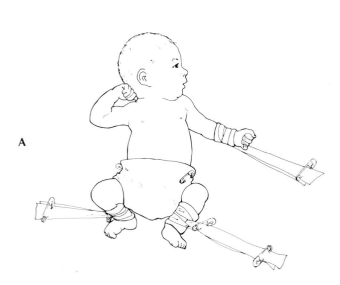

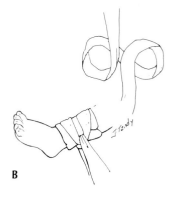

Fig. 37-15. A, Clove-hitch restraints in place. **B,** Clove-hitch device. This restraint does not tighten after its application. Apply padding prior to device.

Assisting with collection of blood specimen

Technique

1. Position and restrain infant.
   a. Femoral venipuncture: Position child in frog posture; place hands over infant's knees. Avoid pressure of fingers over inner aspect of thigh because vein in this area may be occluded.
   b. External jugular venipuncture (Fig. 37-17): "Mummy" infant as necessary. Lower infant's head over rolled towel, edge of table, or your knee, and stabilize.
   c. Handle infant gently; talk quietly to him during procedure.
2. a. After venipuncture, apply pressure over area with sterile gauze for 3 to 5 minutes.
   b. If jugular vein was used, raise infant's head and shoulders while applying pressure.
   c. Comfort infant as necessary.

Rationale

1. Facilitates venipuncture. Prevents tissue trauma. Prevents cold stress.

2. Prevents leakage of additional blood into tissues or formation of hematoma (later this may result in hyperbilirubinemia). If infant is vigorous, direct pressure, restraint, and comforting prevent activity that could initiate or prolong bleeding.

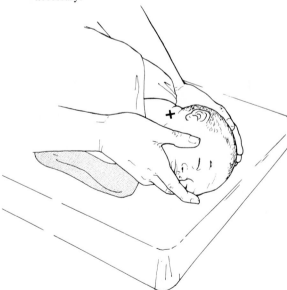

Fig. 37-17. Position for jugular venipuncture. Neonate is "mummied."

Technique—cont'd

3. Observe infant for 1 hour.

4. Record site, amount of blood taken, reason for specimen, infant response.

Rationale—cont'd

3. Can detect further bleeding (oozing, hematoma). Enclosed bleeding can lead to hypovolemic shock, hyperbilirubinemia, or both.

4. Allows ongoing evaluation and adjustment of care plans.

Determining blood pressure: flush method

Some centers are equipped with sophisticated biometric consoles for accurate determination of blood pressure. The flush technique for the determination of blood pressure is imprecise. This provides a rapid rough estimate of the mean diastolic/systolic pressure (the reading is midway between the diastolic and systolic pressures). This often assists in the early detection and proper treatment of the high-risk infant.

Equipment includes a manometer and cuff about 1 inch wide and 3 inches long.

Limitations of the flush method are the following:

1. The normal range for infants of various gestational ages and weights is still unknown.

2. The existing standard for infants weighing 2500 gm or more (5½ pounds) is 30 to 60 mm Hg.

3. The determination requires practice. One should practice this method on normal newborns. Findings must be recorded.

The procedure is as follows:

Technique

1. Infant should be quiet.

2. Wrap cuff around infant's extremity snugly:
   a. Arm—just above wrist.
   b. Leg—just above ankle.
3. With elastic bandage or hand, squeeze extremity below cuff.
4. Simultaneously pump manometer to 120 to 140 mm Hg.
5. Release hand (or elastic wrap) while allowing the manometer gauge to fall 5 mm Hg/sec.
6. Note pressure reading at time extremity flushes.
7. If reading is above or below 30 to 60 mm Hg, repeat procedure on different extremity.
8a. If reading remains low in

Rationale

1. Activity (crying) raises BP.

2. Minimizes error in reading.

3. Blanches area distal to cuff.

4. As above.

5. Perfusion of extremity occurs. Appropriate speed of descent is necessary for accurate reading.
6. Approximate mean diastolic-systolic pressure.
7. Rules out operator error or confirms finding.

8a. Index of suspicion for

Technique—cont'd

b. If there is marked discrepancy between leg and arm readings, record and report to physician.

c. Observe infant for other signs and symptoms while awaiting physician. Check chart for pregnancy history, labor and delivery experience, and condition of infant since birth.

Using urine specimen collectors

A variety of urine specimen collection bags are available, usually with instructions accompanying them. Although the following directions are specific to the U-Bag (Hollister), they are generally applicable to many other types:

Rationale—cont'd

shock, hypovolemia, hypoplastic left heart.

b. Suggests cardiovascular anomaly (e.g., coarctation of aorta).

c. Collect other pertinent data to permit physician to diagnose disorder and initiate appropriate treatments.

Technique

1. Separate infant's legs. Make sure pubic and perineal area is clean, dry, and free from mucus. Do not apply powders, oils, or lotions to skin.

2. Remove protective paper, exposing hypoallergenic adhesive (Fig. 37-18, *A*).

3. For girls, stretch perineum to flatten skin folds. Press adhesive firmly to skin all around vagina. (NOTE: Start with narrow portion of butterfly-shaped adhesive patch.) *Be sure to start at bridge of skin separating rectum from vagina and work upward* (Fig. 37-18, *B*). For boys, tuck penis and scrotum through aperture

Rationale

1. Assures leakproof seal. Decreases chance of contamination.

2. Exposes adhesive. Decreases chance of allergic reaction.

3. Assures leakproof seal. Decreases chance of contamination from urine and stool.

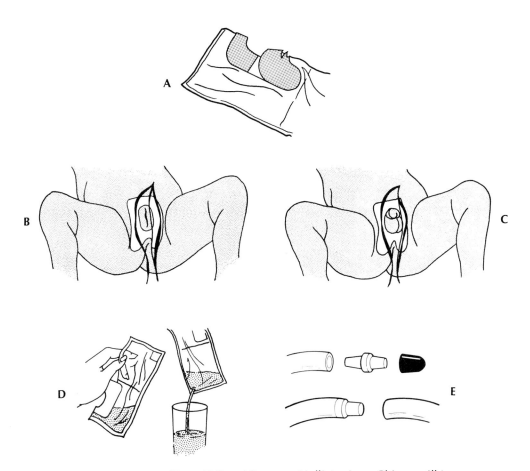

Fig. 37-18. Hollister U-Bag. (Courtesy Hollister Inc., Chicago, Ill.)

Technique—cont'd

of collector before removing protective paper from adhesive. Fit bag over penis, and press flaps firmly to perineum, making sure entire adhesive coating is firmly attached to skin with no puckering of adhesive (Fig. 37-18, *C*).

4. To drain, hold bag in left hand. Tilt bag so urine is away from blue tab. Remove tab and drain in clean receptacle (Fig. 37-18, *D*).

Rationale—cont'd

4. Facilitates emptying without use of scissors, which can contaminate or be contaminated.

Apply the 24-hour U-Bag in the same manner as just described. Direct the drainage into a receptacle. The collection tube can be shortened or capped (Fig. 37-18, *E*). See directions accompanying the bag.

DIAGNOSTIC TESTS

APT. This test is administered prior to delivery to differentiate between maternal and fetal blood when there is vaginal bleeding. It is performed as follows: Add 0.5 ml blood to 4.5 ml of distilled water. Shake. Add 1 ml of 0.25 N sodium hydroxide. Fetal and cord blood remains pink for 1 to 2 minutes. Maternal blood becomes brown in 30 seconds.

"Shake" or "foam" test. This test is administered during pregnancy to ascertain the presence of lecithin (surfactant), an indicator of fetal lung maturity. It is performed as follows: After amniocentesis, dilute amniotic fluid and mix with 95% alcohol (to a final con-

Table 37-1. Diagnostic tests for phenylketonuria*

Test	Method	Use
Urine tests		
Diaper test	10% ferric chloride dropped on freshly wet diaper. Green spot is positive, indicates probable PKU.	Cheap. Useful in screening large groups of infants but not of value until the infant is at least 6 weeks of age.
Phenistix† test	Prepared test stick pressed against wet diaper or dipped in urine. Green color reaction indicates probable PKU.	Simple; more accurate than diaper test. Useful in screening large groups of infants but not of value until after infant is 6 weeks of age.
Dinitrophenyl-hydrazine (DNPH) test‡	0.5 to 1 ml of urine placed in test tube, and equal amount of DNPH solution added. Immediate pale yellow-orange color reaction is negative. Gradual change to opaque bright yellow is positive and indicates probable PKU.	Cheap, accurate but more complicated than diaper test or Phenistix; most useful in clinical setting to confirm these tests.
Blood serum phenylalanine tests		
Guthrie inhibition assay methods§	Drops of blood placed on filter paper. Lab uses a bacterial growth inhibition test. Level above 8 mg phenylalanine/100 ml blood diagnostic of PKU.	Effective in newborn period. Used also to monitor PKU diet. Blood easily obtained by heel or finger puncture. Inexpensive; used for wide-scale screening.
LaDu-Michael method‖	5 ml of blood; serum separated and tested for phenylalanine. Level above 8 mg/100 ml blood indicates PKU. In PKU patients, level above 8 to 12 mg phenylalanine/100 ml blood indicates loss of dietary control.	Useful diagnostic tool and to monitor PKU diet. Requires blood drawn from patient, and lab method is difficult (test not available in many labs).
McCaman and Robins fluorometric method¶	5 ml of blood; serum separated and tested for phenylalanine. Level above 8 mg indicates PKU or loss of dietary control.	Diagnostic and diet monitoring tool. Lab procedure more simple than LaDu-Michael method. Test not available in many labs.

*From Williams, S. 1973. Nutrition and diet therapy (ed. 2). St. Louis, The C. V. Mosby Co., p. 427.
†Manufactured by Ames Company, Elkhart, Ind.
‡Centerwall, W., and Centerwall, S. 1961. Phenylketonuria. U.S. Children's Bureau, Pub. No. 338, Washington, D.C., U.S. Government Printing Office.
§Guthrie, R. 1961. Blood screening for phenylketonuria, J.A.M.A. **178:**863.
‖LaDu, B., and Michael, P. 1960. An enzymatic spectrophotometric method for the determination of phenylalanine in blood. J. Lab. Clin. Med. **55:**491.
¶McCaman, M., and Robins, E. 1962. Fluorometric method for the determination of phenylalanine in the serum. J. Lab. Clin. Med. **59:**885.

centration of 47.5% alcohol). Shake mixture vigorously for 15 seconds; allow to stand for 15 seconds. The test is positive (surfactant is present) if a complete ring of bubbles persists in the 1:2 dilution tube.

Dextrostix. This test screens for levels of glucose in blood from a heel stick or venous sample. To administer, freely apply a large drop of capillary or venous blood sufficient to cover entire reagent area on a printed strip. Wait exactly 60 seconds (use the sweep second hand or stop watch for timing). Quickly wash off blood for 1 to 2 seconds with a sharp stream of water, using a wash bottle. Read the result within 1 to 2 seconds after washing. Hold the strip close to the color chart. Interpolate if necessary.

Hemoglobin electrophoresis. This test is used to diagnose sickle cell disease in newborns. Cord blood is analyzed.

Bac-U-Dip. This is a screening test for bacteria in urine. Dip the lower one fourth of the test strip into the urine and withdraw immediately. Color change requires 2 to 3 minutes. A positive test, presence of bacteria in the urine, is evidenced by a definite pink or a red color of any degree.

Coombs' test. This test is performed to determine the presence of anti-D (Rh-positive) antibody in blood. The direct Coombs' test is done on fetal cord blood (postnatal) and the indirect test, on maternal blood (prenatal).

Indirect. A specimen of maternal blood is obtained. Rh-positive red blood cells are added to maternal serum; if the serum contains antibodies, the Rh-positive red blood cells agglutinate.

Direct. A specimen of fetal cord blood is obtained. Fetal red blood cells are washed and exposed to Coombs' serum. If antibodies are present on the fetal red blood cells, they will agglutinate.

Tests used in phenylketonuria. Table 37-1 summarizes the methods and usefulness of the tests used to diagnose phenylketonuria.

New tests. The tests described in Table 37-2 are currently in the experimental stages.

TREATMENT IN EXPERIMENTAL STAGES

A deficiency of vitamin E in early born infants may be one causal factor in the development and/or severity of retrolental fibroplasia (RLF). Some premature infants develop RLF in the absence of oxygen abuse. Intramuscular injections of vitamin E (α-tocopherol) may reduce the incidence of RLF and its sequelae, deviations from normal vision, and blindness.

Table 37-2. New diagnostic tests

Test	Specimen/method	Purpose/comments
Level of human placental lactogen (HPL): Unfavorable prognosis $\geq 1\ \mu g/ml$ Favorable prognosis $\leq 0.7\ \mu g/ml$	Amniotic fluid	Predictive index of severity of Rh isoimmunization and outcome for fetus/newborn *Comment:* Currently test for bilirubin levels is more reliable
Amount of palmitic acid content in amniotic fluid lecithin: No appearance of RDS if $\geq 20\%$ RDS occurs if $<20\%$	Amniotic fluid	Predictive index of fetal lung maturity regardless of contamination by blood or meconium in specimen *Comment:* Currently this test is time-consuming and requires technicians with considerable expertise
Degree of oxygen saturation in cutaneous vessels	Transcutaneous electrode with heating device to ensure optimal perfusion at site	Predictive index of arterial oxygen tension *Comment:* (1) Discrepancies exist between arterial P_{O_2} values and cutaneous P_{O_2} values in hypoxic infants; (2) there is need to evaluate arterial P_{O_2} as optimal physiologic reference index (e.g., is cutaneous P_{O_2} value more critical indicator of tissue supply of oxygen?)
Determining diameter and length of scalp hair (diameter and length of scalp hair in small-for-date infant is less than that of well-nourished controls)	Electron microscopy	Index of intrauterine nutrition *Comment:* Effective method to evaluate amino acid metabolism without jeopardy to fetus or mother

REFERENCES

Babson, S. G., Benson, R. C., Pernoll, M. L., and Benda, G. I. 1975. Management of high-risk pregnancy and intensive care of the neonate (ed. 3). St. Louis, The C. V. Mosby Co.

Clausen, J., and others. 1976. Maternity nursing today. San Francisco, McGraw-Hill Book Co.

Currents: perinatology, neonatology, pediatric nutrition. Nov. 1975. Columbus, Ohio, Ross Laboratories. Extracted from:

Baum, and others. 1974. Neonatal hair as a record of intrauterine nutrition. Biol. Neonate **25:**208.

Fenner, and others. 1975. Transcutaneous determination of arterial oxygen tension. Pediatrics **55:**224.

Niven, and others. 1974. Human placental lactogen levels in amniotic fluid in Rhesus isoimmunization. J. Obstet. Gynaecol. Br. Commonw. **81:**988.

The premature infant, vitamin E deficiency and retrolental fibroplasia. 1974. Pa. Am. J. Clin. Nutr. **27:**1158.

Russell, and others. 1974. Palmitic acid content of amniotic fluid lecithin as an index to fetal lung maturity. Ohio Clin. Chem. **20:**1431.

Sinnecker, and others. 1974. Herpes simplex infections in the newborn. Berlin **29:**2375.

Dobson, V., and Cowett, R. M. 1974. Long-term effect of phototherapy on visual function (abstract). Second annual meeting, American Society for Photobiology, July.

Dobson, V., Riggs, L., and Siqueland, E. 1974. Electroretinographic determination of dark adaptation functions of children exposed to phototherapy as infants. J. Pediatr. **85:**25.

Elder, R. L. 1973. Ultraviolet light hazards from phototherapy (letter). Bureau of Radiological Health, U.S. Food and Drug Administration.

Emery, J. 1975. How to use the U-Bag. Chicago, Ill. Hollister Incorporated.

Korones, S. B. 1976. High-risk newborn infants: the basis for intensive nursing care (ed. 2). St. Louis, The C. V. Mosby Co.

Letters to the editor: responses to phototherapy for neonatal hyperbilirubinemia. 1974. J. Pediatr. **84:**457.

Lewak, N. Management of idiopathic hyperbilirubinemia in term infants: community practices. Pediatrics **53:**471.

The Lippincott manual of nursing practice. 1974. Philadelphia, J. B. Lippincott Co.

Lucey, F. J. The effects of light on the newly born infant. J. Perinat. Med. **1:**1, 1973.

Lund, H. T., and Jacobsen, J. 1974. Influence of phototherapy on the biliary bilirubin excretion pattern in newborn infants with hyperbilirubinemia. J. Pediatr. **85:**262.

Lund, H. T., and Petersen, I. 1974. Beta-glucuronidase in duodenal bile of jaundiced newborn infants treated with phototherapy. J. Pediatr. **85:**268.

National Research Council. 1974. Preliminary report of the committee on phototherapy in the newborn infant. J. Pediatr. **84:**135.

Oliver, T. K. 1972. The newborn. In Kelley, V. (ed.). Brennemann's practice of pediatrics. New York, Harper & Row, Publishers.

Phototherapy caused increase in blood flow. 1974. Pediat. News **8,** Feb.

Roberts, J. 1973. Suctioning the newborn. Am. J. Nurs. **73:**63.

Rubaltelli, F. F., and others. 1974. Urinary excretion of tryptophan metabolites during phototherapy. Clin. Pediatr. **85:**865.

Silverman, W., and Parke, P. 1965. The newborn: keep him warm. Am. J. Nurs. **65:**81, Oct.

Tucker, S., and others. 1975. Patient care standards. St. Louis, The C. V. Mosby Co.

Warren, F. 1975. Blood pressure readings: getting them quickly on an infant. Nursing **75:**13, April.

Wu, P. Y. K., and Berdahl, M. 1974. Irradiance in incubators under phototherapy lamps. J. Pediatr. **84:**754.

UNIT ELEVEN

Current implications of legal aspects of maternity nursing and problem-oriented system

CHAPTER 38

Legal and ethical aspects of maternity nursing

CHERYL HALL HARRIS

All maternity nurses have a clear responsibility to keep current in all areas of their changing, expanding specialty, including the legal ramifications of their actions. According to Ladimer (1975), legal actions involving maternity and gynecologic patients are fourth in incidence of all malpractice suits. With this in mind, this chapter will review for nurses the current legal attitudes toward major obstetric issues. Some of the concepts to be discussed relate primarily to physicians. However, these are included because nurses frequently are in a position to influence a physician's actions, or lack of action, by reminding the physician of the medicolegal implications inherent in the situation. Since ethical issues are often precursors of law, this chapter will discuss briefly those areas related to maternity care that have significant ethical and sociologic implications.

GENERAL LEGAL CONCEPTS
Malpractice

Anyone who practices nursing is required to fulfill professional responsibilities as well as would another professional with comparable training under the same circumstances. Any failure to meet these standards (either by omission or commission of an act) constitutes negligence, and legal action can be brought against the nurse for that negligent act.

Malpractice is professional negligence and is comprised of four elements: (1) duty to a person, (2) failure to carry out that duty (breach of duty), (3) an injury sustained by that person, and (4) proximate cause—a causal relationship must be established between the breach of duty and the person's injury. If any of these elements is missing, there is no basis for legal action.

The following are examples of negligence within the context of maternity nursing:

1. A patient began premature labor. During the first 1½ hours, the nurses neglected to notify either a house physician or the attending obstetrician. When delivery became imminent, the nurses rushed the mother to the delivery suite. The delivery was unattended by an obstetrician, pediatrician, or nurse. Although the infant later developed spasticity, legal action was not brought by the parents. The nurses and the institution could have been held liable for negligence if a suit had been initiated.

2. A nurse was held liable for administering a lethal (adult dose) injection of digitalis to an infant. Her negligence included administration of the drug and failing to question the dosage and alert the ordering physician to the questionable dosage. Even if she had secured confirmation from the ordering physician, the nurse would still have been negligent in administering a dosage that she should have recognized as incorrect.

3. In a recent case a nurse handed the physician an incorrect strength of silver nitrate solution, which he instilled in an infant's eyes, thereby impairing the infant's vision. The suit was won by the plaintiff because both the nurse and physician were negligent in not checking the strength of the solution prior to its administration.

Various other incidents have been the subject of litigation, such as mistaking the identities of newborns by failing to check the name bands and burns resulting from failure to properly cover a hot water bottle. These examples illustrate the legal duty of nurses to be alert and to possess the necessary expertise to exercise sound professional judgment in the performance of their responsibilities.

One further word of caution concerning negligence and malpractice: nurses in a critical care situation should remember their own physical and mental limitations. If a nurse works additional shifts or on her days off and she commits a negligent act, her fatigue will not excuse her poor performance. She will be held to the same standard of care as any other reasonable professional.

Circumstances arise when a nurse may disagree with a physician's order. If she disagrees, she can and should request that the physician perform the procedure. In addition, there are circumstances wherein a nurse may be expected to perform functions traditionally assumed by a physician, for example, external cardiac massage or resuscitation. The nurse must be properly trained to perform these tasks before she assumes the responsibilities. The appropriateness of nurses performing these tasks has not yet been tested in the courts, however.

A nurse must have sufficient "job knowledge" to perform as a reasonably trained person would. In highly specialized areas such as labor and delivery rooms, specific technical training is required to equip the nurse for the variety of complex situations that may occur during her tour of duty. A thorough orientation program and continuing education courses should be provided by the institution in which the nurse is employed. Moreover, it is the nurse's responsibility to take advantage of the training that is offered. When a nurse has been trained in a specific task, it should be documented in her personnel file so that should a related issue arise, she can prove that she was properly prepared. In this regard, the Nurses' Association of the American College of Obstetricians and Gynecologists (NAACOG) has established (1976) a certification program for nurses who have gained additional training in maternal, gynecologic, and neonatal nursing. To qualify for this certification, nurses will be required to take courses, have work experience, and satisfactorily complete examinations in their particular field of interest.

Standard of care

All persons make mistakes. Some are reasonable mistakes; others are unreasonable mistakes. It is negligent to make an unreasonable mistake, but a person who makes a reasonable mistake is acting as a reasonably prudent person and hence is free from negligence. The test is whether in forming a judgment relating to the adoption of a course of conduct, a person exercised that degree of care which an ordinary and prudent person similarly situated would have exercised under the same or similar circumstances.

Under certain circumstances, injury to the patient will have occurred even though the nurse and/or physician will have met or exceeded the standard of care. Such an incident is termed an *unavoidable accident*.

It is critically important for every nurse to be thoroughly familiar with the policies and procedures of her employing institution, since those policies and procedures constitute the standard of case within that institution.

Generally, negligence in nursing falls into one or more of the following three broad categories: (1) failing to act, (2) having the authority to act but performing the authorized act in an improper manner, and (3) performing an unauthorized act.

Standing and contingency orders

Many nursing units use standing orders for routine procedures. With standing orders in effect, the nurse may perform certain procedures and then chart those procedures indicating to the physician that they have been performed. Standing orders must be reviewed and updated periodically, however.

Contingency orders are a more complex form of standing orders. In this instance, nurses should be given a detailed list of patient problems and procedures, including laboratory values, in a notebook format. On the basis of their assessment of patients' conditions and laboratory studies, they then may be directed to provide necessary treatment before notifying physicians. Physicians must determine which portions of the contingency orders they wish to have in effect by means of their signatures in appropriate sections. This system probably will provide the most efficient and rapid treatment of the patient without constant physician attendance while assuring legal protection of the nurse.

Charting

The legal significance of charting by the nurse cannot be overemphasized. Many malpractice suits have been decided on the basis of information contained in the nurse's record. The best way nurses can prove that they did perform a certain task is by written documentation in their notes. In addition, there is legal significance attached to nursing observations of a patient's condition at a particular time.

In many instances, a suit may not be initiated for a number of years. For this reason, nurses cannot rely on their memory to recall their actions in a specific instance. Although the statute of limitations usually restricts a plaintiff from filing suit after a given number of years, a minor may delay until he reaches the age of majority before filing an action, since the statute does not begin to run its course until the patient reaches majority. Therefore nurses, physicians, and hospitals are vulnerable for many years to legal action concerning patient care, the only complete record of which is the patient's chart.

Equipment

Fetal monitors are now used widely in labor and delivery units. The nurse must be able to attach the leads of a monitor to a patient, and she must be able to interpret the tracings produced by the machine. Nurses must check equipment frequently for accuracy. If there is an alarm system or a monitoring device to alert the nurse to patient problems, the alarm should not be turned off for convenience. If an alarm is deactivated and the patient develops a problem, the nurse may be found guilty of negligence.

Some qualified person whose direct responsibility is to check equipment for proper functioning and to detect any electrical hazards produced by the equipment should be hired by the institution. Monitors usually are attached to a patient with a gel that improves electrical conduction. A patient may receive an electrical shock or a burn at the site of electrode placement if the equipment is malfunctioning.

Informed consent

All patients imply their consent to routine treatment when they place themselves under a physician and nurse's care in an institution. In emergency situations, consent is implied, unless the patient offers evidence to the contrary (e.g., refusing a blood transfusion for religious reasons). For potentially hazardous procedures, consent must be obtained preferably in writing. Oral consent is sufficient, provided it is witnessed by a reliable individual. It is the physician's responsibility to obtain the patient's informed consent; it is the nurse's responsibility to confirm that this consent has been obtained.

Informed consent means that the significant benefits and risks inherent in the procedure have been explained to the patient, as well as alternative methods of treatment, that the physician has answered the patient's questions concerning the procedure, and that the patient has then agreed to have the procedure performed.

If consent is not obtained, legal action for battery can be initiated. If additional surgery not clearly specified in the original consent form is performed, the physician is liable for battery, unless the consent form provides for reasonable and necessary extensions. To give legal consent, a patient must be mentally and physically competent; otherwise, consent must be obtained from an immediate family member or other person accompanying the patient. If a patient refuses to give consent for treat-

ment, the physician must explain the risks of refusal to the patient and ask the patient to sign a form stating that she refuses therapy even though she is aware that her refusal may prove detrimental to her health or life.

Maternal rights

A recent innovation in maternity care is "The Pregnant Patient's Bill of Rights" by Doris B. Haire, the coordinator of the Committee on Patients' Rights (Appendix A). The essence of this document is that the pregnant patient deserves as much information as possible about the effects of any drugs or treatment on herself or her infant, since she or her baby may suffer from any adverse sequelae to the drugs or treatment she receives. The general public is now aware that although the U.S. Federal Drug Administration may approve a particular drug and a physician then prescribe it, it may not be safe for every woman or her baby. Furthermore, the bill of rights argues that a maternity patient has the right to have someone for whom she cares accompany her through labor and delivery. Although this issue is not yet settled, many couples are turning to other alternatives than hospitals as the setting for childbirth. If health professionals wish to make childbirth a satisfying rather than a threatening experience for parents, they should attempt to incorporate the reasonable wishes of patients into institutional procedures whenever possible.

Insurance

Nurses must carry professional liability insurance for their own protection. Even if an institution provides insurance coverage, it generally only applies while the nurse is on duty at the institution. In the event of negligence or malpractice during other times of the nurses' professional practice, the nurse would not be covered by the employer's policy. As Grace Barbee, former lawyer for the California Nurses' Association, once remarked, "It can be expensive to prove your innocence." Reasonably priced insurance policies, which are well worth the expense, are available to nurses.

There are two types of professional liability insurance for nurses: claims-made policies and occurrence policies. *Claims-made policies* provide protection for the nurse only if the policy is in force at the time that the claim is made. Thus if legal action was brought against a nurse in 1976 for an incident that occurred in 1975, a claims-made policy would need to be in force in 1976 to afford protection. *Occurrence policies* provide protection for a given period of time and include coverage of any incidents that may occur within that period, regardless of the date of legal action concerning those incidents. Any nurse having an occurrence policy covering the period of 1970 to 1976 would be protected against legal action concerning incidents occurring during those years, even though suit was not brought until 1977.

ISSUES FOR NURSE-MIDWIVES

In the United States, nurse-midwives do not function as independent practitioners but rather as part of a health care team directed by a physician. Whether a nurse-midwife can practice is determined by licensure within the legal jurisdiction in which she is employed. Nurse-midwives are trained to perform normal deliveries and to give care to mothers and infants at the time of delivery and during the ensuing weeks. The nurse-midwife can provide care for mothers throughout a *normal* pregnancy, labor, and delivery. If abnormalities are discovered, patients must be transferred to the care of a physician.

In 1976 there were thirteen approved programs of study, with three additional programs awaiting approval (Appendix M). In addition, nurse-midwives function in some midwifery capacity in almost all fifty states. There is one private obstetric practice that includes three obstetricians and six nurse-midwives in Springfield, Ohio. Contrary to expectations, the nurse-midwives were well accepted by the private and/or middle-class patients. In the future, it is expected that nurse-midwives will be used by private obstetricians on an associate or referral basis in other cities.

LEGAL AND ETHICAL CONCEPTS FOR PRECONCEPTIONAL PATIENTS
Sexual counseling

Discussion of sexual matters has become more open during recent years. This frankness has led to a rise in the number of self-styled sexual counselors, who may even be charlatans. Sexual counseling should be done by trained personnel who are interested and skilled in helping people with sexual problems. There are currently few statutes that regulate this field. In the future, licensure probably will be required for sexual counselors.

With regard to minors, many state laws are being liberalized to permit counseling and treatment of minors for pregnancy, venereal disease, and contraception without the requirement of prior parental consent. No matter who receives counseling on sexual matters, they have a right to privacy and confidentiality.

Sterilization

Either men or women may be candidates for sterilization, but for the purpose of this discussion, only female sterilization will be considered. Sterilization is only occasionally essential for the patient's health. Hence most sterilization operations are elective. For voluntary sterilization, the patient must give her informed consent. The explanations given to obtain the consent must explain the major alternatives to sterilization, including the principal benefits and risks involved. The psychologic risks should be mentioned also; most individuals who later regret their decision for sterilization are those who are young, made their decision during periods of stress, or made the decision on the advice of a physician who may suggest the procedure at the last minute. Mc Garrah (1974) lists the following guidelines for those who are involved in obtaining consent for sterilizations:

1. The patient should realize that essentially all sterilization operations are permanent and irreversible.

2. If sterilization is being chosen because the woman is under emotional or financial stress, she should realize that these conditions may improve at a later date.

3. The woman should try other methods of contraception before selecting permanent sterilization.

4. The physician should rarely recommend sterilization but should await the request from the patient.

5. The patient should not be allowed to make a hasty decision; ideally there should be a waiting period of a week or more between the time consent is first given and the operation is performed.

6. The patient should be aware that sterilization is not problem-free and that there are occasional failures resulting in pregnancy.

Certain legal questions surround the sterilization of mentally retarded or incompetent women. These are considered involuntary sterilizations, since the woman is legally incapable of granting consent. Noon (1975) cites a case in England involving an 11-year-old girl who was ruled "dull-normal" in intelligence with a level of understanding of a 9- to 9½-year-old child. Her mother requested her sterilization, even though the headmaster of the girl's school and a psychologist disapproved of the sterilization because they believed she was improving. She was made a ward of the court, and the judge decided against sterilization until she was older and could make her own choice. In a case in the United States, a 20-year-old woman was diagnosed as mentally incompetent by two psychiatrists who believed she would never be mentally competent. Sadoff (1975) suggested that she should have had the sterilization procedure explained to her, even though her consent to the operation would not be legally binding (because of her mental incompetence). He held that the best way to handle this case was to have had a court hearing to decide her mental competency for the future and to have legal approval for the sterilization.

At least 300,000 sterilizations are performed in North America each year. Hospitals that are supported entirely by taxation cannot refuse to perform sterilizations. However, there are "conscience" clauses that allow physicians and institutions other than these to refuse to perform sterilizations on moral, religious, or medical judgment grounds.

Genetic counseling

Genetic counseling is often given after the birth of an infant with a defect. Before counseling sessions can be held, an accurate diagnosis must be made. A thorough physical examination, laboratory studies, x-ray examination, and a complete family history are therefore essential to document the cause of the defect. The physician must utilize personal knowledge and published data to aid in making the diagnosis and explaining the prognosis to the family. The purpose of counseling is to enable the couple to understand the recurrence risk and prognosis for other possibly affected children. Based on that information, the couple must then decide whether to have additional children.

Most genetic counseling is done by informed pediatricians; however, perhaps the most successful counseling is that done by a person whose specialty is medical genetics. Another solution is the training of obstetricians in genetic counseling because they are the ones who see patients most frequently. They can choose the time to do the initial counseling and can pursue the problem with additional information at a later time. Certainly the only individuals who should do genetic counseling are those who have received specialized training in this field. Currently programs are available on a graduate level to train nurses in the techniques of genetic counseling. This will enable them to work in a medically directed genetic counseling center.

Parents who receive genetic counseling have a right to privacy concerning these matters as with other privileged information. However, there is an ethical question to be answered when one parent is found to be a carrier of a lethal disease: who should inform other potential carriers in the extended family? The parents may be unwilling to inform these individuals because of guilt or embarrassment, even though they do have an ethical obligation to notify their relatives. If the physician notifies other family members without consent from the parents, he may breach the laws concerning privileged information.

There are several ethical issues in the genetics of the future. The fertilization of a human ovum in vitro with subsequent transplantation into the mother's uterus has been accomplished by Steptoe (1976). In England, a couple with a poor reproductive history consented to this experimental technique. An egg from the mother was fertilized in vitro and at 4½ days of development was introduced into her uterus through the cervix. The subsequent pregnancy was terminated spontaneously at 13 weeks of gestation because of the death of the fetus, which had developed as a tubal pregnancy. This raises the question of whether fertilized eggs from one couple could be transplanted into a surrogate mother who would serve as a human incubator.

Artificial insemination

Numerous legal problems stem from the practice of artificial insemination. There are two types of artificial insemination: artificial insemination of the patient with her husband's sperm (AIH) to fertilize her egg in vivo and artificial insemination of the patient with a donor's sperm (AID). AID will be considered here because it alone has serious legal ramifications. The probability of an increase in the incidence of AID is significant as adoptions become more difficult to arrange. The primary indications for AID are male infertility or genetic reasons.

Five people are involved in AID: the husband, wife, donor, physician and the resultant child. Several issues have been identified by Richardson (1975):

1. Is the child conceived illegitimate?

2. Does AID constitute criminal adultery or adultery that could lead to divorce on those grounds?

3. Could the donor be held liable for rape if the woman denies she gave consent?

4. Does the child produced as a result of AID have legal rights to the donor's estate if the donor leaves his estate to his children?

5. What are the AID child's rights to his mother's husband's estate?

Legal obligations can be met by ensuring that the husband, wife, and donor all give written consent to the procedure. The donor should not know the identity of the husband and wife and vice versa. The physician should be given permission to select the donor. The consent may also include a clause to remove liability from the physician if the infant should be abnormal. The best way to assure that the AID child is legitimate is for the couple to adopt him formally. However, many states are considering legislation giving such a child rights as a legitimate heir to the husband and wife. Legislation must be carefully drawn to prevent children produced by AID from initiating legal action against the physician, according to Edwards (1973). The basis for these suits includes withholding information from these children concerning the donor's identity, thereby preventing the child from claiming natural rights as the donor's child.

Antenatal diagnosis

Do parents have the right and responsibility to assure that their children will have no genetic defects? With all the advances in antenatal diagnosis, including mass screening and amniocentesis, fetoscopy, and amnioscopy, this goal is becoming more realistic. These techniques increase the freedom of parents by giving them more information with which to make decisions. In some cases, parents may have an obligation to society to prevent the production of children with severe genetic defects. In fact, society may eventually decide to legislate active prevention of specific birth defects.

Mass screening. The ultimate goal of mass screening is to detect carriers of genetic diseases *before* the birth of an affected infant. Mass screening should provide individuals with the information to decide whether to have children based on the knowledge of their genetic status. Informed consent from those tested is essential, and total confidentiality must be respected. All results must be reported to the person who has undergone the screening procedures.

Screening is not feasible for the general public, so there must either be (1) a specific group at risk (e.g., sickle cell anemia among blacks or Tay-Sachs disease among Ashkenazi Jews), (2) definite knowledge of inheritance patterns for a specific disease, or (3) an inexpensive, accurate test for detection of the carrier. There are problems even with a specific population to be screened; for example, the population may not appreciate or understand the screening procedure or the results. In any event, the persons doing the screening must have expertise in cell biology and biochemistry to provide accurate, reliable test results from the sample. Since accuracy is of the utmost importance, screening programs should be regionalized to assure the high quality control that is necessary for the sophisticated techniques required.

Amniocentesis. The routine use of amniocentesis for all mothers at risk is rapidly becoming available. More than sixty hereditary metabolic diseases can now be diagnosed in utero. There are categories of women who are at risk, including women over 35 years of age and those who have had infants with Down's syndrome, a history of specific genetic disease, fetal irradiation, or elevated toxoplasmosis titers. Amniocentesis is reasonably safe for the mother, and it carries less than 5% risk to the fetus. There are increased dangers when the procedure is done in the third trimester, however. The moth-

er should be given this information when she is asked to sign the consent form for the procedure.

Amniocentesis and subsequent abortion of affected fetuses can help reduce the incidence of birth defects. The need for absolute accuracy in diagnosis by amniocentesis cannot be overstressed; from a legal standpoint this is paramount. If a mother is told that her fetus is normal and she later delivers a defective infant with a disease that could have been detected by amniocentesis, the physician who performed the amniocentesis could be held liable.

Many physicians will not perform an amniocentesis unless the parents agree to an abortion when an abnormal fetus is detected. Milunsky (1974), disagrees with this practice, however. He believes the physician would be imposing his philosophy on the parents and argues that they have a right to know if their infant is normal. In his experience, based on 500 high-risk cases in which amniocentesis was done, 95% of studies showed fetal normalcy. Milunsky further suggests that it is the physician's duty to inform high-risk patients of the availability of, risks of, and indications for amniocentesis and to refer patients elsewhere if his beliefs prevent him from doing the procedure.

Amniocentesis may also be used to determine fetal sex. If amniocentesis is performed and a sex-linked disease is diagnosed, such as hemophilia, then an elective abortion can prevent the birth of the defective male infant. On the other hand, if the parents prefer an infant of one sex rather than the other and choose to abort fetuses of the "wrong" sex, this is an inappropriate use of amniocentesis in Steinfels' opinion (1974). Stenchever (1972) described a case of a 38-year-old woman who had 3 children, one boy and two girls. She requested an amniocentesis to rule out Down's syndrome. She was found to be carrying a normal female fetus, but she requested an abortion because she desired a male child. The request was denied. Because of the risks involved, it is ethically inappropriate to use amniocentesis merely to determine the sex of children. Actually laboratories will not be capable of handling all such tests. Stenchever and others suggest that the sex of the fetus not be reported unless it is crucial to the medical management of the case.

Amniocentesis may be used also to determine fetal gestational age in cases in which early elective delivery is indicated such as Rh sensitization. The L/S ratio in amniotic fluid is an index of fetal lung maturity. With this and related information, an obstetrician often can delay the elective delivery of an immature infant with the potential for developing idiopathic RDS, one of the most severe diseases of premature infants. An interesting question can be asked in the event of early elective delivery of an infant who subsequently develops RDS: Is the delivering physician liable for the injuries caused to the infant? This has not been tested in the courts.

Fetoscopy. The experimental procedure of transuterine fetoscopy may provide an improvement in antenatal diagnosis through direct vision aspiration of fetal blood. With a proper sample, a karyotype could be obtained within 5 days instead of the 2 to 6 weeks required with amniotic fluid. If an abortion were necessary, the reduced time required for the studies could be beneficial. The other useful aspect of aspiration of fetal blood is the detection of fetal metabolic diseases. The legal implications of fetoscopy and aspiration of fetal blood involve risks to the mother and fetus from abortions or premature delivery, infection, or hemorrhage.

Amnioscopy. Direct visualization of amniotic fluid through the intact membranes with a vaginal speculum can be used to detect meconium staining of the fluid, indicative of fetal distress or fetal death. The need for accuracy once again becomes apparent because of the legal sequelae of inappropriate action based on false information obtained by this technique.

• • •

Antenatal diagnosis employing ultrasonography or radiologic examination deserves comment. The use of ultrasound to ascertain fetal size is helpful, in cases of postmaturity when an enlarged fetus is suspected and before abortion (as described later). Ultrasound probably is neither a hazard for the mother nor fetus. Radiologic examination is most frequently used to determine fetal presentation or position and to diagnose fetopelvic disproportion. The danger of this procedure is fetal irradiation. Both of these tests must be done accurately, and the information obtained should lead to appropriate action to avoid legal complications.

In summary, antenatal diagnosis is fraught with difficulties through errors of omission or commission. Accuracy in performing the tests, appropriate action after the results are known, and confidentiality are important legal precepts relating to antenatal diagnosis. If a physician does not wish to perform an abortion when the fetus is diagnosed as defective because of his own religious or moral beliefs, he is obligated to refer the patient to another physician.

Fetal research

There have been many questions regarding fetal research since the Supreme Court's decision on abortion in 1973, which rules that the fetus is not a person before a vaguely described state of viability. In November,

1973, the U.S. Department of Health, Education, and Welfare proposed stringent prohibitions against fetal research. This document prevents experimentation to prolong the life of the nonviable fetus, as well as experimentation that involves a pregnant woman about to undergo abortion if such experimentation might injure the fetus. For example, one cannot study the effects of rubella vaccine on a fetus to be aborted. It should be remembered that experimentation which might prove injurious is allowed once a human has been delivered. Fost believes that the trend to protect the fetus from experimentation is a logical continuation of society's concern about utilizing human subjects for research.

In June, 1974, Massachusetts passed legislation making fetal research a felony, with a penalty of up to 5 years' imprisonment. This law prohibits experimentation on live fetuses either within the uterus or after delivery. A live fetus was defined as one showing evidence of life. Studies may be done to ascertain fetal viability, to preserve the life of the fetus, to preserve the life of the mother, or, when the procedure will not jeopardize the life of the fetus, providing the fetus is not to be the subject of a planned abortion. Curran (1975) is dissatisfied with this law because many of the key phrases are not well defined. He is also concerned that violation of the law is classified as a felony with severe penalties. Moreover, Massachusetts is one state with a law that requires hospitals to provide resuscitation equipment in the room where therapeutic abortions are performed, and the physician is required to take reasonable steps to preserve the life of aborted fetuses who are developed beyond the level of 24 weeks' gestation.

Research must not be permitted on fetuses if the investigators offer to perform the abortion to obtain the fetus for research. This is to prevent those who do research from offering free abortions to women in exchange for fetuses to be used as research subjects, including some in utero. Interesting questions regarding fetal research and abortion have been posed by Hirsch (1975): May an abortion patient consent to experimentation of the fetus in utero? Does the woman having the abortion have a legal right to the disposition of fetal remains? Can an aborted fetus be kept alive for experimental purposes? These and numerous other questions have not yet been thoroughly scrutinized legally, but indications are that they will be.

ETHICAL AND LEGAL ISSUES OF ABORTION

The controversy over abortion continues and probably always will, since neither side is willing to accept the precepts of the other. In this section, the arguments of both sides will be presented, including the legal issues surrounding this problem.

As a result of the Supreme Court decision of January, 1973, abortion is legal anywhere in the United States. In the momentous seven to two decision, the Court declared the following:

1. During the first trimester, the state cannot bar any woman from obtaining an abortion from a licensed physician.

2. In the second trimester, the state can regulate the performance of an abortion if such regulation relates to the preservation and protection of the woman's health.

3. In the third trimester, the state can regulate and even prohibit abortions, except those deemed necessary to protect the woman's life and health, and the state may impose safeguards for the fetus.

The essence of the Court's decision is that existing state abortion control laws were found to be unconstitutional on the basis that they invaded the privacy of the mother. One of the major problems with the decision is that the Court did not decide the issue of when life begins. The Court reasoned that since physicians, theologians, and philosophers were unable to decide this issue, neither could be judiciary. However, the Court did define *viability* as that point of development when the fetus can survive outside the uterus (perhaps with artificial aid) at about 22 to 23 weeks' gestational age. The decision also included the concept that the fetus is not a person, for purposes of protection under the Fourteenth Amendment, and that neither the woman's spouse nor the father of the fetus has any rights to prevent an abortion.

The Supreme Court decision did not provide for abortion on demand; the physician still has the right and the obligation to exercise his professional judgment. Moreover, the decision did not mention pregnant minors. In most states, however, minors can obtain an abortion without the consent of their parents. One issue is whether a minor is classified as having the rights of majority, and many states grant a female these rights when she is married or pregnant.

Provisions termed *conscience clauses* are found in most state laws. These stipulations allow physicians, institutions, and other personnel to refuse to assist in abortions if it is against their moral, ethical, or religious principles, without fear of reprisal. Nonetheless, public hospitals (city, county, and state) must permit their facilities to be used for abortions.

Now that abortion laws have been liberalized, difficulties arise in estimating gestational age because a patient may not accurately report her LMP if she is seeking an abortion. Stubblefield (1975) suggests that if the uterine fundus is above the umbilicus, an ultrasound study should be done to determine the biparietal diameter. If the fetal biparietal diameter is larger than the mean for 22.5 weeks' gestation in that hospital's sample, the abortion should be refused. Infants who are born after a mother has been refused abortion may be placed for adoption. If the abortion must be done to save the mother's life or because of a grossly anomalous fetus, then the decision of whether to use the neonatal intensive care unit (NICU) should be made before the abortion is done. Clearly the obstetrician's dilemma is to determine when a fetus is viable. Most states require a death certificate for a fetus aborted after 20 weeks' gestation. If abortion is by hysterotomy, the fetus may have a chance for survival, but this operation carries more complications for the mother.

In two prominent abortion cases, a primary dispute was the determination of the point at which an aborted fetus becomes a separate individual. Was this at the time it was separated from the mother (but still physically in utero), or when it was physically outside the mother's body? After summarizing these two cases, Wecht (1975) offered suggestions for physicians who perform abortion to terminate late pregnancy. First, there should be documentation of any signs of fetal life either before or after delivery, especially at the point at which the fetus is considered a person, and second, emergency resuscitation should be accomplished for any liveborn fetus as defined in the state's statutes. Wecht further surmises that prosecutors could conceivably attempt indirect control over therapeutic abortions by producing fear in physicians about possible manslaughter-murder charges. He believes that the Supreme Court should further clarify its ruling.

Is it appropriate to utilize a NICU to treat an aborted fetus? With the significant improvements in neonatal care, there are improved chances for survival of even 700 to 800 gm infants. Naturally this raises the issue of efficient utilization of the NICU: if an infant with a poor prognosis is admitted, there will be a reduction in the facilities for an infant with better chances. This could be viewed as inappropriate use of resources. The issue is further complicated if one contrasts the situation wherein an unwanted fetus produced by an abortion competes for care with a fetus delivered after spontaneous abortion to a couple with a poor reproductive history who desperately want a baby. Avery (1973) suggests that the parents should make the decision of whether to use the NICU.

From an ethical standpoint, abortion is essentially the removal of the woman's support for the fetus, leading to loss of fetal survival, since it cannot sustain its own life without the mother. Bok (1974) suggests that if an abortion is performed after the diagnosis of a defective fetus, then the parents have consented to remove support for that particular fetus. This raises the issue of abortion for the fetus' own sake.

Camenisch (1976) concludes that one does not have the right to inflict the pain and tragic consequences of certain detectable serious diseases on an innocent infant. In his view, this argument for abortion is not offered as a mask for other motives, for example, the economic and psychologic difficulties parents of such an infant would face, but rather to alleviate the suffering of the child. By this reasoning, the fetus receives "nothingness" rather than abnormality and therefore no suffering because of its own malformation. If we could, we should choose health, normalcy, and lack of suffering for ourselves, so why not for another? Society needs productive persons and has limited resources to care for the congenitally handicapped. If a damaged fetus is aborted, there should be more room for a normal one. This raises the questions of what is normal and healthy and who should make that decision.

It is difficult to summarize the abortion controversy, but basically the "pro-abortionists" believe that the mother's rights take precedence and that abortion should be performed to allow the mother her freedom of privacy. Most "anti-abortionists" believe that the fetus is human from the moment of conception and as such should be protected from abortion, which ends life. Many pro-abortionists believe that abortions should be used only as a last resort, with contraception and adoption to be used as other alternatives.

Fetal rights

The abortion ruling of the Supreme Court did not discuss the quality of fetal life that is not aborted. Therefore society may still recognize a fetus' right to be well born, with a sound mind and body as mentioned in the "Declarations of the Rights of the Child," a resolution adopted by the United Nations General Assembly (Appendix B). Embryonic development may be affected by numerous teratogenic circumstances, such as viruses, drugs, and environmental hazards. The number of drugs ingested by pregnant women, including even aspirin and prescription drugs, has increased. Hence a fetus may be at greater risk than ever from well-intentioned administration of medications. For example, progestin, which is given to prevent a threatened spontaneous abortion, may masculinize a female fetus.

The *right to be well born* is a concept that provides the infant with necessary antenatal care to ensure him the greatest possible quality of life. Ament (1974) suggests the following measures to effect this right to be well born:

1. Maternal immunity to rubella to protect against the anomalies caused by that disease
2. Pregnancy testing for all females in their childbearing years who are admitted to hospitals, so that no drugs will inadvertently be given to a pregnant woman who is not yet aware of her pregnancy
3. Adequate medical care for all mothers, including informing a mother of the risks and dangers of heavy medication during labor and delivery
4. Treatment of pregnant drug addicts
5. Reporting all birth anomalies to a central agency to facilitate research on the incidence of anomalies
6. Care for aborted fetuses born alive (in New York City, at least one fetus that lived was placed for adoption)

Legally, from the time of conception, a fetus can inherit property and be the beneficiary of a trust. If a child is born alive and then dies of antenatal injuries, a wrongful death action may be brought if the antenatal injuries occurred after the fetus reached viability. Some courts have upheld fetal rights in utero: in the case in which the mother, a Jehovah's Witness, refused a blood transfusion, the court ordered the transfusion because otherwise the infant might have died. Legally a fetus is not considered a person until it is born, but in the case of *Smith* v. *Brennan* reported by Ament, "justice requires that the principle be recognized that a child has a legal right to begin life with a sound mind and body."

LEGAL CONCEPTS DURING LABOR

Nurses who are involved in the care of patients in labor have numerous legal responsibilities to their patients. They must be knowledgeable about fetal monitoring and the proper actions that they must take in maternal, fetal, or neonatal emergencies. In addition, nurses have a legal obligation to inform the attending physician of their observations of the patient during the physician's absence through careful, accurate charting.

Fetal monitoring

See the discussion on equipment (p. 639).

Anesthetics

During labor and delivery, anesthetics are given for the mother's comfort, even though there are risks to the mother and infant. Nurse anesthetists must be aware of the correct procedures for administering anesthetics, and nurse attendants must also ensure the patient's safety. Ladimer (1975) describes two suits in which the administration of spinal anesthetic resulted in paralysis of the mother. In the first case, no pillow was placed under the mother's head during the administration of a saddle block anesthetic agent while she was in a side-lying position, resulting in the mother's subsequent paralysis. In the second case, leg paralysis was a result of improper stirrup adjustment during delivery.

Anesthetic risks to the infant should also be considered because all inhalant or intravenous anesthetic drugs promptly cross the placenta. The infant should be observed carefully after delivery if a general anesthetic is given, since the drugs used may have severe depressing effects on the infant. Gottschalk (1975) observes that because of possible serious complications which may accompany administration of anesthetics, anesthesiologists probably should administer these drugs, thus minimizing negligence related to the administration of the anesthetic.

Complications

Maternal. Numerous maternal complications may occur during the period of labor and delivery. Patients should not be left unattended during labor, and frequent physical assessment of the patient's condition should be made and charted. If the proper standard of care is not followed and the patient develops a complication, a case for negligence could be made.

If nurses detect signs of fetal distress, for example, meconium staining of the amniotic fluid, or if they should detect a prolapsed cord, they must notify the physician immediately and prepare for emergency treatment. If a cesarean section is likely, all details relevant to the operation should be observed, such as the patient's condition, observance of sterile technique, or counting sponges.

Neonatal. A series of initial care steps should be completed for all neonates. These include providing a patent airway, clamping the umbilical cord, and careful examination of the infant while providing a warm environment. Emergency resuscitation equipment for the infant must be available. Because birth is an extremely stressful situation for a newborn, a trained person whose sole responsibility is the care of the infant should be in the delivery room. Often the obstetrician, anesthesiologist, and nurse are all involved with the care of the mother, and the infant is placed off to one side with no one to even observe him. This is negligent care.

Cold stress, or subjecting an infant to an environmental temperature below his thermoneutral environmental level, can produce acidosis even in a healthy newborn and can also lead to respiratory problems. Therefore it is essential that the infant be kept warm in an incubator or under a radiant heating device where he can be observed until his temperature stabilizes. Since the evidence in current literature demonstrates that preventing cold stress is important and is therefore an accepted standard of care, the nurse has a legal responsibility to provide this care (Chapters 30 and 33).

In all states, careful identification of the infant is required. Fingerprints of the mother and handprints or footprints of the infant must be obtained by the nurse. In addition, arm bands must be affixed to the mother and infant. For legal reasons, it is important that the infant be identified as quickly as possible, preferably in the presence of the mother.

Stillborns

In an instance in which an infant is born dead, there must be careful documentation of the events surrounding the delivery. Even though the birth of a stillborn is disquieting, the nurse must carefully chart the events as they occur. Stillborns should be examined for congenital anomalies, using x-ray and laboratory studies, including chromosome studies when possible. This will provide essential documentation concerning reasons for fetal death, as well as facilitate genetic counseling for the parents.

Defective infants

Many infants require resuscitation at birth, and decisions must be made immediately as to whether resuscitation is necessary. Is it ethically and legally permissible to withold resuscitation from small preterm infants and/or infants with congenital anomalies? This may be ethically appropriate, but the omission may lead to legal complications. Some of these issues are discussed below.

LEGAL ISSUES IN POSTNATAL UNIT

Nursing care of postnatal patients involves legal obligations also. If a postnatal patient convulses or hemorrhages, the nurse must take the responsibility of notifying the physician and must take appropriate supportive action. Suits have been initiated because of postnatal infection. If a patient can prove that incorrect technique was the cause of the infection, she may have a legal right to claim negligence. If a patient is discharged early from the hospital and later develops a problem, she may sue the physician, claiming abandonment.

ETHICAL ISSUE OF EUTHANASIA IN NICU

The controversial issue of euthanasia deserves special attention. In October, 1973, Duff and Campbell broke the silence of the taboo subject of euthanasia in special care nurseries. They described 43 patients who were the subjects of passive euthanasia after intensive considerations by the staff and parents. In the background information for their report, Duff and Campbell (1973) stated that some parents believed "their child had a right to die since he could not live well or effectively." The physicians sometimes concluded that, "the parents' or siblings' rights to relief from the seemingly pointless, crushing burdens were important considerations." For these and other reasons, "As a result, some treatments were withheld or stopped with the knowledge that earlier death and relief from suffering would result." The parents gave informed consent for the withdrawal of treatment. In these instances, the personnel who were involved with these severely affected hopeless infants believed that the infants had acquired the right to die.

These infants present problems that are highly controversial and emotionally charged. Although those involved in the care of these infants reluctantly reach the inevitable conclusion that the infant should expire, the decision is never an easy one. There are some who argue that these decisions are illegal, and Duff and Campbell conclude, "If working out these dilemmas in ways such as we suggest is in violation of the law, we believe the law should be changed."

Waldman (1976) deplores the actions of physicians who decide that certain patients should be allowed to die, although he concedes the ethical situations are extremely difficult to resolve. He states, "Decisions to withhold extraordinary care must be limited to those patients who have zero potential and zero prognosis." The Committee on Ethics and Survival of the Nassau Pediatric Society (of which Waldman was chairman) adopted the following resolutions: (1) that a committee be formed in each hospital, including persons from health and legal professions, clergy, social workers, geneticist, and lay persons, to be involved in the decision-making process of allowing the withdrawal of extraordinary measures to continue life and that (2) "all resuscitative measures necessary for the survival of the newborn infant, regardless of weight or condition, should be employed in the immediate neonatal period."

The right to die for infants must be decided for the individual, not dogmatically by category, and the ultimate decision is the responsibility of the attending physician, asserts McCormick (1974). He suggests that criteria should be set to determine infants who should be saved despite illness or deformity and those who should be allowed to die. The sophistication of modern medicine has produced this dilemma: many infants who would have died quickly a few years ago now may be saved.

Robertson (1975) reviews the practice of passive, involuntary euthanasia from a legal standpoint. He stresses that infants cannot give consent, and if the parents consent to withholding lifesaving treatment, the infant cannot demand his rights.

Are there criteria that can be used for decision making, for example, no treatment for anencephalics but treatment for hydrocephalics? Robertson (1975) states: "Since the power to cause the death of a defective newborn is an awesome one, it is essential that such decision be carefully confined by law." He further concluded, "Such decisions are made by people trying to do what they think is best under extremely difficult circumstances. The suggestion that such sincere and well-intended decisions might be criminal is offensive." Robertson does not believe criminal charges should be filed, but he suggests that charges *could* be brought. This does not mean that prosecution would lead to conviction, however.

Parents, nurses, and physicians may be risking criminal liability unless they are aware of the legal ramifications of their actions. Parents must be informed that they risk criminal liability for child neglect by consenting to withhold treatment. Robertson insists that "Nurses who participate or acquiesce in parental decisions to withhold treatment may also be at risk." In the case of a defective infant, withholding essential care presents a possible case of homicide by omission against the parents, physicians, and nurses, with the degree of homicide dependent on the extent of premeditation. The courts have not ruled directly on the criminal liability of personnel who refuse extraordinary lifesaving care for defective infants; however, parents have been prosecuted for directly killing defective children.

Robertson supports the suggestion by Duff and Campbell that parents and physicians making the decision to withhold essential treatment is inappropriate. He suggests that a better alternative would be to have a committee serve as the patient advocate. He does not want this controversy to be resolved by criminal proceedings but rather that decisions be made outside the courts, providing there are safeguards to the decision-making process. Finally, he states: "The existence of potential criminal liability is no guarantee that parents, physicians, nurses, and hospitals will in fact be prosecuted, nor that any prosecution would be successful."

SUMMARY

A wide variety of ethical and legal issues arise in the multifaceted field of maternity care. This chapter has presented a review of current legal attitudes toward several of the issues a nurse may encounter in her care of maternity patients. Perinatal nursing is a rapidly developing subspecialty, and the continued emergence of nurse-midwifery promises to be an exciting trend of the future.

Genetics not only presents legal problems today, but
more legal issues will arise in the years to come. The
abortion issue remains controversial and probably always
will. The concepts inherent in the practice of euthanasia
in the NICU raise many ethical and legal questions.
Legal aspects of maternity nursing are fascinating and
essential knowledge for all nurses who plan to care for
new mothers and infants.

REFERENCES

Ament, M. 1974. The right to be well-born. J. Leg. Med. **2:**
24, Nov.-Dec.

Avery, M. E. 1975. Considerations on the definition of viability. N. Engl. J. Med. **292:**206.

Bok, S. 1974. Ethical problems of abortion. Hastings Cent.
Rep. **2,** Jan.

Camenisch, P. F. 1976. Abortion: for the fetus' own sake.
Hastings Cent. Rep. **6:**38, April.

Creighton, H. 1974. The malpractice problem. Nurs. Clin.
North Am. **9:**425.

Curran, W. J. 1973. The abortion decision: the Supreme Court
as moralist, scientist, historian, and legislator. N. Engl. J.
Med. **228:**950.

Curran, W. J. 1975. Experimentation becomes a crime: fetal
research in Massachusetts. N. Engl. J. Med. **292:**300.

Duff, R. S., and Campbell, A. G. 1973. Moral and ethical
dilemmas in the special care nursery. N. Engl. J. Med. **281:**
890.

Edwards, R. G. 1973. The problem of compensation for antenatal injuries. Nature **246:**54, Nov.

Fost, N. 1974. Our curious attitude toward the fetus. Hastings
Cent. Rep. **4:**4, Feb.

Gottschalk, W. 1975. Problems and risks of obstetrical anesthesia. In Aladjem, S. (ed.). Risks in the practice of modern
obstetrics. St. Louis, The C. V. Mosby Co.

Hirsch, H. L. 1975. Legal guidelines for the performance of
abortions. Am. J. Obstet. Gynecol. **122:**679.

Ladimer, I. 1975. Risks in the practice of modern obstetrics—
a legal point of view. In Aladjem, S. (ed.). Risks in the
practice of modern obstetrics. St. Louis, The C. V. Mosby
Co.

McCormick, R. A. 1974. To save or let die—the dilemma of
modern medicine. J.A.M.A. **229:**172.

McGarrah, R. E. 1974. Voluntary female sterilization: abuses,
risks and guidelines. Hastings Cent. Rep. **4:**5, June.

Milunsky, A. 1974. Prenatal diagnosis of genetic abnormalities. Clin. Perinatol. **1:**25.

Noon, C. 1975. The right to reproduce. Lancet **2:**625.

Richardson, D. W. 1975. Artificial insemination in the human.
In Emery, A. E. H. (ed.). Modern trends in human genetics. London, Butterworths.

Robertson, J. A. 1975. Involuntary euthanasia of defective
newborns: a legal analysis. Stanford Law Review **27:**269.

Robertson, J. A., and Fost, N. 1976. Passive euthanasia of
defective newborn infants: legal considerations. J. Pediatr.
88:883.

Sadoff, R. 1975. Questions and answers. J. Leg. Med. **3:**9.

Steinfels, P. 1974. Choosing the sex of our children. Hastings
Cent. Rep. **4:**3, Feb.

Stenchever, M. A. 1972. An abuse of prenatal diagnosis.
J.A.M.A. **221:**408.

Steptoe, P. C. 1976. Reimplantation of a human embryo with
subsequent tubal pregnancy. Lancet **1:**880.

Stubblefield, P. J. 1975. Abortion vs. manslaughter, Arch.
Surg. **110:**790.

Waldman, A. M. 1976. Medical ethics and the hopelessly ill
child. J. Pediatr. **88:**891.

Wecht, C. H. 1975. A comparison of two abortion-related
legal inquiries. J. Leg. Med. **3:**26.

CHAPTER 39

Problem-oriented system

HELEN READEY

Maternity patients represent typical consumers of health care services in that they are now more aware of what constitutes quality health care and more likely to demand greater accountability of the health care team. Concurrent with this attitude toward accountability, patients also have the right to full and complete disclosure of the medical record documenting their care.

In response to these events and in an effort to improve patient care, Weed (1969, 1970) introduced a new system of compiling and using medical-related data. For the maternity patient as well as other patients, it reflects a plan of management of the whole patient with a succinct list of all problems—physical, psychologic, socioeconomic, and demographic. No one problem is treated out of context or in direct opposition to other existing problems. The problem-oriented system as it is known is a threefold system that includes (1) a problem-oriented record (POR), (2) a process of auditing to detect deficiencies, and (3) techniques for correcting these deficiencies.

The components of the POR are the data base, problem list, initial plan, and progress notes. (See examples of POR on pp. 652 and 653.)

DATA BASE

The data base encompasses the sum total of all information gathered about any one patient on admission. Included in the data base are the patient's past history, present medical and nursing history, personal and psychosocial history, family history, physical examination and review of systems, laboratory findings, and patient profile. The patient profile is a brief narrative about the patient's life-style and that of the family.

Data should not be collected haphazardly but should be the result of preliminary decisions about the information needed. If the collection of data cannot be made initially, perhaps because of the patient's presenting problem, which may be of an emergency nature, then the first problem on the problem list becomes "incomplete data base."

If a patient is readmitted who has previously been evaluated with a POR, it is only necessary to write an interval note that relates the previous admission to the current admission.

The information collected must be scrutinized and condensed to synthesize a problem list. Conclusions as to the nature of problems are supported by the information accumulated in the data base. The data base continues to grow as more information is added, and it is out of the data base that problems continue to emerge.

PROBLEM LIST

A problem may be defined as a "patient's unmet need or lack of observable and/or nonobservable elements which a human being must have for physical and psychological homeostasis or equilibrium" (Berni and Readey, 1974). The problem list becomes the index to the patient's health record and represents an updated synoptic overview of information available about any one patient.

The problem list is frequently referred to as the "kingpin" of the system because it allows one to see clearly the relationship between all the patient's problems by encouraging the tagging of physical, psychologic, socioeconomic, and demographic problems. This approach assures a more humanistic manner of delivering health care. The health professional will continuously be reminded that derangements other than those of a physical nature may seriously impede the patient's ability to function.

All health care personnel are invited to add to the problem list, but the problem should be stated at a level of refinement in keeping with the understanding of the recorder. For example: "persistent vomiting" defined by the nurse may be redefined as "hyperemesis gravidarum'' by the physician. Caution must be used in making an assessment without substantiating evidence. It is suggested that a problem be listed as a symptom until diagnostic studies or other significant new information permits refining that symptom to a diagnosis. However, the system is open and permits the simple and complex, the ill-defined and well-established diagnosis to be used as problems.

Because the problem list summarizes all the known problems of the patient, it is usually the first page of the patient's chart. A number is affixed to each problem so that all subsequent plans and progress notes can use this identifying number. Problems are updated as evidence permits, and an arrow is used to indicate the level of resolution of that problem as shown in the following example:

5. 3/1/75 Hypertension $\xrightarrow{3/2/75}$ Preeclampsia-eclampsia

These arrows preserve the chronologic order the system dictates. A problem that is resolved will not necessitate the use of arrows, and the ultimate degree of resolution is considered to be a diagnosis. After the problem is resolved, its identifying number is no longer reassigned. The number assigned to a problem serves to trace the course of a single problem through the patient's chart.

The problem list often enables the medical practitioner to discern a constellation of problems that may resemble a well-defined syndrome. When this occurs, the numbers assigned to problems that are now included in the syndrome will no longer be used.

In the psychiatric adaptation of the Weed system, an inventory of the patient's assets and resources is included. The rationale is that these assets are necessary to develop a reasonable treatment plan that will reestablish the state of homeostasis. Problems here are also expressed in their own observational terms. That is, ''spends most of her time alone'' or ''cries easily'' would be preferred to a diagnosis of ''depression.''

Minor episodes that are of a self-limiting or temporary nature are simply designated as tentative problems and included in the progress notes. If the problem continues for a period exceeding 72 hours, it should be added to the current problem list. This approach simply eliminates a cluttered problem list. The problem list then summarizes at a glance all the problems of any one patient and designates their state of resolution. Weed (1969) remarked, ''The length of the problem list is the Lord's business, the quality of it is yours.''

INITIAL PLAN

The initial plan includes the physician's orders or medical directives. These are numbered and titled cor-

respondingly to problems on the problem list. Some of these directives are aimed at establishing a diagnosis and include all the necessary studies. They represent an orderly approach to the acquisition of the requisite information. Rule outs (R/O) belong here. An example follows:

R/O multiple pregnancy—do a scanogram.

Other directives are related to the management prescribed as therapy and still others to patient education. These latter include the precise directions given to the patient and her family regarding the management of her problem(s). This minimizes conflicting information dispensed by the health team personnel. Patient education often serves to transform the patient into an intelligent partner in her own care. She should understand that she possesses the power to influence the course and outcome of her pregnancy.

PROGRESS NOTES

Numbered and titled progress notes constitute the follow-up phase of the problem-oriented approach. They coincide with the problem list and enable any team member to read all data collected regarding any one problem without having to search through a multiplicity of information pertaining to other problems. This accumulation of data specific to each problem provides the health professional with a more reliable basis for formulating a meaningful therapeutic strategy. Progress notes include narrative notes, flow sheets, and discharge summary.

Narrative notes. The acronym SOAP has proved a useful reminder of the four elements of the narrative notes: Subjective, Objective, Assessment, and Plan. The SOAP format is used as a framework for organized documentation and is compatible with the problem-solving approach as used in the nursing process. This suggested format includes a narrative account of observations, an assessment, and plan(s) regarding the possible solution of the problem. Separate SOAPs are constructed for each problem. The system suggests that this SOAP format be used when writing narrative progress notes and discharge summaries and when consultations are indicated.

Data collected is divided into two parts, subjective and objective. *Subjective* refers to the problem from the patient's point of view. Using quotation marks is recommended so that all disciplines reading the quotation can draw their own conclusions as to what the patient is implying. It is not necessary to use all four components of the SOAP format, so if the patient does not contribute to defining the problem, the ''S'' is simply followed by ''none.'' *Objective* findings include clinical observations made or specific information collected that relates to the problem on hand such as pertinent laboratory findings. The *assessment* is the conclusion that one reaches after analyzing the subjective and objective findings. Assessment may connote progression or regression in relation to the problem. The *plan* signifies in detail the course to be followed regarding the problem. As designated under initial plans, this aspect is written as a threefold plan in light of diagnostic plans, therapeutic plans, and plans for patient education.

Nursing personnel usually are expected to write at least one SOAP note every 24 hours. This does not mean, however, that each item on the problem list must be discussed with such frequency. All disciplines associated with patient care should contribute to the progress notes so that a chronologic sequence is preserved.

Examples of narrative notes are on pp. 654 and 655.

Flow sheets. Flow sheets are an excellent way to follow the course of any disease process to identify parameters and to monitor rapidly changing or complex problems as in the delivery unit. Flow sheets can be used in lieu of narrative progress notes, but a summary of change, stability, or progress should appear periodically in SOAP format on the progress sheet. The flow sheet readily reveals relationships between many variables and indicates the patient's progress at a glance. The labor or newborn record is an excellent example of a flow sheet.

Discharge summary. The general format for the discharge summary is problem oriented and includes all problems listed on the problem list. The focus is on providing for continuity of care and an overall assessment of accomplishments of hospitalization or care given. Active and inactive problems are designated, and each is discussed in SOAP fashion. The plan should include proposed follow-up, and any prescribed regimen should be spelled out in detail. Active problems not considered during hospitalization are enumerated, along with a statement regarding the reason for nonintervention.

Consultations are requested in reference to a specific problem and its corresponding number, but it is essential that the consultant is aware of all problems so as to avoid treatment out of context. The discussion appears in SOAP format and should support decisions reached and recommendations made. New problems may be added to the problem list as a result of a consultation.

The process of auditing the POR as a means of correcting deficiencies in patient care requires adopting standards of care, evaluating the care given in light of these standards to detect deficiencies, recommending

action to correct acknowledged deficiencies, and assessing the effectiveness of the approaches selected for corrective action. Regarding the process of audit, Weed (1969) emphasizes the need for thoroughness, reliability, analytic sense, and efficiency. Audit illuminates the logic used in the reasoning process and determines the proficiency of one's course of action to measure performance. Evaluation of the quality of patient care is a prerequisite to determining where improvement and alteration in the delivery of care must take place.

The problem-oriented system acts as a tool for quality control of medical care, since documentary proof regarding patient problems is now readily available. Allied health personnel become directly accountable to the patient for the quality of care rendered. The problem-oriented system provides a method of coping with the weaknesses and capitalizing on the strengths of our health care system.

Advantages of the problem-oriented system may be summarized as follows:

1. Simplifies search for data by providing a means of cataloging information on a problem list, serving as a summary or index to the patient's chart
2. Facilitates the coordination of medical care with nursing care, since both disciplines are permitted to use the same chart forms
3. Does not in itself guarantee delivery of better health care, but it does facilitate sharing of expertise among all multidisciplinary health personnel caring for the same patient
4. Replaces a memory-oriented system with a documented system
5. Converts a source-oriented, disorganized, unindexed patient medical record to a well-organized, indexed record of information that is clearly visible and retrievable
6. Provides a means of cross-indexing of plans and progress notes, since they are keyed to the numbered problems as they are seen on the problem list
7. Supports the need to spend more time with patients so that the patient's milieu is clearly apparent before an attempt is made to define problems
8. Encourages an orientation to preventive, health-oriented care, as well as illness care, by documenting patient education
9. Assists in determining professional accountability with regard to the current concerns of licensure, peer review, and professional certification
10. Focuses on the patient as an individual when it

encourages the identification of physical, psychologic, socioeconomic, and demographic problems

11. Enhances the communication process among all team members, encouraging genuine cooperation and exchange of philosophies
12. Provides a framework for professional growth
13. Elevates the patient's record to the level of a scientific manuscript and stimulates critical thinking by advocating use of the problem-solving process
14. Lends itself to computerization and research endeavors
15. Serves as a teaching document and is considered to be the key to continuing education
16. Permits information concerning a specific problem to be released while confidentiality of the remainder of the record is assured
17. Provides a continuing chronologic sequence of developments regarding health care
18. Encourages the use of clinical algorithms (a pre-agreed-on sequence of events used in the management of certain common problems)
19. Permits nursing care plans to become part of the patient's permanent record and encourages the use of the nursing process
20. Encourages patients to keep a list of their problems on their person at all times, thereby assuring that the treatment of one problem will not prove detrimental to others
21. Problem list provides for successful continuity from one shift to another and for "float" personnel because it quickly acquaints all team members with the whole gamut of problems listed on any one patient's chart
22. Facilitates audit by providing a feedback loop that helps to continually upgrade the quality of care, interpret the activities of all disciplines, and compare the patient's care to established standards of practice

---

POR: FAMILY RELATIONSHIPS—FATHER*

Data base	Problem list (unmet needs)	Initial plans (possible solutions)	Progress notes
May 10: "She acts so crazy. Crying all the time. Too tired to do anything. What's wrong?"	1.† Needs information regarding normal changes of pregnancy.	1. Discuss changes of pregnancy (physical, emotional, sexual) and father's feelings regarding these.	1. Resolved.
"She wants to breast-feed. I can't stand the thought. It's so animal-like."	2. Difference between husband and wife preferences on method of feeding newborn.	2. Encourage couple to discuss feelings about breast/bottle–feeding openly. Meet with both again; at subsequent meeting; stat after delivery.	2. Unresolved.
Wife is Rh negative.	3. Possibility of isoimmunization.	3. Take blood specimen. Determine type, Rh and inform couple at next visit.	3. Unresolved.
"I want to get her there (hospital) on time. I don't want to look stupid."	4. Needs information regarding signs of labor, other occurrences. Wants to perform adequately.	4. Refer to expectant parents' class, or meet with nurse to discuss signs of labor, who to call, what to report, where to go. Give printed sheet with above information on it.	4. Will think about classes and check some out. Unresolved.
July 22: Lost his job. Short on savings.	8. Needs financial assistance.	8. Refer to social worker for food stamps, etc.	8. Unresolved.
Dec. 17, after baby: "When the baby cries, I get so mad, so frustrated. Sometimes I get up and go for a walk."	11. Difficulty coping with infant's crying.	11. Discuss feelings about crying. Discuss infant crying as a form of communication. Discuss methods of coping with crying. Give telephone number of place to call if frustration builds too high. Arrange to meet with couple regarding this at subsequent visits.	11. Unresolved.

*Exerpts from a patient's record.
†Numbers correspond to those on patient's record.

POR: BIRTH OF INFANT WITH DOWN'S SYNDROME*

Data base	Problem list (unmet needs)	Initial plans (possible solutions)	Progress notes
April 12: Mother weeping frequently, pacing floor, keeps face to wall when in bed, nibbles at food.	1.†Grief work.	1. Plan times to be available to parent(s). Initiate discussion about infant.	1. Mother's rest and diet improved somewhat. Weeps frequently especially when viewing infant.
April 13: Mother and father hesitant to hold infant. Refer to child as "it."	2. Establishing a positive mother-child-father relationship.	2. Allow and encourage parent(s) to visit and hold infant when ready. Refer to infant by name. Point out and explain physical and behavioral characteristics while holding infant.	2. Mother held infant; father not ready yet. Both hesitantly referred to her by name.
April 14: 22-year-old primipara who has had uneventful pregnancy and labor.	3. Diagnosis of etiology of Down's syndrome.	3. Construct pedigree, do karyotype on mother; dermatoglyphics. Explain procedures to mother and discuss her reactions to them. Make appointment for couple at genetics clinic next week.	3. Mother listened quietly, nodding head occasionally. No questions at this time.
Dec. 20: Infant has been irritable and uninterested in food for 2 days, temperature of 101° F, runny nose.	7. Upper respiratory tract infection.	7. Diagnosis: viral infection. Treatment: cough suppressant; antibiotics, postural drainage. Parent education: postural drainage, medications. Parents to call back in 2 days.	7. Mother learned how to do postural drainage quickly; gave medication under supervision; feels comfortable about daughter's care.
June, 2 years later: Parents think mother needs some time to herself and child needs additional social stimulation and special training. Mother also wants to learn more about teaching her daughter.	20. Entry into school system.	20. Give list of available schools in area for children with special problems. Parents to see social worker regarding financial arrangements and transportation.	20. Parents seemed agreeable and interested in implementing plan.
Mother complains of inability to deny child anything and frustration by child's slow learning. Parents express hesitance in disciplining child with "her problem."	21. Discipline.	21. Exploration of parental feelings and ideas regarding discipline. Development of an acceptable, consistent approach to discipline. Appointment with pediatric nurse specialist in a week.	21. Parents discussed ideas regarding discipline and decided on a short-term goal: setting limits at bedtime.

*Excerpts from a patient's record.
†Numbers correspond to those on patient's record.

NARRATIVE NOTES: NAUSEA AND VOMITING IN ANTENATAL PERIOD*

Subjective data	Objective data	Assessment	Plan
Example I: First trimester			

Comes on early in morning on rising and late in afternoon. Cannot face making dinner.	1. No history of flu or contact with persons with stomach upsets.
	2. Bouts daily and intermittent.
	3. Pregnancy 5 weeks' duration.
	4. Temperature normal.
	5. Pulse: 80/min.
	6. BP: 110/80.
	7. No proteinuria or glycosuria.
	8. Embarrassed at work by nausea.
		Diagnosis: nausea and vomiting associated with pregnancy.	1. Instruct patient concerning following:
			  a. Probable cause: normal response to pregnancy; may be expected to last about 4 more weeks.
			  b. Diet: small frequent feedings, some carbohydrates (e.g., crackers and milk) before rising and as afternoon snack.
			  c. Motion: Discuss ways of rising slowly to minimize sudden hypotension.
			  d. Telephoning in progress report in 1 week's time.

Example II: Second trimester			

All food is nauseating. Cannot keep anything down. Feels ill and desperate.	1. Patient appears dehydrated, has lost weight (10 pounds), is tense and nervous.
	2. Vomiting persists after every meal. Did not stop after third month of pregnancy.
	3. No history of colds or contacts with persons with flu.
	4. Pregnancy 14 weeks' duration.
	5. Uncommunicative about family situation.
	6. Temperature: 99.6° F, not above 100.4° F.
	7. Pulse: 90/min usual.
	8. BP: 105/70.
	9. No proteinuria or glycosuria.
	10. No abdominal tenderness.
	11. No jaundice.
		Diagnosis: possible hyperemesis gravidarum.	1. Notify physician of findings.
			2. Give recognition to patient of seriousness of condition for self and baby.
			3. Prepare patient for possible hospitalization for following:
			  a. Correction of dehydration and malnourishment by special diet and if necessary IV therapy.
			  b. Rest and relief from active participation in daily activities of home and/or work.
			  c. Further medical investigation (e.g., blood tests, etc.).
			  d. Supportive therapy for any psychosocial problems.

*Examples of recordings in patient's records.

NARRATIVE NOTES: PAIN IN POSTNATAL PERIOD*

Subjective data	Objective data	Assessment	Plan
Problem: Headache			
Example I			

1. "Generalized headache."
2. "Persistent and severe."
	1. Delivery 72 hours ago.
	2. BP 130/90.
	3. Urinalysis +3 protein.
	4. Edema—face puffy.
	5. No anesthesia at delivery.
	6. No record of elevated BP.
		Possible postnatal pre-eclampsia.	1. Notify physician immediately.
			2. Meanwhile
			  a. Confine to bed; ensure rest.
			  b. Repeat BP q ½ hour.
			  c. Begin I and O sheet.
			  d. Have medications, padded tongue blade, O_2, and suction accessible.

*Examples to illustrate differing assessments of a problem and differing plans of care.

Subjective data	Objective data	Assessment	Plan
Problem: Headache—cont'd			
Example I—cont'd			
	7. Up and about; appears anxious, fretful.		e. Stay with mother when infant is with her. 3. Record findings immediately.
Example II 1. "Generalized headache." 2. "Persistent and severe." 3. "Feels like vomiting."	1. Delivery 36 hours ago. 2. BP 105/70, same as prenatal baseline BP. 3. Spinal anesthesia for delivery. 4. Headache worse when up.	Spinal headache.	1. Best rest, supine position. 2. Head elevation <8 inches. 3. Medication as ordered. 4. Force fluids. 5. Ice bag to head. 6. Record and report to physician on next rounds.

Example III
1. "Generalized headache."
2. "Comes and goes."
3. "No one pays any attention to me"; "I hate it here."
	1. Delivery 24 hours ago.
	2. BP 110/70, same as prenatal baseline BP.
	3. Local anesthesia for delivery.
	4. Crying, face tense, hands clenched, hostile remarks regarding care.
		Stress headache. Anxiety level high.	1. Comfort measures, bath, rub back, clean linen, etc.
			2. Medication if ordered and wanted.
			3. Listen to patient for cues as to source of discomfort.
			4. If mood and/or headache persist
			  a. Notify physician.
			  b. Involve family.
			  c. Alert community agency.

Problem: Breast tenderness			
Example I 1. "Generalized tenderness extending into armpit." 2. "Constant, increases with pressure or touch; breasts feel hot."	1. 48 hours after delivery. 2. Breasts feel tense, are swollen, feel warm to touch, veins are prominent, ipsilateral axillary adenopathy. 3. Tender to touch. 4. Not breast-feeding. 5. Refused Tace after delivery. 6. Temperature 98.8° F.	Engorgement prior to drying up of breasts.	1. Firm breast binder, ice bag to breast. 2. Information regarding length of time discomfort may be expected to last (48 hours). 3. Medication for discomfort as ordered. 4. Avoid allowing hot shower water run on breasts. 5. Do not express milk.

Example II
1. "Nipples sore when baby sucks."
	1. 3 days after delivery.
	2. Nipples macerated and fissured.
	3. Allows baby to suck as long as he wants.
	4. Mother fair-skinned.
	5. Temperature 98° F.
		Nipples damaged by too lengthy sucking of infant.	1. Decrease sucking time to 4 to 5 min/breast for 3 days.
			2. Expose nipple to air, wash after feeding, dry carefully.
			3. Suggest
			  a. Using nipple shield.
			  b. Expressing milk and feeding by bottle for 1 or 2 days.
			4. After 3 days gradually increase sucking time 1 min/feeding/day. Increase number of feedings (every 2 hours) if necessary.

Example III 1. "One part of breast very tender and enlarged." 2. "Having chills, feels feverish." 3. "Rash over breast area."	1. 3 weeks after delivery. 2. Erythema over infected and undated segment. 3. Ipsilateral axillary adenopathy. 4. Breast painful to touch. 5. Temperature 102° F.	Possible mastitis.	1. Notify physician of findings immediately. 2. Nursing can be continued until medical advice received. 3. If nursing discontinued, pump breast if wishes to breast-feed again. 4. Firm supportive brassiere. 5. Force fluids. 6. Medication as ordered for discomfort.

REFERENCES

Berni, R., and Readey, H. 1974. Problem-oriented medical record implementation: allied health peer review. St. Louis, The C. V. Mosby Co.

Bjorn, J. C., and Cross, H. D. 1970. The problem oriented practice of private medicine. New York, McGraw-Hill Book Co.

Bloom, J., and others. 1971. Problem-oriented charting, Am. J. Nurs. **71:**2144.

Brubacker, J. S. 1962. Modern philosophies of education. New York, McGraw-Hill Book Co.

Hurst, J. W. 1971. How to implement the Weed system. Arch. Intern. Med. **128:**456.

Schell, P., and Campbell, A. T. 1972. POMR—not just another way to chart. Nurs. Outlook **20:**510.

Weed, L. 1969. Medical records, medical education, and patient care. Chicago, Year Book Medical Publishers, Inc.

Weed, L. 1970. Medical records, medical education and patient care: the P-O record as a basic tool. Chicago, Year Book Medical Publishers, Inc.

Woody, M., and Mallison, M. 1973. The problem-oriented system for patient-centered care. Am. J. Nurs. **73:**1168.

APPENDIXES

APPENDIX A

The Pregnant Patient's Bill of Rights*

The Pregnant Patient has the right to participate in decisions involving her well-being and that of her unborn child, unless there is a clearcut medical emergency that prevents her participation. In addition to the rights set forth in the American Hospital Association's "Patient's Bill of Rights" (which has also been adopted by the New York City Department of Health), the Pregnant Patient, because she represents *two* patients rather than one, should be recognized as having the additional rights listed below.

1. *The Pregnant Patient has the right,* prior to the administration of any drug or procedure, to be informed by the health professional caring for her of any potential direct or indirect effects, risks or hazards to herself or her unborn or newborn infant which may result from the use of a drug or procedure prescribed for or administered to her during pregnancy, labor, birth or lactation.

2. *The Pregnant Patient has the right,* prior to the proposed therapy, to be informed, not only of the benefits, risks and hazards of the proposed therapy but also of known alternative therapy, such as available childbirth education classes which could help to prepare the Pregnant Patient physically and mentally to cope with the discomfort or stress of pregnancy and the experience of childbirth, thereby reducing or eliminating her need for drugs and obstetric intervention. She should be offered such information early in her pregnancy in order that she may make a reasoned decision.

3. *The Pregnant Patient has the right,* prior to the administration of any drug, to be informed by the health professional who is prescribing or administering the drug to her that any drug which she receives during pregnancy, labor and birth, no matter how or when the drug is taken or administered, may adversely affect her un-

born baby, directly or indirectly, and that there is no drug or chemical which has been proven safe for the unborn child.

4. *The Pregnant Patient has the right* if cesarean section is anticipated, to be informed prior to the administration of any drug, and preferably prior to her hospitalization, that minimizing her and, in turn, her baby's intake of nonessential pre-operative medicine, will benefit her baby.

5. *The Pregnant Patient has the right,* prior to the administration of a drug or procedure, to be informed if there is *no* properly controlled follow-up research which has established the safety of the drug or procedure with regard to its direct and/or indirect effects on the physiological, mental and neurological development of the child exposed, via the mother, to the drug or procedure during pregnancy, labor, birth or lactation—(this would apply to virtually all drugs and the vast majority of obstetric procedures).

6. *The Pregnant Patient has the right,* prior to the administration of any drug, to be informed of the brand name and generic name of the drug in order that she may advise the health professional of any past adverse reaction to the drug.

7. *The Pregnant Patient has the right* to determine for herself, without pressure from her attendant, whether she will accept the risks inherent in the proposed therapy or refuse a drug or procedure.

8. *The Pregnant Patient has the right* to know the name and qualifications of the individual administering a medication or procedure to her during labor or birth.

9. *The Pregnant Patient has the right* to be informed, prior to the administration of any procedure, whether that procedure is being administered to her for her or her baby's benefit (medically indicated) or as an elective procedure (for convenience or teaching purposes).

10. *The Pregnant Patient has the right* to be accom-

---

*From Haire, D. B. 1975. The Pregnant Patient's Bill of Rights. J. Nurse-Midwifery **20**:29, Winter. This article is not reproduced here in its entirety.

panied during the stress of labor and birth by someone she cares for, and to whom she looks for emotional comfort and encouragement.

11. *The Pregnant Patient has the right* after appropriate medical consultation to choose a position for labor and for birth which is least stressful to her baby and to herself.

12. *The Obstetric Patient has the right* to have her baby cared for at her bedside if her baby is normal, and to feed her baby according to her baby's needs rather than according to the hospital regimen.

13. *The Obstetric Patient has the right* to be informed in writing of the name of the person who actually delivered her baby and the professional qualifications of that person. This information should also be on the birth certificate.

14. *The Obstetric Patient has the right* to be informed if there is any known or indicated aspect of her or her baby's care or condition which may cause her or her baby later difficulty or problems.

15. *The Obstetric Patient has the right* to have her and her baby's hospital medical records complete, accurate and legible and to have their records, including Nurses' Notes, retained by the hospital until the child reaches at least the age of majority, or, alternatively, to have the records offered to her before they are destroyed.

16. *The Obstetric Patient,* both during and after her hospital stay, has the right to have access to her complete hospital medical records, including Nurses' Notes, and to receive a copy upon payment of a reasonable fee and without incurring the expense of retaining an attorney.

It is the obstetric patient and her baby, not the health professional, who must sustain any trauma or injury resulting from the use of a drug or obstetric procedure. The observation of the rights listed above will not only permit the obstetric patient to participate in the decisions involving her and her baby's health care, but will help to protect the health professional and the hospital against litigation arising from resentment or misunderstanding on the part of the mother.

APPENDIX B

United Nations Declaration of the Rights of the Child

PREAMBLE

Whereas the peoples of the United Nations have, in the Charter, reaffirmed their faith in fundamental human rights, and in the dignity and worth of the human person, and have determined to promote social progress and better standards of life in larger freedom,

Whereas the United Nations has, in the Universal Declaration of Human Rights, proclaimed that everyone is entitled to all the rights and freedoms set forth therein, without distinction of any kind, such as race, color, sex, language, religion, political or other opinion, national or social origin, property, birth or other status,

Whereas the child, by reason of his physical and mental immaturity, needs special safeguards and care, including appropriate legal protection, before as well as after birth,

Whereas the need for such special safeguards has been stated in the Geneva Declaration of the Rights of the Child of 1924, and recognized in the Universal Declaration of Human Rights and in the statutes of specialized agencies and international organizations concerned with the welfare of children,

Whereas mankind owes to the child the best it has to give

NOW THEREFORE THE GENERAL ASSEMBLY PROCLAIMS

This Declaration of the Rights of the Child to the end that he may have a happy childhood and enjoy for his own good and for the good of society the rights and freedoms herein set forth, and calls upon parents, upon men and women as individuals and upon voluntary organizations, local authorities and national governments to recognize these rights and strive for their observance by legislative and other measures progressively taken in accordance with the following principles:

PRINCIPLE 1

The child shall enjoy all the rights set forth in this Declaration. All children, without any exception whatsoever, shall be entitled to these rights, without distinction or discrimination on account of race, color, sex, language, religion, political or other opinion, national or social origin, property, birth or other status, whether of himself or of his family.

PRINCIPLE 2

The child shall enjoy special protection, and shall be given opportunities and facilities, by law and by other means, to enable him to develop physically, mentally, morally, spiritually and socially in a healthy and normal manner and in conditions of freedom and dignity. In the enactment of laws for this purpose the best interests of the child shall be the paramount consideration.

PRINCIPLE 3

The child shall be entitled from his birth to a name and a nationality.

PRINCIPLE 4

The child shall enjoy the benefits of social security. He shall be entitled to grow and develop in health; to this end special care and protection shall be provided both to him and to his mother, including adequate pre-natal and post-natal care. The child shall have the right to adequate nutrition, housing, recreation and medical services.

PRINCIPLE 5

The child who is physically, mentally or socially handicapped shall be given the special treatment, education and care required by his particular condition.

PRINCIPLE 6

The child, for the full and harmonious development of his personality, needs love and understanding. He shall, wherever possible, grow up in the care and under the responsibility of his parents, and in any case in an atmosphere of affection and of moral and material security; a child of tender years shall not, save in exceptional circumstances, be separated from his mother. Society and the public authorities shall have the duty to extend particular care to children without a family and to those without adequate means of support. Payment of state and other assistance toward the maintenance of children of large families is desirable.

PRINCIPLE 7

The child is entitled to receive education, which shall be free and compulsory, at least in the elementary stages. He shall be given an education which will promote his general culture, and enable him on a basis of equal opportunity to develop his abilities, his individual judgment, and his sense of moral and social responsibility, and to become a useful member of society.

The best interests of the child shall be the guiding principle of those responsible for his education and guidance; that responsibility lies in the first place with his parents.

The child shall have full opportunity for play and recreation, which shall be directed to the same purposes as education; society and the public authorities shall endeavor to promote the enjoyment of this right.

PRINCIPLE 8

The child shall in all circumstances be among the first to receive protection and relief.

PRINCIPLE 9

The child shall be protected against all forms of neglect, cruelty and exploitation. He shall not be the subject of traffic, in any form.

The child shall not be admitted to employment before an appropriate minimum age; he shall in no case be caused or permitted to engage in any occupation or employment which would prejudice his health or education, or interfere with his physical, mental or moral development.

PRINCIPLE 10

The child shall be protected from practices which may foster racial, religious and any other form of discrimination. He shall be brought up in a spirit of understanding, tolerance, friendship among peoples, peace and universal brotherhood and in full consciousness that his energy and talents should be devoted to the service of his fellow men.

APPENDIX C

Joint statement on maternity care (1971) and supplementary statement (1975)

JOINT STATEMENT ON MATERNITY CARE (1971)

The American College of Obstetricians and Gynecologists, The Nurses Association of The American College of Obstetricians and Gynecologists and the American College of Nurse-Midwives recognize the increasing needs for general health care and, more specifically, the deficits in availability and quality of maternity care. The latter, which are not confined to any social class, can best be corrected by the cooperative efforts of teams of physicians, nurse-midwives, obstetric registered nurses and other health personnel. The composition of such teams will vary and be determined by local needs and circumstances. The functions and responsibilities of team members should be clearly defined according to the education and training of the individuals concerned.

To achieve the aims of providing optimal maternity care for all women the following recommendations are made:

1. The health team organized to provide maternity care will be directed by a qualified obstetrician-gynecologist.

2. In such medically-directed teams, qualified nurse-midwives may assume responsibility for the complete care and management of uncomplicated maternity patients.

3. In such medically-directed teams, obstetric registered nurses may assume responsibility for patient care and management according to their education, training and experience.

4. In such medically-directed teams, other health personnel who have been trained in specific areas of maternity care may participate in the team functions according to their abilities and within the definitions of responsibility established by the team.

5. Written policies describing the specific functions of each of the team members should be prepared. They should be reviewed and revised periodically according to changing needs.

In endorsing the above statement, The American College of Obstetricians and Gynecologists, The Nurses Association of The American College of Obstetricians and Gynecologists and the American College of Nurse-Midwives recognize as their common goal the need for improvement and expansion of health services now being provided for women.

In order to maintain a continuing evaluation of the health services being provided for women and to plan for needed improvements and expansion, a mechanism for continued communication between all the organizations responsible for their provision is being developed.

The American College of Nurse-Midwives
1000 Vermont Avenue N.W.
Suite 500
Washington, D.C. 20005

The American College of Obstetricians and Gynecologists
One East Wacker Drive
Chicago, Illinois 60601

The Nurses Association of The American College of Obstetricians and Gynecologists
One East Wacker Drive
Chicago, Illinois 60601

SUPPLEMENTARY STATEMENT (1975)

Many questions have arisen concerning the meaning of the recommendation in the Joint Statement on Maternity Care (1971) that the health care team be "directed by a qualified obstetrician-gynecologist." These questions are justified and are accentuated by other developments in the specialty of obstetrics-gynecology which include the changing birth rate, formalization of new roles for personnel, emphasis on preventive care, HMO's, plans for national health insurance, PSRO, and regionalization of health services.

It is recognized that the obstetrician-gynecologist cannot under all circumstances be physically present to direct the health team; therefore it is essential that mechanisms of communication be clearly established for him or her to provide direction. Thus, the nature of the direction of the health team indeed becomes crucial.

The obstetrician-gynecologist working within a team giving health care to women has many responsibilities. These range from the direct provision of services to community health efforts and include:

a. The supervision of the medical care provided by all team members.

b. The direct provision of care for complications of pregnancy and for complex medical and surgical gynecological conditions.

c. The setting of medical care standards.

d. The provision of consultation to other team members.

e. The surveillance of task distribution within the team.

f. Participation in the ongoing educational activities of the team.

g. The introduction of new medical techniques as they become available.

h. The development of medical research.*

---

*From "Medical Practice in the Obstetric-Gynecologic Health Care Team." Interorganizational Committee on Ob/Gyn Health Personnel, September, 1973.

In view of the diversity of health care systems in which the obstetric-gynecologic health team currently functions, no universal systems model can be applied. Generally, however, the team is found in the following broad contexts:

1. Urban (intramural, on site, immediate referrals)
2. Rural (with institutional affiliation)
3. Rural (without institutional affiliation but with obstetric consultation available)
4. Private office (urban or rural)

The logistics of consultation and referral may vary with geographic and climatic conditions, but the following basic principles of team interaction are valid regardless of these conditions:

1. There must be a written agreement among members of the team clearly specifying consultation and referral policies and standing orders. The representatives of each practice discipline should participate in the development of and be signatory to the agreement.

2. The obstetrician-gynecologist, upon signing protocols, must accept full responsibility for direction of medical care rendered by the team in accordance with his or her orders.

3. In circumstances wherein the functions of the team leader are necessarily performed by physicians without specialty training in obstetrics-gynecology, medical direction should be provided through a formal consultative arrangement with a qualified obstetrician-gynecologist who is available to team members for continuing consultation and assurance of quality care.

APPENDIX D

Pregnancy diagnostic tests

BIOLOGIC TESTS

HCG produced by the chorionic villi appears in the blood and urine of pregnant women by the tenth day after conception. This hormone produces characteristic hemorrhagic changes in the ovaries of mice within 96 hours after injection (Aschheim-Zondek test) and of rabbits, within 48 hours (Friedman test).

HCG causes extrusion of ova in the female toad, ejection of sperm in the male frog or toad (Galli Mainini test), and ovarian hyperemia in the immature rat within 2 to 6 hours (Kupperman test).

IMMUNOLOGIC TESTS

These biologic tests have been largely superseded by immunologic bioassay tests for HCG: hemagglutination-inhibition (most sensitive test, fewer false negatives, but results are not obtained for 2 hours), complement-fixation test, and precipitation-reaction test. Pregnosticon* is a commonly used hemagglutination-inhibition test.

A simple (Latex inhibition) slide test using Gravidex†

---

*Organon Inc., West Orange, N.J.
†Ortho Pharmaceutical Corp., Raritan, N.J.

produces more rapid results, although it is less sensitive. In this procedure, a drop of antiserum (antihuman chorionic gonadotropin serum) is mixed on a slide with a drop of urine for 30 seconds. Then 2 more drops of antigen indicator are added and mixed by rocking the slide for 2 minutes. Visible agglutination is indicative of a *negative* reaction (pregnancy is unlikely). Absence of agglutination constitutes a *positive* test (pregnancy is likely).

OTHER TESTS

Other tests currently being used are ultrasonogram visualization of the conceptus and hormone-induced withdrawal bleeding test. The first can diagnose a pregnancy in the first 6 weeks and is harmless to mother and embryo. The second is performed immediately after the first missed menstrual period. A combination of progesterone and estrogen is taken orally for 2 to 3 days. On withdrawal of the medication, menstruation will occur in the nonpregnant woman within 2 weeks. In the pregnant woman, the production of the hormones by the corpus luteum and placenta is sufficient to maintain the pregnancy and no bleeding occurs.

APPENDIX E

Obstetric presentations, positions, and cervical dilatation

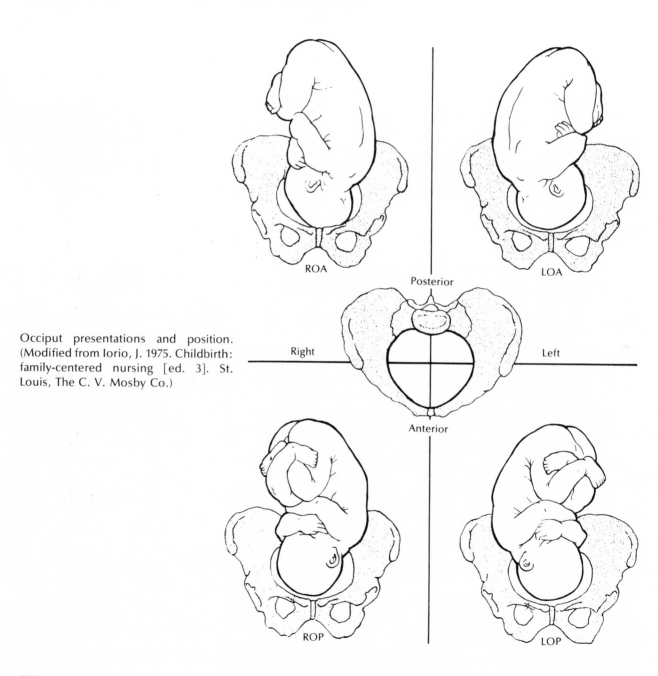

Occiput presentations and position. (Modified from Iorio, J. 1975. Childbirth: family-centered nursing [ed. 3]. St. Louis, The C. V. Mosby Co.)

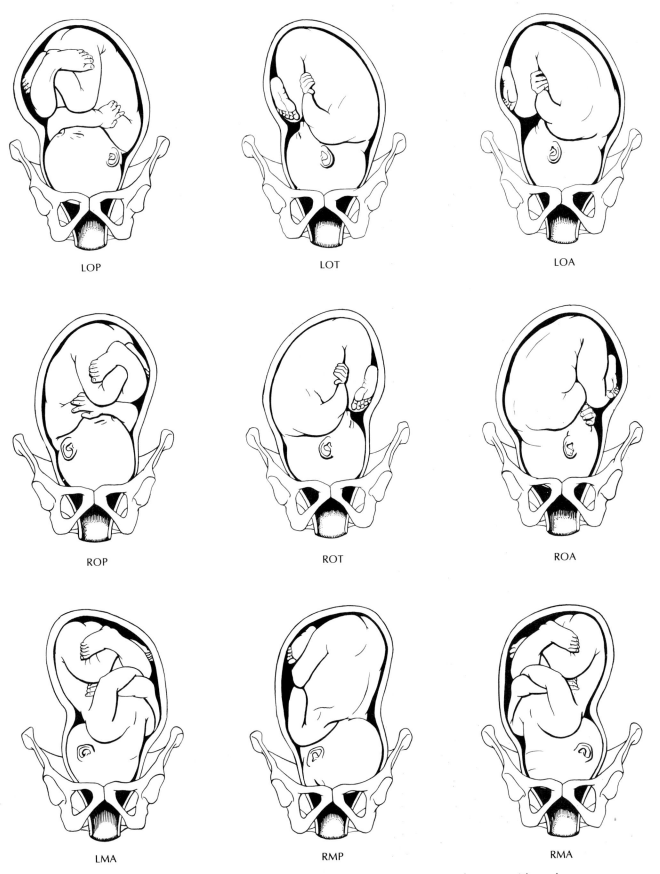

LOP   LOT   LOA

ROP   ROT   ROA

LMA   RMP   RMA

Categories of presentation and positions. Note outer contours of uterus with each presentation. (Courtesy Ross Laboratories, Columbus, Ohio.)

Continued.

Categories of presentation and positions.

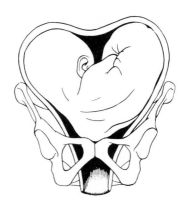

Shoulder presentation

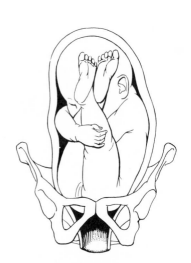

Frank breech
(complete breech)

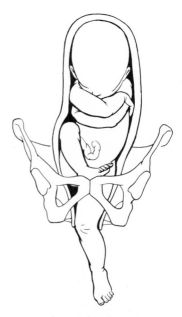

Incomplete breech
(single footling breech)

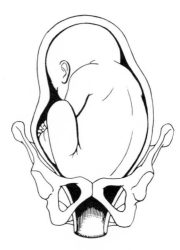

LSA

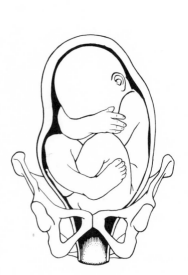

LSP

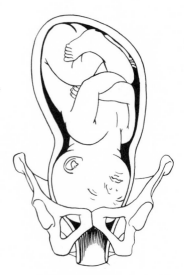

Brow presentation

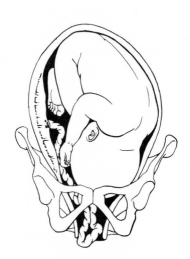

Prolapse of cord

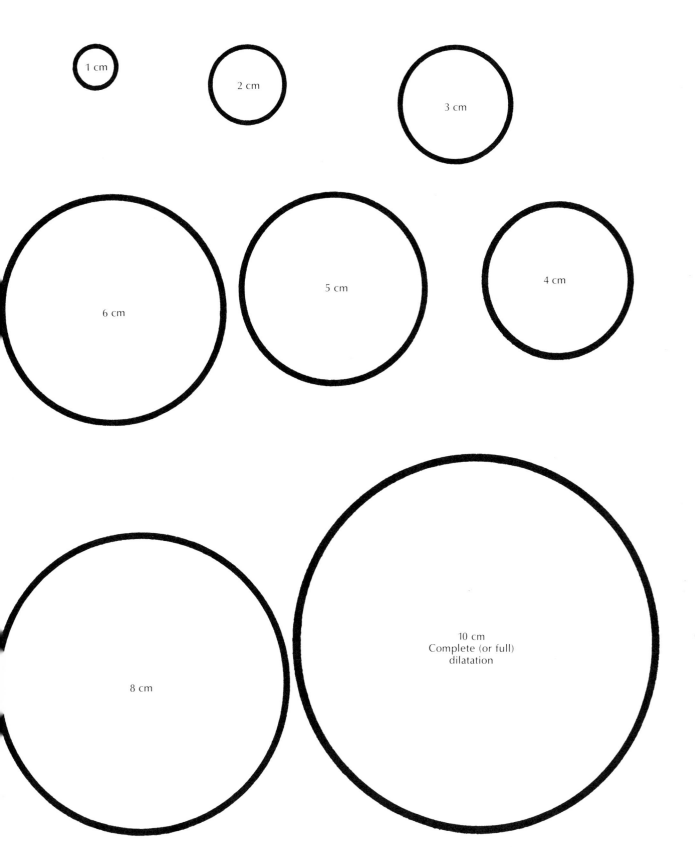

Aid for visualization of cervical dilatation.

APPENDIX F

Nutrition

STANDARD WEIGHT FOR HEIGHT (FEMALE)*

Height without shoes plus 1 inch	Standard weight
4' 10"	104
4' 11"	107
5' 0"	110
5' 1"	113
5' 2"	116
5' 3"	118
5' 4"	123
5' 5"	128
5' 6"	132
5' 7"	136
5' 8"	140
5' 9"	144
5' 10"	148
5' 11"	152
6' 0"	156

*The above weights were taken from Metropolitan Life Insurance Company, Actuarial Tables, 1959, and adjusted to comply with instructions appearing on the Gain in Weight Grid: height in inches without shoes plus 1 inch to establish a standard for heels. Patients should be weighed with shoes as normally worn. The table above is for medium body build and, except for extreme body build deviations, these figures should be used.

For example, a patient whose height, measured without shoes, is 5 feet 4 inches would have 1 inch added; therefore, her standard weight for height would be 128 pounds.

Ranges are not acceptable in estimating standard weight, since this is an objective observation and represents the midpoint. This midpoint must be used for recording purposes.

For patients under age 25, 1 pound should be deducted for each year.

FOOD LISTS FOR USE WITH LOW PHENYLALANINE DIET *

Food	Amount	Phenylalanine (mg)	Protein (gm)	Calories
Vegetables				
(each serving listed contains approximately 15 mg phenylalanine)				
Baby and Junior				
Beets	7 tbsp	15	1.1	35
Carrots	7 tbsp	15	0.7	28
Creamed spinach	1 tbsp	16	0.4	6
Green beans	2 tbsp	15	0.3	7
Squash	4 tbsp	14	0.4	14
Sweet potato	4 tbsp	15	0.7	42
Table vegetables				
Asparagus, cooked	1 stalk	12	0.6	4
Beans, green, cooked	4 tbsp (¼ cup)	14	0.6	9
Beans, yellow, wax, cooked	4 tbsp (¼ cup)	15	0.6	9
Bean sprouts, mung, cooked	2 tbsp	18	0.6	5
Beets, cooked	8 tbsp (½ cup)	14	0.8	34
Beet greens, cooked	1 tbsp	14	0.2	3
Broccoli, cooked	1 tbsp	11	0.3	3
Brussels sprouts, cooked	1 medium	16	0.6	5
Cabbage, raw, shredded	8 tbsp (½ cup)	15	0.7	12
Cabbage, cooked	5 tbsp (⅓ cup)	16	0.8	12
Carrots, raw	⅙ large (¼ cup)	16	0.5	16
Carrots, cooked	8 tbsp (½ cup)	17	0.5	23
Cauliflower, cooked	3 tbsp	18	0.6	6
Celery, cooked, diced†	4 tbsp (¼ cup)	15	0.4	6
Celery, raw†	1 8-inch stalk	16	0.5	7
Chard leaves, cooked	2 tbsp	19	0.6	6
Collards, cooked	1 tbsp	16	0.5	5
Cucumber slices, raw	8 slices, ⅛ inch thick	16	0.7	12
Eggplant, diced, raw	3 tbsp	18	0.4	9
Kale, cooked	2 tbsp	20	0.5	5
Lettuce†	3 small leaves	13	0.4	5
Mushrooms, cooked†	2 tbsp	14	0.4	35
Mushrooms, fresh†	2 small	16	0.5	3
Mustard greens, cooked	2 tbsp	18	0.6	6
Okra, cooked†	2 3-inch pods	13	0.4	7
Onion, raw, chopped	5 tbsp (⅓ cup)	14	0.5	20
Onion, cooked	4 tbsp (¼ cup)	14	0.5	19
Onion, young scallion	5 5-inch long	14	0.5	23
Parsley, raw, chopped†	3 tbsp	13	0.4	5
Parsnips, cooked, diced†	3 tbsp	13	0.3	18
Peas	1 tbsp	15	0.4	5
Peppers, raw, chopped†	4 tbsp	13	0.4	12
Pickles, dill	8 slices, ⅛ inch thick	16	0.7	12
Pumpkin, cooked	4 tbsp (¼ cup)	14	0.5	16
Radishes, red, small†	4	13	0.4	8
Rutabagas, cooked	2 tbsp	16	0.3	10
Spinach, cooked	1 tbsp	15	0.4	3
Squash, summer, cooked	8 tbsp (½ cup)	16	0.6	16
Squash, winter, cooked	3 tbsp	16	0.6	14
Tomato, raw	½ small	14	0.5	10

*Modified from Bureau of Public Health Nutrition of the California State Department of Public Health. 1961 revision. PKU, a diet guide for parents of children with phenylketonuria. Berkeley, Calif., pp. 7-11.
†Phenylalanine calculated as 3.3% of total protein.

Continued.

FOOD LISTS FOR USE WITH LOW PHENYLALANINE DIET—cont'd

Food	Amount	Phenylalanine (mg)	Protein (gm)	Calories
Vegetables—cont'd				
Table vegetables—cont'd				
Tomato, cooked	4 tbsp (¼ cup)	15	0.6	10
Tomato juice	4 tbsp (¼ cup)	17	0.6	12
Tomato catsup	2 tbsp	17	0.6	34
Turnip greens, cooked	1 tbsp	18	0.4	4
Turnips, diced, cooked	5 tbsp (⅓ cup)	16	0.4	12
Soups (condensed)				
Asparagus	1½ tbsp	16	0.5	14
Beef broth	1 tbsp	14	0.5	3
Celery	2 tbsp	18	0.4	19
Minestrone	1 tbsp	17	1.5	25
Mushroom	1 tbsp	11	0.2	17
Onion	1 tbsp	14	0.6	8
Tomato	1 tbsp	11	0.2	11
Vegetarian vegetable	1½ tbsp	17	0.4	14
Fruits				
(each serving listed contains approximately 15 mg phenylalanine)				
Baby and Junior				
Applesauce	11 tbsp	15	0.3	137
Applesauce and apricots	10 tbsp	15	0.4	128
Applesauce and pineapple	10 tbsp	15	0.3	110
Apricots with tapioca	12½ tbsp	15	0.5	146
Bananas	8 tbsp (½ cup)	14	0.6	97
Bananas and pineapple	10 tbsp	14	0.4	117
Peaches	9½ tbsp	16	0.7	117
Pears	14 tbsp	15	0.6	136
Pears and pineapple	14 tbsp	15	0.8	146
Plums with tapioca	11 tbsp	15	0.5	149
Prunes with tapioca	9½ tbsp	14	0.4	119
Fruit juices				
Apricot nectar	6 ounces (¾ cup)	14	0.6	102
Cranberry juice	12 ounces (1½ cup)	15	0.6	39
Grape juice	4 ounces (½ cup)	14	0.5	80
Grapefruit juice	8 ounces (1 cup)	16	1.2	104
Orange juice	6 ounces (¾ cup)	16	1.2	84
Peach nectar	5 ounces (⅔ cup)	15	0.5	75
Pineapple juice	6 ounces (¾ cup)	16	0.6	90
Prune juice	4 ounces (½ cup)	16	0.5	84
Table fruits				
Apple, raw	2 medium (2½-inch diameter	16	0.6	160
Applesauce	16 tbsp (1 cup)	16	0.6	273
Apricots, raw	1 medium	12	0.5	25
Apricots, canned	2 medium in 2 tbsp syrup	14	0.6	80
Avocado, cubed or mashed‡	5 tbsp (⅓ cup)	16	0.6	80
Banana, raw, sliced	5 tbsp (¼ cup)	15	0.5	66
Blackberries, raw‡	5 tbsp (⅓ cup)	14	0.6	25
Blackberries, canned in syrup‡	5 tbsp (⅓ cup)	13	0.5	55
Blueberries, raw or frozen‡	12 tbsp (¾ cup)	16	0.6	60

‡Phenylalanine calculated as 2.6% of total protein.

FOOD LISTS FOR USE WITH LOW PHENYLALANINE DIET—cont'd

Food	Amount	Phenylalanine (mg)	Protein (gm)	Calories
Fruits—cont'd				
Table fruits—cont'd				
Blueberries, canned in syrup‡	10 tbsp	16	0.6	140
Boysenberries, frozen, sweetened‡	8 tbsp (½ cup)	16	0.6	72
Cantaloupe, diced	⅙ medium	13	0.4	19
Cherries, sweet, canned in syrup‡	8 tbsp (½ cup)	16	0.6	104
Dates, pitted, chopped	3 tbsp	18	0.7	96
Figs, raw‡	1 large	18	0.7	40
Figs, canned in syrup‡	2 figs in 4 tsp syrup	16	0.6	90
Figs, dried‡	1 small	16	0.6	40
Fruit cocktail‡	12 tbsp (¾ cup)	16	0.6	120
Grapefruit, raw	½ medium	11	0.5	41
Grapes, American type	8 grapes	14	0.5	24
Grapes, American slipskin	5 tbsp (⅓ cup)	16	0.6	25
Grapes, Thompson seedless	8 tbsp (½ cup)	13	0.8	64
Guava, raw‡	½ medium	13	0.5	35
Honeydew melon‡	¼ small 5-inch melon	13	0.5	32
Mango, raw‡	1 small	18	0.7	66
Nectarines, raw	1 to 2 inches high (2-inch diameter)	15	0.4	45
Oranges, raw	1 medium (3-inch diameter) or ⅔ cup sections	15	1.5	73
Papayas, raw‡	¼ medium or ½ cup	14	0.6	36
Peaches, raw	1 medium	15	0.5	46
Peaches, canned in syrup	2 medium halves	18	0.6	88
Pears, raw	1 (3 × 2½ inches)	14	1.3	100
Pears, canned in syrup	2 medium halves in 2 tbsp syrup	14	1.3	78
Pineapple, raw‡	16 tbsp (1 cup)	16	0.6	80
Pineapple canned in syrup‡	2 small slices	13	0.5	93
Plums, raw	½ (2-inch plum)	12	0.3	15
Plums canned in syrup	3 in 2 tbsp syrup	16	0.5	91
Prunes, dried	2 large	14	0.4	54
Raisins, dried seedless	2 tbsp	14	0.5	54
Raspberries, raw‡	5 tbsp (⅓ cup)	13	0.5	25
Raspberries, canned in syrup‡	6 tbsp	14	0.5	78
Strawberries, raw‡	10 large	16	0.6	32
Strawberries, frozen‡	6 tbsp	14	0.5	108
Tangerines	1½ large	15	1.2	66
Watermelon‡	½ cup cubes	13	0.5	28
Breads and cereals				
(each serving listed contains approximately 30 mg phenylalanine)				
Baby and Junior				
Cereals, ready to serve				
Barley	3 tbsp	32	0.8	24
Oatmeal	2 tbsp	35	1.2	28
Rice	5 tbsp (⅓ cup)	30	0.6	40
Wheat	2 tbsp	30	0.6	17
Creamed corn	3 tbsp	30	0.5	27
Sweet potatoes (Gerber's)	3 tbsp	32	0.5	31
Table foods				
Cereals, cooked				
Cornmeal	4 tbsp (¼ cup)	29	0.6	29

Continued.

FOOD LISTS FOR USE WITH LOW PHENYLALANINE DIET—cont'd

Food	Amount	Phenylalanine (mg)	Protein (gm)	Calories
Breads and cereals—cont'd				
Table foods—cont'd				
Cream of rice	4 tbsp (¼ cup)	35	0.7	34
Cream of Wheat	2 tbsp	27	0.6	16
Farina	2 tbsp	25	0.5	18
Malt-o-Meal	2 tbsp	27	0.5	17
Oatmeal	2 tbsp	32	0.7	18
Pettijohns	2 tbsp	24	0.5	19
Ralston	2 tbsp	34	0.7	18
Rice, brown or white	4 tbsp (¼ cup)	35	0.7	34
Wheatena	2 tbsp	27	0.5	19
Cereals, ready to serve				
Alpha Bits	4 tbsp (¼ cup)	32	0.6	28
Cheerios	3 tbsp	32	0.6	20
Corn Chex	7 tbsp	31	0.7	39
Cornfetti	5 tbsp (⅓ cup)	31	0.6	46
Cornflakes	5 tbsp (⅓ cup)	29	0.6	30
Crispy Critters	4 tbsp (¼ cup)	30	0.6	28
Kix	5 tbsp (⅓ cup)	28	0.6	31
Krumbles	3 tbsp	32	0.7	26
Rice Chex	6 tbsp	32	0.7	49
Rice flakes	5 tbsp (⅓ cup)	33	0.6	32
Rice Krispies	6 tbsp	30	0.6	40
Rice, puffed	12 tbsp (¾ cup)	30	0.6	38
Sugar Crisp, puffed wheat	4 tbsp (¼ cup)	30	0.6	46
Sugar Frosted Flakes	5 tbsp (⅓ cup)	29	0.6	55
Wheat Chex	10 biscuits	30	0.6	22
Wheaties	3 tbsp	26	0.5	20
Wheat, puffed	6 tbsp	30	0.6	16
Crackers				
Barnum Animal	5	30	0.6	45
Arrowroot cookies	1½	33	0.7	31
Graham (65 per pound)	1	26	0.5	30
Ritz (no cheese)	2	24	0.5	34
Saltines (140 per pound)	2	29	0.6	28
Tortilla, corn	½ (6-inch diameter)	32	0.8	32
Wheat Thins (248 per pound)	5	30	0.6	45
Zweiback	⅔ biscuit	30	0.6	21
Corn, cooked	2 tbsp	32	0.7	17
Hominy	2 tbsp	32	0.7	17
Macaroni, cooked	1½ tbsp	34	0.6	19
Noodles, cooked	1½ tbsp	30	0.6	19
Popcorn, popped	5 tbsp (⅓ cup)	31	0.6	17
Potato chips	6 (2-inch diameter)	29	0.7	68
Potato, Irish, cooked	3 tbsp	33	0.8	31
Spaghetti, cooked	2 tbsp	33	0.6	21
Sweet potato, cooked	2 tbsp	25	0.4	31
Fats				
(each serving listed contains approximately 5 mg phenylalanine)				
Butter	1 tbsp	5	0.1	100
French dressing, commercial	1 tbsp	5	0.1	59
Margarine	1 tbsp	5	0.1	100
Mayonnaise, commercial	½ tbsp	5	0.1	30
Olives, green or ripe	1 medium	5	0.1	12

FOOD LISTS FOR USE WITH LOW PHENYLALANINE DIET—cont'd

Food	Amount	Phenylalanine (mg)	Protein (gm)	Calories
Desserts				

(each serving listed contains approximately 30 mg phenylalanine)

Food	Amount			
Cake§	¹/₁₂ of cake			
Cookies				
Rice flour§	2			
Corn starch§	2			
Arrowroot	1½			
Ice cream				
Chocolate§	⅔ cup			
Pineapple§	⅔ cup			
Strawberry§	⅔ cup			
Jello	⅓ cup			
Puddings§	½ cup			
Sauce, Hershey	2 tbsp			
Wafers, sugar, Nabisco	5			

Free foods
Apple juice
Beverages, carbonated
Gingerbread§
Guava butter
Candy
   Butterscotch
   Cream mints
   Fondant
   Gumdrops
   Hard
   Jelly beans
   Lollipops
Cherries, maraschino
Fruit ices (if no more than ½ cup
   used daily)
Jell-Quik
Jellies
Kool-Aid
Lemonade
Molasses
Oil
Pepper, black, ground
Popsicles, with artificial fruit flavor
Rich's Topping
Salt
Shortening, vegetable
Soy sauce
Sugar, brown, white, or confectioner's
Syrups, corn or maple
Tang

§Low phenylalanine recipes in Phenylalanine-restricted diet recipe book. 1972. Berkeley, State of California Department of Public Health.

APPENDIX G

Conversion tables and equivalents*

METRIC SYSTEM

The units of measurement in the metric system are as follows:

meter (m) for length
gram (gm) for weight
liter (ℓ)   for capacity or volume
(Note: cubic centimeter [cc] also indicates volume.)

With these units the following prefixes are used:

micro   1/1,000,000 of a unit
milli   0.001 (1/1000) of a unit
centi   0.01 (1/100) of a unit
deci   0.1 (1/10) of a unit
deka   10 times the unit
hekto   100 times the unit
kilo   1000 times the unit
cubic   the total area covered, measured in square lengths

Thus:

1 kilogram (kg) = 1000 grams (gm)
1 gram (Gm) = 1000 milligrams (mg)
1 milligram (mg) = 1000 micrograms (μg)

AVOIRDUPOIS AND IMPERIAL SYSTEMS

Weight
    1 pound (lb) = 16 ounces (oz)
    1 ounce = 437.5 grains (gr)
Height
    1 yard (yd) = 3 feet (ft)
    1 foot (ft) = 12 inches (in)
Capacity
    1 gallon = 4 quarts = 8 pints
    1 quart = 2 pints
    1 pint = 20 fluid ounces
    1 fluid ounce = 8 drams (or drachm)
    1 dram = 60 minims

APPROXIMATE METRIC AND IMPERIAL EQUIVALENTS

Useful approximate metric and imperial equivalents

1 cm = 0.39 inch	1 inch = 2.54 cm
1 meter = 1.1 yards	1 foot = 30.48 cm

To convert centimeters to inches
    Divide the length in centimeters by 2.54.
    Example: The average newborn infant measures 50.8 cm:
    $$= \frac{50.8}{2.54} = 20 \text{ inches}$$

To convert inches to centimeters
    Multiply the length in inches by 2.54.
    Example: The average newborn infant measures 20 inches:
    $$= 20 \times 2.54 = 50.8 \text{ cm}$$

Weight	
30 gm = 1 ounce	30 mg = $\frac{1}{2}$ grain
15 gm = $\frac{1}{2}$ ounce	20 mg = $\frac{1}{3}$ grain
8 gm = 120 grains	15 mg = $\frac{1}{4}$ grain
4 gm = 60 grains	10 mg = $\frac{1}{6}$ grain
2 gm = 30 grains	7.5 mg = $\frac{1}{8}$ grain
1 gm = 15 grains	6 mg = $\frac{1}{10}$ grain
600 mg = 10 grains	3 mg = $\frac{1}{20}$ grain
450 mg = $7\frac{1}{2}$ grains	1 mg = $\frac{1}{60}$ grain
300 mg = 5 grains	(1000 μg)
250 mg = 4 grains	0.6 mg = $\frac{1}{100}$ grain
200 mg = 3 grains	0.5 mg = $\frac{1}{120}$ grain
150 mg = $2\frac{1}{2}$ grains	0.3 mg = $\frac{1}{200}$ grain
100 mg = $1\frac{1}{2}$ grains	0.2 mg = $\frac{1}{300}$ grain
60 mg = 1 grain	0.1 mg = $\frac{1}{600}$ grain
50 mg = $\frac{3}{4}$ grain	

*From Chinn, P. L., and Leitch, C. J. 1974. Child health maintenance. St. Louis, The C. V. Mosby Co.

CONVERSION OF POUNDS AND OUNCES TO GRAMS FOR NEWBORN WEIGHTS

Pounds	\ Ounces 0	1	2	3	4	5	6	7	8	9	10	11	12	13	14	15
0	—	28	57	85	113	142	170	198	227	255	283	312	430	369	397	425
1	454	482	510	539	567	595	624	652	680	709	737	765	794	822	850	879
2	907	936	964	992	1021	1049	1077	1106	1134	1162	1191	1219	1247	1276	1304	1332
3	1361	1389	1417	1446	1474	1503	1531	1559	1588	1616	1644	1673	1701	1729	1758	1786
4	1814	1843	1871	1899	1928	1956	1984	2013	2041	2070	2098	2126	2155	2183	2211	2240
5	2268	2296	2325	2353	2381	2410	2438	2466	2495	2523	2551	2580	2608	2637	2665	2693
6	2722	2750	2778	2807	2835	2863	2892	2920	2948	2977	3005	3033	3062	3090	3118	3147
7	3175	3203	3232	3260	3289	3317	3345	3374	3402	3430	3459	3487	3515	3544	3572	3600
8	3629	3657	3685	3714	3742	3770	3799	3827	3856	3884	3912	3941	3969	3997	4026	4054
9	4082	4111	4139	4167	4196	4224	4252	4281	4309	4337	4366	4394	4423	4451	4479	4508
10	4536	4564	4593	4621	4649	4678	4706	4734	4763	4791	4819	4848	4876	4904	4933	4961
11	4990	5018	5046	5075	5103	5131	5160	5188	5216	5245	5273	5301	5330	5358	5386	5415
12	5443	5471	5500	5528	5557	5585	5613	5642	5670	5698	5727	5755	5783	5812	5840	5868
13	5897	5925	5953	5982	6010	6038	6067	6095	6123	6152	6180	6209	6237	6265	6294	6322
14	6350	6379	6407	6435	6464	6492	6520	6549	6577	6605	6634	6662	6690	6719	6747	6776
15	6804	6832	6860	6889	6917	6945	6973	7002	7030	7059	7087	7115	7144	7172	7201	7228

CONVERSION OF INCHES TO CENTIMETERS

Inches	Centimeters
10	25.40
10½	26.67
11	27.94
11½	29.21
12	30.48
12½	31.75
13	33.02
13½	34.29
14	35.56
14½	36.83
15	38.10
15½	39.37
16	40.61
16½	41.91
17	43.18
17½	44.45
18	45.72
18½	46.99
19	48.26
19½	49.58
20	50.80
20½	52.07
21	53.34
21½	54.61
22	55.88
22½	57.15
23	58.42
23½	56.69
24	60.96

APPROXIMATE WEIGHT EQUIVALENTS

Apothecary	Metric
$\frac{1}{320}$ grain	0.2 mg
$\frac{1}{210}$ grain	0.3 mg
$\frac{1}{160}$ grain	0.4 mg
$\frac{1}{100}$ grain	0.65 mg
$\frac{1}{64}$ grain	1.0 mg
$\frac{1}{32}$ grain	2.0 mg
$\frac{1}{16}$ grain	4.0 mg
$\frac{1}{12}$ grain	5.4 mg
$\frac{1}{10}$ grain	6.5 mg
$\frac{1}{8}$ grain	8.0 mg
$\frac{1}{6}$ grain	11.0 mg
$\frac{1}{4}$ grain	16.0 mg
$\frac{1}{3}$ grain	22.0 mg
$\frac{3}{8}$ grain	24.0 mg
$\frac{1}{2}$ grain	32.0 mg
$\frac{3}{4}$ grain	50.0 mg
1 grain	65.0 mg
1½ grains	0.1 gm
2 grains	0.13 gm
2½ grains	0.16 gm
3 grains	0.2 gm
5 grains	0.32 gm
7½ grains	0.5 gm
10 grains	0.65 gm
15 grains	1.0 gm
1 dram	4.0 gm
1 ounce	30.0 gm

FLUID VOLUME

Useful approximate metric and imperial equivalents

1 liter	= 1.75 pints
1 oz	= 30 ml
1 pint	= 0.568 liters or 568 ml
1 gallon	= 4.55 liters

Conversion table

Liters		Pints
0.28	0.5	0.88
0.57	1	1.75
1.14	2	3.50
1.70	3	5.28
1.28	4	7.04
2.85	5	8.80
3.42	6	10.50
3.99	7	12.30
4.55	8	14.08

To read the table: 3 liters = 5.28 pints
3 pints = 1.70 liters

MEASUREMENTS

Domestic	Apothecary	Metric
1 teaspoon	1 dram	4 ml
1 tablespoon	½ fluid ounce	15 ml
1 teacup	4 ounces	120 ml
1 tumbler	8 ounces	240 ml

TEMPERATURE EQUIVALENTS

Centigrade	Fahrenheit	Centigrade	Fahrenheit
34.0	93.2	38.6	101.4
34.2	93.6	38.8	101.8
34.4	93.9	39.0	102.2
34.6	94.3	39.2	102.5
34.8	94.6	39.4	102.9
35.0	95.0	39.6	103.2
35.2	95.4	30.8	103.6
35.4	95.7	40.0	104.0
35.6	96.1	40.2	104.3
35.8	96.4	40.4	104.7
36.0	96.8	40.6	105.1
36.2	97.1	40.8	105.4
36.4	97.5	41.0	105.8
36.6	97.8	41.2	106.1
36.8	98.2	41.4	106.5
37.0	*98.6*	41.6	106.8
37.2	98.9	41.8	107.2
37.4	99.3	42.0	107.6
37.6	99.6	42.2	108.0
37.8	100.0	42.4	108.3
38.0	100.4	42.6	108.7
38.2	100.7	42.8	109.0
38.4	101.1	43.0	109.4

To convert Fahrenheit to centigrade

(Temperature minus 32) $\times$ $\frac{5}{9}$

Example: To convert 98.6° Fahrenheit to centigrade

98.6 − 32 = 66.6 $\times$ $\frac{5}{9}$ = 37° centigrade

To convert centigrade to Fahrenheit

$\frac{9}{5}$ $\times$ temperature + 32

Example: To convert 40° centigrade to Fahrenheit

$\frac{9}{5}$ $\times$ 40 = 72 + 32 = 104° Fahrenheit

CONVERTING FRENCH SIZE INTO MILLIMETERS OR INCHES*

French size	Diameter (mm)	Diameter (inches)
1	⅓	0.013
2	⅔	0.026
3	1	0.039
4	1⅓	0.052
5	1⅔	0.065
6	2	0.078
7	2⅓	0.091
8	2⅔	0.104
9	3	0.118
10	3⅓	0.131
11	3⅔	0.144
12	4	0.157
13	4⅓	0.170
14	4⅔	0.183
15	5	0.196
16	5⅓	0.209
17	5⅔	0.223
18	6	0.236
19	6⅓	0.249
20	6⅔	0.262
21	7	0.275
22	7⅓	0.288
23	7⅔	0.301
24	8	0.314
25	8⅓	0.328
26	8⅔	0.341
27	9	0.354
28	9⅓	0.367
29	9⅔	0.380
30	10	0.393

Since many catheters are labeled in French sizes, the above table is presented to aid the nurse in selecting the most appropriate size catheter for use.

*Courtesy Sterilon Corporation, Buffalo, N.Y.

APPENDIX H

Standard parameters in the neonatal period*

1. Hematologic

Clotting factors

Activated clotting time (ACT)	2 min
Bleeding time (Ivy)	1-8 min
Clot retraction	Complete 1-4 hr
Clotting time	
2 tubes	5-8 min
3 tubes	5-15 min
Fibrinogen	150-300 mg/dl†
Fibrinolysin (plasminogen)	Lysis of clot
Partial thromboplastin time (PTT)	<90-120 sec
Prothrombin time, one-stage (PT)	12-21 sec
Thromboplastin generation test (TGT)	8-24 sec in 6 min tube

	Term	Preterm
Hemoglobin (gm/dl)	17-19	15-17
Hematocrit (%)	57-58	45-55
Sedimentation rate (ESR) mm/hr	0-2	1-5
Reticulocytes (%)	3-7	Up to 10
Fetal hemoglobin (% of total)	40-70	80-90
Nucleated RBC/mm³ (per 100 RBC)	200 (0.05)	(0.2)
Platelet count/mm³	100-300,000	120-180,000
WBC/mm³	15,000	10,000-20,000
Neutrophils (%)	45	47
Eosinophils and basophils (%)	3	
Lymphocytes (%)	30	33
Monocytes (%)	5	4
Immature WBC (%)	10	16

2. Biochemical

Alpha-l-fetoprotein	0
Ammonia	100-150 μg/dl
Amylase	0-1000 IU/hr
Antistreptolysin O titer, group B	
Normal	12-100 Todd units
Recent streptococcal infection	200-2500 Todd units

*1 to 6 from Pierog, S. H., and Ferrara, A. 1976. Medical care of the sick newborn (ed. 2). St. Louis, The C. V. Mosby Co.; 7 courtesy Ross Laboratories, Columbus, Ohio.

†dl refers to deciliter (1 deciliter = 100 ml); this conforms to the SI system: international measurements that have been standardized.

2. **Biochemical**—cont'd

Bilirubin, direct		0-1 mg/dl
Bilirubin, total	Cord:	<2 mg/dl
	Peripheral blood: 0-1 day	6 mg/dl
	1-2 day	8 mg/dl
	3-5 day	12 mg/dl
Blood gases	Arterial:	pH 7.31-7.45
		Pco_2 33-48 mm Hg
		Po_2 50-70 mm Hg
	Venous:	pH 7.28-7.42
		Pco_2 38-52 mm Hg
		Po_2 20-49 mm Hg
Calcium, ionized		2.1-2.6 mEq/ℓ
Calcium, total		4-7.0 mEq/ℓ

Catecholamines (μg/24 hr)
    Neonatal: norepinephrine, 2-12; epinephrine, 1-2
    Newborn: norepinephrine, 2-4; epinephrine, 0-1

Ceruloplasmin (p-phenylenediamine dihydrochloride, 37° C)	1-30 mg/dl
Chloride	95-110 mEq/ℓ
Cholesterol, esters	42-71% of total
Cholesterol, total	45-170 mg/dl
Copper	20-70 μg/dl
Cortisol	
AM specimen	15-25 μg/dl
PM specimen	5-10 μg/dl
C-reactive protein (CRP)	0
Creatine	0.2-1 mg/dl (higher in females)
Creatine phosphokinase (CPK) (creatine phosphate, 30° C)	10-300 IU/ℓ
Creatinine	0.3-1 mg/dl
Electrophoresis, total protein	Preterm: 4.3-7.6 gm/dl
	Newborn: 4.6-7.4 gm/dl

    Preterm: albumin, 3.1-4.2; α_1-globulin, 0.1-0.5; α_2-globulin,
        0.3-0.7; β-globulin, 0.3-1.2; γ-globulin, 0.3-1.4
    Newborn: albumin, 3.6-5.4; α_1-globulin, 0.1-0.3; α_2-globulin,
        0.2-0.5; β-globulin, 0.2-0.6; γ-globulin, 0.2-1.2

Fatty acids, free	0.4-1 mg/ℓ
Fibrinogen	150-300 mg/dl
Glucose, fasting (FBS)	
Hepatitis-associated (Australia) antigen	0
Immunoglobulin levels, serum, newborn	660-1.439 mg/dl
IgG 645-1.244	
IgM 5-30	
IgA 0-11	
Iodine, butanol extractable (BEI)	3-13 μg/dl
Iodine, T_4-by-column (thyroxine)	3-12 μg/dl
Iodine, T_4 (competitive protein binding thyroxine)	3-12 μg/dl
Iodine, total serum organic (PBI)	4-14 μg/dl
Iron	100-200 μg/dl
Iron-binding capacity (IBC)	60-175 μg/dl
17-Ketogenic steroids (17-KGS)	2.4 mg/24 hr
17-Ketosteroids (17-KS)	0.5-2.5 mg/24 hr
Lactic dehydrogenase (LDH) (pyruvate, 30° C)	300-1500 IU/ℓ
Lipids, total	170-450 mg/dl
Lipoproteins, newborn (mg/dl)	
Alpha 70-180	

2. **Biochemical**—cont'd   **Preterm**

Beta 50-160	
Chylo 50-110	
Magnesium	1.4-2.9 mEq/ℓ
Malic dehydrogenase (MDH) (oxalacetic acid, 37° C)	41-68 IU/ℓ
Phosphatase, acid	10.4-16.4 IU/ℓ
Phosphatase, alkaline	50-275 IU/ℓ
Phospholipids	75-170 mg/dl
Phosphorus	3.5-8.6 mg/dl
Potassium	4-7 mg/ℓ
Pregnanetriol	0 mg/24 hr
Protein, total	4.3-7.6 gm/dl
Sodium	140-160 mEq/ℓ
Transaminases, serum	
Glutamic-oxalacetic (SGOT) (aspartate, 30° C)	5-70 IU/ℓ
Glutamic-pyruvic (SGPT)	5-50 IU/ℓ
Triglycerides	5-40 mg/dl
Urea nitrogen (BUN)	5-15 mg/dl
Vanillylmandelic acid (VMA)	0-1 mg/24 hr

3. **Urinalysis**

Volume: 20 to 40 ml excreted daily in the first few days; by 1 week, 24-hour urine volume close to 200 ml

Protein: may be present in the first 2 to 4 days

Casts and WBCs: may be present in the first 2 to 4 days

Osmolarity (mOsm/ℓ): 100 to 600

pH: 5 to 7

Specific gravity: 1.001 to 1.020

4. **Cerebrospinal fluid**

Calcium	2-3 mg/ℓ
Cell count	WBCs/mm³ 0-15
	RBCs/mm³ 0-500
Chloride	110-120 mg/ℓ
Color	May be xanthochromic
Glucose	24-40 mg/dl
Lactic dehydrogenase (LDH)	5-80 IU/ℓ
Magnesium	3-3.3 mg/dl
Pandy's test (for excess globulins)	Negative
pH (37° C)	7.33-7.42
Pressure	50-80 mm Hg
Protein, total	20-120 mg/dl
Sodium	130-165 mg/ℓ
Specific gravity	1.007-1.009
Transaminase, glutamic-oxalacetic (GOT)	2-10 IU/ℓ
Volume	5 ml

5. **Cardiorespiratory**

Blood pressure at birth

  Term: systolic, 70 mm Hg; diastolic, 45 mm Hg

  Preterm: systolic, 50-60 mm Hg; diastolic, 30 mm Hg

Respiratory rate: 30-40/min

Heart rate, fetus

  Baseline: 120-160/min

    Tachycardia: >160/min (with maternal complication)

    Bradycardia: <120/min (with maternal hypotension and hypoxia)

    Acceleration: tachycardia >160/min with uterine contraction—normal

  Beat-to-beat variability: disappears with fetal distress

5. **Cardiorespiratory**—cont'd
    With uterine contraction
        Early deceleration: bradycardia with onset of contraction—benign
        Variable deceleration: bradycardia due to cord compression—usually benign
        Late deceleration: bradycardia after lag period due to fetal hypoxia—ominous sign
    Heart rate, term infant: 140 ± 20/min

6. **Urine screening tests for inborn errors of metabolism**
    Benedict's test: for reducing substances in the urine—glucose, galactose, fructose, lactose; phenylketonuria, alkaptonuria, tyrosyluria, and tyrosinosis *may* give positive Benedict's test.
    Ferric chloride test: an immediate, green color for phenylketonuria, histidinemia, and tyrosinuria; a gray to green color for presence of phenothiazines, isoniazid; red to purple color for presence of salicylates or ketone bodies.
    Dinitrophenylhydrazine test: for phenylketonuria, maple-syrup urine disease, Lowe's syndrome.
    Cetyltrimethyl ammonium bromide test: for mucopolysaccharides: immediate positive reaction in gargoylism (Hurler's syndrome); delayed, moderately positive reaction for Marfan's, Morquio-Ullrich, and Murdoch syndromes.
    Metachromatic stain (of urine sediment): Granules (free or as inclusion bodies in cells) are seen in metachromatic leukodystrophy; may also be seen rarely in Tay-Sachs and other lipid diseases of the central nervous system.
    Amino acid chromatography: Aminoaciduria may be normal in newborns; chromatography may be helpful to detect hypophosphatasia and argininosuccinicaciduria.

7. **Growth and development**
    See pp. 684 to 687.

**GIRLS: BIRTH TO 36 MONTHS
PHYSICAL GROWTH
NCHS PERCENTILES***

NAME _____ RECORD # _____

*Adapted from: National Center for Health Statistics: NCHS Growth Charts, 1976. Monthly Vital Statistics Report. Vol. 25, No. 3, Supp. (HRA) 76-1120. Health Resources Administration, Rockville, Maryland, June, 1976. Data from The Fels Research Institute, Yellow Springs, Ohio.

© 1976 ROSS LABORATORIES

DATE	AGE	LENGTH	WEIGHT	HEAD C.
	BIRTH			

DATE	AGE	LENGTH	WEIGHT	HEAD C.

From Birth
SIMILAC® WITH IRON
Infant Formula

For Milk Sensitivity
ISOMIL®
Soy Isolate Formula

After Formula . . . Before Milk
ADVANCE®
Nutritional Beverage

ROSS LABORATORIES
COLUMBUS, OHIO 43216
DIVISION OF ABBOTT LABORATORIES, USA

48110.2/AUGUST, 1976

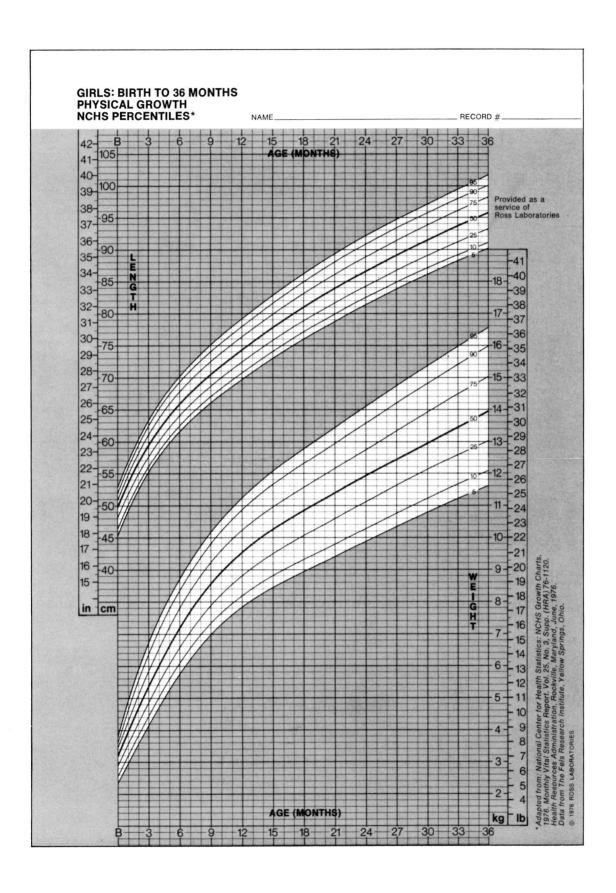

GIRLS: BIRTH TO 36 MONTHS
PHYSICAL GROWTH
NCHS PERCENTILES*

NAME _____ RECORD # _____

Provided as a
service of
Ross Laboratories

*Adapted from: National Center for Health Statistics: NCHS Growth Charts, 1976. Monthly Vital Statistics Report. Vol. 25, No. 3, Supp. (HRA) 76-1120. Health Resources Administration, Rockville, Maryland, June, 1976. Data from The Fels Research Institute, Yellow Springs, Ohio.

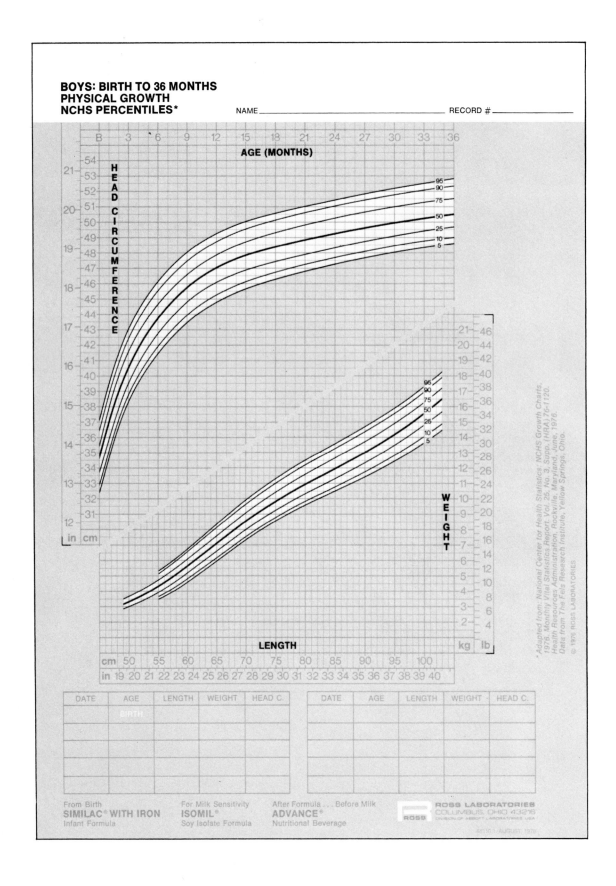

BOYS: BIRTH TO 36 MONTHS
PHYSICAL GROWTH
NCHS PERCENTILES*

NAME _____ RECORD # _____

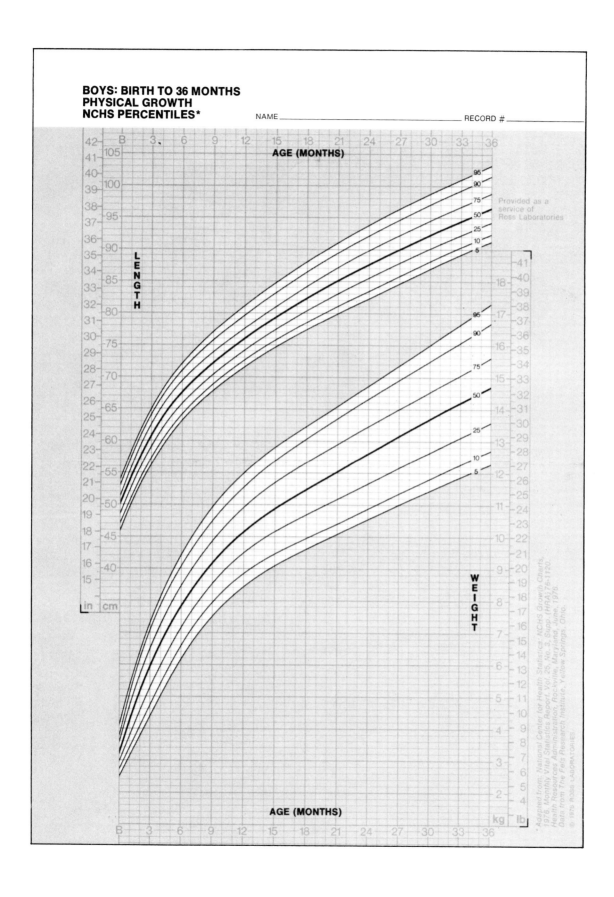

BOYS: BIRTH TO 36 MONTHS
PHYSICAL GROWTH
NCHS PERCENTILES*

NAME_____ RECORD #_____

APPENDIX I

Recommended schedule for active immunization of normal infants and children*

	Diphtheria-tetanus-pertussis	Polio	Measles	TB test	Rubella	Mumps	Tetanus-diphtheria
2 months	✔	✔					
4 months	✔	✔					
6 months	✔						
1 year				✔			
15 months			✔		✔	✔	
1½ years	✔	✔					
4 - 6 years	✔	✔					
14 - 16 years							✔

*From American Academy of Pediatrics. 1977. You and your pediatrician: common childhood problems. Evanston, Ill., The Academy.

APPENDIX J

Patient record forms

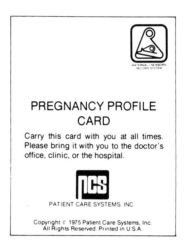

Identification Data

Patient's name: Mrs. Alice Kramer

Physician or clinic: Revere Medical Center

Tel. no. 617 438-9926 Chart no. 87507

Delivery hospital: Revere Memorial Hosp.

Tel. no. 617 827-6613 Data on file: ☒ Yes ☐ No

In emergency please notify: Harold Kramer

Tel. no. 617 738-4073

WARNING!

I (am) (have) _____

PREGNANCY PROFILE CARD

Carry this card with you at all times. Please bring it with you to the doctor's office, clinic, or the hospital.

PCS
PATIENT CARE SYSTEMS, INC.

Prob. No.	Medications	Dosage	Dates
	Natalins	Tabs ī od	5/9 —
	Bendectin #20	Tabs ī tid	7/4 11/5
			:
			:
			:
			:

Sensitivities to medication: None

Blood Type	LMP	EDD	GTPAL
O+	3-27-74	12-26-74	4 2 1 0 2

Prob. No.	Significant Problems	Status A	Status R
	None		

Physician's Signature: Michael Barber, M.D.

Pregnancy Profile Record
Part I

MATERNAL / NEWBORN RECORD SYSTEM

Patient's name _Alice Kramer_ No. _87507_
Date of birth _11-22-44_ Age _30_ Soc. Sec. number _156-43-1178_
Marital status _Married_ Race _Black_ Relig. _Prot._ Last grade _12th_
Physician _Micheal Barber, M.D._ Tel. no. _438-9926_

Patient's address _417 South Maple St., Revere, Mass. 02614_ Tel. no. _738-4073_
Name of child's father _Harold Kramer_ Emergency name _____ Relation to pt. _Husband_ Tel. no. _____
Referring physician _____ Office address _____ Tel. no. _____
Newborn's physician _Robert Washington, M.D._ Office address _29-63 Terrace Drive, Revere, Mass._ Tel. no. _735-1127_

Pregnancy History Grav _4_ Term _2_ Prem _1_ Abort _0_ Live _2_ **Periods** Interval between _30_ days Duration _5_ days LMP _3-27-74_ EDC _12-26-74_

No.	Date (mo/yr)	Wks. gest.	Labor (hrs)	Spont.	Ind.	Type of delivery	Alive/ Dead	Baby's weight	Complications (both maternal and neonatal)
1	10/67	40	14	✓		PLFD	A	6-11	None
2	8/70	37	10	✓		PLFD	A	6-9	None
3	3/72	32	4	✓		NSD	A	3-6	Neonatal death - RDS
4									
5									
6									
7									
8									
9									

Initial Physical Examination Date _5-9-74_ B.P. _110/70_ Pulse _80_ Height _5'3"_ Weight _118_ Weight @ LMP _115_

SYSTEM	Normal	Selected Abnormalities				Other	Detail All Positive Findings Below
SKIN	1 ✓	☐ Rashes	☐ Eruptions	☐ Pallor	☐ Jaundice	☐	10. Appendectomy 1960
EYES	2 ✓	☐ Lid lag	☐ Unequal pupils	☐ <Light reflex	☐ >Light reflex	☐	
ENT	3 ✓	☐ Abn. mucosa	☐ Exudates	☐ Obstructions	☐ Hearing loss	☐	
MOUTH	4 ✓	☐ Poor teeth	☐ Gingivitis	☐ Sores		☐	
NECK	5 ✓	☐ Asymmetry	☐ Pulsations	☐ Adenopathy	☐ Enlarged thyroid	☐	
CHEST	6 ✓	☐ Asymmetry	☐ >A-P diameter	☐ Rub		☐	
LUNGS	7 ✓	☐ <Sounds	☐ >Sounds	☐ Rales	☐ Wheezing	☐	
BREASTS	8 ✓	☐ Asymmetry	☐ Enlarged	☐ Discharge	☐ Tenderness	☐	
HEART	9 ✓	☐ Abnormal size	☐ Arrhythmias	☐ Murmurs	☐ Sounds	☐	
ABDOMEN	10 ☐	☐ Tenderness	☐ Rigidity	☐ Masses	☐ Herniation	☐	
		☑ Scars	☐ Obesity				
EXTREMITIES	11 ✓	☐ Varicosities	☐ Ulcerations	☐ Edema	☐ Deformations	☐	
REFLEXES	12 ✓	☐ Unequal	☐ Hypoactive	☐ Hyperactive	☐ Absent		

Pelvic Examination

VULVA	13 ✓	☐ Varicosities	☐ Vulvitis	☐ Condyloma	☐ Skin lesions	☐	
PERINEUM	14 ✓	☐ Lacerated	☐ Relaxed	☐ Scarring		☐	
VAGINA	15 ✓	☐ Discharge	☐ Varicosities	☐ Cystocele	☐ Rectocele	☐	
CERVIX	16 ✓	☐ Open	☐ Inflamed	☐ Bleeding	☐ Lesions	☐	
ADNEXA: LEFT	17 ✓	☐ Not palpable	☐ Thickened	☐ Tender	☐ Masses	☐	
ADNEXA: RIGHT	18 ✓	☐ Not palpable	☐ Thickened	☐ Tender	☐ Masses	☐	
UTERUS	19 ✓	Size _7 wks_		☐ Small for dates	☐ Large for dates	☐	
RECTUM	20 ✓	☐ Masses	☐ Hemorrhoids			☐	

Bony Pelvis 21 Prediction: ☑ Adequate ☐ Borderline ☐ Inadequate ☐

22 Diag. conj. _12 cm_ 24 IT-diameter _9 cm_ 26 Shape sacrum _Angul_ 28 S.S. notch _2½ FB_ 30
23 Pubic arch _Avg._ 25 Post sag. diam. _9 cm_ 27 Ischial spines _Blunt_ 29 Coccyx _Mobile_ 31

☐ See additional progress notes
Exam by: _M. Barber, M.D._

Prenatal Flow Record

Part I

MATERNAL / NEWBORN RECORD SYSTEM

Patient's name	Alice Kramer
Date of birth	11-22-44 Age 30 No. 87507

LMP 3-27-74 Date	PMP 2-25-74 Date	Interval between periods	30 Days	EDC 12-26-74 Date	Profile Card given to pt. 12-2-74 Date	This form sent to hospital 12-2-74 Date

Blood type and Rh	Patient	O +	Hct/Hgb	34	31		Rh titres				VDRL	Neg	
	Baby's father	A +	Date	5/9	11/19		Date				Date	5/9	
Rubella titre	< 8	Pap test	I										
Date	5/9	Date	5/9	Date				Date			Date		

Visit date 1974		5/9	6/7	7/4	8/2	9/6	10/4	11/5	11/19	12/2	12/10	12/16	12/23						
Wks. gestation by dates		7	11	15	19	24	28	32	34	36	37	38	39						
Wks. gestation by size		7			20			32		36	—								
WEIGHT Pre-gravid 115	This visit	118	119	122	125	128	132	134	136	139	140	141	141						
	Cumulative	3	4	7	10	13	17	19	21	24	25	26	26						
Blood pressure		110/70	110/75	110/70	115/75	115/70	115/75	120/80	120/80	115/80	120/80	125/80	115/80						
Edema		—	—	—	—	—	—	—	+	+	+	++	+						
URINE Sugar		—	—	—	—	—	—	—	—	—	—	—	—						
URINE Albumin		—	—	—	—	—	—	—	—	—	—	+	—						
SYMPTOMS Bleeding																			
SYMPTOMS Discharge																			
SYMPTOMS Dizziness/Fainting				✓															
SYMPTOMS Headache				✓							✓	✓							
SYMPTOMS Leg cramps								✓	✓	✓		✓							
SYMPTOMS Nausea/Vomiting			✓	✓	✓	✓													
OPTIONAL Engagement										dip	dip	dip							
OPTIONAL																			
OPTIONAL																			
FETUS Heart rate or tones				✓	✓			✓			✓	✓	✓						
FETUS Uterine growth				✓				✓			✓		✓						
FETUS Movement					✓			✓					✓						
FETUS Est. presentation											Vtx		Vtx						
Pregnancy Risk Level		None									None		None						
New problems		✓		✓								✓							
Medication changes		✓		✓				✓											
Next appointment (wks)		4	4	4	4	4	4	2	2	2	1	1	1						
Initials		MB	RT	EC	RT	MB	EC	RT	RT	MB	EC	RT	MB						

Initial	Signature	Initial	Signature	Initial	Signature	Initial	Signature	Initial	Signature
MB	M. Berber, MD	RT	R. Taggert, MD	JF	Joan Ferguson, RN	EC	C. Coopersmith, MD		

Physician's Record Copy

Pregnancy Profile Record
Part II

MATERNAL / NEWBORN
RECORD SYSTEM

LEAVE THIS AREA
FOR HOSPITAL
NAMEPLATE

Patient's name *Alice Kramer*	Date of birth *11-22-44*	
Marital status *Marr.* Religion *Protestant* Age *30* Ht. *5'3"* Wt. *141*		
Physician *Micheal Barber*	Tel. no. *438-9926*	
Husband [ ] *Harold Kramer*	Tel. no. *734-4073*	

Summary Information Describe the final status of all patient's prenatal problems including listed Risk Indicators and any additional relevant data.

Normal multigravid 3 complications

Plans for Labor, Delivery, and Aftercare

Delivery	☒ Vaginal ☐ Cesarean	Rubella Ig	☐ No ☒ Yes
Anesthesia: *Regional*		Rh₀ (D) Ig	☒ No ☐ Yes
In delivery room: *Husband*		Nursing baby	☐ No ☒ Yes
Sterilization	☐ No ☒ Yes → *p.p. tubal ligation*		
Rooming in	☐ No ☒ Yes *circumcision if boy*		

Baby's physician *Robert Washington* Tel. no. *735-1127*
Date *12-2-74* Signature *Michael Barber, MD*

Admitting Information and Physical Examination LMP *3-27-74*

Grav *4*	Term *2*	Prem *1*	Abort *O*	Live *2*	EDC *12-26-74*

	Date	Time	Weeks Gestation *39*
Admitted at	*12-26-74*	*8:40* ᴬ/P	B. P. *120/80*
Membranes rupt.		*4:00* ᴬ/P	Temp. *99°*
Labor started		*5:00* ᴬ/P	Pulse *85*
Last meal		*1:30* ᴬ/P	Resp. *16*

☐ Recent URI ☐ Dentures ☐ Contacts Fundal ht. *39*

☐ Presented Profile Card Admitted by: *Patricia Dunfee, R.N.*

Hct/Hgb *32*	Urine sugar *Neg.*	Urine albumin *Neg.*

Prenatal Medications List all medications prescribed or taken during this pregnancy. Use Function Codes on the reverse side to define the purpose of medications. ☐ **None**

Code	Medications	Dosage	Start	Stop
23	*Natalins Rx*	*Tabs ī od*	*5/9*	—
05	*Bendectin #20*	*Tabs ī tid*	*7/4*	*11/5*
			:	
			:	
			:	
			:	
			:	

Sensitivities (food and medications)   ☒ None

Lab Values Enter the values and dates of the latest test results obtained. Use blank areas for any additional tests.

Blood type and Rh	Patient *O +*	Hct/Hgb *31*	Rh titre
	Baby's father *A +*	date *11/19*	date

VDRL *Neg* date *5/9*	Rubella titre *< 8* date	Pap *I* date	Urine sugar *Neg* date *11/19*

Urine albumin *Neg* date *11/19*	date	date	date

date	date	date	date

Admission Complications ☐ None

- ☐ No prenatal data available
- ☐ No prenatal care received
- ☐ Premature labor (< 35 weeks)
- ☐ Overdue EDC (>41 weeks)
- ☐ Medical induction requested
- ☐ Pronounced vaginal bleeding
- ☒ Membranes ruptured pre-admit
- ☐ Meconium noted in fluid
- ☐ Fluid had noticeable odor
- ☐ _____
- ☐ _____

Abdomen ☒ WNL
- ☐ Abn.
RLQ scar appendectomy

Fetal presentation
- ☒ Vertex   ☐ Floating
- ☐ Breech   ☐ Dipping
- ☐ Face/Brow   ☒ Engaged
- ☐ Transverse
- ☐ Other_____

Extremities ☐ WNL
- ☒ Abn.
Pre tibial trace edema

Head and Neck ☒ WNL
- ☐ Abn.

Other Findings
Reflexes - WNL

Heart and Lungs ☒ WNL
- ☐ Abn.
RSR - no murmurs
Lungs - clear

Exam by: *Michael Barber, MD*

Patient transferred to: *Delivery room*   Time *7:15* ᴬ/P
Date *12-27-75* Signature *Cheryl Bonner, R.N.*

Prenatal Flow Record
Part II

MATERNAL / NEWBORN
RECORD SYSTEM

Patient's name __Alice Kramer__

Date of birth __11-22-44__ Age __30__ No. __87507__

Date	Progress Notes
5/9	27 yr. old grav 4 para 3 c̄ adequate. pelvis Prognosis good for vaginal delivery. Rx: Bloods + urine done. Coverage agreed to for Drs. Barber, Taggert, Coopersmith. Natalins, diet and book given. M. Barber, M.D
7/4	Bendectin for nausea Tabs ī tid. E. Coopersmith, M.D
11/5	Nausea stopped Bendectin withdrawn. R. Taggert, M.D.
12/2	Pt. reports slight vaginal itching. Culture neg. MB
12/16	Slightly elevated alb. c̄ 2+ ankle pitting. Pt. cautioned re: fluid + salt. intake. RT

☐ See additional progress notes.

Pregnancy Risk Indicators

1. Examine patient
2. Develop/update problem list
3. Mark corresponding indicators ⦿

■ = High risk indicator
■ = Medium risk indicator
■ = Low risk indicator
☐ = No risk

NO YES
☐ ■ Drug dependencies
☐ ■ Habitual smoker (≥1 pack per day)
☐ ■ Less than eighth grade education
☐ ■ Pregnancy without family or partner's support

☐ ■ Prior transfusions
☐ ■ Incompetent cervix
☐ ■ Uterine or cervical malformations
☐ ■ Contracted pelvis
☐ ■ Height under 5 feet tall
☐ ■ Overweight (>15%) for height
☐ ■ Underweight (>15%) for height
☐ ■ Underage (<18) or overage (>33)
☐ ■ Uterine surgery (noncesarean)
☐ ■ Primigravida (if YES skip to "Diabetes")

☐ ■ Cesarean section
☐ ■ Induced abortions
☐ ■ Habitual abortions
☐ ■ Grand multipara (≥6 births)
☐ ■ Multiparous before age 20
☐ ■ Second pregnancy in 12 months

☑ ■ Fetal deaths
☐ ⊙ Neonatal deaths
☑ ■ Premature or LBW infants
☑ ■ Congenital or chromosomal anomalies
☑ ■ H.B.W. infants (≥10 pounds)

☐ ■ Diabetes
☐ ■ Heart disease : class 2, 3, or 4
☐ ■ Hemoglobinopathy
☐ ■ Thyroid disease
☐ ■ Anemia (unresponsive to Fe)
☐ ■ Heart disease : class 1
☐ ■ Epilepsy
☐ ■ Tuberculosis

1st Tri	2nd Tri	3rd Tri	
NO YES	NO YES	NO YES	
☐ ■	☐ ■	☐ ■	Hypertension
☐ ■	☐ ■	☐ ■	Renal disease
☐ ■	☐ ■	☐ ■	Herpes
☐ ■	☐ ■	☐ ■	Pyelonephritis
☐ ■	☐ ■	☐ ■	Cystitis
☐ ■	☐ ■	☐ ■	Thromboembolic disease
☐ ■	☐ ■	☐ ■	Venereal disease
☐ ■	☐ ■	☐ ■	Rh, ABO, or other blood sensitivities
☐ ■	☐ ■	☐ ■	Vaginal bleeding
	☐ ■	☐ ■	Abnormal presentation ———
	☐ ■	☐ ■	Failure to gain weight
	☐ ■	☐ ■	Hydramnios
	☐ ■	☐ ■	Intrauterine growth retardation
	☐ ■	☐ ■	Toxemia : moderate/severe
	☐ ■	☐ ■	Multiple pregnancy
	☐ ■	☐ ■	Toxemia : mild
		☐ ■	Post-term pregnancy (≥41 weeks)

Other indicators:

Physician's Record Copy

Weight Change and Urine Estriol Curves

(See reverse side for tables of standard values)

MATERNAL / NEWBORN
RECORD SYSTEM

Patient name _Alice Kramer_

Date of birth _11-22-44_ Age _30_ No. _87507_

Change in Weight Curve (black)

Immediate pregravid weight _115_

Height (in.) _63_
(without shoes plus one inch)

Standard weight _118_
(record wt. with shoes)

Urine Estriol Curves (green)
Upper curve = average excretion
Lower curve = 95% confidence limit
Values below this curve are considered to be critical.

Cumulative Weight Change (lb)

Urine Estriol (mg. per 24 hrs.)

Weeks of Gestation

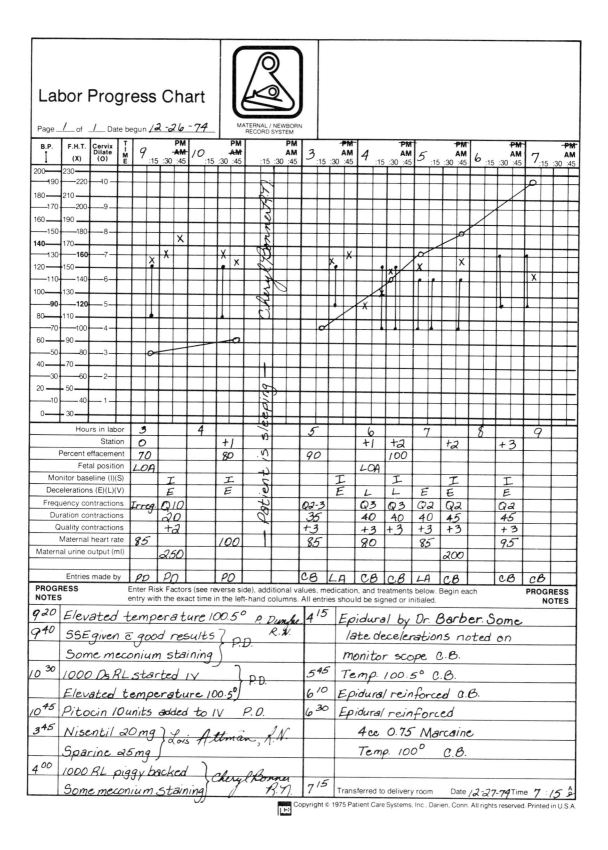

Labor Progress Chart

Page _1_ of _1_ Date begun _12-26-74_

MATERNAL / NEWBORN RECORD SYSTEM

B.P.	F.H.T. (X)	Cervix Dilate (O)	TIME
200	230		
190	220	10	
180	210		
170	200	9	
160	190		
150	180	8	
140	170		
130	160	7	
120	150		
110	140	6	
100	130		
90	120	5	
80	110		
70	100	4	
60	90		
50	80	3	
40	70		
30	60	2	
20	50		
10	40	1	
0	30		

	9	10		3	4	5	6	7

Cheryl Bonner R.N.
Patient is sleeping

Hours in labor	3	4		5	6	7	8	9			
Station	0	+1			+1	+2	+2	+3			
Percent effacement	70	80		90	100						
Fetal position	LOA				LOA						
Monitor baseline (I)(S)		I	I		I	I	I	I			
Decelerations (E)(L)(V)		E	E		E	L	L	E	E	E	
Frequency contractions	Irreg.	Q10		Q2-3	Q3	Q3	Q2	Q2	Q2		
Duration contractions		20		35	40	40	40	45	45		
Quality contractions		+2		+3	+3	+3	+3	+3	+3		
Maternal heart rate	85		100	85	80		85		95		
Maternal urine output (ml)		250					200				
Entries made by	PD	PD	PD	CB	LA	CB	CB	LA	CB	CB	CB

PROGRESS NOTES

Enter Risk Factors (see reverse side), additional values, medication, and treatments below. Begin each entry with the exact time in the left-hand columns. All entries should be signed or initialed.

9²⁰	Elevated temperature 100.5° P. Dumke	4¹⁵	Epidural by Dr. Barber. Some
9⁴⁰	SSE given c̄ good results ⎫ R.N.		late decelerations noted on
	Some meconium staining ⎭ P.D.		monitor scope. C.B.
10³⁰	1000 D₅RL started IV ⎫ P.D.	5⁴⁵	Temp. 100.5° C.B.
	Elevated temperature 100.5° ⎭	6¹⁰	Epidural reinforced C.B.
10⁴⁵	Pitocin 10 units added to IV P.D.	6³⁰	Epidural reinforced
3⁴⁵	Nisentil 20 mg ⎫ Lois Attman, R.N.		4 cc 0.75 Marcaine
	Sparine 25 mg ⎭		Temp. 100° C.B.
4⁰⁰	1000 RL piggy backed ⎫ Cheryl Bonner	7¹⁵	Transferred to delivery room Date 12-27-74 Time 7:15 ᴬ/ₚ
	Some meconium staining ⎭ R.N.		

Labor and Delivery Summary

MATERNAL / NEWBORN
RECORD SYSTEM

Infant's physician Robert Washington, M.D.
(please print)

Labor Summary

	DATE	TIME
MEMBRANES RUPTURED	12-26-74	4 00 P
ONSET OF LABOR		5 00 P
ADMITTED TO HOSPITAL		8 40 P
COMPLETE CERVICAL DIL.	12-27-74	7 00 A

☒ Augmentation (ARM) (Oxytocin)
☒ Monitoring (Internal) (External)

Labor Risk Factors   ☐ None

☐ Abruption
☐ Bleeding of unknown origin
☐ Cord prolapse
☐ Decreased FHT baseline
☒ Elevated temp. (>100°F)
☐ Extended fetal bradycardia
☐ Extended fetal tachycardia
☐ Hydramnios
☐ Meconium staining
☐ Multiple late decelerations
☐ Multiple variable decelerations
☐ Placenta previa
☐ Precipitous labor (<3 hrs)
☐ Prolonged labor (>20 hrs)
☐ Prolonged latent phase
☐ Prolonged 2nd stage (>2.5 hrs)
☐ Protracted active phase
☐ Secondary arrest of dilatation
☐ Seizure activity
☐ Tetanic contractions
☐ Toxemia (mild)
☐ Toxemia (moderate/severe)
☐ _____
☐ _____

Medications

	Total dosage
Niscntil	20 mg
Sparine	25 mg
Marcaine	4cc .75mg

TIME OF LAST NARCOTIC   3 45 P

Presenting Position

☒ Vertex LOA
☐ Breech
☐ Transverse lie
☐ Face or brow _____
☐ Compound _____
☐ Unknown

Delivery Summary

	DATE	TIME
DELIVERY OF INFANT	12-27-74	7 35 A

Method of Delivery

Cephalic
☐ Spontaneous   Type
☒ Low forceps ⎤ Simpson
☐ Mid forceps ⎦
☐ Vacuum extraction
☐ Rotation _____ to _____
Breech
☐ Spontaneous
☐ Partial extraction (assisted)
☐ Total extraction
☐ Forceps to A.C. head
Cesarean (details in operative notes)
☐ Low cervical: transverse
☐ Low cervical: vertical
☐ Classical
☐ Cesarean hysterectomy

Delivery Anesthesia

☐ None
☐ Local
☐ Pudendal
☐ Paracervical
☒ Epidural (pre-del 3 hrs 30 min)
☐ Spinal
☐ General (pre-del ___ hrs ___ min)

Placenta and Cord

Expulsion at   7 45 A
☐ Spontaneous
☒ Expressed   Blood loss
☐ Manual   ☒ Normal
☐ Adherent   ☐ >500 ml
☐ Curettage
Configuration
☒ Normal
☐ Abn. _____
Weight 500 gm
② ③ Umbilical vessels
☒ Cord blood to (lab) (refrig.)

Episiotomy

☐ None   Suture
☐ Median
☒ Mediolateral   3-0 chromic
☐ Other

Laceration

☒ None
___ Degree perineal
☐ Vaginal
☐ Cervical
☐ Uterine rupture
☐ Other

Delivery Summary (cont.)

Surgical Procedures

☐ Tubal ligation
☐ Other _____

Medications   ☒ None

Drug	Dose	Rt	Time
Deladumone	2ml	IM	7 20 A
Pitocin	0.12	IV	7 50 A
			A/P
			A/P
			A/P
			A/P

Sig: Michael Barber, M.D.

Infant Data

_1_ of ① ② _____ births
☐ Male ☒ Female ☐ Ambiguous

Weight 30.90 gm
                lb   oz
Length 49 cm
                in
ID Number 8163
Record Number 31063

Apgar Scores

	Heart rate	Respiration	Muscle tone	Reflex irritation	Skin color	Totals
1 min	1	1	2	1	1	6
5 min	2	2	2	2	1	9

Resuscitation

☐ Spontaneous
☒ Free oxygen
☐ Intubation
☐ Bag and mask
☐ Cardiac
☐ Other _____
_2_ Mins. to sustained respiration

Medications

☒ None
☐ Glucose
☐ Sodium bicarbonate
☐ Drug antagonists
☐ Umbilical catheter
☐ Scalp care
☐ Other _____

Infant Data (cont.)

Congenital Defects

☒ None   ☐ Skin   ☐ Skeletal
☐ CNS   ☐ GI   ☐ GU
☐ Cardiopulmonary ☐ Other

Describe: _____
_____
_____

Birth Trauma

☐ None   ☐ Fracture
☐ Nerve injury   ☐ Bruise
☒ Molding   ☐ Other
Describe: Deformed
right foot
_____
_____

Abn. Intrauterine Conditions

☐ None
☐ Rash/petechiae
☐ Hepatosplenomegaly
☒ Meconium staining
☒ (<) ☐ (>) subcut. fat
☐ Other _____

Output

☒ Urine
☒ Stool mec.
☒ Gastric 15 (ml)

☒ AgNO₃ 1% or _____
Sig: C. Bonner, R.N.
☒ Living at transfer to:
Newborn nursery
Deceased   Date
☐ antepartum   12-27-74
☐ intrapartum   Time
☐ postpartum   8 00 A

Delivered by
Michael Barber, M.D.
Assisting
N. Ricardo, 4 NS
Anesthetist
_____

Circulating nurse
Cheryl Bonner R.N.
Eliz. Beasley, LPN

Initial Newborn Profile

MATERNAL / NEWBORN
RECORD SYSTEM

1. Basic Data (entered by nursing personnel)

G	T	P	A	L
4	2	1	O	2

Mother's name *Alice Kramer*

LMP *3-27-74*

EDC *12-26-74*   Delivery date *12-27-74*   Time of birth *7:35* A

Apgar at: *6* 1 min. *9* 5 min.   ☐ Male ☒ Female ☐ Ambiguous

2. Physical Examination

Date of exam *12-27-74*   Time of exam *10:30* P   Baby's age at exam *3* hrs.

Rectal temperature *97.9°*   Respiration rate *55*   Pulse rate *135*

Femoral pulse: ☒ Normal   ☐ Absent/weak   ☐ Delayed

(Code: ☒ = No abnormalities   ▣ = Abnormalities present)

1 ☒ Reflexes	6 ☒ Thorax	11 ☒ Genitals
2 ▣ Skin: color, lesions	7 ☒ Lungs	12 ☒ Anus
3 ☒ Head/Neck	8 ☒ Heart	13 ☒ Trunk/Spine
4 ☒ Eyes	9 ☒ Abdomen	14 ▣ Extremities/Joints
5 ☒ ENT	10 ☒ Umbilicus	15 ☐ Tone/Appearance

Description of abnormal findings — Please describe your findings objectively. Reserve your impressions or diagnoses for part 3 below. Please begin your findings with the reference number preceding each category.

② *Skin dry and peeling. Somewhat jaundiced c̄ decreased subcutaneous fat. Some meconium staining*

⑭ *Right foot in marked varus position Possible dislocation*

3. Impressions and Diagnosis

Initial Risk Estimate	☐ No risk	☒ Low risk	☐ Medium risk	☐ High risk

1. Jaundiced at 3 hrs. of age. Possible RO-ABO incompatibility and sepsis
2. Right metatarsus varus

Newborn Risk Indicators — the signs and observations listed below are known to be highly predictive of morbidity and mortality in the newborn. Please review them, along with the prior risk information available to you, in order to arrive at your Initial Risk Estimate in part 3.

Observable at birth
Abnormal presentation
Multiple birth
Low birth weight
✓Resuscitation at birth
1 min. Apgar ≤5
5 min. Apgar ≤7
Placental abnormalities
Two cord vessels
Difficult catheterization
≥20ml. of gastric aspirate
Small mandible with cleft palate
Grunting
Deep retractions
Imperforate anus
Pallor
✓Jaundice
Plethora
Convulsions
Decreased tone
✓Congenital malformations

Within 24 hrs. postpartum
Abdominal distension
Vomiting
Failure to pass meconium (if skin not stained)
Melena
Apneic episodes
Tachypnea (transient)
See-saw breathing
Cyanosis
Petechiae/Ecchymoses
✓Jaundice
Pallor
Plethora
Fever
Hypothermia
Arrhythmias
Murmur
Lethargy
Tremors (jitters)
Convulsions

4. Maturity Evaluation

Gest. age by dates *39* wks.	Weight *3090* gms.⊠/ozs.	Chest circ. *32* cm.
Gest. age by exam *37* wks.	Length *49* cm.	Head circ. *34* cm.

This infant is classified as:
☐ Pre-term (<37 weeks)   ☒ Term (37-42 weeks)   ☐ Post-term (>42 weeks)
☐ SGA   ☒ AGA   ☐ LGA

5. Plans: diagnostic and therapeutic

1. Obtain MBR now. Do type and Rh, Coombs, Hgb, and retic. count.
2. Observe right foot. Hold X-ray for now.

Signature: *Robert Washington, M.D.*

Nursery Flow Record

Page _1_ of _2_ Date begun _12-27-74_

MATERNAL / NEWBORN RECORD SYSTEM

Birthdate _12-27-74_ Time _7:35 A_

Sex _Female_ ID/Band no. _8163_

Delivered by: _Micheal Barber, M.D._

Admit to nursery _12-27-74_ Time _8:05 P_

Admitted by: _Mabel Grossman, R.N._

Aquamephyton 1 mg IM _1 amp_ Time _7:45 A_

by: _Cheryl Bonner, R.N._

Blood type and Rh Results _A+_ Date _12-28-74_

Serology _Neg_

Coombs' (Dir) (Indir) _Neg_

PKU _Spec. given_ _12-31-74_

Infant's physician _Robert Washington, M.D._ Tel. no. _617-735-1127_

Mother's name _Mrs. Alice Kramer_ Chart no. _31062_ Room no. _417_

Blood Type and _O+_ Antibody screen ☐ Neg ☐ Pos VDRL ☒ Neg ☐ Pos

Physician's Initial Risk Estimate ☐ No risk ☒ Low risk ☐ Medium risk ☐ High risk

Gest. age = 39 wks Ped. called by Mabel Grossman, R.N.

Doctor ordered Coombs, Hgb, Retic count on 12/27

12/28 1 p.m. Spit up old, bloody mucous

Slight bleeding from cord due to clamp irritation – M.G.

Pt's parents have father's visiting nights

Date	12-27	→	→	12-28	→	→	→	→	→	→	→	12-29	→
Time/Shift	8-10	12-2	4-6	8-10	12-2	4-6	8-10	12-2	4-6	8-10	12-2	4-6	8-10
Baby's age	NB	3	6	11	16	20	25	29	34	38	43	2d.	2d.
Incubator/Warmer temp.				82		81			81		82		81
Baby's temperature	97⁹		97⁹		99⁰		97⁹		97⁹		97⁸		97⁶
Rate of respiration	55		55		60		60		55		50		60
Quality of respiration	wheeze	normal		normal			normal						normal
Apical pulse	135		130		135		130		130		135		140
Muscle tone	decreased	normal		normal			normal						normal
Skin tone	peeling	jaun.	jaun.	jaun.	jaun.		jaun.		jaun.		jaun.		jaun.
Umbilical stump			moist		moist		bleeding		bleeding				moist
Baby's weight	3070						2930						2985
INTAKE G/H₂O (oz)	NPO	NPO	NPO	³/₄	—	¼							
Enf. c̄ fe x 6							³/₄	1½	1	1¼	1¼	½	1½
Toleration				sips	sips	sips	fair	poor	well	well	well	fair sleepy	well
OUTPUT Urine	—	—	—	✓	—	—	✓	✓	✓	✓	✓	✓	✓
Stool	—	—	—	mec	—	mec	mec	—	—	s. mec	mec	mec	mec
Gastric (ml)	—	—	—	spit up	mucous	—	spit up	vomit	—	—	—	—	—
ADDITIONAL INFORMATION Phototherapy			✓	✓	✓	✓	✓	✓	✓	✓	✓	✓	✓
MBR			10.3		11.1		10.5	13.6		12.6	13.0		14.7
Dr. visited			✓		✓		✓		✓				✓
Entries by:	MG	MG	SC	SC	F.J.	F.J.	MG	MG	SC	SC	F.J.	F.J.	MG

MG _Mabel Grossman, R.N._ SC _Sealy Childs, R.N._ F.J. _Florence Jacobs, R.N._

Newborn Discharge Summary

MATERNAL / NEWBORN
RECORD SYSTEM

Physical Examination

Date of exam 12-31-74	Time of exam 10 30 A/P	Baby's age at exam 4 hours days
Temperature 99°	Respiration rate 60	Pulse rate 130

(Code ✓ = No abnormalities ⊙ = Abnormalities present)

1 ✓ Reflexes   6 ✓ Thorax   11 ✓ Genitals
2 ⊙ Skin: color, lesions   7 ✓ Lungs   12 ✓ Anus
3 ✓ Head/Neck   8 ✓ Heart   13 ✓ Trunk/Spine
4 ✓ Eyes   9 ✓ Abdomen   14 ⊙ Extremities/Joints
5 ✓ ENT   10 ✓ Umbilicus   15 ✓ Tone/Appearance

Description of abnormal findings — Please describe your findings objectively. Reserve your impressions or diagnoses for the Discharge section below. Please begin your findings with the reference number preceding the circled category.

② Mild icterus
⑭ Flexion deformity rt. foot

Discharge Status

— Use this section to summarize the baby's present condition. Describe briefly existing and resolved neonatal problems. If the baby is deceased, explain the reasons for death.

Problem: (1) Hyperbilirubinemia
Developed: 1 ☐ At birth   2 ✓ In nursery
Status: 1 ✓ Resolved   3 ☐ Stable
     2 ☐ Diminished   4 ☐ Accelerated

Problem (2) Flexion deformity rt. foot
Developed: 1 ✓ At birth   2 ☐ In nursery
Status: 1 ☐ Resolved   3 ✓ Stable
     2 ☐ Diminished   4 ☐ Accelerated

Problem (3)
Developed: 1 ☐ At birth   2 ☐ In nursery
Status: 1 ☐ Resolved   3 ☐ Stable
     2 ☐ Diminished   4 ☐ Accelerated

Problem (4)
Developed: 1 ☐ At birth   2 ☐ In nursery
Status: 1 ☐ Resolved   3 ☐ Stable
     2 ☐ Diminished   4 ☐ Accelerated

Basic Data

Infant's name: Kramer (last)   Sue Anne (first)

Discharge weight 3030 gms/ozs

Mother's record number 31062
Infant's record number 31063
Infant's ID number 8163

Tests	Results	Date
Blood Type	O+	12-28
Coombs (dir)	Neg	↓
Serology (blood)	Neg	
PKU urine	Spec	12-31
Hgb	14	12-28
Retic	1.2	12-28

Sex ☐ Male ✓ Female ☐ Ambiguous
Race ☐ Caucasian ✓ Black ☐ Other

Date of birth 12-27-74
Time of birth 7:35 A/P

Place of birth
✓ In hospital   ☐ En route
☐ At home   ☐ Unknown
☐ Other hospital _____

If baby died note: Age at death ___ days ___ hrs   Autopsy ☐ Yes ☐ No

Newborn in discharged on 12-31-74   Time 11:00 A/P
✓ With mother (or with _____)
☐ To another service _____
☐ To another hospital _____
☐ Against advice

Follow-up visit scheduled for 1-14-75
☐ With private physician
✓ At clinic: Revere Medical Center
Note: Formula prep + feeding inst. given

Date 12-31-74   Nurse's Signature Mabel Grossman   RN

Course of treatment & impressions — Please refer to problem (1), (2), (3), or (4) in your summary. Note also your final impression of the baby at discharge.

Full term, newborn female
1. Hyperbilirubinemia 2nd to ABO incompatibility. Phototherapy begun 12-27. Stopped 12/29. Check Hgb next clinic visit.
2. Continue foot stretching exercises at home. Cast later if necessary.
Prognosis good for listed complications.

Date 12-31-74   Physician's Signature Robert Washington, MD

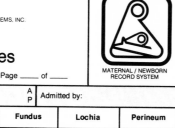

PATIENT CARE SYSTEMS, INC.

Postpartum
Nurses' Notes

Page _____ of _____

MATERNAL / NEWBORN
RECORD SYSTEM

Time admitted to postpartum unit		A P	Admitted by:				Patient's physician _Please Print_

Date	Hour		Fundus	Lochia	Perineum	Breasts	Progress Notes
	. .	A P					
	. .	A P					
	. .	A P					
	. .	A P					
	. .	A P					
	. .	A P					
	. .	A P					
	. .	A P					
	. .	A P					
	. .	A P					
	. .	A P					
	. .	A P					
	. .	A P					
	. .	A P					
	. .	A P					
	. .	A P					
	. .	A P					
	. .	A P					
	. .	A P					
	. .	A P					
	. .	A P					
	. .	A P					
	. .	A P					
	. .	A P					
	. .	A P					

Please sign all notes

Postpartum Progress Notes

Page _1_ of _2_

MATERNAL / NEWBORN
RECORD SYSTEM

Time admitted to postpartum unit	9:45 A/P	Admitted by: L. Clayton, R.N.		Patient's physician Micheal Barber, M.D.

Date	Hour	Fundus	Lochia	Perineum	Breasts	Progress Notes
1-27	9:50 A/P	Firm @ u over to right side	mod. Rubra	Clean Ice glove	Soft	BP 110/70 P80 Husb. at bedside L.C.
	10:30 A/P	↓				BP 110/70 P80 L. Clayton, R.N.
	11-2 A/P					BP 110/80 P70
	9:30 A/P	Firm over to right side Unt	mod. Rubra			OOB to bathroom - voided small amount L.C.
	10:30 A/P	↓				Abd. prep done. Voided small amt. in bathroom L.C.
1-27	11:15 A/P	F @ u				Cath: 1000 cc. obtained L.C.
1-28	11-7 A/P	F @ u				NPO for surgery in AM R. Gasewski, R.N.
	5:30 A/P					Inst: care of perineum Voided X1 ǫs R.G.
	7-9 A/P	Firm u + 2	mod.	clean	soft	Pre-op for TL Pt. OOB + voided Prepared for surgery BP 110/70 T 99⁶ P80 R 18
	A/P					TO OR @ 9AM S. Prestwick, R.N.
	12:10 A/P					Returned from OR fully reacted but sleepy BP 120/90 P76 R20
	A/P					Band-aid on abd. clean and intact Pt. restless M. Miller, R.N.
	2:00 A/P	Firm	mod. Rubra	clean	soft	Pt. encouraged to move S.P.
1-28	3-11 A/P	↓ u abd. soft	M.R.			OOB → BR voided ǫs Band-aid dry M. Ledecky, R.N.
1-29	11-7 A/P	abd. soft	mod. Rubra			Slept well voiding ǫs
	7-3 A/P	↓	↓	clean	soft	Pt. encouraged to force fluids + lie flat. Pt. complaining of spinal headache. OOB very little S. Prestwick, R.N.
	A/P					
1-29	3-11 A/P	Abd. soft				OOB voiding ǫs c/o headache M. Ledecky, R.N.
1-30	7-3 A/P	↓	mod. Serosa	clean	soft erect	Incision clean. Force fluids Sub-sternal binder applied by
	A/P					Dr. Thompson. Binder removed, uncomfortable because of abd.
	A/P					incision. Headache when OOB Dr. Peterson visited about baby.
	A/P					Bottle fed baby 2X S. Prestwick, R.N.
1-30	3-11 A/P	Abd. soft	mod. Serosa	clean	firm leaking	Bra pads given. Inst to use cold socks → breasts
	A/P					Medicated for headache c̄ some relief. M. Ledecky, R.N.
	A/P					

Please sign all notes

Obstetric Discharge Summary

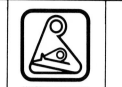

MATERNAL / NEW BORN
RECORD SYSTEM

Reasons For Admission

Admission date _12-27-74_   Weeks gestation _39_

☐ Risk pregnancy (list indicators below)   Code

1 _Normal multigravid without_   _____
2 _complications_   _____
3 _____   _____
4 _____   _____
5 _____   _____
6 _____   _____

☒ Ruptured membranes   ☐ Threatened abortion
☐ Bloody show   ☐ Mid-trimester abortion
☐ Free bleeding   ☐ Induction for labor
☒ Contractions   ☐ For cesarean section
☐ Other _____

Labor and Delivery: a brief description of labor, anesthesia, delivery procedures, the placenta and cord, and any resulting complications. Note: for more complete details, refer to the *Labor and Delivery Summary* record.

Outcome of this pregnancy

☐ Undelivered   ☒ Delivered at this hospital
☐ Aborted   ☐ Delivered at: _____

Rapid labor progress c̄ IV pitocin
Epidural, vertex OA low forceps c̄
mid-line episiotomy 3-0 chromic.
Est. blood loss 200 c.c. Cervix
inspected. Uterus intact

_____
_____
_____

Puerperium

Surgical procedures

☒ Sterilization (define) _p.p. tubal ligation_
☐ Other _____

Summary of postpartum complications

Problem list	Act.	Res.	Code
1 _Anemia_	☒	☐	_____
2 _Mastalgia_	☐	☒	_____
3 _____	☐	☐	_____
4 _____	☐	☐	_____
5 _____	☐	☐	_____
6 _____	☐	☐	_____
7 _____	☐	☐	_____

Additional notes: _General condition good. Fundus_
firm, non-tender. Lochia clear.
Episiotomy clean c̄ slight swelling.
Breasts neg.

Puerperium (cont.)

Discharge status of patient

☒ Alive   ☐ Deceased   Autopsy ☐ Yes ☐ No   Code

Reasons for death _____

Patient is discharged on _12-31-74_

☐ To a private physician
☒ To a postpartum clinic _Revere Medical Center_
☐ To another service _____
☐ To another hospital _____
☐ Against advice

Plans for follow-up visit on _1-8-75_
Return in 1 week for stitch removal

Return in 6 weeks for p.p. follow-up

_____
_____

Discharge Summary of the Newborn

Name _Sue Anne_   Apgar _6_ 1 min _9_ 5 min
Record no. _31063_   Birthweight _3090_ gm
Birth _1_ of ①②   Computed gest. age
☐ Male ☒ Female ☐ Ambiguous   _37_ wks = _AGA_

Summary of neonatal complications

Problem list	Act.	Res.
1 _Jaundice_	☐	☒
2 _Dislocation rt. foot_	☒	☐
3 _____	☐	☐
4 _____	☐	☐
5 _____	☐	☐
6 _____	☐	☐
7 _____	☐	☐

Discharge status of newborn

☒ Alive   ☐ Neonatal death ____ days ____ hrs postpartum
☐ Stillborn   ☐ Autopsy   ☐ No autopsy

Reasons for death _____

Newborn is discharged on _12-31-74_

☒ With mother (or with _____)
☐ To another service _____
☐ To another hospital _____
☐ Against advice

Summary by _Micheal Barber, M.D._

Completed on _12-31-74_   Time _3:30_ P

Assessment forms: high-risk and normal neonates

See pp. 704 to 713.

State of California - Health and Welfare Agency

INFANT TRANSPORT FORM PART 1

Department of Health

REFERRING

HOSPITAL _____

CITY _____

CODE [ ][ ][ ][ ][ ] PHONE _____ _____

RECEIVING

HOSPITAL _____

CITY _____

CODE [ ][ ][ ][ ][ ] PHONE _____ _____

PATIENT'S NAME _____

BIRTHDATE [ ][ ][ ][ ][ ][ ] TIME [ ][ ][ ][ ]

FATHER'S NAME _____

OCCUPATION _____

AREA CODE _____ BUS PHONE _____

MOTHER'S NAME _____

MAIDEN NAME _____ PLACE OF BIRTH _____

ADDRESS _____

_____

AREA CODE _____ PHONE _____

PERTINENT HISTORY, MOTHER

AGE [ ][ ] GR [ ][ ] PARA [ ][ ] SAB [ ] TAB [ ]

PRIOR FD [ ] NND [ ] LBW [ ]

RACE [ ]

		BLOOD TYPE [ ]			VDRL
1	WHITE				
2	MEXAM	1 O+	6 O-		0 NEG
3	BLACK	2 A+	7 A-		1 POS
4	CHINESE	3 B+	8 B-		
5	JAPANESE	4 AB+	9 AB-		
6	OTHER	5 "+"	0 "-"		

HISTORY OF

DIABETES	1	OTHER, SPECIFY
3RD TRI BLEEDING	2	
PLACENTA PREVIA	3	
ABRUPTIO PLACENTA	4	
ECLAMPSIA	5	
TOXEMIA	6	
RH SENSITIZATION	7	
AMNIONITIS	8	ICDA CODES
DRUG ABUSE	9	[ ][ ][ ][ ][ ] [ ][ ][ ]

RX DURING PREGNANCY

TYPE   DOSAGE   TRIMESTER

_____

_____

RX DURING LABOR & DELIVERY (INCLUDE OXYTOCIC)

AGENT   ROUTE   HRS ẋ DELIVERY

_____

_____

_____

LABOR 1ST STAGE [ ][ ] HRS 2ND [ ][ ] MINS

ROM [ ][ ] HRS BEFORE DELIVERY [0] SPONTANEOUS

[1] ARTIFICIAL

PRESENTATION

[ ]   DELIVERY [ ]

0 VERTEX	0 SPONTANEOUS	PLACENTA
1 BREECH	1 MID FORCEPS	0 NORMAL
2 OTHER	2 C/S REPEAT	1 ABNORMAL SPECIFY
	3 " ELECT	
	4 " EMERG	
	5 OTHER	

TO BE FILLED OUT BY

LABOR & DELIVERY (CONT)

IN TRACHEA

MECONIUM STAINED AMNIOTIC FLUID [ ] [ ]

	NONE 0	0 No
RESUSCITATION	THIN 1	1 YES
	THICK 2	9 UNK

0	NONE	
1	CATHETER SUCTION	
2	OXYGEN	FETAL MONITOR [ ]
3	BAG & MASK	0 No
4	INTUBATION	1 EXTERNAL
5	POSITIVE PRESSURE	2 INTERNAL
6	UMBILICAL CATHETER	
7	DRUGS	
8	CARDIAC MASSAGE	FETAL DISTRESS [0] No
9	OTHER	[1] YES

AMNIOCENTESIS [0] No   FETAL SCALP BLOOD [0] No

[1] YES   SAMPLING [1] YES

IF ANSWER IS YES TO EITHER OF ABOVE GIVE RESULTS

REFERRING HOSPITAL

LOW- AND MEDIUM-RISK NURSERIES*	Date
Symptoms of illness	Ward
	Hosp. No.
	Name

Birth Wt _____ gm Birth date _____ Address

Date													
Time													
Hour of age													
Fed poorly													
Sucked poorly													
Gagged													
Drooled													
Regurgitated													
Hiccoughs													
Mucus (specify site)													
Abdominal distention													
Abnormal stools													
Sore buttocks													
Weight loss													
Convulsions													
Rigid													
Opisthotonus													
Twitching													
Irritable													
Hyperactive													
Tires easily													
Less active													
Lethargic													
Weak cry													
Shrill cry													
Pulse rate													
Respiratory rate													
Shallow respirations													
Deep respirations													
Irregular respirations													
See-saw respirations													
Intercostal retractions													
Zyphoid retractions													
Dilated alae nasi													
Grunting													
Rest periods <10 secs													
Rest periods 10-25 secs													
Apnea (25 secs or more)													
Cough													

+ = Mild a = ac
++ = Moderate p = pc
+++ = Severe r = Rest
$\bar{c}$ = With handling or feeding only

*From Newborn Service, Division of Perinatal Medicine, University of Colorado Medical Center, Denver, Colo.

LOW- AND MEDIUM-RISK NURSERIES—cont'd
Symptoms of illness—cont'd

Date

Ward

Name

Hosp. No.

Address

Date													
Time													
Hour of age													
Sneeze													
Stuffy nose													
Wheezing													
Body temperature													
Incubator temperature													
Cyanosis, circumoral													
Cyanosis, circumocular													
Cyanosis, extremities													
Cyanosis, generalized													
Pallor													
Plethora													
Mottled													
Jaundice													
Petechiae (specify area)													
Ecchymoses (specify area)													
Bleeding (specify area)													
Edema (specify area)													
Sclerema													
Umbilical redness													
Umbilical oozing													
Alcohol to cord													
Pustular rash													
Other rash													
Abscess													
Skin irritated (specify area)													
Skin dry or peeling													
Eye discharge													
Other													
Eyes open													
Yawn													
Demanding													
Hungry													
Sucks well													
Weight gain													
Strong cry													
Active													
Color stable													

INTENSIVE CARE NURSERY*
Symptoms of illness

Date

Ward

Name

Hosp. No.

Birth Wt _____ gm   Birth date _____   Address

Date													
Time													
Hour of age													
Gavaged poorly													
Sucked poorly													
Gagged													
Drooled													
Regurgitated													
Hiccoughs													
Mucus on tube													
Mucus, other													
Abdominal distention													
Abnormal stools													
Sore buttocks													
Weight loss													
Convulsions													
Rigid													
Opisthotonus													
Twitching													
Irritable													
Hyperactive													
Tires easily													
Less active													
Lethargic													
Weak cry													
Shrill cry													
Pulse rate													
Oxygen, liters													
Oxygen concentration (%)													
Respiratory rate													
Shallow respirations													
Deep respirations													
Irregular respirations													
Rest periods <10 secs													
Rest periods 10-25 secs													
Apnea (25 secs or more)													
Intercostal retractions													
Zyphoid retractions													
See-saw respirations													
Dilated alae nasi													
Grunting													
Cough													

+ = Mild   a = ac
++ = Moderate   p = pc
+++ = Severe   r = Rest
                              $\bar{c}$ = With handling or feeding only

*From Newborn Service, Division of Perinatal Medicine, University of Colorado Medical Center, Denver, Colo.

INTENSIVE CARE NURSERY—cont'd
Symptoms of illness—cont'd

Date

Ward

Name

Hosp. No.

Address

Date													
Time													
Hour of age													
Sneeze													
Stuffy nose													
Body temperature													
Incubator temperature													
Cyanosis, circumoral													
Cyanosis, circumocular													
Cyanosis, extremities													
Cyanosis, generalized													
Pallor													
Plethora													
Mottled													
Jaundice													
Petechiae (specify area)													
Ecchymoses (specify area)													
Bleeding (specify area)													
Edema (specify area)													
Sclerema													
Umbilical redness													
Umbilical oozing													
Alcohol to cord													
Pustular rash													
Other rash													
Abscess													
Skin irritated (specify area)													
Skin dry or peeling													
Eye discharge													
Other													
Eyes open													
Yawn													
Demanding													
Hungry													
Sucks well													
Weight gain													
Strong cry													
Active													
Color stable													

CHILDREN'S HOSPITAL OF SAN FRANCISCO

NEW BORN I.C.U.

TREATMENT AND ACTIVITY RECORD

SIGNATURES

0730 - 1600

1530 - 2400

2345 - 0745

TIME	TEMPERATURE			OXYGEN	RESP RATE ①	APNEA	POSTURAL DRAINAGE	SUCTION ② RESULT	APICAL	BRADY	BLOOD PRESSURE		COLOR ③	EDEMA ④	ACTIVITY ⑤	TONE ⑥	POSITION ⑦	PHOTO THERAPY	LAB WORK			X - RAYS	SPECIAL PROCEDURES DR 'S VISITS
	ISO HOOD ¹Nₐₛₐₗ		AX		RESP						CUFF	ARTER							BLOOD	URINE	CULTURE		
0800																							
0900																							
1000																							
1100																							
1200																							
1300																							
1400																							
1500																							
1600																							
1700																							
1800																							
1900																							
2000																							
2100																							
2200																							
2300																							
2400																							
0100																							
0200																							
0300																							
0400																							
0500																							
0600																							
0700																							

EXPLANATION OF CODES

① RESP. CODE: A=APNEA   P=PERIODIC   R=RETRACT   1=MILD   2=MODERATE   3=SEVERE   G=GRUNT   F=FLARE   C=CRYING   S=SHALLOW

② RESULT CODE: S=SCANT   M=MODERATE   L=LARGE

③ COLOR CODE: A=ASHEN   C=CYANOTIC   CC=CIRCUMORAL CYANOSIS   AC=ACROCYANOSIS   D=DUSKY   J=JAUNDICE   M=MOTTLED   P=PINK   PL=PLETHORIC   PP=PALE

④ EDEMA COLOR: N=NONE   M=MILD   MM=MODERATE   S=SEVERE

⑤ ACTIVITY CODE: A+++=ACTIVE   AS=ACTIVE c̄ STIMULATION   I=IRRITABLE   J=JITTERY   H=HYPERACTIVE   L=LETHARGIC   N=NON-REACTIVE

⑥ TONE CODE: P=POOR   A=APPROPRIATE   E=EXAGGERATED   Q=QUIET

⑦ POSITION CODE: R=RIGHT SIDE   L=LEFT SIDE   P=PRONE   S=SUPINE   S=◄HEAD ELEVATED

SIGNATURES

CHILDREN'S HOSPITAL OF SAN FRANCISCO

NEW BORN I.C.U.

RESPIRATORY FLOW RECORD

0730-1600

1530-2400

2345-0755

DATE

DATE OF RESPIRATORY THERAPY

TIME	OXYGEN		① SIGHING		E.T. TUBE IRRIGATION	CPAP PRESSURE	BABY BIRD				② CHEST TUBE	③ SITE	BLOOD GASES				
	ISOLETTE	BABY	METHOD				VENT. RATE	BABY RATE	PEAK PRESSURE	END PRESSURE			PH	PCO2	PO2	HCO3	BE

EXPLANATION OF CODES

① METHOD CARE: N= NASAL   T= ENDOTRACHEAL TUBE   M= MASK   H = HOOD

② CHEST TUBE CODE: M= MILKED   F = FLUCTUATING   SS = SEROSANGUINOUS DRAINAGE   B = BLOODY DRAINAGE   S = SERIOUS DRAINAGE

③ SITE CODE: UA = UMBILICAL ARTERY   TA = TEMPORAL ARTERY   RA = RADIAL ARTERY   HS = HEEL STICK   V = VENOUS

CHILDREN'S HOSPITAL OF SAN FRANCISCO

NEONATAL

24 HOUR INTAKE/OUTPUT RECORD

DATE | PREVIOUS WEIGHT | CURRENT WEIGHT

		INTAKE						ORAL/TUBE			OUTPUT				LAB STIX				
		PARENTERAL								ACTIVITY						SUGAR	ACETONE	PROTEIN	ph	BLOOD
08	BASIC SOLUTION	ADDI-TIVES	DES. VOL. /HR	AMT. IN CHAMBER	ACT. VOL. /HR.	HOURLY FLUID BALANCE +	-	TYPE	AMT. TAKEN		U R.	SPECIFIC GRAVITY	NG	STOOL AND OTHER						

DAY 08 09 10 11 12 13 14 15 — TOTAL DAY (A.M.)

P M 16 17 18 19 20 21 22 23 — TOTAL (P.M.)

NIGHT 24 01 02 03 04 05 06 07 — TOTAL NIGHT

TOTAL FOR 24 HOURS

TOTAL I.V. / TOTAL BLOOD / TOTAL ORAL / GRAND TOTAL

TOTAL I.V. / TOTAL NG / TOTAL OTHER & STOOL / GRAND TOTAL

CODE:
NW - NIPPLED WELL
NF - NIPPLED FAIR
NP - NIPPLED POOR
G - GAVAGED

CHILDREN'S HOSPITAL OF SAN FRANCISCO

NEONATAL BALANCE RECORD

DATE	TIME	HGB GMS	HCT %	TSP GM%	DEXTRO STIX MG%	BLOOD SUGAR MG%	NA MEQ	K MEQ	CL MEQ	BUN MG%	CA MG%	BILIRUBIN			BLOOD GASES	BLOOD BALANCE			OTHER
												DIR MG%	IN MG%	TOTAL MG%		IN	OUT	BAL.	

CHILDREN'S HOSPITAL OF SAN FRANCISCO

MEDICATION RECORD
(INFANTS)

MEDICATION DOSAGE—ROUTE—SCHEDULE	DATE		07-15	15-23	23-07	07-15	15-23	23-07	07-15	15-23	23-07	07-15	15-23	23-07
CONTROLLED DRUGS	TIME													
	SITE													
	INTLS													
	TIME													
	SITE													
	INTLS													
	TIME													
	SITE													
	INTLS													
	TIME													
	SITE													
	INTLS													
	TIME													
	SITE													
	INTLS													
	TIME													
	SITE													
	INTLS													
	TIME													
	SITE													
	INTLS													
	TIME													
	SITE													
	INTLS													
	TIME													
	SITE													
	INTLS													
	TIME													
	SITE													
	INTLS													
	TIME													
	SITE													
	INTLS													

SITE OF INJECTION CODE:
RQ = RIGHT UPPER OUTER QUADRANT   RD = RIGHT DELTOID   RAT = RIGHT ANTERIOR THIGH   RLT = RIGHT LATERAL THIGH
LQ = LEFT UPPER OUTER QUADRANT   LD = LEFT DELTOID   LAT = LEFT ANTERIOR THIGH   LLT = LEFT LATERAL THIGH
RVG = RIGHT VENTRO GLUTEAL   LVG = LEFT VENTRO GLUTEAL

INITIALS	SIGNATURE	INITIALS	SIGNATURE	INITIALS	SIGNATURE

APPENDIX L

A parents' guide to the Newborn Intensive Care Unit (NBICU)*

I. Why do babies come to the NBICU?

The Newborn Intensive Care Unit is a special unit of the hospital designed and equipped to care for babies who are sick when they are born and during the first few weeks of life. Those babies who need special watching are also brought here. Some of these babies are born at Children's Hospital; some are transferred from other hospitals or from home.

This pamphlet was written to help parents who have babies in the NBICU understand our procedures and services at Children's Hospital. We have tried to answer some of your questions about your baby's hospitalization.

II. How do I get to the NBICU?

A. See attached map.

B. *Parking* is available on the street near the hospital.

There is also a parking lot on Cherry Street between Sacramento and California Streets, off the Emergency Entrance to the hospital. The parking lot charge is 50¢ an hour, $2.00 maximum a day.

C. *Services in the hospital:* On the ground floor of the hospital are located the gift shop, coffee shop and cafeteria. There are rest rooms on the ground floor across from the public telephones in the main corridor. Gift Shop hours are 10:00 AM-4:00 PM and 6:00 PM-8:00 PM weekdays, and 1:00 PM-4:00 PM on weekends. Coffee Shop hours are from 11:00 AM-3:30 PM. The cafeteria serves breakfast from 6:00-10:30 AM, lunch from 11:30 AM-1:30 PM, and dinner from 4:15 PM-7:00 PM. Vending machines are located in the cafeteria also.

D. *Newborn ICU:* The NBICU is located on the second floor of the hospital beyond the regular nursery. There are public telephones located near the elevators on the second floor.

*From Children's Hospital and Medical Center, San Francisco, Calif.

III. When can I visit?

A. *Visiting hours:* The NBICU is open 24 hours a day and you are invited to visit at any time. Since morning hours are often busy with doctors' rounds, we ask that you plan your visit after this time. Occasionally an emergency will arise while you are visiting; at this time the nurse or doctor may ask you to wait outside the unit until the emergency is over.

B. *Who can visit?* Parents and grandparents can visit in the NBICU, but due to our lack of space we ask that visitors be limited to two at a time.

C. *Can I touch my baby?* Certainly! To maintain cleanliness we ask that you wear a nursery gown, which you can get from the nurse, and that you wash your hands first (and also upon leaving the nursery, after you have removed the gown). Only you, the parents, may touch your baby.

If the baby or the mother are in isolation, ask your doctor before you visit.

If you have a cold, a skin infection, or diarrhea, you may not be able to visit. It is best to check with your doctor first.

D. *Surgery:* It is not possible to accompany your baby to surgery. However, you may wait in the waiting rooms near the nursery or on the ground floor. We will ask you to sign a permit for surgery and for special procedures, such as a lumbar puncture (also called a spinal tap or an LP).

IV. To whom can I talk?

Telephone calls from parents are welcome 24 hours a day. The NBICU number is _____.

A. *Physicians: Your private doctor is the best source of information about your baby's condition and medical information.* If your baby has been transferred from another hospital or if you belong to the Children's Hospital Clinic, Dr. _____ or Dr. _____,

Directors of the nursery, are available to give you medical information.

A pediatric intern or resident (housestaff) is assigned to care for your baby. They, too, are available to help answer your questions. The residents and interns are in the nursery 24 hours a day. You will be introduced to your housestaff doctor when you visit the NBICU.

B. _____ (name) is the Head Nurse in the NBICU.

Every baby is assigned one nurse every 8 hours around the clock. The nurses are specially trained for working with small or ill babies. They are a valuable source of information for baby care and are glad to help you learn about your baby.

Often additional nursing care is desirable after the baby's discharge. Please ask your doctor or the nurse in charge about this.

C. *Social worker:* _____ (name) is the social worker for the NBICU. Since the birth of a baby who is small or ill is so unexpected, parents often need someone to talk to about their emotional and family concerns. The social worker can also help you prepare for the baby's discharge. If you wish to talk to the social worker, please ask your doctor, the nurse in charge, or call her directly at _____. It is valuable to talk with her at least once before you leave the nursery.

D. *Business office.* Financial concerns also contribute to the crisis of having your baby in the NBICU. Sometimes if you enroll the baby on your insurance policy when he or she is born, the insurance will cover part or all of the baby's hospital bill. Check on your policy to see what coverage you have.

If you have no insurance, California Medical Assistance Program—Medically Needy Only can be checked out through your county welfare department.

Crippled Children's Services are available for a limited time for some illnesses. Check with your doctor about this program. If appropriate, he will direct you to the CCS office in your county.

If you have questions, _____ (name) or _____ (name) in the Business Office are happy to help you. Their number is _____.

V. What is all that equipment?

When you first visit your baby he or she will probably be in an *isolette* or *incubator*. An isolette is an environment that provides constant warmth and cleanliness through the course of the baby's illness.

If your baby has respiratory lung disease, extra oxygen will be pumped into the isolette to help him breathe.

Sometimes a ventilator (breathing machine) may be used to help the baby breathe better.

If your baby is too small or too ill to eat he may have *intravenous* feeding (IV), (this means feeding through the veins) or he may be *gavage-fed* (this means a tube is passed into the baby's stomach). Some medicines are given through the IV.

Some babies have heart monitor wires taped to their arms, legs, or chest. The heart monitor tells the doctor and the nurse how your baby's heart is beating. In addition, babies often have *monitor leads* to watch their breathing. Some babies forget to breathe for awhile; when this happens a beeper on the monitor goes off to alert the nurse.

The nurse at your baby's isolette will be glad to explain this equipment to you.

VI. What is hyaline membrane disease? Respiratory distress syndrome?

Hyaline membrane disease (HMD) is a disease of the lungs which affects many premature babies. This happens because the lungs are still immature. Some babies are much sicker than others; we do not know why.

Babies with HMD breathe with great difficulty. They need extra oxygen, mist and intravenous fluids. They must be kept very warm and they may need help with their breathing with a bag and mask or a ventilator.

The disease may go on for days or sometimes for many weeks. It will *not* hurt your baby to touch him. The nurses often stimulate the baby to breathe more or to help clear the mucus from the lungs.

VII. What does it mean if my baby is premature?

A premature baby is generally an unexpected event for everyone concerned. Parents are not ready to receive the baby at home and babies are not mature enough to live outside the womb without some help.

There are many reasons why babies are born prematurely, but some are born early without a known cause. Your doctor may or may not be able to tell you the direct cause.

VIII. What is hyperbilirubinemia (jaundice)?

Your body and your baby's body are constantly producing new red blood cells and getting rid of old red blood cells. Hyperbilirubinemia occurs when your baby's body can't get rid of old red blood cells fast enough. The accumulation of old red blood cells is seen in the yellowish color of your baby's skin. Hyperbilirubinemia is sometimes called *jaundice,* but this is *not* the same as adult jaundice.

We treat hyperbilirubinemia with light. If your baby needs light treatment, he will wear a cap and goggles to keep the bright light out of his eyes.

IX. Can I feed my baby?

As your baby gets better, we will encourage you to feed him or her. This helps both of you learn about each other and helps bring you, the parents and your baby, closer together. Since babies' schedules change, a call to the nursery ahead of time will help you plan your visit around feeding time.

X. How can I breast-feed my baby?

It is advisable to check with your doctor before breast-feeding. If it's all right with your doctor and your baby is still in an isolette, the nurse will instruct you on how to pump your breasts and save the milk for the baby. If possible, we prefer to use breast milk for babies who weigh less than 3½ pounds. If you aren't planning to breast feed or if you don't have enough milk, we can use milk from the Mother's Milk Bank located here at Children's Hospital. The Mothers' Milk Bank will accept donations of any extra breast milk you might have.

XI. Is it normal to feel my emotions more at this time?

Yes. Since your baby is in the hospital you may feel down or depressed at this time. It is also normal to feel like eating less and to sleep irregularly. These feelings are temporary and should improve as you feel better about your baby. If they do not go away, be sure to contact your doctor.

XII. Don't babies go home when they weigh five pounds?

Weight is not the only indicator of whether a baby is healthy and ready to go home.

In the NBICU when a baby is:

1. Free of illness
2. Able to maintain his or her own temperature
3. Eating well
4. Gaining weight regularly, and
5. If the parents are comfortable feeding and handling the baby and things are ready at home

then your baby is ready to be discharged.

XIII. The follow-up clinic

_____ (name) and _____ (name) (Coordinator of the Follow-Up Clinic) will invite certain babies back to Children's Hospital to be evaluated at 6 months of age and intervals after that.

APPENDIX M

Nurse-midwife education

When a nurse-midwife is certified by the American College of Nurse-Midwives, she is entitled to use the initials C.N.M. after her name.

Institutions offering ACNM approved basic education in nurse-midwifery, internship programs, or refresher programs are listed below. Approval status is subject to change periodically. This information is current as of March, 1976.

Booth Maternity Center   R,I
6051 Overbrook Ave.
Philadelphia, Pa. 19131

In affiliation with
Maternity Center Association
48 E. 92nd St.
New York, N.Y. 10028

College of Medicine and Dentistry of   CB
New Jersey
School of Allied Health Professions
Nurse-Midwifery Program
100 Bergen St.
Newark, N.J. 07103

Columbia University Graduate Program in   MB
Maternity Nursing and Nurse-Midwifery
Department of Nursing, Faculty of Medicine
Columbia-Presbyterian Medical Center
622 W. 168th St.
New York, N.Y. 10032

Frontier School of Midwifery and Family   CB
Nursing
Wendover
Leslie County, Ky. 41775

Georgetown University School of Nursing   CB
3700 Reservoir Rd., N.W.
Washington, D.C. 20007

The Johns Hopkins University   MB
School of Hygiene and Public Health
Nurse-Midwifery Program
615 North Wolfe St.
Baltimore, Md. 21205

Medical University of South Carolina   CB
Nurse-Midwifery Program, College of Nursing
80 Barre St.
Charleston, S.C. 29401

St. Louis University   MB
Department of Nursing
Graduate Program in Nurse-Midwifery
1401 South Grand Blvd.
St. Louis, Mo. 63104

Simpson Center for Maternal Health   R,I
The Community Hospital of Springfield,
   Clark County
350 South Burnett Rd.
Springfield, Ohio 45505

State University of New York   CB,R,I
College of Health Related Professions
Nurse-Midwifery Program
Box 1216
450 Clarkson Ave.
Brooklyn, N.Y. 11203

United States Air Force   CB
Nurse-Midwifery Program
Malcolm Grow USAF Medical Center
Andrews Air Force Base, Md. 20331

The University of Illinois at the Medical Center MB
College of Nursing, Department of Maternal-
   Child Nursing
Nurse-Midwifery Program
P.O. Box 6998
Chicago, Ill. 60680

University of Kentucky   MB
College of Nursing
Albert B. Chandler Medical Center
Lexington, Ky. 40506

University of Mississippi   *CB,R
Nurse-Midwifery Program
2500 North State St.
Jackson, Miss. 39216

---

*   = Graduate credit offered.

717

University of Utah   MB,R
College of Nursing
Graduate Major in Maternal and Newborn
   Nursing and Nurse-Midwifery
25 South Medical Dr.
Salt Lake City, Utah 84112

Yale University School of Nursing   *MB
Graduate Program in Maternal and Newborn
   Nursing and Nurse-Midwifery
38 South St.
New Haven, Conn. 06510

R   = Refresher program; for nurse-midwives who have not prac-
      ticed in recent years and want to update their knowledge and
      clinical practice and/or take the National Certification Exam to
      become a certified nurse-midwife. Length varies according to
      needs of the individual, but usually a minimum of 12 weeks is
      necessary to fulfill requirements for certification.
I   = Internship; for recent graduates of CB and MB programs who
      desire additional clinical experience prior to entering the pro-
      fession of nurse-midwifery. Length varies according to indi-
      vidual's needs.
CB = Certificate basic program. Prerequisite is R.N. Length is 8
      months to 1 year.
MB = Masters' basic program. Prerequisite is R.N. plus bachelors
      degree. Length is 1 to 2 years.
*   = 3-year program for nonnurse college graduates.

APPENDIX N

Community resources*

American Academy of Pediatrics

P.O. Box 1034
Evanston, Ill. 60204

Provides literature for families, parents, and health profession groups related to child health, illness, and welfare.

American Academy of Husband-Coached Childbirth

P.O. Box 5224
Sherman Oaks, Calif. 91413

Teaches Robert A. Bradley's method of "Husband-Coached Childbirth," an off-shoot of Grantly Dick-Head method.

American National Red Cross

17th and D St., N.W.
Washington, D.C. 20006

Provides service to the armed forces and their families; service to the veterans and their families; disaster services; blood services; health and community services.

American Society for Psychoprophylaxis in Obstetrics (ASPO)

1523 L St., N.W.
Washington, D.C. 20005

Teaches Lamaze technique of prepared childbirth to interested couples; prepares qualified people for teaching this method.

Association for the Aid of Crippled Children

345 East 46th St.
New York, N.Y. 10017

Devoted to the prevention of crippling diseases and conditions and to improvement in the care of disabled children and youth and in their adjustment in society.

Child Study Association of America

9 East 89th St.
New York, N.Y. 10028

Provides parent education materials.

Child Welfare League of America, Inc.

44 East 23rd St.
New York, N.Y. 10010

Develops standards of service for the protection and care of children in their own homes or away from home through boarding home care, institutional care, adoption, day care,

or homemaker service; and in community programs through the following means: cooperation with governmental departments of child welfare, publications, information exchange service, loan library and record forms, case record collection, and general information and education in the field service consultation and regional agencies.

Family Service Association of America, Inc.

44 East 23rd St.
New York, N.Y. 10010

Provides counseling and mental health services to families under stress, preventing family breakdown and promoting the development of family social work and wholesome family life through the following means: field service for family service agencies, assistance in development of qualified personnel in family casework, and information and research on family life.

Florence Crittenton Association of America

608 South Dearborn St.
Chicago, Ill. 60605

Unites in forming an effective and continuing organization; develops and maintains standards of service; in general, assists in bringing about a greater understanding of factors relating to unmarried mothers and adolescent girls with other problems in adjustment.

International Childbirth Education Association (ICEA)

P.O. Box 5852
Milwaukee, Wisconsin 53220

Assists individuals and childbirth groups who are interested in family-centered maternity. ICEA is a worldwide organization.

ICEA Supplies Center

P.O. Box 70258
Seattle, Wash. 98107

Provides books and pamphlets (e.g., *Bookmarks* is an annotated catalogue of resources available that is published several times a year and is available free of charge).

La Leche League International, Inc.

9616 Minneapolis Ave.
Franklin Park, Ill. 60131

Provides support for nursing mothers.

Maternity Center Association, Inc.

48 East 92nd St.
New York, N.Y. 10028

---

*Modified from Chinn, P. L. 1974. Child health maintenance: concepts in family-centered care. St. Louis, The C. V. Mosby Co.

719

National Academy of Sciences

2101 Constitution Ave.
Washington, D.C. 20418

Provides recommended dietary allowance and other nutrition resources.

National Clearinghouse for Drug Abuse Information

Box 1701
Washington, D.C. 20013

Provides educational and informational materials related to drug use and abuse to professional and lay groups.

National Committee on Homemaker Services

1790 Broadway
New York, N.Y. 10019

Promotes improvement in the quality of homemaker services and stimulates the extension of services under both voluntary and public auspices in communities throughout the country.

National Conference of Catholic Charities

1346 Connecticut
Washington, D.C. 20036

Gives particular emphasis to service for children and youth; i.e., foster care, counseling (unmarried parents), adoption services (statewide), short-term counseling to families and youth, emergency material assistance.

National Foundation/March of Dimes

1275 Mamaroneck Ave.
White Plains, N.Y. 10605

Seeks to improve the level of care for all patients with arthritis and birth defects by national grant support of clinical study centers throughout the United States. Grants are made to teaching institutions to conduct clinical research and teaching and to provide patient care.

National Society for Crippled Children and Adults, Inc.

2023 West Ogden Ave.
Chicago, Ill. 60612

Carries out the following three point program: (1) education of the public, professional workers, and parents; (2) research to provide increased knowledge of the causes of handicapping conditions and their prevention and of improved methods of care, education, and treatment; and (3) direct services for crippled children and adults in the fields of health, welfare, education, recreation, rehabilitation, and employment; also charters and develops state and territorial societies to implement the program at state and local levels.

National Society for the Prevention of Blindness, Inc.

16 East 40th St.
New York, N.Y. 10016

Studies causes of blindness or impaired vision; advocates measures leading to the elimination of such causes.

National Tuberculosis Association, Inc.

1790 Broadway
New York, N.Y. 10019

Studies tuberculosis and other respiratory diseases and disseminates information and stimulates the programs of its 2,000 affiliated state and local associations for the prevention, treatment, and control of tuberculosis and other respiratory diseases.

Nurses' Association of the American College of Obstetricians and Gynecologists

1 East Wacker Drive
Chicago, Illinois 60601

Parents Without Partners, Inc.

80 Fifth Ave.
New York, N.Y. 10011

Develops and provides a broad comprehensive program for the enlightenment and guidance of parents without partners and their children on the special problems they encounter and for assistance on the various readjustments involved.

Planned Parenthood Federation of America, Inc.

501 Madison Ave.
New York, N.Y. 10022

Provides leadership for universal acceptance of family planning as an essential element of responsible family life through education, service, and research.

Save the Children Federation, Inc.

345 East 46th St.
New York, N.Y. 10017

Helps eliminate the causes of poverty among children in the United States and overseas while maintaining efforts to ameliorate the effects of poverty in those areas where the needs are greatest.

Travelers Aid and International Social Services Association (TAISSA)

345 East 46th St.
New York, N.Y. 10017

Assists youths and adults with problems related to travel, including returning to former residence, assistance in obtaining employment, and counseling for personal problems.

United Cerebral Palsy Associations, Inc.

321 West 44th St.
New York, N.Y. 10036

Promotes research through a grant program; provides treatment, education, and rehabilitation of persons with cerebral palsy; subsidizes through grants in aid professional training programs of all types related to the problem of cerebral palsy; furthers, by professional and public education, information concerning all aspects of the problem of cerebral palsy; promotes better techniques and facilities for the diagnosis and treatment of persons with cerebral palsy; acts as a source of information on law and legislation in the field of the handicapped, including those disabled by cerebral palsy; cooperates with governmental and private agencies concerned with the welfare of the handicapped.

For genetics clinics and treatment centers in area, contact the following organizations:

National Genetics Foundation, Inc.

250 West 57th St.
New York, N.Y. 10019

National Foundation/March of Dimes*

1275 Mamaroneck Ave.
White Plains, N.Y. 10605

Other resources include the following:

1. State Department of Public Health
2. Bureau of Maternal-Child Health of the United States Department of Health, Education, and Welfare in Washington, D.C.
3. Local organizations: National Society for Crippled Children and Adults, Inc.; National Cystic Fibrosis Society; Muscular Dystrophy Association of America; organizations for parents of children with Tay-Sachs disease, sickle cell anemia, or crippling diseases; pediatric units in local hospitals and medical centers; city and county services (e.g., mental retardation).

---

*The National Foundation/March of Dimes publishes a directory of genetic services. It is involved in professional education, as well as research of genetic defects. The Foundation also sponsors programs for the purpose of teaching and disseminating information to the general public.

APPENDIX O

Magazines and publications

Birth and Family Journal: quarterly publication, sponsored by International Childbirth Education Association (ICEA) and American Society of Psychoprophylaxis in Obstetrics (ASPO)
110 El Camino Real
Berkeley, Calif. 94705

MCN The American Journal of Maternal Child Nursing
10 Columbus Circle
New York, N.Y. 10019

Journal of Nurse Midwifery: official publication of the American College of Nurse Midwives
1000 Vermont Avenue N.W.
Washington, D.C. 20005

Maternal/Newborn Advocate: quarterly publication of the National Foundation/March of Dimes
The National Foundation/March of Dimes
Box 2000
White Plains, N.Y. 10602 (complimentary)

Bookmarks: annotated catalogue of book reviews published several times per year
ICEA Supplies Center
P.O. Box 70258
Seattle, Wash. 98107 (complimentary)

Briefs—Footnotes on Maternity Care: a publication of the Maternity Center Association
48 East 92 St.
New York, N.Y. 10028

Glossary

abdominal Belonging or relating to the abdomen and its functions and disorders.

   a. delivery Birth of a child through a surgical incision made into the abdominal wall and uterus; cesarean section.

   a. gestation Implantation of a fertilized ovum outside the uterus but inside the peritoneal cavity.

   a. hysterectomy The surgical removal of the uterus through an abdominal wall incision.

   a. pregnancy See *abdominal gestation.*

ablatio placentae See *abruptio placentae.*

abortion Termination of pregnancy before the fetus is viable and capable of extrauterine existence, usually less than 21 to 22 weeks' gestation (or when the fetus weighs less than 600 gm).

   complete a. Fetus and all related tissue has been expelled from the uterus.

   elective a. Termination of pregnancy chosen by the woman that is not required for her physical safety.

   habitual a. (recurrent) Loss of three or more successive pregnancies for no known cause.

   incomplete a. Loss of pregnancy in which some but not all the products of conception have been expelled from the uterus.

   induced a. Intentionally produced loss of pregnancy by patient or others.

   inevitable a. Threatened loss of pregnancy that cannot be prevented or stopped and is imminent.

   missed a. Loss of pregnancy in which the products of conception remain in the uterus after the fetus dies.

   septic a. Loss of pregnancy in which there is an infection of the product of conception and the uterine endometrial lining, usually resulting from attempted termination of early pregnancy.

   spontaneous a. Loss of pregnancy that occurs naturally without interference or known cause.

   therapeutic a. Pregnancy that has been intentionally terminated for medical reasons.

   threatened a. Early symptoms of a possible abortion are present (e.g., the cervix begins to dilate).

   voluntary a. See *abortion, elective.*

abruptio placentae Partial or complete premature separation of a normally implanted placenta.

abstinence Refraining from sexual intercourse periodically or permanently.

accreta, placenta See *placenta accreta.*

acidosis Increase in hydrogen ion concentration resulting in a lowering of blood pH below 7.35.

   metabolic a. Result of increased nonudatile acids from (1) abnormal metabolism (too many acids produced), (2) renal malfunction (acids not being excreted), or (3) excessive loss of base (diarrhea).

acme Highest point (e.g., of a contraction).

acrocyanosis Peripheral cyanosis; blueing of hands and feet in most infants at birth that may persist for 7 to 10 days.

acromion Projection of the spine of the scapula (forming the point of the shoulder) used to explain the presentation of the fetus.

adenomyoma Type of tumor affecting glandular and smooth muscle tissue, such as uterine musculature.

adnexa Adjacent or accessory parts of a structure.

   uterine a. Ovaries and fallopian tubes.

afibrinogenemia Absense or decrease of fibrinogen in the blood such that the blood will not coagulate. In obstetrics, this condition occurs from complications of abruptio placentae or retention of a dead fetus.

afterbirth Lay term for the placenta and membranes expelled after the birth or delivery of the child.

afterpains Painful uterine cramps that occur intermittently for approximately 2 to 3 days after delivery resulting from contractile efforts of the uterus to return to its normal involuted condition.

agalactia Absence or failure of milk secretion after childbirth.

alae nasi Nostrils.

albuminuria Presence of readily detectable amounts of albumin in the urine.

allantois Tubular diverticulum of the posterior part of the embryo's yolk sac that passes into the body stalk, accompanied by the allantoic blood vessels that develop and become the umbilical vein and paired umbilical arteries; later, after fusing with the chorion, it helps to form the placenta.

alveoli, fetal Terminal pulmonary sacs that in fetal life are filled with fluid. This fluid is a transudate of fetal plasma.

ambient Surrounding; around.

amenorrhea Absence or suppression of menstruation.

amnesia Loss of memory.

amnii, liquor See *liquor amnii.*

amniocentesis Procedure in which a needle is inserted through the abdominal and uterine walls into the amniotic fluid. This procedure is used for assessment of fetal health and maturity and for therapeutic abortion.

amniography Procedure used primarily to detect placenta previa by x-ray examination, entailing injection of radiopaque dye into amniotic fluid.

amnion Inner membrane of two fetal membranes that forms the sac and contains the fetus and the fluid which surrounds it in utero.

amnionitis Infected amniotic fluid, occurring most frequently after early rupture of membranes.

amniotic Pertaining or relating to the amnion.

   a. sac Membrane "bag" that contains the fetus before delivery.

   a. fluid Fluid surrounding fetus derived primarily from maternal serum and fetal urine.

anaerobic catabolism In the absence of free oxygen, the breakdown of organized substances into simpler compounds, with the resultant release of energy.

analgesic Any drug or agent that will relieve pain.

android pelvis Male type of pelvis.

androgen Substance that produces masculinizing effects (e.g., testosterone).

anencephaly Congenital deformity that is characterized by the absence of cerebrum, cerebellum, and flat bones of skull.

anesthesia Partial or complete absence of sensation with or without loss of consciousness.

anomaly Organ or structure that is malformed or in some way abnormal with reference to form, structure, or position.

anovular menstrual period When cyclic uterine bleeding is not accompanied by the production and discharge of an ovum.

anoxia Absence of oxygen.

antenatal Occurring before or formed before birth.

antepartal Before labor.

anterior Pertaining to the front.

   a. fontanel See *fontanel, anterior.*

anteroposterior repair Operation in which the upper and lower walls of the vagina are reconstructed to correct relaxed tissue.

antibody Specific protein substance developed by the body that exerts restrictive or destructive action on specific antigens such as bacteria or toxins.

anthropoid pelvis Pelvis in which the anteroposterior diameter is equal to or greater than the transverse diameter.

apnea Cessation of respirations for more than 10 seconds associated with generalized cyanosis.

areola Pigmented ring of tissue surrounding the nipple.

   secondary a. During the fifth month of pregnancy, a second faint ring of pigmentation is seen around the original areola.

articulation Fastening together or connection of the various bones of the skeleton, a joint. The articulations of the bones are classified as (1) immovable (synarthrosis), (2) slightly immovable (amphiarthrosis), and (3) freely movable (diarthrosis).

artificial insemination introduction of semen by instrument injection into the vagina or uterus for impregnation.

Aschheim-Zondek test Pregnancy test in which a woman's urine is injected into a mouse. The animal is sacrificed and its ovaries examined after 5 days. Enlarged ovaries and maturing follicles indicate a positive test.

asphyxia Decreased oxygen and/or excess of carbon dioxide in the body.

   fetal a. Condition occurring in utero, with the following biochemical changes: hypoxemia (lowering of Po_2), hypercapnia (increase in Pco_2), and respiratory and metabolic acidosis (reduction of blood pH).

   a. livida Condition in which the infant's skin is characteristically pale, pulse is weak and slow, and reflexes are depressed or absent; also known as *blue asphyxia.*

   a. pallida Condition in which the infant appears pale and limp and suffers from bradycardia (80 beats/min or less) and apnea.

aspiration syndrome Function of fetal hypoxia: with hypoxia, the anal sphincter relaxes and meconium is released; reflex gasping movements draw meconium and other particulate matter in the amniotic fluid into the bronchial tree, obstructing the air flow after birth.

asynclitism Oblique presentation of the fetal head at the superior strait of the pelvis; the pelvic planes and those of the fetal head are not parallel.

atelectasis Pulmonary pathology involving alveolar collapse.

atony Without muscle tone.

atresia Absence of a normally present passageway.

   biliary a. Absence of the bile duct.

   choanal a. Complete obstruction with membranous or bony tissue of the posterior nares, which open into the nasopharynx.

   esophageal a. Congenital anomaly in which the esophagus ends in a blind pouch or narrows into a thin cord, thus failing to form a continuous passage to the stomach.

attitude Body posture or position.

   fetal a. Relation of fetal parts to each other in the uterus (e.g., all parts flexed, all parts flexed except neck is extended, etc.).

auscultation Process of listening for sounds produced within the body.

autosomes Any of the paired chromosomes other than the sex (X and Y) chromosomes.

axis Line, real or imaginary, about which a part revolves or that runs through the center of a body.

   pelvic a. Imaginary curved line that passes through the centers of all the anteroposterior diameters of the pelvis.

azoospermic Absence of sperm in the semen.

bag of waters Lay term for the sac containing amniotic fluid and fetus.

ballottement (1) Movability of a floating object (e.g., fetus). (2) Diagnostic technique using palpation: a floating object, when tapped or pushed, moves away and then returns to touch the examiner's hand.

Bandl's ring Abnormally thickened ridge of uterine musculature between the upper and lower segments that follows a mechanically obstructed labor, with the lower segment thinning abnormally.

Barr body or sex chromatin Chromatin mass located against the inner surface of the nucleus in females, possibly representing the inactive X chromosome.

Bartholin's glands Two small glands situated on either side of the vaginal orifice that secrete small amounts of mucus during coitus, which are homologous to the bulbourethral glands in the male.

basalis, decidua See *decidua basalis.*

Bell's palsy See *palsy, Bell's.*

bicornuate uterus Anomalous uterus that may be either a double or single organ with two horns.

biliary atresia See *atresia, biliary.*

bilirubin Yellow- or orange-colored pigment that is a breakdown product of hemoglobin. It is carried by the blood to the liver where it is chemically changed in the liver and excreted in the bile or is conjugated and excreted by the kidneys.

bimanual Performed with both hands.

   b. palpation Examination of a woman's pelvic organs done by placing one hand on the abdomen and one or two fingers of the other hand in the vagina.

biopsy Removal of a small piece of tissue for microscopic examination and diagnosis.

blastoderm Germinal membrane of the ovum.

   b. vesicle Stage in the development of a mammalian embryo that consists of an outer layer, or trophoblast, and a hollow sphere of cells enclosing a cavity.

bleeding diathesis See *diathesis, bleeding.*

born out of asepsis (BOA) When the birth takes place without the use of sterile technique.

Braxton Hicks sign Mild, intermittent, painless uterine contractions that occur during pregnancy. These contractions occur more frequently as pregnancy advances but do not represent true labor.

Braxton Hicks version One of several types of maneuvers designed to turn the fetus from an undesirable position to a more acceptable one to facilitate delivery.

breast milk jaundice Pregnandiol in mother's milk inhibits enzyme (glucuronyl transferase) necessary for the conjugation of bilirubin, resulting in yellowing of infant's skin.

breech presentation When the buttocks and/or feet are nearest the cervical opening and are born first. This occurs in approximately 3% of all deliveries.

   complete b. Buttocks, legs, and feet present simultaneously.

   footling (incomplete) b. One or both feet present.

   frank b. Buttocks present, with hips flexed so that thighs are against abdomen.

bregma Point of junction of the coronal and sagittal sutures of the skull; the area of the anterior fontanel of the fetus; the brow.

brim Edge of the superior strait of the true pelvis; the inlet.

brown fat Source of heat unique to neonates that is capable of greater thermogenic activity than ordinary fat. Deposits are found around the adrenals, kidneys, and neck, between the scapulas, and behind the sternum for several weeks after birth.

caked breast See *engorgement.*

calcemia Amount of serum calcium.

capsularis, decidua See *decidua capsularis.*

caput Occiput of fetal head appearing at the vaginal introitus preceding delivery of the head.

   c. succedaneum Swelling of the tissue over the presenting part of the fetal head caused by pressure during labor.

carrier Individual who carries a gene that does not exhibit itself in physical or chemical characteristics but that can be transmitted to children (e.g., a female carrying the trait for hemophilia, which is expressed in male offspring).

catamenia Menses.

caudal anesthesia Type of regional anesthesia used in childbirth in which the anesthetic agent is injected into the caudal area of the spinal canal through the sacral hiatus, affecting the caudal nerve roots and thereby anesthetizing the cervix, vagina, and perineum.

caul Hood of fetal membranes covering fetal head during delivery.

cautery Method of destroying tissue by the use of heat, electricity, or chemicals.

cephalhematoma Extravasation of blood from ruptured vessels between a skull bone and its external covering, the periosteum. Swelling is limited by the margins of the cranial bone affected (usually parietals).

cephalic Pertaining to the head.

   c. presentation Any part of the fetal head is presenting.

cephalopelvic disproportion (CPD) When the infant's head is of such a shape, size, or position that it cannot pass through the mother's pelvis.

cervical amputation Neck of the uterus is removed.

cervical cauterization Destruction (usually by heat or electric current) of the superficial tissue of the cervix.

cervical conization Excision of a cone-shaped section of tissue from the endocervix.

cervical erosion Alteration of the epithelium of the cervix caused by chronic irritation or infection.

cervical polyp Small tumor on a stem (pedicle) attached inside the cervix.

cervical stenosis Narrowing of the canal between the body of the uterus and the cervical os.

cervicitis Cervical infection.

cervix Lowest and narrow end of the uterus; the "neck"; between the external os and the body or corpus of the uterus. The lower end of the cervix extends into the vagina.

cesarean hysterectomy Removal of the uterus immediately after the delivery of an infant by cesarean section.

cesarean section Delivery of a fetus by an incision through the abdominal wall and uterus.

Chadwick's sign Increased vascularity of the vagina gives the mucous membrane a violet color that is visible from about the fourth week of pregnancy.

change of life See *climacteric.*

chloasma Increased pigmentation over bridge of nose and

cheeks of pregnant women and some women taking oral contraceptives; also known as *mask of pregnancy*.

choanal atresia See *atresia, choanal*.

chorioamnionitis Stimulated by organisms in the amniotic fluid, an inflammatory response in the amniotic membranes, which then become infiltrated with polymorphonuclear leukocytes.

chorioepithelioma Carcinoma of the chorion; rapid malignant proliferation of the epithelium of the chorionic villi.

chorion Fetal membrane closest to the intrauterine wall that gives rise to the placenta and continuing as the outer membrane surrounding the amnion.

chorionic villi See *villi, chorionic*.

chromosome Element within the cell nucleus carrying genes and composed of DNA and proteins.

circumcision Excision of the newborn male's prepuce (foreskin).

cleft palate Incomplete closure of the palate or roof of mouth; a congenital fissure.

climacteric (change of life) Period when the human body undergoes significant psychologic and physiologic changes such as the termination of reproductive function in the female.

clitoris Female organ homologous to male penis; a small, ovoid body of erectile tissue situated at the anterior junction of the vulva.

  prepuce of the c. See *prepuce of the clitoris*.

coccyx Small bone at the base of the spinal column.

colostrum Yellowish secretion from the breast containing mainly serum and white blood corpuscles preceding the onset of true lactation 2 or 3 days after delivery.

colpectomy Surgical excision of the vagina.

colporrhaphy (1) Procedure of suturing the vagina. (2) Procedure whereby the vagina is denuded and sutured for the purpose of narrowing the vagina.

colpotomy Any surgical incision into the wall of the vagina.

communicating hydrocephalus See *hydrocephalus, communicating*.

complete abortion See *abortion, complete*.

complete breech presentation See *breech presentation, complete*.

complementary feeding Supplemental feeding given to the infant if he is still hungry after breast-feeding.

compliance, lung Degree of distensibility of the lung's elastic tissue.

conception Union of the sperm and ovum resulting in fertilization.

conceptional age In fetal development, the number of completed weeks since the moment of conception. Because the moment of conception is almost impossible to determine, conceptional age is estimated at 2 weeks less than gestational age.

concurrent sterilization Method of preparing formula in which all the ingredients and equipment are sterilized prior to mixing.

condyloma Wartlike growth on the skin usually seen near

the anus or external genitals. There is a pointed type and the flat, broad, moist papule of secondary syphilis.

confinement Term applied to the period of childbirth and early puerperium.

congenital Present or existing before birth.

conjoined twins See *twins, conjoined*.

conjugate Diameter of the pelvis as measured from the center of the promontory of the sacrum to the back of the symphysis pubis.

conjunctivitis Inflammation of the mucous membrane that lines the eyelids and that is reflected onto the eyeball.

consanguinity Existing blood relationship between people.

contraception Prevention of impregnation or conception.

contraction ring See *Bandl's ring*.

Coombs' test Indirect: test for Rh-positive antibodies in maternal blood; direct: test for maternal Rh-positive antibodies in fetal cord blood. A positive test indicates the presence of antibodies or titer.

copulation Coitus; sexual intercourse.

corpus luteum Yellow body. After rupture of the graafian follicle at ovulation, the follicle develops into a yellow structure that secrets progesterone in the second half of the menstrual cycle, atrophying about 3 days before sloughing of the endometrium in menstrual flow. Should impregnation occur, this structure continues to produce progesterone until the placenta can take over this function.

cotyledon One of the fifteen to twenty-eight visible segments of the placenta on the maternal surface, each comprised of fetal vessels, chorionic villi, and an intervillous space.

Couvelaire uterus See *uterus, Couvelaire*.

Crede's method Obsolete method by which the placenta is expelled by downward manual pressure on the uterus through the abdominal wall. The thumb is placed on the posterior surface of the fundus of the uterus and the flat of the hand on the anterior surface. Pressure is applied in the direction of the birth canal.

Crede's prophylaxis Instillation of 1% silver nitrate solution into the conjunctivas of newborn infants immediately after birth to prevent ophthalmia neonatorum, particularly that caused by gonorrheal organisms.

crepitus (1) Noise produced when pressure is applied to tissues containing abnormal amounts of air. (2) Grating sound heard when broken bone ends are moved. (3) Noise of gas being expelled from the intestines.

crowning Stage of delivery when the top of the fetal head can be seen at the vaginal orifice.

cul-de-sac of Douglas Pouch formed by a fold of the peritoneum dipping down between the anterior wall of the rectum and the posterior wall of the uterus; also called *Douglas's cul-de-sac, pouch of Douglas,* and *rectouterine pouch*.

curettage Scraping of the endometrium lining of the uterus with a curette to remove the contents of the uterus (as is done after an inevitable or incomplete abortion) or to obtain specimens for diagnostic purposes.

cutis marmorata Transient vasomotor phenomenon occurring

primarily over extremities when the infant is exposed to chilling. It appears as a pink or faint purple capillary outline on the skin. Occasionally it is seen if the infant is in respiratory distress.

cyesis Pregnancy.

cystocele Bladder hernia; injury to the vesicovaginal fascia during labor and delivery may allow herniation of the bladder into the vagina.

cytogenics Branch of genetics concerned primarily with the study of chromosomes and correlations with associated gene behavior.

decidua Mucous membrane, lining of uterus, or endometrium of pregnancy that is shed after giving birth.

   d. basalis Maternal aspect of the placenta comprised of uterine blood vessels, endometrial stroma, and glands. It is shed in lochial discharge after delivery.

   d. capsularis That part of the decidua membranes surrounding the chorionic sac.

   d. vera Nonplacental decidual lining of the uterus.

decrement Decrease or stage of decline, as of a contraction.

delivery, abdominal See *abdominal delivery.*

dermatoglyphics Study of skin ridge patterns on fingers, toes, palms of hands, and soles of feet.

desquamation Shedding of epithelial cells of the skin and mucous membranes.

diaphragmatic hernia Congenital malformation of diaphragm that allows displacement of the abdominal organs into the thoracic cavity.

diastasis recti abdominis Separation of the two recti abdominis muscles along the median line. This is often seen in women with repeated childbirths or with a multiple gestation (triplets, etc.). In the newborn it is usually due to incomplete development.

diathesis Hereditary condition, tendency, or susceptibility of an individual to some abnormality or disease.

   bleeding d. Predisposition to abnormal blood clotting.

dilatation of cervix Stretching of the external os from an opening a few millimeters in size to an opening large enough to allow the passage of the infant.

dilatation and curettage (D and C) Vaginal operation in which the cervical canal is stretched enough to admit passage of an instrument called a *curette.* The endometrium of the uterus is scraped with the curette to empty the uterine contents or to obtain tissue for examination.

discordance Discrepancy in size (or other indicator) between twins.

disparate twins See *twins, disparate.*

dizygotic Related to or proceeding from two zygotes (fertilized ova).

dizygous twins See *twins, dizygous.*

delivery Expulsion of the child with placenta and membranes by the mother or their extraction by the obstetric practitioner.

   d. abdominal See *abdominal delivery.*

deoxyribonucleic acid (DNA) Intracellular complex protein that carries genetic information, consisting of two purines

(adenine and quanine) and two pyrimidines (thymine and cystosine).

Döderlein bacillus Gram-positive bacteria occurring in normal vaginal secretions.

dominant trait Gene that is expressed whenever it is present in the heterozygous gene state (e.g., brown eyes are dominant over blue).

Douglas's cul-de-sac See *cul-de-sac of Douglas.*

Down's syndrome Abnormality involving the occurrence of a third chromosome, rather than the normal pair (trisomy 21), that characteristically results in a typical picture of mental retardation and altered physical appearance. This condition was formerly called *mongolism* or *mongoloid idiocy.*

dry labor Lay term referring to labor in which amniotic fluid has already escaped. A "dry birth" does not exist.

ductus arteriosus In fetal circulation, an anatomic shunt between the pulmonary artery and arch of the aorta. It is obliterated after birth by a rising Po_2 and change in intravascular pressures in the presence of normal pulmonary function. Normally, it becomes a ligament after birth but in some instances remains patent.

ductus venosus In fetal circulation, a blood vessel carrying oxygenated blood between the umbilical vein and the inferior vena cava, bypassing the liver. It is obliterated and becomes a ligament after birth.

Duncan mechanism Placenta is delivered with the maternal surface presenting rather than the shiny fetal surface.

dyscrasia Incompatible mixture (e.g., fetal and maternal blood incompatibility).

dysfunction, placental See *placental dysfunction.*

dysfunctional uterine bleeding Abnormal bleeding from the uterus for reasons that are not readily established.

dysmaturity See *intrauterine growth retardation.*

dysmenorrhea Difficult or painful menstruation.

dyspareunia Painful sexual intercourse.

dystocia Prolonged, painful, or otherwise difficult delivery or birth due to mechanical factors produced by either the passenger (the fetus) or the passage (the pelvis of the mother) or due to inadequate powers (uterine and other muscular activity).

   placental d. Difficulty in the delivery of the placenta.

ecchymosis Bruises; bleeding into tissue caused by direct trauma, serious infection, or bleeding diathesis.

eclampsia Severe complication of pregnancy of unknown cause and occurring more often in the primigravida, characterized by tonic and clonic convulsions, coma, high blood pressure, albuminuria, and oliguria occurring during pregnancy or shortly after delivery.

ectoderm Outer layer of embryonic tissue giving rise to skin, nails, and hair.

ectopic Out of normal place.

   e. pregnancy Implantation of the fertilized ovum outside of its normal place in the uterine cavity. Locations include the abdomen, fallopian tubes, and ovaries.

effacement Thinning and shortening or obliteration of the cervix that occurs during late pregnancy and/or labor.

effleurage Gentle stroking used in massage.

ejaculation Sudden expulsion of semen from the male urethra.

elective abortion See *abortion, elective.*

embolus Any undissolved matter (solid, liquid, or gaseous) that is carried by the blood to another part of the body and obstructs a blood vessel.

embryo Conceptus from the second or third week of development until 5 to 8 weeks' gestation when mineralization (ossification) of the skeleton begins. This period is characterized by cellular differentiation and predominantly hyperplastic growth.

empathy Projection of one's own consciousness and awareness onto that of another so as to obtain an objective awareness of and insight into the emotions, feelings, and behavior of another person and their meaning and significance. Empathy may be distinguished from sympathy in that sympathy is usually nonobjective and noncritical, and the state of empathy includes relative freedom from emotional involvement.

endocervical Pertaining to the interior of the canal of the cervix of the uterus.

endocrine glands Ductless glands that secrete hormones into the blood or lymph.

endometriosis Tissue closely resembling endometrial tissue but aberrantly located outside the uterus in the pelvic cavity. Symptomatology may include pelvic pain or pressure, dysmenorrhea, dyspareunia, abnormal bleeding from the uterus or rectum, and sterility.

endometrium Inner lining of the uterus that undergoes changes due to hormones during the menstrual cycle and pregnancy; decidua.

engagement In obstetrics, refers to the entrance of the fetal presenting part into the superior pelvic strait and the beginning of the descent through the pelvic canal.

engorgement Distention or vascular congestion. In obstetrics, it is the process of swelling of the breast tissue and is brought about by an increase in blood and lymph supply to the breast, which precedes true lactation. It lasts about 48 hours and usually reaches a peak between the third and fifth postnatal day.

entoderm Inner layer of embryonic tissue giving rise to internal organs such as the intestines.

enzygotic Developed from one fertilized ovum.

epicanthus Fold of skin covering the inner canthus and caruncle that extends from the root of the nose to the median end of the eyebrow which is characteristically found in certain races but may occur as a congenital anomaly.

episiotomy Surgical incision of the perineum at the end of the second stage of labor to facilitate delivery and to avoid laceration of the perineum. (See *perineotomy.*)

epispadias Urethral canal terminates on dorsum of penis or above the clitoris (rare).

Epstein's pearls Small, white blebs found along the gum margins and at the junction of the soft and hard palates. They are a normal manifestation and are commonly seen in the newborn.

Erb's palsy See *palsy, Erb's.*

ergot Drug obtained from *Claviceps purpurea,* a fungus, which stimulates the smooth muscles of blood vessels and the uterus, causing vasoconstriction and uterine contractions.

erythema toxicum Innocuous pink papular rash of unknown cause with superimposed vesicles appearing within 24 to 48 hours after birth and resolving spontaneously within a few days.

erythroblastosis fetalis Hemolytic disease of the newborn caused by isoimmunization due to Rh incompatibility or ABO incompatibility.

escutcheon Pattern of distribution of pubic hair.

esophageal atresia See *atresia, esophageal.*

estrangement, psychologic Reaction to the birth of and subsequent separation from a sick and/or premature infant whereby the mother is diverted from establishing a normal relationship with her baby.

estriol Major metabolite of estrogen that increases during the second half of pregnancy with an intact fetoplacental unit (normal placenta, normal fetal liver, and adrenals) and normal maternal renal function.

estrogen Female sex hormone produced by the ovary and placenta.

estrus Cyclic period of sexual activity in mammals other than primates; in heat.

eugenics Science that deals with the improvement of the human race through control of hereditary (genetic) factors by voluntary social action.

euthenics Science that deals with the improvement of the human race through the control of environmental factors (pollution, drugs, prevention of malnutrition and disease).

exchange transfusion Replacement of 70% to 80% of circulating blood by withdrawing the recipient's blood and injecting a donor's blood in equal amounts, the purposes of which are to prevent an accumulation of bilirubin in the blood above a dangerous level and to prevent the accumulation of other byproducts of hemolysis in hemolytic disease.

exostosis Benign cartilage-covered hump on the surface of a bone often resulting from chronic irritation.

expulsive Having the tendency to drive out or expel.

　e. contractions Labor contractions that are characteristic of the second stage of labor.

extraperitoneal Occurring or located outside of the peritoneal cavity.

extrauterine Occurring outside the uterus.

　e. pregnancy Ectopic pregnancy in which the fertilized ovum implants itself outside of the uterus.

facies Pertaining to the appearance or expression of the face; certain congenital syndromes typically present with a specific facial appearance.

fallopian tubes Two canals or oviducts extending laterally from each side of the uterus through which the ovum travels after ovulation to the uterus.

false labor Those uterine contractions that do not result in cervical dilatation, are irregular, felt more in front, often do not last more than 20 seconds, and do not become longer or stronger.

failure to thrive Neonate or infant whose growth and development pattern is below the norms for age.

fecundation Act of fertilization or impregnation.

fertility Quality of being able to reproduce.

fertilization Union of an ovum and sperm.

fetal Pertaining or relating to the fetus.

    f. attitude See *attitude, fetal.*

    f. asphyxia See *asphyxia, fetal.*

    f. death Death of the developing fetus after 20 weeks' gestation.

    f. distress Evidence such as a change in the fetal heart beat or activity indicating that the fetus is in jeopardy.

fetofetal transfusion See *parabiotic syndrome.*

fetotoxic Poisonous or destructive to the fetus.

fetus Child in utero from the seventh to ninth week of gestation until birth.

fibroid Fibrous, encapsulated connective tissue tumor especially of the uterus.

fimbria Structure resembling a fringe, particularly the fringe-like end of the fallopian tube.

fissure Groove or open crack in tissue.

fistula Abnormal tubelike passage that forms between two normal cavities, possibly congenital or caused by trauma, abscesses, or inflammatory processes.

flaccid Having relaxed, flabby, or absent muscle tone.

flaring of nostrils Widening of nostrils (alae nasi) during inspiration in the presence of air hunger; sign of respiratory distress.

flexion In obstetrics, resistance to the descent of the baby down the birth canal causes the head to flex, or bend, so that the chin approaches the chest, thus reducing the diameter of the presenting part.

fluid, amniotic See *amniotic fluid.*

follicle Small secretory cavity or sac.

    graafian f. Mature, fully developed ovarian cyst containing the ripe ovum. The follicle secretes estrogens, and after ovulation, the corpus luteum develops within the ruptured graafian follicle and secretes estrogen and progesterone.

follicle-stimulating hormone (FSH) Hormone produced by the anterior pituitary during the first half of the menstrual cycle. Stimulates development of the graafian follicle.

fontanel Broad area, or soft spot, consisting of a strong band of connective tissue contiguous with cranial bones and located at the junctions of the bones.

    anterior f. Diamond-shaped area between the frontal and two parietal bones just above the baby's forehead.

    posterior f. Small, triangular area between the occipital and parietal bones.

footling (incomplete) breech presentation See *breech presentation, footling.*

foramen ovale Septal opening between the atria of the fetal heart. The opening normally closes shortly after birth,

but if it remains patent, surgical repair usually is necessary.

foreskin Prepuce, or loose fold of skin covering the glans penis.

fornix Any structure with an arched or vaultlike shape.

    f. of the vagina Anterior and posterior spaces, formed by the protrusion of the cervix into the vagina, into which the upper vagina is divided.

fossa Shallow depression.

fourchette Tense band of mucous membranes at the posterior angle of the vagina connecting the posterior ends of the labia minora.

frank breech presentation See *breech presentation, frank.*

fraternal twins Nonidentical twins that come from two separate fertilized ova.

frenulum Thin ridge of tissue in midline of undersurface of tongue extending from its base to varying distances from the tip of the tongue.

Friedman's test Modification of the Aschheim-Zondek pregnancy test: the urine of a woman suspected of pregnancy is injected into a mature, unmated female rabbit. If at the end of 2 days of these injections, the ovaries of the rabbit contain fresh corpora lutea or hemorrhagic corpora, the test is positive, signifying that the woman is pregnant.

FSH See *follicle-stimulating hormone.*

fundus Dome-shaped upper portion of the uterus between the point of insertion of the fallopian tubes.

funic souffle See *souffle, funic.*

funis Cordlike structure, especially the umbilical cord.

galactagogue Any agent that causes the flow of milk to increase.

galactorrhea Excessive flow or secretion of milk.

gamete Mature male or female germ cell; the mature sperm or ovum.

gastrula Early embryonic stage of development that follows the blastula.

gavage To feed by means of a tube passed to the stomach.

gene Factor on a chromosome responsible for hereditary characteristics of offspring.

generative Capable of reproduction.

genetics Biologic science that deals with the genetic transmission of physical and chemical characteristics from parents to offspring, as well as the influence of environmental agents on genes and genetic expression.

genitals Organs of reproduction.

genotype Hereditary combinations in an individual determining his physical and chemical characteristics. Some genotypes are not expressed until later life (e.g., Huntington's chorea); some hide recessive genes, which can be expressed in offspring; and others are expressed only under the proper environmental conditions (e.g., diabetes appearing under the stresses of obesity or pregnancy).

gestation Period of intrauterine fetal development from conception through birth; the period of pregnancy.

    abdominal g. See *abdominal gestation.*

gestational age In fetal development, the number of completed weeks counting from the first day of the last normal menstrual cycle.

glycosuria Presence of glucose (a sugar) in the urine.

Goodell's sign Softening of the cervix, a probable sign of pregnancy, occurring during the second month.

gonad Gamate-producing or sex gland; the ovary or testis.

gonadotropin hormone Hormone that stimulates the gonads.

graafian follicles or *vesicles* See *follicles, graafian.*

gravid Pregnant.

grunt, expiratory Sign of respiratory distress (hyaline membrane disease or advanced pneumonia) indicative of the body's attempt to hold air in the alveoli for better gaseous exchange.

gynecoid pelvis Pelvis in which the inlet is round instead of oval or blunt; heart-shaped. Typical female pelvis.

gynecology Study of the diseases of the female, especially of the genital, urinary, or rectal organs.

habitual (recurrent) abortion See *abortion, habitual.*

habitus Indications in appearance of tendency or disposition to disease or abnormal conditions.

harlequin sign Rare color change of no pathologic significance occurring between the longitudinal halves of the neonate's body. When placed on one side, the dependent half is noticeably pinker than the superior half.

Hegar's sign Softening of the lower uterine segment that is classified as a probable sign of pregnancy and that may be present during the second and third month of pregnancy and is palpated during bimanual examination.

hematoma Collection of blood in a tissue; a bruise or blood tumor.

hemoconcentration Increase in the number of red blood cells resulting from either a decrease in plasma volume or increased erythropoiesis.

hemorrhagic disease of newborn Bleeding disorder during first few days of life based on a deficiency of vitamin K.

heterozygous Two dissimilar genes at the same site or locus on paired chromosomes (e.g., at the sites for eye color, one chromosome carrying the gene for brown, the other for blue).

high risk That which has an increased possibility of suffering harm, damage, loss, or death; for example, a high-risk pregnancy is one that is complicated by a condition such as preeclampsia-eclampsia from which the mother and child have a greater possibility of damage or death than in a more normal pregnancy.

hirsutism Condition characterized by the excessive growth of hair or the growth of hair in unusual places.

Homan's sign Early sign of phlebothrombosis of the deep veins of the calf in which there are complaints of pain when the leg is in extension and the foot is dorsiflexed.

homoiothermic Refers to the ability of certain animals to maintain internal temperature at a specified level regardless of the environmental temperature; a warm-blooded animal. This ability is not fully developed in the human neonate.

homologous Similar in structure or origin but not necessarily in function.

homozygous Two similar genes at the same locus or site on paired chromosomes.

hormone Chemical substance produced in an organ or gland that is conveyed through the blood to another organ or part of the body, stimulating it to increased functional activity or secretion. See specific hormones.

human chorionic gonadotropin (HCG) See *prolan.*

hyaline membrane disease (HMD) Disease characterized by interference with ventilation at the alveolar level theoretically due to the presence of fibrinoid deposits lining alveolar ducts. Membrane formation is related to prematurity (especially with fetal asphyxia) and insufficient surfactant production (L/S ratio less than 2:1). Otherwise known as *respiratory distress syndrome (RDS).*

hydatidiform mole Degenerative process in the chorionic villi that produces multiple cysts and rapid growth of the uterus with hemorrhage. Signs and symptoms include vaginal bleeding, the discharge containing some of the grapelike vesicles.

hydramnios or *polyhydramnios* Amniotic fluid in excess of 1.5ℓ; often indicative of fetal anomaly and frequently seen in diabetic pregnant women even if there is no coexisting fetal anomaly.

hydrocele Collection of fluid in a saclike cavity, especially in the sac that surrounds the testicle causing the scrotum to swell.

hydrocephalus Excessive accumulation of cerebrospinal fluid within the ventricles of the brain resulting from interference with normal circulation and absorption of the cerebrospinal fluid and especially from the destruction of the foramens of Magendie and Luschka due to congenital anomalies, infection, injury, or brain tumors. In infants, the increased head diameter is possible because the sutures of the skull have not closed.

    communicating h. Normal communication between the fourth ventricle and the subarachnoid space is maintained, allowing cerebral fluid to circulate into the lumbar thecal space.

    noncommunicating h. Ventricular fluid does not empty into the lumbar thecal space.

hydrops fetalis Most severe expression of Rh isoimmunization; infants exhibit gross edema (anasarca) and profound pallor and seldom survive.

hymen Membranous fold that normally partially covers the entrance to the vagina in the virgin.

hymenal tag Normally occurring redundant hymenal tissue protruding from the floor of the vagina that disappears spontaneously in a few weeks after birth.

hyperbilirubinemia Elevation of unconjugated serum bilirubin concentrations, which is indicative of hemolytic processes due to blood incompatibility (Rh, ABO), intrauterine infection, septicemia, neonatal renal infection, enzymatic deficiencies in erythrocytes, and drugs (e.g., large doses of vitamin K or maternal ingestion of salicylates or sulfisoxazole [Gantrisin]).

hypercapnia Excessive arterial Pco₂ caused by inadequate ventilation. In excessive amounts it acts as a respiratory depressant.

hyperemesis gravidarum Excessive vomiting during pregnancy leading to starvation and dehydration.

hypermagnesemia Excessive amount of serum magnesium; in obstetrics, it occurs in the mother and/or fetus after the mother is treated with magnesium sulfate for preeclampsia-eclampsia.

hyperplasia Increase in number of cells; formation of new tissue.

hypersomnia Excessive need for sleep.

hypertrophy Enlargement or increase in size of existing cells.

hypofibrinogenemia Deficient level of fibrinogen in the blood, a substance that is necessary for normal clotting of the blood; in obstetrics, it occurs following complications of abruptio placentae or retention of a dead fetus.

hypogalactia Deficient secretion of milk.

hypogastric arteries Branches of the right and left iliac arteries carrying deoxygenated blood from the fetus through the umbilical cord where they are known as *umbilical arteries,* to the placenta.

hypomagnesemia Abnormally low amount of serum magnesium that may occur after blood transfusions.

hypospadias Anomalous positioning of the male urinary meatus on the undersurface of the penis.

hypotensive drugs Drugs that lower the blood pressure.

hypoxemia Reduction in arterial Po₂ resulting in metabolic acidosis by forcing anaerobic glycolysis, pulmonary vasoconstriction, and direct cellular damage.

hypoxia Insufficient availability of oxygen to meet body tissue metabolic needs.

hysterectomy Surgical removal of the uterus.

   abdominal h. See *abdominal hysterectomy*

   panhysterectomy Entire uterus, ovaries, and tubes are removed.

   subtotal h. Fundus and body of the uterus are surgically removed, but the cervial stump remains.

   total h. Entire uterus, including the cervix, is removed but the ovaries and tubes remain.

hysterotomy Surgical incision into the uterus.

icterus neonatorum Jaundice in the newborn.

idiopathic respiratory distress syndrome (hyaline membrane disease) Severe respiratory condition found almost exclusively in premature infants.

iliopectineal line Bony ridge on the inner surface of the ilium and pubes that divides the true and false pelvis; the brim of the true pelvic cavity; the inlet.

immature baby Infant usually weighing less than 1134 gm (2½ pounds) and who is considerably underdeveloped at birth.

implantation Embedding of the fertilized ovum in the uterine mucosa.

impotence Male's inability, partial or incomplete, to perform sexual intercourse or to achieve orgasm.

impregnation To fertilize or make pregnant.

inanition Pathophysiologic condition of the body resulting from lack of food and water; starvation.

inborn error of metabolism Hereditary deficiency of a specific enzyme needed for normal metabolism of specific chemicals (e.g., deficiency of phenylalanine hydroxylase results in PKU; a deficiency of hexosaminidase results in Tay-Sachs disease).

incompetent cervix Cervix is unable to remain closed until a pregnancy reaches term due to a mechanical defect in the cervix, causing dilatation and effacement usually during the second or early third trimester of pregnancy.

incomplete abortion See *abortion, incomplete.*

increment To increase or build up, as of a contraction.

incubator Apparatus that is used for an infant in which the temperature may be regulated.

induced abortion See *abortion, induced.*

inertia Sluggishness or inactivity; in obstetrics, refers to the absence or weakness of uterine contractions during labor.

inevitable abortion See *abortion, inevitable.*

infant Any child that is under 1 year of age.

infantile uterus Condition in which the uterus fails to attain adult characteristics.

infertility Decreased capacity to conceive.

infiltration Process by which a substance such as a local anesthetic drug is deposited within the tissue.

inlet Passage leading into a cavity.

   pelvic i. Upper brim of the pelvic cavity.

innominate Without a name.

   i. bone Refers to the hip bone.

internal os Inside mouth or opening.

intervillous space Irregular spaces in the maternal portion of placenta filled with maternal blood, serving as sites of maternal-fetal gas, nutrient, and waste exchange.

intrathecal Within the subarachnoid space.

intrauterine device (IUD) Small plastic or metal forms placed in the uterus to prevent implantation of a fertilized ovum.

intrauterine growth retardation Fetal undergrowth of any etiology such as deficient nutrient supply or intrauterine infections, or associated with congenital malformations.

introitus Entrance into a canal or cavity such as the vagina.

intromission Insertion of one part or object into another (e.g., introduction of penis into vagina).

in utero Within or inside the uterus.

inversion Turning end for end, upside down, or inside out.

   i. of the uterus Condition in which the uterus is turned inside out so that the fundus intrudes into the cervix or vagina, caused by a too vigorous removal of the placenta before it is detached by the natural process of labor.

involution (1) Rolling or turning inward. (2) Reduction in size of the uterus after delivery and its return to its normal size and condition.

ischium Lower lateral two-fifths of the acetabulum and the short stout column of bone that supports it.

jaundice Yellow discoloration of the body tissues caused by the deposit of bile pigments (unconjugated bilirubin); icterus.

breast milk j. See *breast milk jaundice.*

pathologic j. Jaundice noticeable before 24 hours after birth caused by some abnormal condition such as an Rh or ABO incompatibility.

physiologic j. Jaundice usually occurring 48 hours or later after birth, reaching a peak at 5 to 7 days, gradually disappearing by the seventh to tenth days, and caused by the normal reduction in the number of red blood cells. The infant is otherwise well.

Kahn test Precipitation or flocculation test for the diagnosis of syphilis.

kalemia Amount of serum potassium.

karyotype Schematic arrangement of the chromosomes within a cell to demonstrate their numbers and morphology.

kernicterus Bilirubin encephalopathy involving the deposit of unconjugated bilirubin in brain cells, resulting in death or impaired intellectual, perceptive, or motor function, and adaptive behavior.

Kernig's sign Stiffness of the neck; nuchal rigidity.

labia Lips or liplike structures.

l. majora Two folds of skin containing fat and covered with hair that lie on either side of the vaginal opening and form each side of the vulva.

l. minora Two thin folds of delicate skin inside the labia majora.

labor Series of processes by which the fetus is expelled from the uterus; parturition; childbirth.

laceration Irregular tear of wound tissue; in obstetrics, it usually refers to a tear in the perineum, vagina, or cervix caused by childbirth.

lactation Function of secreting milk or period during which milk is secreted.

lactogenic That which stimulates the production of milk.

l. hormone Gonadotropin produced by anterior pituitary and responsible for promoting growth of breast tissue and lactation; prolactin; luteotropin.

lactosuria Presence of lactose in the urine during late pregnancy and lactation. Must be differentiated from glycosuria.

lambdoid Having the shape of the Greek letter lambda.

l. suture Suture line extending across the posterior third of the skull, separating the occipital bone from the two parietal bones and forming the base of the triangular posterior fontanel.

lanugo Downy, fine hair characteristic of the fetus between 20 weeks' gestation to birth that is most noticeable over the shoulder, forehead, and cheeks but found on nearly all parts of the body except the palms of the hands, soles of the feet, and the scalp.

laparotomy Incision into the abdominal cavity.

large for date or *large for gastational age (LGA)* Excessive growth for gestational age.

lavage Washing out of a cavity such as the stomach.

leukorrhea White or yellowish mucous discharge from the cervical canal or the vagina that may be normal physiologically or due to pathologic states of the vagina and endocervix (e.g., *Trichomonas vaginalis* infections).

lie Relationship existing between the long axis of the fetus and the long axis of the mother. In a longitudinal lie, the fetus is lying lengthwise or vertically, whereas in a transverse lie the fetus is lying crosswise or horizontally in the mother's abdomen.

LH See *luteinizing hormone.*

ligation To suture, sew, or otherwise tie shut.

tubal l. Abdominal operation in which the fallopian tubes are tied off and a section removed to interrupt tubal continuity and thus sterilize the patient.

lightening Sensation of decreased abdominal distention produced by uterine descent into the pelvic cavity due to the settling of the fetal presenting part into the pelvis and usually occurring 3 weeks before the onset of labor in primigravidas.

linea nigra Line of darker pigmentation seen in some pregnant women during the latter part of term that appears on the middle of the abdomen and extends from the pubis toward the umbilicus.

lingua Tongue or tonguelike structure.

l. frenata Tongue with a very short frenum, resulting in tongue-tie, an extremely rare condition.

liquor Any fluid liquid.

l. amnii Amniotic fluid that surrounds the fetus within the amniotic sac.

lithotomy position Position in which the patient lies on her back with her knees flexed and abducted thighs drawn up toward her chest.

live birth Birth in which the fetus, regardless of gestational age, manifests any heartbeat, breathes, or displays voluntary movement.

livida, asphyxia See *asphyxia livida.*

lochia Vaginal discharge during the puerperium consisting of blood, tissue, and mucus.

l. alba Thin, yellowish to white, vaginal discharge that follows lochia serosa on about the tenth postnatal day and that may last from the end of the third to the sixth postnatal week.

l. rubra Red, distinctly blood-tinged vaginal flow that follows delivery and lasts 2 to 4 days after delivery.

l. serosa Serous, pinkish brown, watery vaginal discharge that follows lochia rubra until about the tenth postnatal day.

lunar month Four weeks (28 days).

lutein Yellow pigment derived from the corpus luteum, egg yolk, and fat cells.

l. cells Ovarian cells involved in the formation of the corpus luteum and that contain a yellow pigment.

luteinizing hormone (LH) Hormone produced by the anterior pituitary that stimulates ovulation and the development of the corpus luteum.

luteotropin (LTH) Lactogenic hormone; prolactin; an adenohypophyseal hormone.

lysis of adhesions Operation to free adhesions, or bands of tissue, that have caused organs to be abnormally drawn or tied to each other.

lysozyme Enzyme with antiseptic qualities that destroys foreign organisms and that is found in blood cells of the granulocytic and monocytic series and is also normally present in saliva, sweat, tears, and breast milk.

maceration (1) Process of softening a solid by soaking it in a fluid. (2) Softening and breaking down of fetal skin from prolonged exposure to amniotic fluid as seen in a postterm infant. Also seen in a dead fetus.

macroglossia Hypertrophy of tongue or tongue large for oral cavity seen in some preterm neonates and in neonates with Down's sydrome.

macrosomia Large body size as seen in neonates of diabetic or prediabetic mothers.

magnesemia Amount of serum magnesium.

mammary glands Two compound glands of the female breast that are made up of lobes and lobules that secrete milk for nourishment of the young. Mammary glands exist in a rudimentary level in the male.

mask of pregnancy See *chloasma*.

mastalgia Breast soreness or tenderness.

mastectomy Excision, or removal, of the breast.

mastitis Inflammation of mammary tissue of the breasts.

maturation (1) Process of attaining maximal development. (2) In biology, a process of cell division during which the number of chromosomes in the germ cells (sperm or ova) is reduced to one half the number characteristic of the species.

meatus Opening from an internal structure to the outside (e.g., urethral meatus).

mechanism Instrument or process by which something is done, results, or comes into being; in obstetrics, labor and delivery.

meconium First stools of infant: viscid, sticky, dark greenish brown, almost black; sterile, odorless.

meconium-stained fluid In response to hypoxia, fetal intestinal activity increases and anal sphincter relaxes, resulting in the passage of meconium.

meiosis Process by which germ cells divide and decrease their chromosomal number by one half.

-melia Pertaining to a limb or part of a limb or extremity as in amelia (absence of a limb) or phocomelia (absence of part of arms or legs).

membrane Thin, pliable layer of tissue that lines a cavity or tube, separates structures, or covers an organ or structure; in obstetrics, the amnion and chorion surrounding the fetus.

menarche Onset or beginning of menstrual function.

menopause Permanent cessation of ovarian function and menstrual activity.

menorrhagia Abnormally profuse or excessive menstrual flow.

menses (menstruation) Periodic vaginal discharge of bloody fluid from the nonpregnant uterus that occurs from the age of puberty to menopause.

mentum Chin.

mesoderm Embryonic middle layer of germ cells giving rise to all types of muscles, connective tissue, bone marrow, blood lymphoid tissue, and all epithelial tissue.

metabolic acidosis See *acidosis, metabolic*.

metrorrhagia Abnormal bleeding from the uterus, particularly when it occurs at any time other than the menstrual period.

microcephalic Having or pertaining to an abnormally small head.

micrognathia Abnormally small mandible or chin.

midwife Female who practices the art of helping and aiding the delivery of neonates.

migration In obstetrics, the passage of the ovum from the ovary into the fallopian tubes and into the uterus.

milia Unopened sebaceous glands appearing as tiny, white, pinpoint papules on forehead, nose, cheeks, and chin of a neonate that disappear spontaneously in a few days or weeks.

milk-leg See *phlegmasia alba dolens*.

miscarriage Spontaneous abortion; lay term usually referring specifically to the loss of the fetus between the fourth month and viability.

missed abortion See *abortion, missed*.

mitochondria Slender microscopic filaments or rods found in the cell cytoplasm, which are the principle sites of oxidative reactions by which the cell is provided with energy.

mitosis Process of somatic cell division in which a single cell divides, but both of the new cells have the same number of chromosomes as the first.

molding Overlapping of cranial bones or shaping of the fetal head to accommodate and conform to the bony and soft parts of the mother's birth canal during labor.

mongolian spot Bluish gray or dark nonelevated pigmentation area over the lower back and buttocks present at birth in some infants, primarily nonwhite. The spot fades by school age in black or Oriental infants and within the first year or two of life in other infants.

mongolism See *Down's syndrome*.

moniliasis Infection of the skin or mucous membrane by yeastlike fungi, *Candida albicans*.

monozygotic Originating or coming from a single fertilized ovum, such as identical twins.

monozygous twins See *twins, monozygous*.

Montgomery's glands Small, nodular prominences on the areolas around the nipples of the breasts that enlarge during pregnancy and lactation.

mons veneris Pad of fatty tissue and coarse skin that overlies the symphysis pubis in the woman and that, after puberty, is covered with short curly hair.

morning sickness Nausea and vomiting that affect some women during the first few months of their pregnancy; may occur at any time of day.

morbidity (1) Condition of being diseased. (2) Number of cases of disease or sick persons in relationship to a specific population; incidence.

mortality rate Death rate; number of deaths in relation to a specific population; incidence.

morula Developmental stage of the fertilized ovum in which there is a solid mass of cells resembling a mulberry.

mosaicism Condition in which some somatic cells are normal, whereas others show chromosomal aberrations.

mucous membrane Specialized thin layer tissue lining certain cavities and passages that is kept moist by the secretion of mucus.

mucous-trap suction apparatus. Device consisting of a catheter with a mucous trap that prevents mucus aspirated from the newborn infant's nasopharynx and trachea from being sucked or drawn into the operator's mouth.

mucus Viscid fluid secreted by the mucous membranes.

multigravida Woman who has been pregnant two or more times.

multipara Woman who has had two or more pregnancies in which the fetuses reached viability, without regard to their being alive or dead at the time of birth.

multiple pregnancy Pregnancy in which there is more than one fetus in the uterus at the same time.

mutation Change in a gene or chromosome in gametes that may be transmitted to offspring.

natal Relating or pertaining to birth.

navel Depression in the center of the abdomen where the umbilical cord was attached to the fetus; umbilicus.

neonatal mortality rate Number of neonatal deaths per 1000 live births.

neonate Newborn from birth through the twenty-eighth day of life.

neutral temperature range That grouping of environmental conditions in which the neonate's oxygen consumption is at a minimum and his temperature is within normal limits.

nevus Natural blemish or mark; a congenital circumscribed deposit of pigmentation in the skin; mole.

n. flammeus Port wine stain; reddish, usually flat, discoloration of the face or neck. Due to its large size and color, it is considered a serious deformity.

nidation Implantation of the fertilized ovum in the endometrium, or lining, of the uterus.

noncirculating hydrocephalus See *hydrocephalus, noncommunicating*.

nulligravida Woman who has never been pregnant.

nullipara Woman who has not yet delivered a viable fetus.

nystagmus Constant, involuntary, rhythmic oscillation of the eyeball. The movements may be in any direction.

obstetrix Midwife; Latin, from *obstare*, to stand before.

occiput Back part of the head or skull.

occipitobregmatic Pertaining to the occiput (the back part of the skull) and the bregma (junction of the coronal and sagittal sutures).

oligohydramnios Abnormally small amount or absence of amniotic fluid often indicative of fetal urinary tract defect.

oliguria Diminished secretion of urine by the kidneys.

omphalic Concerning or pertaining to the umbilicus.

omphalitis Infection of the umbilical stump characterized by redness, edema, and purulent exudate in severe infections.

omphalocele Congenital defect resulting from failure of closure of abdominal wall or muscles leading to hernia of abdominal contents through the navel.

oocyesis Ectopic ovarian pregnancy.

oophorectomy Excision or removal of an ovary.

operculum Plug of mucus that fills the cervical canal during pregnancy.

ophthalmia neonatorum Infection in the neonate's eyes usually resulting from gonorrheal infection contracted when the fetus passes through the birth canal (vagina).

orifice Normal mouth; entrance of opening to any aperture.

os Mouth or opening.

external o. (o. externum) External opening of the cervical canal.

internal o. (o. internum) Internal opening of the cervical canal.

o. uteri Mouth or opening of the uterus.

ossification Mineralization of fetal bones.

outlet Opening by which something can exit.

pelvic o. Inferior aperture or opening of the true pelvis.

ovarian follicle See *follicle, ovarian*.

ovary One of two glands in the female situated on either side of the pelvic cavity that produces the female reproductive cell, the ovum, and two known hormones, estrogen and progesterone.

ovulation Periodic ripening and discharge of the unimpregnated ovum from the ovary, usually 14 days prior to the onset of menstrual flow.

ovum Female germ or reproductive cell produced by the ovary; egg.

oxygen toxicity Oxygen overdosage that results in pathologic tissue changes.

oxytocics Those drugs that stimulate uterine contractions, thus accelerating childbirth and preventing postnatal hemorrhage. They may be used to increase the let-down reflex during lactation.

oxytocin Hormone produced by the posterior pituitary that stimulates uterine contractions and the release of milk in the mammary gland (let-down reflex).

pains, expulsive See *expulsive contractions*.

pallida, asphyxia See *asphyxia pallida*.

palpation Examination performed by touching the external surface of the body with the fingers or palmar surface of the hand.

bimanual p. See *bimanual palpation*.

palsy Permanent or temporary loss of sensation or ability to move and control movement; paralysis.

Bell's p. Peripheral facial paralysis due to lesion of the facial nerve, causing the muscles of the unaffected side of the face to pull the face into a distorted position.

Erb's p. Paralysis of the deltoid, biceps, long supinator, and anterior brachial muscles due to injury of the brachial plexus (as might occur during birth) or due to injury of the fifth and sixth cervical nerves.

panhysterectomy See *hysterectomy.*

Papanicolaou (Pap) smear Microscopic examination using scrapings from the cervix, endocervix, or other mucous membranes that will reveal, with a high degree of accuracy, the presence of malignant cells.

para Refers to past pregnancies that have produced a viable infant, whether the infant is dead or alive at birth.

parabiotic syndrome Fetofetal blood transfer due to placental vascular anastomoses occurring in a small percentage of identical twins, resulting in one plethoric twin (polycythemia) and one pale twin (anemia).

parametritis Inflamed condition of the cellular tissue or parametrium of the uterus; pelvic cellulitis.

parametrium Fat, smooth muscle and loose connective tissue around the uterus that extends laterally between the layers of the broad ligaments.

parenteral Administration or injection of nutrients, fluids, or drugs into the body by any way other than the digestive tract.

parity Number of liveborn or stillborn infants having reached the age of viability that a woman has delivered.

parovarian Pertaining to the residual structure in the broad ligament between the fallopian tubes and the ovary.

parturient Woman giving birth.

parturition Process or act of giving birth.

pathognomonic Characteristic or distinctive symptom or sign of a disease that facilitates the recognition or differentiation of that disease from other conditions.

pathologic jaundice See *jaundice, pathologic.*

patulous Open or spread apart.

pedigree Shorthand method of depicting family lines of individuals who manifest a physical or chemical disorder.

pelvic Pertaining or relating to the pelvis.

　p. axis See *axis, pelvic.*

　p. inlet See *inlet, pelvic.*

　p. outlet See *outlet, pelvic.*

pelvimeter Device for measuring the diameters and capacity of the pelvis.

pelvimetry Measurement of dimensions and proportions of the pelvis to determine its capacity and ability to allow the passage of the fetus through the birth canal.

pelvis Bony structure formed by the sacrum, coccyx, innominate bones, symphysis pubis, and ligaments that unite them.

　android p. See *android pelvis.*

　anthropoid p. See *anthropoid pelvis.*

　gynecoid p. See *gynecoid pelvis.*

　platypelloid p. See *platypelloid pelvis.*

pemphigus neonatorum Neonatal impetigo.

penis Male organ used for urination and copulation.

perforation of the uterus Accidental puncture of the uterus, usually with a curette.

perinatal period Period extending from the twenty-eighth week of gestation through the end of the twenty-eighth day after birth.

perinatologist Physician who specializes in fetal and neonatal care.

perineorrhaphy Suture or operation used in repairing a laceration of the perineum, usually following labor.

perineotomy Surgical incision into the perineum. In obstetrics the perineotomy is usually called an *episiotomy* and is done at the end of the second stage of labor to avoid laceration of the perineum and to facilitate delivery.

perineum Area between the vagina and rectum in the female and between the scrotum and rectum in the male.

periodic breathing Sporadic episodes of cessation of respirations for periods of 10 seconds or less not associated with cyanosis commonly noted in premature infants.

peritoneum Strong serous membrane reflected over the viscera and lining the abdominal cavity.

pessary Device placed inside the vagina to function as a supportive structure for the uterus or a contraceptive device.

petechiae Pinpoint hemorrhagic areas caused by numerous disease states involving infection and thrombocytopenia and occasionally found over the face and trunk of the newborn due to increased intravascular pressure in the capillaries during delivery.

phenotype Expression of certain physical or chemical characteristics in an individual resulting from interaction between genotype and environmental factors.

phenylketonuria Recessive hereditary disease that results in a defect in the metabolism of the amino acid phenylalanine due to the lack of an enzyme, phenylalanine hydroxylase, which is necessary for the conversion of the amino acid phenylalanine into tyrosine. If not treated, brain damage may occur, causing severe mental retardation.

phimosis Tightness of the prepuce or foreskin of the penis.

phlebitis Inflammation of a vein with symptoms of pain and tenderness along the course of the vein, inflammatory swelling and acute edema below the obstruction, and discoloration of the skin due to injury or bruise to the vein, possibly occurring in acute or chronic infections or after operations or childbirth.

phlebothrombosis Formation of clots or thrombi in the vein; inflammation of the vein with secondary clotting.

phlegmasia alba dolens Phlebitis of the femoral vein with thrombosis leading to a venous obstruction, causing acute edema of the leg, and occurring occasionally after delivery; also called *milk-leg.*

phototherapy Utilization of intense (200 to 400 footcandles) fluorescent lights to reduce serum bilirubin levels.

physiologic jaundice See *jaundice, physiologic.*

pinna Ear cartilage.

placenta Latin, flat cake; afterbirth; specialized vascular disc-shaped organ for maternal-fetal gas and nutrient exchange. Normally it implants in the thick muscular wall of the upper uterine segment.

　abruptio p. See *abruptio placentae.*

p. accreta Invasion of the uterine muscle by the placenta, thus making separation from the muscle difficult if not impossible.

p. previa Placenta that is abnormally implanted in the thin, lower uterine segment and that is typed according to proximity to cervical os: total—completely occludes os, partial—does not occlude os completely, and marginal—placenta encroaches on margin of internal cervical os.

placental Pertaining or relating to the placenta.

p. dysfunction Placenta that is failing to meet fetal needs and requirements; placental insufficiency.

p. dystocia See *dystocia, placental.*

p. souffle See *souffle, placental.*

platypelloid pelvis Shape of a broad pelvis; shortened in the anteroposterior diameter and having a flattened oval, transverse shape.

plethora Deep beefy red coloration ("boiled lobster" hue) of a newborn due to an increased number of blood cells (polycythemia) per volume of blood.

pneumomediastinum Accumulation of air around the heart and vena cava.

pneumothorax Escaped air from affected lung into the pleural space, displacing the heart and mediastinum toward the unaffected side of the chest.

podalic Concerning or pertaining to the feet.

p. version Shifting the position of the fetus so as to bring the feet to the outlet in labor.

polycythemia Increased number of erythrocytes, which may be due to large placental transfusion, fetofetal transfusion, or maternal-fetal transfusion.

polydactyly Excessive number of digits, fingers or toes.

polygenic Pertaining to the combined action of several different genes.

polyhydramnios See *hydramnios.*

polyuria Excessive secretion and discharge of urine by the kidneys.

position Relationships of an arbitrarily chosen spot such as the occiput, sacrum, chin, or scapula on the presenting part of the fetus to the front, back, or sides of the maternal pelvis.

positive sign of pregnancy Definite sign of pregnancy (e.g., hearing the fetal heartbeat, visualization and palpation of fetal movement by the examiner, sonographic examination).

posterior Pertaining to the back.

p. fontanel See *fontanel, posterior.*

postmature infant Postterm; infant born at the beginning of forty-second week of gestation or later.

postnatal Happening or occurring after birth.

postpartum Happening or occurring after birth.

precipitate delivery Rapid or sudden labor of less than 3 hours' duration.

preeclampsia Disease encountered during pregnancy or early in the puerperium characterized by increasing hypertension, albuminuria, and generalized edema.

pregnancy Period between conception through complete delivery of the products of conception. The usual duration of pregnancy in the human is 280 days, 9 calendar months, or 10 lunar months.

abdominal p. See *abdominal gestation.*

ectopic p. See *ectopic pregnancy.*

extrauterine p. See *extrauterine pregnancy.*

premature infant Infant born before completing the thirty-seventh or thirty-eighth week of gestation, irrespective of birth weight; preterm infant.

premonitory Early symptom or warning.

prenatal Occurring or happening before birth.

prepuce Fold of skin or foreskin covering the glans penis of the male.

p. of the clitoris Fold of the labia minora that covers the glans clitoris.

presentation That part of the fetus which first enters the pelvis and lies over the inlet: may be head, face, breech, or shoulder.

breech p. See *breech presentation.*

cephalic p. See *cephalic presentation.*

presenting part That part of the fetus which lies closest to the internal os of the cervix.

pressure edema Edema of the lower extremities caused by pressure of the heavy pregnant uterus against the large veins.

presumptive signs Manifestations that suggest pregnancy but that are not absolutely positive. These include the cessation of menses, Chadwick's sign, morning sickness, and quickening.

preterm infant See *premature infant.*

previa, placenta See *placenta previa.*

priapism Continuous erection of the penis, not usually accompanied by sexual feeling, which may appear in conjunction with leukemia, renal calculi, and spinal cord lesions.

primigravida Woman who is pregnant for the first time.

primipara Woman who has delivered one child who had reached viability without regard to the child's being dead or alive at the time of birth.

primordial Existing first or existing in the simplest or most primitive form.

probable signs Manifestations or evidence that indicate that there is a definite likelihood of pregnancy. Among the probable signs are enlargement of the abdomen, Goodell's sign, Hegar's sign, Braxton Hicks sign, and positive hormonal tests for pregnancy.

proband Individual in a family who comes to the attention of a genetic investigator because of the occurrence of a trait; the index case, or propositus.

prodromal Early symptom or warning of the approach of a disease or condition (e.g., prodromal labor).

progesterone Hormone produced by the corpus luteum and placenta whose function is to prepare the endometrium of the uterus for implantation of the fertilized ovum, develop the mammary glands, and maintain the pregnancy.

projectile vomiting Extremely forceful, expulsive vomiting.

prolactin See *lactogenic hormone.*

prolan Hormone produced by chorionic villi, now called *human chorionic gonadotropin (HCG)*, that is found in the urine of pregnant women and forms the basis of the biologic and immunologic pregnancy tests.

prolapsed cord Protrusion of the umbilical cord in advance of the presenting part.

promontory of the sacrum Superior projecting portion of the sacrum when in situ in the pelvis at the junction of the sacrum and the L5.

prophylactic Pertaining to prevention or warding off of disease.

propositus See *proband*.

proteinuria Excretion of protein, usually albumin, into urine.

pseudocyesis Condition in which the patient has all the usual signs of pregnancy, such as enlargement of the abdomen, cessation of menses, weight gain, and morning sickness, but is not pregnant; phantom or false pregnancy.

pseudopregnancy See *pseudocyesis*.

pseudoprematurity See *intrauterine growth retardation*.

psychologic miscarriage Absence or lack of love for the infant.

psychoprophylaxis Mental and physical education of the parents in preparation for childbirth, with the goal of minimizing the fear of pain and promoting positive family relationships.

puberty Period in life in which the reproductive organs mature and one becomes functionally capable of reproduction.

pubic Pertaining to the pubis.

pubis Pubic bone forming the front of the pelvis.

pudendal block Injection of a local anesthetizing drug at the pudendal nerve root so as to produce numbness of the genitals and perianal region.

pudendum External genitals of either sex.

puerperal sepsis Infection of the pelvic organs during the postnatal period; childbed fever.

puerperium Period of time following the third stage of labor and lasting until involution of the uterus takes place, usually about 3 to 6 weeks.

quickening Maternal perception of fetal movement which usually occurs between the sixteenth and twentieth weeks of gestation.

rabbit test See *Friedman's test*.

radium insertion Introduction of metallic element radium (Ra) into the uterus or cervix to treat cancer.

rales Crackling sounds heard as air passes through the fluid present within the terminal bronchioles and alveoli.

RDS See *respiratory distress syndrome*.

recessive trait Gene that is expressed only when present in the homozygotic state.

rectocele Herniation or protrusion of the rectum into the posterior vaginal wall.

reflex Automatic response built into the nervous system that does not need the intervention of conscious thought (e.g., in the newborn, rooting, gagging, grasp).

regurgitate Vomiting or spitting up of solids or fluids.

residual urine Urine that remains in the bladder after urination.

respiratory distress syndrome (RDS) Condition resulting from decreased pulmonary gas exchange, leading to retention of carbon dioxide (increase in arterial P_{CO_2}). Commonest neonatal causes are prematurity and perinatal asphyxia; hyaline membrane disease.

restitution In obstetrics, the turning of the fetal head to the left or right after it has completely emerged from the introitus as it assumes a normal alignment with the infant's shoulders.

resuscitation Restoration of consciousness or life in one who is apparently dead or whose respirations have ceased.

retained placenta All or part of the placenta remains in the uterus after delivery.

retraction (1) Indrawing or sucking in of soft tissues of chest, indicative of an obstruction at any level of the respiratory tract from the oropharynx to alveoli. (2) Retraction of uterine muscle fiber. After contracting, the muscle fiber does not return to its original length but remains slightly shortened, a unique attribute of uterine muscle that aids in preventing postnatal hemorrhage.

retroflexion Bending backward.

r. of the uterus Condition in which the body of the womb is bent backward at an angle with the cervix, whose position usually remains unchanged.

retrolental fibroplasia Retinopathy of prematurity associated with hyperoxemia, resulting in eye injury and blindness.

retroversion Turning or a state of being turned back.

r. of the uterus Displacement of the uterus; the body of the uterus is tipped backward with the cervix pointing forward toward the symphysis pubis.

Rh factor Inherited antigen present on erythrocytes. The individual with the factor is known as *positive* for the factor.

rhonchi Coarse, snorelike sounds produced as air passes through the fluid in the large bronchi, frequently heard after aspiration of oral secretions or feedings.

rhythm method Contraceptive method in which a woman abstains from sexual intercourse during the ovulatory phase of her menstrual cycle and at least 3 days before and 1 day after the ovulation date.

ribonucleic acid (RNA) Element responsible for transferring genetic information within a cell; a template or pattern.

Ritgen maneuver Procedure used to control the delivery of the head.

rooming-in unit Maternity unit which is designed so that the newborn baby's crib is at the mother's bedside or in a nursery adjacent to the mother's room.

rotation In obstetrics, the turning of the fetal head as it follows the curves of the birth canal downward.

Rubin's test Transuterine insufflation of the fallopian tubes with carbon dioxide to test their patency.

sac, amniotic See *amniotic sac*.

sacroiliac Of or pertaining to the sacrum and ilium.

sacrum Triangular bone composed of five united vertebras and situated between L5 and the coccyx; forms the posterior boundary of the true pelvis.

saddle block anesthesia Type of regional anesthesia produced by injection of a local anesthetic solution into the cerebrospinal fluid intrathecal space in the spinal canal.

sagittal suture Band of connective tissue separating the parietal bones, extending from the anterior to posterior fontanel.

salpingo-oophorectomy Removal of a fallopian tube and ovary.

scaphoid abdomen Abdomen with a sunken interior wall.

Schultze's mechanism Delivery of the placenta with the fetal surfaces (shiny in appearance) presenting.

sclerema Hardening of skin and subcutaneous tissue that develops in association with such life-threatening disorders as severe cold stress, septicemia, and shock.

sebaceous glands Oil-secreting glands found in the skin.

secondary areola See *areola, secondary.*

secundines Fetal membranes and placenta expelled after childbirth; afterbirth.

segmentation Process of cleavage or division by which the fertilized ovum multiply before differentiation into layers occurs.

semen Thick, whitish, viscid secretion discharged from the urethra of the male at orgasm; the transporting medium of the sperm.

sensitization Development of antibodies to a specific antigen.

septic abortion See *abortion, septic.*

singleton Pregnancy with a single fetus.

small for date or *small for gestational age (SGA)* Inadequate growth for gestational age.

souffle Soft, blowing sound or murmur heard by auscultation.

  funic s. Soft, muffled, blowing sound produced by blood rushing through the umbilical vessels and synchronous with the fetal heart sounds.

  placental s. Soft, blowing murmur caused by the blood current in the placenta and synchronous with the maternal pulse.

  uterine s. Soft, blowing sound made by the blood in the arteries of the pregnant uterus and synchronous with the maternal pulse.

spermatogenesis Process by which mature spermatozoa are formed, during which the diploid chromosome number is reduced by half.

spermatozoon Mature male sex or germ cell formed within the testes.

spina bifida occulta Congenital malformation of the spine in which the posterior portion of laminas of the vertebras fails to close but there is no herniation or protrusion of the spinal cord or meninges through the defect. The newborn may have a dimple in the skin or growth of hair over the malformed vertebras.

spontaneous abortion See *abortion, spontaneous.*

station Relationship of the presenting fetal part to an imaginary line drawn between the ischial spines of the pelvis.

sterility (1) State of being free from living microorganisms. (2) Complete inability to reproduce offspring.

stillborn Fetus that is born dead.

striae gravidarum ("stretch marks") Shining reddish lines caused by stretching of the skin, often found on the abdomen, thighs, and breasts during pregnancy. These streaks turn to a fine pinkish white or silver tone in time in fair-skinned women and brownish in darker skinned women.

subinvolution Failure of a part (e.g., the uterus) to reduce to its normal size and condition after enlargement from functional activity (e.g., pregnancy).

subluxation Incomplete dislocation.

subtotal hysterectomy See *hysterectomy, subtotal.*

succedaneum Localized edema of scalp of no clinical significance resulting from obstructed venous return caused by pressure from the dilating cervix.

superfecundation Successive fertilization of two or more ova formed during the same menstrual cycle by the sperm of the same or different fathers.

superfetation Fertilization of an ovum when the woman is already pregnant.

supernumerary nipples Excessive number of nipples varying in size from small pink spots to the size of normal nipples and usually not associated with underlying glandular tissue.

suppuration Process by which pus is formed.

surfactant Lipoprotein necessary for normal respiratory function that stabilizes the alveolar sacs by lowering surface tension, thus preventing alveolar collapse (atelectasis).

suture (1) Junction of the adjoining bones of the skull. (2) Operation uniting parts by sewing them together.

symphysis pubis Fibrocartilaginous union of the bodies of the pubic bones in the midline.

syndactyly Malformation of digits, commonly seen as a fusion of two or more toes to form one structure.

tachypnea Excessively rapid respiratory rate (e.g., in neonates, respiratory rate of 60/minute or more).

telangiectatic nevi ("stork bites") Clusters of small, red, localized areas of capillary dilatation commonly seen in neonates at the nape of the neck or lower occiput, upper eyelids, and nasal bridge that can be blanched with pressure of a finger.

teratogenic agent Any drug, virus, or irradiation, the exposure to which can cause malformation of the fetus.

teratogens Nongenetic factors that cause malformations and disease syndromes in utero.

term infant Live infant born between the thirty-eighth and forty-second week of completed gestation.

testicle One of the glands contained in the male scrotum that produces the male reproductive cell or sperm and the male hormone testosterone.

tetany, uterine Extremely prolonged uterine contractions.

tetralogy of Fallot Congenital cardiac malformation consisting of pulmonary stenosis, intraventricular septal defect, dextroposed aorta that receives blood from both ventricles, and hypertrophy of the right ventricle.

therapeutic abortion See *abortion, therapeutic.*

thermogenesis Creation or production of heat, especially in the body.

threatened abortion See *abortion, threatened.*

thrombocytopenic purpura Hematologic disorder characterized by prolonged bleeding time, decreased number of platelets, increased cell fragility, and purpura, which result in hemorrhages into the skin, mucous membranes, organs, and other tissue.

thromboembolus Obstruction of a blood vessel by a clot that has become detached from its site of formation.

thrombophlebitis Inflammation of a vein with secondary clot formation.

thrombus Blood clot obstructing a blood vessel that remains at the place it was formed.

thrush Fungus infection of the mouth or throat characterized by the formation of white patches on a red, moist, inflamed mucous membrane and caused by *Candida albicans.*

toco, toko Combining form that means childbirth or labor.

tongue-tie Congenital shortening of the frenulum, which, if severe, may interfere with sucking and articulation and is a rare condition.

torticollis Congenital or acquired stiff neck caused by shortening or spasmodic contraction of the neck muscles that draws the head to one side with the chin pointing in the other direction; wryneck.

total hysterectomy See *hysterectomy, total.*

toxemia Term previously used for disorders occurring during pregnancy or early puerperium, now known as *preeclampsia-eclampsia,* that are characterized by one or all of the following: edema, hypertension, albuminuria, and, in severe cases, convulsion and coma.

tracheoesophageal fistula Congenital malformation in which there is an abnormal tubelike passage between the trachea and esophagus.

translocation Condition in which a chromosome breaks and all or part of that chromosome is transferred to a different part of the same chromosome or to another chromosome.

trauma Physical or psychic injury.

Trichomonas vaginitis Inflammation of the vagina caused by *Trichomonas vaginalis,* a parasitic protozoa, and characterized by persistent burning and itching of the vulvar tissue and a profuse, frothy, white discharge.

trimester Time period of 3 months.

trisomy Condition whereby any given chromosome exists in triplicate instead of the normal duplicate pattern.

trophectoderm See *trophoblast.*

trophoblast Outer layer of cells of the developing blastodermic vesicle that develops the trophoderm, or feeding layer, which will establish the nutrient relationships with the uterine endometrium.

tubal ligation See *ligation, tubal.*

twins Two neonates from the same impregnation developed within the same uterus at the same time.

　conjoined t. Twins who are physically united; Siamese twins.

　disparate t. Twins who are different (e.g., in weight) and distinct from one another.

　dizygous t. Twins developed from two separate ova fertilized by two separate sperm at the same time; fraternal.

　monozygous t. Twins developed from a single fertilized ovum; identical.

undergrown baby See *intrauterine growth retardation.*

umbilical cord Structure connecting the placenta and fetus and containing two arteries and one vein encased in a tissue called *Wharton's jelly.* The cord is ligated at birth and severed; the stump falls off in 4 to 10 days.

umbilical vasculitis Inflammation of the umbilical cord and its blood vessels.

umbilicus Navel or depressed point in the middle of the abdomen that marks the attachment of the umbilical cord during fetal life.

urachus Epithelial tube connecting the apex of the urinary bladder with the allantois. Its connective tissue forms the median umbilical ligament.

urinary frequency Need to void occurs often or at close invervals.

urinary meatus Opening or mouth of the urethra.

uterine Referring or pertaining to the uterus.

　u. adnexa See *adnexa, uterine.*

　u. souffle See *souffle, uterine.*

uterus Hollow muscular organ in the female designed for the implantation, containment, and nourishment of the fetus during its development until birth.

　Couvelaire u. Interstitial myometrial hemorrhage following premature separation (abruptio) of placenta causes a purplish-bluish discoloration of the uterus. Boardlike rigidity of the uterus is noted.

　inversion of the u. See *inversion of the uterus.*

　retroflexion of the u. See *retroflexion of the uterus.*

　retroversion of the u. See *retroversion of the uterus.*

vagina Normally collapsed musculomembranous tube that forms the passageway between the uterus and the entrance to the vagina.

varices or varicose veins Swollen, distended, and twisted veins that may develop in almost any part of the body but are most commonly seen in the legs, caused by pregnancy, obesity, congenital defective venous valves, and occupations requiring much standing.

vasectomy Ligation or removal of a segment of the vas deferens usually done bilaterally to produce sterility in the male.

venous Pertaining or relating to the veins.

vera, decidua See *decidua vera.*

vernix caseosa Protective gray-white fatty substance of cheesy consistency covering the fetal skin.

version Act of turning the fetus in the uterus to change the presenting part and facilitate delivery.

　p. version See *podalic version.*

vertex Crown or top of the head.

　v. presentation When the fetal skull is nearest the cervical opening and born first.

vesicle, blastoderm See *blastoderm vesicle.*

vestibule Area at the entrance to another structure.

　v. of vagina Space between the labia minora where the urinary meatus and vaginal introitus are located.

viable Capable of living, such as a fetus that has reached a stage of development, usually 28 weeks or older, which will permit it to live outside the uterus.

villi Short, vascular processes or protrusions growing on certain membranous surfaces.

chorionic v. Tiny vascular protrusions on the chorionic surface that project into the maternal blood sinuses of the uterus and that help to form the placenta and secrete HCG.

voluntary abortion See *abortion, elective.*

vulva External genitals of the female that consist of the labia majora, labia minora, clitoris, urinary meatus, and vaginal introitus.

vulvectomy Removal of the external genitals of the female.

well-baby clinics Those clinics which offer medical supervision and services to healthy infants.

Wharton's jelly White, gelatinous material surrounding the umbilical vessels within the cord.

witch's milk Secretion of a whitish fluid for about a week after birth from enlarged mammary tissue in the neonate, presumably resulting from maternal hormonal influences.

womb See *uterus.*

X chromosome Sex chromosome in humans existing in duplicate in the normal female and singly in the normal male.

X linkage Genes located on the X chromosome.

Y chromosome Sex chromosome in the human male necessary for the development of the male gonads.

zero fluid balance Amount of intake equals the amount of output.

zona pellucida Inner, thick, membraneous envelope of the ovum.

zygote Cell formed by the union of two reproductive cells or gametes; the fertilized ovum resulting from the union of a sperm and ovum.

Index